Paracetamol (Acetaminophen)

A Critical Bibliographic Review

Paracetamol (Acetaminophen)

A Critical Bibliographic Review

LAURIE F. PRESCOTT

Professor of Clinical Pharmacology,
University of Edinburgh

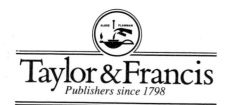

Taylor & Francis
Publishers since 1798

UK   Taylor & Francis Ltd, 1 Gunpowder Square, London, EC4A 3DE
USA   Taylor & Francis Inc., 1900 Frost Road, Suite 101, Bristol, PA 19007

British Library Cataloguing in Publication Data

A catalogue record for this book is available from the British Library.

ISBN 0-7484-0136-9 (cased)

Library of Congress Cataloguing Publication data are available

Cover design by Hybert Design & Type, Waltham St Lawrence, Berks

Typeset in Times 10/12 pt by Santype International Ltd, Salisbury, Wiltshire

Printed in Great Britain by T. J. Press (Padstow) Ltd

Contents

Contents

Contents

Contents

Preface

My interest in analgesic drugs was kindled in 1963 when I was a Research Fellow with Professor Louis Lasagna at The Johns Hopkins Hospital, Baltimore, Maryland, USA. Since that time I have been involved continuously with studies on paracetamol (acetaminophen), and over this period its use worldwide has increased dramatically to the extent that it is now one of the most commonly taken of all drugs. In many areas it has become the most popular non-prescription drug for the treatment of fever, minor aches and pains and the symptomatic relief of common ailments. Some of the actions of paracetamol seem to be related to inhibition of prostaglandin synthesis, but it differs in many important respects from aspirin and the non-steroidal anti-inflammatory drugs and it has proved to be remarkably safe when used properly. The realization that it could cause acute hepatic necrosis when taken in overdosage came as a bombshell more than 70 years after it was first used in clinical medicine and this marred its otherwise exemplary safety record. The subsequent frequent use of paracetamol for self-poisoning resulted in notoriety and attracted much adverse publicity. More than 20 years ago, Jerry Mitchell and his colleagues elucidated the mechanism whereby paracetamol causes acute liver injury, and provided a rational basis for the introduction of effective antidotes for the prevention of liver damage following overdosage. Paracetamol has since been used increasingly as a model compound for producing experimental hepatic necrosis.

In this book, I have attempted to summarize the important properties and actions of paracetamol in the form of a critical bibliographic review. The motivation for this was to add to the original series of monographs on antipyrine, acetanilide, phenacetin and the salicylates written by Martin Gross, Leon Greenberg and Paul Smith nearly half a century ago. I hope that the present review will be as valuable to investigators and clinicians today as these monographs were to me many years ago when I first became interested in this fascinating group of drugs.

Laurie Prescott
Edinburgh, 1995

Acknowledgements

I gratefully acknowledge the assistance provided by Professor E. Muscholl and Dr J. H. Shelley with translation and research into the history of paracetamol and related drugs. I am indebted to Dr J. B. Spooner and Group Medical Services, Sanofi Winthrop Ltd for valuable assistance with the bibliography and I must also thank Ms E. R. Shields and Mrs M. A. Stirling for their continuing help and encouragement.

The History of Paracetamol

Paracetamol (acetaminophen) was a product of the rapidly developing chemical industry in Germany towards the end of the nineteenth century. At that time, prevailing medical opinion held that fevers were harmful, and that the temperature should be lowered by whatever means possible. The only available agents that were capable of reducing fever were naturally occurring quinine and salicylates, and otherwise fevers had to be 'cured' by primitive and now long discredited treatments such as bleeding, purging and sweating. Newly synthesized compounds such as antipyrine (phenazone), acetanilide, acetophenetidin (phenacetin) and acetylsalicylic acid (aspirin) effectively lowered the body temperature in patients with fever and it is easy to understand their immediate and enthusiastic acceptance by the medical profession. Antipyrine was first synthesized by Knorr in 1884 from phenylhydrazine and ethyl acetoacetate, and although it was mistakenly thought to be structurally related to quinine, it was nevertheless found to be an effective antipyretic and soon gained wide usage. Acetanilide was synthesized much earlier by the reaction of aniline with acetyl chloride or acetic anhydride (Gerhardt, 1853), and the accidental discovery of its therapeutic properties in 1886 has become one of the classical stories in the history of drug development. According to Gross (1946), Cahn and Hepp, two physicians in Strasbourg, were using naphthalene to treat intestinal worms, and a new supply, provided by a recently employed pharmacist, did not perform at all as anticipated but was noted instead to produce a marked fall in temperature in a febrile patient. They investigated this unexpected result and discovered that, by mistake, the pharmacist had given them acetanilide instead of naphthalene. Gross cited an obscure monthly magazine for women as the source of this story and the original reports of the clinical use of acetanilide by Cahn and Hepp (1886, 1887a,b) described only its remarkable antipyretic action and ability to reduce the pain of rheumatism with no mention of any accidental discovery. In their first paper they remarked that by lucky chance they were presented with a substance which demonstrated outstanding antipyretic activity, and that this same material was investigated by Dr E. Hepp in Biebrich and identified as a long-known chemical which would conventionally be described as acetanilide or phenylacetamide (Cahn and Hepp, 1886). Many years later, Venzmer (1932) described the strange and momentous incident in Kopp's pharmacy in Strasbourg in some detail and he likened the subsequent extensive use of acetanilide to an avalanche started by a rolling snowball.

He also drew attention to the happy coincidence of the manufacture of phenacetin in quantity from p-nitrophenol that had accumulated as a byproduct of the burgeoning German dye industry. The real question is why did it take 45 years for this story to be published, and why did it appear in such an unlikely place? There was no mention of the pharmacist's mistake in contemporary reports of the introduction of acetanilide in Lyon (Lepine, 1886) and New York (Shrady, 1886), or in later reviews (Sharp, 1915; Wood, 1931). Phenacetin was introduced into medical practice a year after acetanilide (Hinsberg and Kast, 1887), and like acetanilide and antipyrine, it rapidly gained wide popularity. Although these drugs were originally introduced to reduce fever, their ability to ameliorate mild to moderate pain was soon recognized and eventually this became the primary indication for their therapeutic use.

The synthesis of paracetamol by reduction of p-nitrophenol to p-aminophenol with tin and glacial acetic acid and its subsequent (inadvertent) acetylation was described by Morse in 1878. Its first clinical use is attributed to von Mering (1893), although he gave only the following scanty details: 'After these experiments had shown that p-aminophenol was an unsatisfactory drug because of its marked side effects, acetylaminophenol, i.e. p-aminophenol acetylated on the amino group, was investigated. This drug produces the same side effects as p-aminophenol, albeit weaker, so that its medical use is not recommended despite its prompt antipyretic and antineuralgic potency.' Hinsberg and Treupel (1894) gave the first detailed account of the properties and clinical use of paracetamol. They showed that an oral dose of 500 mg was as effective in reducing fever as 700 mg of phenacetin or 1 g of antipyrine, and a comparison of paracetamol and antipyrine in one of their patients, named Veit, is reproduced in Figure 1.1. Aspirin, phenacetin, acetanilide and antipyrine quickly became established as effective antipyretic analgesics, but paracetamol made little impression and it was soon abandoned. This is surprising because it was soon discovered to be an important metabolite of both acetanilide and phenacetin, and it was even known to be excreted in the form of etheral sulphate and glucuronide conjugates (Jaffe and Hilbert, 1888; Mörner, 1889; Sharp, 1915).

Many years later, paracetamol was rediscovered as the major metabolite of acetanilide and phenacetin in man (Brodie and Axelrod, 1948a,b, 1949) and rabbits (Smith and Williams, 1948, 1949). This resulted in a sudden renewal of interest and paracetamol was marketed in the USA in 1950 as a combination with aspirin and caffeine ('Triogesic'). It was withdrawn one year later following three reports of agranulocytosis, but a review of these cases made a causal relationship unlikely and it was reintroduced as a prescription drug. It subsequently became available without prescription in 1955 and was first marketed in the United Kingdom in 1956 (Spooner and Harvey, 1976; Ameer and Greenblatt, 1977). In a series of studies over the next decade, it was generally found to be as effective as aspirin and nonprescription combination analgesics for reducing fever (Cornely and Ritter, 1956; Colgan and Mintz, 1957) and for the relief of pain caused by radiant heat (Flinn and Brodie, 1948), cancer (Wallenstein and Houde, 1954), dental surgery (Boréus et al., 1956) and arthritis (Newton and Tanner, 1956). Paracetamol became available in France in 1957, but was little used (Garnier et al., 1982) and its adoption by other countries was slow. In Sweden it did not become available without prescription until 1974 (Bengtsson and Lindholm, 1977), and the unrestricted sale of paracetamol in Spain, Norway and Denmark was delayed until 1976, 1982 and 1984, respectively (Jakobsen et al., 1984; Bodd et al., 1985; Manrique Larralde et al., 1988). During the

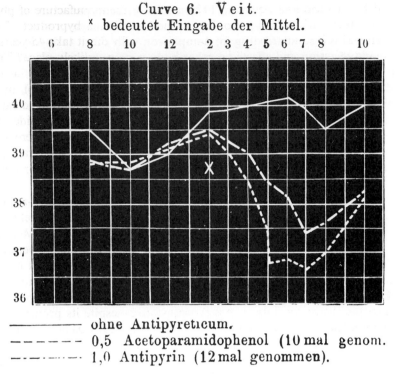

Curve 6. Veit.

ˣ bedeutet Eingabe der Mittel.

——————— ohne Antipyreticum.

— — — — — 0,5 Acetoparamidophenol (10 mal genom.

—·—·——·— 1,0 Antipyrin (12 mal genommen).

Figure 1.1 Reduction in fever in patient 'Veit' following administration of 500 mg of paracetamol and 1 g of antipyrine on different days. The temperature (°C) is displayed on the 'y' axis and the time of day in hours appears at the top of the graph. The control temperature on a day without drug therapy is shown as a continuous line (from Hinsberg and Treupel, 1894).

1960s and 1970s, the toxicity of non-prescription analgesics and analgesic combinations was a cause for concern but in normal use paracetamol proved to be very safe. In particular, it did not share the formidable gastrointestinal toxicity and adverse effects on haemostasis of aspirin, it did not cause methaemoglobinaemia and haemolysis as did acetanilide and phenacetin, and there was few, if any, reports of analgesic abuse and nephropathy involving paracetamol alone. As a consequence, the use of paracetamol has increased steadily, and in some countries it is the leading non-prescription antipyretic analgesic. With this degree of success and universal availability, it was inevitable that paracetamol would be used increasingly for the fashionable habit of self-poisoning, and hitherto unsuspected liver damage following overdosage was first reported in 1966 in Scotland (Davidson and Eastham, 1966; Thomson and Prescott, 1966). Other reports soon appeared from other countries and severe liver damage, and less commonly acute renal failure, following paracetamol poisoning became a major cause for concern. In an elegant series of studies, Mitchell and his colleagues showed that hepatic necrosis induced by toxic doses of paracetamol was caused by its conversion to a reactive metabolite that depleted protective glutathione and became bound covalently to vital cell constituents (Jollow *et al.*, 1973; Mitchell *et al.*, 1973b,c; Potter *et al.*, 1973). These findings resulted in the development of N-acetylcysteine as a safe effective antidote (Prescott

3

et al., 1977b; Rumack and Peterson, 1978) and at present, paracetamol is involved in about one-third of adult self-poisonings in the United Kingdom.

Paracetamol is a standard drug for comparison with other antipyretic analgesics and its mode of action and effects on other body systems continue to attract attention. It is now used extensively as a model compound for the study of acute drug-induced liver injury and there has been intense interest in its metabolism and the mechanisms of hepatotoxicity. Meanwhile, its popularity as a mild analgesic and over-the-counter remedy remains undiminished.

Physicochemical Properties and Prodrugs of Paracetamol

Physicochemical Properties

Paracetamol is known as acetaminophen in North America and in several other countries. Other names include N-acetyl-p-aminophenol, acetamidophenol, 4-hydroxyacetanilide, N-(4-hydroxyphenyl) acetamide, APAP and NAPAP. It is a white odourless crystalline powder with a melting point of 169–171°C and a molecular weight of 151.2. The partition coefficient in octanol and pH 7.2 buffer is 6.24. The empirical formula is $C_8H_9NO_2$ and the Chemical Abstracts Service Registry Number is 103-90-2 (IARC Monograph, 1990). The structural formula is shown in Figure 2.1.

Paracetamol is a weak organic acid with a pKa value of 9.5 (Prescott and Nimmo, 1971). It is moderately soluble in hot water, alkaline aqueous solutions and more polar organic solvents such as methanol and acetone. The physicochemical properties of paracetamol have been reviewed in detail by Fairbrother (1974) and El-Obeid and Al-Badr (1985). There are official standards for the identification, purity and stability of paracetamol in many Pharmacopoeias, including those of Britain, Europe and the United States of America (*British Pharmacopoeia*, 1988; Martindale, 1993).

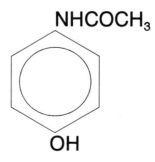

Figure 2.1 Paracetamol

Paracetamol is available in a large number of official and proprietary products alone and in combination with other analgesics and drugs such as caffeine, antihistamines and sympathomimetics. It is taken orally as tablets, capsules and elixirs, and rectally in suppository form. It was listed as an ingredient in more than 850 proprietary and official products (Martindale, 1993). It was suggested that paracetamol might occur naturally in man (Montegue *et al.*, 1994).

Prodrugs of Paracetamol

Acetanilide and phenacetin were the classical prodrugs of paracetamol but others have been developed and some have had limited clinical use.

Benorylate

Benorylate (4-acetamidophenyl-O-acetylsalicylate) is an ester of paracetamol and acetylsalicylate. It is a poorly soluble prodrug, which was rapidly hydrolyzed to paracetamol and salicylic acid after absorption. Its actions and uses were those of the constituent drugs (Robertson *et al.*, 1972; Moore *et al.*, 1989; Williams *et al.*, 1989a). A cyclic paracetamol-acetylsalicylic acid prodrug has also been described (Marzo *et al.*, 1990).

Paracetamol-N-acetyl-DL-methionate

Studies have been reported with the N-acetyl-DL-methionine ester of paracetamol (p-acetamidophenyl-2-carbamoyl-4-methylthiobutanoate). This prodrug was also poorly soluble and it was absorbed slowly and hydrolyzed rapidly *in vivo* to the parent drug and racemic methionine. As paracetamol-induced hepatic necrosis could be prevented by l-methionine taken at the same time (McLean, 1974; Neuvonen *et al.*, 1985; Neuvonen *et al.*, 1986), it was hoped that this form of the drug would be safe if taken in overdose. The paracetamol-methionine ester was as effective an analgesic as conventional paracetamol, but it had a longer duration of action (Skoglund and Skjelbred, 1984; Skoglund *et al.*, 1992).

Propacetamol

Propacetamol is the N,N-diethylglycine ester of paracetamol and it is marketed in France and Belgium as a formulation for intramuscular or intravenous use. It was rapidly and quantitatively hydrolyzed to paracetamol and its therapeutic indications were essentially the same as for paracetamol (Moreau *et al.*, 1990; Bannwarth *et al.*, 1992; Depré *et al.*, 1992; Autret *et al.*, 1993; Beaulieu, 1994).

Other prodrugs

Other prodrugs of paracetamol include eterylate (Priego *et al.*, 1983), 1-(p-acetamin-ophenoxy)-1-ethoxyethane (Hussain *et al.*, 1978), 4-acetamidophenyl-2-(5-p-toluyl-1-methylpyrrole) acetate (Sabater *et al.*, 1993), and fatty acid (Bauguess *et al.*, 1975a,b), sulphate (Williams *et al.*, 1983), aminoacid (Kovach *et al.*, 1981), carbonate (Dittert *et al.*, 1968), carboxylic acid (Rattie *et al.*, 1970), thiophene carboxylic acid (Spano and Stacchino, 1979) and aminoalkylbenzoate (Jensen *et al.*, 1991) esters.

Analytical Methods for the Assay of Paracetamol and its Metabolites in Biological Fluids

Introduction

Many methods have been described for the assay of paracetamol in biological samples, and with rapid advances in analytical technology there have been great improvements over the years. The older methods are now of historical interest only and the choice of method depends ultimately on the purpose for which it is required. Most published methods were based on conventional colorimetry, spectrophotometry, thin layer-, gas liquid-, and high performance liquid chromatography, while more recently introduced techniques for routine analyses included enzyme-mediated immunoassay and polarization fluoroimmunoassay. In addition, there have been many reports of non-biological methods such as those that have been developed for the quality control of pharmaceutical products containing paracetamol (Chafetz *et al.*, 1971; Davis *et al.*, 1974b; Ellcock and Fogg, 1975; Lau *et al.*, 1989; Issopoulos, 1990; El-Din *et al.*, 1991; Milch and Szabó, 1991; Bozdogan *et al.*, 1992; Verma *et al.*, 1992, and others). These will not be considered further unless relevant. There were no technical difficulties with the assay of paracetamol. It has a rather small distribution volume of about one 1 kg^{-1} and as it was given in gram doses, the concentrations in biological fluids were high and remained in the mg 1^{-1} range for many hours after a therapeutic dose. It was not extensively bound to plasma proteins and had potentially reactive phenolic and acetamido groups for derivatization if necessary. It was stable and had a moderately high ultraviolet optical extinction coefficient. The ideal analytical method would be simple, quick, cheap, reliable, sensitive, specific and would not require the use of complex or expensive equipment. For most biopharmaceutic and pharmacokinetic applications, some form of solvent extraction or chromatographic separation was considered to be essential to minimize interference by endogenous compounds and other drugs and metabolites. In some methods, the drug was extracted with organic solvents from a solid phase produced by addition of anhydrous sodium sulphate, florisil, activated charcoal or a borate/celite mixture to the sample (Gwilt *et al.*, 1963b; Hackett and Dusci, 1977; Jeevanandam *et al.*, 1980; Pegon and Vallon, 1981; Vila-Jato *et al.*, 1981; Mathis and Budd, 1988) and by solid-phase column extraction using supports such as octadecylsilica (Schmid *et al.*, 1980; To and Wells, 1985; El Mouelhi and Buszewski,

1990; Lillsunde and Korte, 1991). Prior clean-up has also been achieved by double solvent extraction (Palmer, 1986). The [^{14}C]- labelled drug in blood and tissue homogenates has been assayed directly following benzene extraction to reduce interference and precipitation of proteins (Davison *et al.*, 1961). It was important to recognize that the plasma and urine concentrations of paracetamol conjugates often greatly exceeded those of paracetamol itself and this was an important potential source of interference (Stewart *et al.*, 1979). A chromatographic separation was usually necessary for the proper measurement of paracetamol metabolites.

In general, the same methodology could be applied to the measurement of paracetamol in different body fluids, although modification might be necessary to reduce interference and increase sensitivity. For obvious reasons plasma was usually used rather than whole blood, and the first step in many assays consisted of the removal of the proteins by precipitation. There was little site-dependent variation in arterial and venous blood concentrations of paracetamol at postmortem examination (Jones and Pounder, 1987) and it has been estimated in bone marrow and tissue from a severely decomposed body (Bal *et al.*, 1989). Some investigators claim to have found a good correlation between the concentrations of paracetamol in plasma and saliva (Glynn and Bastian, 1973; Dechtiaruk *et al.*, 1976; Adithan and Thangam, 1982; Cardot *et al.*, 1985b; Galinsky *et al.*, 1987b; Kamali *et al.*, 1987a; Nakano *et al.*, 1988; Shim *et al.*, 1990b), and in milk and saliva (Berlin *et al.*, 1980). Salivary concentrations were measured in a number of kinetic and metabolic studies (Mucklow *et al.*, 1980; Miners *et al.*, 1983, 1984c, 1986; Kamali *et al.*, 1985, 1987b, 1992; Ray *et al.*, 1985, 1986; Klein *et al.*, 1986; Back and Tjia, 1987; Galinsky *et al.*, 1987b; Hagenlocher *et al.*, 1987; Pradeep Kumar *et al.*, 1987; Somaja and Thangam, 1987; Sommers *et al.*, 1987; Adithan *et al.*, 1988; Borin and Ayres, 1989; Griener *et al.*, 1990; Ali and Sharif, 1993), but this could not be recommended as major discrepancies have been noted. The concentrations in saliva may be spuriously high during the first three hours after dosing (Lowenthal *et al.*, 1976) and the ratio between salivary and plasma concentrations was influenced by salivary flow rate (Kamali *et al.*, 1992). In one study, the salivary:serum paracetamol concentration ratio was highly dependent on the sampling time (Adithan and Thangam, 1982), and in another, mean concentrations of paracetamol in saliva were almost double those measured in plasma (Kamali *et al.*, 1992). Multiple and variable peaks have been observed in the concentrations of paracetamol in saliva following oral administration and these could not be attributed to enterohepatic recycling (Shim *et al.*, 1990b; Shim and Jung, 1992a,b). Despite these shortcomings, the assay of paracetamol in saliva may be justified in circumstances where blood sampling was impracticable as in the case of pharmacokinetic studies during spaceflight (Putcha and Cintrón, 1991).

Paracetamol and its major metabolites have been measured without difficulty in bile using established analytical and preparative high performance liquid chromatographic methods (Hinson *et al.*, 1982; Siegers *et al.*, 1983b; Hidvegi and Ecobichon, 1986; Jayasinghe *et al.*, 1986; Madhu *et al.*, 1989; Gregus *et al.*, 1990). In one report the conjugates of [^{14}C]-paracetamol in bile were assayed by a combination of paper, Sephadex gel column, and high performance liquid chromatography (Wong *et al.*, 1979). The direct analysis of paracetamol and its glutathione and glucuronide conjugates in bile by high performance liquid chromatography and mass spectrometry has been reported (Betowski *et al.*, 1987) and the biliary excretion of paracetamol conjugates has been studied using high performance liquid and thin layer chromatography followed by nuclear magnetic resonance analysis (Hinson *et al.*, 1982; Spurway *et al.*, 1990; Seddon *et al.*, 1994).

High performance liquid chromatography met most general research requirements for sensitivity, precision and specificity, and was the most favoured technique at the present time. However, the requirements for emergency assay of plasma paracetamol in hospital patients admitted with an overdose were quite different. In such circumstances, an assay was needed that could provide rapid and reliable results under emergency conditions with simple apparatus, and which could possibly be performed by a relatively unskilled operator. Sensitivity was not an issue. Simple rapid colorimetric methods were popular for this application but there was always a risk of interference from other substances. For routine indications, the use of expensive or complex methodology such as polarization fluoroimmunoassay (Coxon *et al.*, 1988; Edinboro *et al.*, 1991) and high resolution proton nuclear magnetic resonance (Bales *et al.*, 1988) was rather taking a sledge hammer to crack a nut, but sensitive and highly specific methods were necessary for identification and quantitation of minor metabolites. Methods for the routine assay of paracetamol have been reviewed by Wiener (1978) and Stewart and Watson (1987), and external quality control schemes were established for hospital laboratories (Epton, 1979; Wiener, 1980). Minor modifications of previously published methods have often been described (sometimes without acknowledgement) and these will not be discussed. The methods of assay of paracetamol in biological fluids have been reviewed in detail by Fairbrother (1974) and El-Obeid and Al-Badr (1985).

Colorimetry

In colorimetric assays of paracetamol the chromogens were developed from reactions involving

1. the phenolic group of the parent drug:
    - alkaline hypobromite – the Folin Ciocalteau reagent (Meola, 1978),
    - nitrite and 2-nitroso-1-naphthol-4-sulphonic acid (Shihabi and David, 1984),
    - ferric reduction with 2,4,6-tris(2-pyridyl)-S-triazine (Liu and Oka, 1980),
2. the amino group of p-aminophenol formed by acid hydrolysis of paracetamol:
    - diazotization and coupling with α-naphthol (Brodie and Axelrod, 1948a),
    - production of an indophenol blue by direct coupling with alkaline α-naphthol (Lester and Greenberg, 1947) or o-cresol (Tompsett, 1969),
    - the original Bratton-Marshall reaction with N-(1-naphthyl) ethylenediamine (Heirwegh and Fevery, 1967),
    - coupling with phenol in the presence of hypobromite or hypochlorite (Welch and Conney, 1965; Davis *et al.*, 1974b),
    - reaction with vanillin (Plakogiannis and Saad, 1978) or p-dimethylaminocinnamaldehyde (Liu and Skale, 1985),
3. direct nitrosation of the aromatic ring with nitrous acid to give 2-nitro-4-acetamidophenol (Le Perdriel *et al.*, 1968; Chafetz *et al.*, 1971) and
4. quenching of the violet colour of the free 2,2-diphenyl-1-picrylhydrazyl radical by its reaction with the secondary amine function of the acetamido group of paracetamol to form the yellow diphenylpicrylhydrazine (Routh *et al.*, 1968), quenching of the green colour of an established method for determination of glucose

(Clothier *et al.*, 1981), and reaction with molybdenatophosphoric acid to give 'molybdenum blue' (Issopoulos, 1990).

The first practical methods for measurement of paracetamol in blood and urine were based on colour reactions with p-aminophenol. In the method described by Lester and Greenberg (1947), plasma proteins were precipitated and the paracetamol extracted into ethylene dichloride and back-extracted into alkaline solution prior to hydrolysis to p-aminophenol by heating with hydrochloric acid. The intensity of the blue colour obtained by adding α-naphthol and sodium hydroxide was measured at 635 nm. A similar approach was described by Brodie and Axelrod (1948a) using ether extraction followed by diazotization of the p-aminophenol and coupling with α-naphthol to give a red diazo dye, which was read at 510 nm. These original methods have since been modified extensively, usually with the object of making them more simple and sensitive, and other colour reactions have also been used. In some procedures, precipitation of plasma proteins and solvent extraction have been omitted. Details of some of these methods are summarized in Table 3.1.

The use of colorimetric methods is now largely restricted to the emergency determination of plasma paracetamol in hospital laboratories. One formerly popular assay was based on the methods of Le Perdriel *et al.* (1968), Chafetz *et al.* (1971) and Daly *et al.* (1972) as modified by Glynn and Kendal (1975). Paracetamol was reacted directly with nitrous acid to give yellow 2-nitro-4-acetamidophenol and all that was required was the addition of reagents to the sample. There was good agreement with a standard differential absorbance method (Wiener, 1977) and between manual and kit versions of this method (Braiotta and Buttery, 1982). One problem was interference by salicylate giving spuriously high results (Hill, 1983; Badcock *et al.*, 1984), and various correction factors and modifications (such as measurement at a higher wavelength or solvent extraction) were proposed to minimize this (Mace and Walker, 1976; Walberg, 1977; Archer and Richardson, 1980; Barker and Jacobs, 1982; Buttery *et al.*, 1982a; Longlands and Wiener, 1982; Swanson and Walters, 1982; Mezei *et al.*, 1983). Details of some modifications are shown in Table 3.2. In one procedure, which was based on a centrifugal analyser, interference by salicylate was virtually eliminated and only a 50 μl sample was required (Shihabi and David, 1984). However, salicylate interference in some commercial kits for the colorimetric assay of paracetamol caused major discrepancies, which would influence management decisions in overdose patients (Rosenbaum *et al.*, 1980; Reed *et al.*, 1982; Jenny, 1985). There was considerable interference with the method of Glynn and Kendal in patients with uraemia (Dinwoodie, 1978), but this could be reduced by prior ether extraction (Bailey, 1982). In patients with jaundice there was interference with the ferric reduction method of Liu and Oka (1980) in proportion to the plasma bilirubin concentration and this was reduced by the use of protein-free filtrates (Kellmeyer *et al.*, 1982). The ferric reduction method was modified as a rapid screening test (Tulley, 1985) and it was said not to be subject to interference from salicylate (Liu and Bigler, 1983). Bilirubin also interfered with methods based on the Folin-Ciocalteau reagent, but this was minimized by prior treatment with p-diazobenzene sulphonic acid, which formed a non-extractable red dye (Swanson and Walters, 1982). It must be assumed that salicylate and other phenolic drugs would interfere with all the indophenol blue reactions, and the potential for interference was a serious disadvantage of colorimetric methods. In one report, it was claimed that salicylate did not interfere with the indophenol reaction, but in the quoted pro-

Table 3.1 Colorimetric assays for paracetamol.

Colour reaction	Wavelength (nm)	Prior solvent extraction	Interference from conjugates	Reference
(1) *Indophenol Blue*				
(a) Phenolic group of paracetamol reacts with phenol in presence of alkaline hypobromite (Folin-Ciocalteau reagent)	620	No	Yes	Welch and Conney, 1965
	660	Yes	No	Meola, 1978
	660	Yes	No	Gupta, 1982
	660	Yes	No	Swanson and Walters, 1982
	660	Yes	No	Gupta *et al.*, 1983
(b) Acid hydrolysis to p-aminophenol then reaction with alkaline phenol, α-naphthol or o-cresol	635	Yes	No	Lester and Greenberg, 1947
	635	Yes	No	Gwilt *et al.*, 1963b
	620	No	Yes	Tompsett, 1969
	620	No	Yes	Wilkinson, 1976
	615	No	Yes	Love, 1977
	620	No	Yes	Frings and Saloom, 1979
	615	No	Yes	Miceli *et al.*, 1979b
	615	No	Yes	Adithan and Thangam, 1982
	620	No	Yes	Novotony and Elser, 1984
	620	No	Yes	Patel and Morton, 1988
	620	Yes	No	Shannon *et al.*, 1990
(2) *Diazotization*				
Acid hydrolysis to p-aminophenol which is diazotized and coupled with α-naphthol or N-(1-naphthyl) ethylenediamine	510	Yes	No	Brodie and Axelrod, 1948a
	578	Yes	No	Heirwegh and Fevery, 1967
(3) *Reaction with vanillin*	395	No	Yes	Plakogiannis and Saad, 1978
(4) *Reaction with p-dimethylaminocinnamaldehyde*	520	Yes	No	Liu and Skale, 1985
(5) *Reaction with diphenylpicrylhydrazyl*	527	Yes	No	Routh *et al.*, 1968
(6) *Reaction with 2-nitroso-1-naphthol-4-sulphonic acid*	530	No	No	Shihabi and David, 1984
(7) *Reaction with molybdenophosphoric acid*	695	No	Unknown	Issopoulos, 1990
(8) *Ferric reduction*				
Reduction of ferric to ferrous iron by paracetamol then reaction with 2,4,6-tris(2-pyridyl)-S-triazine	593	Yes	No	Liu and Oka, 1980

13

Table 3.2 Colorimetric assays for paracetamol based on aromatic nitrosation.

Colour reaction	Wavelength (nm)	Comments	Reference
Direct reaction with HCl and nitrite to form 2-nitro-4-acetamidophenol followed by alkalinization	430	Original method	Le Perdriel *et al*, 1968
	430	Most popular modification	Glynn and Kendal, 1975
	450	Reduced interference by salicylate	Mace and Walker, 1976
	430	Increased sensitivity	Walberg, 1977
	430	Reduced interference by salicylate	Archer and Richardson, 1980
	430	Reduced interference in uraemia	Bailey, 1982
	430	Reduced interference by salicylate	Barker and Jacobs, 1982
	450	Reduced interference by salicylate	Longlands and Wiener, 1982
Reaction with 2-nitroso-1-naphthol-4-sulphonic acid and nitrite	530	Reduced interference by salicylate	Shihabi and David, 1984

cedure the conjugates of paracetamol were hydrolyzed to p-aminophenol causing gross interference anyway, irrespective of any contribution from salicylate (Miceli and Aravind, 1980). Unexpected (but in retrospect predictable) problems have arisen with false positive results from samples taken with blood gas syringes containing heparin preserved with cresol (Pitts, 1979) and false negative results in patients who have ingested large amounts of ascorbic acid, which inhibited the indophenol blue reaction (Swale, 1977). This reaction was also inhibited by tetracycline and chloramphenicol (Chakrabarty, 1979), while levodopa and related compounds could give false positive results (Andrews *et al.*, 1982).

The most serious source of error with some colorimetric (and other simple) methods was the omission of the organic solvent extraction of paracetamol before acid hydrolysis to p-aminophenol. In such circumstances, paracetamol glucuronide and paracetamol sulphate (often present in much higher concentrations in the sample than the parent drug) would also be hydrolyzed to p-aminophenol, leading to gross overestimation of the paracetamol. This would not be recognized during method development if (as was usually the case) standards were prepared simply by weighing in paracetamol because the false high values would only occur in the presence of the conjugates. The enormity of the errors (which may result in four- to seven-fold mean overestimates of the true concentration of paracetamol) would not be appreciated unless the method was compared with a specific procedure using real samples from individuals who have taken paracetamol. The clinical consequences of the use of such unsatisfactory procedures were disturbing (Stewart *et al.*, 1979; Buttery *et al.*, 1982b). For these reasons, the methods of Tompsett (1969), Dolegeal-Vendrely and Guernet (1976), Wilkinson (1976), Love (1977), Plakogiannis and Saad (1978), Frings and Saloom (1979), Miceli *et al.* (1979b), Adithan and Thangam (1982), Novotony and Elser (1984) and Patel and Morton (1988) are not suitable for the estimation of paracetamol in biological samples. Novotony and Elser compounded the errors by stating incorrectly that the treatment nomogram for poisoned patients was based on total free and conjugated paracetamol, and that total drug should be measured.

In other comparisons, good correlations have been obtained with plasma samples containing paracetamol conjugates analysed by the nitrosation method of Glynn and Kendal (1975) and specific gas liquid and high performance liquid chromatographic methods (Chambers and Jones, 1976; Stewart *et al.*, 1979; Buttery *et al.*, 1982b), and with samples made up with weighed-in paracetamol only (Archer and Richardson, 1980; Bridges *et al.*, 1983; Hale and Poklis, 1983). On the other hand, in one report, the Glynn and Kendal method gave much higher values than high performance chromatography in the analysis of samples from two patients who had taken paracetamol in overdosage and the discrepancies were greatest at low concentrations (Duffy and Byers, 1979). It was not stated whether the ingestion of other drugs by these patients had been excluded. The cysteine and mercapturic acid conjugates of paracetamol could contribute to the colour reaction, but their concentrations in plasma were not high enough to cause clinically significant errors. Blank sera could give apparent concentrations of paracetamol of 10–20 mg l^{-1} (Walberg, 1979; Alkhayat, 1986b). Screening tests for the intake of phenacetin and paracetamol were based on acid hydrolysis of urine followed by the indophenol reaction (Dubach, 1967a; Simpson and Stewart, 1973; Padmore and Padmore, 1987). Urine screening has very limited value in the management of overdose patients and false negative results have been obtained (Ray *et al.*, 1987). Major interference could also be caused by the presence in the urine of ascorbate (Buttery *et al.*, 1988) and N-acetylcysteine (Davey and Naidoo, 1993). Methods have been described again for the estimation of total free and conjugated paracetamol in urine by acid hydrolysis followed by the indophenol reaction (Moës, 1974a; Chang *et al.*, 1993). Microwave heating was recommended for the rapid hydrolysis of paracetamol and its conjugates prior to the formation of indophenol blue (Dasgupta and Kinnaman, 1993).

Ultraviolet (UV) Spectrophotometry

Relatively few spectrophotometric methods for the estimation of paracetamol have been based on its native UV absorbance. The drug was extracted from the sample (usually plasma), using ether, ethyl acetate or chloroform, and either back-extracted into weak alkali or the solvent evaporated and the residue taken up in sodium bicarbonate solution or methanol. In the most popular method (Routh *et al.*, 1968), the differential absorbance spectrum of paracetamol was measured at 266 nm. This corresponded to the isobestic points of both acetylsalicylate and salicylate, and interference by these drugs, therefore, was conveniently avoided. However, phenylbutazone caused serious interference (Wiener *et al.*, 1976). Similar methods were described in which the differential absorbance was measured at 266 and 290 nm (Scemama, 1972; Knepil, 1974). It was claimed that there was no interference from salicylate in these methods but the assays were performed on standards with weighed-in paracetamol rather than samples from real patients or volunteers. In one very simple method, the optical density of an ether extract of plasma was determined directly at 250 nm (Dordoni *et al.*, 1973). As the authors admitted, this method was not specific and many drugs were shown to cause interference (Spooner *et al.*, 1976). More recently, a procedure based on the second derivative spectrum of paracetamol in methanol has been described (Dingeon *et al.*, 1988). The spectrum was scanned from 300 to 216 nm, and the second derivative was taken as the difference between the absorbance at the maximum peak at 262 nm and the minimum at 241 nm. The lower limit of reliability was only 10 mg l^{-1} but there was no interference by salicylate. The method gave good correlations with an indophenol blue method (Gupta, 1982) using both weighed-in standards and samples from overdose patients. In another study, there was a good correlation between the assay of weighed-in standards by second derivative spectrophotometry and high performance liquid chromatography but the performance of the former method deteriorated at concentrations below 50 mg l^{-1} (Edinboro *et al.*, 1991). A combined second derivative spectroscopic assay of plasma paracetamol and salicylate has been described. However, prior hydrolysis to p-aminophenol was required and, as it was therefore non-specific, it would have very limited application (Bermejo *et al.*, 1991).

Paper, Thin Layer and Column Chromatography

Early chromatographic methods for the estimation of paracetamol and its metabolites were based on paper chromatography (Jollow *et al.*, 1974; Smith and Timbrell, 1974) and conventional thin layer chromatography using different solvents with colour reagents and fluorescence quenching to develop the spots (Büch *et al.*, 1966b, 1967c; Cummings *et al.*, 1967; Klutch and Bordun, 1968; Goenechea, 1969; Gmyrek *et al.*, 1971; Gupta *et al.*, 1977; Concheiro *et al.*, 1982; Degen *et al.*, 1982; Lohse, 1985; Kahela *et al.*, 1987). A rapid thin layer chromatographic method has been described for the assay of paracetamol in saliva (Drehsen and Rohdewald, 1981) and a thin layer procedure for the emergency estimation of paracetamol following over-dosage has been developed in which the drug is detected by its reaction with ferric iron and 2,4,6-tris(2'pyridyl)-S-triazine to give an intense blue colour (Kelly *et al.*, 1984). Thin layer chromatography was also used for urine screening to detect the intake of phenacetin and paracetamol (Kobbe and Goenechea, 1982). In metabolic studies with $[^3H]$- and $[^{14}C]$-paracetamol using paper or thin layer chromatog-raphy, the drug and its metabolites have been determined by cutting the paper into strips or scraping the spots from the plates and measuring the radioactivity by scin-tillation spectrometry after elution with methanol (Mitchell *et al.*, 1974; Thomas *et al.*, 1974; Smith and Griffiths, 1976; Pang and Gillette, 1978b; Warrander *et al.*, 1985; Spurway *et al.*, 1990). Another approach was a preliminary thin layer chro-matographic separation followed by reversed phase high performance liquid chro-matography with electrochemical detection (Hamilton and Kissinger, 1982). Two-dimensional thin layer chromatography has been used to facilitate the separa-tion of paracetamol and its metabolites (Imashuku and LaBrosse, 1971; Andrews *et al.*, 1976; Davis *et al.*, 1976b). Paracetamol and its metabolites have also been separated by Sephadex gel column chromatography but this technique was very time-consuming (Jagenburg *et al.*, 1968). DEAE cellulose anion exchange resin columns have also been used to separate $[^3H]$-paracetamol and its conjugates in urine with measurement of radioactivity in fractions of the eluate (Grantham *et al.*, 1972, 1974). Although some of the early methods were developed primarily for the isolation of acetanilide and phenacetin metabolites, they did provide for the first time a means for reasonably specific, if laborious, determination of paracetamol. Although these older methods have now been largely superseded, simple rapid assays for paracetamol in plasma have been developed using high performance thin layer chromatography with densitometry (Berner *et al.*, 1985; Kosmeas and Clerc, 1989). Thin layer chromatography has been combined with gas chromatography and mass spectrometry to provide a rapid and sensitive system for comprehensive drug screening in urine (Lillsunde and Korte, 1991).

Gas Liquid Chromatography

In gas liquid chromatographic methods the drug or derivative was vaporized and carried by an inert gas through a heated column packed with a support material, which was coated with a thin layer of a stationary liquid phase. Liquid phases differ in polarity and so compounds were retained according to their affinity as they parti-tioned between them and the carrier gas. Paracetamol eluting from the column could be measured by flame ionization detection (Prescott, 1971a), nitrogen-phosphorus sensitive flame ionization detection (Kinsella *et al.*, 1979), electron capture detection (Chan and McCann, 1979), or mass spectrometry (Murray and Boobis, 1991).

There were problems with the direct gas chromatography of paracetamol due to its polarity and this caused obvious 'tailing' with serious adsorption losses even on polar liquid phases. The losses were most marked at low concentrations and the response was not linear. Several investigators have described simple methods using underivatized paracetamol (Grove, 1971; Windorfer and Röttger, 1974; Stewart and Willis, 1975; Chambers and Jones, 1976; Kinsella *et al.*, 1979; Jeevanandam *et al.*, 1980), but these will be subject to adsorption losses that would undoubtedly increase unpredictably as the columns age. In the report by Grove (1971) there was clear evidence of adsorption as the calibration graph did not pass through the origin. It was necessary, therefore, to form less polar derivatives prior to chromatography and the trimethylsilyl (Prescott, 1971a), acetyl (Prescott, 1971b), benzoyl (Street, 1975), methyl (Garland *et al.*, 1977), O-heptyl-N-methyl (Dechtiaruk *et al.*, 1976), trifluoromethylbenzoyl (Murray and Boobis, 1986), pentafluorobenzyl (Chan and McCann, 1979) and trifluoroacetyl (Kaa, 1980; Murray and Boobis, 1991) derivatives of paracetamol have been synthesized for this purpose (Table 3.3).

The general method for the assay of paracetamol consisted of addition of the internal standard (commonly N-propionyl- or N-butyryl-p-aminophenol) to the buffered sample, which was then extracted into an organic solvent such as ether or ethyl acetate. The solvent was removed by evaporation, and the residue redissolved in a small volume. The derivatizing reagents were added and when the reaction was complete an aliquot of up to 10 μl was injected into the chromatograph. A variety of liquid phases have been used, and in most reports the response has been measured with a flame ionization detector. The concentration of paracetamol in the original sample was calculated from the peak area or height ratio of the unknown to the internal standard relative to a known standard response.

In the first practical method for the assay of plasma and urine paracetamol by gas liquid chromatography after therapeutic doses, the drug was converted to the trimethylsilyl derivative (Prescott *et al.*, 1970). There have been many subsequent modifications and improvements, and details of some published methods are set out in Table 3.3. Capillary gas chromatography was used for toxicological analysis of paracetamol and other agents in fatal poisoning with multiple drugs (Klys and Brandys, 1988). Gas liquid chromatography was an excellent technique for the assay of drugs such as paracetamol but its popularity has waned in recent years because of the invariable need for solvent extraction and derivatization. However, when combined with mass spectrometry and fragmentography, it retained an eminent position in a very powerful technique for the identification and trace analysis of paracetamol and its metabolites (Baty *et al.*, 1976; Garland. *et al.*, 1977; Murray and Boobis, 1991). With this combination, as little as 1 pg of paracetamol was detected (Murray and Boobis, 1986, 1991). Capillary gas chromatography was used with mass spectrometry and stable isotopes to determine the extent of acetylation and deacetylation of paracetamol (Baty *et al.*, 1988) and synthetic N-acetyl-p-benzoquinoneimine was also analysed by gas chromatography and mass spectrometry (Huggett and Blair, 1983b). Trace residues of paracetamol after handling tablets were detected by surface sampling and ion mobility spectrometry (Lawrence, 1987).

High Performance Liquid Chromatography

High performance liquid chromatography has developed in recent years to the point where it is now the technique of choice for most drug analyses. Unlike gas liquid chromatography, it was not limited by considerations of volatility, temperature stability, molecular weight or polarity and derivatization was not normally necessary.

Table 3.3 Details of some gas liquid chromatographic assays of paracetamol.

Derivative	Extracting solvent	Liquid phase	Column temp °C	Detector*	Internal standard	Reference
Trimethylsilyl	Ethyl acetate	5%OV1	150–160	FID	p-Bromacetanilide	Prescott et al., 1970
None	Ether	2%FFAP	240	FID	Diphenylphthalate	Grove, 1971
Trimethylsilyl	Ethyl acetate	10%OV1	200	FID	p-Chloracetanilide	Prescott, 1971a
Acetyl	Ethyl acetate	3%OV1	220	FID	N-Butyryl-p-aminophenol	Prescott, 1971b
Trimethylsilyl	Ether	3%OV1	160	FID	p-Bromacetanilide	Thomas and Coldwell, 1972
None	Chloroform	3%HI-EFF 8BP	240	FID	N-Butyryl-p-aminophenol	Stewart and Willis, 1975
Benzoyl	Ether	SE52	220	FID	N-Butyryl-p-aminophenol	Street, 1975
Trifluoroacetyl	Ethyl acetate	3%OV17	120	FID	3-Hydroxyacetanilide	Alván et al., 1976
Trimethylsilyl	Ethyl acetate	3%OV17	160	MS	d_2-Paracetamol	Baty et al., 1976
None	Ether	3%HI-EFF 8BP	225	not stated	N-Butyryl-p-aminophenol	Chambers and Jones, 1976
Heptyl-methyl	Ether	3%OV17	150–260	FID	N-Propionyl-p-aminophenol	Dechtiaruk et al., 1976
Butyryl	Ethyl acetate	3%OV17	200	FID	N-propionyl-p-aminophenol	Serfontein et al., 1976
Methyl	Ether	3%SP2250	165	FID	p-Bromacetanilide	Evans and Harbison, 1977
Methyl	Benzene/CH_2Cl_2	3%OV17	180–195	MS	d_3-Paracetamol	Garland et al., 1977
Acetyl	Ether	3%OV17	190	FID	Diphenylpyraline	Hackett and Dusci, 1977
Trimethylsilyl	Ether	3%OV1	210	FID	p-Bromacetanilide	Kalra et al., 1977
Methyl	Ethyl acetate	3%SE30	210	N-P FID	Theobromine	Siegers et al., 1978
Acetyl	CH_2Cl_2	3%SP225-DA	180	FID	2-Hydroxyacetanilide	Thoma et al., 1978
Methyl	Ether	3.8%SE30	145	FID	N-Butyryl-p-aminophenol	Wahl and Rejent, 1978
Pentafluorobenzyl	Ether/CH_2Cl_2	3%SP2100	200	ECD	N-Butyryl-p-aminophenol	Chan and McCann, 1979
None	Ethyl acetate	3%OV17	190	N-P FID	Barbiturate	Kinsella et al., 1979
Trifluoroacetyl	Ethyl acetate	OV210/OV1	120	FID	2-Hydroxyacetanilide	Kaa, 1980
Trifluoroacetyl	Ethyl acetate	3%OV17	130	FID/MS	N-Butyryl-p-aminophenol	Bitzén et al., 1981
Acetyl	Pyridine	3%OV17	190	FID	N-Butyryl-p-aminophenol	Pegon and Vallon, 1981
Methyl	Ether	3%OV225	225	N-P FID	N-Butyryl-p-aminophenol	Sharman, 1981
Methyl	Ethyl acetate	3%OV17	190	FID	Phenobarbitone	Becherucci et al., 1981
Acetyl	Chloroform	3%Apolane 87	235	FID	N-Butyryl-p-aminophenol	Huggett et al., 1981
CF_3methylbenzoyl	Ether	SE54	160–280	MS	$[^2H_3]$-Paracetamol	Murray and Boobis, 1986
Trifluoroacetyl	Ether	Capillary	210	MS	$[^2H_4]$-Paracetamol	Murray and Boobis, 1991

* FID = flame ionization detector, N-P FID = nitrogen/phosphorus-sensitive flame ionization detector, ECD = electron capture detector, MS = mass spectrometry

Early methods for the assay of paracetamol in blood plasma and urine by this technique employed conventional chromatographic materials such as silica and ion exchange resins (Wong *et al.*, 1976a; Blair and Rumack, 1977). However, separations were greatly improved with the introduction of reverse-phase supports such as C_{18} hydrocarbon bonded to silanized spherical silica (octadecylsilica, ODS) used in conjunction with polar mobile phases such as methanol/water with or without buffers or ion pairing or suppressing agents. With minor modification it was possible to separate and measure multiple metabolites simultaneously (Knox and Jurand, 1977, 1978). Chromatography was usually carried out under isocratic conditions, but the composition of the mobile phase could be varied with programmed gradient elution for more complex analyses involving the estimation of multiple metabolites (Figure 3.1) (Mrochek *et al.*, 1974; Hart *et al.*, 1981; Aguilar *et al.*, 1988). Detection was usually by ultraviolet spectrophotometry and this was often adequate for measurement of paracetamol concentrations following a therapeutic dose without the need for an organic solvent extraction to clean up and concentrate the sample. The effects of eluant pH on the ionic and molecular forms of paracetamol and on its chromatographic properties were reported (Nivaud-Guernet *et al.*, 1994).

Mrochek *et al.* (1974) and Katz *et al.* (1975) reported the comprehensive and lengthy separation and identification of paracetamol and many of its metabolites in urine by high resolution anion exchange chromatography, and Knox and Jurand (1977, 1978) described in detail more practical procedures for the determination of paracetamol and its important metabolites using reverse-phase bonded supports and ion-pair systems. Riggin *et al.* (1975) first reported the use of a sensitive electrochemical detector for the assay of paracetamol, and soon after, a number of simple specific methods appeared in which the drug was chromatographed on silica gel (Wong *et al.*, 1976a), cation exchange resin (Blair and Rumack, 1977) and reverse-phase octadecylsilica (Gotelli *et al.*, 1977; Horvitz and Jatlow, 1977; Howie *et al.*, 1977; Adriaenssens and Prescott, 1978). The C_{18} bonded silica supports were clearly superior to previously available materials, and these methods were developed and refined in many subsequent reports. Thus, by modifying an earlier method, Buchanan *et al.* (1979) estimated plasma paracetamol in a 100 μl sample within five minutes with a coefficient of variation of 2.3–3.6 per cent. With electrochemical detection, concentrations could be measured down to 20–50 μg l^{-1} (Riggin *et al.*, 1975; Miner and Kissinger, 1979a), and microvolumetric methods have been developed for repeated sampling in small animals (To and Wells, 1985).

In its simplest form, the general method for the assay of paracetamol in plasma consisted of addition of internal standard (commonly N-propionyl- or N-butyryl-p-aminophenol), precipitation of plasma proteins with trichloracetic or perchloric acid, centrifugation, and injection of an aliquot of the clear supernatant onto a reverse-phase 5 or 10 μ octadecylsilica column. The mobile phase may be a buffered water-methanol mixture and the column effluent was monitored with a UV detector at 254 nm. Some investigators included a solvent extraction with ether or ethyl acetate before chromatography. Details of some published reports are summarized in Table 3.4. The simplest methods were usually adequate for the measurement of paracetamol following therapeutic doses, and with the more complex procedures, metabolites could also be determined. Reverse-phase high performance liquid chromatography has been employed for the investigation of a cyclic acetylsalicylate-paracetamol prodrug (Marzo *et al.*, 1990) and combined with mass spectrometry, for detailed metabolic studies of 3-hydroxyacetanilide, a regioisomer of paracetamol

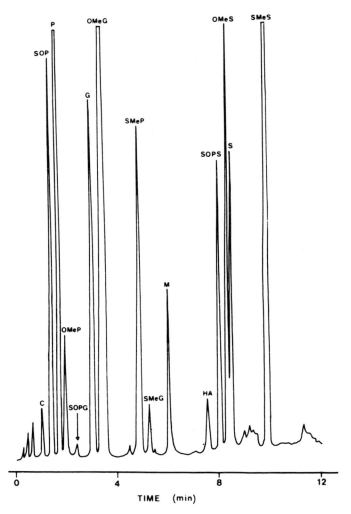

Figure 3.1 Gradient-programmed ion-pair separation of paracetamol and its metabolites in urine on a reverse phase 5 μ C_{18} column with UV detection at 254 nm. The mobile phase was 0.02 M tetrabutylammonium, 0.01 M Tris, pH 5.0 (phosphoric acid) programmed from 15 to 50 per cent acetonitrile over 11 min after a delay of 1 min at a flow rate of 2 ml min^{-1}, 1.0 AUFS. The peak identities were as follows: P = paracetamol, C = paracetamol cysteine conjugate, SOP = 3-thiomethylparacetamol sulphoxide, OMeP = 3-methoxyparacetamol, SOPG = 3-thiomethylparacetamol sulphoxide glucuronide, G = paracetamol glucuronide, OMeG = 3-methoxyparacetamol glucuronide, SMeP = 3-thiomethylparacetamol, SMeG = 3-thiomethylparacetamol glucuronide, M = paracetamol mercapturic acid conjugate, HA = hippuric acid, SOPS = 3-thiomethylparacetamol sulphoxide sulphate, OMeS = 3-methoxyparacetamol sulphate, S = paracetamol sulphate, SMeS = 3-thiomethylparacetamol sulphate. (Reproduced from Aguilar *et al.*, 1988, with permission.)

(Rashed and Nelson, 1989b). It has also been used for the purification of $[^{14}C]$-paracetamol for metabolic studies (Devalia and McLean, 1982). Methods have been described for the automated on-line extraction of paracetamol from serum followed by liquid chromatographic assay (van der Wal *et al.*, 1982).

Table 3.4 Details of some high performance liquid chromatographic assays of paracetamol.

Column	Mobile phase	Solvent extraction	Internal standard	Detector and wavelength (nm)	Metabolites measured	Reference
Anion exchange	Gradient elution	No	None	UV 254	Yes	Mrochek et al., 1974
Polyamide	PO_4 buffer	Ethyl acetate	None	EC	No	Riggin et al., 1975
Silica	TF, $CHCl_3$, HAc	Ether	None	UV 247	No	Wong et al., 1976a
Cation exchange	$NH_4H_2PO_4$ buffer	No	NBA	UV 247	No	Blair and Rumack, 1977
Reverse phase	MeOH, HAc	No	None	UV 254	Yes	Buckpitt et al., 1977
Reverse phase	Acetonitrile, PO_4 buffer	Ethyl acetate	Acetoacetanilide	UV 254	No	Gotelli et al., 1977
Reverse phase	Acetonitrile, PO_4 buffer	Ether	NPA	UV 250	No	Horvitz and Jatlow, 1977
Reverse phase	HAc, ethyl acetate	No	4-Fluorophenol	UV 250	Yes	Howie et al., 1977
Reverse phase	MeOH, HF	No	None	UV 254	Yes	Knox and Jurand, 1977
Reverse phase	HF, isopropanol, PO_4 buffer	No	NPA	UV 254	Yes	Adriaenssens and Prescott, 1978
Reverse phase	Acetonitrile, acetate buffer	No	HET	UV 254	No	Black and Sprague, 1978
Reverse phase	Acetonitrile, acetate buffer	No	None	UV 254	No	Fowler and Altmiller, 1978
Reverse phase	MeOH, HF	No	None	UV 254	Yes	Knox and Jurand, 1978
Reverse phase	Gradient elution	No	4-Fluorophenol	UV 250	Yes	Moldéus, 1978
Polyamide	MeOH, PO_4 buffer	Ethyl acetate	Butoxyphenol	EC	No	Munson et al., 1978
Reverse phase	HF, isopropanol, PO_4 buffer	No	NPA	UV 250	No	Buchanan et al., 1979
Silica	$CHCl_3$, heptane, EtOH, HAc	Ethyl acetate	3-Hydroxyacetanilide	UV 254	No	Fletterick et al., 1979
Reverse phase	Acetonitrile, water	Ethyl acetate	3-Hydroxyacetanilide	UV 254	No	Lo and Bye, 1979
Reverse phase	Isopropanol, phosphoric acid	$CHCl_3$, IP	8-Chlorotheophylline	UV 248	No	Miceli et al., 1979a
Reverse phase	MeOH, HAc	DM, ether, IP	NPA	EC	No	Miner and Kissinger, 1979a
Reverse phase	Acetonitrile, HPS	Ethyl acetate	^{3}H-paracetamol	UV 254/280	Yes	Pang et al., 1979b
Reverse phase	MeOH, PO_4 buffer	Acetonitrile	Salicylamide	UV 254	No	Wilson, 1979
Reverse phase	MeOH, HAc	No	None	Rad	Yes	Wong et al., 1979
Reverse phase	Acetonitrile, acetate buffer	No	NBA	Not stated	No	Berlin et al., 1980
Reverse phase	MeOH, PO_4 buffer	No	None	UV 248	No	Ebel et al., 1980
Reverse phase	MeOH, water	Ether	Vanillin	UV 254	No	Imamura et al., 1980
Reverse phase	MeOH, PO_4 buffer	No	None	UV 254/280	No	Nielsen-Kudsk, 1980
Reverse phase	MeOH, PO_4 buffer	No	None	EC	No	Surmann, 1980
Reverse phase	Acetonitrile, MeOH, water	Ethyl acetate	2-Hydroxyacetanilide	UV 254	No	Ameer et al., 1981
Reverse phase	Various	PGC	None	UV 254	Yes	Gemborys and Mudge, 1981
Reverse phase	Gradient elution	No	None	UV 254	Yes	Hart et al., 1981
Reverse phase	Acetonitrile, acetate buffer	No	HET	UV 254	No	Manno et al., 1981

						Reference
Reverse phase	Acetonitrile, HAc, TEA	Ethyl acetate	HET	UV 204	No	Quattrone and Putnam, 1981
Reverse phase	MeOH, phosphate buffer	No	Salicylamide	UV 240	No	Uges et al., 1981
Reverse phase	MeOH, HF	Na_2SO_4, MeOH	None	UV 254	No	Vila-Jato et al., 1981
Reverse phase	MeOH, HAc	Ethyl acetate	Acetanilide	UV 250	No	West, 1981
Silica	$CHCl_3$, heptane, EtOH, HAc	Ethyl acetate	3-Hydroxyacetanilide	UV 248	No	Buskin et al., 1982
Reverse phase	Acetonitrile, PO_4 buffer	Ethyl acetate	None	UV 237	No	Douidar and Ahmed, 1982
Reverse phase	MeOH, HAc	No	Diethyltoluamide	UV 248	No	Ferrel and Goyette, 1982
Reverse phase	MeOH, acetate buffer	TLC	None	EC	Yes	Hamilton and Kissinger, 1982
Reverse phase	MeOH, acetate buffer	DM, IP	8-Chlorotheophylline	UV 280	No	Kinberger and Holmén, 1982
Reverse phase	Dioxane, TBA	No	None	UV 254	Yes	Newton et al., 1982b
Reverse phase	MeOH, water	No	None	UV 240	No	O'Connell and Zurzola, 1982
Reverse phase	Acetonitrile, PO_4 buffer	Ethyl acetate	HET	UV 254	No	Ou and Frawley, 1982
Silica	MeOH, PO_4 buffer, TEA	$CHCl_3$, IP	HET	UV 254	Yes	van der Wal et al., 1982
Reverse phase	MeOH, HAc, PO_4 buffer	No	None	UV 270	Yes	Wilson et al., 1982a
Reverse phase	MeOH, PO_4 buffer	Ether	NBA	EC	No	Borm et al., 1983
Reverse phase	Gradient elution	No	None	None	Yes	Glazenburg et al., 1983
Reverse phase	Ethanol, water	Ethyl acetate	Salicylamide	UV 254	Yes	Hikal et al., 1983
Reverse phase	MeOH, HAc, HPS	Ethyl acetate	3-Hydroxyacetanilide	UV 254	No	Villeneuve et al., 1983
Reverse phase	MeOH, PO_4 buffer, TBA	No	Sulphacetamide	UV 250	Yes	Watari et al., 1983
Reverse phase	MeOH, HF, water	Ethyl acetate	NPA	UV 254	No	Wong, 1983
Reverse phase	Acetonitrile, acetate buffer	No	None	UV 254	Yes	Ameer et al., 1984
Reverse phase	Acetonitrile, acetate buffer	Ether	HET	UV 254	No	Demotes-Mainard et al., 1984
Reverse phase	MeOH, water	Acetonitrile	NPA	UV 254	No	Korduba and Petruzzi, 1984
Reverse phase	Acetonitrile, PO_4 buffer	No	None	UV 254	Yes	Miners et al., 1984a
Reverse phase	Acetonitrile, PO_4 buffer	No	Theophylline	UV 254	Yes	Jung and Zafar, 1985
Reverse phase	AN, MeOH, PO_4 buffer	$CHCl_3$, AN	None	UV 234	No	Tebbett et al., 1985
Reverse phase	Gradient elution	No	Acetanilide	UV 248	Yes	To and Wells, 1985
Reverse phase	Tetrahydofuran, water	Ethyl acetate	Propophylline	UV 254	No	Willems et al., 1985
Reverse phase	Acetonitrile, TBA	No	p-OH-benzoic acid	UV 245	Yes	Colin et al., 1986b
Reverse phase	MeOH, PO_4 buffer	Ethyl acetate	HET	UV 250	No	Hannothiaux et al., 1986
Reverse phase	MeOH, HAc	No	None	UV 254	Yes	Hidvegi and Ecobichon, 1986
Reverse phase	HAc, PO_4 buffer	No	4-Fluorophenol	UV 254	Yes	Mineshita et al., 1986
Reverse phase	MeOH, NH_4Ac, NaAc	Ethyl acetate	NPA	EC	No	Palmer, 1986
Reverse phase	MeOH, acetate buffer	No	Benzoic acid	UV 249	No	Starkey et al., 1986
Reverse phase	IP, HF, PO_4 buffer	No	NPA	UV 240	Yes	Stevens and Gill, 1986
Reverse phase	IP, HF, PO_4 buffer	No	3-Hydroxyacetanilide	UV 254	Yes	Tredger et al., 1986b

(cont.)

Table 3.4 (cont.)

Column	Mobile phase	Solvent extraction	Internal standard	Detector and wavelength (nm)	Metabolites measured	Reference
Reverse phase	MeOH, HAc, PO$_4$ buffer	No	None	UV 254	Yes	Vila-Jato et al., 1986b
Reverse phase	MeOH, NH$_4$COOCH$_3$	No	None	Mass spectrometry	Yes	Betowski et al., 1987
Reverse phase	Acetonitrile, water	Acetonitrile, IP	Sulphamerazine	UV 254	No	Colin et al., 1987
Reverse phase	Gradient elution	No	None	UV 254/SS	Yes	Dolphin et al., 1987
Reverse phase	MeOH, KH$_2$PO$_4$	Ethyl acetate	Salicylamide	UV 254	No	Kinney and Kelly, 1987
Reverse phase	Gradient elution	No	3-Hydroxyacetanilide	UV 254	Yes	Ladds et al., 1987
Reverse phase	Acetonitrile, Na$_2$SO$_4$, H$_3$PO$_4$	No	Theophylline	UV 254	Yes	Nakamura et al., 1987a
Reverse phase	MeOH, PO$_4$ buffer	No	3-Hydroxyacetanilide	UV 254	Yes	Sood and Green, 1987
Reverse phase	Gradient elution	No	None	UV 254/280	Yes	Aguilar et al., 1988
Reverse phase	MeOH, HAc, PO$_4$ buffer	No	Theobromine	UV 242	Yes	Bhargava et al., 1988
Reverse phase	Acetonitrile, NaAc buffer	No	Propoxyphylline	UV 280	No	Cociglio and Alric, 1988
Reverse phase	MeOH, PO$_4$ buffer	No	Benzoic acid	UV 240	No	Dawson et al., 1988b
Reverse phase	Gradient elution	No	None	UV 254/EC	Yes	Debets et al., 1988
Reverse phase	MeOH, acetonitrile, PO$_4$ buffer	CH$_3$Cl, IP	IBX	UV 273	No	Meatherall and Ford, 1988
Reverse phase	Acetonitrile, HAc, AHP	No	8-Chlorotheophylline	UV 254	No	Osterloh and Yu, 1988
Reverse phase	Acetonitrile, water	No	2-Hydroxyacetanilide	UV 254	No	Salvadó et al., 1988
Silica	Heptane, CH$_2$Cl$_2$, IP, MeOH	Acetonitrile	Phenacetin	UV 266	No	Avramova, 1989
Reverse phase	MeOH, PO$_4$ buffer	No	4-Fluorophenol	UV 254	No	Kotal et al., 1989
Reverse phase	MeOH, water, isopropanol	No	None	UV 254	No	Mancilla et al., 1989
Reverse phase	MeOH, PO$_4$ buffer, TBA	No	None	UV 250	No	Rustum, 1989
Reverse phase	MeOH, HAc, TBA, K$_2$SO$_4$	CHCl$_3$, IP	HET	UV 254	Yes	Kamali and Herd, 1990
Reverse phase	MeOH, acetonitrile, HAc	Ether/EtAc	TMB	UV 238	Yes	Marzo et al., 1990
Reverse phase	Gradient elution	No	None	F, UV 254	Yes	McCormick and Shihabi, 1990
Reverse phase	Acetonitrile, HAc	Ethyl acetate	p-anisamide	UV 280	No	Mizuta et al., 1990b
Reverse phase	MeOH, water	Ethyl acetate	3-Hydroxyacetanilide	UV 254	No	Rónai et al., 1990
Reverse phase	MeOH, PO$_4$ buffer	No	None	EC	No	Zhou and Wang, 1990
Reverse phase	IP, HF, PO$_4$ buffer	No	Metacetamol	UV 254	Yes	Blackledge et al., 1991
Reverse phase	Trimethylamine, IP, PO$_4$ buffer	No	None	UV 280	No	Curtis et al., 1991
Reverse phase	Acetonitrile, PO$_4$ buffer, IBA	No	None	EC	No	van Bommel et al., 1991a
Reverse phase	Gradient elution	No	Theophylline	UV 254	Yes	Esteban et al., 1992
Reverse phase	Acetonitrile, water	No	None	UV 245	No	Shim and Jung, 1992a
Reverse phase	IP, HF, PO$_4$ buffer	No	3-Hydroxyacetanilide	UV 254	Yes	Skoglund et al., 1992

Reverse phase	Acetonitrile, PO$_4$ buffer	No	NPA	EC	No	Whelpton *et al.*, 1993
Reverse phase	HAc, IP, PO$_4$ buffer	No	2-Hydroxyacetanilide	UV 254	Yes	Lau and Critchley, 1994

AHP = aminohydroxymethylpropanediol, AN = acetonitrile, DM = dichloromethane, EC = electrochemical, F = fluorescence detection, HET = β-hydroxyethyltheophylline, HF = formic acid, HPS = heptanesulphonic acid, IBA = isobutylamine, IBX = isobutylmethylxanthine, IP = isopropanol, NBA = N-butyryl-p-aminophenol, NPA = N-propionyl-p-aminophenol, PGC = prior gel filtration chromatography, Rad = radioactivity measured in eluant fractions, SS = scintillation spectrometry, TBA = tetrabutylammonium phosphate, TEA = triethylamine, TLC = prior thin layer chromatography, TMB = trimethoxybenzaldehyde, UV = ultraviolet spectrophotometry.

Electrochemical Detection

The electrochemical detection of paracetamol was first described by Riggin (1975) and this method was subsequently developed by other investigators (Table 3.4). Although electrochemical detection was more difficult to set up, it was more selective and could be much more sensitive than UV detectors for paracetamol and phenolic metabolites such as the cysteine and mercapturic acid conjugates. Paracetamol was measured electrochemically in cerebrospinal fluid (Walsh *et al.*, 1982) and the sensitivity of electrochemical detection was such that it could be measured directly in blood, tissue fluids and brain tissue even *in vivo* (Munson and Abdine, 1978; Falkowski and Wei, 1981; Cheney-Thamm *et al.*, 1987; Sabol and Freed, 1988). In one simple direct reagentless electrochemical method, a permselective cellulose acetate membrane was used with an outer diffusion-limiting microporous polycarbonate membrane (Christie *et al.*, 1993). After precipitation of proteins and conversion to the nitroso derivative, as little as 0.6 mg l^{-1} of paracetamol could be measured directly using pulse polarography (Alkayer *et al.*, 1981). Paracetamol has also been used as an internal standard for calibrating *in vivo* electrochemical electrodes for the direct assay of brain catechols (Morgan and Freed, 1981). With electrochemical measurement of paracetamol by differential pulse voltammetry, the concentration was indicated by the current flow rate and the specificity was determined by the redox potential. A detailed investigation of the voltammetry of paracetamol and its metabolites revealed good agreement between cyclic voltammograms of millimolar solutions and hydrodynamic voltammograms from nanogram quantities studied by chromatographically assisted hydrodynamic voltammetry (Miner *et al.*, 1981). The sensitivity of amperometric detectors for paracetamol was such that it could cause serious errors in the estimation of other analytes. Interference with glucose analysis was reduced by the use of a permselective electropolymerized film (Groom and Luong, 1993) and in another approach, paracetamol was removed biocatalytically with surface bound tyrosinase (Wang *et al.*, 1993).

Microdialysis

Microdialysis is a method for the continuous sampling of small molecules in tissue fluids. Fluid was circulated through an implanted tube containing a semipermeable membrane across which the drug diffused. The fluid was collected for analysis, which was usually performed by liquid chromatography combined with electrochemical detection. The metabolism and pharmacokinetics of paracetamol in brain tissue have been studied electrochemically with direct *in vivo* microdialysis (Hsiao *et al.*, 1990; Scott *et al.*, 1990, 1991; Morrison *et al.*, 1991; De Lange *et al.*, 1993, 1994), and the mathematical description of the performance of a microdialysis probe *in vivo* was validated by the results of a pharmacokinetic study of paracetamol in rat brain and plasma (Morrison *et al.*, 1991). In other studies, the effects of different microdialysis membranes on the transport of paracetamol were reported (Hsiao *et al.*, 1990; Linhares and Kissinger, 1992). Microdialysis with liquid chromatography was used to determine the extent of protein binding of paracetamol (Sarre *et al.*, 1992) and to investigate the effects of ethanol on its disposition and kinetics in conscious rats (Linhares and Kissinger, 1994). Capillary ultrafiltration was another method for continuous sampling of tissue fluids *in vivo* and it was used in the same way as microdialysis for the pharmacokinetic monitoring of paracetamol in subcutaneous tissue in rats (Linhares and Kissinger, 1992, 1993).

Enzymatic Methods

The development of enzyme-based assays of paracetamol has been driven by the need for precise specific emergency measurement of plasma concentrations in routine hospital laboratories for the management of paracetamol overdosage. Several methods have been described in which paracetamol was hydrolyzed enzymatically to p-aminophenol by aryl acylamidases of bacterial origin. The liberated p-aminophenol could then be quantitated electrochemically (Bramwell *et al.*, 1990; Shannon *et al.*, 1990) or by colorimetry using the well-established colour reaction with o-cresol (Hammond *et al.*, 1981, 1984; Price *et al.*, 1983). The latter method compared well with standard gas liquid and high performance liquid chromatographic methods and there were no serious problems with interference (Brown *et al.*, 1983; Price *et al.*, 1983, 1986a; Hucker *et al.*, 1984; Starkey *et al.*, 1986). However, lower values were obtained with the enzymic method on postmortem blood samples than with a chemical method (Dawson *et al.*, 1988a). The method was available commercially in kit form (Braiotta and Buttery, 1985; Slater, 1987), but the costs of analysis could be greatly reduced if volumes were reduced and standard reagents were used (Alkhayat, 1986a). The method was readily automated and was adapted to centrifugal and other analysers (Campbell *et al.*, 1983; Hallworth, 1983; Sullivan and Kenny, 1985; Jefferson, 1986; Higgins, 1987; Kenny and Ward, 1987). Enzymatic hydrolysis followed by the o-cresol colour reaction was one of the most frequently used procedures for the emergency estimation of paracetamol in hospital laboratories in the United Kingdom. The method was modified for the measurement of therapeutic plasma concentrations of paracetamol (Roberts *et al.*, 1985; Edwardson *et al.*, 1989) but heat treatment of samples to inactivate the HTLV-III virus caused a significant increase in concentrations, presumably as a result of partial hydrolysis of conjugates (Houssein *et al.*, 1985). Recently, an improved enzyme method was reported in which the p-aminophenol reacted with 8-hydroxyquinoline in the presence of manganese ions to give a stable blue colour that was measured at 600 nm. There appeared to be no serious interference and, as only two working reagents were required, the method could readily be adapted to a wide range of clinical analysers (Morris *et al.*, 1990).

The enzyme-based paracetamol assay with electrochemical detection of the p-aminophenol has been developed as a bedside assay. One drop of blood was applied to a disposable reagent strip where the paracetamol was hydrolyzed by the acylamidase. The strip also functioned as an electrochemical sensing and reference electrode, and its conductivity was measured and displayed digitally on a meter or printed out. The method took less than one minute and compared satisfactorily with high performance liquid chromatography (Jones *et al.*, 1990), polarization fluoroimmunoassay (Shannon *et al.*, 1990) and enzymic hydrolysis followed by colorimetry (Bramwell *et al.*, 1990). N-Acetylcysteine could cause interference but this could be prevented by the incorporation of glutathione into the electrode strip to cause saturating elevation of charge values (Vaughan *et al.*, 1991).

Immunoassay

A homogenous enzyme multiplied immunoassay (EMIT), using glucose-6-phosphate dehydrogenase catalyzed conversion of NAD to NADH, has also been developed for paracetamol (DeLaurentis *et al.*, 1982; Hepler *et al.*, 1984). This technique has been exploited commercially and is now a popular method for emergency assay in hospitals in the USA. Interference has been reported with lipaemic and haemolyzed samples (Bridges *et al.*, 1983). Another commercial system based on the same method required modification but gave good correlations with an enzyme-colorimetric method and was not subject to interference by metabolites, other drugs, haemoglobin, bilirubin or lipaemic samples (Campbell and Price, 1986). The method has been adapted for use with a micro centrifugal analyser (Bradley *et al.*, 1983). EMIT assays were successfully adapted to the Technicon RA-1000 random access analyser (Boyd *et al.*, 1985; Hallbach and Guder, 1991). A particle concentration fluorescence immunoassay was developed for the detection of 3-(cystein-S-yl)-paracetamol adducts (Benson *et al.*, 1989).

Polarization Fluoroimmunoassay

The technique of polarization fluoroimmunoassay (Abbott TDx) has been applied to the emergency estimation of paracetamol and, although expensive, it was also widely used in the USA. Good correlations have been reported with enzyme immunoassay and high performance liquid chromatographic methods (Keegan *et al.*, 1984; Edinboro *et al.*, 1991). The design of immunogens and suitable labels has been described, together with a technique based on a fluorescein-labelled analogue and sheep antisera. The rapid dissociation kinetics allowed the combination of the label and antiserum in one reagent. The procedure only required 5 μl of serum and, following addition of the reagent, the fluorescence polarization could be read after a short incubation period (Coxon *et al.*, 1988; Gallacher *et al.*, 1988).

Other Methods

Several other techniques have been adapted for the assay of paracetamol and many procedures have been automated. Paracetamol has no useful native fluorescence, but it could be converted to fluorescent derivatives. The limit of sensitivity claimed for a method based on the native fluorescence of p-aminophenol formed by acid hydrolysis was said to be 0.5 mg l^{-1} but it would be non-specific as the conjugates would be included (Dolegeal-Vendrely and Guernet, 1976). In another method, paracetamol in whole blood was extracted into ether, back-extracted into alkali and reacted with potassium ferricyanide to form fluorescent 2,2-dihydroxy-5,5'-diacetylaminobiphenyl, which was measured at activation and emission wavelengths of 337 and 425 nm respectively (Kaito *et al.*, 1974; Shibasaki *et al.*, 1980). An automated flow-injection technique was based on the same method with the ferricyanide immobilized on an exchange resin column and the fluorescence was also enhanced by the presence of dimethylformamide (Calatayud and Benito, 1990). Other fluorometric assays involved hydrolysis to p-aminophenol followed by reaction with benzylamine (Kaito and Sagara, 1974) and oxidation with ceric ammonium sulphate and reaction with 3-amino 2(1H)-quinolinethione (Yoshida *et al.*, 1980). An improved fluorescence assay was based on the reaction of paracetamol and its conjugates with 1-nitroso-2-naphthol in the presence of nitrite with activation and fluorescence wavelengths of 467 and 552 nm (Shibasaki *et al.*, 1982).

Paracetamol has been estimated using a fluoride-selective electrode to monitor the products of the reaction of paracetamol with 1-fluoro-2,4-dinitrobenzene in a flow-injection system (Apostolakis *et al.*, 1991), and another automated fast flow injection method has been described in which paracetamol was reacted with 1-nitroso-2-naphthol in the presence of cerium, and the resulting chromogen was measured at 540 nm (Georgiou and Koupparis, 1990). Micellar electrokinetic chromatography, capillary zone electrophoresis and capillary isotachophoresis were proposed for rapid confirmation of the presence of paracetamol following overdosage although precise quantitation was not possible (Caslavska *et al.*, 1993).

Paracetamol Metabolites

Early methods for the estimation of paracetamol metabolites were limited to acid hydrolysis of the glucuronide and sulphate conjugates to p-aminophenol, which was assayed colorimetrically and expressed as 'total paracetamol' (Brodie and Axelrod, 1948a). In subsequent developments, these conjugates were determined separately or together following hydrolysis to the parent drug by incubation with aryl sulphatase and β-glucuronidase. The paracetamol was then determined by a variety of methods. With separate use of the enzymes, the concentration of each conjugate could be determined from the total by subtraction (Welch *et al.*, 1966; Kampff-meyer, 1971; Prescott, 1971a; Smith and Timbrell, 1974; Borm *et al.*, 1983). The sulphate and glucuronide conjugates were also separated by paper and thin layer chromatography, and quantitated independently as above after elution from the stationary phase (Büch *et al.*, 1967c; Cummings *et al.*, 1967; Smith and Timbrell, 1974; Andrews *et al.*, 1976). Jagenburg and Toczko (1964) isolated and identified the cysteine conjugate of paracetamol using cation exchange chromatography, and subsequently the separation and quantitation of paracetamol and its glucuronide, sulphate, cysteine and mercapturic acid conjugates in urine by paper chromatography and Sephadex gel filtration chromatography was described (Jagenburg *et al.*, 1968). Soon after, 3-methoxy-4-hydroxyacetanilide was identified by anion exchange chromatography as a urinary metabolite of paracetamol formed from phenacetin given to a two-year-old girl with a neuroblastoma (Burtis *et al.*, 1970). A very detailed analysis of metabolites of paracetamol in urine and serum, following administration of the drug in man, was reported using high resolution ion exchange chromatography. The compounds in urine were identified as 2-methoxyparacetamol with its glucuronide and sulphate conjugates, the glucuronide, sulphate, cysteine and mercapturic acid conjugates of paracetamol and the sulphate conjugate of 2-hydroxyparacetamol (Mrochek *et al.*, 1974). These and other minor metabolites of paracetamol were later separated by two-dimensional thin layer chromatography and substitutions were identified in the 3- rather than the 2-position (Andrews *et al.*, 1976). The high performance liquid chromatography of paracetamol metabolites in plasma and urine on reverse phase bonded (octadecylsilica) supports with ion pairing was a major advance, and for the first time the simultaneous analysis of paracetamol and many of its metabolites became possible (Knox and Jurand, 1977,

1978). The assay of minor paracetamol metabolites in urine was facilitated by the combination of thin layer and liquid chromatography with electrochemical detection (Hamilton and Kissinger, 1982).

From a quantitative point of view the most important metabolites of paracetamol were the glucuronide, sulphate, cysteine and mercapturic acid conjugates and there have been many subsequent reports of their rapid and convenient measurement of by modification and development of these methods (Buckpitt *et al.*, 1977; Howie *et al.*, 1977; Adriaenssens and Prescott, 1978; Pang *et al.*, 1979b; Jung and Zafar, 1985; Hidvegi and Ecobichon, 1986; Bhargava *et al.*, 1988; Kamali and Herd, 1990; Esteban *et al.*, 1992). For determination of these metabolites in urine, all that was usually necessary was addition of a suitable internal standard and injection onto the analytical column. The sensitivity for phenolic metabolites has been increased by the use of electrochemical detection, and urinary metabolites could be quantitated according to the number of coulombs transferred, assuming that it was a two-electron oxidation (Lunte *et al.*, 1990). Other minor metabolites of paracetamol that have been measured include 3-methoxy- and 3-thiomethyl- derivatives and their glucuronide and sulphate conjugates, 3-thiomethylparacetamol sulphoxide and the glutathione conjugate (Buckpitt *et al.*, 1977; Knox and Jurand, 1977; Gemborys and Mudge, 1981; Hart *et al.*, 1981; Wilson *et al.*, 1982a; Miners *et al.*, 1984a; To and Wells, 1985; Ladds *et al.*, 1987; Aguilar *et al.*, 1988). Gradient elution was usually necessary to facilitate the separation of paracetamol and its metabolites in one chromatographic run, and an example is shown in Figure 3.1. The N-hydroxy metabolites of paracetamol and related compounds were selectively estimated as their ferric chelates at 546 nm (Hinson *et al.*, 1980a) and gel filtration and thin layer chromatography have been used prior to liquid chromatography (Gemborys and Mudge, 1981; Hamilton and Kissinger, 1982). The formation of paracetamol glucuronide *in vitro*, and the activities of glucuronyl transferase and sulphotransferase with paracetamol as substrate were measured directly by high performance liquid chromatography (Knight and Skellern, 1980; To and Wells, 1984). The potentially toxic reactive intermediate metabolite of paracetamol, N-acetyl-p-benzoquinoneimine, could be determined *in vitro* by high performance liquid chromatography with electrochemical detection, and it could also be generated electrochemically from paracetamol (Miner and Kissinger, 1979b; Getek *et al.*, 1989). Liquid chromatography with electrochemical detection was also used to study the metabolism of 2- and 3-hydroxyacetanilide (Hamilton and Kissinger, 1986). Many investigators have adapted existing high performance liquid chromatographic methods for the estimation of [³H]- and [¹⁴C]-paracetamol and its metabolites. The eluate was usually collected in fractions and the radioactivity measured by liquid scintillation spectrometry (Massey and Racz, 1981; Corcoran *et al.*, 1985b; Dolphin *et al.*, 1987; McLaughlin and Boroujerdi, 1987; Tee *et al.*, 1987).

The optical molar extinction coefficients for paracetamol and its glucuronide, sulphate, cysteine and mercapturic acid conjugates were very similar but several investigators have calculated the relative response factors to enhance the precision of quantitative studies (Hart *et al.*, 1981; Miners *et al.*, 1984a). In addition, a method has been described for establishing the calibration curves for assay of the glucuronide and sulphate conjugates without the need for authentic standards (Nakamura *et al.*, 1987a). High performance liquid chromatography has been used to monitor the reaction of paracetamol with hydrogen peroxide in the presence of horseradish peroxidase to form fluorescent polymers of the drug (McCormick and Shihabi,

1990). In addition, methods have been developed for the separation and identification of the oxidation, polymerization and glutathione conjugation products of these reactions with peroxidase using high performance liquid chromatography, mass spectrometry and magnetic resonance spectroscopy (Potter *et al.*, 1985, 1986).

Other more sophisticated techniques for the analysis of paracetamol metabolites included preparation of alkoxycarbonyl derivatives for mass spectral analysis (Hoffmann and Baillie, 1988), combined gas chromatography and mass spectrometry with oxygen-18 or deuterium labelled drug (Hoffmann *et al.*, 1990), electron impact, chemical ionization and field desorption mass spectrometry (Nelson *et al.*, 1981b), thermospray liquid chromatography/mass spectrometry (Betowski *et al.*, 1987; Reid *et al.*, 1990), fast atom bombardment mass spectrometry (Ackermann *et al.*, 1984; Lay *et al.*, 1987; Haroldsen *et al.*, 1988), spin-trapping of the free radical of paracetamol (Nelson *et al.*, 1981a) and metabolic profiling and mapping with proton nuclear magnetic resonance (Bales *et al.*, 1984a, 1985, 1988; Spurway *et al.*, 1990). The glutathione and cysteine conjugates of paracetamol have been generated on line in a liquid chromatography system by interfacing an electrochemical cell with a thermospray mass spectrometer in a flow-injection system. The conjugates appeared after the electrochemical formation of N-acetyl-p-benzoquinoneimine and reaction with glutathione and cysteine (Getek *et al.*, 1989). High resolution nuclear magnetic resonance spectroscopy was used to detect paracetamol and its metabolites directly in urine (Bales *et al.*, 1984b) and in hepatocytes isolated from rat liver (Nicholson *et al.*, 1985).

4

The Absorption of Paracetamol

Mechanism and Sites of Absorption

Paracetamol is absorbed from the gastrointestinal tract by passive non-ionic diffusion (Bagnall *et al.*, 1979) and the rate of transfer depends, therefore, on factors such as the concentration gradient between the gastrointestinal lumen and the circulation, aqueous and lipid solubility and mucosal blood flow, permeability and surface area. The rate also depends on formulation factors because paracetamol must dissolve in gastrointestinal fluids before it can be absorbed. Paracetamol is a weak acid with a pKa value of 9.5 (Prescott and Nimmo, 1971) and as it was therefore largely unionized over the physiological range of pH, the rate of mucosal transfer would be independent of pH. Its water and lipid solubilities were such that rapid and complete absorption would be anticipated, and this has been confirmed in many studies. The intestinal absorption of paracetamol was almost complete in rabbits (Nakamura *et al.*, 1987b) and most of an oral dose was rapidly excreted in the urine in rats (Miller and Fischer, 1974), mice (Corcoran *et al.*, 1985b), cats and dogs (Savides *et al.*, 1984; Podder *et al.*, 1988). A toxic oral dose of 500 mg kg^{-1} was absorbed very rapidly in mice with 70 per cent disappearing from the gastrointestinal tract in 30 min (Fischer *et al.*, 1981). In man, approximately 75–95 per cent of a therapeutic oral dose of paracetamol was recovered in the urine in 24 h as unchanged drug and metabolites (Cummings *et al.*, 1967; Prescott *et al.*, 1968; Nimmo *et al.*, 1973b; Levy and Houston, 1976; Holt *et al.*, 1979; Prescott, 1980; Thomas *et al.*, 1980; Critchley *et al.*, 1983, 1986; Kamali *et al.*, 1987b; Kaniwa *et al.*, 1988; Hekimoglu *et al.*, 1991; Pantuck *et al.*, 1991; Rose *et al.*, 1991; and others). In studies in which paracetamol was given to rats with a non-absorbable marker, the most efficient site of absorption was found to be the mid-small intestine (Weikel and Lish, 1959). Bagnall *et al.* (1979) showed that paracetamol was absorbed by passive transport over a wide range of concentrations and pH according to first-order kinetics. Absorption was greatest from the small intestine where 70 per cent of the dose was absorbed in 30 min compared with 29 per cent from the colon and 22 per cent from the stomach over the same period of time. In dogs, 89 per cent of a dose placed into a closed intestinal sac was absorbed in one hour (Podder *et al.*, 1988). With the *in situ* perfused rat intestine preparation, the absorption of paracetamol was biphasic and although the rate of absorption was fastest from the first segment of the small intestine, the extent of absorption was greatest from the middle segment and was independent of the dose (Pang *et al.*, 1986). In another study, the absorption of paracetamol from the isolated perfused rat small intestine was rapid and dose dependent (Sakai *et al.*, 1980). In man, dose had no significant effect on the overall absorption of paracetamol (Gwilt *et al.*, 1963a; Seideman *et al.*, 1980; Critchley *et al.*, 1983; Clements *et al.*, 1984; Borin and Ayres, 1989). The small intestinal absorption of paracetamol was studied in four healthy volunteers using a segmental steady-state perfusion technique with a triple lumen tube. Absorption was similar from proximal and distal sites, and the rate was directly related to the amount infused per unit time and the transmucosal water flux (Gramatté and Richter, 1993).

The absorption of paracetamol from the rat small intestine was inhibited by polyvinylpyrrolidone, and this effect was reversed by urea (Sekikawa *et al.*, 1979). Intestinal absorption was not enhanced by taurine (Kimura *et al.*, 1981), or by the solubilization of paracetamol with taurocholate/oleic acid and taurocholate/ lysophosphatidyl choline (Poelma *et al.*, 1990, 1991). In another report, several drugs including caffeine, diazepam and phenylbutazone were said to decrease the absorption of paracetamol across the everted rat intestine, but no mechanism was proposed (Eswarasankaran *et al.*, 1982). Studies of the transport of paracetamol in the rabbit jejunum, ileum and distal colon showed that both unidirectional fluxes were not saturable with concentrations up to 4500 mg l^{-1} (Swaan *et al.*, 1994). There was negligible lymphatic absorption of paracetamol in rats but about 15 per cent of the glyceryl decyl ether, with and without modification by an *n*-alkyl chain, appeared in thoracic duct lymph after oral administration (Sugihara *et al.*, 1988). The glucose-stimulated absorption of water increased the uptake of paracetamol in chronic isolated jejunal loops in rats (Lu *et al.*, 1992a,b).

The faster uptake of paracetamol from the small intestine than from the stomach was attributed to the greater surface area and hence absorptive capacity at the former site. An important consequence was that unless the rate of absorption of paracetamol was normally very slow, it would be determined by the rate at which the drug was transferred from the stomach to the site of rapid absorption in the upper small intestine. Absorption also involved the process of dissolution from a solid dosage form and either of these two steps could be rate-limiting. Measures of absorption obtained by conventional pharmacokinetic analysis, such as mean absorption times and rate constants, therefore were usually hybrid terms that included dissolution, gastric emptying and uptake from the small intestine. Heading *et al.* (1973) found that rapid gastric emptying in 14 convalescent patients was associated with the early appearance of high peak plasma paracetamol concentrations whereas peak concentrations were low and appeared late when gastric emptying was slow. This relationship between gastric emptying and paracetamol absorption has been confirmed in many subsequent studies (see below). Paracetamol was absorbed very rapidly when it was given under conditions where gastric emptying was rapid such as in the fasting state with a large volume of fluid or an effervescent solution (Figure 4.1). In such circumstances there was little or no lag time and peak plasma concentrations could occur within 15 min of ingestion (Carlo *et al.*, 1955; Prescott, 1980; Dougall *et al.*, 1983; Borin and Ayres, 1989) with absorption half times as short as 6–8 min (Divoll *et al.*, 1982c; Ameer *et al.*, 1983). In six healthy subjects the absorption of paracetamol appeared to be dose dependent and was slower after a dose of 2 g than after 1 and 0.5 g (Rawlins *et al.*, 1977), and

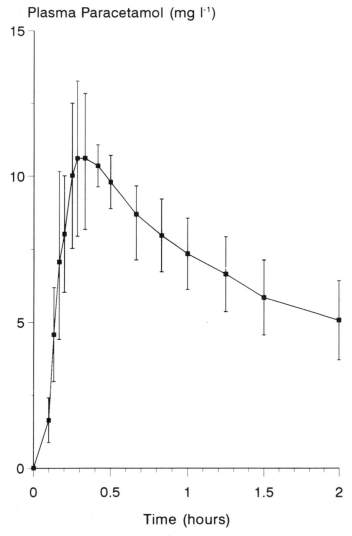

Plasma Paracetamol (mg l⁻¹)

Time (hours)

Figure 4.1 Rapid oral absorption of 12 mg kg^{-1} of paracetamol given in solution to four fasting healthy volunteers. The plasma concentrations are expressed as means $\pm$ standard deviation.

similar findings were reported in another study where a dose of 1 g appeared to be absorbed more slowly than a dose of 0.5 g (Liedtke *et al.*, 1979). These results could conceivably be explained by paracetamol-induced inhibition of gastric emptying as proposed by Weikel and Lish (1959) but they were not confirmed in other studies with doses of 5 and 20 mg kg^{-1} given orally in solution over 2 h (Clements *et al.*, 1984) and 0.5 and 1 g given as tablets (Seideman *et al.*, 1980). In a study in which 15 subjects were given oral doses of 325, 500, 1000, 1500 and 2000 mg of paracetamol, there was no significant effect of dose on absorption (Borin and Ayres, 1989). Furthermore, paracetamol was absorbed very rapidly when it was taken in overdose, and peak concentrations invariably occurred well within 4 h (Prescott *et al.*, 1971). In a comparative study of plasma drug concentrations, 1 g of paracetamol produced

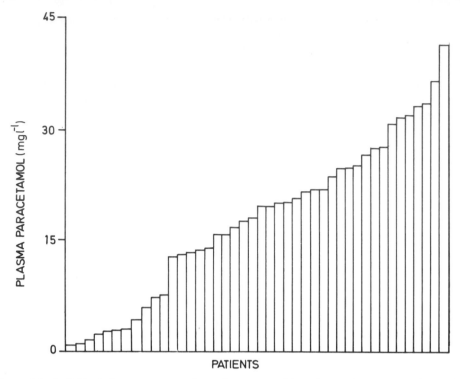

Figure 4.2 Individual plasma concentrations of paracetamol in 43 hospital patients one hour after an oral dose of 1.5 g (redrawn from Prescott, 1974, with permission).

a much earlier but lower peak than the same dose of acetylsalicylic acid (Weikel, 1958).

In practice, the rate of paracetamol absorption is subject to many variables and a range of values will be obtained depending on the circumstances. For example, in a survey of 43 fasting convalescent hospital patients, there was an 80-fold range in plasma paracetamol concentrations one hour after administration of three 500 mg tablets (Figure 4.2) (Prescott, 1974). In a study in healthy volunteers, in which paracetamol was taken orally in solution under different conditions with simultaneous isotopic measurement of gastric emptying, the absorption curves and emptying patterns indicated negligible absorption from the stomach. A pharmacokinetic model was proposed in which the conventional single compartment used to represent the gastrointestinal tract was replaced by two compartments, one representing the stomach and the other the small intestine from which the drug was absorbed rapidly. With this model there was good agreement between experimental and observed values, and the mean first-order rate constant for direct transfer of paracetamol from the intestinal lumen to the systemic circulation was equivalent to an absorption half time of 6.8 ± 0.9 min. As expected, this was shorter than the corresponding half time of gastric emptying (Clements *et al.*, 1978).

First Pass Metabolism of Paracetamol

Paracetamol is absorbed rapidly and essentially completely from the gastrointestinal tract, but the whole dose was not available to the systemic circulation because a variable fraction was lost by first pass metabolism in the gastrointestinal tract and liver. There was no appreciable presystemic loss in the lung (Bhargava and Hirate, 1989; Hirate *et al.*, 1990). Paracetamol was eliminated largely by glucuronide and sulphate conjugation and, although β-glucuronidase and aryl sulphatase were present in the gastrointestinal mucosa, only a small fraction of the dose was conjugated by these enzymes in the gut during absorption (Grafström *et al.*, 1979b; Nakamura *et al.*, 1987b). In experiments with rat intestinal loops, 3 per cent and 1.4 per cent of a tracer dose were absorbed in 30 min as the glucuronide and sulphate conjugates respectively (Josting *et al.*, 1976), and in another study in dogs the corresponding recoveries in one hour were 5.4 per cent and 8.1 per cent of the total absorbed (Podder *et al.*, 1988). The intestinal glucuronide and sulphate conjugation of paracetamol in rats was concentration dependent and saturable (Goon and Klaassen, 1990; Tone *et al.*, 1990). In the recirculating perfused rat intestine preparation, about 5.5 per cent of a dose of 15 mg of paracetamol was recovered in 2 h as the glucuronide and 2.3 per cent as the sulphate conjugate and there was no increase in the absolute amounts of conjugates formed when the dose was increased to 60 mg (Pang *et al.*, 1986). Vascular intestinal perfusion studies in mice confirmed the formation of the sulphate conjugate and it was shown to be actively transported into the circulation (Wollenberg and Rummel, 1984). Isolated rat small intestinal cells metabolized paracetamol to its glucuronide, sulphate, glutathione and cysteine conjugates (Grafström *et al.*, 1979a).

In rats given 40 mg kg^{-1} of paracetamol, the oral bioavailability was 40 per cent and the liver was the primary site of extraction with little intestinal metabolism (Bélanger *et al.*, 1987). In rats given 15 mg kg^{-1} of intravenous and intraperitoneal paracetamol, only 34 per cent of the dose reached the systemic circulation unchanged by the latter route. The hepatic clearance of paracetamol was dose dependent and in the isolated perfused rat liver, the fractions extracted were 27, 36, 47 and 52 per cent at concentrations of 50, 10, 5 and 1 mg l^{-1} respectively (Cohen *et al.*, 1974). The authors suggested that individual differences in the peak concentrations of paracetamol after oral administration might reflect variation in this dose-dependent first pass loss as a result of differences in gastric emptying and hence absorption rate. In another study, rats were given tracer doses of [^{14}C]- and [^{3}H]-paracetamol intravenously, intraportally and intraperitoneally, and the mean first pass losses varied from 27 to 44 per cent (Pang and Gillette, 1978b). In dogs, first pass metabolism accounted for about 20 per cent of oral doses of 30 and 50 mg kg^{-1} of paracetamol (Olling and Rauws, 1986; Podder *et al.*, 1988).

Although the liver has been the primary site of the first pass metabolism of paracetamol in most reports, some workers have reported otherwise. Thus, when rats were given 200 mg kg^{-1} of paracetamol by different routes, the total body extraction following oral administration was 49 per cent and the major contribution was intestinal sulphate conjugation (Bhargava and Hirate, 1989). These workers also reported extensive, dose dependent and largely intestinal first pass loss of 34–50 per cent of doses of 15–300 mg kg^{-1} of paracetamol in rats (Hirate *et al.*, 1990). There was also an age effect. In rats aged 10 weeks and 1 year the first pass loss of an oral dose of 30 mg kg^{-1} was 46 per cent (again mostly intestinal) while the corresponding fraction at 3 weeks of age was only 10 per cent (Hirate *et al.*, 1991). In another report, the first pass metabolism of paracetamol in rats was also due largely to sulphate conjugation and again this was dose dependent (Tone *et al.*, 1990). Oral paracetamol was completely absorbed in rats and the extent was not influenced by treatment with thyroxine although this reduced the gastrointestinal extraction ratio (Zhu *et al.*, 1991). As pointed out by Pang and Gillette (1978b), errors in estimates of first pass loss may arise because of the effects of drugs themselves on liver blood flow, reliance on plasma rather than blood concentrations, non-selective absorption of drugs given intraperitoneally and problems caused by enterohepatic circulation.

There were species differences in the extent of first pass metabolism and it was estimated that 10 per cent of a therapeutic dose of paracetamol would be lost in this way in man (Chiou, 1975). A comparison of the extent of sulphate conjugation after oral and intravenous administration of doses of 5 and 20 mg kg^{-1} in healthy subjects showed no effect of route of administration at either dose level, indicating insignificant gastrointestinal sulphate conjugation of the drug. There was also no significant dose dependence and the fractions lost on oral administration were 20 and 19 per cent at both dose levels (Clements *et al.*, 1984). The latter result is perhaps surprising because partial saturation of sulphate conjugation may occur within the therapeutic dose range (Levy and Yamada, 1971). In studies of the human intestinal metabolism of paracetamol (50 ng) in Ussing chambers, only about 4 per cent was conjugated in 2 h. When the drug concentration was increased 1000-fold, there was a decrease in the fraction appearing as sulphate, and an increase in glucuronide conjugate (Rogers *et al.*, 1987a). A comparison of oral and intravenous paracetamol in six healthy volunteers appeared to show that first pass metabolism was dose-dependent with the loss decreasing from 37 per cent after a dose of 500 mg to 11 and 13 per cent after doses of 1 and 2 g (Rawlins *et al.*, 1977). Unfortunately, this conclusion was not justified because three different oral doses were compared with only one intravenous dose of 1 g. Other investigators have reported first pass losses varying from 11 to 41 per cent and there was no obvious effect of dose (Table 4.1). Mean plasma concentrations of paracetamol following oral and intravenous doses of 12 mg kg^{-1} in four healthy subjects are shown in Figure 4.3 and in this case the mean first pass loss was 24 per cent and the bioavailability 76 per cent. The comparative systemic availability of paracetamol was essentially the same when it was given as such, and when it was given as phenacetin (Levy, 1971). The first pass metabolism of paracetamol was inducible. In six normal subjects and six epileptic

Table 4.1 Pre-systemic or first pass loss of paracetamol during oral absorption in healthy subjects.

Oral dose	Intravenous dose	Fraction of dose lost (%)	Reference
500 mg	1000 mg	37	Rawlins *et al.*, 1977
1000 mg	1000 mg	11	Rawlins *et al.*, 1977
2000 mg	1000 mg	13	Rawlins *et al.*, 1977
500 mg	1000 mg	38	Douglas *et al.*, 1978
1000 mg	1000 mg	11	Perucca and Richens, 1979
12 mg kg^{-1}	12 mg kg^{-1}	24	Prescott, 1980
650 mg	650 mg	25	Ameer *et al.*, 1981
650 mg	650 mg	13–21	Ameer *et al.*, 1983
5 mg kg^{-1}	5 mg kg^{-1}	20	Clements *et al.*, 1984
20 mg kg^{-1}	20 mg kg^{-1}	19	Clements *et al.*, 1984
1000 mg	600 mg	37–41	Eandi *et al.*, 1984
500 mg	Not stated	28	Tukker *et al.*, 1986

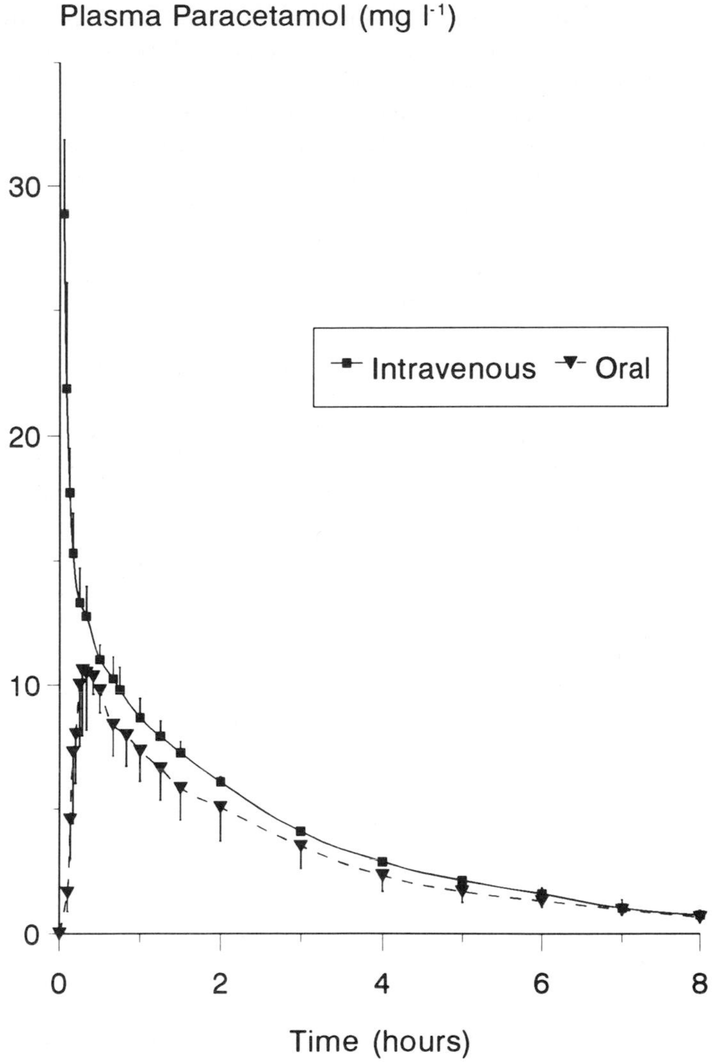

Plasma Paracetamol (mg l⁻¹)

Figure 4.3 Plasma concentrations of paracetamol following administration of 12 mg kg⁻¹ intravenously and orally on separate occasions in four fasting healthy volunteers. The concentrations are expressed as means ± standard deviation.

patients taking anticonvulsants, which cause induction of drug metabolizing enzymes, the first pass losses following oral and intravenous doses of 1 g of paracetamol were 11 and 23 per cent respectively (Perucca and Richens, 1979). Paracetamol increased the bioavailability of ethinyl oestradiol by competing with it for intestinal sulphate conjugation (Back *et al.*, 1990; Orme and Back, 1991).

Formulation and Bioavailability

The dissolution of a drug from a solid dosage form is an essential prerequisite for absorption and assessment of *in vitro* dissolution characteristics may be a useful guide to physiological availability (Sotiropoulos *et al.*, 1981). However, discrepancies have been noted between *in vitro* findings and the *in vivo* absorption of paracetamol (Mwangi and Sixsmith, 1982). Three simple dissolution procedures applied to eight different lots of commercial paracetamol tablets showed that dissolution was slow from tablets that were several years old, while 50 per cent dissolution of recently manufactured tablets occurred in less than 15 min. As judged by the 24 h urinary recovery, the relative bioavailability ranged from 85 to 98 per cent in comparisons with a control solution (Mattock *et al.*, 1971b). Gwilt *et al.* (1963a) reported that about 25 per cent of subjects were 'low absorbers' of paracetamol tablets as shown by blood concentrations of less than 10 mg l^{-1} at 45 min after oral doses of 1 g taken as a reference tablet and seven commercial formulations. There were differences between brands, and a tablet containing sorbitol was claimed to be better absorbed than a standard tablet taken whole or crushed. Similar findings were reported by Grove (1971) but it was subsequently shown that sorbitol had no effect on the aqueous solubility of paracetamol or on its partition between water and octanol, and there was no obvious explanation for the claimed effect of improvement in paracetamol absorption (Walters, 1968). It was necessary to standardize conditions for comparative absorption studies and a protocol was devised for this purpose (Mattock *et al.*, 1971a). The absorption of 1 g of paracetamol given as eight lots of tablets, an elixir and a control aqueous solution were compared in 10 subjects. There was considerable individual variation in blood concentrations, and absorption was fastest with the solution. The relative bioavailability based on urinary recovery ranged from 85 to 98 per cent (McGilveray *et al.*, 1971). Many other studies have revealed similar variation in the rate of paracetamol absorption as shown by the maximum plasma concentrations, lag times, times to maximum concentrations and plasma concentration–time curves following administration as solid and liquid dosage forms taken alone and in combination with other drugs. However, according to the urinary recovery, there were no important differences between the various preparations in the total amount absorbed (Carlo *et al.*, 1955; Hedges and Kaye, 1973; Albert *et al.*, 1974b; Richter and Smith, 1974; Nimmo *et al.*, 1979b; Divoll *et al.*, 1982c; Dougall *et al.*, 1983; Fritz *et al.*, 1984; Persaud *et al.*, 1985; Tukker *et al.*, 1986; Hekimoglu *et al.*, 1987, 1991; Ali *et al.*, 1988; Parier *et al.*, 1988; Pedraz *et al.*, 1988a; Walter-Sack *et al.*, 1989b). Absorption varied from time to time in the same individual (Richter and Smith, 1974; Schurizek *et al.*, 1988), and absorption was invariably faster from liquid formulations (especially effervescent solutions) than from solid dosage forms (Carlo *et al.*, 1955; Hedges and Kaye, 1973; Hedges *et al.*, 1974; Fascetti Testi *et al.*, 1975; Windorfer and Vogel, 1976; Liedtke *et al.*, 1979; Wójcicki *et al.*, 1980; Divoll *et al.*, 1982c; Ameer *et al.*, 1983; Dougall *et al.*, 1983; Eandi *et al.*, 1984; Walter-Sack *et al.*, 1989b). The systemic availability of paracetamol may be greater from liquid than from solid dosage forms (Ameer *et al.*, 1983). In one study, absorption from an effervescent formulation was said to be no faster than from conventional tablets. However, the method used for the assay of plasma paracetamol was unsuitable because it also included metabolites (Saano *et al.*, 1983b).

In bioavailability studies, the absorption of the test formulations should ideally be compared with a standard oral solution as well as an intravenous dose so that relative and absolute bioavailabilities can be calculated (Olling and Rauws, 1986). Sampling was often terminated prematurely, but the errors caused by truncated blood concentration curves usually had little effect on the final result (Lovering *et al.*, 1975). Paracetamol bioavailability studies have been carried out using salivary paracetamol concentrations but there was more variability than with plasma sampling (Cardot *et al.*, 1985b, 1986). The Weibull function was applied to the *in vitro* dissolution data and the predicted kinetic data from salivary concentration measurements following oral administration of paracetamol (Rodriguez *et al.*, 1990). Bioavailability studies were carried out using 'monkey's bread', the dried pulp of the baobab fruit, as the sole hydrophilic matrix-type excipient in the manufacture of paracetamol tablets (Arama *et al.*, 1989). Some antacids retarded the dissolution of paracetamol from commercial tablets *in vitro* (Iwuagwu and Aloko, 1992) but propylene glycol had no effect on the absorption of paracetamol from solutions or solid dispersions (Vila-Jato *et al.*, 1986a; Prakongpan *et al.*, 1993).

The relationship between pharmacodynamic response and kinetic characteristics was used to develop a coated bead dosage form of paracetamol giving zero-order controlled release over 12 h to produce a theoretically optimum antipyretic response in children (Hossain and Ayres, 1992). Another controlled release formulation of paracetamol was based on a gradient matrix system and gave a prolonged release pattern with low plasma concentrations extending over many hours. This pattern was maintained with repeated twice daily dosing and a pseudo steady state was reached within two or three days (van Bommel *et al.*, 1991a,b). Other controlled and delayed release forms of paracetamol were based on incorporation into egg albumin microspheres (Torrado *et al.*, 1990), and the use of polyvinyl chloride membrane-coated tablets (Shim *et al.*, 1990a), amylodextrin (van der Veen *et al.*, 1994) and an organic acid-induced sigmoidal release system (Narisawa *et al.*, 1994).

Paracetamol Absorption and Gastric Emptying

The dependence of paracetamol absorption on gastric emptying described by Heading *et al.* (1973) has been the subject of many subsequent reports. Gastric emptying in a group of hospital patients was delayed by intravenous injection of propantheline, and there was a corresponding marked slowing of the absorption of paracetamol. Conversely, its absorption was accelerated by intravenous metoclopramide, a drug which stimulates gastric emptying (Nimmo *et al.*, 1973b). The close relationship between gastric emptying and paracetamol absorption was strengthened further when it was shown that narcotic analgesics strongly inhibited gastric emptying and grossly impaired the absorption of paracetamol given at the same time (Figure 4.4) (Nimmo *et al.*, 1975a). Individual variation in the times of peak concentrations following administration of a standard formulation was attributed to individual variation in the rate of gastric emptying (Letley *et al.*, 1980). Further confirmatory studies included the reversal by naloxone of the inhibition of gastric emptying and paracetamol absorption induced by pentazocine (Nimmo *et al.*, 1979a), the slowing of gastric emptying and paracetamol absorption by guar gum and pectin gel fibre (Holt *et al.*, 1979), the inhibition of gastric emptying and paracetamol absorption by levodopa in young and elderly subjects (Robertson *et al.*, 1990, 1992), and the delaying effects of intravenous atropine on gastric emptying and paracetamol absorption, also in young and fit elderly volunteers (Rashid and Bateman, 1990). In the above studies, the paracetamol was taken as tablets or in solution, but a good correlation was also demonstrated between gastric emptying

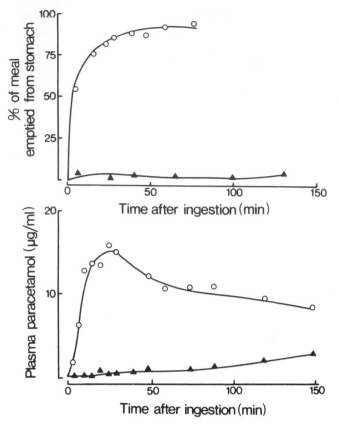

Figure 4.4 The effect of diamorphine (10 mg by intramuscular injection) (▲), compared with placebo (○) on gastric emptying (top panel) and absorption of 20 mg kg^{-1} of paracetamol in solution (lower panel) in a fasting healthy subject (reproduced with permission from Nimmo *et al.*, 1975a).

and the absorption of paracetamol taken with food (Koizumi *et al.*, 1988b). A significant relationship was also found between the absorption of paracetamol taken in liquid and solid form with different liquid diets and gastric emptying as assessed by changes in blood glucose and gallbladder emptying (Walter-Sack *et al.*, 1989b). Other investigators have confirmed a significant correlation between the emptying of radionuclide-labelled test meals from the stomach and the plasma and saliva concentrations of simultaneously administered paracetamol (Harasawa *et al.*, 1982; Maddern *et al.*, 1985; Koizumi *et al.*, 1988a). In 9 of 11 patients in an intensive care unit, the pattern of gastric emptying as shown by plasma paracetamol concentrations following an oral dose correlated well with measurements of emptying made by gastric impedance monitoring (Columb *et al.*, 1992). In all of these reports, there was a significant relationship between different measures of gastric emptying and paracetamol absorption, and an example is shown in Figure 4.5. In another report, an undefined mathematical model was used with a unique equation for curve-fitting of gastric emptying data and paracetamol concentrations in healthy subjects (Palmas *et al.*, 1985, 1986). Unfortunately, details were inadequate and the unique equation was not specified.

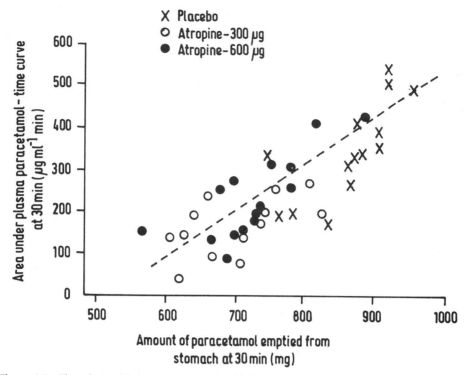

X Placebo
O Atropine–300 μg
● Atropine–600 μg

Figure 4.5 The relationship between paracetamol absorption as shown by the area under the plasma concentration–time curve, and amount of drug emptied from the stomach determined by ultrasound, 30 min after ingestion of 1 g of paracetamol in solution in seven healthy young and seven healthy elderly volunteers. Gastric emptying was modified by intravenous injection of 300 and 600 μg of atropine 10 min before the paracetamol was taken (reproduced with permission from Rashid and Bateman, 1990).

In contrast to this weight of evidence, Petring *et al.* (1986, 1990) were unable to demonstrate a significant correlation between gastric emptying of semisolid oatmeal in healthy volunteers of both sexes and any measure of the absorption of paracetamol incorporated into the meal. It was often assumed that gastric emptying and paracetamol absorption were simple exponential processes but this was not necessarily the case. Even under carefully controlled conditions there was considerable individual variation and both processes may be irregular with variable lag periods and marked short-term deviations from linearity as shown by irregular gastric emptying and early multiple peaks in plasma and salivary paracetamol concentrations (Clements *et al.*, 1978; Robertson *et al.*, 1990, 1992; Shim and Jung, 1992a). The multiple plasma peaks observed in rats given oral paracetamol were not related to enterohepatic cycling of the drug and were essentially abolished by intravenous administration (Shim and Jung, 1992b). However, the combined oral administration of paracetamol and ranitidine in rats resulted in multiple plasma concentration peaks but these were not correlated for the two drugs, raising doubts that irregular gastric emptying was the cause (Shim and Suh, 1992). Liquid and solid meals emptied from the stomach at different rates and paracetamol absorption seemed to be more closely related to the emptying of liquids than solids (Petring *et al.*, 1986;

Petring and Flachs, 1990). Different patterns were likely when the paracetamol was taken in solution, in tablets and in a meal. The indices of paracetamol absorption that have been employed in correlations with gastric emptying rates included the peak plasma concentration (Cmax), the time to peak concentration (Tmax) and area under the plasma concentration–time curve (AUC). These were indirect measures and alternative indices of paracetamol absorption were the cumulative fraction absorbed with time profile (van Wyk *et al.*, 1990) and comparisons of the proportional areas under the plasma concentration–time curves (van Wyk *et al.*, 1993c). A hold-up of paracetamol tablets in the oesophagus added to the delay in absorption caused by the time taken for gastric emptying. Thus, when 11 supine patients took a tablet of paracetamol with 15 ml of water oesophageal transit was delayed and the peak plasma concentration occurred 70 min later than in 9 patients who took the tablet while standing (Channer and Roberts, 1985).

Many other investigators have used the kinetics of paracetamol absorption as a simple indirect non-invasive measure of gastric emptying and there has been particular interest in the effects of analgesia and anaesthesia on this process (Nimmo, 1984; Schurizek, 1991). Other circumstances included assessment of the effects on gastric emptying of cold pain stress (Thorén *et al.*, 1989a,b), gastrointestinal symptoms in patients with gastritis (Tatsuta *et al.*, 1989), peptic ulcer disease (Harasawa *et al.*, 1979), oesophagectomy (Goldstraw and Bach, 1981), pain and anxiety before elective and emergency surgery (Marsh *et al.*, 1984), Colles's fracture (Steedman *et al.*, 1991), brief anaesthesia for cystoscopy (Reilly and Nimmo, 1984), minor gynaecological surgery and termination of pregnancy (Simpson *et al.*, 1988), hysterectomy with epidural anaesthesia (Nimmo *et al.*, 1978), cardiac surgery (Wilkinson *et al.*, 1994; Goldhill *et al.*, 1995), abstention from smoking cigarettes (Petring *et al.*, 1985) and ingestion of a protein meal (Robertson *et al.*, 1991). In addition to the studies mentioned above, many workers have investigated the effects that other drugs, which might influence gastric emptying under different conditions, have on the absorption of paracetamol (see below).

Studies in Animals

The kinetics of paracetamol absorption could also be used to assess gastric emptying in conscious rats (Hatanaka *et al.*, 1994). The mean absorption time of paracetamol was used to assess the effects of size of dosage form and food on gastric emptying in man and dogs (Kaniwa *et al.*, 1988), and it has also been used as a marker for gastrointestinal transit in dogs where a good correlation was demonstrated with the bioavailability of chlorothiazide (Mizuta *et al.*, 1990b). In a double marker technique, paracetamol absorption was used to estimate the rate of gastric emptying and salicylazosulphapyridine was used to determine gastrointestinal transit time in dogs. This method was used to study the effect of meals on gastric emptying and gastrointestinal transit times (Mizuta *et al.*, 1990a) and to investigate the relationship between transit time and the absorption of nitrofurantoin (Mizuta *et al.*, 1991) and a new non-steroidal anti-inflammatory drug (Mizuta *et al.*, 1990c). An alternative method for the measurement of small bowel transit time in dogs with an ileostomy was oral administration of paracetamol and indocyanine green. Gastric emptying was assessed by the kinetics of paracetamol absorption and small intestinal transit time by the appearance of the indocyanine green at the ileostomy (Yamaki *et al.*, 1992).

Factors Influencing Paracetamol Absorption

Effects of Food and Diet

By slowing the rate of gastric emptying, food generally delayed the absorption of drugs, and this principle applied to paracetamol. The magnitude of the effect seemed to depend on the nature of the meal, and, to a lesser extent, the dosage form of the drug. Jaffe *et al.* (1971) compared the effects of high carbohydrate, high protein and high fat meals, a balanced meal and different amounts of pectin on the absorption of a single 325 mg tablet of paracetamol as judged by the urinary excretion rates of total drug over a period of 9 h. The initial excretion rate was reduced by the high carbohydrate meal, and this was attributed to an interaction with pectin. Otherwise there was little difference between meals in the total amounts excreted. In another study, blood concentration and urinary excretion data following ingestion of 1 g of paracetamol tablets indicated that the absorption rate was up to five times faster when taken fasting than with a substantial high carbohydrate breakfast. There were no significant differences in the total amounts recovered in the urine (McGilveray and Mattock, 1972; Mattock and McGilveray, 1973). As shown by salivary concentrations, the absorption of paracetamol was greatly slowed when it was taken with different meals, and absorption was slowest with a high protein meal (Cardot *et al.*, 1985a). Somewhat different results were observed when 1 g of paracetamol was taken as tablets by South African ethnic subjects fasting or with breakfasts consisting primarily of cereal, maize porridge or bacon and eggs. Absorption was most rapid in the fasting state and although it was influenced most by the high fat meal, the greatest delay in absorption occurred with the high fibre cereal breakfast (Wessels *et al.*, 1992). In another report, the absorption of paracetamol from a liquid formulation was not influenced by balanced diets containing different amounts of nutrients and fibre, but when it was taken as tablets the rate of systemic availability was reduced more than with the liquid dosage form, and there was a further delay when the tablets were taken with a meal rich in dietary fibre (Walter-Sack *et al.*, 1989b). Dietary gel fibre significantly delayed the absorption of paracetamol (Holt *et al.*, 1979), and this may have been due in part to the effect of the increased viscosity on gastric emptying. Dietary fibre in the form of guar gum and sugar beet fibre had variable effects on paracetamol absorption and gastric emptying in healthy volunteers following meals of different composition. Paracetamol absorption was slower after high fat than after high protein meals, and it was also slowed by intravenous injection of glucose, especially in subjects who had previously been maintained on a low fat diet (Morgan *et al.*, 1985, 1988, 1990). On the other hand, dietary fibre given as pectin, but not bran, seemed to accelerate paracetamol absorption in rats by a mechanism independent of effects on gastric emptying (Brown *et al.*, 1979). Divoll *et al.* (1982c) found that a standard breakfast significantly reduced the rate of absorption of paracetamol given as tablets or a liquid formulation in both young and elderly subjects, and similar findings have been reported in young adults given tablets (Eandi *et al.*, 1984). The absorption of paracetamol was incomplete and abnormally slow in healthy Thai vegetarians, possibly because of the increased fibre content of their diet (Prescott *et al.*, 1993). In another study absorption was significantly retarded when paracetamol powder was taken with a standard meal (Kaniwa *et al.*, 1988).

Although these reports gave a fairly consistent picture of slower absorption of paracetamol taken with food or fibre, a few investigators have reported different results. Some 25 per cent of subjects were classed as 'low absorbers' of 1 g of paracetamol given as tablets 1–2 h after a standard breakfast of cereal and toast. This was to be expected in the light of the above findings, but when tablets were formulated with sorbitol, the absorption was said to be better, and not to be influenced by food (Gwilt *et al.*, 1963a). In one recent study, bran appeared to have no important effect on paracetamol absorption as judged by plasma concentrations although it reduced the 24 h urinary recovery of total drug and metabolites (Holt *et al.*, 1992). Isocaloric meals containing 10.5 or 30.5 g of protein and 64.3 and 43.5 g of carbohydrate were reported to have no significant effect on the absorption of 1.5 g of paracetamol given in solution (Robertson *et al.*, 1991) and, similarly, there was no effect when paracetamol was taken in combination with tryptophan and glycine (Waller *et al.*, 1991b). In contrast, the bioavailability of paracetamol in rabbits was reduced by arginine, tryptophan, and histidine, but not by glycine given in solution at the same time (Deshpande, 1980), and 10-fold dilution of an aqueous solution of paracetamol resulted in a reduced rate of absorption in rabbits (De Beer *et al.*, 1985).

Effects of Age, Sex and Body Weight

In an absorption study, a significant relationship was claimed between blood concentrations of paracetamol and age but this was probably due to age-related changes in body weight as a fixed dose was given (Gwilt *et al.*, 1963a). The absolute systemic bioavailability of paracetamol tablets and elixir tended to be less in fasting elderly than fasting young subjects, but there were no differences between the age groups when the drug was taken with food (Divoll *et al.*, 1982b,c). The pattern of absorption of paracetamol taken in solution with and without levodopa appeared to be the same in healthy young and elderly subjects (Robertson *et al.*, 1990, 1992). There were no significant differences in the absorption of 20 mg kg^{-1} of paracetamol given as tablets to 19 fit elderly and 19 young subjects (Gainsborough *et al.*, 1993a,b). The pre-systemic gastrointestinal conjugation of paracetamol was less in rats aged 3 weeks than in those aged 10 weeks and 1 year (Hirate *et al.*, 1991).

There was no clear evidence for any sex difference in paracetamol absorption. The maximum plasma concentrations and areas under the plasma concentration–time curves following oral doses of 1 g tablets were reported to be significantly higher during the luteal and follicular phases of the ovulatory cycle in females than in males (Wójcicki *et al.*, 1979a). Although a fixed dose was given, the body weights were not specified and it seems unlikely that the differences were due to changes in absorption. Petring and Flachs (1990) found that the rate of gastric emptying of a semisolid meal decreased linearly in females during the menstrual cycle, but the lag period and absorption of paracetamol were not related to the day of the cycle.

As expected on the basis of distribution, blood concentrations were higher in subjects of lighter than heavier body weight given a fixed dose of paracetamol (Gwilt *et al.*, 1963a). As judged by the maximum plasma concentrations and the time to reach peak concentrations, the absorption of 650 mg of paracetamol as tablets was apparently slower in morbidly obese individuals than in healthy control subjects of normal weight and the overall disposition of the drug in the obese subjects was not affected when they lost 8–30 kg in weight (Lee *et al.*, 1981b).

Effects of Time of Day, Sleep and Posture

The absorption of 1 g of paracetamol tablets taken after a meal at 11.00 pm, just prior to sleep, was reduced compared with a similar control study when the drug was taken at 8.30 am. The mean total paracetamol excreted in the urine in 8 h during the day was 517 ± 50 mg and 336 ± 59 mg during the night. The urine flow rate was greater by day, but these findings were attributed to slower and reduced absorption during sleep (McGilveray and Mattock, 1972; Mattock and McGilveray, 1973). In a more recent study, 500 mg of paracetamol was given during normal daytime activity, during bedrest by day and before sleep at night. The mean maximum plasma concentration was lower and the time to reach peak concentrations was longer during sleep than during the day but the differences were not statistically significant (Rumble *et al.*, 1991). In six healthy volunteers, the time of day had no effect on the absorption of 1 g of paracetamol given as tablets at 8.00 am, 2.00 pm and 8.00 pm (Malan *et al.*, 1985). Kamali *et al.* (1987b) gave six healthy subjects 1.5 g of paracetamol as tablets on six different occasions at 4.00 am, 8.00 am, 12.00 noon, 4.00 pm and 8.00 pm. Unspecified main meals were taken at 7.30 am, 12.00 noon and 7.30 pm, but the breakfast meal was stated to be much lighter than the evening meal. The 4 h urinary excretion of the major metabolite, paracetamol glucuronide, was less after the dose at 8.00 pm than at 8.00 am. There was no significant temporal variation in the excretion of parent drug or other metabolites. In another group of subjects, salivary concentrations of paracetamol were lower during the first 90 min after administration at 8.00 am than at 8.00 pm. No information was given about posture and activity at these times. There were no other changes in paracetamol disposition after dosing at different times and these findings could be explained by slower gastric emptying and absorption of paracetamol when it was taken after a large meal in the evening than after a light breakfast in the morning. In another report, paracetamol was said to be absorbed faster in 10 geriatric patients when it was taken at 7.00 pm than at 7.00 am but the mean plasma concentration–time curves for the two studies were almost superimposable (Bruguerolle *et al.*, 1990).

Posture and activity can influence gastric emptying and hence paracetamol absorption, but, despite their importance, these factors were rarely mentioned. Eight subjects took 1.5 g of paracetamol tablets on two occasions, once when ambulant and once when lying on the left side. There was a highly significant delay in absorption in the left lateral position which was attributed to effects on gastric emptying (Nimmo and Prescott, 1978). In another study, paracetamol was absorbed more slowly when it was taken in the lying position than when the subjects were ambulant (Gawronska-Szklarz *et al.*, 1985). As judged by saliva concentrations, the absorption of paracetamol during spaceflight was slow and variable in comparison with pre-flight control studies and this might have been related to weightlessness and motion sickness during the flight (Putcha and Cintrón, 1991).

Effects of Disease

As expected, there was marked impairment of paracetamol absorption in gastric outlet obstruction and pyloric stenosis (Prescott, 1974; Gabriel *et al.*, 1985). Compared with studies carried out just before surgery, the absorption of paracetamol was markedly impaired in patients four weeks after partial gastrectomy for gastric and duodenal ulcer, as shown by decreased maximum plasma concentrations and areas under the plasma concentration–time curves (Wójcicki *et al.*, 1984). Three months after pancreatoduodenectomy with selective proximal vagotomy, paracetamol absorption and gastric emptying were delayed in patients with total gastric preservation (Watanabe *et al.*, 1992) and there was also a delay in absorption in patients who had had a subtotal colectomy (Kayama and Koh, 1991). Studies in patients with surgical resection of the gastrointestinal tract indicated that most absorption of paracetamol occurred distal to the duodenojejunal flexure (Ueno *et al.*, 1995). The paracetamol absorption rate apparently increased in some patients with duodenal ulcer and slowed in others, and absorption was delayed in patients with gastric ulcer (Wójcicki and Gawronska-Szklarz, 1984). Similar findings were noted in another study in patients with active peptic ulcers, and paracetamol absorption seemed to be related to gastric acid secretion (Harasawa *et al.*, 1979). The basis for these findings is obscure. Gastric acid output would not be expected to have an effect, and, indeed, paracetamol absorption was essentially normal in patients with achlorhydria (Pottage *et al.*, 1974). Its absorption was delayed in patients with gastric ulcer (Harasawa *et al.*, 1982), chronic gastrointestinal symptoms and endoscopic appearances of fundal gastritis (Tatsuta *et al.*, 1989) and gastric cancer (Gawronska-Szklarz *et al.*, 1988; Tatsuta *et al.*, 1990). It was also abnormally slow in patients with coeliac disease and Crohn's disease, and this was largely a consequence of slower gastric emptying (Holt *et al.*, 1981). Paracetamol absorption was normal following small intestinal bypass surgery for obesity (Terry *et al.*, 1982) and after administration via a feeding jejunostomy (Nelson *et al.*, 1986). It was normal in malnourished children (Mehta *et al.*, 1982), but abnormally slow in patients with morbid obesity (Lee *et al.*, 1981b).

Variable effects have been reported in other disease states. Paracetamol absorption was delayed after minor gynaecological surgery (Mushambi *et al.*, 1992) but surgery itself delayed gastric emptying, and the most important cause was the use of narcotic analgesics (Nimmo, 1982). Anxiety was also a factor, and paracetamol absorption was delayed and reduced in patients with a low predisposition to anxiety who became very anxious before surgery (Simpson and Stakes, 1987). Paracetamol absorption was faster in patients with hyperthyroidism and slower in patients with hypothyroidism but the differences were not great (Forfar *et al.*, 1980). In children with fever, rapid and possibly dose-dependent absorption of paracetamol was noted (Wilson *et al.*, 1982b), and in another study a disproportionate increase in the area under the plasma concentration–time curve with dose was observed (Windorfer and Vogel, 1976). Paracetamol absorption was not impaired in patients with severe burn injury (Hu *et al.*, 1993b), or acute uncomplicated falciparum malaria (Wilairatana *et al.*, 1995). In nine patients with an acute migraine attack, absorption was slower as shown by the peak concentrations and areas under the plasma concentration–time curves than in a subsequent study when they were free of headache. The decrease in area under the curve was correlated with the severity of nausea during the attack, and this was thought to be related to delayed gastric emptying (Tokola and Neuvonen, 1981, 1984; Tokola, 1988). Marked impairment of paracetamol absorption was reported in 20 patients given 1 g of paracetamol tablets two weeks after suffering a stroke. Similar, more marked changes, with a significant reduction in the areas under the plasma concentration–time curves, were found when the studies were repeated after six weeks (Stankowska-Chomicz and Gawronska-Szklarz, 1987). Paracetamol absorption was impaired in elderly patients with cerebrovascular disease, especially those who were in coma (Inoue *et al.*, 1993) and also in patients with spinal cord injury (Halstead *et al.*, 1985). Absorption was also abnormally slow in patients with head injury, and the delay was related to the severity of the injury (Power *et al.*, 1989). As shown by the kinetics of paracetamol absorption, there was a delay in the gastric emptying of solids, but not liquids, in diabetic patients with autonomic neuropathy (Cavallo-Perin *et al.*, 1991) and the paracetamol absorption method for assessment of gastric emptying was validated for studies of the glycaemic response to food (Bijlani *et al.*, 1992). Decreased absorption of paracetamol was also observed in dogs with streptozotocin-induced diabetes (Koizumi *et al.*, 1989) and in mice with endotoxin-induced diarrhoea (Sakurai *et al.*, 1985). Paracetamol absorption was said to be decreased in a 33-year-old woman with Behçet's syndrome. No drug could be detected in the blood after she was supposed to have taken 500 mg three times a day as an outpatient and, similarly, there was said to be no absorption of diazepam, carbamazepine and diphenylhydantoin given under the same conditions (Chaleby *et al.*, 1987). Despite a previous psychiatric history in this patient, the possibility of lack of compliance was not considered as the cause of this remarkable inability to absorb drugs and the defect was attributed instead to inflammatory changes in the duodenum associated with the Behçet's syndrome.

Pregnancy and Labour

Paracetamol absorption has been used as a convenient measure of gastric emptying during the various stages of pregnancy and labour (Nimmo, 1978). The absorption of paracetamol was slower and less complete in a 27-year-old woman on the last day of pregnancy than on a repeat study 38 days later, and this was attributed to delayed gastric emptying in late pregnancy (Galinsky and Levy, 1984b). In one study, paracetamol was absorbed more slowly during the first trimester of pregnancy than in non-pregnant control women (Clark and Seager, 1983) but in others, its absorption was normal during the first, second and third trimesters of pregnancy (Macfie *et al.*, 1991; Whitehead *et al.*, 1993). Absorption was delayed in mothers within 2 h of delivery but drugs given for analgesia were not specified and the possibility that gastric emptying might have been inhibited by narcotic analgesics was not mentioned (Whitehead *et al.*, 1993). This inhibitory effect was of relatively short duration and subsequent absorption was rapid with no differences between the first and third days after delivery (Gin *et al.*, 1991).

Effects of Drugs on Paracetamol Absorption

Gastric emptying was influenced by many drugs, and as it was such an important determinant of the rate of paracetamol absorption, it is not surprising that there were many interactions based on this mechanism. Where the urinary excretion of paracetamol has been measured in these absorption interaction studies, there has usually been no significant change in the total amount recovered. Anticholinergic agents inhibited gastric emptying and accordingly the rate of paracetamol absorption was reduced by drugs such as propantheline (Nimmo *et al.*, 1973b), desmethylimipramine (Hall *et al.*, 1976a) and atropine (Imbimbo *et al.*, 1990; Rashid and Bateman, 1990; van Wyk *et al.*, 1990). In one study pirenzepine reduced salivary flow rate without decreasing the absorption of paracetamol tablets (Kamali *et al.*, 1992), and in another it did not prevent an increased rate of paracetamol absorption when given in combination with neostigmine and metoclopramide (van Wyk *et al.*, 1990). As might be anticipated from effects on gastric emptying, oral isoprenaline caused a significant dose-dependent delay in the absorption of crushed paracetamol tablets, and this effect was blocked by propranolol. Salbutamol also delayed paracetamol absorption while propranolol given by itself had the opposite effect. Propranolol had no significant effect on the urinary recovery of paracetamol (Clark *et al.*, 1980). Gastric emptying was strongly inhibited by narcotic analgesics, and heroin, pethidine and pentazocine greatly delayed emptying and paracetamol absorption in healthy subjects (Nimmo *et al.*, 1975a; Clements *et al.*, 1978) (Figure 4.4). Similar results were observed following administration of pethidine, heroin and pentazocine to women in labour, and this effect was not reversed by metoclopramide (Nimmo *et al.*, 1975b). However, narcotic-induced inhibition of gastric emptying and paracetamol absorption was reversed by naloxone in healthy subjects (Nimmo *et al.*, 1979a) and by cisapride in patients prior to surgery (Rowbotham and Nimmo, 1987; Rowbotham *et al.*, 1988). The effects of morphine were partially reversed by intramuscular metoclopramide (Rowbotham *et al.*, 1988). In one report, gastric emptying and paracetamol absorption were said to be delayed in patients undergoing surgery (Simpson *et al.*, 1988) but this was probably caused by unstated drugs given for premedication, anaesthesia, and analgesia. Other investigators have demonstrated inhibition of paracetamol absorption (and by implication, gastric emptying) by narcotic analgesics (Nimmo *et al.*, 1978; Todd and Nimmo, 1983; Murphy *et al.*, 1984a; Rowbotham and Nimmo, 1987; Rowbotham *et al.*, 1988; Schurizek *et al.*, 1989d; Thorén *et al.*, 1989a; McNeill *et al.*, 1990). In contrast to the marked effects of drugs such as morphine, therapeutic doses of codeine, loperamide and diphenoxylate with atropine did not inhibit paracetamol absorption (Bajorek *et al.*, 1978; Nimmo *et al.*, 1979b; Holt *et al.*, 1992). Other treatments that slowed down the absorption of paracetamol included levodopa (Waller *et al.*, 1991a), nefopam (Todd and Nimmo, 1983), terbinafine (Sommers *et al.*, 1992), rectally administered prochlorperazine in patients with acute migraine attacks (Tokola, 1988) and antacids containing aluminium and magnesium hydroxides (Albin *et al.*, 1985). Paracetamol absorption was not delayed or reduced by sucralfate (a sulphated disaccharide aluminium compound) (Kamali *et al.*, 1985) or by intravenous diazepam (Adelhøj *et al.*, 1985a). The inhibitory effects of glucagon and butropium on paracetamol absorption and gastric emptying were associated with endoscopic evidence of reduced gastric peristalsis (Kawamoto *et al.*, 1985).

Drugs that stimulated gastric emptying accelerated paracetamol absorption. Thus, in healthy subjects taking paracetamol tablets, intravenous metoclopramide (10 mg) increased maximum plasma concentrations from 12.5 to 20.5 mg l^{-1} and reduced the time to reach peak concentrations from 120 to 48 min (Nimmo *et al.*, 1973b). Intravenous metoclopramide had a similar effect in reversing the decreased rate of paracetamol absorption induced by narcotic analgesics (Murphy *et al.*,

1984a; McNeill *et al.*, 1990), but in another study it had no effect when given alone (van Wyk *et al.*, 1990). Oral cisapride increased the rate of paracetamol absorption in healthy subjects (van Wyk *et al.*, 1992), and given intramuscularly it was more effective than intramuscular metoclopramide in reversing the delay in paracetamol absorption induced by morphine in patients before surgery (Rowbotham *et al.*, 1988). Other drugs that have been reported to increase the rate of paracetamol absorption include chloroquine (Adjepon-Yamoah *et al.*, 1986), domperidone (Tatsuta *et al.*, 1989) and neostigmine (van Wyk *et al.*, 1990). The combination of paracetamol with domperidone was more effective in shortening the duration of migraine attacks than paracetamol alone and it was possible that this was due in part to more reliable absorption (MacGregor *et al.*, 1993). Guaiphenesin in a combination tablet seemed to increase the rate of paracetamol absorption and availability but these effects were antagonized by inclusion of caffeine into the formulation (Perlík *et al.*, 1988). Other drug interactions involving gastric emptying and paracetamol absorption in man and animals are summarized in Table 4.2.

Although in general the effects of different drugs on gastric emptying and paracetamol absorption have been according to their expected pharmacological actions, there have been several inconsistent and negative reports. In some cases, such as with oral and rectal metoclopramide, this was probably due to slow absorption of the primary drug itself, while with others, a lack of efficacy in reversing potent inhibitory effects on gastric emptying of drugs such as narcotic analgesics does not mean that the expected response would not occur under other circumstances. Nevertheless, unexpected failure to influence the rate of paracetamol absorption has been reported with cisapride (Rowbotham *et al.*, 1992), carisoprodol, chlormezanone and orphenadrine (Saano *et al.*, 1990), amantidine (Aoki and Sitar, 1992), cimetropium (Imbimbo *et al.*, 1990), diazepam (Todd and Nimmo, 1983; Adelhøj *et al.*, 1985a; Schurizek *et al.*, 1988), loperamide (Kirby *et al.*, 1989; van Wyk *et al.*, 1992), bethanecol (Kirby *et al.*, 1989) and metoclopramide given by the oral (Dougall *et al.*, 1983; Galinsky *et al.*, 1986; Kirby *et al.*, 1989; Manara *et al.*, 1990; van Wyk *et al.*, 1992), rectal (Tokola, 1988), intramuscular (McNeill *et al.*, 1990) and intravenous routes (van Wyk *et al.*, 1990). Paracetamol and metoclopramide seemed to be absorbed normally from a combination capsule in healthy volunteers (Becker *et al.*, 1992).

Reduction of Paracetamol Absorption Following Overdosage

Because of the potential problems of hepatotoxicity after overdosage of paracetamol, considerable attention has been given to the use of oral activated charcoal in attempts to reduce absorption in poisoned patients. The binding of paracetamol to charcoal *in vitro* was independent of pH and varied according to the ratio of drug to charcoal. At least four times as much charcoal as paracetamol was required for effective adsorption and the maximum adsorption capacity was 234 mg of paracetamol per gram of charcoal (Bainbridge *et al.*, 1977). Although the *in vitro* capacity for adsorption of paracetamol varied greatly with different charcoals (Boehm and Oppenheim, 1977; van de Graaff *et al.*, 1982) this was not always the case (Al-Shareef *et al.*, 1990). When 1 g of paracetamol in solution was taken with 5 g and 10 g of activated charcoal at the same time, the total excreted in the urine was reduced to 52.8 and 38.5 per cent of the recovery without charcoal. When 10 g of charcoal

Table 4.2 Some drug interactions involving gastric emptying and paracetamol absorption.

Species	Drug(s) given with paracetamol (route)[1]	Effect on rate of paracetamol absorption	Reference
Rat	caffeine (oral)	decreased	Siegers, 1973
Mouse	aspirin (oral)	decreased	Whitehouse *et al.*, 1977
Man	atropine (im)	decreased	Wójcicki *et al.*, 1977a
Man	atropine (oral)	increased	Kazmierczyk, 1979
Man	neostigmine (oral)	increased	Kazmierczyk, 1979
Man	papaverine (oral)	no change	Kazmierczyk, 1979
Man	post. pituitary extract (oral)	no change	Kazmierczyk, 1979
Man	hydrochloric acid (oral)	no change	Kazmierczyk, 1979
Man	$CaCO_3$ (oral)	no change	Kazmierczyk, 1979
Man	ethanol (20% oral)	no change	Kazmierczyk, 1979
Man	ethanol (40% oral)	decreased	Kazmierczyk, 1979
Man	atropine (im)	increased	Wójcicki *et al.*, 1979b
Man	neostigmine (im)	increased	Wójcicki *et al.*, 1979b
Man	hydrochloric acid (oral)	decreased	Wójcicki *et al.*, 1979b
Man	$CaCO_3$ (oral)	increased	Wójcicki *et al.*, 1979b
Man	atropine (im)	decreased	Wójcicki *et al.*, 1979c
Man	papaverine (im)	no change	Wójcicki *et al.*, 1979c
Rabbit	chlorpromazine (ip)	decreased	Imamura *et al.*, 1980
Rabbit	atropine (ip)	decreased	Imamura *et al.*, 1980
Rat	aspirin (oral)	decreased	Seegers *et al.*, 1980b
Man	ketamine (im)	no change	Grant *et al.*, 1981
Rabbit	diphenhydramine (oral)	decreased	Imamura *et al.*, 1981
Rabbit	$Al(OH)_3$ (oral)	no change	Chen *et al.*, 1983
Man	glycopyrrolate (iv)	decreased	Clark and Seager, 1983
Man	atropine (iv)	no change	Clark and Seager, 1983
Man	halothane anaesthesia	decreased	Adelhøj *et al.*, 1984
Man	diazepam (oral)	no change	Adelhøj *et al.*, 1984
Man	pethidine (im)	decreased	Frame *et al.*, 1984
Man	pethidine + naloxone (im)	decreased	Frame *et al.*, 1984
Man	morphine (oral)[2]	minor decrease	Park and Weir, 1984
Man	morphine (im)	decreased	Park and Weir, 1984
Man	diazepam (oral)	no change	Petring *et al.*, 1984
Man	mepivacaine (epidural)	no change	Petring *et al.*, 1984
Man	diazepam (oral)	no change	Shah *et al.*, 1984
Man	nalbuphine (im)	decreased	Shah *et al.*, 1984
Man	morphine (im)	decreased	Shah *et al.*, 1984
Man	buprenorphine (iv)	decreased	Adelhøj *et al.*, 1985b
Rabbit	domperidone (oral)	no change	Kaka and Al-Khamis, 1986
Man	morphine (im)	decreased	Nimmo *et al.*, 1986
Man	meptazinol (im)	decreased	Nimmo *et al.*, 1986
Man	bupivacaine (spinal)	decreased	Adelhøj *et al.*, 1987
Man	chlorpromazine (iv)	no change	Petring *et al.*, 1987
Man	methotrexate (iv)[3]	no change	Kamali *et al.*, 1988
Man	fentanyl (not stated)	decreased	Milligan *et al.*, 1988
Man	alfentanil (not stated)	decreased	Milligan *et al.*, 1988
Man	fentanyl (iv)	decreased	Petring *et al.*, 1988
Man	fentanyl + droperidol (iv)	decreased	Petring *et al.*, 1988
Man	atropine (im) + hexamethonium (im)	decreased	Chen *et al.*, 1988

Table 4.2 *(cont.)*

Species	Drug(s) given with paracetamol (route)[1]	Effect on rate of paracetamol absorption	Reference
Man	morphine (epidural)	decreased	Thorén and Wattwil, 1988
Man	bupivacaine (epidural)	no change	Thorén and Wattwil, 1988
Man	morphine (oral)[2]	no change	Clyburn and Rosen, 1989
Man	metoclopramide (iv)	increased	Sánchez *et al.*, 1989
Man	propantheline (oral)	decreased	Sánchez *et al.*, 1989
Man	enflurane anaesthesia	decreased	Schurizek *et al.*, 1989b
Man	halothane anaesthesia	decreased	Schurizek *et al.*, 1989c
Man	bupivacaine (epidural)	decreased	Thorén *et al.*, 1989b
Man	lignocaine (spinal)	no change	Thorén *et al.*, 1989b
Man	bupivacaine (epidural)	no change	Geddes *et al.*, 1991
Man	fentanyl (epidural)	decreased	Geddes *et al.*, 1991
Rat	morphine (sc, oral)	decreased	Janicki *et al.*, 1991
Man	cisapride (oral)[4]	increased	Kasai *et al.*, 1991
Man	morphine (im)	decreased	Kluger *et al.*, 1991
Man	cisapride (rectal) + morphine (im)	decreased	Kluger *et al.*, 1991
Rat	tolmetin (oral)	increased	Sabater *et al.*, 1991
Man	disopyramide (oral)	control	Kuroda *et al.*, 1992
Man	disopyramide (oral) + cisapride (oral)	increased	Kuroda *et al.*, 1992
Man	morphine (epidural)	decreased	Thörn *et al.*, 1992
Man	bupivacaine (epidural)	no change	Thörn *et al.*, 1992
Man	bupivacaine (extradural)	control	Wright *et al.*, 1992
Man	bupivacaine + fentanyl (extradural)	decreased	Wright *et al.*, 1992
Man	bupivacaine (epidural)	control	Ewah *et al.*, 1993
Man	fentanyl (epidural)	decreased	Ewah *et al.*, 1993
Man	diamorphine (epidural)	decreased	Ewah *et al.*, 1993
Man	zingiber officinale (oral)	no change	Phillips *et al.*, 1993
Man	metoclopramide (iv)	increased	Sommers *et al.*, 1993
Man	octreotide (sc)	decreased	Sommers *et al.*, 1993
Man	Liu-Jun-Zi-Tang (oral)	increased	Tatsuta and Iishi, 1993
Man	metoclopramide (iv)	control	van Wyk *et al.*, 1993a
Man	metoclopramide (iv) + fluoxetine (oral)	decreased	van Wyk *et al.*, 1993a
Man	metoclopramide (iv) + meterogoline (oral)	decreased	van Wyk *et al.*, 1993a
Man	metoclopramide (iv) + pizotifen (oral)	decreased	van Wyk *et al.*, 1993a
Man	metoclopramide (iv) + methysergide (oral)	decreased	van Wyk *et al.*, 1993a
Man	metoclopramide (iv)	no change	van Wyk *et al.*, 1993b
Man	neostigmine (sc)	increased	van Wyk *et al.*, 1993b
Man	granisetron (iv)	no change	Sommers *et al.*, 1994
Man	ondansetron (iv)	no change	Sommers *et al.*, 1994
Man	metoclopramide (iv)	no change	Sommers *et al.*, 1994

[1] Routes of administration: im = intramuscular, ip = intraperitoneal, iv = intravenous, sc = subcutaneous, [2] controlled delayed release, [3] concentrations measured in saliva, [4] diabetes.

was taken 30 min after paracetamol taken as elixir, suspension and tablets, the urinary recoveries were 68.9, 49.7 and 46 per cent of the control values. With a constant ratio of charcoal to drug of 10 : 1, absorption decreased as the dose of charcoal increased (Levy and Houston, 1976). The efficient adsorption of paracetamol to charcoal *in vitro* and *in vivo* has been confirmed by many investigators (Dordoni *et al.*, 1973; Bainbridge *et al.*, 1977; Boehm and Oppenheim, 1977; Neuvonen *et al.*, 1983; Galinsky and Levy, 1984a; Neuvonen and Olkkola, 1988; Al-Shareef *et al.*, 1990).

To effectively reduce paracetamol absorption after overdosage, however, the charcoal must be given as soon as possible. It was claimed that administration of charcoal one hour after paracetamol in starved pigs achieved considerable reduction in drug concentrations but no data were provided. In any event, the pig model would be inappropriate as gastric emptying was greatly delayed in this species and the pattern was quite different from that in man (Lipscomb and Widdop, 1975). With the simultaneous ingestion of 2 g of paracetamol and 10 g of activated charcoal, absorption was reduced by 63 per cent but when the administration of charcoal was delayed for one hour the reduction was only 23 per cent (Dordoni *et al.*, 1973). In another study, 10 volunteers were given a potentially hepatotoxic overdose of 5 g of paracetamol on four occasions, once for a control study and three times following 30 g of charcoal given after 15, 30 or 120 min. The urinary recovery of drug was reduced by 48, 44 and 33 per cent respectively but there was no mention of adverse effects or monitoring of liver function tests (Rose *et al.*, 1991). There was always a delay before poisoned patients arrived at hospital, and the usefulness of activated charcoal in reducing absorption, therefore, was limited despite anecdotal accounts of efficacy after late administration (Mofenson and Caraccio, 1992). As might be expected, a rapid and profuse catharsis induced by ingestion of 70 per cent sorbitol solution increased the misery but did not increase the efficacy of charcoal in reducing paracetamol absorption in healthy volunteers (McNamara *et al.*, 1988), and in another study, intervention one hour after ingestion of paracetamol with a charcoal–sorbitol mixture had no advantage over ipecac in reducing absorption of the drug (McNamara *et al.*, 1989). Neither method had any great effect in reducing paracetamol absorption. Catharsis induced by a polyethylene glycol and electrolyte solution reduced the peak plasma concentrations of paracetamol following an oral dose of 4 g (but not 2 g) in healthy volunteers but charcoal given with or without whole bowel lavage had no effect on the absorption of the higher dose of paracetamol (Hassig *et al.*, 1993). In dogs, oral activated charcoal was much more effective in reducing paracetamol absorption than catharsis induced by several agents (van de Graaff *et al.*, 1982). Despite these unimpressive and inconsistent findings, the combination of charcoal and sorbitol was still recommended as first aid for paracetamol poisoning (Eyer and Sprenger, 1991). Syrup of ipecac was often given to induce vomiting in poisoned patients in the hope that absorption would be limited but efficacy depended on the time interval between ingestion and emesis (Bond *et al.*, 1993). In a comparative study of activated charcoal and syrup of ipecac given 5 and 30 min after a dose of 1 g of paracetamol in six volunteers, charcoal was more effective in reducing absorption than the ipecac even though this caused vomiting on each occasion (Figure 4.6) (Neuvonen *et al.*, 1983).

The anion exchange resins cholestyramine and colestipol also bind paracetamol strongly (Siegers *et al.*, 1983b; Al-Shareef *et al.*, 1990). When given in a dose of 12 g immediately after ingestion of 2 g of paracetamol, cholestyramine reduced absorp-

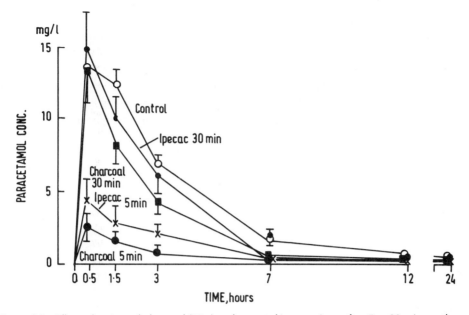

Figure 4.6 Effect of activated charcoal (50 g) and syrup of ipecac given after 5 or 30 min on the absorption of paracetamol tablets (1 g) taken with 100 ml of water in six fasting healthy subjects (redrawn from Neuvonen *et al.*, 1983).

tion by 62 per cent but when administration was delayed for one hour, the corresponding reduction was only 16 per cent (Dordoni *et al.*, 1973). Cholestyramine may adsorb paracetamol and its conjugates secreted into the gastrointestinal tract as a result of enterohepatic circulation. In rats, cholestyramine given 4 and 24 h after paracetamol completely prevented hepatic and renal toxicity, and greatly reduced the urinary recovery of the drug and its conjugates (Siegers and Möller-Hartmann, 1989).

Rectal Absorption of Paracetamol

Paracetamol was fairly well absorbed from the rectum but the rate was usually slower than with the oral route (Moolenaar *et al.*, 1979a; Kummer and Mehlhaus, 1984) and differences in the rectal absorption of paracetamol and phenacetin were related to their lipid solubility (Häuser and Pfleger, 1965). The release processes that preceded absorption depended on the composition and age of solid dosage forms (Höbel and Talebian, 1960; Moës, 1974b; Moës and Jaminet, 1976; Djimbo and Moës, 1986; Hagenlocher *et al.*, 1987; Kahela *et al.*, 1987; Lauroba *et al.*, 1990). When given as an enema, absorption was independent of pH and dose, but the rate increased with increasing volume (Moolenaar *et al.*, 1979a; Moolenaar, 1980). The absorption of paracetamol from a suppository that also contained codeine and buclizine was not impaired after storage for two years (Burgess *et al.*, 1985). It was also dependent on the particle size of the drug suspended in the fatty suppository base (Moolenaar *et al.*, 1979b). Children undergoing tonsillectomy or adenoidectomy were given 20 mg kg^{-1} of paracetamol rectally in an aqueous suspension and the mean maximum plasma concentration of 10.9 mg l^{-1} did not occur until after

? h. Analgesia was unsatisfactory, possibly because of the delay in absorption (Gaudreault *et al.*, 1988). Rectal suppositories and oral paracetamol syrup were compared in two groups of 15 children with fever. Paracetamol syrup was absorbed much faster and better than the suppositories and it produced the greatest fall in temperature 2 h earlier than the rectal form (Keinänen *et al.*, 1977). In children recovering from enteric fever, the absorption of rectal paracetamol was slow and incomplete compared with that from a syrup. Plasma concentrations following the administration of the suppositories were consistently below the minimum therapeutic concentration and the relative bioavailability was only about 30 per cent (Dange *et al.*, 1987). In a comparison of nasogastric and rectal paracetamol in neonates following cardiac surgery, plasma concentrations were lower with rectal administration but there were no significant differences between the routes in antipyretic effects (Hopkins *et al.*, 1990). In another similar study in young children, rectal paracetamol was ineffective in lowering temperature (Mitchell *et al.*, 1991). In other reports, paracetamol given as 0.5 and 1 g suppositories was absorbed very slowly with low plasma concentrations that did not reach a maximum for 3–4 h (Figure 4.7) (Liedtke *et al.*, 1979) and absorption was faster from tablets and micro-enemas than from suppositories (Paulsen and Kreilgård, 1984). The absorption of paracetamol from suppositories continued to be slow with repeated dosing in healthy volunteers (Liedtke *et al.*, 1980). The absorption of paracetamol from lipophilic and hydrophilic suppositories was slow but similar in children with postoperative fever and there were significant correlations between peak plasma concentrations and the maximum antipyretic response (Cullen *et al.*, 1989). In a comparison of oral tablets and rectal suppositories containing 0.5 and 1 g of parace-

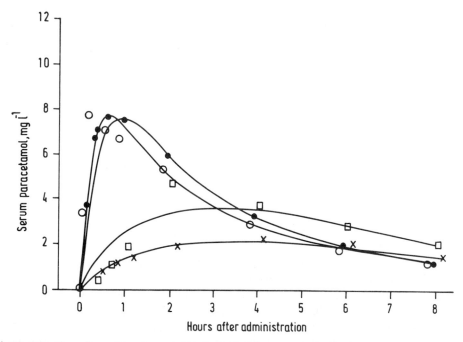

Figure 4.7 Slow absorption of rectal paracetamol. Serum concentrations in 10 subjects after administration of doses of 1 g given different formulations orally as tablets (○, ●) and rectally as suppositories (□, ×) (redrawn from Liedtke *et al.*, 1979).

tamol, the mean time to reach maximum concentrations was 2–3 h, and the maximum concentrations and areas under the plasma concentration–time curve were less with rectal than oral administration. The relative bioavailability from the suppositories was 60–90 per cent (Seideman *et al.*, 1980; Salvadó *et al.*, 1990; Blume *et al.*, 1994). Similar relative bioavailability was observed in another study when paracetamol was given as a suppository and as solid and liquid oral dosage forms. Again, absorption was delayed after rectal administration (Walter-Sack *et al.*, 1989a). The rate of absorption and bioavailability of paracetamol suppositories was highly dependent on the formulation (Moolenaar and Cox, 1980; Kahela *et al.*, 1987), and rather slow and incomplete absorption has been reported by other investigators with different preparations depending on factors such as size and weight of the suppositories, dielectric properties, melting characteristics, viscosity and lipid and surfactant content (Höbel and Talebian, 1960; Shangraw and Walkling, 1971; Moës, 1974b; Pagay *et al.*, 1974; Feldman, 1975; Munson *et al.*, 1978; Degen *et al.*, 1982; Abd Elbary *et al.*, 1983; Degen and Maier-Lenz, 1984; Eandi *et al.*, 1984; Müller *et al.*, 1984; Djimbo and Moës, 1986; Klein *et al.*, 1986; Hagenlocher *et al.*, 1987; Gjellan *et al.*, 1994). In other reports, the 24 h urinary recovery following administration of suppositories containing 500 and 1000 mg of paracetamol was only 46 per cent of the dose (Anania *et al.*, 1976), and in a comparison with the intravenous route the absolute bioavailability of rectal paracetamol only amounted to 30–40 per cent (Eandi *et al.*, 1984). There was considerable variation in the absorption of paracetamol from different brands of suppositories in some studies (Saano *et al.*, 1983a,c) but less in others (Concheiro *et al.*, 1984). Not surprisingly, the absorption of paracetamol from suppositories was impaired in geriatric patients with rectal faecal accumulation (Hagen *et al.*, 1991). Paracetamol absorption from different types of suppository, and *in vitro* and *in vivo* correlations have been investigated in experimental animals (Golovkin, 1980; Regdon *et al.*, 1994) and the isolated rat rectum preparation was used for permeation studies (Lin and Yang, 1990).

Other Routes of Administration

Intramuscular Absorption

Unspecified formulations containing 300 and 600 mg of paracetamol in volumes of 2 and 4 ml were injected intramuscularly into the gluteal region in six subjects on separate occasions. No information was provided concerning posture, activity or the precise site and depth of the injections. In three subjects absorption of the 300 mg dose was fairly rapid with a mean time to peak concentrations of 0.8 h while in the other three absorption was delayed with a corresponding time of 2.5 h. Following the 600 mg dose, absorption was also slow but was less variable and a mean peak concentration of 7.5 mg l^{-1} was reached in 1.7 h (Figure 4.8). Unfortunately, no comparisons were made with other routes of administration, and as the authors admitted, the slow absorption in some cases was probably the result of injection into fat rather than muscle. There was no mention of adverse effects or pain at the injection sites (Macheras *et al.*, 1989). Paracetamol appeared to be well absorbed after intramuscular injection of 50 mg kg^{-1} in buffalo calves and the mean maximum plasma concentration (Cmax) and time to maximum concentration (Tmax) were 42 mg l^{-1} and 1.5 h respectively (Sidhu *et al.*, 1993).

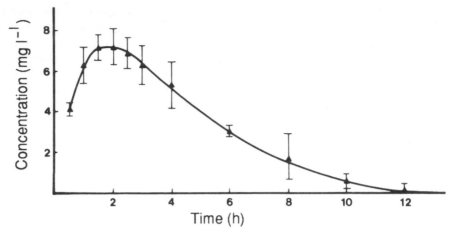

Figure 4.8   Plasma concentrations of paracetamol following intramuscular injection of 600 mg in six volunteers (reproduced with permission from John Wiley & Sons Ltd, from Macheras *et al.*, 1989).

Dermal Absorption

A transdermal therapeutic system containing paracetamol was based on a thermo-responsive membrane containing monooxyethylene trimethylolpropane tristearate which had a phase transition temperature of 38°C. Paracetamol was released from the temperature-activated system and shown to permeate excised hairless rat skin (Nozawa *et al.*, 1991). The penetration enhancers azone and lauryl alcohol increased the transport of paracetamol through shed snake skin and this effect was related to changes in the partition coefficient rather than to changes in the diffusion coefficient (Bhatt *et al.*, 1991).

Absorption as a Function of Therapeutic Efficacy

Paracetamol given in suppositories reduced fever in rats (Lock *et al.*, 1979). When it was given intraperitoneally in solution, it produced approximately twice the anti-pyretic response as the same dose given as a suspension and this was attributed to better absorption (Stolar *et al.*, 1973). In another report, a syrup formulation of paracetamol produced more consistent and longer-lasting analgesia in rats than an elixir containing 9.5 per cent ethanol even though serum concentrations were similar with both dosage forms (Babhair and Tariq, 1990).

There have been few studies of the role of absorption as a determinant of the therapeutic response to paracetamol in man. On the basis of pharmacodynamic and pharmacokinetic modelling, a dosage form was developed to produce optimum analgesic and antipyretic activity in children. A plot of plasma concentrations against antipyretic response gave a counterclockwise hysteresis loop consistent with a delay between equilibration of drug concentrations and the site of action, which was presumed to be in the central nervous system (Hossain and Ayres, 1992). In keeping with these predictions, there was considerable delay in maximum lowering of temperature in children with fever given paracetamol in rapidly absorbed liquid preparations (Windorfer and Vogel, 1976). Paracetamol suppositories with a lipophilic base produced higher plasma concentrations and a significantly greater antipyretic response in febrile children than a suppository with a hydrophilic base (Cullen *et al.*, 1989), while a rapidly absorbed paracetamol syrup was more effective in children with fever than a suppository (Keinänen *et al.*, 1977). A similar relationship between the absorption of oral and rectal paracetamol and analgesia has been described (Gaudreault *et al.*, 1988). Slow release and plain tablets of paracetamol produced different plasma concentration patterns in healthy volunteers but there was no difference in analgesic efficacy against laser-induced pain (Nielsen *et al.*, 1991). In another report by the same workers, immediate release, but not sustained release, paracetamol had an analgesic effect greater than that of placebo (Nielsen *et al.*, 1992).

Absorption of Paracetamol Prodrugs

The absorption of acetanilide and phenacetin was essentially complete (Greenberg and Lester, 1946; Brodie and Axelrod, 1948b, 1949; Prescott *et al.*, 1968). Benorylate has poor aqueous solubility and although gastrointestinal absorption was slow, it was rapidly hydrolyzed to salicylate and paracetamol by plasma and liver esterases. Following an oral dose of 4 g, peak plasma paracetamol concentrations were delayed for 1.5–4 h (Robertson *et al.*, 1972; Williams *et al.*, 1989a). A cyclic open ester paracetamol-acetylsalicylic acid prodrug was absorbed in rats more rapidly and completely than benorylate (Marzo *et al.*, 1990). Fatty acid ester prodrugs of paracetamol have been prepared and as the chain length increased, there was a corresponding decrease in aqueous solubility, absorption and bioavailability (Bauguess *et al.*, 1975a,b).

5

The Distribution of Paracetamol

Introduction

Paracetamol crosses cell membranes readily, and unlike salicylate, it has little effect on conductance and proton transport through phospholipid bilayer and mitochondrial membranes (Gutknecht, 1992). It was thought to cross cell membranes by diffusion, but at low concentrations a saturable component was identified in isolated rat liver cells (McPhail et al., 1993). At the subcellular level, paracetamol was distributed to a greater extent in lysosomes than in nuclear, mitochondrial, microsomal and cytosolic fractions (Studenberg and Brouwer, 1993a). In man, paracetamol had a distribution volume of about 0.9 l kg^{-1} and similar values have been reported in animals (see Chapter 10). The concentrations of paracetamol in different organs two hours after administration of 2.7 g of phenacetin in a dog showed a relatively even distribution with tissue:plasma concentration ratios close to unity. Concentrations were lowest in fat and cerebrospinal fluid and highest in liver and kidney (Brodie and Axelrod, 1949). In another study in dogs, the findings were generally similar with a mean tissue water to plasma water concentration ratio of about 1.1 (Gwilt et al., 1963b). Concentrations were low in lung tissue in rats, cats and monkeys, and there was no marked localization of paracetamol in different parts of the brain except for high concentrations in the pituitary gland in rats (Davison et al., 1961). Following administration of benorylate and a cyclic paracetamol-acetylsalicylate ester in rats, the highest concentrations of paracetamol were observed in liver and kidney (Marzo et al., 1990) and similar findings in respect of total radioactivity were reported after the administration of [^{14}C]-paracetamol in guinea pigs, hamsters, neonatal rats and mice (Whitehouse et al., 1975, 1977; Wong et al., 1976b, 1980b; Green and Fischer, 1984; Skoglund et al., 1987). Very high concentrations of radioactivity appeared in the bile (Wong et al., 1980b) and high concentrations were subsequently found in the intestine and faeces reflecting the extensive biliary excretion of paracetamol metabolites (Harvison et al., 1986b). Following oral administration of a toxic dose of 500 mg kg^{-1} of paracetamol in mice, peak concentrations were high in all tissues and were higher in liver and kidney than in plasma (Fischer et al., 1981). In other reports, paracetamol concentrations were somewhat higher in the kidney than in plasma (Newton et al., 1985a; Tarloff et al., 1989b) and it was not concentrated in the tubular fluid to the same extent as the glucuronide and sulphate conjugates to which the tubules were impermeable (Mudge, 1982).

In studies carried out in a 25-year-old woman who died after overdosage with multiple drugs including paracetamol, the concentrations of unchanged drug were similar in arterial and venous blood taken from several sites and in lung, spleen, myocardium and skeletal muscle. Concentrations were lower in cerebrospinal fluid, vitreous humour, fat and brain, and higher in liver and kidney (Jones and Pounder, 1987). Paracetamol was introduced into the trachea in five human cadavers and, when blood was sampled from different sites 48 h later, the concentrations were high in the pulmonary artery and veins but there was only limited diffusion into the heart and other major vessels (Pounder and Yonemitsu, 1991).

Tissue Distribution

Distribution into Red Blood Cells

The mean red blood cell to plasma paracetamol concentration ratio in horses was 0.74 (Engelking *et al.*, 1987a), and in man the mean concentrations were also somewhat greater in whole blood than in plasma at various times after dosing (Lester and Greenberg, 1947; Gwilt *et al.*, 1963b). There was no appreciable binding of paracetamol to red blood cells (Gazzard *et al.*, 1973).

Brain and Cerebrospinal Fluid

In rats aged 11 and 33 days, the plasma and brain concentrations of paracetamol were similar (Green and Fischer, 1984), and, in another study, the concentrations in brain were similar to those in other tissues although the time of the peak was delayed (Fischer *et al.*, 1981). Concentrations were somewhat higher in brain than in serum in rats given doses of 30 and 50 mg kg^{-1} (Ara and Ahmad, 1980) and 2 h after toxic doses of 750–1250 mg kg^{-1}, mean brain concentrations in young rats were 200–300 mg l^{-1} (Green and Fischer, 1984). Microdialysis has been used to monitor brain concentrations of paracetamol and the time of the peak concentration lagged behind the time of the peak in plasma (Cheney-Thamm *et al.*, 1987). Microdialysis was also employed for studies of the effects of changing conditions of the blood brain barrier on the transport of paracetamol (De Lange *et al.*, 1993) and for the analysis of transients in the tissue and brain concentrations of the drug following bolus intravenous injection in rats (Morrison *et al.*, 1991). Confluent monolayers of bovine cerebrovascular cells were cultured to investigate the characteristics of the blood–brain barrier, and a relationship was established between the endothelial permeability to paracetamol and other drugs, and lipophilicity (van Bree *et al.*, 1988). The uptake of paracetamol into the cerebrospinal fluid had previously been shown to be related to its lipid solubility (Ochs *et al.*, 1985), and a linear process for its transport into brain indicated a mechanism based on passive diffusion (van Bree *et al.*, 1989a). In patients with rheumatic and nerve root compression pain, paracetamol appeared rapidly in the cerebrospinal fluid following intravenous administration of its prodrug propacetamol. Concentrations increased to a maximum at 4 h, after which time the concentrations in the cerebrospinal fluid remained higher than those in plasma (Bannwarth *et al.*, 1992; Bannwarth and

Netter, 1994). Similar findings were reported in patients with continuous spinal anaesthesia given intravenous paracetamol (Moreau *et al.*, 1993).

Saliva

The average concentrations of paracetamol in plasma and saliva were generally similar but quantitative measurement in saliva was not reliable. Substantial discrepancies were noted during the first few hours after oral administration (Lowenthal *et al.*, 1976; Kamali *et al.*, 1987a; Nakano *et al.*, 1988) and in addition, saliva concentrations depended on the flow rate (Rashid and Bateman, 1990). Equilibration could occur between the concentrations of paracetamol in plasma and saliva under basal conditions, but this relationship could not be maintained when saliva flow was stimulated because rapid transfer was prevented due to its limited lipid solubility (Feller and le Petit, 1977).

Breast Milk

A pharmacokinetic model was developed to describe the passage of paracetamol into the milk in lactating goats. The milk to plasma concentration ratio was not constant and the pattern varied according to the route and duration of dosing (Figure 5.1) (Wilson *et al.*, 1987). In lactating rabbits given paracetamol intravenously, the concentrations in milk eventually fell in parallel with serum concentrations and as shown by the ratio of the areas under the concentration curves, the mean milk to serum concentration ratio was 0.58 (McNamara *et al.*, 1991). In man, paracetamol passed readily into breast milk, but concentrations were less than those

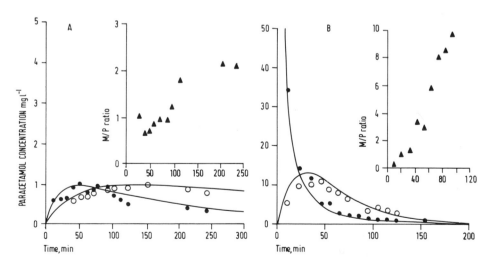

Figure 5.1 Effects of route of administration and time on the milk (○) and plasma (●) concentrations of paracetamol, and the derived milk : plasma concentration ratios (▲), (insets) in (A) a lactating goat given 60 mg kg^{-1} orally and (B) another lactating goat given the same dose by intravenous infusion over 2 min (redrawn with permission from S. Karger AG, Basel, from Wilson *et al.*, 1987).

in plasma (Berlin *et al.*, 1980; Hurden *et al.*, 1980; Bitzén *et al.*, 1981; Notarianni *et al.*, 1987). In one study, the partition ratio between milk and plasma was 0.81 (Bitzén *et al.*, 1981) while in another, the mean ratio of the areas under the milk and plasma concentration–time curves was 0.94 (Beaulac-Baillargeon *et al.*, 1994). The half life of paracetamol in milk was longer than the half life in plasma (Findlay *et al.*, 1981). Although only about 2 per cent of a normal therapeutic dose of paracetamol in an infant was transferred in a single feed 4 h after ingestion of 1 g by the mother, the occurrence of a skin rash in an infant was attributed to sensitivity following transfer of small amounts in milk feeds in this way (Matheson *et al.*, 1985).

Transplacental Transfer

In pregnant sheep, paracetamol passed freely to and from the maternal and fetal circulations, and the placental and non-placental clearances of the drug from the latter increased with gestational age (Wang *et al.*, 1986a). The transplacental transfer of paracetamol was demonstrated in a woman who had taken phenacetin just before delivery (Levy *et al.*, 1975a) and in 10 normal women who were given 1 g of paracetamol at the onset of the second stage of labour, there were significant differences after delivery between mean maternal and fetal concentrations (5.9 and 7.9 mg l^{-1} respectively) (Naga Rani *et al.*, 1989). In postpartum perfusion studies, there was no human placental metabolism of paracetamol (Wiegand *et al.*, 1984).

Distribution in the Eye

Paracetamol diffused readily across haemo-ocular barriers in rabbits following intravenous administration and the time course of paracetamol concentrations in the aqueous humour and plasma were similar. The uptake into, and elimination from, other ocular tissues was slower and the penetration into the lens was very poor. There were relatively low concentrations of paracetamol glucuronide and sulphate conjugates in the aqueous humour (Romanelli *et al.*, 1991).

Synovial Fluid

Five patients with rheumatoid arthritis and joint effusions were given paracetamol by intra-articular injection into the knee joint in amounts to give concentrations of about 20 mg l^{-1}. The paracetamol was cleared rapidly with a mean half life of 1.1 h, indicating its rapid transfer between blood and the synovial fluid in inflamed joints (Owen *et al.*, 1994).

Effects of Physiological and Pathological Factors

Following intravenous injection of paracetamol, the initial distribution phase was rapid with a half time of less than 20 min (Clements and Prescott, 1976; Rawlins *et al.*, 1977). The distribution volume corrected for body weight was similar in young and elderly subjects of either sex (Briant *et al.*, 1976; Divoll *et al.*, 1982a,b) but in one study a decrease with age was reported (Bedjaoui *et al.*, 1984). There was no temporal variation (Shively and Vesell, 1975; Kamali *et al.*, 1987b). No significant abnormalities were found in the distribution of paracetamol in patients with renal failure (Lowenthal *et al.*, 1976), epilepsy (Perucca and Richens, 1979) or thyroid disease (Forfar *et al.*, 1980). In one report, the volume of distribution of paracetamol was reduced in patients with congestive cardiac failure (Ochs *et al.*, 1983) while in another it was said to be increased (Pradeep Kumar *et al.*, 1987). However, in the latter study, paracetamol was measured in saliva and the pharmacokinetic calculations were unsound. Abnormal distribution of intravenous paracetamol has been observed in patients with Gilbert's syndrome in whom the disposition kinetics were more in keeping with a one-compartment rather than the expected two-compartment pharmacokinetic model (Douglas *et al.*, 1978). In obese subjects the volume of distribution corrected for body weight was smaller in both males and females compared with controls of normal body weight (Abernethy *et al.*, 1982a). The weight-adjusted volume of distribution of paracetamol in children with fever was similar to that observed in adults (Wilson *et al.*, 1982b).

Minor age-related changes have been observed in the renal distribution of paracetamol (Tarloff *et al.*, 1989b) and aspirin appeared to alter the relative tissue concentrations of total radioactivity following oral administration of [^{14}C]-paracetamol in different ways in guinea pigs, hamsters and mice (Whitehouse *et al.*, 1975, 1977; Wong *et al.*, 1976b). Fasting did not affect the distribution of paracetamol in horses (Engelking *et al.*, 1987a). The distribution volume was similar in adult non-pregnant and pregnant ewes and in neonatal lambs, but it was apparently decreased in fetal lambs (Wang *et al.*, 1990). In another study, there was no change in the volume corrected for body weight in pregnant rats (Lin and Levy, 1983b). The dynamics of the distribution of paracetamol were analysed in terms of the second and third moments as applied to systems with and without an elimination phase (Weiss and Pang, 1992).

Plasma Protein Binding

Paracetamol was not extensively bound to plasma proteins and it was less strongly bound than salicylate (Davison *et al.*, 1961). No binding could be detected by ultra-filtration or equilibrium dialysis at concentrations of 60–80 mg l^{-1} and at total concentrations ranging from 90 to 280 mg l^{-1} the fraction bound ranged from 8 to 43 per cent (Gazzard *et al.*, 1973). In another study, about 20 per cent was bound over the concentration range of 15–174 mg l^{-1} and binding was largely independent of drug concentration (Morris and Levy, 1984). Other investigators have reported plasma protein binding to the extent of 5–20 per cent (Lowenthal *et al.*, 1976; Ebel *et al.*, 1980; Hurden *et al.*, 1980; Bitzén *et al.*, 1981; Kamali *et al.*, 1987a) and there was little or no binding of paracetamol to the proteins in milk (Hurden *et al.*, 1980; Bitzén *et al.*, 1981) or saliva (Kamali *et al.*, 1987a). In overdose and spiked uraemic plasma samples the mean fraction of paracetamol bound was 24.1 per cent (Milligan *et al.*, 1994). In healthy subjects and *in vitro* there was no binding of paracetamol glucuronide to plasma proteins, but more than 50 per cent of the sulphate conjugate was bound (Morris and Levy, 1984). There was no significant plasma protein binding of either conjugate in anephric patients (Lowenthal *et al.*, 1976).

In animals, the plasma protein binding of paracetamol was also independent of concentration and it varied from 10 to 43 per cent. The glucuronide and sulphate conjugates were bound to the extent of 0–10 and 12–64 per cent respectively (Brodie and Axelrod, 1949; Duggin and Mudge, 1975; Hekman *et al.*, 1986; Wang *et al.*, 1986a; Ecobichon *et al.*, 1988; McNamara *et al.*, 1991; Studenberg and Brouwer, 1993a) and the sulphate conjugate was bound less in fetal lambs than in adult sheep (Wang *et al.*, 1986a). The binding of paracetamol and its glucuronide and sulphate conjugates to the proteins of hepatocyte cytosol amounted to 10, 3 and 12 per cent respectively (Studenberg and Brouwer, 1993a). Microdialysis has been used to determine the extent of plasma protein binding of paracetamol (Herrera *et al.*, 1990; Sarre *et al.*, 1992).

Distribution of Paracetamol Conjugates

The polar conjugates of paracetamol have a much more restricted distribution than the parent drug. Thus the glucuronide and sulphate conjugates did not enter red blood cells (Lester and Greenberg, 1947) and they were virtually excluded from the central nervous system (Davison *et al.*, 1961; Fischer *et al.*, 1981; Green and Fischer, 1984; Romanelli *et al.*, 1991). Considerable amounts of glucuronide conjugate were found in the liver and kidney in rats (Davison *et al.*, 1961; Green and Fischer, 1984) and in mice tissue concentrations of all the conjugates of paracetamol were low except for higher concentrations of paracetamol glucuronide in liver, and higher concentrations of the cysteine conjugate in kidney (Fischer *et al.*, 1981). In another investigation, the renal concentrations of glucuronide and sulphate conjugates were 5–10 times higher than in plasma, while the renal cortical concentrations of the mercapturic acid conjugate were 10–20 times higher (Newton *et al.*, 1985a). Autoradiographic studies with [^{14}C]-paracetamol in mice given toxic doses of 400 and 800 mg kg^{-1} showed the highest and most persistent concentrations of radioactivity in the liver and kidney (Skoglund *et al.*, 1987). As might be expected, neither the glucuronide nor sulphate conjugates of paracetamol passed from the maternal into the fetal circulation (Wang *et al.*, 1986a) or into breast milk (Notarianni *et al.*, 1987).

Following the intravenous injection of the glucuronide and sulphate conjugates of paracetamol in rats, there was a rapid equilibration phase followed by an exponential decline in plasma concentrations (Tone *et al.*, 1990). The respective volumes of distribution of these conjugates in rats varied from 0.18 to 0.49 and 0.21 to 0.34 l kg^{-1} (Galinsky and Levy, 1981; Lin and Levy, 1983b; Tone *et al.*, 1990). Following the intravenous injection of paracetamol glucuronide and sulphate in fetal lambs *in utero*, both conjugates exhibited biphasic elimination curves. The clearance was almost exclusively by renal excretion and the distribution volumes and total clearances increased with gestational age of the fetuses. Neither conjugate was subject to systemic hydrolysis or transplacental transfer (Wang *et al.*, 1985). In man, the distribution volume of the glucuronide and sulphate conjugates combined was calculated as 14.1–19.1 l per 1.73 m^2 body surface area in patients with renal failure (Lowenthal *et al.*, 1976) and 0.24 l kg^{-1} in overdose patients (Prescott and Wright, 1973). In another study in patients with renal failure, the volumes of distribution of the glucuronide and sulphate conjugates were estimated at 0.28 and 0.29 l kg^{-1} respectively (Prescott *et al.*, 1989b).

6

The Metabolism of Paracetamol

Historical Survey

Following the introduction of acetanilide and phenacetin towards the end of the last century, there were several reports of the fate of these precursors of paracetamol in the body. Although the analytical methods available at that time were crude and non-specific, it was thought that these drugs were excreted in urine in animals as sulphate and glucuronic acid conjugates of p-aminophenol (Jaffe and Hilbert, 1888). Mörner (1889) isolated the double potassium salt of oxalate and the sulphate conjugate of paracetamol from the urine of patients treated with acetanilide and suggested that a glucuronide conjugate was also formed because partly purified extracts were optically active and reduced alkaline copper salts. He also showed that when the urine from patients treated with acetanilide was hydrolyzed with acid in the presence of phenol and chromic acid, it gave a positive indophenol reaction when made alkaline with ammonia. He even mentioned the possibility of the formation of a mercapturic acid metabolite. Subsequently it was accepted that acetanilide and phenacetin were excreted as sulphate and glucuronic acid conjugates of paracetamol, and reports of these early metabolic studies were reviewed by Gross (1946) and Smith (1958).

Following the development of more specific methods for the assay of free and conjugated paracetamol in biological fluids, Greenberg and Lester (1946) reported the rapid urinary excretion of 70–90 per cent of therapeutic doses of acetanilide in man as conjugated p-aminophenol. Of this amount, some 96 per cent appeared as O-conjugates and 4 per cent as N-conjugates (i.e. paracetamol). In a subsequent study in subjects given acetanilide, no p-aminophenol was found in the blood, but there was rapid conversion of acetanilide to paracetamol, which in turn was conjugated and then rapidly excreted in the urine. Approximately two-thirds of the urinary conjugate was etheral sulphate and one-third 'glycuronate' (glucuronide) (Lester and Greenberg, 1947). Similar results were reported by Brodie and Axelrod (1948b). In two subjects, each given 1 g of acetanilide, plasma concentrations of paracetamol rose to 8–10 mg l^{-1} with subsequent higher concentrations of conjugated paracetamol. Following administration of 1 g of paracetamol itself, 85 per cent was recovered in the urine as conjugates and about 3 per cent as unchanged drug. Plasma concentrations of paracetamol were similar following administration of equimolecular doses of acetanilide and paracetamol, and the question was raised as to whether the analgesic effects of acetanilide could be explained by its rapid conversion to paracetamol. Smith and Williams (1948) found that about 70 and 10 per cent of doses of acetanilide and paracetamol were excreted in the urine of rabbits as the glucuronide and sulphate conjugates of paracetamol respectively.

Virtually identical findings were reported with phenacetin, which was also shown to be almost quantitatively converted to paracetamol in man. Unlike acetanilide and phenacetin, paracetamol was shown not to cause methaemoglobinaemia in man and again it was suggested that the therapeutic effects of phenacetin might be mediated by its conversion to paracetamol (Brodie and Axelrod, 1949). At the same time, paracetamol glucuronide and sulphate were shown to be major urinary metabolites of phenacetin in rabbits (Smith and Williams, 1949). Vest *et al.* (1959) measured the glucuronide conjugate of paracetamol in serum and showed that its formation was greatly depressed in infants during the first few weeks of life. More definitive studies of the isolation and quantitation of the urinary glucuronide and sulphate conjugates of paracetamol were reported by Büch *et al.* (1966a, 1967a,b,c, 1968) and Cummings *et al.* (1967) using thin layer chromatography, and by Jagenburg *et al.* (1968) using gel filtration chromatography. The extensive conversion of paracetamol to glucuronide and sulphate conjugates has since been confirmed repeatedly, and in most species these two metabolites together accounted for some 70–90 per cent of a dose (see below).

In recent years the biotransformation of paracetamol has been a subject of intense interest and several new metabolites have been identified. This renewed interest arose from the discovery of the metabolic activation of paracetamol by cytochrome P450-dependent mixed function oxidase to a reactive arylating intermediate that became bound covalently to hepatocytes causing necrosis when the drug was taken in overdosage (Jollow *et al.*, 1973; Mitchell *et al.*, 1973b,c; Potter *et al.*, 1973). Paracetamol was also shown to bind covalently to human liver microsomes (Dybing, 1977). The potentially toxic metabolite was thought to be N-acetyl-p-benzoquinoneimine and it was normally inactivated by preferential conjugation with reduced glutathione (Mitchell *et al.*, 1974; Gemborys *et al.*, 1978; Healey *et al.*, 1978; Corcoran *et al.*, 1980; Dahlin *et al.*, 1984; Nelson *et al.*, 1991; Vermeulen *et al.*, 1992). The glutathione conjugate was secreted into bile (Wong *et al.*, 1981; Hinson *et al.*, 1982; Siegers *et al.*, 1984; Gregus *et al.*, 1988b), and in the gut it was hydrolyzed to the cysteine derivative, which was reabsorbed and then excreted in the urine together with the acetylated form, the mercapturic acid conjugate (Mitchell *et al.*, 1974; Grafström *et al.*, 1979b).

A cysteine conjugate of paracetamol had been isolated previously by Jagenburg and Toczko (1964) during the investigation of a previously unknown ninhydrin-positive compound found in the urine of patients taking phenacetin, and subsequently Jagenburg *et al.* (1968) identified the cysteine and mercapturic acid conjugates of paracetamol as minor urinary metabolites of paracetamol in man. At the time, the toxicological significance of these metabolites was not appreciated. The mercapturic acid conjugate of paracetamol was found as a metabolite of acetanilide, and its formation from a glutathione conjugate via an epoxide intermediate was proposed (Grantham *et al.*, 1974). In 1972, a new urinary metabolite of phenacetin in dogs was identified by Focella *et al.* as a thiomethyl conjugate of paracetamol, and its formation via N-acetyl-p-benzoquinoneimine was suggested (Calder *et al.*,

1974). Subsequently, 3-thiomethylparacetamol and its oxidation product paracetamol 3-methylsulphoxide were confirmed as minor urinary metabolites of paracetamol (Klutch *et al.*, 1978; Gemborys and Mudge, 1981; Warrander *et al.*, 1985; Epstein *et al.*, 1991). 3-Thiomethylparacetamol was also excreted as its glucuronide and sulphate conjugates (Hart *et al.*, 1982b). Other minor metabolites of paracetamol have been described in several species and these included 3-hydroxy- and 3-methoxyparacetamol and their glucuronide and sulphate conjugates (Andrews *et al.*, 1976; Knox and Jurand, 1977, 1978; Gemborys and Mudge, 1981; Anderson *et al.*, 1983; Dolphin *et al.*, 1987; Factor *et al.*, 1989; Epstein *et al.*, 1991), and methoxy derivatives of the cysteine and mercapturic acid conjugates of paracetamol (Knox and Jurand, 1977, 1978). In animals (but apparently not in man), a minor pathway of paracetamol metabolism involved deacetylation to p-aminophenol (Smith and Griffiths, 1976; Carpenter and Mudge, 1981; Gemborys and Mudge, 1981; Newton *et al.*, 1983a) and this agent could then be subject to metabolic activation resulting

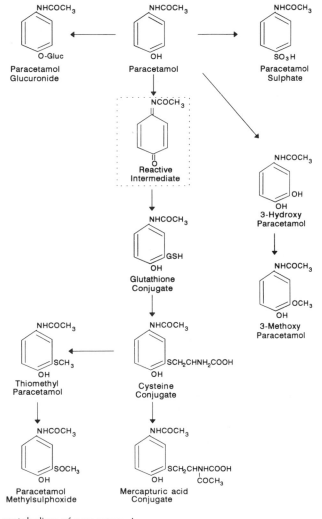

Figure 6.1. The metabolism of paracetamol.

in the formation of cysteine and mercapturic acid conjugates of hydroquinone (Pascoe *et al.*, 1988; Rashed *et al.*, 1990).

From a quantitative point of view, the most important urinary metabolites of paracetamol in man were the glucuronide, sulphate, cysteine and mercapturic acid conjugates, while other metabolites (and their glucuronide and sulphate conjugates), including those derived from the glutathione conjugate and 3-hydroxyparacetamol, seemed to be of little practical significance. There were considerable species differences in the extent of biliary and renal excretion of the different metabolites of paracetamol, and an overall scheme for its metabolism is shown in Figure 6.1. The sulphate conjugate of paracetamol was excreted rapidly and it produced no pharmacological effects (Williams *et al.*, 1983) but the 3-thiomethyl metabolite has analgesic activity that was comparable to that of the parent drug but of shorter duration (Hertz and Deghenghi, 1983). N-hydroxyparacetamol was proposed as a toxic metabolite of paracetamol (Calder *et al.*, 1981a). It was cytotoxic to rat kidney cells and it caused chromosomal damage together with dose-dependent inhibition of DNA synthesis (Djordjevic *et al.*, 1986; Dunn *et al.*, 1987). It was also hepatotoxic and nephrotoxic (see below). The 3-hydroxy- and 3-methoxy-derivatives were hepatotoxic in mice (Forte *et al.*, 1984) and they could also cause abnormal neurulation in cultured rat embryos (Harris *et al.*, 1989; Stark *et al.*, 1990). p-Aminophenol was more active than paracetamol in inhibiting prostaglandin synthesis in mouse neuronal and rat renal medullary tissues (Bruchhausen and Baumann, 1982).

Glucuronide Conjugation

In most species paracetamol was converted extensively to the O-glucuronide conjugate, and this product was a major urinary metabolite of the drug in man (Cummings *et al.*, 1967; Levy and Regårdh, 1971; Mrochek *et al.*, 1974; Prescott, 1980; Prescott *et al.*, 1981; Critchley *et al.*, 1983, 1986; Clements *et al.*, 1984; Mitchell *et al.*, 1984b; Sonne *et al.*, 1986; Galinsky *et al.*, 1987b; Thomas *et al.*, 1988; Lee *et al.*, 1992), mice (Wong *et al.*, 1981; Miners *et al.*, 1984a; Gregus *et al.*, 1988b), hamsters (Jollow *et al.*, 1974; Wong *et al.*, 1976b; Gregus *et al.*, 1988b), rabbits (Smith and Timbrell, 1974; Gregus *et al.*, 1988b; Smolarek *et al.*, 1990), guinea pigs (Smith and Timbrell, 1974; Whitehouse *et al.*, 1975; Gregus *et al.*, 1988b), ferrets (Smith and Timbrell, 1974), dogs (Savides *et al.*, 1984; Podder *et al.*, 1988; Smolarek *et al.*, 1990), sheep (Wang *et al.*, 1986a, 1990), baboons (Altomare *et al.*, 1984a), monkeys (Smolarek *et al.*, 1990) and ponies (Greenblatt and Engelking, 1988). At low doses, paracetamol glucuronide was only a minor metabolite in the rat (Miller and Fischer, 1974) and the overall extent of its formation varied from none in some amphibia (Clothier *et al.*, 1981) and less than 2 per cent in cats (Welch *et al.*, 1966; Savides *et al.*, 1984), to more than 90 per cent in guinea pigs (Whitehouse *et al.*, 1975). The glucuronide conjugation of paracetamol occurred primarily in the liver, and the fraction of the dose recovered in the urine was largely independent of the route of administration (Miller and Fischer, 1974; Clements *et al.*, 1984; Thomas *et al.*, 1988). Some glucuronide conjugation of paracetamol occurred in the gastrointestinal tract (Josting *et al.*, 1976; Watari *et al.*, 1984; Nelson *et al.*, 1986; Pang *et al.*, 1986; Rogers *et al.*, 1987a; Podder *et al.*, 1988; Gregus *et al.*, 1988a; Ramakrishna *et al.*, 1989; Goon and Klaassen, 1990; Hirate *et al.*, 1990,

1991; Tone *et al.*, 1990), kidney (Jones *et al.*, 1979; Ross *et al.*, 1980; Emslie *et al.*, 1981a, 1982; Newton *et al.*, 1982a; Bock *et al.*, 1993), and spleen and lung (Hirate *et al.*, 1990; Bock *et al.*, 1993). Isolated rat intestinal cells metabolized paracetamol to its glucuronide conjugate (Grafström *et al.*, 1979a) and the intestinal glucuronidation of paracetamol was inducible with butylated hydroxyanisole (Hjelle *et al.*, 1985b). The extrahepatic metabolism of paracetamol was of little quantitative significance, and route of administration had little effect on the fractional excretion of metabolites (Clements *et al.*, 1984; Tone *et al.*, 1990).

Glucuronide conjugation is catalyzed by a family of glucuronyltransferases and uridine 5'-diphosphoglucuronic acid (UDP-GA) is an essential co-substrate. The specific enzyme for paracetamol has been characterized in human liver microsome fractions. The reaction proceeded according to Michaelis-Menten kinetics and the isozyme appeared to be distinct from those which catalyzed the glucuronidation of substrates such as morphine and 4-methylumbelliferone (Miners *et al.*, 1990; Miners and Lillywhite, 1991). The effects of detergents and factors such as incubation time, protein concentration and pH on the activity of human liver glucuronyltransferase have been described with paracetamol as the substrate (Pacifici *et al.*, 1988). In different systems, paracetamol appeared to be an overlapping substrate of several glucuronyltransferases and inducible forms of the enzymes were demonstrated in rat kidney, lung and spleen, and in human kidney (Bock *et al.*, 1993). The glucuronidation of paracetamol was inducible by agents such as butylated hydroxyanisole (Moldéus *et al.*, 1982b) and phenobarbitone (Prescott *et al.*, 1981; Bock and Bock-Hennig, 1987; Studenberg and Brouwer, 1993b) and it was subject to dose-dependent competitive inhibition by other substrates such as the metabolites of phenobarbitone and antipyrine (Douidar and Ahmed, 1987; Monshouwer *et al.*, 1994). In man, the glucuronide conjugation of paracetamol was co-regulated with cytochrome P450 isoforms such as CYP1A2, and the capacity for glucuronide conjugation was affected by gender, the use of oral contraceptives and smoking (Bock *et al.*, 1994). As shown by antegrade and retrograde perfusion of the isolated rat liver, the lobular distribution of paracetamol glucuronide conjugation activity was reported to be dose-dependent with a greater capacity in periportal than centrilobular zones (Mitchell *et al.*, 1989). Similar periportal dominance of the glucuronide conjugation of paracetamol was reported in rat hepatocytes separated by density gradient centrifugation (Araya *et al.*, 1986). However, in another study in isolated hepatocytes, glucuronide conjugation was faster at high drug concentrations in perivenous than periportal cells (Anundi *et al.*, 1993).

Paracetamol analogues such as 2-hydroxy- and 3-hydroxyacetanilide also formed glucuronide conjugates (Hamilton and Kissinger, 1986). The glucuronide conjugation of paracetamol was demonstrated in isolated rat hepatocytes (Moldéus *et al.*, 1982b; Dawson *et al.*, 1990, 1992), rat liver snips and slices (McPhail *et al.*, 1990; Miller *et al.*, 1993a), cultured rat hepatocytes (Kane *et al.*, 1990b), dog hepatocytes (Bolcsfoldi *et al.*, 1981) and also in primary cultures of human hepatocytes (Koebe *et al.*, 1994). Direct proton nuclear magnetic resonance spectroscopy was used to monitor the excretion of the glucuronide conjugate following therapeutic doses of paracetamol in man (Bales *et al.*, 1984b) and to study its formation by isolated hepatocytes (Nicholson *et al.*, 1985). The glucuronide conjugation of paracetamol was used as a probe for the non-invasive investigation of glucose and galactose metabolism in man (Hellerstein and Munro, 1988) and for studies of glycogen repletion (Shulman *et al.*, 1990). In another report, the rate of paracetamol glucuronide conjugation by rat hepatocytes was assessed by the kinetics of incorporation of label from [C^{14}]-fructose (Dawson *et al.*, 1992).

Compared with sulphate conjugation, the glucuronidation of paracetamol was characterized by low affinity and high capacity (Jollow *et al.*, 1974; Moldéus, 1978; Siegers *et al.*, 1978; Watari *et al.*, 1983; Hjelle and Klaassen, 1984; Miners *et al.*, 1984a). It has been claimed that the glucuronide conjugation of paracetamol was saturated in man following overdosage, and that this caused liver damage because a disproportionately large fraction of the dose was then shunted towards the pathway of toxic metabolic activation (Davis *et al.*, 1976b; Slattery and Levy, 1979a; Slattery *et al.*, 1981). While this might be the case in rats where glucuronide conjugation was not the dominant route of elimination (Davis *et al.*, 1976a; Poulsen *et al.*, 1985c), there was undisputable clinical evidence that glucuronidation of paracetamol was not readily saturated in man, even in severely poisoned patients (Prescott, 1983, 1984). The reported K_m values for paracetamol glucuronidation *in vitro* were in the range of 4–10 mM in rats and mice (Bolanowska and Gessner, 1978; Moldéus, 1978; McPhail *et al.*, 1990) and man (Miners *et al.*, 1990), and again this suggests that saturation would be unlikely unless drug concentrations were very high. In keeping with these findings, saturation of glucuronidation could not be demonstrated in the isolated perfused rat liver or with isolated dog hepatocytes even at paracetamol concentrations of 10 mM (i.e. more than 1500 mg l^{-1}) (Grafström *et al.*, 1979b; Bolcsfoldi *et al.*, 1981), and in mice there was no evidence of saturation as the dose increased from 50 to 400 mg kg^{-1} (Figure 6.2) (Miners *et al.*, 1984a).

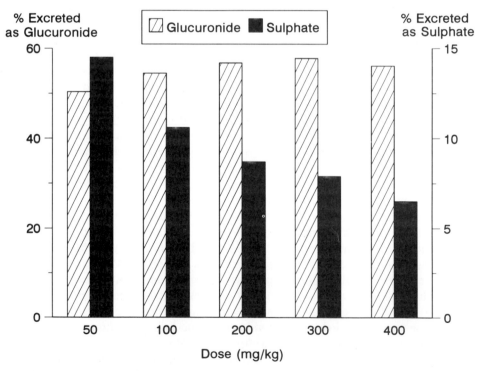

Figure 6.2. Reduction in the sulphate conjugation of oral paracetamol with increasing dose in the male C3H mouse. The results are expressed as percentage of the dose recovered in 24 h (from Miners *et al.*, 1984a).

Nevertheless, capacity-limited glucuronide conjugation of paracetamol has been reported in rats (Jollow *et al.*, 1974; Siegers *et al.*, 1978) and the mechanism was probably depletion of the co-substrate (Price and Jollow, 1984). Hepatic UDP-GA was reduced to 15, 23 and 42 per cent of control values at 0.5, 1 and 2 h after an intraperitoneal dose of 600 mg kg^{-1} of paracetamol (Hjelle *et al.*, 1985a). The rapid depletion was not caused by a decrease in UDP-glucose, but was probably related to inhibition of the dehydrogenase secondary to accumulation of cytoplasmic NADH (Hjelle, 1986). The depression of glucuronidation of a toxic dose of paraceta-mol produced by fasting in rats was associated with decreased production of UDP-GA (Price and Jollow, 1988). The formation of paracetamol glucuronide was reduced in rats with hereditary deficiency of bilirubin glucuronyl transferase (Gunn rats) (de Morais *et al.*, 1992a) and in the much less affected human equivalent of patients with Gilbert's disease (de Morais *et al.*, 1992b). This impairment of conjuga-tion was associated with increased metabolic activation of paracetamol and enhanced hepatic and renal toxicity in rats (de Morais and Wells, 1988, 1989). In isolated kidneys from Gunn rats perfused with unrealistically high concentrations of paracetamol (about 2000 mg l^{-1}), glucuronide conjugation was greatly reduced in heterozygotes and none was detected in homozygotes (Emslie *et al.*, 1982). Glucuro-nide conjugation in man was reviewed recently by Miners and MacKenzie (1991).

Sulphate Conjugation

Sulphate conjugation is a major parallel route of non-toxic elimination of paraceta-mol in many species and there was usually a reciprocal relationship with the extent of glucuronide conjugation. The capacity for conjugation by these safe pathways of elimination corresponded to the susceptibility to toxicity in different species as shown by effects on cultured isolated hepatocytes and liver slices (Green *et al.*, 1984a; Smolarek *et al.*, 1990; Miller *et al.*, 1993a). Sulphate conjugation was the dominant route of paracetamol metabolism in rats (Galinsky *et al.*, 1986; Brouwer and Jones, 1990; Miller *et al.*, 1993a) and cats (Savides *et al.*, 1984), while it accounted for less than 10 per cent of a dose in guinea pigs (Whitehouse *et al.*, 1975; Ecobichon *et al.*, 1989). Büch *et al.* (1968) showed that paracetamol decreased the urinary excretion of free sulphate, and that the excretion of its sulphate conjugate was limited by the availability of inorganic sulphate. They also showed that the sulphate conjugation of paracetamol could be stimulated by the addition of sodium sulphate or thiosulphate. Sulphoconjugation became capacity-limited at relatively low dose levels and an important limiting factor was the availability of the co-substrate adenosine 3-phosphate-5-phosphosulphate (PAPS). This in turn depended on the provision of inorganic sulphate derived from dietary intake and aminoacids such as methionine and cysteine (Cocchetto and Levy, 1981; Levy *et al.*, 1982; Gla-zenburg *et al.*, 1983; Morris and Levy, 1983b; Levy, 1986). A diet deficient in sul-phate decreased inorganic sulphate concentrations and the formation of paracetamol sulphate in rats but it did not reduce the concentration of PAPS, whereas treatment with molybdate decreased the concentrations of inorganic sul-phate and PAPS, and reduced the sulphate conjugation of paracetamol (Gregus *et al.*, 1994b). Dietary deficiencies of sulphate and cysteine alone had no major effect on the sulphate conjugation of paracetamol but there was a significant decrease with their combined deficiency (Gregus *et al.*, 1994a). With isolated rat hepatocyte preparations, the formation of paracetamol sulphate depended on the presence of cofactors and the availability of PAPS was related to concentrations of inorganic sulphate (Sweeny and Reinke, 1988). Paracetamol markedly depleted PAPS in the liver (but not in the kidney) and drastically reduced blood and tissue inorganic sulphate concentrations (Kim *et al.*, 1992).

Aryl sulphotransferases are ubiquitous cytosolic enzymes, and although the sulphate conjugation of paracetamol occurred primarily in the liver, small amounts could be formed in other tissues as noted above for glucuronidation. The sulphate conjugation of paracetamol was demonstrated in human colonic mucosa (Ramakrishna *et al.*, 1989) and in fetal lung cytosol (Jones *et al.*, 1992a). Purified paracetamol sulphotransferase in rat liver was active at pH 9.0 and had a molecular weight of 35 kD. It appeared to be distinct from other sulphotransferases and was only expressed in liver (Coughtrie and Sharp, 1990; Coughtrie *et al.*, 1990). Other investigators have described a multiplicity of different forms of phenol sulphotransferase active against paracetamol in rat liver cytosol and different forms were involved in the reaction at high and low concentrations of the drug (Mizuma *et al.*, 1984). In the rat, dose-dependent saturable sulphate conjugation in the gut and liver accounted for most of the first pass metabolism of paracetamol (Tone *et al.*, 1990). At higher doses, the capacity for intestinal conjugation with sulphate exceeded that for glucuronide conjugation, which was readily saturated (Goon and Klaassen, 1990). In mice, selective active transport systems for removal of the conjugate have been demonstrated in the brush border and basolateral membranes of enterocytes (Wollenberg and Rummel, 1984). Intestinal bacterial flora may contribute to sulphate conjugation, and in rats the urinary excretion of paracetamol sulphate was significantly reduced by pretreatment with antibiotics (Kim and Kobashi, 1986). The sulphate conjugate of paracetamol was taken up into isolated rat hepatocytes by carrier-mediated transport, and the conjugate formed intracellularly was released rapidly into the medium (Iida *et al.*, 1989). Hepatic uptake was influenced by the presence of albumin, and studies with a barrier-limited space-distributed variable time transit model showed low liver cell permeability and a small binding space for the unbound fraction (Goresky *et al.*, 1992). In the once-through perfused rat liver preparation, the greater the hepatocellular activity for the formation of paracetamol from tracer doses of acetanilide and phenacetin, the greater the extent of paracetamol sulphate conjugation. This was thought to be related to the effect of times of formation and transit through the liver (Pang *et al.*, 1982). Retrograde perfusion studies showed that the sulphate conjugation of paracetamol occurred predominantly in the periportal region of the liver (Pang and Terrell, 1981a) and the zonal activity of rat paracetamol sulphotransferase was not distributed evenly as shown by combined hepatic arterio-portal venous and hepatic arterial-hepatic venous perfusion studies (Pang *et al.*, 1988a). There was good agreement between the kinetics of the sulphate conjugation of paracetamol in isolated rat hepatocytes, 9000 g supernatant fractions of liver and the perfused rat liver preparation (Pang *et al.*, 1985). The dominance of paracetamol sulphate conjugation in periportal rather than centrilobular areas was thought to be due to regional differences in the V_{max} values (Araya *et al.*, 1986). In contrast to these findings, others were not able to confirm the periportal dominance of the sulphate conjugation of paracetamol (Anundi *et al.*, 1993). Kinetic modelling was used to study the effects of phenobarbitone induction on the sulphate conjugation of paracetamol in rats (Studenberg and Brouwer, 1993b).

Human platelet phenol sulphotransferase activities towards paracetamol and 3-methoxy-4-hydroxyphenylglycol were correlated (Anderson *et al.*, 1981) and paracetamol was a substrate for the thermolabile and thermostable forms of human platelet sulphotransferase. Both enzymes were regulated independently (Reiter and Weinshilboum, 1982b) and of the two functional forms of human platelet sulphotransferase, paracetamol was conjugated primarily by the 'M' form (Bonham Carter *et al.*, 1983). In isolated rat hepatocytes, inhibition of glutathione synthesis with buthionine sulphoximine did not reduce the sulphate conjugation of paracetamol but there was a marked reduction following exposure to 2,6-dichloro-4-nitrophenol (Dalhoff and Poulsen, 1993b). Toxic doses of paracetamol decreased the synthesis of PAPS but did not reduce glutathione synthesis (Dalhoff and Poulsen, 1992) while cysteine stimulated the synthesis of PAPS in hepatocytes previously depleted of glutathione by diethyl maleate and incubated with toxic concentrations of paracetamol. However, cysteine did not increase the formation of the sulphate conjugate (Dalhoff and Poulsen, 1993c). A simple method for determination of the rate of formation of the sulphate conjugate of paracetamol was based on the use of [^{35}S]-sulphate (Dawson *et al.*, 1991).

Saturation of Sulphate Conjugation

The sulphate conjugation of paracetamol in rats could be described by Michaelis-Menten kinetics, and *in vivo* the K_m was only about 100 μM. In the absence of inorganic sulphate depletion, paracetamol was eliminated largely by this route, and the total clearance of a small dose (less than 15 mg kg^{-1}) depended on hepatic blood flow while the elimination of large doses was limited by the conjugation capacity (Lin and Levy, 1986). Similar K_m values have been proposed for the sulphate conjugation of paracetamol in man (Slattery and Levy, 1979a) and saturation occurred in mice at 0.25 mM concentrations (Moldéus, 1978). A progressive reduction in the fractional sulphate conjugation with increasing dose of paracetamol in the mouse is shown in Figure 6.2. Early saturation of the sulphate conjugation of paracetamol was shown in rat liver snips and isolated hepatocytes (McPhail *et al.*, 1990), cultured rat hepatocytes (Kane *et al.*, 1990b) and isolated dog hepatocytes (Bolcsfoldi *et al.*, 1981). In primary cultures of human liver cells, the capacity for the sulphate conjugation of paracetamol was reduced after incubation for 16 days (Koebe *et al.*, 1994). Reduction in the availability of inorganic sulphate by dietary restriction of protein and sulphur-containing aminoacids was associated with a marked decrease in the sulphate conjugation of paracetamol (Krijgsheld *et al.*, 1981; Glazenburg *et al.*, 1983), and administration of paracetamol itself produced an acute dose-related reduction in plasma inorganic sulphate concentrations, which in turn reduced the extent of sulphoconjugation (Krijgsheld *et al.*, 1981; Lin and Levy, 1981, 1982, 1983a; Levy *et al.*, 1982; Kim *et al.*, 1992). The consequences in terms of the elimination kinetics and metabolic fate of paracetamol depended on whether sulphate conjugation was a major or a minor route for its removal. In rats given 150 mg kg^{-1} of paracetamol intravenously, the serum inorganic sulphate concentration was reduced to 10 per cent of control values (Lin and Levy, 1983a). In this species, sulphate conjugation was the dominant route of elimination, and sulphate depletion caused dose-dependent reduction in clearance, an increase in the half life of the drug, a compensatory increase in glucuronide conjugation and increased susceptibility to hepatotoxicity (Levy *et al.*, 1982; Price and Jollow, 1989b).

There was no significant reduction in plasma inorganic sulphate concentration in mice following oral administration of 190 mg kg^{-1} of paracetamol (de Vries *et al.*, 1990) and in man, a single dose of 1.5 g of paracetamol produced a small reduction in the plasma concentrations and urinary excretion of inorganic sulphate (Morris and Levy, 1983b). There was a circadian rhythm of serum sulphate concentrations in man, and levels were lowest in the morning and highest in early evening. During administration of 650 mg of paracetamol four times a day for four days, this rhythm was preserved but concentrations were decreased (Hoffman *et al.*, 1990, 1991). With single and multiple doses of 650 mg there were fluctuations in serum inorganic sulphate, but as expected there was no change in the paracetamol half life. Paradoxically, serum inorganic sulphate levels were elevated in patients who were taking the drug regularly (Hendrix-Treacy *et al.*, 1986). In another study in which patients took doses of 2–12 g of paracetamol daily for prolonged periods, there was an increase in plasma concentrations of inorganic sulphate and a decrease in its urinary excretion. Overall, the urine sulphate to glucuronide conjugate ratios were low (Blackledge *et al.*, 1991). Paracetamol-induced inorganic sulphate depletion in rats inhibited the synthesis of cartilage glycosaminoglycans (van der Kraan *et al.*, 1988). Although there was a significant decrease in serum sulphate levels during the first four weeks of administration of 200 mg kg^{-1} of paracetamol twice daily, subsequently the change was diminished only to a small and insignificant extent. There was a corresponding fall and return to normal in glycosaminoglycan content of cartilage (van der Kraan *et al.*, 1990). Depleted inorganic sulphate could be replenished by administration of sodium sulphate, sulphite and thiosulphate and N-acetylcysteine, and depending on the circumstances and species, this might increase sulphate conjugation and accelerate the elimination of paracetamol (Büch *et al.*, 1968; Galinsky *et al.*, 1979; Lin and Levy, 1981; Galinsky and Levy, 1984a; Miller and Jollow, 1986b; Sun *et al.*, 1989). The administration of paracetamol in the form of its N-acetyl-DL-methionate ester in mice did not influence the plasma concentrations of the sulphate (or glucuronide) conjugates (Skoglund *et al.*, 1992). Inorganic sulphate was retained in chronic renal failure where its greater availability compared with normal controls resulted in greater fractional sulphate conjugation and reduced plasma concentrations of paracetamol during continuous infusion of the drug (Lin and Levy, 1982). Depletion of sulphur aminoacids by chronic administration of paracetamol in the diet retarded growth in rats, and this effect could be reversed with methionine and cysteine (McLean *et al.*, 1989). The extent of metabolism of paracetamol by glucuronide and sulphate conjugation depended on many factors including species and dose, and fractional urinary excretion data for man and laboratory animals are summarized in Table 6.1.

Metabolic Activation of Paracetamol

The mechanism of the hepatotoxicity of paracetamol by its conversion to a reactive intermediate metabolite by NADPH-dependent microsomal cytochrome P450

Table 6.1 Fractional urinary excretion of the glucuronide and sulphate conjugates of paracetamol in different species.

Species	Dose (mg kg^{-1})	Route	% excreted as glucuronide conjugate	% excreted as sulphate conjugate	Reference
Man	12	oral	63.3	32.0	Cummings *et al.*, 1967
Man	15	oral	66.9	28.8	Levy and Ragårdh, 1971
Man	15	oral	61.4	25.8	Levy and Yamada, 1971
Man	10	oral	57.6	38.2	Amsel and Davison, 1972
Man	30	oral	65.8	31.2	Robertson *et al.*, 1972
Man	23	oral	58.7	29.2	Mrochek *et al.*, 1974
Man[1]	8.3	oral	39.0	27.0	Smith and Timbrell, 1974
Man	14–57	oral	50.0	20.0	Davis *et al.*, 1976b
Man[2]	53	oral	64.1	16.9	Davis *et al.*, 1976b
Man[2]	137	oral	64.1	15.6	Davis *et al.*, 1976b
Man[2]	157	oral	61.6	14.6	Davis *et al.*, 1976b
Man[3]	214	oral	41.2	10.0	Davis *et al.*, 1976b
Man	15	oral	46.2	33.3	Houston and Levy, 1976
Man	10	oral	60.4	36.4	Miller *et al.*, 1976b
Man	21	oral	54.0	33.0	Forrest *et al.*, 1979
Man[4]	21	oral	59.0	29.0	Forrest *et al.*, 1979
Man[5]	21	oral	50.0	35.0	Forrest *et al.*, 1979
Man	20	oral	54.7	32.3	Prescott, 1980
Man[6]	150	oral	75.3	9.3	Prescott, 1980
Man[3]	170	oral	66.5	9.7	Prescott, 1980
Man	10	oral	64.7	28.4	Thomas *et al.*, 1980
Man	20	oral	57.0	30.0	Prescott *et al.*, 1981
Man	10	oral	55.7	41.5	Reiter and Weinshilboum, 1982a
Man	20	oral	59.0	28.8	Critchley *et al.*, 1983
Man	15	oral	59.1	26.2	Miners *et al.*, 1983
Man[7]	22	oral	56.4	32.6	Mitchell *et al.*, 1983
Man	12	oral	57.3	33.3	Villeneuve *et al.*, 1983
Man[8]	12	oral	53.0	31.5	Villeneuve *et al.*, 1983
Man[5]	12	oral	51.7	37.1	Villeneuve *et al.*, 1983
Man	5	oral	46.6	36.9	Clements *et al.*, 1984
Man	5	iv	47.6	38.4	Clements *et al.*, 1984
Man	20	oral	53.2	30.0	Clements *et al.*, 1984
Man	20	iv	50.4	33.7	Clements *et al.*, 1984
Man	15	oral	50.4	44.2	Galinsky and Levy, 1984a
Man	15	oral	58.7	27.2	Miners *et al.*, 1984c
Man	22	oral	59.7	28.2	Mitchell *et al.*, 1984b
Man	21	oral	64.2	28.6	Pantuck *et al.*, 1984
Man	22	oral	53.8	31.2	Critchley *et al.*, 1986
Man[9]	22	oral	58.2	32.0	Critchley *et al.*, 1986
Man[10]	22	oral	57.9	28.9	Critchley *et al.*, 1986
Man	15	oral	57.4	31.0	Jayasinghe *et al.*, 1986
Man[7]	15	oral	58.1	27.3	Miners *et al.*, 1986
Man	16	oral	55.1	33.5	Rayburn *et al.*, 1986
Man	7.5	iv	49.2	24.9	Sonne *et al.*, 1986
Man	15	oral	59.5	30.7	Amouyal *et al.*, 1987
Man	15	oral	53.2	35.3	Bock *et al.*, 1987
Man	15	oral	52.3	17.2	Galinsky *et al.*, 1987b
Man	22	iv	51.9	42.8	Kamali *et al.*, 1987b
Man	15	oral	40.3	37.2	Ladds *et al.*, 1987

(cont.)

Table 6.1 *(cont.)*

Species	Dose (mg kg^{-1})	Route	% excreted as glucuronide conjugate	% excreted as sulphate conjugate	Reference
Man	15	oral	52.1	35.1	Notarianni *et al.*, 1987
Man	7	oral	51.6	30.6	Slattery *et al.*, 1987
Man	42	oral	59.5	23.5	Slattery *et al.*, 1987
Man	15	oral	56.0	36.0	Ullrich *et al.*, 1987
Man[11]	15	oral	56.0	36.0	Ullrich *et al.*, 1987
Man[12]	20	oral	59.8	30.2	Kamali *et al.*, 1988
Man	15	oral	55.4	30.4	Miners *et al.*, 1988
Man[13]	15	oral	63.0	25.4	Miners *et al.*, 1988
Man	15	iv	51.9	26.0	Sonne *et al.*, 1988
Man	15	oral	54.2	29.5	Thomas *et al.*, 1988
Man	15	iv	53.1	29.5	Thomas *et al.*, 1988
Man	14	oral	60.7	28.1	Prescott *et al.*, 1989b
Man[14]	15	oral	46.8	26.4	Slattery *et al.*, 1989
Man	14	oral	46.0	48.0	Venkataramanan *et al.*, 1989
Man[15]	14	oral	36.0	56.0	Venkataramanan *et al.*, 1989
Man	8	iv	57.4	38.9	Wynne *et al.*, 1990
Man[13,16]	8	iv	58.2	36.4	Wynne *et al.*, 1990
Man[13,17]	9	iv	46.3	48.3	Wynne *et al.*, 1990
Man	7.5	oral	46.6	31.5	Epstein *et al.*, 1991
Man	10	oral	51.3	34.5	Hindmarsh *et al.*, 1991
Man	26	oral	58.0	31.0	Leung and Critchley, 1991
Man	15	oral	53.2	33.2	Osborne *et al.*, 1991
Man	7.5	iv	44.4	29.5	Poulsen *et al.*, 1991
Man[4,5]	7.5	iv	37.4	21.7	Poulsen *et al.*, 1991
Man	10	oral	56.9	32.7	Veronese and McLean, 1991
Man	20	iv	64.2	30.0	de Morais *et al.*, 1992b
Man[18]	15.5	oral	54.5	35.9	Lee *et al.*, 1992
Man[19]	15.5	oral	62.2	28.9	Lee *et al.*, 1992
Man	10	oral	51.5	44.1	Patel *et al.*, 1992
Man[20]	10	oral	51.8	44.0	Patel *et al.*, 1992
Man	20	oral	56.2	33.3	Esteban and Pérez-Mateo, 1993a
Man	20	oral	55.7	39.0	Kamali, 1993
Man	20	oral	50.4	37.6	Prescott *et al.*, 1993
Man	7.5	oral	50.1	31.7	Roos *et al.*, 1993
Mouse	50	ip	48.8	27.3	Jollow *et al.*, 1974
Mouse	400	ip	60.7	19.5	Jollow *et al.*, 1974
Mouse	150	oral	45.3	16.0	Whitehouse *et al.*, 1977
Mouse	250	ip	37.2	19.3	Wong *et al.*, 1980b
Mouse	150	oral	47.6	14.3	Wong *et al.*, 1981
Mouse	50	oral	50.4	14.5	Miners *et al.*, 1984a
Mouse	400	oral	56.1	6.5	Miners *et al.*, 1984a
Mouse	200	oral	58.9	9.0	Miners *et al.*, 1984b
Mouse	1000	oral	42.3	8.7	Corcoran *et al.*, 1985b
Mouse	350	oral	39.1	19.6	Whitehouse *et al.*, 1985
Mouse	500	oral	52.3	7.8	Corcoran and Wong, 1986
Mouse	600	ip	59.0	11.0	Hazelton *et al.*, 1986b
Mouse	300	ip	61.0	12.0	Larrey *et al.*, 1986
Mouse[21]	300	ip	52.0	21.0	Larrey *et al.*, 1986
Mouse	600	ip	67.3	7.9	Letteron *et al.*, 1986
Mouse	20	ip	45.9	22.7	Miller and Jollow, 1986a

Table 6.1 *(cont.)*

Species	Dose (mg kg^{-1})	Route	% excreted as glucuronide conjugate	% excreted as sulphate conjugate	Reference
Mouse	400	oral	64.7	10.4	Tredger *et al.*, 1986b
Mouse	100	oral	55.6	9.0	Dolphin *et al.*, 1987
Mouse	100	ip	53.1	8.7	Price and Gale, 1987
Mouse	300	ip	65.6	14.8	Reicks and Hathcock, 1987
Mouse[22]	300	ip	71.5	11.6	Reicks and Hathcock, 1987
Mouse	150	iv	74.3	5.9	Gregus *et al.*, 1988b
Mouse	200	ip	57.6	9.9	Mikov *et al.*, 1988
Mouse	200	ip	43.5	7.8	Pascoe *et al.*, 1988
Mouse	50	ip	64.3	10.7	Adamson *et al.*, 1991
Rat	300	ip	48.3	33.5	Büch *et al.*, 1967c
Rat	600	ip	16.7	22.5	Büch *et al.*, 1967c
Rat	50	ip	35.2	47.6	Jollow *et al.*, 1974
Rat	1200	ip	54.8	16.1	Jollow *et al.*, 1974
Rat	25	ip	3.8	68.6	Miller and Fischer, 1974
Rat	25	oral	4.8	77.0	Miller and Fischer, 1974
Rat	25	ip	2.7	68.9	Miller and Fischer, 1974
Rat[1]	125	oral	14.0	44.0	Smith and Timbrell, 1974
Rat	495	oral	33.3	35.2	Davis *et al.*, 1976a
Rat	1485	oral	35.6	29.5	Davis *et al.*, 1976a
Rat	2492	oral	31.5	32.4	Davis *et al.*, 1976a
Rat	3503	oral	27.5	20.4	Davis *et al.*, 1976a
Rat[23]	211	oral	5.0	52.0	Smith and Griffiths, 1976
Rat[7]	211	oral	22.0	40.0	Smith and Griffiths, 1976
Rat	10	iv	5.8	89.3	Cotty *et al.*, 1977
Rat	320	iv	24.5	34.8	Cotty *et al.*, 1977
Rat	150	oral	18.9	50.8	Thomas *et al.*, 1977b
Rat	tracer	iv	3.4	90.4	Pang and Gillette, 1978b
Rat	150	iv	25.8	60.6	Galinsky and Levy, 1979
Rat	tracer	iv	3.1	94.3	Pang *et al.*, 1979a
Rat	150	oral	16.7	72.2	Thomas *et al.*, 1980
Rat	25	ip	10.0	60.0	Green and Fischer, 1981
Rat	250	ip	20.0	20.0	Green and Fischer, 1981
Rat	500	ip	50.4	15.5	Sato and Lieber, 1981
Rat	30	iv	5.3	86.9	Galinsky and Levy, 1982
Rat[7]	150	iv	37.4	49.6	Hart *et al.*, 1982a
Rat[7]	300	iv	23.5	52.7	Hart *et al.*, 1982a
Rat[7]	300	iv	49.2	33.7	Hart *et al.*, 1982a
Rat[23]	1500	oral	41.9	23.0	Hart *et al.*, 1982a
Rat[7]	1500	oral	54.6	21.7	Hart *et al.*, 1982a
Rat	300	oral	42.8	43.0	Hart *et al.*, 1982a
Rat	750	oral	45.0	33.5	Hart *et al.*, 1982a
Rat	2250	oral	55.4	17.1	Hart *et al.*, 1982a
Rat	3000	oral	53.4	19.8	Hart *et al.*, 1982a
Rat	300	ip	45.7	39.3	Hart *et al.*, 1982a
Rat[7,24]	750	oral	54.6	26.5	Hart *et al.*, 1982a
Rat[7,24]	1500	oral	59.9	16.1	Hart *et al.*, 1982a
Rat[7,24]	2250	oral	59.3	12.1	Hart *et al.*, 1982a
Rat	20	ip	13.7	81.0	Price and Jollow, 1982
Rat	200	ip	32.2	57.7	Price and Jollow, 1982
Rat	600	ip	57.5	26.4	Price and Jollow, 1982

(cont.)

Table 6.1 (*cont.*)

Species	Dose (mg kg^{-1})	Route	% excreted as glucuronide conjugate	% excreted as sulphate conjugate	Reference
Rat	100	iv	9.2	70.6	Siegers *et al.*, 1983b
Rat	15	iv	14.6	77.1	Lin and Levy, 1983b
Rat	800	ip	55.7	25.8	Price and Jollow, 1983
Rat[23]	1000	oral	27.9	37.2	Raheja *et al.*, 1983b
Rat[7]	1000	oral	43.6	22.0	Raheja *et al.*, 1983b
Rat	10	iv	5.8	89.3	Watari *et al.*, 1983
Rat	20	iv	4.6	86.9	Watari *et al.*, 1983
Rat	40	iv	6.2	86.2	Watari *et al.*, 1983
Rat	80	iv	14.3	80.4	Watari *et al.*, 1983
Rat	160	iv	24.2	43.1	Watari *et al.*, 1983
Rat	320	iv	24.5	34.8	Watari *et al.*, 1983
Rat	50	icd	6.4	71.0	Griffeth *et al.*, 1985
Rat	37.5	iv	17.0	67.0	Hjelle and Klaassen, 1984
Rat	600	iv	12.3	6.6	Hjelle and Klaassen, 1984
Rat	68	id	4.5	62.1	Watari *et al.*, 1984
Rat	68	iileal	10.8	51.4	Watari *et al.*, 1984
Rat	68	icaecal	6.4	52.0	Watari *et al.*, 1984
Rat	100	iv	12.3	70.1	Jung, 1985
Rat[25]	100	iv	34.6	41.0	Jung, 1985
Rat	4250	oral	26.9	11.7	Poulsen *et al.*, 1985b
Rat	1000	oral	28.9	47.0	Raheja *et al.*, 1985
Rat	100	oral	10.0	52.8	Colin *et al.*, 1986a
Rat	100	ip	14.8	76.8	Colin *et al.*, 1986a
Rat	750	oral	14.4	35.8	Colin *et al.*, 1986a
Rat	750	ip	29.0	19.4	Colin *et al.*, 1986a
Rat	300	iv	37.6	45.3	Dills and Klaassen, 1986
Rat	300	iv	16.5	31.9	Galinsky and Corcoran, 1986
Rat	30	iv	19.4	69.1	Galinsky *et al.*, 1986
Rat	600	ip	52.4	29.1	Price and Jollow, 1986
Rat	300	iv	33.3	31.1	Wong *et al.*, 1986b
Rat[26]	300	iv	30.7	30.3	Wong *et al.*, 1986b
Rat[27]	300	iv	35.6	33.0	Wong *et al.*, 1986b
Rat	710	ip	20.2	15.8	Corcoran and Wong, 1987
Rat[26]	710	ip	21.7	8.5	Corcoran and Wong, 1987
Rat[27]	710	ip	20.1	3.9	Corcoran and Wong, 1987
Rat	287	ip	30.5	47.6	Corcoran *et al.*, 1987c
Rat	30	iv	13.4	82.2	Galinsky *et al.*, 1987a
Rat	100	iv	7.9	60.4	Zafar *et al.*, 1987
Rat	30	iv	7.4	76.1	Galinsky and Chalasinka, 1988
Rat	30	iv	2.7	80.8	Galinsky and Corcoran, 1988
Rat	150	iv	20.3	60.6	Galinsky and Corcoran, 1988
Rat	150	iv	34.5	47.7	Gregus *et al.*, 1988b
Rat	30	iv	20.5	66.8	Kane *et al.*, 1989
Rat[28]	700	ip	74.3	18.0	Price and Jollow, 1989a
Rat[29]	700	ip	65.3	18.8	Price and Jollow, 1989a
Rat	150	iv	18.3	71.6	Svensson and Chong, 1989
Rat	250	ip	19.5	57.9	Tarloff *et al.*, 1989a
Rat	1000	ip	59.0	21.5	Tarloff *et al.*, 1989a
Rat	250	ip	27.7	48.4	Tarloff *et al.*, 1989a
Rat	1000	ip	49.7	19.2	Tarloff *et al.*, 1989a
Rat[30]	150	iv	40.3	54.4	Galinsky *et al.*, 1990
Rat	150	iv	46.8	45.5	Galinsky *et al.*, 1990

Table 6.1 *(cont.)*

Species	Dose (mg kg⁻¹)	Route	% excreted as glucuronide conjugate	% excreted as sulphate conjugate	Reference
Rat[13]	150	iv	45.8	45.8	Galinsky *et al.*, 1990
Rat	150	iv	24.5	68.0	Gregus *et al.*, 1990
Rat	30	iv	1.8	77.1	Shrewsbury and White, 1990
Rat	50	iv	4.5	95.1	Tone *et al.*, 1990
Rat	50	oral	5.4	93.8	Tone *et al.*, 1990
Rat	50	id	7.0	92.3	Tone *et al.*, 1990
Rat	200	iv	5.9	92.8	Tone *et al.*, 1990
Rat	200	id	11.5	87.9	Tone *et al.*, 1990
Rat[23]	15	ip	4.8	91.4	Kane *et al.*, 1991
Rat[23]	125	ip	17.5	67.6	Kane *et al.*, 1991
Rat[23]	300	ip	24.9	41.7	Kane *et al.*, 1991
Rat[7]	15	ip	16.4	74.9	Kane *et al.*, 1991
Rat[7]	125	ip	32.2	50.3	Kane *et al.*, 1991
Rat[7]	300	ip	45.1	27.7	Kane *et al.*, 1991
Rat	150	iv	17.6	60.3	Manning *et al.*, 1991
Rat[30]	150	iv	18.0	48.4	Galinsky *et al.*, 1992
Rat[13]	150	iv	31.9	35.1	Galinsky *et al.*, 1992
Rat	50	iv	15.9	79.9	Watkins and Sherman, 1992
Rat	100	iv	9.9	48.3	Brouwer, 1993
Rat[31]	30	iv	13.3	58.3	Chaudhary *et al.*, 1993
Rat[32]	30	iv	19.4	59.0	Chaudhary *et al.*, 1993
Rat	50	iv	32.5	43.3	Ismail *et al.*, 1994
Rat	100	iv	15.0	67.8	Jang *et al.*, 1994
Hamster	50	ip	39.8	38.0	Jollow *et al.*, 1974
Hamster	150	oral	40.0	25.0	Wong *et al.*, 1976b
Hamster	150	ip	40.0	20.0	Wong *et al.*, 1976b
Hamster	200	ip	52.4	15.6	Miller and Jollow, 1984
Hamster	150	iv	45.3	20.2	Gregus *et al.*, 1988b
Guinea pig[1]	125	oral	74.5	4.2	Smith and Timbrell, 1974
Guinea pig	150	oral	90.0	6.0	Whitehouse *et al.*, 1975
Guinea pig	100	oral	89.0	7.0	Hidvegi and Ecobichon, 1986
Guinea pig	150	iv	90.2	7.0	Gregus *et al.*, 1988b
Rabbit	23	oral	86.0	7.0	Davison *et al.*, 1977
Rabbit[33]	23	oral	77.0	13.0	Davison *et al.*, 1977
Rabbit	150	iv	76.6	16.3	Gregus *et al.*, 1988b
Ferret[1]	125	oral	25.0	10.0	Smith and Timbrell, 1974
Cat	20	oral	1.3	92.0	Savides *et al.*, 1984, 1985
Cat	60	oral	4.9	78.3	Savides *et al.*, 1984, 1985
Cat	120	oral	16.1	57.0	Savides *et al.*, 1984, 1985
Dog	100	oral	76.4	17.3	Savides *et al.*, 1984
Dog	500	oral	75.0	10.4	Savides *et al.*, 1984
Pony	10*	iv	60.6	37.3	Greenblatt and Engelking, 1988
Sheep	15	iv	64.0	30.0	Wang *et al.*, 1990
Sheep[33]	15	iv	46.0	40.0	Wang *et al.*, 1990

(cont.)

Notes to Table 6.1 *(cont.)*

Dose in man based on body weight of 70 kg; * = estimated dose; id = intraduodenal; iileal = intraileal; icaecal = intracaecal; ip = intraperitoneal; iv = intravenous; icd = intracardiac.

[1] given as phenacetin; [2] overdose, moderate liver damage; [3] overdose, severe liver damage; [4] mild chronic liver disease; [5] severe chronic liver disease; [6] overdose, no liver damage; [7] female; [8] chronic alcoholics; [9] Ghanaians; [10] Kenyans; [11] Gilbert's disease; [12] patients with bladder cancer; [13] elderly; [14] N-acetylcysteine given; [15] liver transplant patients; [16] fit; [17] frail; [18] Chinese; [19] Indian; [20] Oriental; [21] pregnant; [22] methionine-deficient diet; [23] male; [24] weanling; [25] protein deficiency; [26] energy-dense diet – lean; [27] energy-dense diet – obese; [28] fed; [29] fasted; [30] young; [31] lean Zucker; [32] obese Zucker; [33] neonatal.

mixed function oxidase was established by Mitchell and his colleagues more than 20 years ago. The covalent binding of paracetamol to cellular constituents and its toxicity were increased when the activity of these enzymes was stimulated by prior treatment with inducing agents such as phenobarbitone and 3-methylcholanthrene, and decreased when their activity was reduced by inhibitors such as cobaltous chloride and piperonyl butoxide (Mitchell *et al.*, 1973b; Potter *et al.*, 1973). Hepatic reduced glutathione was shown to play a crucial protective role by rapid preferential conjugation with the reactive metabolite to prevent covalent binding and tissue arylation (Jollow *et al.*, 1973; Mitchell *et al.*, 1973c; Potter *et al.*, 1974). The metabolic activation of paracetamol and other drugs was increasingly recognized as an important cause of liver toxicity (Mitchell *et al.*, 1973a, 1974; Mitchell, 1975a,b).

The toxic metabolite of paracetamol is widely accepted to be N-acetyl-p-benzoquinoneimine but its precise mode of formation and the mechanisms of toxicity are uncertain (Calder *et al.*, 1974; Mitchell *et al.*, 1974; Gemborys *et al.*, 1978, 1980; Moldéus, 1978; Healey and Calder, 1979; Hinson *et al.*, 1979b, 1981, 1990; Miner and Kissinger, 1979b; Blair *et al.*, 1980; Corcoran *et al.*, 1980; Hinson, 1980; Nelson *et al.*, 1980b; Corcoran and Mitchell, 1981; de Vries, 1981; Nelson, 1982, 1990; Huggett and Blair, 1983a; Savides and Oehme, 1983; Dahlin *et al.*, 1984; Powis *et al.*, 1984; Holme and Jacobsen, 1986; Potter and Hinson, 1986a; Seddon *et al.*, 1987; Tee *et al.*, 1987; Monks and Lau, 1988; Thummel *et al.*, 1988; Andersson *et al.*, 1989; Prasad *et al.*, 1990; Rashed *et al.*, 1990; Holme *et al.*, 1991; Vermeulen *et al.*, 1992; Brent and Rumack, 1993). Initially, by analogy with other hepatotoxins such as bromobenzene, it was thought that the reactive intermediate might be a 2,3- or 3,4-epoxide (Notarianni *et al.*, 1981). There was some support for this theory insofar as an end-product of such a reaction might be 3-hydroxyparacetamol which was a urinary metabolite of paracetamol. However, the generation of an epoxide was excluded by metabolic studies with p-[^{18}O]-paracetamol in which there was no loss of the radiolabel, whereas 50 per cent should have been exchanged during formation of the epoxide (Hinson *et al.*, 1979a, 1980b; Hoffmann *et al.*, 1990). 3-Hydroxyparacetamol seemed to be formed by mechanisms other than direct insertion or epoxidation (Forte *et al.*, 1984) and further proof was provided by Hinson *et al.* (1980b, 1981), who showed that glutathione and ascorbic acid prevented the covalent binding of paracetamol to microsomal protein but had no effect on the formation of 3-hydroxyparacetamol. In addition, the covalent binding of paracetamol was not inhibited by epoxide hydrolase (Steele *et al.*, 1983).

N-hydroxyparacetamol

An alternative route for the formation of the toxic metabolite was N-hydroxylation followed by spontaneous dehydration to yield N-acetyl-p-benzoquinoneimine (Mitchell *et al.*, 1973a; Potter *et al.*, 1973; Davis *et al.*, 1974a; Jollow *et al.*, 1974; Mitchell, 1975b; Hinson *et al.*, 1977; Hinson, 1980; Corcoran and Mitchell, 1981). N-hydroxyparacetamol has been synthesized and it was stable in acid solution but relatively unstable at physiological pH and temperature, forming equimolecular amounts of p-nitrosophenol and paracetamol (Gemborys *et al.*, 1978; Calder *et al.*, 1981a). Under physiological conditions *in vitro* it has a half life of 20–80 min and in the presence of cysteine, N-acetylcysteine and glutathione it formed the corresponding 3-substituted conjugates of paracetamol (Gemborys *et al.*, 1978, 1980; Healey *et al.*, 1978; Healey and Calder, 1979; Corcoran *et al.*, 1980). In aqueous solution above pH 7, N-hydroxyparacetamol rapidly dehydrated to N-acetyl-p-benzoquinoneimine and this reaction was decreased by ascorbic acid and cysteine, which reduced it back to paracetamol (Corcoran *et al.*, 1980).

Exposure of suspensions of isolated rat hepatocytes to N-hydroxyparacetamol for 30 min resulted in depletion of cellular glutathione and cytotoxicity, and this could be inhibited by ascorbic acid, menadione, thiol containing amino acids and glutathione (Holme *et al.*, 1982a,b). N-hydroxyparacetamol also depleted glutathione and caused hepatic and renal necrosis in mice and rats (Healey *et al.*, 1978). It was cytotoxic to renal fibroblasts in culture (Dunn *et al.*, 1987), and it caused a dose-dependent decrease in DNA synthesis in rat kidney cells (Djordjevic *et al.*, 1986). It was more toxic to hamsters than paracetamol and all animals given a dose of 300 mg kg^{-1} intraperitoneally died within 24 h (Gemborys and Mudge, 1981). Genetically determined differences in susceptibility to hepatotoxicity in mice correlated highly with inducible aryl hydrocarbon hydroxylase and acetylarylamine N-hydroxylase activities (Thorgeirsson *et al.*, 1975). Despite these findings, N-hydroxyparacetamol was unlikely to be the precursor of N-acetyl-p-benzoquinoneimine since, although it could be formed from N-hydroxyphenacetin, it was not a metabolite of paracetamol (Hinson *et al.*, 1979b, 1981; Hinson, 1980, 1983; Calder *et al.*, 1981a). A small fraction of a dose of injected N-hydroxyparacetamol survived long enough *in vivo* to be excreted unchanged and in conjugated form (Gemborys and Mudge, 1981), and this kinetic evidence together with the results of trapping studies with a carrier pool of N-hydroxyparacetamol made it an unlikely candidate for the precursor of the arylating metabolite of paracetamol (Hinson *et al.*, 1979b; Nelson *et al.*, 1980b).

One or Two Electron Microsomal Oxidation of Paracetamol?

Evidence for and against the formation of labile epoxy and N-hydroxy intermediates has been reviewed and more recent studies suggested a direct one or two electron oxidation of paracetamol by cytochrome P450 to give N-acetyl-p-benzo-semiquinoneimine or the corresponding benzoquinoneimine (Vermeulen *et al.*, 1992). A mechanism involving electron transfer and production of the more reactive semiquinone radical was proposed (de Vries, 1981), and a series of reactions, possibly coupled with the formation of catechol metabolites via a phenoxyl radical, was supported by nuclear magnetic resonance relaxation measurements and the selectivity of different isoenzymes of cytochrome P450 (van de Straat *et al.*, 1987a; Harvison *et al.*, 1988b; Koymans *et al.*, 1989; Nelson, 1990). N-acetyl-p-benzoquinoneimine and its 3,5-dimethyl analogue were converted by liver microsomes and NADPH to the corresponding 4-aminophenoxyl free radicals, and the final reaction products were purple indophenols (Fischer *et al.*, 1985c). The one electron oxidation of paracetamol by mixed function oxidase would generate hydrogen peroxide and a phenoxy radical (de Vries, 1981; Rosen *et al.*, 1983; Fischer and Mason, 1984), and the phenoxy radical could donate a free electron to molecular oxygen to form superoxide anion and reactive N-acetyl-p-benzoquinoneimine (Kyle *et al.*, 1987).

Although there was some support for the one electron reduction of the quinoneimine with redox cycling as a mechanism of paracetamol toxicity (van de Straat *et al.*, 1987d), in subsequent studies the N-acetyl-p-benzosemiquinoneimine radical could not be detected by electron spin resonance spectroscopy. There was hardly any conjugation of this postulated intermediate with glutathione and it was concluded that paracetamol was oxidized by a direct two electron transfer (van de Straat *et al.*, 1988b). A scheme involving the two electron oxidation of paracetamol by a cytochrome P450-generated caged oxygen-centred radical species has been proposed by which subsequent reactions could account for the known oxidative metabolites of the drug (Hoffmann *et al.*, 1990). The semiquinoneimine radical of paracetamol formed by one electron oxidation was generated by pulse radiolysis, and the properties of the anion form were consistent with oxidation by thiyl radicals (Bisby *et al.*, 1985; Bisby and Tabassum, 1988). It was proposed that the oxidation of paracetamol by cytochrome P450 proceeded by sequential one electron oxidation steps involving hydrogen abstraction, spin delocalization and radical recombination (Koymans *et al.*, 1993). The possible role of free radicals in the toxicity of paracetamol was reviewed (Brent and Rumack, 1993).

Specificity of Cytochrome P450 Isoenzymes

Highly purified forms of cytochrome P450 had different activities for the metabolic activation of paracetamol (Steele *et al.*, 1983) and it could have different effects on these forms by causing induction or inhibition (Ioannides *et al.*, 1984). Earlier spectral and kinetic studies with mouse liver microsome suspensions had suggested that paracetamol was bound to more than one site on cytochrome P450, or that it was bound to two different forms of the enzyme (Aikawa *et al.*, 1977). Different ethanol-inducible isoenzymes of rabbit cytochrome P450 have been isolated, which also activated paracetamol and resulted in the formation of a glutathione conjugate (Morgan *et al.*, 1983; Coon *et al.*, 1984). It was suggested that the glutathione conjugate of paracetamol and 3-hydroxyparacetamol could be formed from N-acetyl-p-benzoquinoneimine as a common precursor by its reaction with glutathione and water respectively. However, the specificity of the isoenzymes of cytochrome P450 involved in the formation of these metabolites in rats indicated that they arose primarily from different intermediates (Harvison *et al.*, 1988b; Nelson, 1990). Nuclear magnetic resonance relaxation studies indicated that the cytochrome P450 isozyme CYP1A1 produced N-acetyl-p-benzoquinoneimine preferentially while CYP2B1 was responsible for the preferential production of 3-hydroxyparacetamol (Myers, 1994). A number of different isoforms of cytochrome P450 were involved in the activation and covalent binding of paracetamol in rats, and the most active appeared to be CYP3A1 (Harvison *et al.*, 1988b; Prasad *et al.*, 1990; Lee *et al.*, 1991a). Cytochrome CYP2E1 played a major role in the microsomal bioactivation of paracetamol in mice but direct extrapolation to toxicity in the whole animal was not possible (Jeffery *et al.*, 1991). In studies with different inducing agents in mice, it was shown that CYP2E1 was important for the metabolic activation of paracetamol at low doses while CYP1A2 was more active at higher toxic doses (Snawder *et al.*, 1994b). In another study, CYP2E1 accounted for about 50 per cent of the activity in the metabolic activation of paracetamol in mouse liver and kidney. There was a correlation between the localization of CYP2E1 in the proximal renal tubules and acute tubular necrosis produced by very large doses of paracetamol. It was concluded that CYP2E1 played an important role in the metabolic activation of paracetamol in mice and that it was a key factor in renal toxicity in this species (Hu *et al.*, 1993a). In trout liver, CYP1A1 was involved in the metabolic activation of paracetamol (Miller *et al.*, 1993c).

The zone-specific generation of the toxic intermediate as mediated by the regional expression of ethanol-inducible cytochrome CYP2E1 could possibly account for the characteristic centrilobular distribution of hepatic necrosis produced by paracetamol (Anundi *et al.*, 1993). Ethanol also induced CYP2E1 in man as shown by the activity of this isoform in liver biopsies (Perrot *et al.*, 1989). The 2E1 and 1A2 forms of cytochrome P450 were said to account for most of the metabolic activation of paracetamol by human liver microsomes at the extraordinarily high concentration of 1500 mg l^{-1} (Raucy *et al.*, 1989), but at lower realistic and therapeutically relevant concentrations, CYP3A4 (the major isoform of P450 in human liver and enterocytes) contributed appreciably to the production of the cytotoxic metabolite (Thummel *et al.*, 1993). The stimulatory and inhibitory effects of different flavonoids on the oxidation of paracetamol by human liver microsomes were related to the activities of CYP1A2, CYP2E1 and CYP3A4 (Li *et al.*, 1994c). It had been thought that omeprazole might potentiate the hepatotoxicity of paracetamol in man through induction of CYP1A2, but this concern was without foundation (Petersen, 1993; Xiaodong *et al.*, 1994). In another report, the cytochrome P450 dependent metabolism of paracetamol was investigated in four human transgenic lymphoblastoid cell lines that expressed the major isozyme activities (Snawder *et al.*, 1994a). In studies with human Hep G2 cells, cytochromes CYP2E1, 1A2 and 3A4 showed substantial activity towards paracetamol (Patten *et al.*, 1993). The multiple isoenzymes of cytochrome P450 involved in the oxidation of paracetamol included CYP1A1, 1A2, 2A1, 2B1, 2C11, 2C12, 2E1, 3A1, 3A2, and 3A4 (Harvison *et al.*, 1988b; Lee *et al.*, 1991a; Miller *et al.*, 1993c) but because of species differences in the expression, activity and inducibility of these isoenzymes, and the effects of dose, extrapolation from the results of studies in animals to real life conditions in man was not possible.

Oxidation of Paracetamol by Peroxidases

In the presence of hydrogen peroxide, paracetamol was converted by horseradish peroxidase to a reactive phenoxyl radical intermediate that had properties similar to the metabolites formed in microsomal incubations. It was bound covalently to mouse liver microsomal protein and albumin, and binding was inhibited by ascorbic acid and catalase but not by superoxide dismutase (Nelson *et al.*, 1981a). Paraceta-mol was converted by peroxidases to the intermediate free radical N-acetyl-4-aminophenoxyl, which was very reactive and formed dimers and ultimately melanin-like polymers (Fischer *et al.*, 1985b; Mason and Fischer, 1986). Glutathione reacted with the products of the oxidation of paracetamol by horseradish peroxidase to reduce the formation of polymers but only minor amounts of the glutathione conju-gate were formed (Potter and Hinson, 1986b). Some of the products were fluores-cent, and they probably resulted from free radical termination reactions (Potter *et al.*, 1985; McCormick and Shihabi, 1990). The generation of a short-lived phenoxyl radical by the oxidation of paracetamol by horseradish peroxidase and lacto-peroxidase was shown by electron spin resonance spectroscopy (West *et al.*, 1984; Fischer *et al.*, 1986), and polymerization was inhibited by reduced glutathione and ascorbic acid, which regenerated the parent compound. 3,5-Dimethylparacetamol formed a more stable phenoxyl radical and this did not form polymers or bind to nucleophiles (Fischer and Mason, 1984; Mason and Fischer, 1986). The oxidation of paracetamol by horseradish peroxidase in the presence of glutathione involved further complex reactions with the glutathionyl radical (Ross and Moldéus, 1985). Glutathione reduced the phenoxy radical to regenerate paracetamol and form its thiyl radical, and the ascorbyl radical was formed similarly in the presence of ascorbate. With ascorbate there was complete reduction of the free radical of para-cetamol (Ramakrishna Rao *et al.*, 1990).

The phenoxyl radical undergoes a rapid electron transfer reaction with NADPH and the NADH formed reacted with oxygen to give superoxide (Keller and Hinson, 1991). Peroxidase probably catalyzed the one electron oxidation of paracetamol to N-acetyl-p-benzosemiquinoneimine (Potter *et al.*, 1986; Potter and Hinson, 1986b, 1987a; Ramakrishna Rao *et al.*, 1990) and reaction thermodynamics calculated for an oxene model for cytochrome P450 indicated the likelihood of the formation of N-acetyl-p-benzoquinoneimine by a peroxidase-like mechanism via radical interme-diates (Loew and Goldblum, 1985). Incubation of paracetamol with horseradish per-oxidase and hydrogen peroxide generated at least three electronically excited species that emitted light (Schmitt and Cilento, 1990). The oxidation of paracetamol by xanthine oxidase in the presence of xanthine also gave rise to polymers and the reaction probably involved a peroxyflavin intermediate (van Steveninck *et al.*, 1989). Highly substituted immunogenic conjugates of paracetamol have been generated with keyhole limpet haemocyanin and bovine serum albumin using horseradish per-oxidase (Chesham and Davies, 1985). Stimulation of the respiratory burst of neu-trophils resulted in the bioactivation and covalent binding of paracetamol to DNA and RNA. Simultaneous labelling with [ring-^{14}C]- and [^{14}C = O]-paracetamol showed binding of the intact drug to DNA but about 50 per cent excess binding of the ring- relative to the carbonyl-labelled form. A significant role for myelo-peroxidase was proposed with one electron oxidation of paracetamol to the phe-noxyl radical (Corbett *et al.*, 1989, 1992). Paracetamol stimulated the chlorinating activity of myeloperoxidase (Marquez and Dunford, 1993) and it was toxic to iso-lated hepatocytes in the presence of myeloperoxidase and bromide ions (O'Brien *et al.*, 1991; Hofstra and Uetrecht, 1993). The oxidation and peroxidation of paraceta-mol, together with the reactions of its intermediates have been reviewed by Potter and Hinson (1989). Horseradish peroxidase catalyzed the one electron oxidation of p-aminophenol, and in the presence of glutathione it formed the corresponding con-jugate (Eyanagi *et al.*, 1991). Paracetamol has been used as a model substrate for biomimetic oxidation reactions using metalloporphyrins with monopersulphate systems acting as catalysts to produce quinoneimines by mimicking the actions of horseradish peroxidase (Bernadou *et al.*, 1991; Vidal *et al.*, 1993).

Prostaglandins and Paracetamol Metabolism in the Kidney

Paracetamol was also subject to metabolic activation in the kidney as shown by studies of its covalent binding and the production of the cysteine and mercapturic acid conjugates (Joshi *et al.*, 1978; Mudge *et al.*, 1978; Jones *et al.*, 1979; Hart *et al.*, 1980; Newton *et al.*, 1982a,b, 1983b). Although there was significant mixed-function oxidase activity in the renal cortex and outer medulla, none was detected in the inner medulla and other mechanisms must be involved in toxicity at this site (Zenser and Davis, 1984). Paracetamol could be metabolized by renal cortical microsomes to an arylating metabolite by the same biochemical mechanism as in the liver (Mitchell *et al.*, 1977; McMurtry *et al.*, 1978; Newton *et al.*, 1983a) but its metabolic activation could also be catalyzed by prostaglandin synthetase and this might be relevant to nephrotoxicity. Moldéus and Rahimtula (1980) showed that microsomes from sheep seminal vesicles rapidly formed the glutathione conjugate of paracetamol when incubated with it in the presence of arachidonic acid, and that the reaction was inhibited by indomethacin. Subsequent studies showed that a similar process occurred in the kidney (Boyd and Eling, 1981), and that whereas the reaction with cytochrome P450 occurred mostly in the renal cortex, the prostaglandin endoperoxide synthetase-dependent cooxygenation of paracetamol took place primarily in the inner medulla (Mohandas *et al.*, 1981b; Zenser and Davis, 1984; Larsson *et al.*, 1985). Glutathione and ascorbic acid inhibited the covalent binding of paracetamol to rabbit renal proteins following its oxidation by both pathways, but only arachidonic acid-dependent cooxidation was inhibited by indomethacin and aspirin (Mohandas *et al.*, 1981a). The activation of paracetamol by prostaglandin synthetase was very rapid, and probably involved a radical species. The reactive intermediate seemed to be the same as that formed via cytochrome P450 since the glutathione conjugates were apparently identical (Moldéus *et al.*, 1982a). The mechanism of oxidation of paracetamol by prostaglandin synthetase probably involved common intermediate enzyme forms for cyclooxygenase- and hydroperoxidase-catalyzed reactions with the production of a free radical (Harvison *et al.*, 1986a). At least one of the intermediate complexes was reduced by low concentrations of the drug and stimulated prostaglandin synthetase while another was reduced with high paracetamol concentrations and inhibited the enzyme (Harvison *et al.*, 1988a). Prostaglandin H synthase probably catalyzed both the one and two electron oxidation of paracetamol leading to polymerization, and in the presence of glutathione, to formation of the corresponding conjugate (Potter and Hinson, 1987b, 1989). Other investigators have favoured a one electron mechanism for the oxidation of paracetamol by horseradish peroxidase and prostaglandin synthase with production of thiyl radicals in the presence of cysteine or N-acetylcysteine (Ross *et al.*, 1984). Aspirin did not inhibit the hydroperoxidase component of prostaglandin endoperoxide synthetase if peroxide cosubstrates were available, and the renal cooxidation of paracetamol could proceed in its presence (Zenser *et al.*, 1983; Zenser and Davis, 1984). The structure-activity relationships for substrates for the cooxidation of arachidonic acid by peroxidase have been reported (Lehmann *et al.*,

1989) and the oxidation of paracetamol by prostaglandin H synthase has been reviewed (Eling *et al.*, 1990).

Paracetamol Analogues

N-acetyl-m-aminophenol (3-hydroxyacetanilide) is a non-hepatotoxic positional isomer of paracetamol that was bound covalently to tissue proteins to a greater extent and was also converted to quinone and hydroquinone metabolites. However, despite this extensive binding, it was less potent in depleting glutathione and less cytotoxic than paracetamol (Nelson, 1980; Streeter *et al.*, 1984a; Streeter and Baillie, 1985; Rashed *et al.*, 1990; Roberts *et al.*, 1990; Tirmenstein and Nelson, 1990; Holme *et al.*, 1991). 3-Hydroxyacetanilide also formed glutathione conjugates analogous to those derived from paracetamol (Rashed and Nelson, 1989a). Unlike 3-hydroxyacetanilide, paracetamol was bound strongly to mitochondrial proteins and it reduced plasma membrane calcium ATPase activity (Tirmenstein and Nelson, 1989). Both parent compounds were less active in inhibiting NADH-linked respiration than their respective quinone derivatives (Ramsay *et al.*, 1989). A dissociation between the covalent binding and cytotoxicity of paracetamol has been noted by other investigators (Gerson *et al.*, 1985; Brady *et al.*, 1991). Thus, agents that reduced paracetamol hepatotoxicity could have little effect on covalent binding (Labadarios *et al.*, 1977; Devalia *et al.*, 1982; Devalia and McLean, 1983), and although the alkylating agent 1,3-bis-(2-chloroethyl)-N-nitrosourea (carmustine, BCNU) inhibited glutathione reductase and potentiated the hepatotoxicity of N-acetyl-p-benzoquinoneimine (Nakae *et al.*, 1988), there was no corresponding increase in covalent binding. Conversely, dithiothreitol protected against toxicity but did not change the extent of binding (Albano *et al.*, 1985). The administration of piperonyl butoxide as late as 2 h after a hepatotoxic dose of paracetamol reduced the severity of liver damage and selective protein arylation, but did not change the total covalent binding (Brady *et al.*, 1991). Similar dissociation between covalent binding and toxicity was observed in studies with dimethyl derivatives of paracetamol (Fernando *et al.*, 1980; Rosen *et al.*, 1984; Fischer *et al.*, 1985c). 3-Monoalkyl substituted paracetamol derivatives were hepatotoxic and the quinoneimine intermediates conjugated with glutathione and also oxidized it to the disulphide. In contrast, the 3,5-dialkyl- substituents were less hepatotoxic, and oxidized glutathione without forming conjugates (van de Straat *et al.*, 1986, 1987a,c). 3,5-Dimethyl-N-acetylbenzoquinoneimine only oxidized thiols and did not bind covalently to hepatocyte protein, but its cytotoxicity was enhanced by pretreatment with BCNU (Rundgren *et al.*, 1988; Andersson *et al.*, 1989). It produced cytotoxicity with the typical blebbing of isolated hepatocytes caused by oxidation of protein thiols, and this was reversed by dithiothreitol (Rundgren *et al.*, 1990). The quinoneimines produced by the oxidation of paracetamol and its 3,5-dimethyl- and 2,6-dimethyl analogues were rapidly reduced to their corresponding semiquinoneimines by NADPH-cytochrome P450 reductase. Glutathione was an excellent nucleophile for the 2,6-dimethylbenzoquinoneimine, but it acted as a one electron reductant with the corresponding 3,5-dimethyl compound. Glutathione acted as both a nucleophile and a reductant with N-acetyl-p-benzoquinoneimine (Rosen *et al.*, 1984). The oxidative and arylating actions of paracetamol could be dissociated in comparative studies with 3,5- and 2,6-dimethylparacetamol (Porubek *et al.*, 1987), and the appearance of high molecular weight protein aggregates that were not linked by disulphide were thought to represent the oxidative properties of these compounds (Birge *et al.*, 1988). In mice and rats, 3,5-dimethylparacetamol showed similar hepatotoxicity but the 2,6-dimethyl isomer produced very little histological evidence of tissue damage (Fernando *et al.*, 1980). N-acetyl-p-benzoquinoncimine could bind covalently to thiols and oxidize thiols while the 2,6-dimethyl and 3,5-dimethyl derivatives bound primarily to thiols and oxidized thiols respectively. The former decreased protein thiols most and inhibited hepatocyte plasma membrane Ca^{2+}-ATPase to the greatest extent whereas the latter was least active in these respects. Arylation of critical thiols appeared to be the most lethal reaction (Nicotera *et al.*, 1989). The arylation and oxidation of thiols, especially in proteins involved with energy metabolism (e.g. ATP and NADPH production), and calcium homeostasis, were early events in damage to hepatocytes exposed to N-acetyl-p-benzoquinoneimine and the dimethyl analogues (Andersson *et al.*, 1989). Of the three monomethylated analogues of paracetamol only 4-hydroxy-N-methylacetanilide was devoid of cytotoxicity in mice, and apart from not being oxidized to a toxic intermediate, its disposition was similar to that of paracetamol. The analgesic activity of the monomethyl compounds parallelled their hepatotoxic potential and both activities parallelled their oxidation potentials (Harvison *et al.*, 1986b). Metabolic alterations caused by aromatic fluorine substitution also modified the toxicity of paracetamol (Barnard *et al.*, 1993b). Introduction at the 2- and 6- positions increased the oxidation potential and this reduced the propensity for oxidative bioactivation and toxicity (Barnard *et al.*, 1993a).

Reactions and Covalent Binding of N-acetyl-p-benzoquinoneimine

N-acetyl-p-benzoquinoneimine has been detected as a direct product of the oxidation of paracetamol formed by incubation with cytochrome P450, NADPH, and NADPH-cytochrome P450 reductase supported by cumene hydroperoxide. It appeared to be a major metabolite of paracetamol but was largely reduced back to the parent compound and was covalently bound to mouse liver microsomal protein with loss of about 20 per cent of the acetyl group as acetamide (Dahlin *et al.*, 1984). In rat and mouse liver microsomes, NADH synergistically enhanced the glutathione conjugation of paracetamol, and this reaction was inhibited by cyanide (Sato and Marumo, 1991). The chemical and electrochemical synthesis of N-acetyl-p-benzoquinoneimine has been described, and it could function both as an oxidizing agent and as an electrophile (Miner and Kissinger, 1979b; Blair *et al.*, 1980). It was moderately stable and, depending on conditions, it could react with nucleophiles such as cysteine, N-acetylcysteine and glutathione to yield paracetamol and the corresponding thiol adducts (Miner and Kissinger, 1979b; Blair *et al.*, 1980; Dahlin and Nelson, 1982; Huggett and Blair, 1982, 1983a,b; Dahlin *et al.*, 1984; Powis *et al.*, 1984). It appeared to react primarily with glutathione, and with [^{14}C]-paracetamol gave a mixture of labelled and unlabelled N-acetyl-p-benzosemiquinoneimine, which then formed paracetamol polymers by radical coupling reactions (Potter and Hinson, 1986a). The spontaneous and glutathione transferase-catalyzed reactions of N-acetyl-p-benzoquinoneimine with glutathione were studied by stop-flow kinetics.

Spontaneous reactions over a wide range of concentrations and pH yielded the glutathione conjugate, paracetamol and glutathione disulphide in the proportions 2 : 1 : 1, while the different isoenzymes of glutathione transferase showed different activities towards conjugation and reduction (Coles *et al.*, 1988). N-acetyl-p-benzoquinoneimine was more toxic than paracetamol (Dahlin and Nelson, 1982) and seemed to kill hepatocytes in culture by a different biochemical mechanism that was more characteristic of a mitochondrial poison (Harman *et al.*, 1991). There was a delay of 10–20 min between exposure of isolated rat hepatocytes to N-acetyl-p-benzoquinoneimine and the onset of toxicity as shown by increased membrane permeability (Holme *et al.*, 1984). It was also cytotoxic to bacteria and caused extensive breaks of single strand DNA in hepatoma cells (Dybing *et al.*, 1984).

Covalent Binding of N-acetyl-p-benzoquinoneimine

Hepatic necrosis induced by paracetamol was closely related to the extent of its covalent binding, which in turn depended on the activity of microsomal cytochrome P450 (Mitchell *et al.*, 1973b; Potter *et al.*, 1973). The reactive metabolite formed *in vivo* and *in vitro*, and synthetic N-acetyl-p-benzoquinoneimine could react with nucleophiles to produce the corresponding adducts and with glutathione the intermediate was rapidly reduced back to paracetamol with formation of the glutathione conjugate. The covalent binding to proteins was inhibited typically by glutathione, other low molecular weight thiols and ascorbic acid (Moldéus, 1978; Buckpitt *et al.*, 1979; Blair *et al.*, 1980; Corcoran *et al.*, 1980; Gemborys *et al.*, 1980; Moldéus and Rahimtula, 1980; Mohandas *et al.*, 1981a; Nelson *et al.*, 1981a; Moldéus *et al.*, 1982a; Huggett and Blair, 1983a; Dahlin *et al.*, 1984; Streeter *et al.*, 1984b; Potter and Hinson, 1986a; Potter *et al.*, 1986; van de Straat *et al.*, 1986, 1988b; Kitteringham *et al.*, 1988). However, in some studies, ascorbic acid has been found not to reduce covalent binding or to protect against hepatotoxicity, and there was no evidence that it reduced the reactive metabolite back to paracetamol (Miller and Jollow, 1984). The major adduct released by the acid hydrolysis of hepatic proteins and bovine serum albumin after exposure to paracetamol was identified as the 3-cysteine conjugate of p-aminophenol, and cysteine residues represented the primary target sites for arylation by the reactive metabolite of paracetamol (Hoffmann *et al.*, 1985a,b). Bovine serum albumin contains one free sulphydryl group per molecule, and it inhibited the covalent binding of the reactive metabolite of paracetamol in a concentration-dependent manner (Streeter *et al.*, 1984b). The conjugation with glutathione (but not other thiols such as cysteine and N-acetylcysteine) was catalyzed by glutathione S-transferases in liver cytosol (Rollins and Buckpitt, 1979). Glutathione reduced the paracetamol phenoxyl radical formed by its oxidation by peroxidase with the regeneration of paracetamol and production of the thiyl radical of glutathione (Ramakrishna Rao *et al.*, 1990). A hepatotoxic dose of paracetamol produced a loss of protein thiols in the liver of mice, and this was probably due to their oxidation (Tirmenstein and Nelson, 1990). Although this depletion of soluble and protein-bound thiols was probably the primary mechanism of the cytotoxicity of N-acetyl-p-benzoquinoneimine (Moore *et al.*, 1985a), marked depletion of protein thiols could occur in the absence of lethal injury to hepatocytes (Kyle *et al.*, 1990).

Target Proteins

The covalent binding of paracetamol to mouse liver proteins *in vivo* was highly selective as shown by immunochemical studies of the centrilobular localization and nature of the binding. Western blot profiles of subcellular fractions indicated that binding was largely restricted to proteins in the 42–44 and 56–58 kD bands (Bartolone *et al.*, 1987; Birge *et al.*, 1991c). In mice, the 58 kD protein was rather evenly distributed whereas cytochrome P450 and the sites of binding of paracetamol were localized to the target cells for toxicity in hepatic, renal and bronchiolar tissue (Emeigh Hart *et al.*, 1990). A different profile of binding was observed when extracts or cells were treated with synthetic N-acetyl-p-benzoquinoneimine, and there was no arylation of the 44 kD protein (Bartolone *et al.*, 1988). The specificity and extent of this selective covalent binding was probably relevant to toxicity because although the binding of the cytotoxic analogue 2,6-dimethylparacetamol to the 44 kD protein was minimal, the 58 kD cytosolic protein was a prominent target (Birge *et al.*, 1989). It was subsequently shown that the same 58 kD protein which was selectively arylated by paracetamol could also be modified by glutathiolation under oxidative conditions (Birge *et al.*, 1991a). Studies with a sensitive immunofluorescence assay and affinity-purified anti-paracetamol antibodies in mice revealed preferential localization of covalent binding to centrilobular regions (Bartolone *et al.*, 1989b). Incubation of cytosolic proteins from mouse liver, lung, kidney, spleen, brain and heart with a paracetamol metabolite generating liver microsomal preparation showed that the cytosolic 58 kD protein was present in all the tissues, but the corresponding paracetamol-protein adducts were only detected in tissues that had been damaged by the drug (Bartolone *et al.*, 1989a). The 44 kD protein was the earliest detectable protein targeted by paracetamol in mouse liver, and 30 min after dosing it was primarily localized in the microsomal fraction (Birge *et al.*, 1991c). The 58 kD paracetamol-binding protein consisted of a cluster of four immunochemically reactive isoforms, and amino acid analysis of the purified protein revealed only eight cysteine residues, raising the possibility of the toxic binding of paracetamol to non-thiol sites on the protein (Bartolone *et al.*, 1992). Electrophoretic analysis of [^{35}S]-labelled proteins following exposure of cultured mouse hepatocytes to toxic concentrations of paracetamol and 3,5-dimethylparacetamol (but not 2,6-dimethylparacetamol) showed progressively decreased synthesis of a 58 kD protein and relatively increased biosynthesis of a 32 kD protein. These effects were attributed to the oxidative properties of the paracetamol and the 3,5-dimethyl derivative (Bruno *et al.*, 1992).

Antiserum from rabbits immunized with the mercapturic acid conjugate of paracetamol covalently bound to keyhole-limpet haemocyanin had specificity for the drug bound to thiols and detected very low concentrations bound to proteins in mouse liver microsomes and cytosol (Roberts *et al.*, 1987a; Potter *et al.*, 1989). With the use of an enzyme-linked immunosorbent assay that was specific for 3-cysteine-paracetamol adducts, it was possible to demonstrate their dose-dependent formation in liver protein in mice at the higher hepatotoxic doses. The 3-cysteine-paracetamol protein adducts were also detectable in serum and were persistent (Pumford *et al.*, 1989). A superior particle concentration fluorescence immunoassay was developed (Benson *et al.*, 1989) and biochemical and histological evidence of hepatotoxicity was related to the localization of the 3-cysteine-paracetamol protein adducts

(Roberts *et al.*, 1989). The most prominent protein containing the 3-cysteine-paracetamol adduct in cytosolic fractions of mouse liver had a relative molecular mass of 55 kD and in fractions purified from a 960 g pellet the protein adduct was present in greatest amounts in plasma membranes and mitochondria. The 55 kD protein from mouse hepatocytes was isolated and amino acid sequencing showed 97 per cent homology with a mouse liver cDNA encoding for a 56 kD selenium binding protein (Pumford *et al.*, 1992). Isolation of genomic DNA recombinants from the mouse cosmid genomic library showed that the paracetamol binding and selenium binding proteins were encoded by two different genes, and their aminoacid sequences differed by only 14 residues (Lanfear *et al.*, 1993). The 3-cysteine-paracetamol protein adducts appeared to be released into the circulation following lysis of hepatocytes and their formation in the liver was a marker of the hepatotoxicity of paracetamol (Ferguson *et al.*, 1990; Hinson *et al.*, 1990; Pumford *et al.*, 1990a; Ramakrishna Rao *et al.*, 1990). The selective arylation of proteins of the same molecular weight by paracetamol was observed in mouse and human liver hepatocyte cultures, and a sample of liver from a patient who had died from paracetamol poisoning (Birge *et al.*, 1990). With a specific immunohistochemical method for the 3-cysteine-paracetamol protein adduct it was possible to demonstrate distinct lobular localization before the onset of centrilobular necrosis, as well as drug binding in the nucleus and binding to hepatocytes at subtoxic doses before glutathione depletion (Roberts *et al.*, 1991b). In mice, radiolabelled paracetamol was bound covalently in a dose-dependent manner to haemoglobin. Degradation of the modified globin revealed the cysteine conjugate as the major radioactive product, and this was consistent with covalent binding mediated largely by N-acetyl-p-benzoquinoneimine. However, approximately 20 per cent of the N-acetyl side chain was lost, and the demonstration of the dihydroxyphenyl cysteine conjugate in the hydrolysate would be in keeping with some binding of p-benzoquinoneimine to haemoglobin (Axworthy *et al.*, 1988).

Glutathione-derived Metabolites of Paracetamol

N-acetyl-p-benzoquinoneimine reacted directly with glutathione under physiological conditions to form the 3-S-glutathionyl conjugate of paracetamol (Miner and Kissinger, 1979b; Dahlin *et al.*, 1984; Potter and Hinson, 1986a) and it reacted similarly with N-acetylcysteine and other thiols *in vitro* to yield the corresponding conjugates (Miner and Kissinger, 1979b; Blair *et al.*, 1980; Huggett and Blair, 1983a). When paracetamol was incubated with mouse liver microsomes it formed adducts directly with glutathione, cysteine, N-acetylcysteine, cysteamine and α-mercaptopropionylglycine, but not with methionine (Buckpitt *et al.*, 1979). The reaction with glutathione (but not the other thiols) was catalyzed by liver cytosolic glutathione-S-transferase (Rollins and Buckpitt, 1979) and the glutathione conjugate was the primary end-product of the metabolic activation of paracetamol. Its formation by isolated hepatocytes was directly related to the loss of intracellular glutathione (Moldéus, 1978). Cysteine stimulated glutathione production in hepatocytes that had been depleted by prior exposure to diethyl maleate in the presence of toxic concentrations of paracetamol, but it did not increase the production of the glutathione conjugate (Dalhoff and Poulsen, 1993c). Paracetamol had a low affinity for glutathione conjugation, and the process was not saturated even at concentrations as high as 10 to 25 mM (1510–3775 mg l^{-1}) (Moldéus, 1978; Grafström *et al.*, 1979b; Moldéus and Gergely, 1980b; Sweeny and Weiner, 1985). The glutathione conjugate of paracetamol was virtually exclusively excreted into bile (Wong *et al.*, 1979; Pang and Terrell, 1981b; Hinson *et al.*, 1982; Siegers *et al.*, 1984; Poulsen *et al.*, 1985c; Lauterburg and Smith, 1986; Gregus *et al.*, 1988b) and concentrations in other body fluids and tissues other than the liver were usually very low. In mice given a toxic dose of 500 mg kg^{-1} of paracetamol, glutathione conjugate concentrations were initially high in the liver, but subsequently fell reflecting acute depletion of hepatic glutathione. Concentrations of the conjugate were very low in blood, brain, kidney and urine (Fischer *et al.*, 1981). Intestinal cells could metabolize paracetamol to the glutathione conjugate (Grafström *et al.*, 1979a).

In the intestine the glutathione conjugate of paracetamol was rapidly hydrolyzed by γ-glutamyltranspeptidase and dipeptidase to the 3-cysteinyl derivative, which was then reabsorbed and excreted in the urine partly unchanged and partly acetylated as the 3-mercapturic acid conjugate (Mitchell *et al.*, 1974; Grafström *et al.*, 1979b; Wong *et al.*, 1981). The cysteine conjugate eventually became the major component in the gastrointestinal tract (Fischer *et al.*, 1981). It could also be formed in the kidney (Moldéus *et al.*, 1978; Jones *et al.*, 1979; Newton *et al.*, 1986) but the high concentrations found there probably indicated active uptake rather than extensive synthesis *in situ* (Fischer *et al.*, 1981). In animals, the cysteine conjugate of paracetamol could be acetylated in the liver, intestine and especially in the kidney (Moldéus *et al.*, 1978; Healey *et al.*, 1980; Fischer *et al.*, 1981; Newton *et al.*, 1986), and the latter was probably an important site of formation of the mercapturic acid conjugate in man (Prescott *et al.*, 1989b). The cysteine and mercapturic acid conjugates of paracetamol in urine were derived almost exclusively from the glutathione conjugate excreted into the bile as they largely disappeared from the urine when the bile duct was cannulated (Wong *et al.*, 1981; Fischer *et al.*, 1985a) and only very small amounts of these conjugates were found in the bile (Grafström *et al.*, 1979b; Glazenburg *et al.*, 1983; Siegers *et al.*, 1983b, 1984; Corcoran *et al.*, 1985b; Colin *et al.*, 1986a; Jayasinghe *et al.*, 1986; Gregus *et al.*, 1988b, 1990; Madhu *et al.*, 1989; Hoffmann *et al.*, 1990; Madhu and Klaassen, 1991). However, the urinary excretion of the cysteine and mercapturic acid conjugates was not altered by bile duct ligation, and biliary excretion was not obligatory for the appearance of these conjugates in the urine (Fischer *et al.*, 1985a). The cysteine and glutathione conjugates of paracetamol administered intraduodenally and intravenously were recovered almost quantitatively in the urine as the cysteine and mercapturic acid conjugates (Wong *et al.*, 1981; Fischer *et al.*, 1985a). The mercapturic acid conjugate was excreted by the kidney by a probenecid-sensitive transport mechanism in the rat (Newton *et al.*, 1986), and in man its renal clearance considerably exceeded those of the other conjugates of paracetamol (Prescott *et al.*, 1989b). Isolated human fetal liver cells could produce the glutathione conjugate of paracetamol (Rollins *et al.*, 1979), and it was converted by γ-glutamyltranspeptidase in human adult and fetal liver to the cysteine conjugate (Moldéus *et al.*, 1980c). Species differences in the biliary excretion of the glutathione conjugate of paracetamol and its hydrolysis products might be related to differences in hepatic γ-glutamyltranspeptidase activity (Gregus *et al.*, 1988b).

In perfused liver and isolated hepatocyte preparations, there was minor conversion of paracetamol to the cysteine (but not usually the mercapturic acid) conjugate (Moldéus, 1978; Moldéus *et al.*, 1980c; Massey and Racz, 1981; Poulsen *et al.*, 1985c; Harman and McCamish, 1986). In the corresponding kidney preparations, a small fraction of the paracetamol appeared as the mercapturic acid conjugate with or without the cysteine conjugate (Jones *et al.*, 1979; Moldéus *et al.*, 1980a; Hart *et al.*, 1980, 1981; Ross *et al.*, 1980; Emslie *et al.*, 1981a; Newton *et al.*, 1982a). In the isolated perfused rat kidney, the glutathione conjugate of paracetamol was rapidly hydrolyzed to the cysteine conjugate, which was then subject to slower acetylation (Newton *et al.*, 1986). The relative fractional urinary recoveries of the cysteine and mercapturic acid conjugates of paracetamol in different species are summarized in Table 6.2. There was considerable variation, which probably reflected differences in the capacity for acetylation. Thus, the cysteine conjugate was elusive in the rat and hamster, but not in the mouse and man (Hart *et al.*, 1981; Jensen *et al.*, 1986), while dogs were poor acetylators and consequently did not form the mercapturic acid conjugate (Savides *et al.*, 1984). Relatively little mercapturic acid conjugate was produced in mice (Table 6.2) and in some studies it was not detected at all (To and Wells, 1985).

Conditions that increased and decreased the metabolic activation of paracetamol had a corresponding effect on the biliary excretion of its glutathione conjugate (Madhu *et al.*, 1989; Gregus *et al.*, 1990; Mansor *et al.*, 1991). Inhibition of the sulphate and glucuronide conjugation of paracetamol had no effect on glutathione conjugation by isolated hepatocytes or the perfused rat liver (Moldéus *et al.*, 1979; Fayz *et al.*, 1984), and its production was maintained even when sulphate conjugation was depressed and hepatic glutathione depleted to 20 per cent of control values by feeding a diet deficient in methionine and cysteine (Glazenburg *et al.*, 1983). Glutathione conjugation in rats was unexpectedly enhanced after prior depletion of hepatic glutathione with a very large hepatotoxic dose of 4250 mg kg^{-1} of paracetamol (Poulsen *et al.*, 1985c). The biliary and renal excretion of the glutathione-derived conjugates was taken to indicate the extent of the metabolic activation of paracetamol and hence risk of toxicity (Jollow *et al.*, 1974; Mitchell *et al.*, 1974; Siegers *et al.*, 1980; Gemborys and Mudge, 1981; Altomare *et al.*, 1984b; Dolphin *et al.*, 1987; Gregus *et al.*, 1987, 1988b; Madhu *et al.*, 1989). In this respect, species differences in the oxidative metabolism of paracetamol corresponded with differences in susceptibility to hepatotoxicity (Davis *et al.*, 1974a; Jollow *et al.*, 1974; Ioannides *et al.*, 1983b; Savides *et al.*, 1984; Boobis *et al.*, 1986; Seddon *et al.*, 1987; Tee *et al.*, 1987; Miller *et al.*, 1993a). However, the relative capacity of parallel detoxification pathways also had to be taken into account (Green *et al.*, 1984a). Thus, the protective effect of oltipraz against hepatotoxicity in hamsters was due not so much to the expected maintenance of liver glutathione as to increased clearance of paracetamol as a result of augmented glucuronide conjugation (Davies and Schnell, 1991).

Thiomethyl Metabolites

Other minor metabolites of paracetamol derived from the glutathione conjugate included 3-thiomethylparacetamol, its oxidation product paracetamol 3-methylsulphoxide, and their glucuronide and sulphate conjugates. These compounds have been confirmed as minor urinary metabolites of paracetamol in man, dogs, hamsters, rats and mice (Klutch *et al.*, 1978; Gemborys and Mudge, 1981; Hart *et al.*, 1981, 1982a; Nelson *et al.*, 1981b; Newton *et al.*, 1983b; Warrander *et al.*, 1985; Miller and Jollow, 1986a; Price and Jollow, 1986; Dolphin *et al.*, 1987; Price and

Table 6.2 Fractional urinary excretion of the cysteine and mercapturic acid conjugates of paracetamol in different species.

Dose (mg kg[-1])	Route	% excreted as cysteine conjugate	% excreted as mercapturic acid conjugate	% excreted as cysteine and mercapturic acid conjugates combined	Reference
Man					
13–26	oral	–	4.0	–	Mitchell *et al.*, 1974
23	oral	3.3	–	–	Mrochek *et al.*, 1974
10	oral	1.9	1.7	3.6	Coldwell *et al.*, 1976
14	oral	–	–	15.0	Davis *et al.*, 1976b
57	oral	–	–	23.0	Davis *et al.*, 1976b
53[1]	oral	–	–	17.3	Davis *et al.*, 1976b
137[1]	oral	–	–	19.8	Davis *et al.*, 1976b
157[2]	oral	–	–	32.5	Davis *et al.*, 1976b
214[2]	oral	–	–	39.2	Davis *et al.*, 1967b
20	oral	–	–	8.0	Prescott, 1980
150[1]	oral	–	–	6.9	Prescott, 1980
170[2]	oral	–	–	15.2	Prescott, 1980
10	oral	1.6	1.4	3.0	Thomas *et al.*, 1980
20	oral	3.7	4.5	8.2	Prescott *et al.*, 1981
20	oral	3.6	4.9	8.5	Critchley *et al.*, 1983
14[3]	oral	–	–	9.1	Miners *et al.*, 1983
15[4]	oral	–	–	9.5	Miners *et al.*, 1983
22[4]	oral	5.5	5.5	11.0	Mitchell *et al.*, 1983
12	oral	1.9	2.7	4.6	Villeneuve *et al.*, 1983
12[5]	oral	5.5	6.4	11.9	Villeneuve *et al.*, 1983
12[6]	oral	2.2	3.9	6.1	Villeneuve *et al.*, 1983
15	oral	5.0	4.0	9.0	Bales *et al.*, 1984b
20	iv	–	–	11.6	Clements *et al.*, 1984
20	oral	–	–	10.7	Clements *et al.*, 1984
5	iv	–	–	10.8	Clements *et al.*, 1984
5	oral	–	–	11.1	Clements *et al.*, 1984
15	oral			10.7	Miners *et al.*, 1984c
21	oral	4.2	–	–	Pantuck *et al.*, 1984
15	oral	4.1	4.6	8.7	Jayasinghe *et al.*, 1986
15[4]	oral	–	–	9.3	Miners *et al.*, 1986
7	iv	6.9	5.7	12.6	Sonne *et al.*, 1986
15	oral	–	–	5.4	Amouyal *et al.*, 1987
15	oral	–	1.5	–	Galinsky *et al.*, 1987b
22	iv	1.2	1.3	2.5	Kamali *et al.*, 1987b
15	oral	4.3	3.1	7.4	Ladds *et al.*, 1987
7–15	oral	–	–	7.4	Notarianni *et al.*, 1987
7	oral	–	–	8.0[7]	Slattery *et al.*, 1987
42	oral	–	–	6.8[7]	Slattery *et al.*, 1987
15	oral	–	–	7.6	Ullrich *et al.*, 1987
15[8]	oral	–	–	7.8	Ullrich *et al.*, 1987
20[9]	oral	–	–	8.2	Kamali *et al.*, 1988
15	oral	–	–	10.8	Miners *et al.*, 1988
15[10]	oral	–	–	9.4	Miners *et al.*, 1988
15	iv	–	4.8	–	Sonne *et al.*, 1988
15	oral	6.4	4.4	10.8	Thomas *et al.*, 1988
15	iv	6.5	4.5	11.0	Thomas *et al.*, 1988
14	oral	3.0	4.1	7.1	Prescott *et al.*, 1989b
15[11]	oral	3.0	2.7	5.7	Slattery *et al.*, 1989
15[12]	oral	3.2	2.6	5.8	Kietzmann *et al.*, 1990
26	oral	4.0	3.0	7.0	Leung and Critchley, 1991
15	oral	–	–	10.0	Osborne *et al.*, 1991
15[11]	oral	–	–	9.2	Osborne *et al.*, 1991
7.5	iv	–	–	1.6	Poulsen *et al.*, 1991
7.5[6]	iv	–	–	2.0	Poulsen *et al.*, 1991
10	oral	2.4	4.1	6.5	Veronese and McLean, 1991
20	iv	0.9	1.2	2.1	de Morais *et al.*, 1992b

(cont.)

95

Table 6.2 *(cont.)*

Dose (mg kg^{-1})	Route	% excreted as cysteine conjugate	% excreted as mercapturic acid conjugate	% excreted as cysteine and mercapturic acid conjugates combined	Reference
15[13]	oral	2.2	3.8	6.0	Lee *et al.*, 1992
15[14]	oral	2.3	3.6	5.9	Lee *et al.*, 1992
15	oral	–	–	9.0	Miners *et al.*, 1992
10	oral	1.5	1.1	2.6	Patel *et al.*, 1992
10[15]	oral	1.1	0.9	2.0	Patel *et al.*, 1992
20	oral	3.7	3.8	7.5	Esteban and Pérez-Mateo, 1993a
20[16]	oral	2.1	2.5	4.6	Prescott *et al.*, 1993
20[17]	oral	2.3	2.5	4.8	Prescott *et al.*, 1993
20	oral	–	–	7.1	Esteban *et al.*, 1994
Mouse					
50	ip		13.3	–	Jollow *et al.*, 1974
150	oral	25.0	3.0	28.0	Coldwell *et al.*, 1976
250	oral	26.4	2.8	29.2	Whitehouse *et al.*, 1976
250	ip	13.8	2.8	16.6	Whitehouse *et al.*, 1976
150	oral	13.6	1.9	15.5	Whitehouse *et al.*, 1977
250	ip	23.9	4.3	28.1	Wong *et al.*, 1980b
150	oral	18.7	2.2	20.9	Wong *et al.*, 1981
50	oral	23.2	<1	–	Miners *et al.*, 1984a
100	oral	23.1	<1	–	Miners *et al.*, 1984a
200	oral	19.9	<1	–	Miners *et al.*, 1984a
300	oral	17.8	1.1	18.9	Miners *et al.*, 1984a
400	oral	14.8	1.3	15.1	Miners *et al.*, 1984a
200	oral	–	–	18.9	Miners *et al.*, 1984b
350	oral	19.4	1.9	21.4	Whitehouse *et al.*, 1985
1000	oral	10.2	2.9	13.1	Corcoran *et al.*, 1985b
500	oral	17.3	0.8	18.1	Corcoran and Wong, 1986
300	iv	–	2.2	–	Galinsky and Corcoran, 1986
600	ip	16.0	3.0	19.0	Hazelton *et al.*, 1986b
300	ip	18.0	2.3	20.3	Larrey *et al.*, 1986
300[18]	ip	19.0	2.5	21.5	Larrey *et al.*, 1986
600	ip	18.0	0.6	18.6	Letteron *et al.*, 1986
400	oral	17.9	0.5	18.4	Tredger *et al.*, 1986b
100	oral	16.5	1.4	17.9	Dolphin *et al.*, 1987
200	ip	22.5	2.7	25.2	Price and Gale, 1987
300	ip	–	14.0	–	Reicks and Hathcock, 1987
300[19]	ip	–	12.9	–	Reicks and Hathcock, 1987
151	iv	13.9	2.0	15.9	Gregus *et al.*, 1988b
200	ip	20.6	0.4	21.0	Mikov *et al.*, 1988
200	oral	25.0	2.0	27.0	Pascoe *et al.*, 1988
50	ip	–	–	8.3	Adamson *et al.*, 1991
Rat					
50	ip	–	3.6	–	Jollow *et al.*, 1974
150	oral	–	6.3	–	Thomas *et al.*, 1974
495	oral	–	–	14.8	Davis *et al.*, 1976a
1485	oral	–	–	12.3	Davis *et al.*, 1976a
2495	oral	–	–	13.9	Davis *et al.*, 1976a
3503	oral	–	–	21.4	Davis *et al.*, 1976a
150	oral	–	6.2	–	Thomas *et al.*, 1977b
500	oral	–	3.9	–	Siegers *et al.*, 1980
500	ip	–	3.0	–	Sato and Lieber, 1981
500	ip	–	1.9	–	Sato *et al.*, 1981a
300[3]	iv	–	4.1		Hart *et al.*, 1982a
300[4]	iv	–	3.1		Hart *et al.*, 1982a
1500[3]	oral	–	9.7		Hart *et al.*, 1982a
1500[4]	oral	–	5.6		Hart *et al.*, 1982a
300[4]	oral	–	5.6		Hart *et al.*, 1982a

Table 6.2 *(cont.)*

Dose (mg kg^{-1})	Route	% excreted as cysteine conjugate	% excreted as mercapturic acid conjugate	% excreted as cysteine and mercapturic acid conjugates combined	Reference
750[4]	oral	–	5.8		Hart et al., 1982a
1500[4]	oral	–	5.6		Hart et al., 1982a
2250[4]	oral	–	6.5		Hart et al., 1982a
3000[4]	oral	–	6.4		Hart et al., 1982a
300[4]	ip	–	2.8		Hart et al., 1982a
150	iv	–	2.2		Hart et al., 1982a
750[4,20]	oral	–	7.2		Hart et al., 1982a
1500[4,20]	oral	–	5.7		Hart et al., 1982a
2250[4,20]	oral	–	4.9		Hart et al., 1982a
20	ip	–	2.6	–	Price and Jollow, 1982
200	ip	–	3.5	–	Price and Jollow, 1982
600	ip	–	4.0	–	Price and Jollow, 1982
800	ip	–	6.2	–	Price and Jollow, 1983
1000[3]	oral	–	3.0	–	Raheja et al., 1983b
1000[4]	oral	–	3.2	–	Raheja et al., 1983b
100	iv	–	1.3	–	Siegers et al., 1983b
1000	oral	–	3.2	–	Raheja et al., 1985
100	oral	–	4.5	–	Colin et al., 1986a
100	ip	–	5.2	–	Colin et al., 1986a
750	oral	–	5.6	–	Colin et al., 1986a
750	ip	–	6.4	–	Colin et al., 1986a
300	iv	–	–	7.0	Dills and Klaassen, 1986
600	ip	–	7.6	–	Price and Jollow, 1986
600	ip	–	4.7	–	Pricc and Jollow, 1986
300	iv	–	–	5.8	Wong et al., 1986b
300[21]	iv	–	–	5.6	Wong et al., 1986b
300[22]	iv	–	–	6.8	Wong et al., 1986b
710	ip	–	–	2.8	Corcoran and Wong, 1987
710[21]	ip	–	–	2.7	Corcoran and Wong, 1987
710[22]	ip	–	–	2.1	Corcoran and Wong, 1987
151	iv	ND	1.2	1.2	Gregus et al., 1988b
700[23]	ip	–	4.3	–	Price and Jollow, 1989a
700[24]	ip	–	5.8	–	Price and Jollow, 1989a
250	ip	2.8[25]	6.2	9.0	Tarloff et al., 1989a
250	ip	5.3[25]	6.0	11.3	Tarloff et al., 1989a
250	iv	7.5[25]	ND	7.5	Tarloff et al., 1989a
250	iv	1.6[25]	3.0	4.6	Tarloff et al., 1989a
150[26]	iv	–	–	7.4	Galinsky et al., 1990
150	iv	–	–	7.9	Galinsky et al., 1990
150[10]	iv	–	–	8.4	Galinsky et al., 1990
Hamster					
50	ip	–	14.2	–	Jollow et al., 1974
150	oral	ND	9.6	–	Coldwell et al., 1976
50	ip	–	17.6	–	Gemborys and Mudge, 1981
150	ip	–	12.6	–	Gemborys and Mudge, 1981
200	ip	–	15.6	–	Gemborys and Mudge, 1981
300	ip	–	14.6	–	Gemborys and Mudge, 1981
425	ip	–	13.9	–	Gemborys and Mudge, 1981
500	ip	–	9.5	–	Gemborys and Mudge, 1981
200	ip	–	8.4	–	Miller and Jollow, 1984
20	ip	–	19.9	–	Miller and Jollow, 1986a
150	ip	–	7.7	–	Miller and Jollow, 1986a
151	iv	2.8	8.4	11.2	Gregus et al., 1988b
Guinea pig					
150	oral	ND	<1.0	–	Coldwell et al., 1976
151	iv	1.0	1.0	2.0	Gregus et al., 1988b

(cont.)

Table 6.2 *(cont.)*

Dose (mg kg⁻¹)	Route	% excreted as cysteine conjugate	% excreted as mercapturic acid conjugate	% excreted as cysteine and mercapturic acid conjugates combined	Reference
Cat					
20	oral	4.7	0.0	4.7	Savides *et al.*, 1984
60	oral	10.7	1.4	12.1	Savides *et al.*, 1984
120	oral	9.7	2.3	12.0	Savides *et al.*, 1984
Dog					
100	oral	4.5	0	4.5	Savides *et al.*, 1984, 1985
200	oral	3.1	0	3.1	Savides *et al.*, 1984, 1985
Rabbit					
151	iv	0.2	6.2	6.4	Gregus *et al.*, 1988b
Baboon					
40	iv	–	0.3	–	Altomare *et al.*, 1984a

If not stated, dose in man estimated assuming body weight of 70 kg; ND = not detected; [1] overdose, no liver damage; [2] overdose, moderate to severe liver damage; [3] male; [4] female; [5] chronic alcoholics; [6] cirrhosis; [7] including thiomethyl metabolites; [8] Gilbert's disease; [9] patients with bladder cancer; [10] elderly; [11] given N-acetylcysteine; [12] intensive care patients; [13] Chinese; [14] Indian; [15] Oriental; [16] Thai; [17] vegetarian; [18] pregnant; [19] methionine-deficient diet; [20] weanling; [21] energy-dense diet, lean; [22] energy-dense diet, obese; [23] fed; [24] fasted; [25] presumed – abbreviations used in original paper not defined; [26] young.

Gale, 1987; Pascoe *et al.*, 1988; Rogers *et al.*, 1988; Slattery *et al.*, 1989; Epstein *et al.*, 1991; Pantuck *et al.*, 1991; Gwilt *et al.*, 1994). Paracetamol 3-methylsulphoxide, and 3-thiomethylparacetamol were formed secondarily from the glutathione conjugate in the enterohepatic circulation as shown by their late appearance in the urine, the effects of bile duct ligation and the metabolism of the minor metabolites administered by themselves (Gemborys and Mudge, 1981). Studies in germ-free mice and mice pretreated with antibiotics showed an important role for the intestinal bacterial flora, and the cysteine conjugate of paracetamol was probably cleaved by cysteine conjugate C-S lyase to 3-thioparacetamol, which was then methylated and excreted in the urine as 3-thiomethylparacetamol (Kim and Kobashi, 1986; Mikov *et al.*, 1988; Mikov and Caldwell, 1990; Mikov, 1994). The methyl group of the thiomethyl metabolites was derived from methionine (Warrander *et al.*, 1985). The glucuronide and sulphate conjugates of the 3-thiomethyl and sulphoxide derivatives have been identified as further minor metabolites of paracetamol in rats and mice (Hart *et al.*, 1981; Mikov *et al.*, 1988). There was considerable interconversion between the 3-thiomethyl and 3-thiomethylsulphoxide metabolites *in vivo* (Gemborys and Mudge, 1981) and their further oxidation to 3-thiomethylparacetamol sulphone has been described in hamsters (Wong *et al.*, 1976b). However, others have not confirmed the existence of a sulphone derivative and its formation was probably a methodological artifact (Gemborys and Mudge, 1981; Warrander *et al.*, 1985). The reported fractional urinary recovery of the thiomethyl and thiomethylsulphoxide metabolites of paracetamol varied considerably between species, and in the hamster at least, their formation was dose-dependent (Table 6.3). In experimental animals these metabolites usually accounted for less than 10 per cent of a dose, and in man the recovery of 3-thiomethylparacetamol was less than 1 per cent. Other possible metabolites of paracetamol derived from the glutathione conjugate included the homocysteine analogues and methoxy derivatives of the cysteine and mercapturic acid conjugates (Knox and Jurand, 1977, 1978).

Other Minor Metabolites

Several other minor metabolites of paracetamol have been described. A small variable fraction of a dose undergoes microsomal ring hydroxylation to a catechol, which may then be O-methylated. Mrochek *et al.* (1974) isolated what was thought to be 2-hydroxyparacetamol sulphate and 2-methoxyparacetamol with its glucuronide and sulphate conjugates in the urine of two volunteers taking paracetamol. Subsequent investigation showed that substitution occurred at the 3-position and the corresponding hydroxy and methoxy derivatives and their glucuronide and sulphate conjugates were established as minor metabolites of paracetamol in man (Andrews *et al.*, 1976; Knox and Jurand, 1977, 1978; Notarianni *et al.*, 1981; Hamilton and Kissinger, 1982; Wilson *et al.*, 1982a; Anderson *et al.*, 1983; To and Wells, 1985; Ladds *et al.*, 1987; Slattery *et al.*, 1987, 1989; Factor *et al.*, 1989; Epstein *et al.*, 1991; Pantuck *et al.*, 1991), mice (Forte *et al.*, 1984; Dolphin *et al.*, 1987; Pascoe *et al.*, 1988; Rashed *et al.*, 1990), rats (Hart *et al.*, 1981; Harvison *et al.*, 1988b) and hamsters (Gemborys and Mudge, 1981). The urinary recoveries of 3-hydroxyparacetamol and 3-methoxyparacetamol in different reports are summarized in Table 6.3 but the values given are not always comparable because in some cases it was not clear whether conjugates of the metabolites were included. There was much variation, and in man for example, the recovery of 3-hydroxyparacetamol ranged from less than 1 per cent to 9.9 per cent. In general, the sum total of these two metabolites accounted for less than 10 per cent of a dose. 4-Hydroxyglycoanilide formed by hydroxylation of the acetamido group was possibly another minor metabolite of paracetamol (Smith and Griffiths, 1976).

Deacetylation

The recent isolation of small amounts of cysteine and mercapturic acid conjugates of hydroquinone as urinary metabolites of paracetamol in mice was consistent with the formation of p-benzoquinoneimine as a secondary, but probably toxicologically insignificant, metabolite of paracetamol (Pascoe *et al.*, 1988; Rashed *et al.*, 1990). p-Aminophenol, from which it could be derived, has been identified as a trace metabolite of paracetamol in hamsters (Gemborys and Mudge, 1981), mice (Carpenter and Mudge, 1981; Rashed *et al.*, 1990) and rats (Hart *et al.*, 1981, 1982a; Newton *et al.*, 1982b, 1983a; Rush *et al.*, 1984; Tarloff *et al.*, 1989b). Paracetamol was deacetylated to a limited extent in rat liver and kidney, but to a much lesser extent in brain (Baumann *et al.*, 1984). However, it was extensively deacetylated in some amphibian species (Clothier *et al.*, 1981, 1982). The hepatotoxicity of N-acetyl-3,5-dimethyl-p-benzoquinoneimine was dependent on its deacetylation (Rossi *et al.*, 1988). p-Aminophenol has not been recognized as a urinary metabolite of paracetamol in man, except in one report in which it was said to be present in brown urine

Table 6.3 Fractional urinary recovery (per cent) of some minor metabolites of paracetemol in different species.

Species	Dose (mg kg^{-1})	Route	3-Hydroxy-paracetamol	3-Methoxy-paracetamol	3-Thiomethyl-paracetamol	Paracetamol 3-thiomethyl-sulphoxide	Reference
Man	23	oral	2.1[1]	2.6[1]	–	–	Mrochek et al., 1974
Man	26	oral	0.66	–	–	–	Klutch et al., 1978
Man	14	oral	7.9	5.7	–	–	Hamilton and Kissinger, 1982
Man	21	oral	–	2.7	–	–	Anderson et al., 1983
Man	14	oral	2.5	–	–	–	Ladds et al., 1987
Man	7	oral	9.9	–	–	–	Slattery et al., 1987
Man	43	oral	6.9	–	–	–	Slattery et al., 1987
Man	14	oral	4.1	3.1	0.84	–	Slattery et al., 1989
Man	7	oral	3.0	2.8	0.64	–	Epstein et al., 1991
Man	21	oral	–	1.7	–	–	Pantuck et al., 1991
Hamster	50	oral	–	0.33	10.3	5.8	Gemborys and Mudge, 1981
Hamster	150	oral	–	0.67	11.4	5.1	Gemborys and Mudge, 1981
Hamster	200	oral	–	0.97	6.3	2.9	Gemborys and Mudge, 1981
Hamster	300	oral	–	1.1	3.7	2.1	Gemborys and Mudge, 1981
Hamster	425	oral	–	1.2	1.1	0.75	Gemborys and Mudge, 1981
Hamster	600	oral	–	1.5	0.71	0.24	Gemborys and Mudge, 1981
Hamster	200	ip	–	–	2.9	2.8	Miller and Jollow, 1984
Hamster	20	ip	–	–	6.0[2]	–	Miller and Jollow, 1986a
Hamster	150	ip	–	–	4.3[2]	–	Miller and Jollow, 1986a
Mouse	500	ip	2.6	0.5	–	–	Forte et al., 1984
Mouse	100	ip	–	<0.1	5.7	1.0	Dolphin et al., 1987

Mouse	200	ip	–	–	5.9^2	–	Price and Gale, 1987
Mouse	200	ip	–	–	5.0^2	–	Mikov et al., 1988
Mouse	200	ip	0.85	1.8	0.3	–	Pascoe et al., 1988
Mouse	250	ip	5.4	4.0	2.4	–	Rashed et al., 1990
Rat[2]	300	iv	–	–	0.8	–	Hart et al., 1982a
Rat[3]	300	iv	–	–	0.7	–	Hart et al., 1982a
Rat[2]	1500	oral	–	–	1.0	–	Hart et al., 1982a
Rat[3]	1500	oral	–	–	3.1	–	Hart et al., 1982a
Rat[3]	300	oral	–	–	1.2	–	Hart et al., 1982a
Rat[3]	750	oral	–	–	2.3	–	Hart et al., 1982a
Rat[3]	2250	oral	–	–	2.0	–	Hart et al., 1982a
Rat[3]	3000	oral	–	–	1.3	–	Hart et al., 1982a
Rat[3]	300	ip	–	–	0.5	–	Hart et al., 1982a
Rat[3]	150	iv	–	–	0.0	–	Hart et al., 1982a
Rat[3,4]	750	oral	–	–	3.3	–	Hart et al., 1982a
Rat[3,4]	1500	oral	–	–	4.5	–	Hart et al., 1982a
Rat[3,4]	2250	oral	–	–	2.1	–	Hart et al., 1982a
Rat	800	ip	–	–	1.5	0.3	Price and Jollow, 1983
Rat	600	ip	–	–	2.4^5	–	Price and Jollow, 1986
Rat	600	ip	1.8^6	–	–	–	Thummel et al., 1988
Rat[7]	700	ip	–	–	1.4^5	–	Price and Jollow, 1989a
Rat[8]	700	ip	–	–	2.3^5	–	Price and Jollow, 1989a
Dog	15	ns	2.8	–	–	–	Klutch et al., 1978
Dog	200	ns	1.3	–	–	–	Klutch et al., 1978

[1] thought to be 2-isomer; [2] male; [3] female; [4] weanling; [5] including sulphoxide metabolite; [6] 3-hydroxy and 3-methoxy metabolites combined; [7] fed; [8] fasted; ns = not stated.

from three patients who had taken multiple drugs including paracetamol in over-dose. Proof of identity was not rigorous and was based on a non-specific colour reaction and thin layer chromatography using only one solvent system (Clark *et al.*, 1986). p-Benzoquinoneimine could be produced by deacetylation of paracetamol to p-aminophenol followed by N-hydroxylation and dehydration to the corresponding imine, or perhaps more likely, the hydrolysis and loss of acetamide from N-acetyl-p-benzoquinoneimine (Dahlin *et al.*, 1984).

p-Aminophenol was considered by some investigators to be implicated in the nephrotoxicity of paracetamol (Mudge, 1982; Newton *et al.*, 1982b, 1983c, 1985a,b; Rush *et al.*, 1984; Zenser and Davis, 1984), and deacetylation increased its experimental embryotoxicity and cytotoxicity (Stark *et al.*, 1989b). Deacetylation was said not to be required for nephrotoxicity in the mouse, and metabolic activation of paracetamol probably occurred *in situ* in renal proximal tubule cell suspensions as shown by selective covalent binding (Emeigh Hart *et al.*, 1991b). It should be noted that extraordinarily high paracetamol concentrations up to 3775 mg l^{-1} were used in this study. In subsequent studies, the *in vitro* binding of paracetamol to rat liver and kidney was found to be dependent on oxidative metabolism and there was no requirement for deacetylation (Mugford and Tarloff, 1995). In rats given [^{14}C-acetyl]-paracetamol, some 6 per cent of the dose was recovered in the expired air (Smith and Griffiths, 1976), and in studies of the loss of deuterated acetyl- labelled paracetamol in nine subjects given 50 mg orally, there was about a 10 per cent exchange of the acetyl group. The acetyl exchange was greater in rats (Baty *et al.*, 1988). In any event, p-aminophenol formed by the deacetylation of paracetamol was unlikely to be relevant to its toxicity because the N-acetyl group and the ring of paracetamol were bound covalently in almost equal amounts and very little acetamide was formed (Hinson and Gillette, 1980; Gillette *et al.*, 1981). Paracetamol reacted with nitrite at low pH (such as is found in the stomach) to give p-benzoquinone, and N-acetyl-p-benzoquinoneimine was identified as an intermediate in its formation (Ohta *et al.*, 1988a).

The relevance of some studies of the metabolism and toxicity of paracetamol must be questioned in the light of the enormous and unrealistic doses and concentrations used. For example, doses of paracetamol as high as 4250 mg kg^{-1} have been given to rats (Poulsen *et al.*, 1985c) and concentrations of 25 and 50 mM (3775 and 7550 mg l^{-1}) have been used in studies with isolated hepatocytes and renal tubule cells (Sweeny and Weiner, 1985; Tee *et al.*, 1987; Emeigh Hart *et al.*, 1991b). Indeed, these concentrations far exceed the aqueous solubility of paracetamol at neutral pH and normal room temperature.

7

Factors Influencing Paracetamol Metabolism

Species Differences

Man and the common laboratory animals seem to share the same major and most minor routes of paracetamol metabolism. However, as shown by variation in the patterns of urinary excretion of metabolites, there are important quantitative species differences involving both toxic metabolic activation and parallel non-toxic conjugation of paracetamol (Davis *et al.*, 1974a; Jollow *et al.*, 1974; Coldwell *et al.*, 1976; Ioannides *et al.*, 1983b; Gregus *et al.*, 1987, 1988b; Seddon *et al.*, 1987; Tee *et al.*, 1987). These differences are summarized in Table 7.1 but it is only possible to make very general comparisons because of intraspecies variation and differences in dose, routes of administration and experimental conditions. To complicate matters further, some investigators have used unnecessarily large and hepatotoxic doses of paracetamol with the result that the different pathways of metabolism would be depressed unpredictably by the effects of dose, depletion of cofactors and acute liver

Table 7.1 Species differences in the metabolism of paracetamol as shown by the average percentage urinary excretion of conjugates.[1]

Species	Conjugates			
	Glucuronide	Sulphate	Cysteine	Mercapturate
Man	50–60	25–35	2–5	2–4
Mouse	50–60	10–20	15–25	1–3
Rat	10–20	40–80	1–5	2–6
Hamster	40–50	20–30	0–2	10–15
Guinea pig	80–90	4–7	1	1
Rabbit	77	16	<1	6
Cat	1–15	60–90	5–10	1–2
Dog	75	15	3–4	0
Pony	60 /	35	–	–
Baboon	–	–	<1	<1

[1] From data in Tables 6.1 and 6.2.

damage. Nevertheless, the dominant route of non-toxic metabolism of paracetamol was clearly glucuronide conjugation in man, guinea pig, mouse, rabbit, dog and pony, while the corresponding major route of elimination in the rat and cat was sulphate conjugation. Cats are deficient in hepatic glucuronyl transferase and were unable to form glucuronides (Welch *et al.*, 1966; Smith and Timbrell, 1974; Savides *et al.*, 1984).

Metabolic Activation

As shown by the combined urinary excretion of the cysteine and mercapturic acid conjugates, the metabolic activation of paracetamol was extensive in the hamster and mouse but minor in the guinea pig, rat and dog (Table 7.1). These differences in metabolism corresponded to species differences in susceptibility to hepatotoxicity (Davis *et al.*, 1974; Jollow *et al.*, 1974a; Ioannides *et al.*, 1983b; Savides *et al.*, 1984; Gregus *et al.*, 1987, 1988b; Seddon *et al.*, 1987; Tee *et al.*, 1987; Liu *et al.*, 1991). There were further species differences in the extent of acetylation of the cysteine conjugate to form the mercapturic acid derivative (Jensen *et al.*, 1986). The cysteine conjugate accounted for most of the glutathione-derived urinary metabolites in the mouse, dog and cat in whom only a minor fraction appeared as the mercapturic acid conjugate. In contrast, the mercapturic acid conjugate was the major component in the hamster while excretion of the cysteine conjugate was minimal (Table 7.1). Little or no mercapturic acid conjugate was found in the urine of dogs (Savides *et al.*, 1984) and this was consistent with their inability to acetylate amino groups (Brodie and Axelrod, 1948b). Paracetamol was extensively deacetylated to p-aminophenol in amphibia (Clothier *et al.*, 1981), but this was only a minor urinary metabolite in mice (Carpenter and Mudge, 1981; Rashed *et al.*, 1990), hamsters (Gemborys and Mudge, 1981) and rats (Smith and Griffiths, 1976; Newton *et al.*, 1982b, 1983a; Tarloff *et al.*, 1989c). It was not confirmed as a metabolite of paracetamol in man. Although it was very difficult to produce renal toxicity with paracetamol in animals, determined efforts have been made to implicate it as a cause of analgesic nephropathy in man. Paracetamol was said to be nephrotoxic in rats by virtue of its renal acetylation to p-aminophenol independent of cytochrome P450, while in mice the mechanism was supposed to be generation of a cytotoxic intermediate metabolite by cytochrome P450 in renal cells *in situ* (Emeigh Hart *et al.*, 1991b). In contrast to findings in other species, the metabolic activation of paracetamol in miniature swine (as judged by the formation of the mercapturic acid conjugate) was demonstrable in microsomal preparations from kidney cortex but not from liver (Peggins *et al.*, 1987). The plasma half life and clearance of paracetamol were similar in dogs, horses and man but its elimination in these species was much slower than in miniature swine (Bailie *et al.*, 1987; Engelking *et al.*, 1987b). There were important species differences in the urinary excretion of paracetamol and its conjugates and examples are shown in Figure 7.1.

Significant species differences in paracetamol metabolism have been demonstrated in hepatocyte cultures and microsomal fractions (Green *et al.*, 1984a; Boobis *et al.*, 1986; Tee *et al.*, 1987; Smolarek *et al.*, 1990; Liu *et al.*, 1991). However, the findings have not necessarily corresponded with those reported by other investigators in intact animals of the same species. Thus, on the basis of the cytotoxicity of paracetamol and N-acetyl-p-benzoquinoneimine in hepatocytes from hamster,

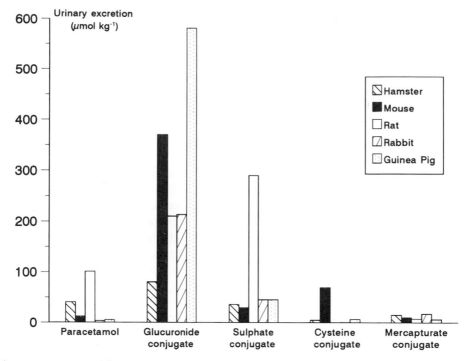

Figure 7.1 Species differences in the urinary excretion of paracetamol and its conjugates during the 2 h after intravenous administration of 150 mg kg^{-1} of paracetamol in animals with bile duct cannulation (data from Gregus *et al.*, 1988a).

mouse, rat and man in relation to their ability to form the glutathione conjugate, Boobis *et al.* (1986) and Tee *et al.* (1987) concluded that man resembled the resistant rat rather than the sensitive mouse in terms of susceptibility to hepatotoxicity. Similar claims were made in studies of the comparative activation of paracetamol by liver microsomal fractions from rat, mouse and man (Seddon *et al.*, 1987). This was clearly not the case in practice as doses of 250–350 and 375 mg kg^{-1} of paracetamol respectively caused severe and fatal liver damage in man (Prescott, 1983) and mice (Mitchell *et al.*, 1973b; Davis *et al.*, 1974a), while on the other hand, rats could survive the enormous dose of 4250 mg kg^{-1} (Poulsen *et al.*, 1985b). Species differences in the extent of depletion of hepatic glutathione produced by paracetamol were related to the amounts of active metabolite covalently bound to liver microsomal proteins (Aikawa *et al.*, 1978b). Rat liver slices were less active than hamster liver slices in forming the toxic metabolite of paracetamol, but they showed greater activity in non-toxic metabolism to the sulphate and glucuronide conjugates. These metabolic differences were associated with much greater susceptibility to hepatotoxicity in the hamster (Miller *et al.*, 1993a). The activity of cytochrome P450 was much less in hepatocytes isolated from the rainbow trout than in those from rats, and glutathione-derived and glucuronide (but not sulphate) conjugates of paracetamol were formed by trout liver (Parker *et al.*, 1981). In other reports, the glucuronide conjugation and metabolic activation of paracetamol were faster in dog than rat hepatocytes (Bolcsfoldi *et al.*, 1981) and paracetamol glucuronyl transferase activity was six to seven times greater in monkey than in human liver (Stevens *et al.*, 1993).

Species differences have also been described in the stimulation and inhibition of paracetamol metabolism. Thus, acetone enhanced the liver microsomal conjugation of paracetamol with glutathione in rats, but had little effect in rabbits and inhibited the reaction in mice (Liu *et al.*, 1991). Similarly, caffeine increased the formation of paracetamol glutathione conjugate by liver microsomes from rats but it had no effect on those from mice (Liu *et al.*, 1992b).

Strain Differences

Substantial strain differences in paracetamol metabolism have also been described and in some cases these corresponded to strain differences in toxicity (Price and Jollow, 1986; Lubek *et al.*, 1988b). In studies with the deacetylation of paracetamol in rats it was not possible to show a convincing relationship with nephrotoxicity (Newton *et al.*, 1983b,c; Tarloff *et al.*, 1989c) although strain differences in susceptibility were associated with differences in arylation of renal macromolecules (Newton *et al.*, 1985b).

Unsuitability of the Rat as a Model for Studies of Paracetamol Metabolism in Man

The metabolism and toxicity of paracetamol in the rat differs greatly from that in man and it is clearly an unsuitable species for studies in which such experimental data are extrapolated to man (Miller and Fischer, 1974). In the circumstances it is difficult to understand why so many investigators have chosen the rat for this purpose.

Dose Dependence

The metabolism of paracetamol was dose dependent even at therapeutic and low subtoxic levels. As the dose increased there was progressive saturation of sulphate conjugation and depletion of inorganic sulphate. At higher doses, the availability of essential cofactors for glutathione and glucuronide conjugation was also reduced. As discussed previously in Chapter 6, sulphate conjugation (but much less so glucuronide conjugation) was readily saturated and as there were marked species differences in the relative importance of these two processes, corresponding differences in dose-dependent metabolism would be anticipated. All other factors being equal, paracetamol elimination, therefore, should be highly dose dependent in the rat and cat where sulphate conjugation was dominant, but much less so in the guinea pig, which depended largely on glucuronidation for its removal. As the dose of paracetamol increased, liver damage would eventually occur and this would further impair its metabolism. The dose dependence of paracetamol metabolism may be manifest by changes in its removal rate, changes in the fractional urinary and biliary excretion of its metabolites and diversion from urinary to biliary elimination. The threshold for the onset of dose-dependent metabolism of paracetamol in man was 10–30 mg kg^{-1} (Reiter and Weinshilboum, 1982a; Clements *et al.*, 1984; Slattery *et al.*, 1987; Griener *et al.*, 1990; Sahajwalla and Ayres, 1991). The corresponding doses in animals have not been well defined but were probably in the ranges of 50–100 mg kg^{-1} in the mouse (Jollow *et al.*, 1974; Miners *et al.*, 1984a), 15–150 mg kg^{-1} in the rat (Galinsky and Levy, 1981; Price and Jollow, 1982; Watari *et al.*, 1983; Hjelle and Klaassen, 1984; Galinsky and Corcoran, 1988; Hirate *et al.*, 1990; Kane *et al.*, 1991) and 20–150 mg kg^{-1} in the hamster (Gemborys and Mudge, 1981; Miller and Jollow, 1986a; Miller *et al.*, 1986).

The uptake of paracetamol by isolated rat hepatocytes was dose dependent and involved a saturable process as well as simple diffusion (Miyazaki *et al.*, 1983). In the isolated perfused rat liver, paracetamol metabolism was dose dependent and as concentrations in the medium increased, the extraction ratio decreased (Cohen *et al.*, 1974; Poulsen *et al.*, 1985c). With increasing paracetamol concentrations there was a decrease in sulphate conjugation with little or no change in glucuronidation and inconstant changes in the production of the glutathione conjugate (Grafström *et al.*, 1979b; Pang and Terrell, 1981b; Fayz *et al.*, 1984; Poulsen *et al.*, 1985c). Sulphate conjugation could be partially restored by the addition of inorganic sulphate (Fayz *et al.*, 1984).

Dose-dependent Elimination

Prolongation of the half life of paracetamol with increasing dose has been observed in the hamster (Miller and Jollow, 1986a; Miller *et al.*, 1986; Lupo *et al.*, 1987), mouse (Siegers *et al.*, 1978) and rat (Davis *et al.*, 1976a; Siegers *et al.*, 1978; Galinsky and Levy, 1981; Price and Jollow, 1982; Lin and Levy, 1983b; Watari *et al.*, 1983; Hjelle and Klaassen, 1984; Galinsky and Corcoran, 1988; Hirate *et al.*, 1990). There was no change in the clearance, half life or composition of urine metabolites in rats as the dose of paracetamol doubled from 15 to 30 mg kg^{-1} (Galinsky and Levy, 1981). As shown in Figure 7.2, the rate of disappearance of paracetamol from the blood of rats following intraperitoneal administration of paracetamol decreased progressively as the dose increased from 50 to 1000 mg kg^{-1}. There was a 10-fold increase in half life from 0.4 to 4.4 h, and at all doses the fall was linear with time (Price and Jollow, 1982). Failure to demonstrate the expected non-linear decline in plasma concentrations of paracetamol indicating saturation kinetics with increasing dose in rats was attributed to restriction of sulphate conjugation caused by depletion of inorganic sulphate (Galinsky and Levy, 1981). In rats, paracetamol caused rapid depletion of hepatic uridine diphosphoglucuronic acid (UDP-GA) and the capacity for glucuronide conjugation at high doses was determined by the flux through the glucuronic acid route and the capacity to synthesize the cosubstrate (Price and Jollow, 1984). A dose-dependent metabolic interaction between antipyrine and paracetamol in pigs was attributed to competition for glucuronide conjugation (Monshouwer *et al.*, 1994).

In man, there are only minor changes in the paracetamol half life at therapeutic and low non-toxic dose levels. There was a small but statistically significant decrease in the plasma clearance of intravenous paracetamol as the dose increased from 5 to 20 mg kg^{-1} (Clements *et al.*, 1984), a minor increase in the saliva half life with the same doses given orally (Griener *et al.*, 1990) and a decrease in clearance of the drug from 22.3 to 17.3 l h^{-1} as the dose was increased from 500 to 3000 mg (Slattery *et al.*, 1987). There were no significant differences in the salivary kinetics of paracetamol, and no evidence of non-linearity following oral doses of 325, 650, 825 and 1000

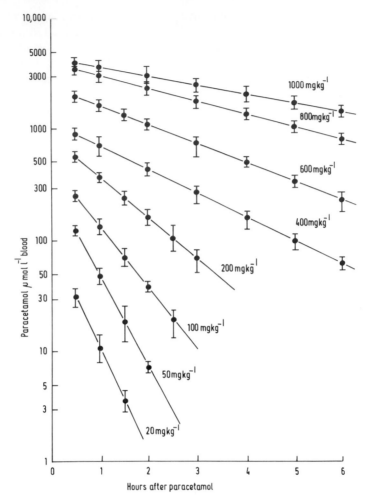

Figure 7.2 The effect of dose on the blood half life of paracetamol following intraperitoneal administration in rats. Values given are means $\pm$ SE (redrawn from Price and Jollow, 1982).

mg in one study in healthy volunteers (Sahajwalla and Ayres, 1991), but in another (also based on measurement of drug in saliva) there were dose-dependent changes in half life and normalized areas under the plasma concentration–time curves in 15 subjects given oral doses of 325, 500, 1000, 1500 and 2000 mg (Borin and Ayres, 1989). Unfortunately, paracetamol concentrations measured in saliva and plasma may differ considerably, and firm conclusions cannot be drawn from these studies. There was no evidence of capacity-limited elimination of paracetamol following rectal administration (Seideman *et al.*, 1980).

Pattern of Urinary Metabolite Excretion

Changes in the pattern of plasma concentrations or urinary excretion of paracetamol metabolites with dose have been described in the mouse (Jollow *et al.*, 1974;

Miners *et al.*, 1984a; Lubek *et al.*, 1988b), hamster (Jollow *et al.*, 1974; Gemborys and Mudge, 1981; Miller and Jollow, 1986a; Miller *et al.*, 1986) and rat (Büch *et al.*, 1967c; Jollow *et al.*, 1974; Davis *et al.*, 1976a; Siegers and Schütt, 1979; Green and Fischer, 1981; Price and Jollow, 1982; Hart *et al.*, 1982a; Lin and Levy, 1983b; Newton *et al.*, 1983b; Watari *et al.*, 1983; Hjelle and Klaassen, 1984; Galinsky and Corcoran, 1988; Tarloff *et al.*, 1989a; Hirate *et al.*, 1990; Tone *et al.*, 1990; Kane *et al.*, 1991). In some reports, the total urinary recovery of paracetamol and metabolites decreased with increasing dose (Newton *et al.*, 1983b; Hjelle and Klaassen, 1984; Tarloff *et al.*, 1989a,c). This may have been due to too short a period of urine collection because as the dose increased above the threshold for hepatic and possibly renal toxicity, metabolism would become impaired and renal excretion would be delayed. Dose-dependent changes in the urinary excretion of unchanged paracetamol and its sulphate and glucuronide conjugates were qualitatively similar in man, mouse, rat and hamster. The proportion appearing as unchanged drug increased with dose as a direct consequence of its slower metabolism and persistence in the body. In addition, there was a marked decrease in the fraction excreted as the sulphate conjugation as a result of saturation, and this was associated with a reciprocal increase in excretion of glucuronide (Kane *et al.*, 1991) (Figure 7.3). The proportions recovered as glutathione-derived conjugates decreased as dose increased in the mouse (Jollow *et al.*, 1974; Miners *et al.*, 1984a) and hamster (Jollow *et al.*, 1974; Gemborys and Mudge, 1981; Miller and Jollow, 1986a), and this was attributed to depletion of hepatic glutathione. The findings in rats have been inconsistent and variable (Jollow *et al.*, 1974; Davis *et al.*, 1976a; Hart *et al.*, 1982a; Price and Jollow,

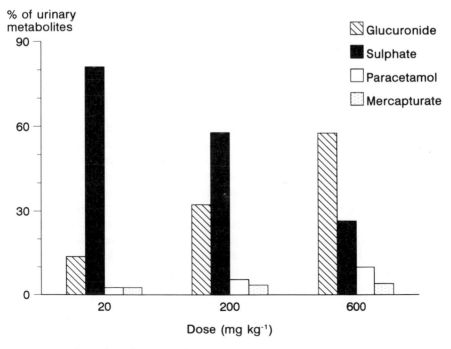

Figure 7.3 Dose-dependent changes in the fractional 24 h urinary recovery of paracetamol and its conjugates following intraperitoneal administration in rats (from Price and Jollow, 1982).

1982; Newton *et al.*, 1983b; Tarloff *et al.*, 1989a). The conversion of paracetamol to p-aminophenol and its conjugates was dose dependent in rats (Hart *et al.*, 1982a; Newton *et al.*, 1983b,c). The dose-related metabolism and toxicity of paracetamol was modified further by the route of administration. Thus, metabolic activation and toxicity were greater following intraperitoneal than oral administration of paracetamol, and with the latter route there was first pass gastrointestinal metabolism of the drug (Colin *et al.*, 1986a; Esteban *et al.*, 1993a,b).

In man, there was a decrease in the urinary excretion of sulphate and an increase in glucuronide conjugate with increasing sub toxic doses of paracetamol (Davis *et al.*, 1976b; Reiter and Weinshilboum, 1982a; Clements *et al.*, 1984; Slattery *et al.*, 1987; Griener *et al.*, 1990). Some investigators have found no increase in glutathione-derived conjugates (Mitchell *et al.*, 1974; Clements *et al.*, 1984), while others have reported both increases (Griener *et al.*, 1990) and decreases (Slattery *et al.*, 1987).

Dose-dependent Biliary Excretion

As the dose increased in rats there was a shift from urinary to biliary excretion of paracetamol and its metabolites. Thus, after a non-toxic dose of 200 mg kg^{-1}, 5.5 per cent was recovered in bile and 72 per cent in urine, while with 1000 mg kg^{-1} dose the corresponding recoveries were 13.5 and 51 per cent (Siegers and Schütt, 1979). With increasing dose, there was increased biliary excretion of unchanged drug and glucuronide conjugate with either no change, or decreased excretion of sulphate conjugate (Watari *et al.*, 1983; Hjelle and Klaassen, 1984). It is not known to what extent these changes reflected a true shift in pathways of excretion or whether they merely represented dose-related changes in plasma concentrations. Paracetamol caused a dose-dependent decrease in biliary glutathione excretion, which was directly related to depletion of hepatic glutathione (Kaplowitz *et al.*, 1983).

Overdosage

Following overdosage of paracetamol in man there was a significant increase in the plasma half life (Figure 7.4). This was of prognostic significance and prolongation of the half life beyond 4 h was usually associated with liver damage (Prescott *et al.*, 1971; Prescott and Wright, 1973; Gazzard *et al.*, 1977). The increase in paracetamol half life after overdosage was related primarily to hepatic injury rather than the dose *per se*. In poisoned patients with similar initial plasma concentrations, the mean half life was 3.4 h in those without liver damage and 6.7 h in those with severe liver damage (Prescott, 1980). In patients who developed fatal liver failure after overdosage the liver was so badly damaged that the conjugation of paracetamol virtually ceased and the plasma half life was grossly prolonged (Prescott and Wright, 1973). A kinetic model of paracetamol elimination based on saturable sulphate and glucuronide conjugation with first-order oxidative metabolism has been proposed (Slattery and Levy, 1979a). Although good agreement was claimed between predicted results and findings in poisoned patients (Davis *et al.*, 1976b; Slattery *et al.*, 1981), this model was not appropriate because the crucial effect of acute liver damage was not taken into account and in any event, as shown in Figure 7.4, there

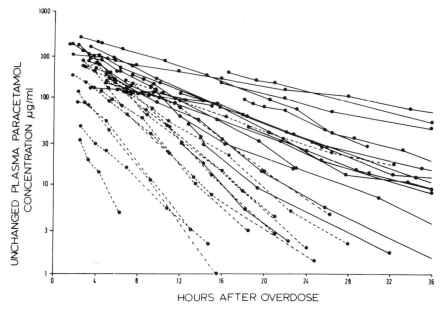

Figure 7.4 Plasma concentrations of paracetamol in 30 patients with and without liver damage following overdosage (redrawn from Prescott *et al.*, 1971).

was no evidence of saturation kinetics in most poisoned patients. Glucuronide conjugation was not usually saturated in man following overdosage, although this could occur rarely at exceptionally high plasma concentrations. Here again, it was not possible to distinguish between the effects of saturation, depletion of cofactors and the consequences of severe intoxication such as reduced liver blood flow, hypothermia, acidosis and other metabolic disturbances (Prescott, 1984). Following overdosage of paracetamol, there were striking changes in the pattern of urinary metabolite excretion as a result of marked saturation of sulphate conjugation with a compensatory increase in glucuronide conjugation. The fractional urinary recovery of the cysteine and mercapturic acid conjugates was also increased (Table 7.2) and this was related to the occurrence and severity of liver damage (Andrews *et al.*, 1976; Davis *et al.*, 1976b; Howie *et al.*, 1977; Prescott, 1980). In animals, toxic doses of paracetamol caused a reduction in hepatic cytochrome P450 content (Aikawa *et al.*, 1978a).

Dose-dependent Extrahepatic Metabolism

Dose-dependent metabolism of paracetamol has been described in the isolated perfused rat kidney (Emslie *et al.*, 1982; Newton *et al.*, 1983b) and the isolated rat intestinal loop (Goon and Klaassen, 1990; Tone *et al.*, 1990). The gastrointestinal metabolism and absorption of paracetamol depended on the dose in rats (Bhargava and Hirate, 1989; Tone *et al.*, 1990). In man, the fractional formation of sulphate conjugate by intestinal mucosa decreased, and glucuronidation increased, as the concentration of paracetamol rose (Rogers *et al.*, 1987a).

Table 7.2 Dose-dependent changes in the urinary recovery of paracetamol and its metabolites in healthy volunteers given an oral dose of 20 mg kg^{-1}, and overdose patients with and without liver damage receiving supportive therapy only.

	No. of subjects or patients	Urinary recovery (%)				Total amount recovered (g)
		Unchanged paracetamol	Sulphate conjugate	Glucuronide conjugate	Mercapturate and cysteine conjugates	
Healthy subjects	8	5.0	32.3	54.7	8.0	1.3
Overdose patients without liver damage	9	8.6	9.3	75.3	6.9	10.3
Overdose patients with severe liver damage	8	8.7	9.7	66.5	15.2	11.8

(From Prescott, 1980)

Repeated Administration

The effects of repeated administration may be considered as related to dose. In rats given acetanilide continuously in their diet for up to four weeks, the fraction recovered as paracetamol glucuronide increased from 4.6 per cent after a single dose to 16 per cent after dosing for one week, while the excretion of paracetamol sulphate decreased from 70 per cent after one day to 43 per cent after dosing for a week (Grantham *et al.*, 1972). In rats given the very large dose of 4250 mg kg^{-1} twice weekly for 18 weeks, prolonged treatment was associated with an increase in the urinary excretion of the glucuronide and mercapturic acid (but not sulphate) conjugates (Poulsen and Thomsen, 1988). In healthy subjects there was no change in the half life of paracetamol after single and multiple doses but less sulphate and more glucuronide conjugate was recovered in the urine on repeated administration (Hendrix-Treacy *et al.*, 1986). There were no consistent changes in steady-state plasma concentrations of sulphate and glucuronide conjugates during repeated administration of paracetamol for 10 days in patients with chronic renal failure, but the concentrations of unchanged drug increased progressively and the concentrations of sulphate conjugate were much lower than predicted (Martin *et al.*, 1991). In some infants and young children with fever there was an increase in the normalized area under the serum concentration–time curve on repeated dosing with paracetamol (Nahata *et al.*, 1984). Differences in kinetics were observed after the first and last doses when healthy volunteers took 325, 650, 825 and 1000 mg of paracetamol every 6 h for five doses on different occasions (Sahajwalla and Ayres, 1991).

Age

Significant changes in the metabolism of paracetamol with age have been reported. In general, glucuronide conjugation was impaired to a greater extent than sulphate conjugation in the very young, while the reverse applied in the elderly.

Fetal Metabolism of Paracetamol

No metabolism of paracetamol could be demonstrated in sheep placenta, and fetal glucuronide and sulphate conjugation activity was lower than in ewes and increased with gestational age (Wang *et al.*, 1986b). The activity of paracetamol glucuronyl transferase was less in fetal than adult sheep and there was evidence for the expression of different forms of the enzyme at different ages (Wang *et al.*, 1986b). The glucuronide and sulphate conjugates of paracetamol were removed largely by renal clearance in fetal lambs. The clearance increased with gestational age and there was no detectable transplacental transfer of these conjugates (Wang *et al.*, 1985). There were significant differences in the total clearance of paracetamol and the renal clearances of the sulphate and glucuronide conjugates in pregnant and non-pregnant ewes, and also in fetal and neonatal lambs (Wang *et al.*, 1990). In pregnant guinea pigs, given paracetamol 50 mg kg^{-1} intravenously at term, almost all of the conjugate in plasma was the glucuronide but in pups delivered by Caesarean section and given the same dose intraperitoneally, there was a much greater proportion of sulphate conjugate (Ecobichon *et al.*, 1989). Human liver and kidney from fetuses aged

18–23 weeks rapidly converted the glutathione conjugate of paracetamol to the cysteine conjugate through the action of γ-glutamyltransferase (Moldéus *et al.*, 1980c). Liver microsomes from fetuses of similar age could oxidize paracetamol and form the glutathione conjugate, but the activity was only about 10 per cent of that in adult microsomes. Sulphate, but not glucuronide conjugation of paracetamol, was demonstrated in isolated fetal hepatocytes (Rollins *et al.*, 1979).

Age Effects in Animals

The metabolic activation of paracetamol seemed to be increased rather than decreased in younger animals, but paradoxically, this was associated with greater resistance to hepatotoxicity. In hepatocytes isolated from 1–3-week-old mice there was greater covalent binding and metabolic activation of paracetamol than in those from adults, but cytotoxicity was similar (Harman and McCamish, 1986). In another study, paracetamol was less hepatotoxic in young than in adult mice, but the partial clearance to glutathione-derived metabolites was greater (Adamson *et al.*, 1991). In mice aged 1, 1.5, 2 and 3 months, 600 mg kg^{-1} of paracetamol produced severe liver damage only in the oldest group. Liver glutathione content and paracetamol concentrations were similar in all age groups but in the 3-month-old mice a greater proportion of the dose appeared in the urine as glucuronide conjugate (Beierschmitt *et al.*, 1989). Paracetamol was nephrotoxic at a dose of 750 mg kg^{-1} in rats aged 9–12 months, but not in those aged 2–3 months. The clearance of paracetamol was less in the older animals but *in vitro* glucuronidation by hepatic microsomes was similar in both age groups (Tarloff *et al.*, 1989b) and there were no differences between the age groups in the pattern of urinary excretion of paracetamol metabolites (Tarloff *et al.*, 1989c). *In vitro* studies in rats showed no age-dependent changes in the activities of hepatic glutathione S-transferase, glucuronyl transferase and sulphotransferase, but renal glutathione S-transferase was less active in 12- and 30-month-old animals than in those aged 3 months (Tarloff *et al.*, 1991). Others have also reported greater nephrotoxicity and slower elimination of paracetamol in older compared with younger rats (Beierschmitt *et al.*, 1986b). In contrast, hepatotoxicity and the production of glutathione-derived conjugates of paracetamol were said to be somewhat reduced in elderly compared with young rats (Rikans and Moore, 1988; Rikans, 1989). The renal oxidative metabolism of paracetamol was reduced in aged rats but there was no decrease in the extent of deacetylation (Beierschmitt and Weiner,1986).

Paracetamol was absorbed and excreted more slowly in neonatal than adult rabbits (Davison *et al.*, 1977) and the gastrointestinal extraction and presystemic metabolism of paracetamol were reduced in rats aged 3 weeks compared with those aged 10 weeks (Hirate *et al.*, 1991). In the younger animals, the plasma half life was shorter than in rats aged 10 weeks and 1 year, and the ratio of glucuronide to paracetamol was greater. As shown by the metabolic ratios of the glucuronide, sulphate and glutathione-derived conjugates in blood, the metabolism of paracetamol was impaired in rats aged 7 and 14 days compared with adults (Prokopczyk *et al.*, 1993). In rats aged from 5 to 90 days the excretion of glucuronide conjugate was increased over the period 11–33 days compared with adults and the excretion of mercapturic acid conjugate decreased with age (Green and Fischer, 1981). Age-related differences were observed in the amounts of glucuronide and sulphate conjugates in the liver and kidney of neonatal and young rats, and the active metabolite of paracetamol appeared to be formed more rapidly by the neonatal rats (Green and Fischer, 1984). In another study, weanling rats tended to produce more glucuronide than sulphate conjugate compared with adults but the recovery of glutathione metabolites was generally similar (Hart *et al.*, 1982a). The total clearance and half life of paracetamol varied little with age in rats aged 5, 14 and 25 months but the urinary excretion of glucuronide conjugate increased and sulphate decreased with age, and the renal clearance of the latter was reduced in the oldest age group. In the latter, the depression of phenol sulphotransferase activity and isozyme pattern parallelled the *in vivo* changes in paracetamol metabolism (Galinsky and Corcoran, 1986; Galinsky *et al.*, 1986). In female rats, ageing decreased the clearance of paracetamol and the formation of its glucuronide, sulphate and glutathione-derived conjugates, and the changes in sulphate conjugation were consistent with age-related changes in the pattern of pituitary secretion of growth hormone (Galinsky *et al.*, 1990). Treatment with buthionine sulphoximine depressed sulphate and increased glucuronide conjugation in young and old rats, but the effect on sulphate conjugation was greater in old rats (Galinsky *et al.*, 1992). In Brown Norwegian rats, age was not a determinant of the glucuronide and sulphate conjugation of paracetamol (Woodhouse and Herd, 1993). There were no differences in the metabolism of paracetamol by isolated hepatocytes in mice aged from 3 to 26 weeks, but in rats of similar age glucuronide conjugation increased and sulphate conjugation decreased as they became older (Sweeny and Weiner, 1985). In dogs, the paracetamol half life was 4.5 times longer in pups aged 4 days than in those aged 40–60 days and sulphate conjugation decreased with age while glucuronide conjugation increased (Ecobichon *et al.*, 1988).

Paracetamol Metabolism in Children

In man the glucuronide conjugation of paracetamol was not well developed in the newborn. Compared with children aged 6–16 years, neonates showed a marked delay in the appearance of paracetamol glucuronide in the serum after a 20 mg kg^{-1} dose of acetanilide (Vest and Streiff, 1959). Similar impairment of glucuronide conjugation was noted in the newborn compared with older children and paracetamol was used as a test drug to assess glucuronidation capacity (Pietsch *et al.*, 1972). In 2–3-day-old infants, given 12 mg kg^{-1} of paracetamol, the mean urinary half life was 3.5 h while considerably more sulphate and less glucuronide conjugate was excreted than in adults (Levy *et al.*, 1975b). Similarly, in urine obtained from a newborn infant whose mother had taken phenacetin ante partum, the sulphate and glucuronide conjugates accounted for 62 and 35 per cent respectively of the total paracetamol metabolites (Levy *et al.*, 1975a). Other investigators have confirmed reversal of the usual adult 2 : 1 ratio of glucuronide to sulphate conjugates of paracetamol in young children and paracetamol glucuronidation appeared to be particularly depressed in a 3-year-old child with progeria (Caldwell *et al.*, 1978). Compared with adults, there was no change in the half life of appearance of paracetamol in the urine in children aged 7–10 years, but again they excreted more sulphate and less glucuronide conjugate (Alam *et al.*, 1977b). In another study, the newborn and children aged 3–9 years also excreted more sulphate and less glucuronide conjugate than adults, but in 12-year-old children the pattern of urinary metabolites of parace-tamol was the same as in adults (Figure 7.5) (Miller *et al.*, 1976b). Paracetamol was excreted into breast milk in concentrations somewhat higher than in plasma and neonates received an estimated maximum of 1.85 per cent of the weight-adjusted maternal dose. However, in this study the pattern of urinary metabolites of parace-tamol in the infants was very atypical with recoveries of unchanged drug, and gluc-uronide, sulphate and cysteine plus mercapturic acid conjugates of 24.9, 54.1, 9.9 and 11.1 per cent respectively (Notarianni *et al.*, 1987). In an infant delivered by Caesarean section following maternal overdosage of paracetamol, the pattern of urinary metabolites was similar to that in the mother but the plasma half life was greatly prolonged at 10 h and there was a marked delay in reaching peak plasma concentrations of the glucuronide and sulphate conjugates. The baby did not develop liver damage (Roberts *et al.*, 1984). The plasma half life of paracetamol was similar in children and adults, and in the former there was no consistent prolonga-tion in the presence of fever (Peterson and Rumack, 1978; Wilson, 1979; Wilson *et al.*, 1982b; Walson and Mortensen, 1989). However, in febrile neonates recovering from cardiac surgery given paracetamol by suppository, the plasma half life was prolonged (Hopkins *et al.*, 1990). The plasma paracetamol half life was considerably increased at 4.33 h in apparently normal Indian children of unstated age who acted as controls in a study of the effect of malnutrition on drug disposition (Mehta *et al.*,

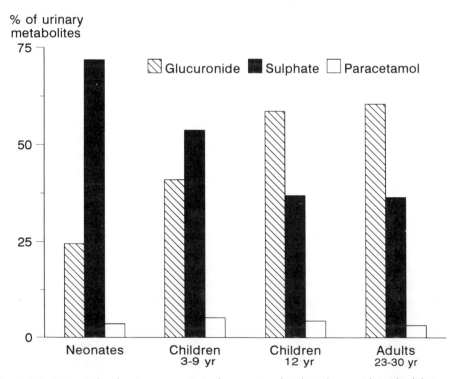

Figure 7.5 Fractional 36 h urinary excretion of paracetamol and its glucuronide and sulphate conjugates in adults and in children of different ages following oral doses of 10 mg kg^{-1} (data from Miller *et al.*, 1976b).

1982). In some young children with fever there may be minor accumulation of paracetamol with repeated dosing (Nahata *et al.*, 1984). The age-dependent disposition of paracetamol has been reviewed in relation to hepatotoxicity in man (Rumore and Blaiklock, 1992).

Metabolism of Paracetamol in the Elderly

Advanced age had only a minor influence on paracetamol metabolism. In human liver microsomal fractions from subjects aged 40–89 years there was no correlation between age and glucuronide and sulphate conjugation activity (Herd *et al.*, 1991). In a comparison of young and elderly subjects with mean ages of 20.8 and 74.9 years given 1000 mg of paracetamol orally, the half life was similar but there was a small decrease in sulphate conjugation in the elderly (Miners *et al.*, 1988). A similar lack of effect of old age on the half life and clearance of paracetamol after an intravenous dose was reported (Divoll *et al.*, 1982a,b). In some studies there was a statistically significant (but clinically unimportant) increase in the plasma paracetamol half life in the elderly (Triggs *et al.*, 1975; Briant *et al.*, 1976; Bedjaoui *et al.*, 1984), while in another paracetamol clearance was actually increased in elderly subjects (Fulton *et al.*, 1979). To some extent a reduced paracetamol clearance in the elderly could be accounted for by the associated reduction in liver volume (Wynne *et al.*, 1990). In the elderly physical frailty was a much more important determinant of paracetamol conjugation than age itself (Wynne *et al.*, 1990; Ellmers *et al.*, 1993).

Sex, Pregnancy and Oral Contraceptives

Sex-related differences have been described in the disposition of several drugs including paracetamol (Wilson, 1984). Male- and female-specific forms of cytochrome P450, which catalyze the glutathione conjugation and 3-hydroxylation of paracetamol, have been identified in rats, and the male isozyme was more active than the female isozyme (Harvison *et al.*, 1988b). Male rats also produced more sulphate and less glucuronide conjugate than females (Smith and Griffiths, 1976; Green and Fischer, 1981; Hart *et al.*, 1982a; Raheja *et al.*, 1983b; Kane and Chen, 1987; Kane *et al.*, 1990b). The same sex differences in the glucuronide and sulphate conjugation of paracetamol were observed *in vitro* with rat liver fractions (Woodhouse and Herd, 1993). Hepatic sulphotransferase activity was greater in male than in female rats and this sex difference persisted in hepatocytes in culture for up to four days (Kane *et al.*, 1990b, 1991). Oophorectomy and castration had no effect on enzyme activity but this was increased by testosterone in oophorectomized females and decreased by ethinyl oestradiol in castrated males (Kane and Chen, 1987). In another study in rabbits the clearance of paracetamol was increased by oophorectomy and reduced by administration of mestranol (Kwiatkowski, 1991). Attempts to 'feminize' gonadal function in male rat pups by perinatal exposure to cimetidine had no effect on the subsequent oxidation or conjugation of paracetamol at the age of 100 days (Kane *et al.*, 1989). The castration of male mice resulted in reduced renal (but not hepatic) metabolic activation of paracetamol but there was no significant effect on the overall rate of its elimination (Emeigh Hart *et al.*, 1994).

The sex difference in sulphotransferase activity in rats disappeared with advancing age (Galinsky *et al.*, 1986) and sex-related changes in the metabolism and kinetics of paracetamol tended to protect female rats against hepatotoxicity (Raheja *et al.*, 1983b). No important sex differences in the metabolism of paracetamol were noted in rats with and without thiamine deficiency (Ruchirawat *et al.*, 1981). Significant sex differences were described in the distribution of cytochrome P450 and the production of the mercapturic acid conjugate of paracetamol by hepatic and renal microsomes from miniature swine (Peggins *et al.*, 1987). Rats pregnant for 20 days and non-pregnant controls were given 15 and 300 mg of paracetamol intravenously. In the high-dose pregnancy group the relative clearance of paracetamol was reduced and the half life was increased, and the relative total clearance decreased as litter size increased. Compared with the controls, the pregnant rats excreted more unchanged paracetamol and less sulphate conjugate in the urine. Paracetamol was cleared very rapidly after the low dose, and its disposition was not influenced by pregnancy (Lin and Levy, 1983b). The renal microsomal metabolic activation of paracetamol was greater in male than in female mice, and this was related to the activity of the CYP2E1 isoform of cytochrome P450. There were no such differences with liver microsomes (Hu *et al.*, 1993a).

Sex Differences in Man

In man sex differences in the metabolism of paracetamol were minor and of no practical significance. Although the elimination rate was found to be independent of sex in several studies (Briant *et al.*, 1976; Abernethy *et al.*, 1982a; Divoll *et al.*, 1982a; Bedjaoui *et al.*, 1984), a lower clearance has been noted in females compared with males (Mucklow *et al.*, 1980; Abernethy *et al.*, 1982a; Miners *et al.*, 1983; Ali and Sharif, 1993). In the study of Mucklow *et al.*, there were multiple confounding factors including race, diet, smoking and the use of ethanol and oral contraceptives. There was a minor reduction in glucuronide conjugation and a corresponding increase in sulphate conjugation in females compared with males (Miners *et al.*, 1983; Rosen *et al.*, 1984), and as shown by the metabolic ratio, there was a greater capacity for glucuronide conjugation in males than in females (Bock *et al.*, 1994). However, in another report, no sex differences were observed in the fractional urinary recoveries of paracetamol and its conjugates (Esteban and Pérez-Mateo, 1993a). A more consistent finding was a smaller volume of paracetamol distribution in females (Wójcicki *et al.*, 1979a; Mucklow *et al.*, 1980; Abernethy *et al.*, 1982a; Divoll *et al.*, 1982a; Miners *et al.*, 1983). Following the oral administration of paracetamol in young females, the area under the plasma concentration–time curve and the maximum plasma concentration were greater, and the half life was longer in the luteal than in the follicular phase of the menstrual cycle, but the differences were not statistically significant (Wójcicki *et al.*, 1979a). In another study, salivary concentrations were measured after oral paracetamol in women on days 3, 10, 14, 20 and 25 of the menstrual cycle. There were no significant differences in half life or clearance but the decline in concentrations was markedly non-linear on each occasion and this could have been a reflection of the unreliability of paracetamol measurement in saliva (Somaja and Thangam, 1987). No sex differences in paracetamol metabolism could be demonstrated in microsomal fractions or isolated hepatocytes prepared from human liver samples obtained at surgery, and the pattern of metabolism was the same as *in vivo* (Kane *et al.*, 1990a; Herd *et al.*, 1991).

Pregnancy and the Use of Oral Contraceptives

The saliva half life of oral paracetamol was compared during the third trimester of pregnancy and in non-pregnant controls. The rate of paracetamol elimination was increased in the pregnant women, and this was associated with increased glucuronide conjugation and oxidative metabolism of the drug (Miners *et al.*, 1986). In one 27-year-old woman there was less pronounced sulphate conjugation one day before parturition than at 38 days after (Galinsky and Levy, 1984b). In another study, a 23-year-old woman took paracetamol before, and at the 12th, 20th and 30th weeks of pregnancy. The apparent clearance of paracetamol was considerably increased during pregnancy but there was no change in the plasma half life (Beaulac-Baillargeon and Rocheleau, 1993). The significance of these findings is uncertain because the clearance of paracetamol cannot be determined following oral administration as the fraction absorbed was not known. In keeping with these observations, the metabolism of paracetamol appeared to be faster in the immediate postpartum period than at six weeks after delivery (Gin *et al.*, 1991). However, an opposite result was obtained in a comparison of the metabolism of paracetamol in six healthy women at 36 weeks of gestation and six weeks after delivery. There were no significant changes in the half life and disposition of paracetamol in late pregnancy apart from the expected minor increase in volume of distribution (Rayburn *et al.*, 1986).

There were no differences in the half life, clearance and distribution of paracetamol in women taking conjugated oestrogen compared with age-matched controls but surprisingly their menopausal status was not mentioned (Scavone *et al.*, 1990b). Drug interactions have been described between paracetamol and oral contraceptives (Fazio, 1991). The clearance of paracetamol was increased in female factory and office workers who took oral contraceptives (Mucklow *et al.*, 1980) and other investigators have demonstrated an increased clearance and a decreased half life of paracetamol with no change in distribution volume in females taking low-dose oestrogen oral contraceptives (Table 7.3) (Abernethy *et al.*, 1982b; Miners *et al.*, 1983; Mitchell *et al.*, 1983; Ochs *et al.*, 1984). The faster elimination of paracetamol was due to increased glucuronide conjugation (Bock *et al.*, 1994). There was also a significant increase in the formation of glutathione derived conjugates but no enhancement of sulphate conjugation (Miners *et al.*, 1983; Mitchell *et al.*, 1983). In contrast to these reports, it was claimed that the sulphate conjugation of paracetamol was impaired in women with high oestrogen states due to pregnancy and the use of oral contraceptive steroids, and that this alleged deficiency in sulphate conjugation might be responsible for the condition of intrahepatic cholestasis of pregnancy (Davies *et al.*, 1994b). It is difficult to accept these findings as urine was only collected for 8 h after the paracetamol was given with a meal, and only a small unspecified fraction of the administered dose was recovered in the urine in this time. In addition, for some reason the method of analysis of the conjugates of paracetamol was indirect and depended on separate enzymic hydrolyses with and without the addition of inhibitors. In pregnant mice the sulphate conjugation of paracetamol was increased and glucuronide conjugation decreased with no change in the production of the glutathione-derived conjugates (Larrey *et al.*, 1986).

Table 7.3 Effects of oral contraceptives on the disposition of paracetamol in female subjects.

	Dose (mg)	Route	Half life (h)	Clearance (ml min^{-1})	Volume of distribution (l)	Source
Oral contraceptive users	650	iv	2.12	339	61	Abernethy et al., 1982b
Controls	650	iv	2.71	229	53	Abernethy et al., 1982b
Oral contraceptive users	1500	oral	1.67	470*	45*	Mitchell et al., 1983
Controls	1500	oral	2.40	287*	42*	Mitchell et al., 1983

* These values are given as $\dfrac{\text{clearance}}{F}$ and $\dfrac{\text{volume of distribution}}{F}$ where F is the unknown fraction of the dose absorbed unchanged

Genetic and Environmental Factors

Genetic deficiencies in bilirubin glucuronyl transferase may influence paracetamol metabolism. The Gunn rat has hereditary hyperbilirubinaemia with impaired ability to form glucuronide conjugates and in homozygous animals no glucuronide conjugation of paracetamol could be demonstrated in the isolated perfused kidney. Nephrotoxicity was enhanced but it was thought not to be due to increased intrarenal formation of the reactive metabolite (Emslie *et al.*, 1982). Compared with Wistar rats, the glucuronide conjugation of paracetamol in heterozygous and homozygous Gunn rats was decreased by 35 and 72 per cent respectively. There was correspondingly increased production of the glutathione-derived metabolites and greater hepatotoxicity and nephrotoxicity in the Gunn rats (de Morais and Wells, 1988, 1989). In congenic RHA rats with normal homozygous, moderately deficient heterozygous and severely deficient homozygous activities of glucuronyl transferase, reduced glucuronide conjugation of paracetamol in the latter groups was associated with increased bioactivation and hepato- and nephrotoxicity (de Morais *et al.*, 1992a).

The human counterparts of the Gunn rat are patients with Gilbert's disease and the Crigler-Najjar syndrome, but the deficiencies in glucuronyl transferase are not so marked. Minor decreases in the glucuronide conjugation of paracetamol were reported in patients with Gilbert's disease and the 24 h urinary recovery of cysteine and mercapturic acid conjugates (3.5 ± 0.4 per cent) was significantly higher than in controls (2.1 ± 0.3 per cent) but still well within the normal range. Among all subjects, glucuronidation correlated inversely with bioactivation (de Morais *et al.*, 1992b). In another study the total clearance of paracetamol following an intravenous dose of 1000 mg was 255 ± 23 ml min^{-1} in patients with Gilbert's disease compared with 352 ± 40 ml min^{-1} in healthy controls. There were no differences between the groups in plasma half life and oral bioavailability (Douglas *et al.*, 1978). In another study in 11 subjects with Gilbert's disease, the metabolism of paracetamol was virtually the same as in control subjects (Ullrich *et al.*, 1987). Although the glucuronide conjugation of paracetamol appeared to be normal in most subjects with Gilbert's disease, in some cases it was impaired with a marked increase in the excretion of metabolites derived from toxic bioactivation (Esteban and Pérez-Mateo, 1993b). There was some evidence for an effect of inheritance on the activity of thermolabile platelet sulphotransferase towards paracetamol in a study of 232 individuals from 49 families (Price *et al.*, 1988). The disposition of paracetamol was normal in subjects with Down's syndrome (Griener *et al.*, 1990). It has been suggested that the variability and changes in the plasma concentrations of paracetamol following administration of diphenylhydantoin might be under genetic control (Cunningham and Price Evans, 1981). However, the metabolic activation and conjugation of paracetamol were unrelated to the debrisoquine oxidation phenotype (Veronese and McLean, 1991).

Geographical and Ethnic Variation

Racial and ethnic variation in paracetamol metabolism has been described but it was often difficult to know whether the changes observed were caused primarily by genetic, dietary or environmental factors. There were no differences in the oral clearance and half life of paracetamol, or in its partial metabolic clearance by glucuronidation, sulphation and oxidation in healthy young Caucasian and Chinese males in South Australia (Osborne *et al.*, 1991). Similar negative findings were noted in rural and westernized Venda and Caucasian subjects in South Africa (Sommers *et al.*, 1987). The half life of paracetamol was essentially the same in Venda villagers as reported elsewhere, but it was claimed that the clearance was greater (Sommers *et al.*, 1985). The salivary clearance of paracetamol was similar in healthy Sudanese and Libyan volunteers (Ali and Sharif, 1993). The clearance of paracetamol was smaller in Asian than in white factory and office workers living in London but there were important differences between the groups in respect of diet and the use of alcohol, tobacco and oral contraceptives (Mucklow *et al.*, 1980). Indians living in Singapore excreted a significantly greater fraction of paracetamol as the glucuronide conjugate and a lesser fraction as the sulphate conjugate than Singapore Chinese, and in both groups the recovery of glutathione-derived conjugates was much less than previously reported in native Scots (Lee *et al.*, 1992). There were no major differences in the glucuronide and sulphate conjugation of paracetamol by Scots and East and West Africans in their own countries. However, there was greatly reduced metabolic activation of paracetamol in the Africans as shown by a very low urinary recovery of cysteine and mercapturic acid conjugates (Critchley *et al.*, 1986). In a comparison of 125 Caucasians and 33 Orientals in Canada, there were no differences in glucuronide and sulphate conjugation but again there was less metabolic activation of paracetamol in the Orientals (Patel *et al.*, 1992). Glucuronide and sulphate conjugation of paracetamol in a Spanish population were similar to that reported in Scotland and Africa but the production of oxidative metabolites was intermediate (Esteban and Pérez-Mateo, 1993a). The metabolism of paracetamol was the same in ethnic Spanish subjects from Alicante and the Basque region (Esteban *et al.*, 1994).

Individual Variation

There was considerable interindividual variation in paracetamol metabolism although the pattern within subjects was relatively constant (Shively and Vesell, 1975; Caldwell *et al.*, 1980; Critchley *et al.*, 1986). In comparisons between normal healthy mono- and di-zygotic twins there was a three-fold range in the rates of paracetamol elimination and glucuronide and sulphate conjugation. Individual variation in paracetamol metabolism arose largely from unidentified environmental rather than genetic factors (Nash *et al.*, 1984a). In Caucasians and Africans the mean urinary paracetamol sulphate to glucuronide ratios were 0.5–0.6, and there was a three-fold intersubject range in glucuronide and sulphate conjugation. As shown in Figure 7.6, the distributions of conjugates were somewhat skewed in Ghanaians but not in Caucasians and Kenyans. In contrast to the relatively uniform glucuronide and sulphate conjugation, there was a 60-fold variation in the urinary recovery of the cysteine and mercapturic acid conjugates and the potentially toxic metabolic activation of paracetamol was extensive in a small minority of individuals, especially Caucasians (Figure 7.7) (Critchley *et al.*, 1986). In a study in 179 healthy subjects there was a 10-fold range in the fraction of paracetamol appearing in the urine as oxidation products but as only a 2 h urine sample was collected, recovery would have been far from complete (Seddon *et al.*, 1987). In Spanish subjects there was an inverse relationship between the formation of the glucuronide and sulphate conju-

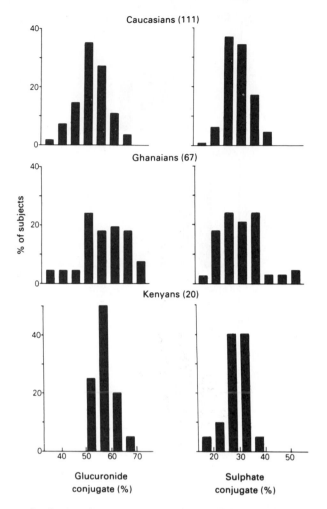

Figure 7.6 Frequency distributions (in 5 per cent increments) of the percentages of the total amounts excreted as paracetamol glucuronide and sulphate conjugates following oral doses of 1.5 g of paracetamol in 111 Caucasian, 67 Ghanaian and 20 Kenyan subjects (reproduced with permission from Critchley *et al.*, 1986).

gates of paracetamol and there was much greater individual variation in its metabolic activation (Esteban and Pérez-Mateo, 1993a). The pattern of urinary excretion of paracetamol glucuronide was thought to be bimodal in Caucasian and Oriental subjects, and there was also a bimodal recovery of the mercapturic acid conjugate relative to the recovery of total glutathione-derived conjugates (Patel *et al.*, 1992). Other investigators have not observed such bimodal distributions (Critchley *et al.*, 1986; Bock *et al.*, 1994).

Temporal Variation

Temporal variation has been noted in the distribution and half life of paracetamol administered at 6.00 am and 2.00 pm but there were no changes in glucuronidation

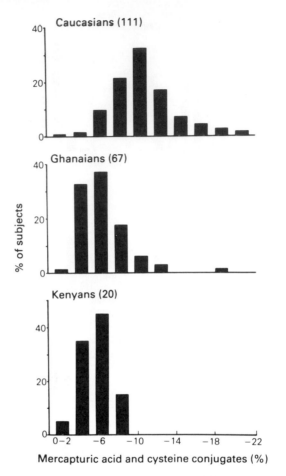

Figure 7.7 Frequency distributions (in 2 per cent increments) of the percentages of the total amounts excreted as the cysteine and mercapturic acid conjugates combined following oral doses of 1.5 g of paracetamol in 111 Caucasian, 67 Ghanaian and 20 Kenyan subjects (reproduced with permission from Critchley *et al.*, 1986).

(Shively and Vesell, 1975). In elderly patients, the paracetamol half life was significantly longer when it was given at 7.00 pm than at 7.00 am (Bruguerolle *et al.*, 1990). In other reports there were no changes in the kinetics of paracetamol given at different times of day (Malan *et al.*, 1985; Kamali *et al.*, 1987b). The latter investigators observed decreased urinary recovery of glucuronide conjugate during the 4 h after the drug was taken orally at 8.00 pm compared with 8.00 am and this was attributed to slower absorption at night. There was a circadian rhythm in hepatic uridine diphosphate (UDP) glucuronic acid in mice which was the reverse of that occurring with glucose and UDP-glucose. However, there were no differences in paracetamol glucuronidation at 8.00 am and 5.00 pm (Howell and Klaassen, 1991). In rats the extra-hepatic metabolism of paracetamol was significant at 9.00 pm, but not at 9.00 am. Thus, the gastrointestinal, pulmonary and hepatic extraction ratios were 0.18, 0.13 and 0.24 at 9.00 pm compared with 0.05, 0.00 and 0.41 respectively at 9.00 am (Bélanger *et al.*, 1987). Posture and sleep seemed to have no significant effect on the kinetics and disposition of paracetamol in man (Rumble *et al.*, 1991).

Smoking

The clearance of paracetamol was said to increase as cigarette consumption rose (Mucklow *et al.*, 1980), and its glucuronide conjugation was increased in heavy smokers as shown by the ratio of urinary metabolites to unchanged paracetamol (Bock *et al.*, 1987, 1994). However, the use of metabolic ratios in this way is not reliable because the renal clearance of paracetamol (but not its conjugates) changes with urine flow rate and the ratios are therefore not constant (Miners *et al.*, 1992). The kinetics and disposition of intravenous paracetamol were said to be the same in smokers and non-smokers (Scavone *et al.*, 1990c) but in another report, smokers eliminated less unchanged drug than non-smokers (Esteban and Pérez-Mateo, 1993a).

Diet and Nutrition

Diet and nutritional state can influence the metabolism of paracetamol but the changes described have not always been consistent and in some cases may have been complicated by dose effects.

Fasting

Fasting produced a paradoxical increase in hepatic glutathione in hamsters and this was associated with decreased production of the glucuronide and mercapturic acid conjugates of paracetamol with the result that the activities of the major pathway of elimination and toxic metabolic activation were decreased to a similar extent (Miller *et al.*, 1986). In rats, fasting decreased the sulphate conjugation of paracetamol and this could be partially restored by the provision of inorganic sulphate (Lauterburg and Mitchell, 1982). With a hepatotoxic dose, fasting decreased the glucuronidation of paracetamol in rats, and although glucuronyl transferase activity was unchanged, the synthetic capacity to form uridine diphosphate glucuronic acid was reduced (Price *et al.*, 1986b; Price and Jollow, 1988). The decrease in glucuronide conjugation induced by fasting could not be reversed by administration of glucose or gluconeogenic substrates (Price and Jollow, 1989a). In another study, the rate of elimination of paracetamol was decreased in fasted compared to fed rats and this was due to reduced conjugation with both glucuronide and sulphate. There was a corresponding increase in the fraction of the dose converted to glutathione-derived conjugates and hepatotoxicity was increased (Price *et al.*, 1987). In fasted (but not fed) rats ethanol produced significant impairment of paracetamol glucuronidation due to failure of compensatory mechanisms to maintain the redox state (Minnigh and Zemaitis, 1982). A three-day fast had only a minor effect on the plasma clearance and half life of paracetamol in horses (Engelking *et al.*, 1987a).

Obesity

Following the intravenous administration of 30 mg kg^{-1} of paracetamol, plasma concentrations were higher, and the clearance and volume of distribution were lower in obese than lean Zucker rats (Blouin *et al.*, 1987). The findings were rather different in another study in rats made obese by feeding an energy-dense diet. The paracetamol half life did not change but the volume of distribution increased and plasma concentrations were lower and less sulphate conjugate was excreted (Corcoran *et al.*, 1987c). The increased glucuronide and decreased sulphate conjugation of paracetamol in overfed obese rats was associated with increased hepato- and nephrotoxicity (Corcoran and Wong, 1987). In another study of obese Zucker rats the capacity for glucuronide conjugation was increased but there was no change in other metabolic pathways (Chaudhary *et al.*, 1993). Obesity, produced by an energy-dense diet in rats, was associated with increased activity of liver microsomal cyto-chrome P450 and the CYP2E1 isozyme, and enhanced oxidation of paracetamol (Raucy *et al.*, 1991). A high fat diet increased the toxic metabolic activation of para-cetamol in ferrets and this was associated with an increase in a protein orthologous to the rat CYP1A1 form of cytochrome P450 (Shavila *et al.*, 1994). Enhanced meta-bolic activation and increased glucuronide and sulphate conjugation of paracetamol was observed in another study in an overfed rat model (Wong *et al.*, 1986b).

Dietary Factors in Animals

Rats were maintained on a diet low in sulphur containing amino acids with methi-onine as the only source of sulphur. Following a low dose of 20 mg kg^{-1}, paraceta-mol was eliminated more slowly than in control animals fed a normal diet, and this was due to a marked reduction in sulphate conjugation. In contrast, after a high dose of 400 mg kg^{-1}, the clearance of paracetamol was increased compared with controls because glucuronide conjugation was enhanced, and this was now the dom-inant pathway of elimination. The formation of mercapturic acid conjugate was also increased (Price and Jollow, 1989b). In rats fed a low protein and low sulphur diet, pretreatment with paracetamol lowered the serum concentration of inorganic sul-phate and decreased the sulphate conjugation of phenol (Krijgsheld *et al.*, 1981). Low methionine and cysteine diets reduced urinary inorganic sulphate and the sul-phate conjugation of paracetamol but its glutathione conjugation was maintained even though hepatic glutathione was reduced (Glazenburg *et al.*, 1983). A low sulphur diet moderately reduced the sulphate conjugation of paracetamol in rats while the administration of molybdate (an alternative substrate for intestinal and renal sulphate transport, and for ATP-sulphurylase) resulted in marked inhibition of paracetamol sulphation (Gregus *et al.*, 1994b). Combined dietary deficiencies of inorganic sulphate and cysteine had a much greater effect in limiting the sulphate conjugation of paracetamol than either deficiency alone (Gregus *et al.*, 1994a). The intracellular concentration of 3-phosphoadenosine-5-phosphosulphate (PAPS) in isolated rat hepatocytes was determined by the concentration of sulphate ion, and the sulphate conjugation of paracetamol increased as this rose to 1 mM after which there was no further increase (Sweeny and Reinke, 1988). The impaired sulphate conjugation of paracetamol caused by reduced availability of sulphate could be alle-viated by administration of inorganic sulphate or a donor such as N-acetylcysteine. The major mechanism of inorganic sulphate homeostasis was non-linear renal clear-ance due to saturable tubular reabsorption (Levy, 1986). Methionine deficiency compromised the normal pathways of paracetamol metabolism in mice, and this effect was potentiated by chronic intake of ethanol, which increased the extent of metabolic activation (Reicks and Hathcock, 1987).

In rats given a diet deficient in thiamine there was an unexpected increase in the elimination rate of paracetamol caused by enhanced glucuronide and sulphate conjugation (Ruchirawat *et al.*, 1981). In a comparison of diets containing 20 per cent fish oil or 20 per cent olive oil, glucuronide conjugation of paracetamol in mice was increased with the fish oil diet while sulphate conjugation and hepatotoxicity were decreased. Fluidization of microsomal membranes was proposed as a mechanism (Speck and Lauterburg, 1991). Protein-calorie malnutrition in rats induced by feeding a diet containing 5 per cent protein resulted in a reduced clearance of paracetamol and excretion of a smaller fraction of the dose as sulphate, and a greater fraction as glucuronide conjugate (Jung, 1985). The induction of a reduced hepatic energy state in rats by treatment with ethionine or fructose impaired the conjugation and oxidative metabolism of paracetamol and reduced the biliary and renal excretion of metabolites (Dills and Klaassen, 1986). Ascorbic acid deficiency in guinea pigs was not associated with decreased hepatic microsomal glucuronidation of paracetamol (Neumann and Zannoni, 1988).

Studies in Man

The sulphate conjugation of paracetamol following a single dose did not differ in healthy subjects from Saskatoon and Rosetown, areas which had low and high concentrations respectively of sulphate in the municipal drinking water. However, during multiple dosing there was a fall in serum sulphate and reduced sulphate conjugation of paracetamol in the volunteers from Saskatoon (Hindmarsh *et al.*, 1991). The mean half life of paracetamol was significantly longer in infants and children with protein-energy malnutrition than in controls (8.14 h compared with 4.33 h), and there was a decrease in half life in the malnourished children after 'nutritional rehabilitation' (Mehta *et al.*, 1982, 1985). However, in another similar study, the half life of paracetamol was not prolonged in malnourished adults (Kohli *et al.*, 1982). The half life of paracetamol was the same in obese and normal subjects, and its overall disposition was not altered by weight loss of 8–30 kg (Lee *et al.*, 1981b). In another study of obese and control subjects given 650 mg of paracetamol intravenously, there were no differences between the groups in the half life or weight-corrected clearance of paracetamol, but the corrected volume of distribution was less in the obese subjects and the clearance of paracetamol in obese subjects was correlated with the clearances of lorazepam and oxazepam (Abernethy *et al.*, 1982a, 1983b). The rate of elimination of paracetamol was not influenced by calorie intake ranging from 21 to 66 kcal kg^{-1} in healthy young male volunteers (Yiamouyiannis *et al.*, 1994). A diet containing charcoal-broiled beef had little or no effect on the metabolism of paracetamol (Anderson *et al.*, 1983), but its glucuronidation was increased by a diet containing brussels sprouts and cabbage (Pantuck *et al.*, 1984). A change from a high-protein, low-carbohydrate to a low-protein, high-carbohydrate diet resulted in a minor increase in the recovery of paracetamol glucuronide with a corresponding decrease in other pathways (Pantuck *et al.*, 1991). A change in parenteral nutrition from dextrose to different branched amino acids had no effect on the metabolic clearance and conjugation of paracetamol in healthy volunteers (Pantuck *et al.*, 1989).

The salivary clearance of paracetamol was greater in Caucasians than in largely vegetarian Asians living in London, but factors other than diet could have been responsible (Mucklow *et al.*, 1980). The saliva clearance of paracetamol in these groups was said to be less than the plasma clearance in black African Venda villagers taking a mainly maize cereal and vegetable diet (Sommers *et al.*, 1985). In another study there were no differences in saliva concentrations of paracetamol, or urinary excretion of glucuronide and sulphate conjugates, in rural Venda villagers taking a traditional largely lactovegetarian diet, Vendas who had adopted a Western lifestyle and diet, and Caucasian students in South Africa (Sommers *et al.*, 1987). Similarly, there were no differences in paracetamol disposition in Caucasian and Thai vegetarians and non-vegetarians (Brodie *et al.*, 1980; Prescott *et al.*, 1993). Ethnic differences have been noted by some (Critchley *et al.*, 1986) but not other investigators (Osborne *et al.*, 1991; Lee *et al.*, 1992), but it has not been possible to define the contribution, if any, of dietary factors. The most significant finding has been a lower fractional urinary recovery of paracetamol cysteine and mercapturic acid conjugates reflecting reduced metabolic activation in Africans (Critchley *et al.*, 1986) and Singapore Indians and Chinese (Lee *et al.*, 1992) compared with Caucasians in Scotland and Australia, and Australian Chinese (Critchley *et al.*, 1986; Osborne *et al.*, 1991). Similar differences were observed between Caucasians and Orientals in Canada but the possible role of dietary factors was not considered (Patel *et al.*, 1992).

Stimulation and Inhibition of Paracetamol Metabolism

Many agents can stimulate or inhibit drug metabolism, and this subject has been of particular interest with paracetamol because changes in the extent of its oxidation by cytochrome P450 have usually been associated with corresponding changes in hepatotoxicity (Mitchell *et al.*, 1973b, 1974; Potter *et al.*, 1973; Davis *et al.*, 1974a; Hinson *et al.*, 1977; Hinson, 1980). However, pretreatment with classical inducing agents such as phenobarbitone did not always potentiate toxicity as expected (Poulsen *et al.*, 1985b) and in some circumstances it even protected against liver damage (Potter *et al.*, 1974; Blouin *et al.*, 1987). The reasons for this paradox are uncertain but the purified isozymes of cytochrome P450 that are inducible by phenobarbitone in animals were not necessarily very active in the oxidation of paracetamol (Ioannides *et al.*, 1983b; Morgan *et al.*, 1983; Steele *et al.*, 1983). In addition, the different pathways of paracetamol metabolism may be affected to a greater or lesser extent by enzyme induction, and toxicity depended on the balance between the activities of the parallel toxic and non-toxic routes of elimination. There have been numerous reports of altered susceptibility to paracetamol hepatotoxicity following pretreatment with a variety of agents. Unfortunately many investigators have made the uncritical and unsubstantiated assumption that the changes observed were the result of induction or inhibition of its metabolism and other mechanisms have not been excluded.

Mechanisms

The repeated administration of many drugs and chemicals results in the induction of paracetamol metabolism and this process involved increased formation of drug metabolizing enzymes over a period of days or weeks as distinct from the immediate increase in enzyme activity that may follow exposure to agents such as detergents. The metabolism of paracetamol was impaired by treatments that caused depletion of essential cofactors (Büch *et al.*, 1966a; Levy *et al.*, 1982; Galinsky, 1986), competitive and non-competitive enzyme inhibition (Bolanowska and Gessner, 1978) and destruction of liver enzymes as a result of hepatotoxicity (Prescott *et al.*, 1971; Siegers *et al.*, 1980). From a mechanistic point of view it was important to differentiate between biochemical and metabolic effects, such as the inhibition of the *in vitro* glutathione conjugation of paracetamol by cyanide (Sato and Marumo, 1991), and toxicological interactions, such as impairment of drug metabolism as a result of hepatic necrosis following paracetamol overdosage (Forrest *et al.*, 1974).

Assessment

An increase or decrease in the overall rate of the disappearance of paracetamol from the circulation can be used as an index of induction or inhibition of major routes of elimination, such as glucuronide conjugation. Pharmacokinetic models have been developed to predict the effects of different inducing agents (Bachmann, 1989) and the consequences of induction on the hepatic disposition of paracetamol and its metabolites (Studenberg and Brouwer, 1993a). The effects of other agents on paracetamol metabolism could usually be demonstrated by changes in the pattern of

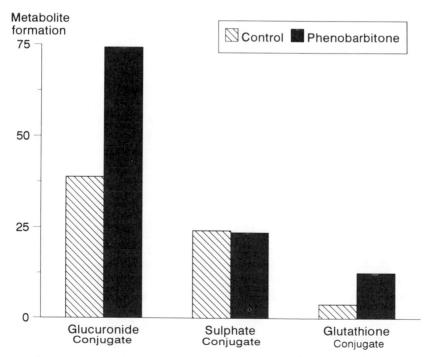

Figure 7.8   Effects of pretreatment with phenobarbitone (80 mg kg^{-1} for three days) on the formation of the glucuronide, sulphate and glutathione conjugates of paracetamol by isolated rat hepatocytes (data from Moldéus, 1978).

129

metabolites excreted in the urine and there were also changes in the pattern of their excretion into bile (Siegers and Schütt, 1979; Loeser and Siegers, 1985; Gregus *et al.*, 1988a, 1990; Madhu *et al.*, 1989; Brouwer and Jones, 1990). These effects on paracetamol metabolism have also been demonstrated in liver microsomal fractions, isolated hepatocytes in culture and perfused liver preparations, and an example of the effect of pretreatment with phenobarbitone on the metabolic activation and glucuronide conjugation of paracetamol by mouse liver microsomes is shown in Figure 7.8.

Induction and Inhibition Studies

Reports of the effects of a variety of drugs and chemicals on the metabolism of paracetamol are summarized in Table 7.4. In general, classical inducers of drug metabolism such as phenobarbitone, 3-methylcholanthrene and polychlorinated biphenyls increased the metabolic activation, covalent binding and toxicity of paracetamol in laboratory animals but the findings cannot be readily extrapolated to man. As shown in Table 7.4, the increase in oxidative metabolism was often associated with increased glucuronide (but not sulphate) conjugation. Indeed, as judged by some studies of urinary recovery, induction seemed to *decrease* sulphate conjugation. However, this is a kinetic artefact because the decrease was only relative to the increased capacity for glucuronide conjugation, which was usually the major pathway of removal. The effects of induction with anticonvulsants or rifampicin on the disposition of paracetamol in man are shown in Figure 7.9. The area under the plasma concentration–time curve and the plasma half life were reduced and production of the glucuronide conjugate was increased (Prescott *et al.*, 1981). Studies of the induction and inhibition of paracetamol metabolism have often yielded conflicting and anomalous results, presumably because of differences in experimental design and conditions. There may also be important species and strain differences in response (Mitchell *et al.*, 1973b; Moldéus and Gergely, 1980b; Lubek *et al.*, 1988b; Liu *et al.*, 1991, 1992b; Madhu *et al.*, 1992b) and other relevant variables included the effects of age (Lee *et al.*, 1991b), duration of treatment (Altomare *et al.*, 1984a) and dose (Roberts *et al.*, 1986). Inducing agents could cause extrahepatic stimulation of paracetamol metabolism in organs such as the kidney, lung and spleen (Emslie *et al.*, 1981a; Newton *et al.*, 1982a,b; Bock *et al.*, 1993).

Isoenzyme Specificity

Some inducers and inhibitors of drug metabolism have selective effects on specific isozymes of cytochrome P450 and this has facilitated the investigation of the different forms of this enzyme that are involved in the metabolic activation of paracetamol (Seddon *et al.*, 1987; Harvison *et al.*, 1988b). In addition, it seemed likely that interactions between paracetamol and drugs such as caffeine and ethanol were isozyme specific (Nouchi *et al.*, 1986; Raucy *et al.*, 1989; Jeffery *et al.*, 1991; Lee *et al.*, 1991a,b; Jaw and Jeffery, 1993). Complex interactions could occur as a result of induction of specific isoforms of cytochrome P450. Thus the glutathione conjugation of paracetamol was increased in mice previously induced with phenobarbitone and dexamethasone, but decreased in mice induced with acetone and β-flavonaphthone (Jaw and Jeffery, 1993). Ethanol induced the perivenous zone-specific oxidation of

(cont.)

Table 7.4 Effects of drugs and chemicals on the rate of paracetamol elimination and on the formation or urinary excretion of paracetamol conjugates.

Agent	Species	Glucuronide conjugate	Sulphate conjugate	Glutathione-derived conjugates	Rate of elimination	Reference
Acetaldehyde	rat*			decreased	decreased	Sato et al., 1991
Acetone	mouse*			no change		Moldéus and Gergely, 1980b
Acetone	rat	no change	decreased	decreased	decreased	Price and Jollow, 1983
Acetone	mouse*			increased	increased	Jeffery et al., 1991
Acetone	rat*			increased		Lee et al., 1991b
Acetone	mouse**			increased		Jaw and Jeffery, 1993
Acetone	man[1]			increased		Roe et al., 1993
N-Acetylcysteine	mouse	no change	decreased	increased	no change	Piperno et al., 1978
N-Acetylcysteine	rat	decreased	increased		increased	Galinsky and Levy, 1979
N-Acetylcysteine	man	decreased	increased	increased		Prescott, 1980
N-Acetylcysteine	mouse**	no change	decreased	increased		Massey and Racz, 1981
N-Acetylcysteine	dog			increased	increased	St Omer and Mohammad, 1984
N-Acetylcysteine	mouse	no change	no change	no change	no change	Corcoran et al., 1985b
N-Acetylcysteine	cat	decreased	increased	no change	increased	Savides et al., 1985
N-Acetylcysteine	mouse	no change	increased	increased	increased	Whitehouse et al., 1985
N-Acetylcysteine	mouse	no change	no change	increased		Corcoran and Wong, 1986
N-D-Acetylcysteine	mouse	no change	increased	no change		Corcoran and Wong, 1986
N-Acetylcysteine	mouse	no change				Wong et al., 1986a
N-Acetylcysteine	man	no change	increased			Reiter and Naudorf, 1987
N-Acetylcysteine	man	no change	increased	increased		Slattery et al., 1987
N-Acetylcysteine	mouse				no change	Peterson and Brown, 1992
Amantidine	man	no change	no change	no change	no change	Aoki and Sitar, 1992
Amiodarone	rat	no change	no change	no change	no change	Svensson and Chong, 1989
Anaesthesia[2]	man				no change	Lewis et al., 1991
Aniline	man*	decreased	increased	decreased		Seddon et al., 1987
Antipyrine	man				decreased	Blyden et al., 1988
Antipyrine	man				decreased	Awni et al., 1990

Table 7.4 *(cont.)*

Agent	Species	Glucuronide conjugate	Sulphate conjugate	Glutathione-derived conjugates	Rate of elimination	Reference
Anti-tuberculous drugs[3]	man				increased	Madhusudanarao et al., 1988a
Ascorbic acid	man	increased	decreased		decreased	Houston and Levy, 1976
Ascorbic acid	hamster	no change	no change		no change	Miller and Jollow, 1984
Borneol	hamster**	decreased	decreased	no change		Smith and Jollow, 1977
Butanediol	rat	no change	decreased	decreased	decreased	Price and Jollow, 1983
Buthionine sulphoximine	mouse	no change	no change	decreased		Drew and Miners, 1984
Buthionine sulphoximine	rat	no change	increased		increased	Galinsky, 1986
Buthionine sulphoximine	rat	increased	decreased		no change	Manning et al., 1991
Butylated hydroxyanisole	rat**	increased	no change			Moldéus et al., 1982b
Butylated hydroxyanisole	mouse*	increased	increased	increased		Hazelton et al., 1985
Butylated hydroxyanisole	mouse	increased	increased		increased	Hazelton et al., 1986b
Butylated hydroxyanisole	man	no change	no change	no change		Verhagen et al., 1989
Butylated hydroxyanisole	rat*	increased				Goon and Klaassen, 1992
Caffeine	rat*			increased		Nouchi et al., 1986
Caffeine	mouse	increased	decreased	decreased	decreased	Price and Gale, 1987
Caffeine	rat**	decreased		increased	no change	Sato and Izumi, 1989
Caffeine	rat*			increased		Lee et al., 1991a
Caffeine	rat*			increased		Lee et al., 1991b
Caffeine	rat			increased		Liu et al., 1992b
Caffeine	mouse			no change		Liu et al., 1992b
Caffeine	rat				no change	Granados-Soto et al., 1993
Caffeine	mouse*			increased		Jaw and Jeffery, 1993
Caffeine	man				no change	Wójcicki et al., 1994
Carbamazepine	man				increased	Perucca and Richens, 1979
Carbamazepine	man	increased	decreased	no change	increased	Prescott et al., 1981
Carbamazepine	man	increased	decreased	increased	increased	Miners et al., 1984c
Carbon tetrachloride	rat	decreased	no change	no change		Siegers and Schütt, 1979
Carbon tetrachloride	rat	no change	no change	no change		Siegers et al., 1980

(cont.)

Factor	Species					Reference
Chloramphenicol	rat	decreased				Bolanowska and Gessner, 1978
Chloroquine	man	no change	no change	no change	no change	Adjepon-Yamoah et al., 1986
Cigarette smoke	man	no change		no change	increased	Mucklow et al., 1980
Cigarette smoke	man	increased	no change	no change	no change	Miners et al., 1984c
Cigarette smoke	man	increased	no change			Bock et al., 1987
Cigarette smoke	man				no change	Scavone et al., 1990c
Cigarette smoke	man	increased				Bock et al., 1994
Cimetidine	man		decreased		no change	Abernethy et al., 1982c, 1983a
Cimetidine	rat	no change	no change	no change	decreased	Galinsky and Levy, 1982
Cimetidine	man	no change	no change	no change	no change	Critchley et al., 1983
Cimetidine	mouse	no change	no change	no change		Miners et al., 1984a
Cimetidine	man	no change		decreased	no change	Miners et al., 1984c
Cimetidine	rat*			no change		Mitchell et al., 1984b
Cimetidine	man*	no change	no change		no change	Mitchell et al., 1984b
Cimetidine	man			no change	no change	Chen and Lee, 1985
Cimetidine	rat	increased	no change			Emery et al., 1985
Cimetidine	man*			no change	no change	Seddon et al., 1987
Cimetidine	man	no change	no change	no change		Vendemiale et al., 1987
Cimetidine	rat			decreased		Bachmann, 1989
Cimetidine	man	no change	no change	no change	no change	Slattery et al., 1989
Cimetidine	rabbit				no change	Ali et al., 1993
Cimetidine	rat**		no change	decreased		Dalhoff and Poulsen, 1993a
Cobaltous chloride	mouse			decreased	no change	Mitchell et al., 1973b
Cobaltous chloride[4]	hamster*	increased	decreased	decreased	increased	Roberts et al., 1986
Cobaltous chloride[5]	hamster*	increased	no change	no change	decreased	Roberts et al., 1986
Cobaltous chloride	hamster**	increased	decreased	decreased		Roberts et al., 1986
Codeine	man	no change	no change	no change	no change	Sonne et al., 1988
+-Cyanidanol	rat	decreased	no change	decreased		Siegers et al., 1980
Cyclosporin	rat	no change	no change		decreased	Galinsky et al., 1987a
Cyclosporin	man			decreased	increased	D'Souza et al., 1989
Cysteamine	mouse*					Buckpitt et al., 1979
Cysteamine	man	no change	no change	no change		Forrest et al., 1982
Cysteamine	hamster	no change	increased	decreased	decreased	Miller and Jollow, 1986a

133

Table 7.4 (cont.)

Agent	Species	Glucuronide conjugate	Sulphate conjugate	Glutathione-derived conjugates	Rate of elimination	Reference
Cysteamine	mouse				no change	Peterson and Brown, 1992
Cysteamine	rabbit				decreased	Ali et al., 1993
Desipramine	man			no change	no change	Mitchell et al., 1974
Dexamethasone	mouse			increased		Jaw and Jeffery, 1993
Dichloronitrophenol	rat	no change	decreased	no change		Fayz et al., 1984
Dicoumarol	rat*	decreased				Bolanowska and Gessner, 1978
Diethyldithiocarbamate	rat	decreased	no change	decreased		Younes et al., 1979
Diethyldithiocarbamate	rat	no change	no change	decreased		Siegers et al., 1980
Diethylether	rat**	decreased	decreased		decreased	Aune et al., 1981
Diethylether	rat	decreased	decreased		decreased	Johannessen et al., 1981
Diethylether	rat**		decreased	increased		Aune et al., 1984
Diethylether	mouse	no change	decreased	no change	decreased	To and Wells, 1986
Diethylmaleate	rat	decreased	no change	decreased		Younes et al., 1979
Diethylmaleate	rat	increased	decreased			Siegers et al., 1980
Diethylmaleate	rat	no change	no change		decreased	Galinsky, 1986
Diftalone	man	no change	no change	no change	no change	Buniva et al., 1977
Dimethylprostaglandin E₂	rat	no change	no change	no change		Raheja et al., 1985
Dimethylsulphoxide	rat	no change	no change	decreased		Younes et al., 1979
Dimethylsulphoxide	rat			decreased		Jeffery et al., 1988
Dimethylsulphoxide	mouse			decreased		Jeffery et al., 1991
Diphenylhydantoin	man				increased	Perucca and Richens, 1979
Diphenylhydantoin	man				increased	Cunningham and Price Evans, 1981
Diphenylhydantoin	man	increased	decreased	no change	increased	Prescott et al., 1981
Diphenylhydantoin	man	increased	decreased	increased	increased	Miners et al., 1984c
Diphenylhydantoin	man*	increased				Bock and Bock-Hennig, 1987
Diphenylhydantoin	man	increased	no change	increased		Bock et al., 1987
Diphenylhydantoin	man	increased	decreased	no change		Dolara et al., 1987
Disulfiram	man	no change	no change	no change	no change	Poulsen et al., 1991

Compound	Species				Reference
Ebselen	mouse**			decreased	Harman et al., 1992a
Enflurane	rat**	no change			Aune et al., 1983
Enflurane	rat			no change	Hanna et al., 1989
Enflurane	rat			no change	Watkins, 1989
Ethanol[c]	man			decreased	Shamszad et al., 1975
Ethanol[a]	man				Wójcicki et al., 1978
Ethanol[a]	man	increased	increased	decreased	Wójcicki et al., 1978
Ethanol[a]	rat	decreased	decreased	decreased	Wójcicki et al., 1978
Ethanol[c]	rat**	increased	no change	increased	Moldéus et al., 1980a
Ethanol[c]	man			increased	Mucklow et al., 1980
Ethanol[a]	rat	decreased	no change	decreased	Siegers et al., 1980
Ethanol[a]	mouse	no change	no change	no change	Wong et al., 1980b
Ethanol[c]	rat	no change	no change	decreased	Sato and Lieber, 1981
Ethanol[c]	rat	no change	no change	increased	Sato et al., 1981a
Ethanol[a]	man		decreased	decreased	Banda and Quart, 1982
Ethanol[c]	man	no change	no change	no change	Critchley et al., 1982
Ethanol[c]	man			no change	Dietz et al., 1982
Ethanol[a]	man	no change	no change	decreased	Critchley et al., 1983
Ethanol[c]	man	no change	no change	increased	Villeneuve et al., 1983
Ethanol[a]	man		decreased	decreased	Altomare et al., 1984a
Ethanol[c]	rat	no change	no change	decreased	Altomare et al., 1984a
Ethanol[a]	baboon	no change	no change	increased	Altomare et al., 1984b
Ethanol[a]	baboon	no change	no change	decreased	Altomare et al., 1984b
Ethanol[c]	man			no change	Dietz et al., 1984
Ethanol[c]	rat	no change	no change	no change	Vendemiale et al., 1984
Ethanol[a]	mouse	decreased	increased	decreased	Tredger et al., 1986b
Ethanol[c]	mouse	increased	no change	no change	Tredger et al., 1986b
Ethanol[a]	rat***	decreased	no change	decreased	Schlager et al., 1987
Ethanol[c]	rat	no change	no change	no change	Thummel et al., 1988
Ethanol[c]	rat		increased	increased	Prasad et al., 1990
Ethanol[a]	man		no change	no change	Skinner et al., 1990
Ethanol[c]	rat*		decreased	decreased	Sato et al., 1991
Ethanol[a]	mouse*		decreased	decreased	Sato et al., 1991

135

Table 7.4 (cont.)

Agent	Species	Glucuronide conjugate	Sulphate conjugate	Glutathione-derived conjugates	Rate of elimination	Reference
Ethanol[a]	rabbit*			decreased	decreased	Sato et al., 1991
Ethanol[a]	rat				decreased	Linhares and Kissinger, 1994
Ethanol[c]	rat				decreased	Linhares and Kissinger, 1994
Flavone	rat*			increased	variable	Lee et al., 1991b
Flavonoids	rat**				variable	Li et al., 1994c
Flavonoids	man**					Li et al., 1994c
5-Fluorouracil	rat	no change	no change		decreased	Bolanowska and Gessner, 1980
Galactosamine	rat	no change	no change		no change	Bolanowska and Gessner, 1980
Galactosamine	rat	decreased	no change	increased	decreased	Gregus et al., 1988a
Galactosamine	rat	decreased	no change	no change	increased	Gregus et al., 1990
Garlic	man	no change	no change	no change	no change	Gwilt et al., 1994
Halothane	rat**				decreased	Aune et al., 1983
Halothane	man				no change	Ray et al., 1986
Halothane	rat				no change	Watkins, 1989
Heparin	rat				no change	Scott et al., 1991
Hydroxyzine	rat*	decreased			no change	Bolanowska and Gessner, 1978
Ibuprofen	man				no change	Wright et al., 1983
Indomethacin	rat				no change	van Kolfschoten et al., 1985
Indomethacin	man				no change	Seideman, 1991
Isoflurane	rat				no change	Watkins, 1989
Isoniazid	man					Ochs et al., 1984
Isoniazid	rat*			increased		Seddon et al., 1987
Isoniazid	man	no change	no change	decreased	decreased	Epstein et al., 1991
Isoniazid	man	increased	increased	decreased		Zand et al., 1993
Ketoconazole	man*				decreased	Seddon et al., 1987
Ketoconazole	mouse*				decreased	Seddon et al., 1987
Methotrexate	man	no change	no change	no change	no change	Kamali et al., 1988
Methoxsalen	mouse	increased	no change	decreased	no change	Letteron et al., 1986

(cont.)

Methoxsalen	man	no change	no change	no change	Amouyal et al., 1987
Methoxsalen	man	no change	no change	no change	Larrey et al., 1987
3-Methylcholanthrene	cat	no change	decreased		Welch et al., 1966
3-Methylcholanthrene	hamster	no change	no change		Jollow et al., 1974
3-Methylcholanthrene	hamster	decreased	no change		Potter et al., 1974
3-Methylcholanthrene	rat	no change	no change		Thomas et al., 1977b
3-Methylcholanthrene	rat	increased	decreased		Coon et al., 1984
3-Methylcholanthrene	mouse	no change	no change		Miners et al., 1984a
3-Methylcholanthrene	hamster	increased	no change		Lupo et al., 1987
3-Methylcholanthrene	rat*	decreased	no change		Seddon et al., 1987
3-Methylcholanthrene	mouse[6]	decreased	increased		Lubek et al., 1988b
3-Methylcholanthrene	mouse[7]	increased	decreased		Lubek et al., 1988b
3-Methylcholanthrene	rat	decreased	decreased		Gregus et al., 1990
3-Methylcholanthrene	mouse*	no change	increased		Jeffery et al., 1991
Metiamide	rat*	increased	decreased	no change	Mitchell et al., 1984b
Metyrapone	man	increased	no change	no change	Galinsky et al., 1987b
Metyrapone	man*		no change	no change	Seddon et al., 1987
Metyrapone	mouse*			increased	Seddon et al., 1987
Metyrapone	rat			no change	Galinsky and Corcoran, 1988
Metyrapone	rat			no change	Lee et al., 1991b
Molybdate	rat			increased	Oguro et al., 1994
Morphine	rat			no change	Bolanowska and Gessner, 1978
β-Naphthoflavone	rat			decreased	Bachmann, 1989
β-Naphthoflavone	mouse			increased	Jaw and Jeffery, 1993
Oestrogen, conjugated	man			decreased	Scavone et al., 1990b
Oleanolic acid	mouse			increased	Liu et al., 1993
Oltipraz	hamster			no change	Davies and Schnell, 1991
Oral contraceptives	man			increased	Mucklow et al., 1980
Oral contraceptives	man			increased	Abernethy et al., 1982b
Oral contraceptives	man			increased	Miners et al., 1983
Oral contraceptives	man			increased	Mitchell et al., 1983
Oral contraceptives	man			increased	Ochs et al., 1984
Oxazepam	mouse	decreased			Dybing, 1976

Table 7.4 (*cont.*)

Agent	Species	Glucuronide conjugate	Sulphate conjugate	Glutathione-derived conjugates	Rate of elimination	Reference
Oxazepam	man	no change	no change	no change	no change	Sonne et al., 1986
Oxytetracycline	goat				decreased	Manna et al., 1994
Pentobarbitone	man*	increased	increased			Bock and Bock-Hennig, 1987
Phenobarbitone	rat	increased	no change			Büch et al., 1966a
Phenobarbitone	rat	increased			increased	Büch et al., 1967a
Phenobarbitone	rat					Mitchell et al., 1973b
Phenobarbitone	mouse				no change	Mitchell et al., 1973b
Phenobarbitone	hamster	increased	decreased	decreased		Jollow et al., 1974
Phenobarbitone	dog				no change	Kampffmeyer, 1974
Phenobarbitone	man			increased	no change	Mitchell et al., 1974
Phenobarbitone	hamster			increased		Potter et al., 1974
Phenobarbitone	rat		decreased			Potter et al., 1974
Phenobarbitone	mouse*	no change				Dybing, 1976
Phenobarbitone	rat	increased	no change	no change	increased	Thomas et al., 1977b
Phenobarbitone	rat**	increased	no change	increased		Moldéus, 1978
Phenobarbitone	man				increased	Perucca and Richens, 1979
Phenobarbitone	rat	increased	decreased	increased		Younes et al., 1979
Phenobarbitone	rat	increased	decreased			Bolanowska and Gessner, 1980
Phenobarbitone	rat	increased	no change	increased		Siegers et al., 1980
Phenobarbitone	man	increased	decreased	no change		Prescott et al., 1981
Phenobarbitone	mouse	no change	no change	increased	increased	Miners et al., 1984a
Phenobarbitone	rat	increased	no change	no change		Poulsen et al., 1985b
Phenobarbitone	man	increased	decreased	no change		Dolara et al., 1987
Phenobarbitone	hamster		no change	no change		Lupo et al., 1987
Phenobarbitone	rat*			increased		Seddon et al., 1987
Phenobarbitone	rat	increased	decreased		increased	Bachmann, 1989
Phenobarbitone	rat	increased	no change	increased	increased	Brouwer and Jones, 1990
Phenobarbitone	rat	increased		increased	increased	Gregus et al., 1990

(cont.)

Compound	Species				Reference
Phenobarbitone	mouse*	increased	no change		Jeffery et al., 1991
Phenobarbitone	rat*	decreased	increased		Lee et al., 1991a
Phenobarbitone	rat*	increased			Goon and Klaassen, 1992
Phenobarbitone	rat	decreased	decreased		Brouwer, 1993
Phenobarbitone	rat	increased	no change	increased	Chaudhary et al., 1993
Phenobarbitone	mouse*	increased	increased		Jaw and Jeffery, 1993
Phenobarbitone	rat**	decreased	decreased		Studenberg and Brouwer, 1993b
Phenylbutazone	man			increased	Gmyrek et al., 1971
Phenolphthalein	rat*	decreased	decreased		Bolanowska and Gessner, 1978
Piperonyl butoxide	mouse	decreased		decreased	Mitchell et al., 1973b
Piperonyl butoxide	hamster	decreased	increased		Jollow et al., 1974
Piperonyl butoxide	hamster			decreased	Potter et al., 1974
Piperonyl butoxide	mouse	no change	no change		Miners et al., 1984a
Piperonyl butoxide	mouse	decreased	no change		Miners et al., 1984b
Piperonyl butoxide	rat			decreased	Bachmann, 1989
Piperonyl butoxide	rat			increased	Bachmann, 1989
Polychlorinated biphenyls	mouse	no change	no change		Dolphin et al., 1987
Poly rI : rC	mouse	no change	no change	increased	Kalabis and Wells, 1990
Poly I-C	man			increased	Smilgin et al., 1993
Polyvinyl chloride	man	decreased	increased	decreased	Abernethy et al., 1985
Probenecid	man	decreased	decreased	decreased	Kamali et al., 1987a
Probenecid	rat	decreased	decreased	no change	Savina and Brouwer, 1992
Probenecid	man	decreased		decreased	Kamali, 1993
Probenecid	mouse*	decreased			von Moltke et al., 1993
Probenecid	rat*	decreased			von Moltke et al., 1993
Probenecid	man*	decreased			von Moltke et al., 1993
Propylene glycol	mouse*		decreased		Snawder et al., 1993
Prednisolone	rat*	decreased			Bolanowska and Gessner, 1978
Prednisolone	rat	decreased	no change		Bolanowska and Gessner, 1980
Prednisone	rat*	decreased			Bolanowska and Gessner, 1978
Prednisone	rat	decreased	no change		Bolanowska and Gessner, 1980
Prednisone	man			increased	D'Souza et al., 1989
PCN[a]	rat		increased		Seddon et al., 1987

139

Table 7.4 (cont.)

Agent	Species	Glucuronide conjugate	Sulphate conjugate	Glutathione-derived conjugates	Rate of elimination	Reference
PCN[8]	rat			increased		Bachmann, 1989
PCN[8]	rat	increased	no change	increased		Gregus et al., 1990
PCN[8]	rat*	increased		increased		Lee et al., 1991a
PCN[8]	hamster	increased	no change	decreased		Madhu and Klaassen, 1991
PCN[8]	rat*	increased				Goon and Klaassen, 1992
Primaquine	man	no change	no change	no change	no change	Back and Tjia, 1987
Primidone	man	increased			increased	Perucca and Richens, 1979
Primidone	man		decreased	no change	increased	Prescott et al., 1981
Propranolol	man	no change			no change	Hayes and Bouchier, 1989
Propranolol		decreased	decreased		decreased	Baraka et al., 1990
Ranitidine	rat		no change	no change		Mitchell et al., 1984b
Ranitidine	rat**	decreased	no change		no change	Emery et al., 1985
Ranitidine	man	no change	increased	no change		Jack et al., 1985
Ranitidine	rat	decreased	no change			Rogers et al., 1985
Ranitidine	rat	decreased	no change	decreased		Rogers et al., 1988
Ranitidine	man	no change	no change	no change	no change	Thomas et al., 1988
Rifampicin	rat	increased	decreased	increased		Younes et al., 1979
Rifampicin	rat	increased	increased	increased		Siegers et al., 1980
Rifampicin	man	increased	decreased	no change	increased	Prescott et al., 1981
Rifampicin	man	increased	no change	no change		Bock et al., 1987
Rifampicin	rat				decreased	Bachmann, 1989
Sacoglottis gabonensis	rat	increased			increased	Madusolumuo and Okoye, 1993
Salicylamide	man	decreased	decreased			Levy and Yamada, 1971
Salicylate	man	no change	no change		no change	Levy and Regårdh, 1971
Salicylate	man	no change	no change			Amsel and Davison, 1972
Salicylate	man	no change	no change			Thomas et al., 1972
Salicylate	rat				no change	Ramachander et al., 1973
Salicylate	rat	increased	decreased	no change		Thomas et al., 1974

Compound	Species					Reference
Salicylate	guinea pig	no change	no change	increased		Whitehouse et al., 1975
Salicylate	mouse	no change	decreased	increased		Whitehouse et al., 1976
Salicylate	hamster	no change	decreased	no change		Wong et al., 1976b
Salicylate	mouse	decreased	no change	no change		Whitehouse et al., 1977
Salicylate	mouse	increased	decreased	increased		Douidar et al., 1985
Selenium	rat			no change		Schnell et al., 1988
Sevoflurane	rat				no change	Watkins, 1989
SKF 525A	dog				no change	Kampffmeyer, 1974
SKF 525A	rat*			no change		Seddon et al., 1987
Stilbene oxide	rat	increased	decreased	increased	increased	Gregus et al., 1990
Sulphate	cat	decreased	increased		increased	Savides et al., 1985
Sulphinpyrazone	man	increased	no change	no change		Miners et al., 1984c
Taurocholate	rat	increased	increased	increased	increased	Galinsky and Chalasinka, 1988
Tetrachlorodibenzodioxin	rat*	increased				Goon and Klaassen, 1992
Tetrachlorodibenzodioxin	rat	increased				Bock et al., 1993
Tetracycline	rat*	decreased				Bolanowska and Gessner, 1978
Thyroxine	rat	no change	no change		no change	Zhu et al., 1991
Trichlorethylene	man				increased	Ray et al., 1993a
Triton X-100	mouse*	increased				Dybing, 1976
Triton X-100	rat*	increased				Bolanowska and Gessner, 1978
UDPAG[9]	rat*	increased				Bolanowska and Gessner, 1978
Valproate	man				no change	Kapetanovic et al., 1981
Zidovudine	rat*	decreased				Ameer et al., 1992
Zidovudine	man				no change	Burger et al., 1994b

* liver microsomes; ** isolated hepatocytes; *** perfused liver preparation; [a] acute; [c] chronic; [1] HEPG2 liver cell cultures; [2] thiopentone, fentanyl, nitrous oxide, halothane; [3] isoniazid + rifampicin + pyrazinamide + ethambutol; [4] 25 mg kg^{-1}; [5] 350 mg kg^{-1}; [6] DBA/2 strain; [7] C57BL/6 strain; [8] pregnenolone-16α-carbonitrile; [9] uridine diphosphate-N-acetylglucosamine

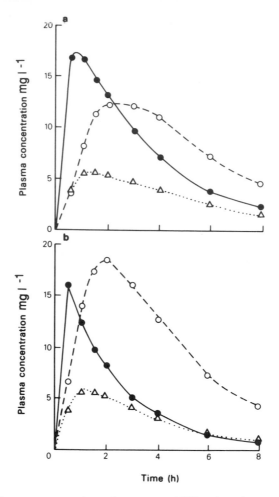

Figure 7.9 Mean plasma concentrations of paracetamol (●) and its glucuronide (○) and sulphate (△) conjugates in (a) 12 healthy volunteers and (b) 15 induced patients following an oral dose of 20 mg kg^{-1} of paracetamol (reproduced with permission from Prescott *et al.*, 1981).

paracetamol through regional expression of cytochrome CYP2E1 in rats (Anundi *et al.*, 1993), and induction of paracetamol metabolism by phenobarbitone in mice resulted in a more rapid onset of cytotoxicity with new sites of protein arylation and adduct formation (Birge *et al.*, 1989). Cytochrome CYP2E1 was also induced in rats, with corresponding enhancement of paracetamol metabolism, by obesity resulting from overfeeding (Raucy *et al.*, 1991). No such effect has been observed in man (Lee *et al.*, 1981b; Abernethy *et al.*, 1982a).

Cytochrome CYP2E1 is inducible by ethanol, and the demonstration that it was particularly active in the oxidation of paracetamol in human liver (Raucy *et al.*, 1989) has been held to support the unproven hypothesis that chronic alcoholics are at greater risk of paracetamol hepatotoxicity because they produce more toxic metabolite (Lieber, 1990a). This theory must be questioned because the K_m for paracetamol oxidation by purified CYP2E1 was about 5 mM, and, therefore, it would only be active at unrealistically high concentrations (Nelson, 1990). In fact, the most active isoform for paracetamol oxidation by human liver at practical therapeutic concentrations was CYP3A4 (Thummel *et al.*, 1993). There seemed to be species differences in the mechanisms of inhibition of paracetamol metabolism by ethanol, and in man the interaction was probably mediated indirectly by depletion of cytosolic NADPH (Thummel *et al.*, 1989). In studies of paracetamol metabolism in healthy subjects with A, B and C subgroups of CYP2E1, elimination was said to be higher in the latter group although this only consisted of two subjects (Tsutsumi *et al.*, 1994). The activity of CYP1A2 as determined by the caffeine metabolic ratio was increased in smokers, and was correlated with the extent of glucuronide conjugation of paracetamol, suggesting an element of co-regulation (Bock *et al.*, 1994).

Duration of Treatment

The duration of exposure to inducing and inhibiting agents is important. Drugs such as ethanol may first inhibit and then stimulate paracetamol metabolism so that acute administration protected, while chronic administration potentiated hepatotoxicity (Wong *et al.*, 1980b; Sato and Lieber, 1981; Sato *et al.*, 1981a,b).

Effects of Disease States

Hepatic and renal disease generally had the expected effects on the metabolism of paracetamol and the excretion of its metabolites respectively, but the changes with other pathology were less predictable. The disposition of paracetamol has been studied in animal models of disease states but these did not necessarily correspond to human disease and the findings could not readily be extrapolated to man. In many cases the mechanisms of reported abnormalities were obscure.

Endocrine Disease

Under certain circumstances, acetone stimulated the metabolic activation of paracetamol (Lee *et al.*, 1991b; Jaw and Jeffery, 1993). However, contrary to expectations, diabetic rats were more resistant to hepatotoxicity than control animals and they metabolized paracetamol faster with enhanced glucuronide and sulphate conjugation. There was no increase in toxic metabolic activation (Price and Jollow, 1982) and diabetes did not alter microsomal glucuronyl transferase activity (Price and Jollow, 1984). Subsequent investigation confirmed the faster conjugation of paracetamol in diabetic rats, but there were strain differences in susceptibility to hepatotoxicity that were related to the capacity for glucuronide conjugation and ability to clear the drug by non-toxic pathways (Price and Jollow, 1986). In mice, diabetes protected against paracetamol hepatotoxicity even though the formation of glutathione conjugate was increased (Jeffery *et al.*, 1991). In rats made diabetic with streptozotocin, the biliary excretion of paracetamol and its glucuronide and sulphate conjugates was decreased (Siegers *et al.*, 1985). Similar results were described in a later study and instead of the expected glutathione conjugate in bile there were comparable levels of cysteine conjugate. The urinary excretion of glucuronide, sulphate and mercapturic acid conjugates was greatly increased and the elimination half life was reduced. These abnormalities were partly reversed by insulin (Watkins and Sherman, 1992). Streptozotocin treatment did not alter the glucuronidation of paracetamol by the phenobarbitone-inducible GT2 form of glucuronyl transferase in rats (Morrison and Hawksworth, 1984). In non-insulin dependent diabetic patients, the metabolism of paracetamol was the same as in healthy control subjects except for a minor increase in partial clearance to the sulphate conjugate (Kamali *et al.*, 1993). In another report, the salivary elimination of paracetamol was said to be reduced in diabetic patients and the half life was correlated with the fasting blood glucose concentration (Adithan *et al.*, 1988). Unfortunately the controls were not well matched in this study and the half life in this group was much shorter than reported in healthy subjects by other investigators.

Hyper- and hypothyroidism had no effect on the pattern of the biliary or urinary excretion of metabolites of paracetamol in rats (Siegers *et al.*, 1980, 1985). On the other hand, the gastrointestinal first pass metabolism of paracetamol in rats was reduced by treatment with thyroxine (Zhu *et al.*, 1991). In hypothyroid patients, the clearance of paracetamol increased significantly after treatment and this was associated with increased glucuronide conjugation of the drug (Sonne *et al.*, 1990). In another study, the plasma half life of paracetamol was decreased in thyrotoxic patients and increased in hypothyroid patients compared with values obtained subsequently in the euthyroid state after treatment (Forfar *et al.*, 1980). These changes could be explained by the effects of thyroid disease on cardiac output and liver blood flow.

Cardiorespiratory Disease

The mean saliva half life of oral paracetamol in nine patients with decompensated congestive cardiac failure due to mitral valve disease was 2.7 h and this was reduced to 1.8 h when five were studied again after treatment. The difference was said to be significant, but both values were well within the range reported by others for healthy subjects. The authors also claimed that the volume of paracetamol distribution was greater in the patients with untreated cardiac failure but such calculations cannot be made after oral administration because the fraction absorbed was not known (Pradeep Kumar *et al.*, 1987). In addition, an unsuitable method of assay was used. It was also claimed that the saliva half life and volume of distribution of paracetamol were increased in patients with rheumatic tricuspid regurgitation, and the same criticisms applied (Pradeep Kumar *et al.*, 1989). In patients with cardiac failure given intravenous paracetamol, there was no change in the half life but total clearance and volume of distribution were reduced compared with healthy control subjects (Ochs *et al.*, 1983). Haemodilution with perfluorochemical emulsions (PFC) or saline reduced the sulphate conjugation of paracetamol in rats, and PFC had opposite effects on the renal clearance of the conjugate at different times (Shrewsbury and White, 1990). In spontaneously hypertensive rats, there was slightly increased sulphate conjugation and slightly decreased glucuronidation of oral and intravenous paracetamol (Jang *et al.*, 1994).

In rats, chronic hypoxia was associated with decreased glutathione conjugation and slower elimination of paracetamol, and the findings were similar in studies with isolated hepatocytes (Aw *et al.*, 1991). The sulphate and glucuronide conjugation of paracetamol by isolated rat hepatocytes was depressed by hypoxia and the oxygen-dependent impairment of glucuronidation was potentiated by fasting (Aw and Jones, 1982, 1984). In another report, however, hypoxia had no significant effect on the total clearance of paracetamol by the perfused rat liver (Studenberg and Brouwer, 1991). The metabolism of paracetamol in rats was not influenced by exposure to high atmospheric pressure at 31 ATA (Aanderud and Bakke, 1983). In five patients with cystic fibrosis given oral paracetamol the plasma half life was similar to that in five healthy controls, but the inappropriately calculated oral clearance was greater in the former, apparently as a result of enhanced sulphate and glucuronide conjugation (Hutabarat *et al.*, 1991).

Gastrointestinal Disease

In two patients with a jejunostomy performed for malignancies that required a gastrectomy, the disposition of oral paracetamol was similar to that observed in four healthy control subjects (Nelson *et al.*, 1986). The plasma concentrations of paracetamol were abnormally low in patients with gastric carcinoma and there was an apparent increase in the total body clearance (Gawronska-Szklarz *et al.*, 1988). As in many other reports, the clearance had been calculated inappropriately after oral administration. Compared with normal subjects, the rate of paracetamol elimination was enhanced in patients with treated and untreated coeliac disease and its glucuronide conjugation was increased in patients with Crohn's disease (Holt *et al.*, 1981).

Liver Disease

Deep X-ray irradiation of the liver reversibly reduced the formation and excretion of the sulphate conjugate of paracetamol in rabbits (Birzle *et al.*, 1967). Acute liver damage produced in rats by administration of carbon tetrachloride markedly reduced the biliary excretion of the glutathione and glucuronide conjugates of paracetamol (Siegers and Schütt, 1979; Loeser and Siegers, 1985) but surprisingly, the paracetamol half life and urinary excretion of metabolites were not influenced by prior treatment with carbon tetrachloride (Siegers *et al.*, 1978, 1980). Partial hepatectomy diminished sulphate and mercapturic acid conjugation in rats, and after seven days glucuronide conjugation was decreased while sulphate and mercapturic acid excretion were enhanced (Siegers *et al.*, 1980). In man, acute hepatic necrosis following overdosage of paracetamol resulted in considerable prolongation of its plasma half life and this was directly related to the severity of liver damage (Prescott *et al.*, 1971; Prescott and Wright, 1973; Gazzard *et al.*, 1977; Hamlyn *et al.*, 1978). There may be virtually complete failure of conjugation of paracetamol in patients who have severe liver necrosis progressing to fatal hepatic failure (Prescott and Wright, 1973). The impairment of drug metabolism caused by mild and moderate liver damage following paracetamol poisoning returned to normal or near normal within 7–21 days (Forrest *et al.*, 1974).

Paracetamol metabolism seemed to be impaired more in patients with liver disease associated with jaundice than in those without jaundice (Fevery and de Groote, 1969) and depression of glucuronide and sulphate conjugation in children with infectious hepatitis was correlated with abnormal liver function tests (Gmyrek and Klimmt, 1971). During the acute phase of viral hepatitis there was a minor but statistically significant increase in the plasma paracetamol half life compared with values observed after recovery and in healthy control subjects. The increase was greatest in patients with severe hepatitis as indicated by prolongation of the pro- thrombin time ratio (Jorup-Rönström *et al.*, 1986). In another study, there was no change in the pattern of 24 h urinary excretion of paracetamol and its conjugates in patients with chronic hepatitis B virus infection (Leung and Critchley, 1991).

There have been several reports of moderately impaired metabolism of para- cetamol in patients with chronic liver disease, including alcoholic cirrhosis, as shown by increased plasma concentrations or half life (Shamszad *et al.*, 1975; Forrest *et al.*, 1977, 1979; Arnman and Olsson, 1978; Andreasen and Hutters, 1979; Siegers *et al.*, 1981; Brazier *et al.*, 1982; Benson, 1983; Villeneuve *et al.*, 1983; Porowski *et al.*, 1988). In some of these reports, an increased paracetamol half life was related to depressed synthetic capacity of the liver as indicated by the plasma albumin concentration and prothrombin time (Forrest *et al.*, 1977, 1979; Andreasen and Hutters, 1979) and elimination was slower in patients with decompensated than compensated liver disease (Brazier *et al.*, 1982). Changes consistent with reduced first pass loss and grossly impaired metabolism of paracetamol were observed in patients with cirrhosis and portosystemic shunting (Forrest *et al.*, 1979). However, some investigators have been unable to show the expected correlations with bio- chemical indices of liver dysfunction (Brazier *et al.*, 1982) and the presence of ascites and portosystemic shunts (Arnman and Olsson, 1978). The elimination of paraceta- mol was impaired in patients admitted for elective portosystemic shunt operations and the impairment was greatly increased five days after surgery (Godellas *et al.*, 1992). There were no significant differences in the overall pattern of urinary excre- tion of glucuronide, sulphate, cysteine and mercapturic acid conjugates in healthy volunteers and patients with mild and severe chronic liver disease (Forrest *et al.*, 1979). Similar negative findings were noted in patients with cirrhosis due to chronic hepatitis B virus infection (Leung and Critchley, 1991). The first pass metabolism of paracetamol was enhanced in chronic alcoholics who did not have biochemical evi- dence of liver damage as shown by a reduced area under the plasma concentration– time curve but there was no significant shortening of the plasma half life (Dietz *et al.*, 1984). In patients with hepatosplenic schistosomiasis and periportal fibrosis there was no prolongation of the paracetamol half life. It was claimed that the maximum plasma concentrations and areas under the plasma concentration–time curves were greater than in healthy controls (El Turabi *et al.*, 1989). This could have been explained simply by the differences between the groups in body weight. There were no obvious abnormalities in paracetamol elimination in patients with hepatic metastases (Arnman and Olsson, 1978), but in patients with untreated primary hepatocellular carcinoma there was enhanced oxidative metabolism as shown by increased urinary excretion of the cysteine and mercapturic acid conjugates (Leung and Critchley, 1991).

Cholestasis produced in rats by administration of taurocholate resulted in a minor increase in paracetamol clearance and sulphate and glucuronide conjugation (Galinsky and Chalasinka, 1988) while extrahepatic cholestasis produced by bile duct ligation in rats resulted in increased glucuronidation (Ouviña *et al.*, 1993, 1994). In man obstructive jaundice was associated with significant prolongation of the plasma paracetamol half life (Brodie *et al.*, 1981). The disposition of oral parace- tamol was normal in patients who had received liver transplants but the time after operation was not mentioned (Venkataramanan *et al.*, 1989).

Renal Disease

In rats with acute renal failure produced by bilateral ureteric ligation, there was increased biliary excretion of paracetamol sulphate but no increase in biliary glucuronide despite marked elevation of the concentrations of this metabolite in plasma (Brouwer and Jones, 1990). In another study in rats with ligated ureters, there was a compensatory increase in biliary excretion of the glucuronide and sulphate (but not glutathione) conjugates of paracetamol (Siegers and Klaassen, 1984). As expected, there was retention of inorganic sulphate with increased sulphate conjugation of paracetamol in rats with acute renal failure and the total clearance of the drug following a dose of 100 mg kg^{-1} (but not 15 mg kg^{-1}) was increased in proportion to the serum sulphate concentrations (Lin and Levy, 1982). Acute water deprivation had no major effect on paracetamol disposition in rats but there was some increase in glucuronide conjugation and the urinary excretion of unchanged drug was reduced (Zafar *et al.*, 1987). This is to be expected as the renal clearance of paracetamol depends on urine flow rate.

The plasma concentrations and half life of paracetamol formed from an oral dose of phenacetin in 11 patients with chronic renal failure (including nine with analgesic nephropathy) were essentially the same as in healthy control subjects but the 24 h excretion of conjugated paracetamol was reduced in the patients according to the extent of renal failure as shown by the creatinine clearance (Prescott, 1969). In another study in patients with chronic renal failure, some of whom had analgesic nephropathy, the 12 h urinary excretion of radioactivity following administration of [^{14}C]-paracetamol was correlated with the creatinine clearance. Paracetamol metabolism appeared to be normal in the patients with renal failure but excretion of the glucuronide, sulphate, cysteine and mercapturic acid conjugates was delayed (Thomas *et al.*, 1980). In patients who developed acute renal failure following paracetamol overdosage there was markedly decreased renal excretion of unchanged and conjugated drug (Prescott and Wright, 1973), while the excretion of paracetamol metabolites was diminished in patients with impaired renal function in an intensive care unit (Kietzmann *et al.*, 1990). It was claimed that the plasma paracetamol half life is abnormally short in renal transplant patients treated with cyclosporin and prednisone. However, blood was sampled hourly for only 4 h, which is not long enough to obtain a reliable estimate of the plasma half life after an oral dose and in any event the mean half life of 2 h was well within the range expected in normal healthy subjects. Inappropriate calculations were also made of the paracetamol clearance and distribution volume (D'Souza *et al.*, 1989). In hospital patients with transitional cell bladder cancer, the 12 h urinary excretion of glucuronide, sulphate and cysteine conjugates of paracetamol was similar to that in control patients with other urological disease but the recovery of the mercapturic acid conjugate was increased (Dolara *et al.*, 1988).

The plasma half life of paracetamol and the fractional urinary recovery of its metabolites were similar in patients with chronic renal failure and healthy control subjects but plasma concentrations of the glucuronide and sulphate conjugates were much higher in the patients, particularly those with end-stage renal disease maintained on regular haemodialysis (Figure 7.10). The late disappearance of paracetamol from the plasma was considerably delayed in the patients with renal failure suggesting augmented enterohepatic circulation of conjugates with regeneration of the parent drug from retained metabolites (Prescott *et al.*, 1989b). Patients with

147

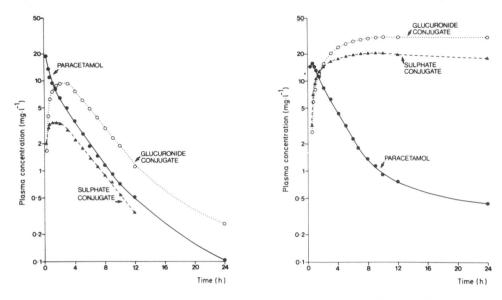

Figure 7.10 Mean plasma concentrations of paracetamol and its glucuronide and sulphate conjugates following an oral dose of 1 g in (left panel) 10 healthy volunteers and six patients with end-stage renal failure on maintenance haemodialysis (right panel) (from Prescott *et al.*, 1989b).

chronic renal failure not requiring treatment by regular dialysis were given paracetamol three times daily for 10 days. The predose plasma concentrations of unchanged drug were greater in the patients than in control subjects with normal renal function and concentrations of glucuronide and sulphate conjugates were greatly elevated in the patients. Predictions of the steady-state plasma concentrations were remarkably accurate for the glucuronide, but not for the sulphate conjugate (Martin *et al.*, 1991). In chronic haemodialysis patients receiving the same paracetamol regimen there was little variation in plasma concentrations of the parent drug and apparent steady-state concentrations of the glucuronide and sulphate conjugates were much lower than expected (Martin *et al.*, 1993). In another study in patients with chronic renal failure receiving regular haemodialysis there was retention of conjugated paracetamol but the half life and volume of distribution of the unchanged drug were the same as in healthy control subjects (Lowenthal *et al.*, 1976). In similar patients, the half life of paracetamol on interdialysis days was within the normal range and it was reduced by 42–53 per cent during dialysis. The extraction ratios during haemodialysis were 0.46 to 0.78 for paracetamol, 0.53 to 0.57 for the glucuronide and 0.13 to 0.60 for the sulphate conjugate (Øie *et al.*, 1975). In a more recent study, the saliva half life of paracetamol was rather short in patients with chronic renal failure (Lee *et al.*, 1990). After extensive investigation, an unknown substance found in the dialysate and serum from patients treated by chronic ambulatory peritoneal dialysis and haemodialysis was identified as paracetamol glucuronide. On the basis of its peritoneal and cuprophan haemodialyzer mass membrane transfer coefficients, the conjugate was proposed as a useful molecular mass marker for peritoneal and haemodialysis (Schoots *et al.*, 1990).

Central Nervous System Disease

There have been several reports of inexplicable major abnormalities of paracetamol disposition in patients with disease of the central nervous system. Patients with Parkinson's disease were said to have a reduced capacity to form the sulphate conjugate of paracetamol as judged by the fraction of an oral dose excreted in the urine in 8 h. The excretion of paracetamol glucuronide was also reduced and there were similar abnormalities in unspecified controls (Steventon *et al.*, 1989, 1990). These findings could be explained by incomplete urine collection, renal impairment or slow or poor absorption of the paracetamol as only 13.6 per cent of the dose appeared in the urine of the Parkinson patients compared with 25.7 per cent in control patients with non-degenerative neurological disease. The same investigators claimed that patients with motor neurone disease also had defective sulphate conjugation of paracetamol (Steventon *et al.*, 1988). Again this may have been related to reduced renal function or impaired absorption as the 8 h urinary recovery in these patients was only 11.2 per cent of the dose instead of the 70–80 per cent expected in healthy subjects. The source of the paracetamol was not disclosed. It was subsequently shown that the sulphate and glucuronide conjugation of paracetamol was not impaired at all in patients with Parkinson's disease and Huntington's chorea, irrespective of other drug therapy (Roos *et al.*, 1993). In another study, there was no evidence for abnormal 3-hydroxylation of paracetamol in patients with Parkinson's disease (Factor *et al.*, 1988, 1989). In patients studied two and six weeks after an acute stroke there was evidence of impaired absorption of paracetamol together with greatly accelerated elimination that was more marked in patients with infarction of the left than the right cerebral hemisphere. There was no obvious explanation for these findings and the kinetic analysis was inappropriate for an orally administered drug (Stankowska-Chomicz and Gawronska-Szklarz, 1987). The serum half life of paracetamol was within the normal range in patients with spinal cord injury (Halstead *et al.*, 1985).

Fever and Infections

Paracetamol is widely used as an antipyretic and the mean plasma half life in children with fever given doses of 5–30 mg kg^{-1} was generally within the range of 1.5–3 h reported for healthy adults (Wilson, 1979; Peterson and Rumack, 1981; Wilson *et al.*, 1982b; Walson and Mortensen, 1989). There was minor but clinically insignificant accumulation of the drug on repeated dosing in febrile infants and children (Nahata *et al.*, 1984) and the elimination of paracetamol as shown by the fall in saliva concentrations was not impaired in patients with active pulmonary tuberculosis (Madhusudanarao *et al.*, 1988b). Malarial infection altered the kinetics of the glucuronide conjugation of paracetamol by rat liver microsomes (Ismail *et al.*, 1992) and decreased glucuronidation *in vivo* was compensated for by increased sulphate conjugation (Ismail *et al.*, 1994). Malaria also decreased paracetamol clearance and the biliary excretion of its glutathione conjugate in rats (Mansor *et al.*, 1991). However, acute uncomplicated falciparum malaria infection had no effect on the disposition and kinetics of paracetamol in Thai patients (Ismail *et al.*, 1995). The rate of elimination of intravenous paracetamol in goats was decreased by

149

endotoxin-induced fever (Manna *et al.*, 1994) and in suspensions of isolated rat hepatocytes, the rate of removal of paracetamol decreased when the temperature was raised from 29 to 39°C (Aarbakke *et al.*, 1978). Treatment of rats with whole cell pertussis-component diphtheria, tetanus and pertussis vaccine two days previously reduced plasma concentrations and increased the clearance of paracetamol. Other vaccines had no such effect (Lin *et al.*, 1989).

Miscellaneous

Chronic treadmill exercise increased the deacetylation of paracetamol in rats (Piatkowski *et al.*, 1993) but physical activity had no effect on the rate of elimination of paracetamol in man (Yiamouyiannis *et al.*, 1994). Traumatic injury produced by hind limb ischaemia in rats was associated with decreased sulphate conjugation of paracetamol (Griffeth *et al.*, 1985). In man general anaesthesia with thiopentone, fentanyl, nitrous oxide and halothane for minor surgical procedures had no clini-cally important effects on paracetamol metabolism (Lewis *et al.*, 1991). In patients undergoing short surgical procedures under halothane anaesthesia (no other drugs were mentioned) the mean saliva half life of paracetamol was said to be reduced from 2.1 h the day before surgery to 0.96 h three days after. The corresponding change in the saliva half life of paracetamol in control patients given epidural ligno-caine anaesthesia was from 2.4 h before to 1.6 h after the operations (Ray *et al.*, 1986). The same data were used in another report where it was claimed that epi-dural anaesthesia given for brief surgery reduced the salivary elimination of parace-tamol (Ray *et al.*, 1985). In both reports the method used for the assay of paracetamol was unsuitable. The disposition of paracetamol in patients in an inten-sive care unit was within normal limits (Kietzmann *et al.*, 1990) but patients with rheumatoid arthritis were said to produce less sulphate conjugate than healthy or hospital patient controls on the basis of the 8 h urinary recovery. The drugs taken previously by the rheumatoid arthritis patients were not mentioned and in these patients the total recovery of paracetamol and metabolites was only 16.4 per cent of the dose (Bradley *et al.*, 1991a). Again, such abnormally low recovery suggests poor absorption, incomplete urine collection or impairment of renal function. Factors influencing the glucuronide conjugation of paracetamol in man have been reviewed (Miners and Mackenzie, 1991; Sonne, 1993).

8

The Biliary Excretion of Paracetamol and its Metabolites

Introduction

The biliary excretion of paracetamol and its metabolites has been studied in the isolated perfused liver and in intact animals. The extent of biliary excretion and fractional recovery of the different metabolites was dose-dependent and there were major species differences (Figure 8.1) (Siegers and Schütt, 1979; Watari et al., 1983; Hjelle and Klaassen, 1984; Gregus et al., 1988b; Madhu et al., 1989). Concentrations were usually higher in bile than in blood (Wong et al., 1981; Jayasinghe et al., 1986), but the total excretion of metabolites into urine was several-fold greater than into bile (Whitehouse et al., 1975; Wong et al., 1981). After oral administration of 200 mg kg^{-1} of paracetamol in rats, only 5.5 per cent of the dose appeared in the bile in 24 h compared with 72 per cent in the urine and when the dose was increased to 1000 mg kg^{-1} the corresponding recoveries were 13.5 and 51 per cent respectively (Siegers and Schütt, 1979). Studies in rats with bile fistulas indicated little biliary excretion or enterohepatic circulation of paracetamol sulphate conjugate. However, there was significant dose-dependent biliary secretion of the glucuronide conjugate that was subject to hydrolysis by gut bacterial flora and subsequently reabsorbed as the parent drug (Watari et al., 1983). The considerable lag time in the enterohepatic circulation of paracetamol glucuronide was due to delay in its transit to the sites of rapid hydrolysis in the ileum and caecum (Watari et al., 1984). As expected, cannulation of the bile ducts reduced the urinary recovery of paracetamol and its metabolites and the intravenous administration of the glutathione conjugate resulted in its appearance in the urine primarily as the cysteine conjugate. The conversion of the glutathione to the cysteine conjugate occurred at multiple sites, but particularly in the intestine and kidney (Fischer et al., 1985a). In intact rats given 100 mg kg^{-1} of paracetamol intravenously, the oral administration of charcoal and cholestyramine interrupted the enterohepatic circulation and reduced the urinary recovery from 91.3 to 72.8 and 59.3 per cent of the dose respectively (Siegers et al., 1983b). The biliary excretion of the glucuronide and sulphate (but not the glutathione) conjugates of paracetamol was increased in rats when renal excretion of the drug and its metabolites was prevented by ligation of the ureters (Siegers and Klaassen, 1984). Following intraperitoneal administration of 50 mg kg^{-1} of paracetamol in newborn

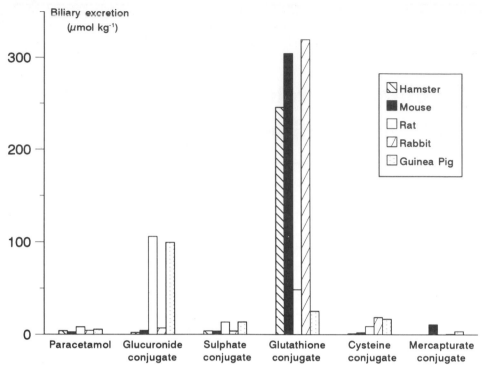

Figure 8.1 Species differences in the biliary excretion of paracetamol and its metabolites during the 2 h following intravenous administration of 150 mg kg^{-1} of paracetamol (data from Gregus *et al.*, 1988b).

guinea-pig pups delivered by Caesarean section, the concentrations of glucuronide and sulphate conjugates were similar in plasma and bile but glutathione and cysteine conjugates were not detected (Ecobichon *et al.*, 1989).

There were marked species differences in the biliary secretion of paracetamol metabolites. As shown in Table 8.1, the glutathione and cysteine conjugates accounted for 70–95 per cent of the total in bile in the hamster, mouse, rabbit and man compared with 25–30 per cent in the rat and guinea pig in whom the glucuronide conjugate was the major biliary metabolite of paracetamol. Little or no mercapturic acid conjugate appeared in bile in any of the species studied, and except in the rat, the sulphate conjugate was a minor biliary metabolite. The relative magnitudes of the toxication pathway of paracetamol (as shown by the combined biliary and urinary excretion of the glutathione, cysteine and mercapturic acid conjugates) and the detoxication pathway (as shown by the corresponding excretion of glucuronide and sulphate conjugates) were compared in relation to susceptibility to hepatotoxicity in different species. The most sensitive species (hamster and mouse) excreted 27–42 per cent of a dose of 150 mg kg^{-1} of paracetamol as toxication metabolites whereas corresponding fraction in the resistant species (rabbit, rat, guinea pig) was only 5–7 per cent. The toxication metabolites appeared mostly in bile as the glutathione conjugate and its hydrolysis products, and their total production was considered to be a good index of the extent of toxic metabolic activation of paracetamol (Gregus *et al.*, 1988b; Madhu *et al.*, 1989). Paracetamol depleted hepatic glutathione, increased its fractional turnover rate and reduced its excretion into bile in both reduced and oxidized forms (Lauterburg and Mitchell, 1982; Lauterburg *et al.*, 1984b). Paracetamol was used as a probe to demonstrate the stimulation of hepatic synthesis and efflux of glutathione produced by methionine and cysteine (Lauterburg and Smith, 1986).

Cannulation of the bile duct in ponies had no significant effect on the plasma kinetics or urinary excretion of paracetamol and its sulphate and glucuronide conjugates, and only about 1 per cent of the dose was recovered in the bile (Greenblatt and Engelking, 1988). In man, the predominant biliary metabolite of paracetamol was the cysteine conjugate, which was probably formed by hydrolysis of the glutathione conjugate as a result of the high γ-glutamyltranspeptidase activity in human bile (Siegers *et al.*, 1984). In healthy volunteers the unchanged drug and its glutathione, mercapturic acid and sulphate conjugates were not detected in bile following oral paracetamol, and a total of less than 1 per cent of the dose was recovered in the bile (Jayasinghe *et al.*, 1986).

In the once-through isolated perfused rat liver preparation, biliary excretion accounted for about 5 per cent of the total dose of paracetamol, and the fractions recovered as unchanged drug, and glutathione, sulphate and mercapturic acid conjugates were 1.8–3.9, 2–3, 57–68 and 6–15 per cent respectively (Pang and Terrell, 1981b). These ratios differed considerably from those observed in intact animals (Table 8.1). In another study in the perfused rat liver, less than 1 per cent of an intraportal dose of [^{3}H]-paracetamol sulphate was recovered in bile (Goresky *et al.*, 1992).

Dose Dependence

The biliary excretion of the glutathione conjugate of paracetamol in hamsters was linear with doses up to 150 mg kg^{-1}, after which there was evidence of saturation kinetics (Madhu *et al.*, 1989). As the dose increased from 37.5 to 600 mg kg^{-1} in rats, the biliary excretion of metabolites rose from 20 to 49 per cent and there was a preferential increase in the output of glucuronide conjugate from 52 to 81 per cent. Paracetamol produced a dose-dependent increase in bile flow rate (Siegers *et al.*, 1983a; Hjelle and Klaassen, 1984) with a decrease in the output of glutathione (Kaplowitz *et al.*, 1983). A reduction in the hepatic energy state produced by ethionine or fructose was associated with a decrease in the biliary excretion of paracetamol and its metabolites (Dills and Klaassen, 1986). Dose-dependent biliary excretion of paracetamol metabolites has also been observed in the isolated perfused rat liver. As concentrations in the perfusate increased from 150 to 1500 mg l^{-1}, the fraction excreted into bile remained relatively constant at 12–14 per cent. However, the proportion recovered as paracetamol sulphate fell from 33 to 14 per cent while the glucuronide and glutathione conjugates increased from 3.2 to 26.8 and from 17 to 39 per cent respectively (Grafström *et al.*, 1979b).

Effects of Induction and Inhibition of Drug Metabolism

In general, pretreatment with agents that stimulated or inhibited microsomal enzyme activity increased or decreased the biliary excretion of the glucuronide and

Table 8.1 Fractional biliary excretion of paracetamol metabolites.

Dose (mg kg⁻¹)	Route	Unchanged paracetamol	Conjugates					% of dose excreted in bile	Reference
			Glutathione	Cysteine	Mercapturic acid	Glucuronide	Sulphate		
Mouse									
250	oral	7.5	61.2	3.4	–	6.9	13.0	18.1	Wong et al., 1979
150	oral	5.7	51.8	2.9	–	18.7	10.8	13.9	Wong et al., 1981
250	oral	2.9	77.6	<0.1	5.7	7.6	5.7	10.5	Fischer et al., 1985a
350	oral	4.7	68.9	–	–	9.4	11.3	10.6	Whitehouse et al., 1985
350	oral[1]	3.8	70.6	–	–	6.9	10.0	16.0	Whitehouse et al., 1985
150	iv[2]	0.8	92.4	0.7	3.3	1.3	1.0	33.0	Gregus et al., 1988b
500	ip	10.1	82.9	–	–	1.2	5.2	–	Jaeschke, 1990
150	iv	0.6	94.3	0.3	1.6	0.8	0.7	–	Madhu et al., 1992b
Rat									
100	iv	4.2	16.4	–	1.1	49.8	28.6	28.7	Siegers et al., 1983b
10	iv	–	–	–	–	6.5	–	–	Watari et al., 1983
40	iv	0.3	–	–	–	5.2	0.6	–	Watari et al., 1983
80	iv	0.6	–	–	–	10.4	1.7	–	Watari et al., 1983
160	iv	0.7	–	–	–	16.5	1.5	–	Watari et al., 1983
320	iv	0.9	–	–	–	24.2	1.9	–	Watari et al., 1983
37.5	iv	2.9	10.9	–	–	52.0	34.7	20.2	Hjelle and Klaassen, 1984
75	iv	3.6	8.4	–	–	49.2	39.5	23.8	Hjelle and Klaassen, 1984
150	iv	4.4	10.7	–	0.46	57.3	26.3	28.1	Hjelle and Klaassen, 1984
300	iv	5.3	8.9	–	0.38	73.0	11.6	29.3	Hjelle and Klaassen, 1984

Dose	Route								Reference
600	iv	7.1	7.9	—	0.57	80.8	6.8	26.5	Hjelle and Klaassen, 1984
100	iv	4.7	16.5	—	—	56.3	28.9	28.4	Siegers and Klaassen, 1984
68	id	0.3	—	—	—	6.1	8.1	—	Watari et al., 1984
68	ii	2.2	—	—	—	16.1	8.8	—	Watari et al., 1984
68	ic	2.1	—	—	—	8.3	8.1	—	Watari et al., 1984
150	ip	3.8	12.6	—	—	54.0	26.4	31.1	Watkins et al., 1984
100	iv	3.7	12.6	—	—	61.4	22.4	24.6	Loeser and Siegers, 1985; Siegers et al., 1985
300	iv	8.2	11.5	5.0	—	62.6	12.3	23.6	Dills and Klaassen, 1986
150	iv	4.4	26.1	4.8	—	56.7	7.2	18.7	Gregus et al., 1988b
100	oral	—	26.0	—	—	54.6	14.6	—	Jeffery et al., 1988
100	oral[2]	—	9.1	—	—	70.1	5.2	—	Jeffery et al., 1988
150	iv	7.6	9.8	0.01	—	59.2	20.5	19.6	Gregus et al., 1990
50	iv	5.1	13.6	—	—	47.8	33.4	15.0	Mansor et al., 1991
100	iv	3.7	—	—	—	66.6	29.8	10.7	Brouwer, 1993
Hamster									
150	iv	1.6	96.1	0.4[3]	—	0.8	1.5	25.6	Gregus et al., 1988b
75	iv	3.4	93.0	1.8[3]	—	2.6	3.9	—	Madhu et al., 1989
Rabbit									
150	iv	6.5	48.2	28.2	7.8	10.6	5.6	6.6	Gregus et al., 1988b
Guinea pig									
150	iv	3.4	15.4	10.2	2.1	60.7	8.3	16.4	Gregus et al., 1998b
Man									
15	oral	2.6	—	61.7	—	13.6	13.6	21.6	Siegers et al., 1984
15	oral	—	—	82.2	—	16.4	—	7.3	Jayasinghe et al., 1986

id = intraduodenal, ii = intra-ileal, ic = intracaecal, [1] with N-acetylcysteine, [2] with dimethylsulphoxide, [3] including cysteinylglycine conjugate glutathione-derived conjugates. The total biliary and urinary excretion of paracetamol and its glutathione-derived and glucuronide (but not sulphate) conjugates was increased in rats by prior treatment with phenobarbitone, 3-methylcholanthrene and pregnenolone-16α-carbonitrile. Trans-stilbene oxide decreased the excretion of the sulphate conjugate. The inducing agents also shifted the excretion of metabolites from bile to urine (Gregus *et al.*, 1990). Some (but not all) of a range of inducers of cytochrome P450 increased the biliary excretion of glutathione conjugates while inhibitors tended to have the opposite effect. Measurement of the biliary excretion of paracetamol glutathione conjugate was proposed as a useful method for detecting changes in cytochrome P450 activity and other factors governing the activation of paracetamol (Madhu *et al.*, 1989). There were species differences in the effects of inducing agents on the biliary excretion of paracetamol glutathione conjugate that were related to differences in susceptibility to toxicity. Thus, pregnenolone-16α-carbonitrile and dexamethasone reduced the biliary excretion of the glutathione conjugate and reduced toxicity in hamsters, but in mice pregnenolone-16α-carbonitrile had no such effect and dexamethasone tended to increase the biliary output of glutathione conjugate and increased toxicity (Madhu *et al.*, 1992a). The effects of inducing agents were not always predictable and in one study treatment with phenobarbitone decreased the biliary excretion of the glucuronide and sulphate conjugates of paracetamol in rats with and without ligation of the renal pedicles (Brouwer and Jones, 1990). The acute administration of phenobarbitone impaired the biliary excretion of paracetamol glucuronide in rats (Brouwer, 1993) and a similar effect was also observed in the isolated perfused rat liver (Studenberg and Brouwer, 1992). Brouwer, 1992).

Other investigators have reported a reduction in the biliary excretion of paracetamol conjugates by chronic ethanol intake (Vendemiale *et al.*, 1984), dimethylsulphoxide (Jeffery *et al.*, 1988; Madhu *et al.*, 1989), butyl-4-hydroxyanisole (McLaughlin and Boroujerdi, 1987), ether (Watkins *et al.*, 1984), other anaesthetics (Watkins, 1989), dithiocarb (Siegers, 1978b), probenecid (Savina and Brouwer, 1992), other inhibitors of cytochrome P450 (Madhu *et al.*, 1989; Jaeschke, 1990; Madhu and Klaassen, 1991; Liu *et al.*, 1993), carbon tetrachloride-induced liver damage (Siegers and Schütt, 1979; Loeser and Siegers, 1985), depletion of hepatic glutathione with phorone (Loeser and Siegers, 1985) and infection with malaria (Mansor *et al.*, 1991). The biliary excretion of the glucuronide and sulphate conjugates of paracetamol was reduced in rats with diabetes induced by treatment with streptozotocin but hyperthyroidism had no effect (Siegers *et al.*, 1985). Exercise increased the biliary clearance of paracetamol and its conjugates in rats (Watkins *et al.*, 1994). Cholestasis induced with taurolithocholate did not impair the glucuronide or sulphate conjugation of paracetamol in rats (Galinsky and Chalasinka, 1988). Depletion of hepatic uridine diphosphate glucuronic acid with galactosamine greatly decreased the biliary excretion of paracetamol glucuronide but there was relatively little effect on its plasma concentrations and urinary excretion, suggesting that the conjugate in bile was largely of hepatic origin (Gregus *et al.*, 1988a). N-acetylcysteine stimulated glutathione synthesis and greatly increased the biliary excretion of the glutathione conjugate of paracetamol in mice (Corcoran *et al.*, 1985b; Whitehouse *et al.*, 1985).

9

Renal Excretion and Other Routes of Removal of Paracetamol and its Metabolites

Mechanisms of the Renal Excretion of Paracetamol

Despite the enormous scale of use of paracetamol and the once widely held suspicion that it might play an important role in the aetiology of analgesic nephropathy, there has been relatively little investigation of the renal distribution and mechanisms of excretion of the drug and its metabolites.

Lester and Greenberg (1947) studied the renal excretion of paracetamol and the combined hydroxy conjugates in two subjects and calculated their renal clearances to be 8–24 and 93–366 ml min^{-1} respectively. The concentrations of paracetamol were higher in the urine than in plasma, and its renal clearance was much less than the glomerular filtration rate as indicated by the clearance of creatinine. As paracetamol was not extensively bound to plasma proteins, it would be filtered freely at the glomerulus and the low renal clearance indicated extensive tubular reabsorption. At the same time, the active tubular secretion of the glucuronide conjugate of paracetamol was inferred because its renal clearance considerably exceeded the creatinine clearance (Mereu *et al.*, 1962). The distribution of paracetamol was studied in kidneys sliced from cortex to papilla from dogs under conditions of water restriction and diuresis. There was as much as a 10-fold increase in the concentrations of unchanged and conjugated drug from cortex to papilla in hydropenic dogs. This concentration gradient resembled the gradient for urea and it disappeared on hydration (Bluemle and Goldberg, 1968). During the transition from water diuresis to vasopressin-mediated antidiuresis in healthy subjects, the urine to plasma concentration ratio of paracetamol rose less than that of creatinine, indicating increased tubular reabsorption of the drug at reduced urine flow rates (Barraclough, 1972).

In studies in dogs, the clearance ratio of unchanged paracetamol remained constant over a wide range of plasma drug concentrations but it increased with increasing urine flow rate. The clearance ratios of the glucuronide and sulphate conjugates did not change with urine flow rate but decreased as their plasma concentrations increased. Probenecid, an inhibitor of the renal tubular transport of many organic acids, had no effect on the renal clearance of paracetamol and the glucuronide conjugate but it significantly reduced the clearance of the sulphate conjugate. Limited stop-flow studies indicated accentuated reabsorption of paracetamol in distal areas of the nephron and net proximal tubular secretion of the sulphate conjugate. There was net reabsorption of glucuronide conjugate but no clear localization of the sites of transport (Duggin and Mudge, 1975). The cortico–medullary concentration gradient of paracetamol glucuronide and sulphate in dogs was inversely related to the urine flow rate, and as with inulin, it developed as a result of their progressive concentration in the tubular fluid in the distal nephron. As expected, the renal clearance of these conjugates was independent of urine flow rate, and the urine to plasma concentration ratio was highest at low flow rates. The concentration of the unchanged drug in the distal nephron increased with dehydration and the reabsorption kinetics were consistent with a process of diffusion (Duggin and Mudge, 1976). With the technique of acute diuresis in dogs, the paracetamol to inulin clearance ratio fell and then increased, as tubular reabsorption of the drug was converted to tubular secretion. The results with the conjugates were less consistent and suggested some degree of intracellular storage (Duggin and Mudge, 1978). The renal clearance of paracetamol glucuronide in dogs following intravenous injection of the glucuronide conjugate was the same as the simultaneously measured inulin clearance, and the role of tubular secretion was questioned (Hekman *et al.*, 1986). After five hours,

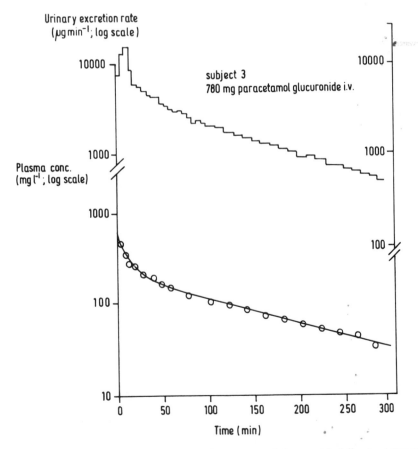

Figure 9.1 Plasma and urinary concentrations of paracetamol glucuronide following intravenous administration of a dose of 780 mg in a Beagle dog (redrawn from Hekman *et al.*, 1986).

98 per cent of the intravenous dose was recovered unchanged in the urine and there was no evidence of deconjugation. The curves of the decline in plasma concentrations and urinary excretion rates of the glucuronide conjugate were virtually superimposable (Figure 9.1).

Overall, these studies indicated that paracetamol was passively reabsorbed, probably throughout the entire nephron, and its clearance increased in a curvilinear fashion with increasing urine flow rate. The renal clearance of the glucuronide and sulphate conjugates was similar to the clearance of inulin but there was active tubular transport that was probably localized to the distal nephron. Their clearance was independent of urine flow rate. The highest urine to plasma concentration ratios of paracetamol and these conjugates occurred at the lowest flow rates.

Effects of Urine Flow Rate and pH

In rats deprived of water for 96 h a decrease in urine volume, from a control value of about 20 ml 24 h^{-1}, to 5 ml 24 h^{-1} was associated with a marked decrease in the renal clearance of paracetamol (Zafar *et al.*, 1987). In man, a clear relationship between urine flow rate and paracetamol clearance was confirmed by several investigators (Prescott and Wright, 1973; Morris and Levy, 1984; Kietzmann *et al.*, 1990; Miners *et al.*, 1992) but in most other studies the urine flow rates were not mentioned. The increase in paracetamol clearance with flow was modest. In one report an increase in urine flow from 1.6 to 13.7 ml min^{-1} resulted in less than a doubling of paracetamol clearance (Prescott and Wright, 1973), while in another, a seven-fold increase in urine flow rate only produced a two- to three-fold increase in clearance (Miners *et al.*, 1992). The renal clearances of the glucuronide and sulphate conjugates of paracetamol were independent of urine flow rate (Prescott and Wright, 1973). In more detailed studies in man the fractional urinary excretion of filtered paracetamol increased with diuresis, and when the clearance studies were repeated after regular administration of paracetamol for one week its excretion was enhanced with a decrease in the extent of back-diffusion (Silberbush *et al.*, 1974).

Paracetamol is a weak organic acid with a pKa value of 9.5. It was largely unionized, therefore, over the physiological range of urine pH and its renal clearance would not be influenced by changes in urine pH. In contrast, the polar glucuronide and sulphate conjugates of paracetamol were extensively ionized in biological fluids irrespective of pH, and their renal clearances would also be independent of urine pH. Urine pH had no clear effect on the renal medullary distribution gradient of paracetamol in dogs (Bluemle and Goldberg, 1968) and the lack of effect of changes in urine pH on the renal clearance of paracetamol and the glucuronide and sulphate conjugates has been confirmed (Barraclough, 1972; Prescott and Wright, 1973; Duggin and Mudge, 1975; Prescott, 1980; Kietzmann *et al.*, 1990).

The Renal Clearance of Paracetamol and its Conjugates

The reported renal clearances of paracetamol and its glucuronide and sulphate conjugates in man and animals are summarized in Tables 9.1 and 9.2. In man the renal clearance of unchanged paracetamol was usually in the range of 10–20 ml min^{-1} in keeping with glomerular filtration and extensive tubular reabsorption while the

Table 9.1 Renal clearances of paracetamol and its conjugates in man (ml min^{-1}).

Subjects	Para-cetamol	Glucuronide conjugate	Sulphate conjugate	Reference
Healthy subjects	12.3	223[1]	–	Lester and Greenberg, 1947
Newborn	2.1[2]	16.2[2]	–	Mereu *et al.*, 1962
Children (school age)	23.9[2]	243[2]	–	Mereu *et al.*, 1962
Overdose patients, no diuresis	12.3	132[1]	–	Prescott and Wright, 1973
Overdose patients, diuresis	23.9	146[1]	–	Prescott and Wright, 1973
Healthy subjects	13	130	166	Prescott, 1980
Healthy subjects	11.9	131	166	Prescott *et al.*, 1981
Induced patients	9.0	116	138	Prescott *et al.*, 1981
Healthy males	19.9	–	–	Miners *et al.*, 1983
Healthy females	17.5	–	–	Miners *et al.*, 1983
Healthy subjects (5 mg kg^{-1})	–	–	273	Clements *et al.*, 1984
Healthy subjects (20 mg kg^{-1})	–	–	205	Clements *et al.*, 1984
Healthy subjects	19.6	–	–	Miners *et al.*, 1984c
Healthy subjects	6.3	100	161	Morris and Levy, 1984
Non-pregnant females	14.8	–	–	Miners *et al.*, 1986
Pregnant females	19.6	–	–	Miners *et al.*, 1986
Healthy females	5.8	–	–	Rayburn *et al.*, 1986
Pregnant females	10.2	–	–	Rayburn *et al.*, 1986
Healthy subjects	10.1	–	–	Kamali *et al.*, 1987b
Healthy subjects (young)	15.7	–	–	Miners *et al.*, 1988
Healthy subjects (elderly)	9.3	–	–	Miners *et al.*, 1988
Healthy subjects	15.7	137	172	Prescott *et al.*, 1989b
Renal failure patients	5.9	14.5	14.8	Prescott *et al.*, 1989b
Healthy subjects	15.2	–	–	Slattery *et al.*, 1989
Healthy subjects	10.7	374	203	Hoffman *et al.*, 1990
Healthy subjects[3]	–	433	906	Pantuck *et al.*, 1991
Healthy subjects[4]	–	236	613	Pantuck *et al.*, 1991
Healthy subjects (fluid restricted)	18.8	–	–	Miners *et al.*, 1992
Healthy subjects (fluid loaded)	47.8	–	–	Miners *et al.*, 1992
Healthy subjects	25.9	–	–	Kamali *et al.*, 1993
Diabetic patients	71.9	–	–	Kamali *et al.*, 1993

[1] glucuronide and sulphate conjugates combined; [2] presumed to be expressed as ml min 1.73 m^2 – no units mentioned by authors; [3] high protein, low carbohydrate diet; [4] low protein, high carbohydrate diet

Table 9.2 Renal clearances of paracetamol and its conjugates in animals (ml min kg^{-1}).

Species	Para-cetamol	Glucuronide conjugate	Sulphate conjugate	Reference
Rat (15 mg kg^{-1})	0.88	4.47	10.2	Galinsky and Levy, 1981
Rat (30 mg kg^{-1})	1.05	4.63	13.2	Galinsky and Levy, 1981
Rat (150 mg kg^{-1})	0.74	4.89	12.2	Galinsky and Levy, 1981
Rat (300 mg kg^{-1})	0.89	5.82	15.4	Galinsky and Levy, 1981
Rat[1]	–	–	14.7	Galinsky and Levy, 1981
Rat[2]	–	13.8	–	Galinsky and Levy, 1981
Rat	0.72	–	–	Galinsky and Levy, 1982
Rat	–	18.8	18.5	Lin and Levy, 1982
Rat (15 mg kg^{-1})	1.5	–	–	Lin and Levy, 1983b
Rat (15 mg kg^{-1}, pregnant)	2.2	–	–	Lin and Levy, 1983b
Rat (300 mg kg^{-1})	1.1	–	–	Lin and Levy, 1983b
Rat (300 mg kg^{-1}, pregnant)	1.2	–	–	Lin and Levy, 1983b
Rat	1.8	6.0	9.8	Jung, 1985
Rat (protein deficiency)	1.6	4.8	6.9	Jung, 1985
Rat	1.27	6.3	20.0	Galinsky, 1986
Rat (diethylmaleate)	1.01	6.3	10.0	Galinsky, 1986
Rat (buthionine sulphoximine)	1.14	5.9	13.6	Galinsky, 1986
Rat (5 months old)	1.2	5.2	15.5	Galinsky and Corcoran, 1986
Rat (14 months old)	1.0	5.5	14.8	Galinsky and Corcoran, 1986
Rat (25 months old)	1.1	5.4	9.7	Galinsky and Corcoran, 1986
Rat (15 mg kg^{-1})	1.3	–	10.9	Lin and Levy, 1986
Rat (30 mg kg^{-1})	1.4	–	10.1	Lin and Levy, 1986
Rat (150 mg kg^{-1})	1.2	–	13.1	Lin and Levy, 1986
Rat (300 mg kg^{-1})	1.2	–	11.8	Lin and Levy, 1986
Rat	0.38	2.2	2.5	Wong *et al.*, 1986b
Rat (energy-dense diet, lean)	0.44	2.2	3.0	Wong *et al.*, 1986b
Rat (energy-dense diet, obese)	0.41	2.9	3.6	Wong *et al.*, 1986b
Rat	2.8	1.5	21.0	Zafar *et al.*, 1987
Rat (water deprived)	1.0	4.6	24.6	Zafar *et al.*, 1987
Rat	2.9	–	–	Galinsky and Chalasinka, 1988
Rat (30 mg kg^{-1})	1.4	–	–	Galinsky and Corcoran, 1988
Rat (150 mg kg^{-1})	0.8	–	–	Galinsky and Corcoran, 1988
Rat	0.9	–	–	Kane *et al.*, 1989
Rat	0.9	–	–	Svensson and Chong, 1989
Rat (5 months old)	1.57	8.42	11.14	Galinsky *et al.*, 1990
Rat (12 months old)	1.21	7.53	8.02	Galinsky *et al.*, 1990
Rat (22 months old)	0.99	5.85	7.28	Galinsky *et al.*, 1990
Rat	3.3	0.8	33.9	Shrewsbury and White, 1990
Rat	1.2	1.3	4.5	Manning *et al.*, 1991
Rat[3]	0.5	6.1	9.3	Savina and Brouwer, 1992
Rat	–	6.63	10.5	Brouwer, 1993
Mouse[4]	0.1	0.4	0.3	Tredger *et al.*, 1986b
Dog[2,4]	–	1.9	–	Hekman *et al.*, 1986

(cont.)

161

Table 9.2 (cont.)

Species	Para-cetamol	Glucuronide conjugate	Sulphate conjugate	Reference
Lamb (neonatal)	–	5.64	4.03	Wang *et al.*, 1985
Sheep (pregnant)	0.3	3.9	4.4	Wang *et al.*, 1986a
Sheep	0.4	5.8	6.8	Wang *et al.*, 1990
Lamb (neonatal)	0.5	3.2	2.2	Wang *et al.*, 1990
Lamb (fetal)	0.6	1.5	1.0	Wang *et al.*, 1990
Baboon	0.74	–	–	Altomare *et al.*, 1984b

[1] intravenous injection of paracetamol sulphate; [2] intravenous injection of paracetamol glucuronide; [3] units not stated; [4] expressed in $1\ h^{-1}$

clearances of the conjugates usually exceeded the normal glomerular filtration rate indicating at least some active tubular secretion. An abnormally high clearance of paracetamol was reported in diabetic patients and although this could have been related to polyuria, no details of urine flow rate were given (Kamali *et al.*, 1993). There was no obvious explanation for the extraordinarily high clearance values quoted for the glucuronide and sulphate conjugates in another report (Pantuck *et al.*, 1991).

The 24 h renal excretion of total paracetamol was correlated with the creatinine clearance in patients with impaired renal function (Dubach, 1967b, 1968) and the renal clearances of paracetamol and its conjugates were all reduced in patients with chronic renal failure (Prescott *et al.*, 1989b). In animals there was no effect of dose on the renal clearance of paracetamol and its sulphate conjugate (Lin and Levy, 1983b, 1986; Galinsky and Corcoran, 1988), and in man the clearance of unchanged drug was the same with overdosage as with therapeutic doses (Prescott and Wright, 1973; Prescott, 1980). In dogs the renal clearances of the glucuronide and particularly the sulphate conjugate of paracetamol were inversely related to their plasma concentrations (Duggin and Mudge, 1975). In man there was a similar inverse relationship between plasma concentrations and the renal clearance of the sulphate conjugate (Clements *et al.*, 1984; Morris and Levy, 1984). Probenecid impaired the renal excretion of the sulphate conjugate in rats, presumably through competition for active transport, but it had no effect on the renal clearance of the glucuronide conjugate (Savina and Brouwer, 1992). As renal function declined with age, the renal clearances of paracetamol and the glucuronide and sulphate conjugates were lower in rats at the age of 12 months than at 5 months, and the clearances were even lower at 22 months (Galinsky *et al.*, 1990).

Paracetamol was converted to the mercapturic acid conjugate in the isolated perfused rat kidney, and it was presumably formed via the glutathione and cysteine conjugates (Healey *et al.*, 1980). Little information was available concerning the renal excretion of the cysteine and mercapturic acid conjugates of paracetamol. In mice clearance values of 1.19 and $0.05\ 1\ h^{-1}$ respectively were quoted (Tredger *et al.*, 1986b). The mean renal clearances of the cysteine and mercapturic acid conjugates in patients with chronic renal failure were 35 and 80 ml min^{-1} respectively and the much greater apparent clearance of the mercapturic acid conjugate raised the possibility of its formation in the kidney by acetylation of the cysteine conjugate. The clearances of the cysteine and mercapturic acid conjugates were much greater than the simultaneously measured clearances of the sulphate and glucuronide conjugates (Prescott *et al.*, 1989b).

Metabolic Ratios

Despite the non-linear formation and clearance kinetics of the sulphate conjugate of paracetamol, the ratios of the amounts of the sulphate and glucuronide conjugates excreted in the urine have been used as an index of the capacities of these two pathways of elimination (Miller *et al.*, 1976b; Caldwell *et al.*, 1980; Critchley *et al.*, 1986; Steventon *et al.*, 1989, 1990). In addition, the proportion of the total excreted as paracetamol and its conjugates in sequential urine samples changed dramatically over time, giving rise to further serious errors unless urine was collected over a long period. As shown in Figure 9.2, during the first 4 h after an oral dose of paracetamol the sulphate conjugate accounted initially for a very high but rapidly falling proportion of the total excreted while there was a corresponding increase in glucuronide

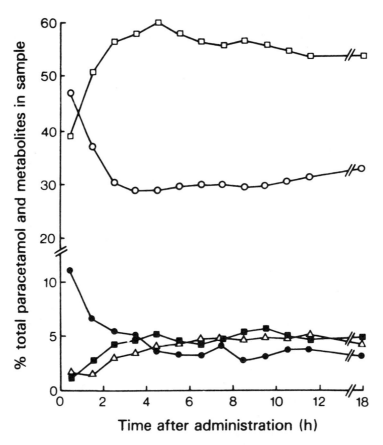

Figure 9.2 Changes in the pattern of the mean fractional urinary excretion of paracetamol (●) and its sulphate (○), glucuronide (□), cysteine (△), and mercapturic acid conjugates (■) with time after an oral dose of 20 mg kg^{-1} in eight healthy subjects (reproduced with permission from Prescott, 1980).

conjugate. Over the same period, the fractional excretion of unchanged drug fell rapidly and the contribution of the cysteine and mercapturic acid conjugates rose progressively. The urinary metabolite to paracetamol ratio has also been proposed as an index of the formation of the different conjugates (Bock *et al.*, 1987). Again, this could introduce unacceptable discrepancies because the metabolic ratios would vary with the urine flow rate. This was the predictable consequence of the flow-dependent renal clearance of paracetamol and flow-independent clearance of its glucuronide and sulphate conjugates (Kietzmann *et al.*, 1990; Miners *et al.*, 1992). There were obvious pitfalls in the interpretation of urinary metabolite excretion data in studies of drug metabolism (Miners and Birkett, 1993).

Elimination of Paracetamol by the Isolated Perfused Kidney

The isolated perfused kidney preparation permitted measurement of virtually any physiological function that could be studied *in vivo*. Over the toxic range of paracetamol concentrations of 150 to 450 mg l^{-1}, the fractional reabsorption by the isolated perfused rat kidney was about 74 per cent irrespective of concentration, and this was similar to values obtained in other species *in vivo*. An apparent maximum rate of reabsorption as the filtered load of paracetamol increased was considered to be an artefact caused by the diuresis induced at high concentrations (Ross *et al.*, 1980).

Extracorporeal Removal

Extracorporeal techniques such as haemodialysis, charcoal haemoperfusion, plasmapheresis and exchange transfusion have been applied in attempts to enhance removal and reduce the toxicity of paracetamol following overdosage. Elimination should be increased because paracetamol was moderately dialyzable, readily adsorbed onto charcoal and it had a relatively small distribution volume. However, these methods of removal were ineffective in preventing paracetamol toxicity and have been abandoned. The probable reason for their failure was that most damage was initiated soon after ingestion when virtually the whole overdose first passed rapidly through the liver during absorption. In addition, paracetamol was normally cleared rapidly and these techniques added relatively little because their clearance was limited by factors such as extraction efficiency, blood flow rate and exchange volumes. More importantly, early specific therapy with N-acetylcysteine was so effective in preventing serious hepatic and renal toxicity that other less certain forms of treatment have become redundant.

Haemodialysis and Peritoneal Dialysis

Paracetamol was dialyzable as it was not extensively bound to plasma proteins and it had a relatively small molecular size. Haemodialysis was carried out in 15 patients with paracetamol poisoning and the clearance by dialysis ranged from about 50 to 150 ml min^{-1} as the flow rate was increased from about 100 to 300 ml min^{-1}. Liver damage was not prevented but haemodialysis was recommended nevertheless as treatment for overdosage (Farid *et al.*, 1972). It was subsequently pointed out that the procedure was performed unnecessarily in at least 11 patients and that only one was at risk of severe liver damage anyway. In one patient there was little more than the equivalent of one tablet of paracetamol in the body before haemodialysis was started (Prescott, 1972). In patients with chronic renal failure the mean clearances of paracetamol and its total conjugates by haemodialysis were 112 and 106 ml min^{-1} respectively. Haemodialysis was advocated for the treatment of paracetamol poisoning on the grounds that it effectively removed the conjugated drug but the logic of this argument is obscure and it was admitted that haemodialysis was not very effective in competing with the liver for removal of the unchanged drug (Lee *et al.*, 1981a). Extraction ratios for paracetamol of 0.46–0.78 were reported in four patients with chronic renal failure during treatment with two dialyzers in series. The corresponding extraction ratios for the glucuronide and sulphate conjugates were 0.53–0.57 and 0.13–0.60. With an average blood flow rate of 250 ml min^{-1}, the whole blood clearance of paracetamol was about 170 ml min^{-1}, and the mean half life fell from a control value of 130 min to 70 min during dialysis (Øie *et al.*, 1975). In another report, the haemodialysis extraction ratio for paracetamol was 0.48 in six patients given a dose of 650 mg, but only about 11 per cent of the dose was removed by the procedure in 3 h (Marbury *et al.*, 1979, 1980). In a severely poisoned 1-year-old child, haemodialysis was started 12 h after the overdose and continued for 6 h. The mean extraction ratio and clearance by dialysis were 0.34 and 18 ml min^{-1} respectively, and the total amount of drug and conjugates removed was 2.8 g. Liver damage was not prevented (Lieh-Lai *et al.*, 1984). A sorbent suspension reciprocating dialyzer incorporating activated charcoal and exchange resins could be used for longer periods than conventional dialyzers but was no more effective in removing paracetamol (Shihab-Eldeen *et al.*, 1988). Peritoneal dialysis has been employed in paracetamol poisoning but no data were given regarding efficacy (MacLean *et al.*, 1968a).

Haemoperfusion

Activated charcoal readily adsorbed paracetamol *in vitro*, and its efficacy and biocompatibility were improved by poly(hydroxyethylmethacrylate) coating (Gazzard *et al.*, 1974c). The extraction of paracetamol during charcoal haemoperfusion in pigs exceeded 90 per cent with removal of about 50 per cent of the dose in 150 min (Willson *et al.*, 1973). Charcoal haemoperfusion enhanced the clearance of paracetamol from the plasma compartment in dogs, and the mean corrected increase was 171 per cent. However, the haemoperfusion clearance decreased markedly after one hour, presumably because of saturation of the charcoal. Failure to take account of the normal processes of drug elimination and distribution resulted in a two-fold overestimate of the efficacy of removal by haemoperfusion (Winchester *et al.*, 1974). In further studies in dogs, charcoal haemoperfusion was considered to be more effective than conventional dialysis for the removal of paracetamol (Widdop *et al.*, 1975; Winchester *et al.*, 1975).

Despite these promising results, a controlled trial of charcoal haemoperfusion in patients with paracetamol poisoning showed no benefit. The plasma clearances of paracetamol were variable and disappointingly low, and only small amounts were removed (Gazzard *et al.*, 1974e). In a case report of combined barbiturate and paracetamol overdosage, an estimated 4.75 g of the latter drug was removed by charcoal haemoperfusion, but this did not prevent liver damage (Helliwell, 1980). There have been other anecdotal claims of the value of haemoperfusion for paracetamol poisoning (Winchester *et al.*, 1981). Haemoperfusion has been advocated for the treatment of late paracetamol poisoning but again this did not prevent severe and fatal liver damage. The amounts removed in some patients were equivalent to less than one tablet of paracetamol (Helliwell and Essex, 1981). In other reports of the use of haemoperfusion for paracetamol poisoning no information was given concerning the efficacy of drug removal (Rigby *et al.*, 1978; Zezulka and Wright, 1982). In a more recent report of the use of charcoal haemoperfusion and daily high-flux dialysis in patients with paracetamol poisoning, the morbidity and mortality were lower in patients who presented within 42 h than in those who presented later. It was implied that the better prognosis in the patients who presented earlier was due to this treatment but no evidence was provided to support this. The haemoperfusion clearance of paracetamol ranged from 120 to 167 ml min^{-1} (Higgins *et al.*, 1993).

Plasmapheresis and Exchange Transfusion

On first principles it is obvious that plasma exchange and exchange transfusion would be even less effective in removing paracetamol than continuous haemodialysis or haemoperfusion. A single oral dose of paracetamol was given to patients with polyarteritis nodosa two hours before plasma exchange. Only 5 per cent of the dose was recovered by the procedure and the plasmapheresis clearance of paracetamol was only 15 per cent of the control clearance (Fauvelle *et al.*, 1988, 1991). Despite a cord blood concentration of paracetamol of only 75 mg l^{-1}, exchange transfusion was performed in a premature neonate born after the mother had taken an overdose of aspirin and paracetamol. As judged by the subsequent blood concentrations of paracetamol, the procedure was of no benefit (Lederman *et al.*, 1983).

Excretion of Paracetamol in Breast Milk

In nursing mothers who had been given paracetamol, concentrations in milk were lower than in plasma. The mean ratio of the milk to plasma area under the concentration–time curve was 0.76 and the half lives in the two fluids were virtually identical. Less than 0.1 per cent of the maternal dose was present in 100 ml of milk (Bitzén *et al.*, 1981). In other studies, paracetamol passed rapidly into milk and concentrations were generally lower than those in plasma and saliva. Only the parent drug was detected in milk and the estimated dose to the suckling infant was a very small fraction of the weight-adjusted maternal dose (Berlin *et al.*, 1980; Matheson *et al.*, 1985; Notarianni *et al.*, 1987). In one report the milk to plasma ratio ranged from 0.2 to 1.9 and the basis for this extreme variation was obscure (Hurden *et al.*, 1980). In eight women given 650 mg of paracetamol the mean milk to plasma concentration ratio was 0.94 and there was a strong correlation with the ratios obtained *in vitro* by equilibrium dialysis (Beaulac-Baillargeon *et al.*, 1994).

10

The Pharmacokinetics of Paracetamol

Model-dependent and Model-independent Analysis

Early studies of the disposition of oral paracetamol in man indicated that it was extensively conjugated and rapidly removed from the body (Brodie and Axelrod, 1948b, 1949; Carlo et al., 1955; Gwilt et al., 1963a) but it was not until 1963 that the first definitive mathematical analysis of the time course of its elimination was described by Nelson and Morioka. They showed that the rate of urinary excretion of paracetamol and total conjugates became first order after absorption and distribution of an oral dose in five healthy subjects, and the mean half life calculated from the excretion data was 1.95 h. A similar more detailed kinetic analysis of the urinary excretion of paracetamol and the glucuronide and sulphate conjugates following administration of 12 mg kg^{-1} in four male subjects was subsequently undertaken by Cummings et al. (1967) according to the scheme shown in Figure 10.1.

In this scheme

D_B = amount of unchanged drug in the body
G_B = amount of glucuronide conjugate in the body
S_B = amount of sulphate conjugate in the body
G_u = amount of glucuronide conjugate excreted in the urine
S_u = amount of sulphate conjugate excreted in the urine
D_u = amount of unchanged paracetamol excreted in the urine
K = overall paracetamol elimination constant
KG_f = glucuronide conjugate formation rate constant
KS_f = sulphate conjugate formation rate constant
K_d = unchanged paracetamol excretion rate constant
KG_u = glucuronide conjugate excretion rate constant
KS_u = sulphate conjugate excretion rate constant

The paracetamol half life calculated from the urinary excretion rate ranged from 2.0 to 2.6 h, and rate constants were derived for the formation and excretion of paracetamol glucuronide and sulphate conjugates. The mean *plasma* half life of paracetamol during the linear elimination phase following an oral dose in healthy

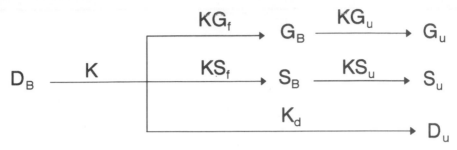

Figure 10.1 A scheme for the metabolism of paracetamol to glucuronide and sulphate conjugates followed by their elimination by renal excretion (from Cummings *et al.*, 1967).

adults was found to be 2.0 h with a range from 1.25 to 3.0 h (Prescott *et al.*, 1968) and this was confirmed in a subsequent study in which paracetamol elimination was compared in healthy subjects taking a therapeutic dose and patients admitted to hospital following acute overdosage (Prescott *et al.*, 1971). The plasma half life of paracetamol was prolonged in the overdose patients who suffered liver damage. At about the same time a mean plasma half life of 3.02 h was reported in healthy subjects in a study of paracetamol absorption from different dosage forms (McGilveray *et al.*, 1971). Pharmacokinetic analysis similar to that described by Cummings *et al.* above was applied in overdose patients to quantify the impairment of paracetamol conjugation and elimination caused by hepatotoxicity and nephrotoxicity. Estimates of the volumes of distribution of paracetamol and the glucuronide and sulphate conjugates were also obtained (Prescott and Wright, 1973).

The model-dependent kinetic analysis of paracetamol disposition in man was developed further by Albert *et al.* (1974a). Plasma paracetamol data from healthy subjects given two oral formulations were simultaneously fitted to an open two-compartment model with a lag time and first-order absorption using the non-linear least squares programme NONLIN to estimate the parameters according to the conventional scheme shown in Figure 10.2.

In this scheme

$$FD = \text{fraction of dose absorbed}$$
$$K_A = \text{absorption rate constant}$$
$$K_{12} \text{ and } K_{21} = \text{transfer rate constants between the compartments}$$
$$K_{el} = \text{elimination rate constant}$$
$$V_1 = \text{volume of central compartment}$$
$$V_2 = \text{volume of peripheral compartment}$$

Unless absorption was rapid the distribution phase was obscured and, as happened in this study, the scheme effectively reduced to a one-compartment model. Equations were presented to indicate when a one-compartment approximation was justified and weighting of the mean plasma concentrations by the reciprocal of their variances gave a more accurate reflection of the disposition in the individual subjects. Following rapid intravenous injection, the distribution of paracetamol from the central to peripheral compartments was shown by the initial very rapid but decreasing rate of fall in plasma concentrations before the final linear elimination phase became established after 45–60 min (Figure 4.3). Data obtained following intravenous administration of 12 mg kg^{-1} of paracetamol in healthy volunteers

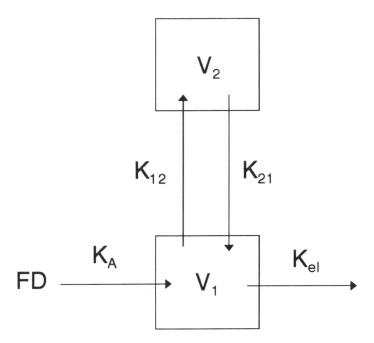

Figure 10.2 A conventional open two-compartment pharmacokinetic model for paracetamol absorption and disposition.

were fitted to a two- or three-compartment model by Clements and Prescott (1976) using a non-linear optimization procedure. For the two-compartment model the plasma concentration–time data were fitted to the following biexponential equation:

$$C_t = Ae^{-\alpha t} + Be^{-\beta t}$$

where C_t is the concentration at time t and A, α, B and β are hybrid constants. The use of different weighting factors resulted in up to a seven-fold variation in paracetamol half life but relatively little variation in predicted mean steady-state plasma concentrations. Conventional model-dependent pharmacokinetic analysis of paracetamol absorption and disposition has since been reported by many investigators in animals and man but it has been necessary to make assumptions about the linearity and structure of the model that have not always been justified. Experimental drug concentration–time data were usually fitted to the chosen model with appropriate weighting factors and estimates of the kinetic variables obtained by iterative curve-fitting.

Non-compartmental methods of analysis have also been used and these were based largely on measurement of the area under the plasma concentration–time curve (AUC) and the area under the first moment curve, which is the total area of the concentration–time × time plot (AUMC). The ratio of the AUMC to the AUC was taken as a measure of the mean residence time (MRT), which, after rapid intravenous injection, was analogous to the drug half life. The clearance and distribution volume were usually calculated from the area measurements as Dose/AUC and Dose(AUMC)/(AUC)² respectively. The biliary and renal clearances of paracetamol and its metabolites were usually calculated as the amounts excreted by these routes in unit time divided by the corresponding AUC. The partial clearances of paracetamol to its different metabolites (also referred to as formation clearances) have been determined as the product of the fractions excreted as the respective metabolites and the total clearance or the amounts recovered in the urine divided by the AUC for paracetamol (Amouyal *et al.*, 1987; Price *et al.*, 1987; Slattery *et al.*, 1987; Thummel *et al.*, 1988; Davies and Schnell, 1991; Howell and Klaassen, 1991; Manning *et al.*, 1991; Studenberg and Brouwer, 1991; and others). Attention was drawn to the interdependence of the different pathways of paracetamol elimination and the misuse of urinary metabolite excretion data in studies of paracetamol metabolism (Miners and Birkett, 1993). The site of sampling was important, and significant differences in paracetamol concentrations and kinetics were found with simultaneous blood sampling from the rat femoral artery and cut tail (Johannessen *et al.*, 1982). Efforts have been made to minimize the sampling required for analysis and both individual and mean values of single sample clearance estimates following intravenous injection of 300 mg kg^{-1} of paracetamol in rats were said to correspond closely to multi-sample clearance estimates (Bachmann, 1989). In another study, pharmacokinetic values derived from multiple samples following a single intravenous administration of 650 mg of paracetamol in 82 volunteers were compared with kinetic estimates based on only two data points at 2 or 3, and 6 h. As expected, the half-life values were highly correlated, but the clearance and volume of distribution were significantly overestimated by the two-point methods (Scavone *et al.*, 1990a). Pharmacokinetic analysis of concentration–time data for paracetamol and its conjugates has been extended to a variety of other circumstances. Examples include paracetamol disposition via biliary excretion and the enterohepatic circulation (Fayz *et al.*, 1984; Gregus *et al.*, 1988b; Studenberg and Brouwer, 1991; Goresky *et al.*, 1992), kinetic studies in perfused intestine and isolated intestinal loops (Pang *et al.*, 1986; Poelma *et al.*, 1990), liver (Pang and Terrell, 1981b; Fayz *et al.*, 1984; Studenberg and Brouwer, 1991, 1992; Goresky *et al.*, 1992), and kidney preparations (Emslie *et al.*, 1981a, 1982), kidney slices (Carpenter and Mudge, 1981), isolated hepatocytes (Aune *et al.*, 1984; Emery *et al.*, 1985; Mizuma *et al.*, 1985; Miller and Jollow, 1986a,b; Iida *et al.*, 1989; Anundi *et al.*, 1993; McPhail *et al.*, 1993) and liver microsomal fractions (Forte *et al.*, 1984; Price and Jollow, 1984; Boobis *et al.*, 1986; Roberts *et al.*, 1986; Seddon *et al.*, 1987; Rogers *et al.*, 1988; Ismail *et al.*, 1992; Bock *et al.*, 1993; Jaw and Jeffery, 1993). Physiologically based pharmacokinetic models were developed for the assessment of paracetamol disposition under conditions of weightlessness in space (Srinivasan *et al.*, 1994) and analyses were extended to describe the behaviour of paracetamol produced from the hydrolysis of prodrugs including propacetamol and eterylate (Priego *et al.*, 1983; Depré *et al.*, 1990; Autret *et al.*, 1993; Sabater *et al.*, 1993).

More complex pharmacokinetic analyses have been reported in special situations. With stepwise increases in the input concentrations of paracetamol in the perfused rat liver, formation of the sulphate conjugate was maximal at less than 1 mg l^{-1} and the relationship between the ratio of steady-state output concentrations of drug to metabolite and the reciprocal of the drug extraction ratio allowed prediction of metabolite concentrations in the liver (Pang and Terrell, 1981b). Other models were developed for the combined hepatic arterial-portal and hepatic arterial-hepatic venous perfusion to investigate paracetamol metabolism in the once-through rat liver preparation (Pang *et al.*, 1988a), and the kinetics of paracetamol formation and sequential first pass elimination from precursors, such as phenacetin and acetanilide, in the perfused rat liver have been reported (Pang and Gillette, 1978a, 1979; Pang *et al.*, 1979a). The kinetics of the sulphate conjugation of paracetamol formed from acetanilide and phenacetin have also been described. The higher the intrinsic clearance for paracetamol formation, the greater was the extent of subsequent sulphate conjugation, and this was explained on the basis of blood transit time and metabolite duration time (Pang *et al.*, 1982). Retrograde perfusion studies with phenacetin and paracetamol in rats gave results that were consistent with a heterogeneous distribution of hepatic drug metabolizing enzymes (Pang and Terrell, 1981a) and in studies in isolated rat hepatocytes, the kinetics of the disappearance of paracetamol formed from phenacetin suggested the lack of a diffusional barrier for preformed drug reaching enzymatic sites (Pang *et al.*, 1985). Attention was drawn to the problems with estimation of the hepatic blood flow rate from *in vivo* pharmacokinetic parameters using tracer doses of paracetamol as a model substrate with intravenous, oral, intraportal and intraperitoneal administration (Pang and Gillette, 1978b), and models were developed to estimate organ clearances for the formation of short-lived metabolites of paracetamol in the hamster liver based on a second-order reaction with a depletable endogenous substance such as glutathione (Chen and Gillette, 1988). The effects of input by the hepatic artery or vein, and the effects of perfusate flow rate and direction on paracetamol conjugation were investigated using the multiple indicator dilution technique (Pang *et al.*, 1988b, 1990, 1994; Pang and Mulder, 1990; Xu *et al.*, 1990). In another report, a dispersion model of the hepatic elimination of paracetamol was based on the spread of residence times of blood flowing through the liver (Roberts and Rowland, 1986). The kinetics of uptake of paracetamol by isolated rat hepatocytes were consistent with diffusion at concentrations above 0.5 mM, but at lower concentrations a saturable process was apparent (McPhail *et al.*, 1993). A two-stage pharmacokinetic model was proposed for the conjugation of paracetamol taken up instantaneously into isolated rat hepatocytes and the membrane transport of the conjugates into the medium. Observed changes in the amount of paracetamol and its glucuronide and sulphate conjugates in the hepatocytes and medium as a function of time agreed well with values obtained by simulation with the model (Iida *et al.*, 1989). The pharmacokinetics of aspirin and paracetamol have been compared by Levy (1981).

Microdialysis

Microdialysis probes have been used increasingly for the pharmacokinetic analysis of paracetamol in different tissues including the brain. This technique allowed for virtually continuous monitoring of paracetamol concentrations over extended periods and was a very powerful tool for pharmacokinetic studies (Morrison *et al.*, 1991; Scott *et al.*, 1991; Linhares and Kissinger, 1993, 1994; De Lange *et al.*, 1994).

Paracetamol Absorption

Simple and reliable measures such as the maximum plasma concentration (C_{max}), the time of the peak concentration (T_{max}) and the AUC have been widely used as indices of paracetamol absorption. The bidirectional transport of paracetamol across different regions of the rabbit intestine was not saturable over the concentration range of

15–4500 mg l^{-1} (Swaan *et al.*, 1994) and the oral absorption of paracetamol was commonly assumed to be first order. Compartmental analysis (with all its limitations) has therefore been used by many investigators to estimate the overall rate constant for drug input (Clements *et al.*, 1978; Forfar *et al.*, 1980; Holt *et al.*, 1981; Divoll *et al.*, 1982b; Mehta *et al.*, 1982; Ameer *et al.*, 1983; Saano *et al.*, 1983b; Tone *et al.*, 1990; Hossain and Ayres, 1992; and others). The optimum choice of model may depend on the different weighting factors used and in one report the uptake of drug into the systemic circulation was described better by two first-order sequential processes than a single process (Pedraz *et al.*, 1988b). The absorption rate constants obtained by these methods were hybrid, and included dissolution of the dosage form, gastric emptying and transfer from the gastro-intestinal tract to the circulation. In practice, dissolution and gastric emptying were the most important rate-limiting steps and they could be included in appropriate pharmacokinetic models. For gastric emptying, the gastrointestinal tract could be considered as two compartments, one representing the stomach from which absorption was negligible, and the other as the small intestine from which absorption was rapid. Analysis with such a model showed good agreement with observed values. The rate of absorption of paracetamol from the intestinal lumen was unrelated to the rate of gastric emptying and the mean half time of transfer to the circulation was only 6.8 min (Clements *et al.*, 1978). It was claimed that the bioavailability of para-cetamol could be estimated reliably with the use of truncated blood concentration–time curves (Lovering *et al.*, 1975) and similar estimates were apparently obtained with sampling from blood and saliva in healthy subjects despite greater variability with saliva concentrations (Cardot *et al.*, 1986; Shim *et al.*, 1990b). Comparisons of *in vitro* and *in vivo* correlations for different slow-release formulations of paraceta-mol were based on the Weibull function calculated from the cumulative dissolution data and plasma and saliva concentrations (Rodriguez *et al.*, 1990).

Comparisons of the mean residence time (MRT) after rapid intravenous and other routes of administration gave the mean absorption time (MAT), and statistical moments have been used as a measure of the absorption rate of different formula-tions of oral and rectal paracetamol (Concheiro *et al.*, 1984; Tukker *et al.*, 1986; Vila-Jato *et al.*, 1986a; Nakae *et al.*, 1988; Pedraz *et al.*, 1988a; Mizuta *et al.*, 1990b; Aw *et al.*, 1991; Depré *et al.*, 1992; Narisawa *et al.*, 1994). The MRT increased as the rate of drug input decreased and could itself be used to give some indication of relative absorption rates. Thus, the MRT in healthy volunteers increased from 5.2 h with an oral solution of paracetamol to 10.2 and 13.3 h after administration of two slowly absorbed controlled-release gradient matrix systems and further comparisons were made of the *in vivo* dissolution times (van Bommel *et al.*, 1991a,b). The MRT has also been used as an index of irregular absorption (Shim and Jung, 1992a). The cumulative fraction of the dose absorbed with time was another convenient measure of the rate of paracetamol absorption and hence, under certain conditions, the rate of gastric emptying (van Wyk *et al.*, 1990, 1992, 1993a,b; Sommers *et al.*, 1994). Both the cumulative fraction absorbed-time profile and the shorter proportional area under the curve method were comparable for assessing the kinetics of paracetamol absorption as a measure of the early phase of gastric emptying of liquids (van Wyk *et al.*, 1993c). Differences in the plasma concentrations of paracetamol after an oral dose in subjects who were recumbent and walking were attributed to changes in the rates of paracetamol absorption and elimination (Gawronska-Szklarz *et al.*, 1985).

The hepatic first pass loss after oral administration can be calculated from area

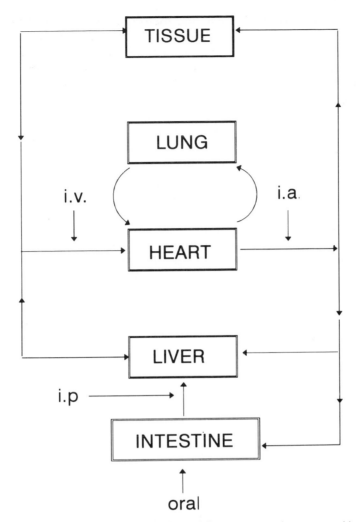

Figure 10.3 A pharmacokinetic model for analysis of the extraction of paracetamol by the gastrointestinal tract, liver and lung following oral, intraperitoneal (i.p.), intravenous (i.v.) and intra-arterial (i.a.) administration (from Bélanger *et al.*, 1987).

measurements and the hepatic blood flow rate if this is known (Chiou, 1975) but the extent of bioavailability has normally been determined as the ratio of the AUCs after extravascular and intravenous administration (Rawlins *et al.*, 1977; Perucca and Richens, 1979; Prescott, 1980; Eandi *et al.*, 1984; Olling and Rauws, 1986; Bhargava and Hirate, 1989; Hirate *et al.*, 1990; and others). The gastrointestinal tract, liver and lung were three potential sites of metabolism of paracetamol, and with a suitable model such as that shown in Figure 10.3, the relative contributions of these organs to the oral extraction ratio have been determined following intra-arterial, intravenous, intraperitoneal, intraportal and oral administration (Bélanger *et al.*, 1987; Bhargava and Hirate, 1989; Hirate *et al.*, 1990, 1991; Zhu *et al.*, 1991). The model was developed further to include the disposition kinetics of the glucuronide and sulphate conjugation of paracetamol to allow calculation of the relative contribution of these processes to the first pass metabolism of the drug in the gastrointestinal tract and liver (Tone *et al.*, 1990). Dilution altered the rate of absorption of a solution of paracetamol in rabbits but did not affect the bioavailability as shown by the area under the plasma concentration–time curve (AUC) (De Beer *et al.*, 1985).

The apparent rate constants for paracetamol absorption following oral administration of different dosage forms in healthy subjects ranged from about 1 to 10 h^{-1} (Clements *et al.*, 1978; Wójcicki *et al.*, 1978; Ameer *et al.*, 1981; Saano *et al.*, 1983b; Hagenlocher *et al.*, 1987; Ali *et al.*, 1988; Kirby *et al.*, 1989; Torrado *et al.*, 1990) and generally similar oral absorption rates were reported in children (Mehta *et al.*, 1982; Wilson *et al.*, 1982b; Brown *et al.*, 1992), the elderly (Divoll *et al.*, 1982b) and patients with peptic ulcer before and after surgery (Wójcicki *et al.*, 1984), right- and left-sided strokes (Stankowska-Chomicz and Gawronska-Szklarz, 1987), Crohn's disease and coeliac disease (Holt *et al.*, 1981), thyroid disease (Forfar *et al.*, 1980), and malnutrition (Mehta *et al.*, 1982). A somewhat wider range of absorption rate constants (0.7–15.8 h^{-1}) was observed with different solid and liquid formulations taken with and without food and dietary fibre (Liedtke *et al.*, 1979; Divoll *et al.*, 1982b,c; Eandi *et al.*, 1984; Walter-Sack *et al.*, 1989b). It was claimed that the rate of oral absorption of paracetamol was dose dependent over the range of 325–2000 mg, but this seemed doubtful. The pharmacokinetic analysis was carried out using saliva and there was difficulty in fitting the data to different models because radical fluctuations in saliva concentrations with time gave illogical profiles (Borin and Ayres, 1989). The rate constants for the rectal absorption of paracetamol depended greatly on formulation and ranged from 0.28 to 7.07 h^{-1} (Liedtke *et al.*, 1979; Degen *et al.*, 1982; Eandi *et al.*, 1984; Müller *et al.*, 1984; Kahela *et al.*, 1987).

The bioavailability of paracetamol in man calculated from the AUC following oral and intravenous administration as shown in Figure 4.3 varied from 95 to 98 per cent to 58 per cent with an average of about 80 per cent (Rawlins *et al.*, 1977; Fulton *et al.*, 1979; Perucca and Richens, 1979; Prescott, 1980; Ameer *et al.*, 1981; Divoll *et al.*, 1982b,c; Eandi *et al.*, 1984; Jack *et al.*, 1985; Depré *et al.*, 1992). The bioavailability of rectal relative to oral paracetamol ranged from 44 to 100 per cent (Moolenaar *et al.*, 1979a,b; Liedtke *et al.*, 1980; Seideman *et al.*, 1980; Degen and Maier-Lenz, 1984; Burgess *et al.*, 1985; Dange *et al.*, 1987; Hagen *et al.*, 1991) but in one report, the absolute bioavailability of rectal paracetamol was less than 40 per cent (Eandi *et al.*, 1984).

Distribution

Information concerning the dynamics of the distribution of paracetamol was obtained using the second and third curve moments, which were related to the variance and skewness of residence time distributions. This method was applied to the mixing and distribution curves in intact and liver-ligated rats (Weiss and Pang, 1992). The peripheral distribution and uptake into the central nervous system of several drugs including paracetamol was determined by their lipid solubility (Ochs *et al.*, 1985) and following the intravenous administration of the prodrug propacetamol in man, paracetamol appeared rapidly in the cerebrospinal fluid (Moreau *et al.*, 1993; Bannwarth and Netter, 1994). The kinetics of the transport of paracetamol across an *in vitro* blood–brain barrier was a function of molecular size and lipophilicity (van Bree *et al.*, 1988), and the unit impulse response procedure was adapted to characterize the transport of paracetamol into and out of the central nervous system (van Bree *et al.*, 1989a). Investigation of the kinetics of the distribution of paracetamol into the eye in rabbits indicated rapid uptake into the aqueous humour but distribution into the other ocular tissues was much slower (Romanelli *et al.*, 1991). The mean clearance of paracetamol from the synovial fluid in patients with rheumatoid arthritis was 40 ml h^{-1} and the half time of removal was about one hour (Owen *et al.*, 1994).

Paracetamol Elimination

Some details of pharmacokinetic data for paracetamol in animals and man are summarized in Tables 10.1 and 10.2. The findings after therapeutic doses in man showed a relatively consistent pattern but there were often major discrepancies in the animal studies. Although species and strain differences may have caused some pharmacokinetic variation in animals, the frequent use of excessive and potentially toxic doses would have been a much more important cause of non-linear kinetics resulting from saturation, depletion of cofactors and liver injury. As shown in Figure 10.4, the total clearance of paracetamol in the rat decreased progressively several-fold as the dose increased from 15 to 1000 mg kg^{-1}. The kinetics of paracetamol elimination were also highly dose dependent in the mouse, hamster, dog and cat (Table 10.1). In all species, the volume of distribution of paracetamol was very similar at 0.8–1.0 l kg^{-1} and the prolongation of half life with increasing dose could be attributed entirely to the decrease in clearance.

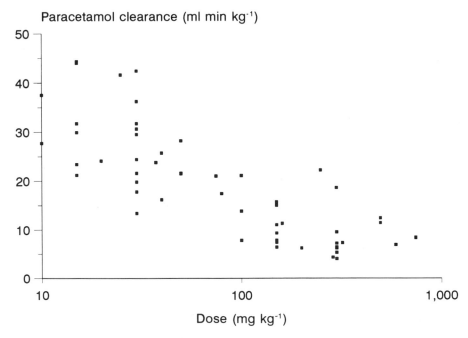

Figure 10.4   The inverse relationship between the dose of paracetamol and its clearance in rats (from data in Table 10.1).

Table 10.1 Pharmacokinetic data following administration of paracetamol in different animal species.

Species	Dose (mg kg^{-1})	Route	Total clearance (ml min^{-1} kg^{-1})	Volume of distribution (l kg^{-1})	Plasma half life (min)	Reference
Rat	15	iv	21.2	1.10	28.5	Cohen *et al.*, 1974
Rat	15	ip			22.8	Cohen *et al.*, 1974
Rat	tracer	iv	33.6	1.77	36.7	Pang and Gillette, 1978b
Rat	tracer	ip	53.7			Pang and Gillette, 1978b
Rat	100	oral			60.6	Siegers *et al.*, 1978
Rat	200	oral			78.6	Siegers *et al.*, 1978
Rat	400	oral			148.8	Siegers *et al.*, 1978
Rat	1000	oral			454.2	Siegers *et al.*, 1978
Rat	100	oral			106.8	Siegers *et al.*, 1978
Rat	400	oral			180.6	Siegers *et al.*, 1978
Rat	600	oral			30.0	Brown *et al.*, 1979
Rat	tracer	iv	40.6		30.0	Pang *et al.*, 1979a
Rat	15	iv	44.3	1.02	16.4	Galinsky and Levy, 1981
Rat	30	iv	42.4	0.88	14.8	Galinsky and Levy, 1981
Rat	150	iv	9.3	0.83	61.7	Galinsky and Levy, 1981
Rat	300	iv	6.4	1.13	122.0	Galinsky and Levy, 1981
Rat	15	iv	44.3	0.97	15.0	Johannessen *et al.*, 1981
Rat	30	iv	33.6	0.74	15.4	Galinsky and Levy, 1982
Rat	150	iv	8.8			Galinsky and Levy, 1982
Rat	15	iv	31.7		17.6	Lin and Levy, 1982
Rat	100	iv	7.8			Lin and Levy, 1982
Rat	20	ip			25.8	Price and Jollow, 1982
Rat	20	ip			25.8	Price and Jollow, 1982
Rat	50	ip			24.0	Price and Jollow, 1982
Rat	100	ip			32.4	Price and Jollow, 1982
Rat	200	ip			38.4	Price and Jollow, 1982
Rat	400	ip			74.4	Price and Jollow, 1982
Rat	600	ip			115.2	Price and Jollow, 1982
Rat	800	ip			181.8	Price and Jollow, 1982
Rat	1000	ip			261.6	Price and Jollow, 1982
Rat	15	iv	27.0	0.67	17.7	Aanderud and Bakke, 1983
Rat[1]	15	iv	39.8	0.89	15.7	Aanderud and Bakke, 1983
Rat	15	iv	29.9	0.89	19.5	Lin and Levy, 1983b
Rat[2]	15	iv	28.5	0.80	21.2	Lin and Levy, 1983b
Rat	300	iv	7.6	0.75	71.0	Lin and Levy, 1983b
Rat[2]	300	iv	5.3	0.78	101.0	Lin and Levy, 1983b
Rat	800	ip			116.0	Price and Jollow, 1983
Rat	10	iv	27.7	0.89		Watari *et al.*, 1983
Rat	20	iv	24.1	0.80		Watari *et al.*, 1983
Rat	40	iv	25.7	1.02		Watari *et al.*, 1983
Rat	80	iv	17.4	1.01		Watari *et al.*, 1983
Rat	160	iv	11.3	1.12		Watari *et al.*, 1983
Rat	320	iv	7.3			Watari *et al.*, 1983
Rat	37.5	iv	23.8	0.82	24.3	Hjelle and Klaassen, 1984
Rat	75	iv	21.0	0.84	27.6	Hjelle and Klaassen, 1984
Rat	150	iv	15.0	0.97	47.1	Hjelle and Klaassen, 1984
Rat	300	iv	9.5	1.10	81.9	Hjelle and Klaassen, 1984
Rat	600	iv	6.9	1.08	114.0	Hjelle and Klaassen, 1984
Rat	50	ic	29.4	0.95	22.4	Griffeth *et al.*, 1985
Rat[3]	50	ic	22.4	0.97	30.1	Griffeth *et al.*, 1985
Rat	100	iv	13.8	0.98	42.9	Jung, 1985
Rat[4]	100	iv	8.8	0.89	67.1	Jung, 1985
Rat	30	iv	30.6	0.78	17.8	Galinsky, 1986
Rat	150	iv	6.4	0.87	95.2	Galinsky, 1986
Rat[5]	300	iv	7.1	0.99	97.2	Galinsky and Corcoran, 1986
Rat[6]	300	iv	6.2	0.92	102.8	Galinsky and Corcoran, 1986
Rat[7]	300	iv	6.5	0.82	87.6	Galinsky and Corcoran, 1986
Rat[5]	30	iv	21.6			Galinsky *et al.*, 1986

Table 10.1   *(cont.)*

Species	Dose (mg kg^{-1})	Route	Total clearance (ml min kg^{-1})	Volume of distribution (l kg^{-1})	Plasma half life (min)	Reference
Rat[6]	30	iv	21.3			Galinsky et al., 1986
Rat[7]	30	iv	23.8			Galinsky et al., 1986
Rat	600	ip	4.0		71	Hazelton et al., 1986b
Rat	20	ip			24.4	Price and Jollow, 1986
Rat	20	ip			25.3	Price and Jollow, 1986
Rat	600	ip			34.8	Price and Jollow, 1986
Rat	600	ip			70.0	Price and Jollow, 1986
Rat	40	iv	16.2	0.86	21.6	Bélanger et al., 1987
Rat	40	oral			22.8	Bélanger et al., 1987
Rat[8]	30	iv	13.4	0.59	30.6	Blouin et al., 1987
Rat[9]	30	iv	10.0	0.44	30.7	Blouin et al., 1987
Rat	750	ip	8.3	1.20	104.0	Colin et al., 1987
Rat	287	ip	4.3		166.0	Corcoran et al., 1987c
Rat[9]	287	ip	2.9		183.0	Corcoran et al., 1987c
Rat	30	iv	27.4			Galinsky et al., 1987a
Rat[10]	30	iv	24.2			Galinsky et al., 1987a
Rat[11]	20	ip			20.4	Price et al., 1987
Rat[12]	20	ip			21.6	Price et al., 1987
Rat[11]	400	ip			56.4	Price et al., 1987
Rat[12]	400	ip			75.0	Price et al., 1987
Rat[11]	700	ip			91.2	Price et al., 1987
Rat[12]	700	ip			118.8	Price et al., 1987
Rat	100	iv	13.8	0.97	45.0	Zafar et al., 1987
Rat	1000	oral			402.0	de Morais and Wells, 1988
Rat[13]	1000	oral			432.0	de Morais and Wells, 1988
Rat[14]	1000	oral			420.0	de Morais and Wells, 1988
Rat	30	iv	31.7	0.82	17.9	Galinsky and Chalasinka, 1988
Rat	30	iv	36.2	0.91	17.3	Galinsky and Corcoran, 1988
Rat	150	iv	7.8	0.81	73.3	Galinsky and Corcoran, 1988
Rat	300	iv	18.6	1.40	156.0	Bachmann, 1989
Rat	200	ia	7.0	0.92	95.3	Bhargava and Hirate, 1989
Rat	200	iv	6.2	0.91	106.5	Bhargava and Hirate, 1989
Rat	200	portal	6.5	0.98	107.5	Bhargava and Hirate, 1989
Rat	30	iv	24.4			Kane et al., 1989
Rat	40	oral	11.5*	0.43*	25.8	Lin et al., 1989
Rat[15]	40	oral	13.1*	0.52*	24.0	Lin et al., 1989
Rat[15]	40	oral	10.5*	0.71*	33.6	Lin et al., 1989
Rat	20	ip			17.0	Price and Jollow, 1989b
Rat	200	ip			39.2	Price and Jollow, 1989b
Rat	400	ip			80.0	Price and Jollow, 1989b
Rat	150	iv	15.7	0.86	40.0	Svensson and Chong, 1989
Rat	250	iv	28.9	2.2	55.4	Tarloff et al., 1989a
Rat	250	iv	22.2	2.0	63.2	Tarloff et al., 1989a
Rat	500	iv	13.0	1.6	94.8	Tarloff et al., 1989a
Rat	500	iv	11.4	1.9	119.7	Tarloff et al., 1989a
Rat	750	iv	8.6	1.8	130.6	Tarloff et al., 1989a
Rat	750	iv	8.4	2.1	170.0	Tarloff et al., 1989a
Rat[16]	500	iv	25.3	1.9	49.9	Tarloff et al., 1989b
Rat[17]	500	iv	12.4	1.0	56.2	Tarloff et al., 1989b
Rat[18]	50	iv	28.2	0.81	27.0	Watkins, 1989
Rat[19]	50	iv	23.9	0.95	32.4	Watkins, 1989
Rat[20]	50	iv	27.8	0.84	26.7	Watkins, 1989
Rat[21]	50	iv	25.7	0.78	24.6	Watkins, 1989
Rat[22]	50	iv	22.2	0.83	31.0	Watkins, 1989
Rat	100	iv	21.1	1.11	38.5	Brouwer and Jones, 1990
Rat	15	ia	23.2	1.1	32.7	Hirate et al., 1990
Rat	15	iv	23.4	0.83	25.3	Hirate et al., 1990
Rat	15	ip			27.1	Hirate et al., 1990
Rat	15	oral			28.0	Hirate et al., 1990

(cont.)

Table 10.1 (*cont.*)

Species	Dose (mg kg[-1])	Route	Total clearance (ml min kg[-1])	Volume of distribution (l kg[-1])	Plasma half life (min)	Reference
Rat	30	ia	22.5	1.20	35.7	Hirate *et al.*, 1990
Rat	30	iv	19.8	0.77	29.7	Hirate *et al.*, 1990
Rat	30	ip			29.0	Hirate *et al.*, 1990
Rat	30	oral			39.1	Hirate *et al.*, 1990
Rat	150	ia	10.6	1.20	78.4	Hirate *et al.*, 1990
Rat	150	iv	11.0	1.00	69.7	Hirate *et al.*, 1990
Rat	150	ip			85.7	Hirate *et al.*, 1990
Rat	150	oral			110.3	Hirate *et al.*, 1990
Rat	300	ia	6.2	1.40	115.6	Hirate *et al.*, 1990
Rat	300	iv	7.2	1.10	115.2	Hirate *et al.*, 1990
Rat	300	ip			132.3	Hirate *et al.*, 1990
Rat	300	oral			192.2	Hirate *et al.*, 1990
Rat	30	iv	43.9	0.89	14.1	Shrewsbury and White, 1990
Rat	50	iv	21.5	0.49[23]		Tone *et al.*, 1990
Rat	10	iv	37.5	0.48[23]		Tone *et al.*, 1990
Rat	30	iv	29.5	0.46[23]		Tone *et al.*, 1990
Rat	70	oral			43.0	Aw *et al.*, 1991
Rat	25	iv	41.6	1.08	17.4	Aw *et al.*, 1991
Rat	30	ia	18.8		34.0	Hirate *et al.*, 1991
Rat[24]	30	ia	4.0	0.63	23.6	Hirate *et al.*, 1991
Rat[24]	30	iv	3.1	0.62	24.7	Hirate *et al.*, 1991
Rat[24]	30	ip			28.2	Hirate *et al.*, 1991
Rat[24]	30	oral			21.6	Hirate *et al.*, 1991
Rat[25]	30	ia	18.8		34.0	Hirate *et al.*, 1991
Rat[25]	30	iv	17.8		30.4	Hirate *et al.*, 1991
Rat[25]	30	ip			27.6	Hirate *et al.*, 1991
Rat[17]	30	ia	10.1		63.1	Hirate *et al.*, 1991
Rat[17]	30	iv	11.7		41.2	Hirate *et al.*, 1991
Rat[17]	30	ip			52.7	Hirate *et al.*, 1991
Rat[17]	30	oral			67.7	Hirate *et al.*, 1991
Rat	150	iv	7.4			Manning *et al.*, 1991
Rat	50	iv	21.6	0.94	30.7	Mansor *et al.*, 1991
Rat	43	iv	24.1	0.62	18.4	Sabater *et al.*, 1991
Rat[26]	43	iv	23.0	0.73	22.9	Sabater *et al.*, 1991
Rat[27]	150	iv	9.0			Galinsky *et al.*, 1992
Rat[28]	150	iv	8.8			Galinsky *et al.*, 1992
Rat	100	iv	21.1	1.12	36.7	Savina and Brouwer, 1992
Rat	50	iv	28.2	0.81	27.0	Watkins and Sherman, 1992
Rat	500	oral	2274.0*		896.4	Madusolumuo and Okoye, 1993
Rat[29]	500	oral	2910.0*		687.6	Madusolumuo and Okoye, 1993
Rat	50	iv	20.3			Ismail *et al.*, 1994
Rat[30]	50	iv	19.9			Ismail *et al.*, 1994
Rat	300	iv	16.9			Ismail *et al.*, 1994
Rat[30]	300	iv	11.9			Ismail *et al.*, 1994
Rat	100	iv	10.3	0.54	41.1	Jang *et al.*, 1994
Rat[31]	100	iv	10.8	0.55	39.2	Jang *et al.*, 1994
Rat	50	iv	12.6	0.80	22.8	Watkins *et al.*, 1994
Rat[32]	50	iv	17.2	0.72	16.7	Watkins *et al.*, 1994
Mouse	500	oral			60.0	Fischer *et al.*, 1981
Mouse	300	ip	18.5	0.90	37.0	Larrey *et al.*, 1986
Mouse[2]	300	ip	16.6	0.94	42.0	Larrey *et al.*, 1986
Mouse	400	oral	22.3*			Tredger *et al.*, 1986b
Mouse	200	ip			21.0	Price and Gale, 1987
Mouse[33]	50	ip	16.5			Adamson *et al.*, 1991
Mouse	50	ip	18.2			Adamson *et al.*, 1991
Mouse	500	ip			68.9	Peterson and Brown, 1992
Hamster[11]	20	ip			19.5	Miller *et al.*, 1986
Hamster[12]	20	ip			21.9	Miller *et al.*, 1986

Table 10.1 *(cont.)*

Species	Dose (mg kg[-1])	Route	Total clearance (ml min kg[-1])	Volume of distribution (l kg[-1])	Plasma half life (min)	Reference
Hamster[11]	75	ip			21.8	Miller *et al.*, 1986
Hamster[12]	75	ip			28.9	Miller *et al.*, 1986
Hamster[11]	150	ip			38.9	Miller *et al.*, 1986
Hamster[12]	150	ip			45.1	Miller *et al.*, 1986
Hamster[11]	200	ip			47.3	Miller *et al.*, 1986
Hamster[12]	200	ip			55.4	Miller *et al.*, 1986
Hamster[11]	350	ip			99.0	Miller *et al.*, 1986
Hamster[12]	350	ip			126.0	Miller *et al.*, 1986
Hamster	100	ip	17.8		24.8	Lupo *et al.*, 1987
Hamster	400	ip	6.3		41.0	Lupo *et al.*, 1987
Guinea pig	100	oral			112.2	Hidvegi and Ecobichon, 1986
Rabbit	100	oral			101	Imamura *et al.*, 1980
Rabbit	100	oral			77	Imamura *et al.*, 1981
Rabbit	100	oral			108	Kaka and Al-Khamis, 1986
Rabbit	30	oral	188.0[34]	0.16[34]	630	Ali *et al.*, 1993
Dog	25	iv			35	Kampffmeyer, 1974
Dog	100	oral			72	Savides *et al.*, 1984
Dog	200	oral			72	Savides *et al.*, 1984
Dog	500	oral			210	Savides *et al.*, 1984
Dog	150	iv	4.04	0.60	107	St. Omer and Mohammad, 1984
Dog[35]	150	iv	6.52	0.59	64	St. Omer and Mohammad, 1984
Dog[36]	50	iv			18	Ecobichon *et al.*, 1988
Dog[4]	50	iv			108	Ecobichon *et al.*, 1988
Dog	10	oral			40	Nakae *et al.*, 1988
Cat	20	oral			36.0	Savides *et al.*, 1984
Cat	60	oral			144.0	Savides *et al.*, 1984
Cat	120	oral			288.0	Savides *et al.*, 1984
Miniature pig[37]	40	iv	9.00	0.76	62.0	Bailie *et al.*, 1987
Baboon	40	iv	6.90	0.83	65.0	Altomare *et al.*, 1984b
Sheep	15	iv	15.30	0.90	58.2	Wang *et al.*, 1990
Sheep[38]	15	iv	3.80	0.88	185.4	Wang *et al.*, 1990
Sheep[2]	15	iv	14.90	0.82	53.4	Wang *et al.*, 1990
Buffalo calves	50	im	1.89	1.22	521.0	Sidhu *et al.*, 1993
Horse[11]	10	iv	4.84	0.83	118.0	Engelking *et al.*, 1987a
Horse[12]	10	iv	3.93	0.81	145.0	Engelking *et al.*, 1987a
Horse	10	iv	5.80	0.80	104.0	Engelking *et al.*, 1987b
Pony	10[39]	iv	4.60	0.75	120.2	Greenblatt and Engelking, 1988

ia = intra-arterial;   iv = intravenous;   ip = intraperitoneal;   ic = intracardiac;   im = intramuscular; * = illegal calculation

[1] at 71 ATA pressure; [2] pregnant; [3] after infrarenal aortic ligation; [4] low protein diet; [5] age 5 months; [6] age 14 months; [7] age 25 months; [8] lean; [9] obese; [10] with cyclosporin; [11] fed; [12] fasted; [13] heterozygous Gunn; [14] homozygous Gunn; [15] after vaccination; [16] age 3 months; [17] age 1 year; [18] urethane anaesthesia; [19] halothane anaesthesia; [20] isoflurane anaesthesia; [21] enflurane anaesthesia; [22] sevoflurane anaesthesia; [23] volume of central compartment; [24] age 3–4 days; [25] age 10 days; [26] with tolmetin; [27] young; [28] old; [29] with *Sacoglottis gabonensis*; [30] malaria infection; [31] spontaneously hypertensive; [32] excercised; [33] age 2 weeks; [34] incorrect units; [35] with N-acetylcysteine; [36] age 60 days; [37] endotoxin fever; [38] neonatal; [39] estimated dose

Table 10.2 Pharmacokinetic data for paracetamol in man.

Dose	Route	Total clearance	Volume of distribution	Half life (min)	Reference
1000 mg	oral[2,3,4]	294 ml min^{-1}	60 l	130	Øie et al., 1975
975 mg 70 kg^{-1}	oral	404 ml min^{-1}*	67 l*	121	Shively and Vesell, 1975
14.3 mg kg^{-1}	oral	477 ml min^{-1}*	1.03 l kg^{-1}*	109	Triggs et al., 1975
14.3 mg kg^{-1}	oral[E]	379 ml min^{-1}*	1.05 l kg^{-1}*	130	Triggs et al., 1975
1000 mg	oral	5.7 ml min kg^{-1}*	0.86 l kg^{-1}*	105	Briant et al., 1976
1000 mg	oral[E]	4.2 ml min kg^{-1}*	0.77 l kg^{-1}*	130	Briant et al., 1976
12 kg^{-1}	iv		0.91 l kg^{-1}	117	Clements and Prescott, 1976
1000 mg	oral[2]		86.1 l*[2]	142	Lowenthal et al., 1976
1000 mg	oral[2,4]		85 l*[2]	134	Lowenthal et al., 1976
1000 mg	oral		120 l*	136	Buniva et al., 1977
1000 mg	iv	352 ml min^{-1}	0.95 l kg^{-1}	150	Rawlins et al., 1977
1000 mg	iv	352 ml min^{-1}	0.95 l kg^{-1}	150	Douglas et al., 1978
1000 mg	iv[5]	255 ml min^{-1}	0.69 l kg^{-1}	134	Douglas et al., 1978
1000 mg	oral	133 ml min^{-1}*	40 l*	29	Wójcicki et al., 1978
1000 mg	oral	355 ml min^{-1}*		126	Andreasen and Hutters, 1979
1000 mg	oral[6]	162 ml min^{-1}*		222	Andreasen and Hutters, 1979
500 mg	iv	364 ml min^{-1}	0.96 l kg^{-1}	74	Fulton et al., 1979
500 mg	iv[E]	241 ml min^{-1}	0.90 l kg^{-1}	83	Fulton et al., 1979
1000 mg	oral	101 ml min^{-1}*	48 l*	343	Kazmierczyk, 1979
500 mg	oral		137 l*	150	Liedtke et al., 1979
500 mg	oral[7]		124 l*	168	Liedtke et al., 1979
500 mg	oral[7]		93 l*	150	Liedtke et al., 1979
1000 mg	oral[7]		112 l*	168	Liedtke et al., 1979
1000 mg	rectal		147 l*	186	Liedtke et al., 1979
1000 mg	rectal		236 l*	432	Liedtke et al., 1979
1000 mg	rectal		108 l*	144	Liedtke et al., 1979
1000 mg	iv	322 ml min^{-1}	0.96 l kg^{-1}	151	Perucca and Richens, 1979
1000 mg	iv[8]	490 ml min^{-1}	1.11 l kg^{-1}	113	Perucca and Richens, 1979
1000 mg	oral	101 ml min^{-1}*	48 l*	343	Wójcicki et al., 1979b

Dose	Route	Clearance	Volume		Reference
1000 mg	oral	115 ml min^{-1}*	39 l*	60	Wójcicki et al., 1979c
1500 mg	oral	4.1 ml min kg^{-1}*		144	Brodie et al., 1980
1500 mg	oral[9]	3.6 ml min kg^{-1}*		168	Brodie et al., 1980
20 mg kg^{-1}	oral[10]	5.4 ml min kg^{-1}*	0.94 l kg^{-1}*	122	Forfar et al., 1980
20 mg kg^{-1}	oral[11]	4.1 ml min kg^{-1}*	0.83 l kg^{-1}*	143	Forfar et al., 1980
20 mg kg^{-1}	oral[12]	3.8 ml min kg^{-1}*	0.83 l kg^{-1}*	166	Forfar et al., 1980
1500 mg	oral[S]	3.9 ml min kg^{-1}*	0.78 l kg^{-1}*	142	Mucklow et al., 1980
1500 mg	oral[S,13]	3.1 ml min kg^{-1}*	0.74 l kg^{-1}*	167	Mucklow et al., 1980
12 mg kg^{-1}	iv	5.45 ml min kg^{-1}	0.90 l kg^{-1}	119	Prescott, 1980
1000 mg	oral	163 ml min^{-1}*	38 l*	254	Wójcicki et al., 1980
650 mg	iv	4.5 ml min kg^{-1}		156	Ameer et al., 1981
20 mg kg^{-1}	oral	4.72 ml min kg^{-1}*	0.82 l kg^{-1}*	124	Holt et al., 1981
20 mg kg^{-1}	oral[14]	6.17 ml min kg^{-1}*	0.74 l kg^{-1}*	91	Holt et al., 1981
20 mg kg^{-1}	oral[15]	5.55 ml min kg^{-1}*	0.86 l kg^{-1}*	108	Holt et al., 1981
650 mg	iv	4.8 ml min kg^{-1}		160	Abernethy et al., 1982a
650 mg	iv[M]	4.55 ml min kg^{-1}	1.02 l kg^{-1}	166	Abernethy et al., 1982b
650 mg	iv[F]	4.16 ml min kg^{-1}	0.93 l kg^{-1}	160	Abernethy et al., 1982b
650 mg	iv[M,16]	3.74 ml min kg^{-1}	1.49 l kg^{-1}	153	Abernethy et al., 1982b
650 mg	iv[F,16]	3.59 ml min kg^{-1}	1.10 l kg^{-1}	139	Abernethy et al., 1982b
650 mg	iv	4.12 ml min kg^{-1}	0.96 l kg^{-1}	163	Abernethy et al., 1982c
650 mg	iv	5.81 ml min kg^{-1}	1.04 l kg^{-1}	127	Abernethy et al., 1982c
650 mg	iv[M]	5.07 ml min kg^{-1}	1.09 l kg^{-1}	156	Divoll et al., 1982a
650 mg	iv[F]	4.08 ml min kg^{-1}	0.94 l kg^{-1}	162	Divoll et al., 1982a
650 mg	iv[M,E]	3.90 ml min kg^{-1}	0.89 l kg^{-1}	162	Divoll et al., 1982a
650 mg	iv[F,E]	3.36 ml min kg^{-1}	0.79 l kg^{-1}	168	Divoll et al., 1982a
650 mg	iv	4.64 ml min kg^{-1}	1.02 l kg^{-1}	156	Divoll et al., 1982b
650 mg	iv[E]	3.74 ml min kg^{-1}	0.86 l kg^{-1}	168	Divoll et al., 1982b
1000 mg	oral	0.21 ml min kg^{-1}*	0.72 l kg^{-1}*	183	Kohli et al., 1982
1000 mg	oral[17]	0.20 ml min kg^{-1}*	0.69 l kg^{-1}*	206	Kohli et al., 1982
9–12 mg kg^{-1}	oral[18]	5.37 ml min kg^{-1}*	0.75 l kg^{-1}*	104	Wilson et al., 1982b
650 mg	iv	4.67 ml min kg^{-1}*	1.05 l kg^{-1}*	191	Ameer et al., 1983
1500 mg	oral	325 ml min^{-1}*	51.8 l*	117	Anderson et al., 1983
1000 mg^{-1}	oral[S,M]	5.62 ml min kg^{-1}*	1.01 kg^{-1}*	125	Miners et al., 1983

Table 10.2 (cont.)

Dose	Route	Total clearance	Volume of distribution	Half life (min)	Reference
1000 mg^{-1}	oral[S,F]	4.61 ml min kg^{-1}*	0.83 l kg^{-1}*	130	Miners et al., 1983
1000 mg^{-1}	oral[S,F,19]	5.62 ml min kg^{-1}*	1.01 l kg^{-1}*	125	Miners et al., 1983
1500 mg	oral[F]	287 ml min^{-1}*	42 l*	144	Mitchell et al., 1983
1500 mg	oral[F,19]	470 ml min^{-1}*	45 l*	100	Mitchell et al., 1983
650 mg	iv	4.59 ml min kg^{-1}	1.02 l kg^{-1}	160	Ochs et al., 1983
650 mg	iv[20]	3.56 ml min kg^{-1}	0.85 l kg^{-1}	171	Ochs et al., 1983
12 mg kg^{-1}	oral	470 ml min^{-1}*		119	Villeneuve et al., 1983
12 mg kg^{-1}	oral[21]	502 ml min^{-1}*		144	Villeneuve et al., 1983
12 mg kg^{-1}	oral[6]	231 ml min^{-1}*		186	Villeneuve et al., 1983
650 mg	oral	298 ml min^{-1}*	86 l*	189	Wright et al., 1983
500 mg	oral	7.8 ml min kg^{-1}*	1.4 l kg^{-1}*	127	Bedjaoui et al., 1984
500 mg	oral[E]	5.1 ml min kg^{-1}*	1.08 l kg^{-1}*	151	Bedjaoui et al., 1984
5 mg kg^{-1}	iv	331 ml min^{-1}			Clements et al., 1984
20 mg kg^{-1}	iv	295 ml min^{-1}			Clements et al., 1984
1000 mg	oral	154 ml min^{-1}*			Dietz et al., 1984
1000 mg	oral[21]	247 ml min^{-1}*			Dietz et al., 1984
600 mg	iv	263 ml min^{-1}	34.9 l	95	Eandi et al., 1984
1000 mg	oral[S,22]	5.78 ml min kg^{-1}*		121	Miners et al., 1984c
1000 mg	oral[S]	5.61 ml min kg^{-1}*		121	Miners et al., 1984c
1000 mg	oral[S,8]	8.32 ml min kg^{-1}*		87	Miners et al., 1984c
1500 mg	oral	442 ml min^{-1}*	78.1 l*	131	Mitchell et al., 1984b
650 mg	iv	4.97 ml min kg^{-1}	1.02 l kg^{-1}	146	Ochs et al., 1984
650 mg	iv[F]	5.19 ml min kg^{-1}	0.98 l kg^{-1}	133	Ochs et al., 1984
650 mg	iv[F,19]	6.12 ml min kg^{-1}	0.98 l kg^{-1}	115	Ochs et al., 1984
1000 mg	oral	8.8*[U]	68*[U]	415	Wójcicki and Gawronska-Szklarz, 1984
1000 mg	oral[23]	6.4*[U]	69*[U]	629	Wójcicki and Gawronska-Szklarz, 1984
1000 mg	oral[24]	3.2*[U]	37*[U]	681	Wójcicki and Gawronska-Szklarz, 1984
1000 mg	oral[23]	6.4*[U]	68.8*[U]	629	Wójcicki et al., 1984
1000 mg	oral[23,24]	8.3*[U]	70.8*[U]	455	Wójcicki et al., 1984

(cont.)

Dose	Route/ref	Clearance	Volume		Reference
1000 mg	oral[25]	3.2*[U]	36.1*[U]	682	Wójcicki et al., 1984
1000 mg	oral[24,25]	5.9*[U]	79.6*[U]	736	Wójcicki et al., 1984
650 mg	iv	329 ml min^{-1}	69 l	151	Abernethy et al., 1985
750 mg	oral	5.57 ml min kg^{-1}*		143	Chen and Lee, 1985
1000 mg	iv	301 ml min^{-1}			Jack et al., 1985
1000 mg	oral[S]	8.8 ml min kg^{-1}*		129	Ray et al., 1985
1000 mg	oral[S,26]	7.6 ml min kg^{-1}*		120	Ray et al., 1985
1000 mg	oral[S,24]	9.7 ml min kg^{-1}*		108	Ray et al., 1985
1500 mg	oral[27]	4.98 ml min kg^{-1}*	0.94 l kg^{-1}*	140	Sommers et al., 1985
1000 mg	oral	284 ml min^{-1}*	48 l*	126	Jorup-Rönström et al., 1986
1000 mg	oral[28]	224 ml min^{-1}*	52 l*	192	Jorup-Rönström et al., 1986
1000 mg	oral[28,29]	353 ml min^{-1}*	67 l*	138	Jorup-Rönström et al., 1986
1000 mg	oral[S]	285 ml min^{-1}*		127	Miners et al., 1986
1000 mg	oral[S,30]	452 ml min^{-1}*		91	Miners et al., 1986
1000 mg	oral[S,26]	7.6 ml min kg^{-1}*		144	Ray et al., 1986
1000 mg	oral[S,31]	9.7 ml min kg^{-1}*		96	Ray et al., 1986
1000 mg	oral[S,26]	8.7 ml min kg^{-1}*		126	Ray et al., 1986
1000 mg	oral[S,32]	17.0 ml min kg^{-1}*		58	Ray et al., 1986
1000 mg	oral[30]	365 ml min^{-1}*		222	Rayburn et al., 1986
1000 mg	oral[33]	257 ml min^{-1}*		186	Rayburn et al., 1986
500 mg	iv	638 ml min		119	Sonne et al., 1986
1000 mg	oral[S]	386 ml min^{-1}*	1.07 l kg^{-1}*	142	Back and Tjia, 1987
650 mg	iv	4.7 ml min kg^{-1}*	1.15 l kg^{-1}	169	Engelking et al., 1987b
1500 mg	iv	4.48 ml min kg^{-1}	1.01 l kg^{-1}	144	Kamali et al., 1987b
1000 mg	oral[S]	4.31 ml min kg^{-1}*	0.69 l kg^{-1}*	96	Pradeep Kumar et al., 1987
1000 mg	oral[S,20]	4.84 ml min kg^{-1}*	1.08 l kg^{-1}*	162	Pradeep Kumar et al., 1987
1000 mg	oral[S,34]	4.54 ml min kg^{-1}*	0.69 l kg^{-1}*	108	Pradeep Kumar et al., 1987
500 mg	oral	372 ml min^{-1}*			Slattery et al., 1987
1000 mg	oral	322 ml min^{-1}*			Slattery et al., 1987
1000 mg	oral[S,35]	2.56 ml min kg^{-1}*		217	Somaja and Thangam, 1987
1000 mg	oral[S,36]	3.17 ml min kg^{-1}*		274	Somaja and Thangam, 1987
1000 mg	oral[S,37]	3.40 ml min kg^{-1}*		119	Somaja and Thangam, 1987
1000 mg	oral[S,38]	2.97 ml min kg^{-1}*		130	Somaja and Thangam, 1987

Table 10.2 (cont.)

Dose	Route	Total clearance	Volume of distribution	Half life (min)	Reference
1000 mg	oral[S,39]	1.58 ml min kg^{-1}*	105*[U]	132	Somaja and Thangam, 1987
1000 mg	oral	9.98*[U]	137*[U]	770	Stankowska-Chomicz and Gawronska-Szklarz, 1987
1000 mg	oral[40]	15.74*[U]	98*[U]	611	Stankowska-Chomicz and Gawronska-Szklarz, 1987
1000 mg	oral[41]	16.98*[U]	107*[U]	661	Stankowska-Chomicz and Gawronska-Szklarz, 1987
1000 mg	oral[42]	24.77*[U]	73*[U]	929	Stankowska-Chomicz and Gawronska-Szklarz, 1987
1000 mg	oral[43]	20.61*[U]		520	Stankowska-Chomicz and Gawronska-Szklarz, 1987
1000 mg	oral[S]	10.4 ml min kg^{-1}*	1.31 l kg^{-1}*	96	Adithan et al., 1988
1000 mg	oral[S,44]	6.0 ml min kg^{-1}*	1.55 l kg^{-1}*	185	Adithan et al., 1988
650 mg	iv	4.84 ml min kg^{-1}	1.14 l kg^{-1}	164	Blyden et al., 1988
1000 mg	oral	201 ml min^{-1}*	70 l*	82	Gawronska-Szklarz et al., 1988
1000 mg	oral[45]	361 ml min^{-1}*	163 l*	61	Gawronska-Szklarz et al., 1988
1500 mg	oral[S,46]	378 ml min^{-1}*	57 l*	144	Kamali et al., 1988
1500 mg	oral[S,46,47]	353 ml min^{-1}*	67 l*	168	Kamali et al., 1988
1000 mg	oral[S,48,49]	17 ml min kg^{-1}*	1.9 l kg^{-1}*	77	Madhusudanarao et al., 1988a
1000 mg	oral[S,48]	9.5 ml min kg^{-1}*	1.9 l kg^{-1}*	134	Madhusudanarao et al., 1988b
1000 mg	oral	6.10 ml min kg^{-1}*		126	Miners et al., 1988
1000 mg	oral[E]	5.61 ml min kg^{-1}*		132	Miners et al., 1988
500 mg	oral[S]	310 ml min^{-1}*	45 l*		Nakano et al., 1988
1000 mg	oral	312 ml min^{-1}*		213	Parier et al., 1988
1000 mg	oral[50]	357 ml min^{-1}*		187	Parier et al., 1988
1000 mg	oral[50]	323 ml min^{-1}*		170	Parier et al., 1988
15 mg kg^{-1}	oral	347 ml min*	29.6 l*	75	Perlik et al., 1988
1000 mg	iv	299 ml min^{-1}	66.9 l	177	Sonne et al., 1988
1000 mg	iv	296 ml min^{-1}		179	Thomas et al., 1988
500 mg	oral	4.43*[I,w]	22.9*[I,w]	214	D'Souza et al., 1989
500 mg	oral[51]	10.2*[I,w]	0.5*[I,w]	120	D'Souza et al., 1989
1000 mg	oral[6]	203 ml min^{-1}*			Hayes and Bouchier, 1989
1000 mg	oral[6]	289 ml min^{-1}*			Hayes and Bouchier, 1989
1625 mg	oral	342 ml min^{-1}	92 l*	192	Pantuck et al., 1989

Dose	Route				Reference
1000 mg	oral^S	4.4 ml min kg^{-1}*	0.69 l kg^{-1}*	96	Pradeep Kumar et al., 1989
1000 mg	oral^{S,52}	4.4 ml min kg^{-1}*	1.04 l kg^{-1}	168	Pradeep Kumar et al., 1989
650 mg	iv	372 ml min^{-1}	68 l	132	Scavone et al., 1989
1000 mg	oral^{53}	405 ml min^{-1}*			Slattery et al., 1989
975 mg	oral	287 ml min^{-1}*		168	Venkataramanan et al., 1989
500 mg	oral^S	5.2 ml min kg^{-1}*	69 l*	132	Verhagen et al., 1989
500 mg	oral^{S,54}	5.4 ml min kg^{-1}*	65 l*	120	Verhagen et al., 1989
650 mg	oral	5.3 ml min kg^{-1}*	1.4 l kg^{-1}×	186	Awni et al., 1990
1500 mg	oral^S	364 ml min^{-1}*	77 l*	162	Baraka et al., 1990
5 mg kg^{-1}	oral^S	3.67 ml min kg^{-1}*	0.59 l kg^{-1}*	107	Griener et al., 1990
5 mg kg^{-1}	oral^{S,55}	4.15 ml min kg^{-1}*	0.74 l kg^{-1}*	125	Griener et al., 1990
10 mg kg^{-1}	oral^S	3.45 ml min kg^{-1}*	0.74 l kg^{-1}*	152	Griener et al., 1990
10 mg kg^{-1}	oral^{S,55}	3.63 ml min kg^{-1}*	0.74 l kg^{-1}*	143	Griener et al., 1990
650 mg	oral^{56}	5.3 ml min kg^{-1}*	1.01 l kg^{-1}×	126	Hoffman et al., 1990
650 mg	oral^{56}	5.9 ml min kg^{-1}*	1.21 l kg^{-1}×	144	Hoffman et al., 1990
1000 mg	oral^{57}	7.7 ml min kg^{-1}*	1.21 l kg^{-1}×	107	Kietzmann et al., 1990
1000 mg	oral^{4,57}	6.9 ml min kg^{-1}*	1.21 l kg^{-1}×	122	Kietzmann et al., 1990
1000 mg	oral^{S,4}	9.5 ml min kg^{-1}*		83	Lee et al., 1990
450 mg	oral	350 ml min^{-1}	44 l*	93	Saano et al., 1990
650 mg	iv		71 l	145	Scavone et al., 1990a
650 mg	iv^F	4.26 ml min kg^{-1}	0.85 l kg^{-1}	144	Scavone et al., 1990b
650 mg	iv^{F,58}	4.61 ml min kg^{-1}	0.82 l kg^{-1}	129	Scavone et al., 1990b
650 mg	iv	5.34 ml min kg^{-1}	1.11 l kg^{-1}	150	Scavone et al., 1990c
650 mg	iv^{59}	5.28 ml min kg^{-1}	1.03 l kg^{-1}	144	Scavone et al., 1990c
750 mg	iv^{11}	4.70 ml min kg^{-1}	0.79 l kg^{-1}	174	Sonne et al., 1990
750 mg	iv^{12}	3.12 ml min kg^{-1}	0.82 l kg^{-1}	198	Sonne et al., 1990
500 mg	iv	4.7 ml min kg^{-1}	0.77 l kg^{-1}	123	Wynne et al., 1990
500 mg	iv^E	3.7 ml min kg^{-1}	0.74 l kg^{-1}	144	Wynne et al., 1990
500 mg	iv^{E,60}	2.5 ml min kg^{-1}	0.61 l kg^{-1}	226	Wynne et al., 1990
650 mg	oral	497 ml min^{-1}*		156	Hindmarsh et al., 1991
650 mg	oral	533 ml min^{-1}*		132	Hindmarsh et al., 1991
16 mg kg^{-1}	oral	4.12 ml min kg^{-1}*		142	Hutabarat et al., 1991
16 mg kg^{-1}	oral^{61}	6.03 ml min kg^{-1}*		117	Hutabarat et al., 1991

185

Table 10.2 (cont.)

Dose	Route	Total clearance	Volume of distribution	Half life (min)	Reference
1000 mg	oral	6.04 ml min kg⁻¹*		138	Osborne et al., 1991
1000 mg	oral[62]	6.15 ml min kg⁻¹*		132	Osborne et al., 1991
1500 mg	oral[63]	443 ml min⁻¹*		132	Pantuck et al., 1991
1500 mg	oral[64]	395 ml min⁻¹		156	Pantuck et al., 1991
500 mg	oral[65]	351 ml min⁻¹*	0.94 l kg⁻¹*	129	Rumble et al., 1991
500 mg	oral[66]	375 ml min⁻¹*	0.92 l kg⁻¹*	123	Rumble et al., 1991
500 mg	oral[67]	332 ml min⁻¹*	1.02 l kg⁻¹*	142	Rumble et al., 1991
325 mg	oral[S]	389 ml min⁻¹*	0.85 l kg⁻¹*	111	Sahajwalla and Ayres, 1991
650 mg	oral[S]	323 ml min⁻¹*	0.95 l kg⁻¹*	109	Sahajwalla and Ayres, 1991
825 mg	oral[S]	328 ml min⁻¹*	0.86 l kg⁻¹*	121	Sahajwalla and Ayres, 1991
1000 mg	oral[S]	307 ml min⁻¹*	0.94 l kg⁻¹*	132	Sahajwalla and Ayres, 1991
650 mg	oral	5.8 ml min kg⁻¹*	1.1 l kg⁻¹*	149	Aoki and Sitar, 1992
12.5 mg kg⁻¹	oral[F,18]	7.18 ml min kg⁻¹*	0.43 l kg⁻¹*	115	Brown et al., 1992
20 mg kg⁻¹	iv	4.7 ml min kg⁻¹		163	de Morais et al., 1992b
500 mg	iv[68]	334 ml min⁻¹	0.93 l kg⁻¹	216	Depré et al., 1992
1000 mg	oral[E,69,70]	576 ml min⁻¹*			Miners et al., 1992
1000 mg	oral[69,71]	607 ml min⁻¹*			Miners et al., 1992
650 mg	oral	5.25 ml min kg⁻¹*	0.84 l kg⁻¹*	110	Beaulac-Baillargeon and Rocheleau, 1993
1500 mg	oral	6.2 ml min kg⁻¹*	1.0 l kg⁻¹*	127	Kamali, 1993
1500 mg	oral[72]	3.4 ml min kg⁻¹*	0.8 l kg⁻¹*	206	Kamali, 1993
500 mg	iv	3.55 ml min kg⁻¹*		162	Kamali et al., 1993
500 mg	iv[44]	3.70 ml min kg⁻¹*		144	Kamali et al., 1993
500 mg	oral[73]		28 l*	181	Prakongpan et al., 1993
500 mg	oral[74]		31 l*	151	Prakongpan et al., 1993
1000 mg	oral[S]	7.6 ml min kg⁻¹*		150	Ray et al., 1993a
1000 mg	oral[S,75]	9.8 ml min kg⁻¹*		90	Ray et al., 1993a
1000 mg	oral[S,31]	14.0 ml min kg⁻¹*		50	Ray et al., 1993a
1000 mg	oral	56 ml min⁻¹*	87 l*	526	Smilgin et al., 1993
1000 mg	oral[76]	95 ml min⁻¹*	72 l*	294	Smilgin et al., 1993

650 mg	oral	87 ml min kg⁻¹*w	0.85 l kg⁻¹*	121	Beaulac-Baillargeon and Rocheleau, 1994
650 mg	oral[30]	119 ml min kg⁻¹*w	0.88 l kg⁻¹*	97	Beaulac-Baillargeon and Rocheleau, 1994
500 mg	oral	6.0 ml min kg⁻¹*	1.10 l kg⁻¹*	156	Burger et al., 1994
1000 mg	oral	461 ml min⁻¹*	0.47 l kg⁻¹*	59	Wójcicki et al., 1994
1000 mg	oral[77]	557 ml min⁻¹*	0.70 l kg⁻¹*	67	Wójcicki et al., 1994
1000 mg	oral	312 ml min⁻¹*		138	Yiamouyiannis et al., 1994
1000 mg	oral	260 ml min⁻¹*		150	Yiamouyiannis et al., 1994

* = illegal calculation; [E] = elderly; [M] = male; [F] = female; [S] = saliva; [I] = inadequate sampling; [U] = unrecognizable units; [w] = wrong units
[2] per 1.73 m²; [3] haemodialysis patients; [4] renal failure; [5] Gilbert's disease; [6] chronic liver disease or cirrhosis; [7] liquid formulation; [8] epileptics or taking anticonvulsants; [9] vegetarian; [10] hyperthyroid; [11] euthyroid; [12] hypothyroid; [13] Asian; [14] Crohn's disease; [15] coeliac disease; [16] obese; [17] malnourished; [18] children; [19] oral contraceptive users; [20] congestive cardiac failure; [21] chronic alcoholics; [22] smokers; [23] gastric ulcer; [24] after surgery; [25] duodenal ulcer; [26] before surgery; [27] African villagers; [28] acute hepatitis; [29] recovered; [30] pregnant; [31] epidural anaesthesia; [32] halothane anaesthesia; [33] 6 weeks postpartum; [34] controlled cardiac failure; [35,36,37,38,39] days 3, 10, 14, 20 and 25 of menstrual cycle; [40,41] right-sided stroke at 2 and 6 weeks; [42,43] left-sided stroke at 2 and 6 weeks; [44] diabetes; [45] gastric cancer; [46] bladder cancer; [47] given with methotrexate; [48] anti-TB therapy; [49] pulmonary TB; [50] different dosage forms; [51] renal transplant patients; [52] tricuspid incompetence; [53] given with 10 g of N-acetylcysteine; [54] after butylated hydroxy-anisole; [55] Down's syndrome; [56] multiple administration; [57] intensive care patients; [58] using conjugated oestrogens; [59] smokers; [60] frail; [61] cystic fibrosis; [62] Chinese; [63] high protein, low carbohydrate diet; [64] low protein, high carbohydrate diet; [65] ambulation; [66] bed rest; [67] sleep; [68] given as propacetamol; [69] three times daily for 4 days; [70] low urine flow rate; [71] high urine flow rate; [72] with probenecid; [73] with ethanol; [74] with polyethylene glycol; [75] with trilene anaesthesia; [76] exposed to polyvinyl chloride; [77] with caffeine

In man, the volume of distribution of paracetamol was also reported as 0.8–1.0 l kg^{-1} by most investigators, and the total clearance and plasma half life with therapeutic doses in healthy subjects were usually about 3–5 ml min kg^{-1} and 1–3 h respectively (Table 10.2). Apart from the studies previously mentioned and those shown in Table 10.2, there have been many other reports of the paracetamol half life in healthy adults and patients with a variety of conditions taking therapeutic doses. In these studies the half life usually fell between 1 h and 3 h with an average of about 2 h (Wójcicki *et al.*, 1979a; Bitzén *et al.*, 1981; Adithan and Thangam, 1982; Saano *et al.*, 1983b; Tokola and Neuvonen, 1984; Albin *et al.*, 1985; Malan *et al.*, 1985; Adjepon-Yamoah *et al.*, 1986; Hendrix-Treacy *et al.*, 1986; Galinsky *et al.*, 1987b; Hagenlocher *et al.*, 1987; Kamali *et al.*, 1987a, 1992; Kinney and Kelly, 1987; Vendemiale *et al.*, 1987; Ali *et al.*, 1988; Kaniwa *et al.*, 1988; Pedraz *et al.*, 1988b; Hekimoglu *et al.*, 1991; Robertson *et al.*, 1991; Seideman, 1991; Becker *et al.*, 1992; Holt *et al.*, 1992). The plasma paracetamol half life has also been reported in children (Levy *et al.*, 1975b; Miller *et al.*, 1976b; Peterson and Rumack, 1978; Wilson, 1979; Nahata *et al.*, 1984; Roberts *et al.*, 1984; Hopkins *et al.*, 1990), vegetarians (Prescott *et al.*, 1993), twins (Nash *et al.*, 1984a) and patients with liver disease (Forrest *et al.*, 1977, 1979; Brazier *et al.*, 1982), obstructive jaundice (Brodie *et al.*, 1981), renal failure (Prescott *et al.*, 1989b), jejunostomy (Nelson *et al.*, 1986), obesity (Lee *et al.*, 1981b), malnutrition (Mehta *et al.*, 1982), enzyme induction (Prescott *et al.*, 1981) and after anaesthesia (Lewis *et al.*, 1991). In most reports the half life has been determined from samples taken for up to 8–10 h after administration, but generally longer half lives have been noted with sampling beyond this time (Clements and Prescott, 1976; Prescott *et al.*, 1989b; van Bommel *et al.*, 1991a). The paracetamol half life has been reported following the administration of different dosage forms (Saano *et al.*, 1983b; Walter-Sack *et al.*, 1989b), different oral doses (Rawlins *et al.*, 1977; Liedtke *et al.*, 1979; Borin and Ayres, 1989; Griener *et al.*, 1990; Sahajwalla and Ayres, 1991) and after rectal administration (Munson *et al.*, 1978; Moolenaar *et al.*, 1979a; Degen *et al.*, 1982; Müller *et al.*, 1984; Klein *et al.*, 1986; Kahela *et al.*, 1987; Walter-Sack *et al.*, 1989a).

Many of the studies summarized in Table 10.2 were performed in healthy young adult volunteers. Data were also obtained from young, elderly, pregnant and obese subjects with a variety of physiological, genetic and pathological conditions, and abnormalities could often be attributed primarily to changes in clearance and distribution volume. Unfortunately, many investigators have attempted to make a pharmacokinetic silk purse out of a sow's ear by forcing the analysis beyond the practical limits imposed by the conditions of the study. This applied particularly to the illegal calculation of total clearance and distribution volume after oral administration in man (Table 10.2). These variables (and, depending on the method of calculation, functions derived from them such as partial clearances) could not be determined properly in such circumstances because the fraction of the dose absorbed and the fraction lost by pre-systemic first pass metabolism were unknown. To add to these difficulties, many workers have used saliva for the kinetic studies and this was not satisfactory because major discrepancies have been observed between paracetamol concentrations in saliva and plasma samples taken at the same time (Lowenthal *et al.*, 1976; Adithan and Thangam, 1982; Kamali *et al.*, 1992). In some studies, results have been expressed in unrecognizable or incorrect units and there have been discordant findings that could not readily be explained within the bounds of physiological reality (Wójcicki and Gawronska-Szklarz, 1984;

Wójcicki *et al.*, 1984; Stankowska-Chomicz and Gawronska-Szklarz, 1987; D'Souza *et al.*, 1989).

Kinetics of Biliary Excretion and Enterohepatic Circulation

Pharmacokinetic models have been developed to describe the biliary excretion and enterohepatic circulation of paracetamol and its conjugates. An additional compartment with a time lag for intestinal transit and hydrolysis of conjugates may be required, and experimental data have been obtained from intact animals and animals with ligated and cannulated bile ducts (Watari *et al.*, 1983, 1984; Studenberg and Brouwer, 1993a). Standard pharmacokinetic methods have also been applied to the kinetics of biliary excretion of paracetamol conjugates in isolated perfused liver preparations (Fayz *et al.*, 1984; Studenberg and Brouwer, 1992). For example, a well-stirred hepatic model with linear processes was developed to describe the concentration–time patterns of paracetamol and its glucuronide and sulphate conjugates in the perfusate and excreted into the bile (Figure 10.5). This model gave results that were inconsistent with the rate of biliary excretion of paracetamol glucuronide in rats but a better fit was obtained when a cytosolic compartment with reversible binding to ligandin was incorporated into the model. However, the physiological relevance of the new model was not supported by subsequent investigation of the protein binding and subcellular distribution of paracetamol and its conjugates (Studenberg and Brouwer, 1993a). A barrier-limited

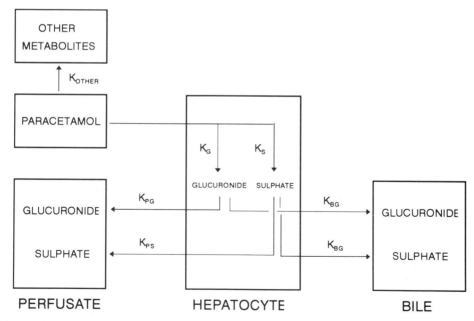

Figure 10.5 A pharmacokinetic model for the uptake, conjugation and hepatobiliary disposition of paracetamol and its glucuronide and sulphate conjugates by the isolated perfused rat liver. The symbols represent the formation (K_G and K_S), biliary excretion (K_{BG} and K_{BS}) and release into the perfusate (K_{PG} and K_{PS}) of the glucuronide and sulphate conjugates respectively (from Studenberg and Brouwer, 1992).

space distributed variable transit time model was proposed for the biliary excretion of paracetamol sulphate by the perfused rat liver (Goresky *et al.*, 1992).

Paracetamol Kinetics in the Materno-fetal-placental Unit and Excretion into Milk

Model-dependent and model-independent methods were used to study the pharmacokinetics of paracetamol in pregnant sheep following infusion to steady state on separate occasions in the mother and fetus. Placental and non-placental clearances were estimated independently and conjugation accounted for most of the non-placental clearance in the mother. Neither the glucuronide nor sulphate conjugates were transferred across the placenta but the parent drug was transferred in both directions by passive diffusion (Wang *et al.*, 1986a). In another report, the pharmacokinetics of intravenous paracetamol were compared in non-pregnant ewes, neonatal lambs, pregnant ewes and their fetal lambs. Placental transfer of paracetamol from the fetus to the mother was the dominant route of fetal clearance of the drug. There have been other reports of the pharmacokinetics of paracetamol in pregnant and non-pregnant animals and humans (Lin and Levy, 1983b; Miners *et al.*, 1986; Rayburn *et al.*, 1986; Ecobichon *et al.*, 1989). The use of a single point estimate of the milk:plasma concentration of paracetamol was liable to error, and simulations of the kinetics of transfer in the goat showed that the variance of the ratio was influenced by the route and duration of administration (Wilson *et al.*, 1987). A diffusional model was used to predict the milk and serum concentrations of paracetamol *in vivo* in adult rabbits and their pups (McNamara *et al.*, 1991). The pharmacokinetic values for paracetamol in plasma and breast milk were similar in postpartum women given an oral dose of 650 mg, and there was good agreement between the milk:plasma concentration ratios observed *in vivo* and the ratios obtained by *in vitro* equilibrium dialysis (Beaulac-Baillargeon *et al.*, 1994).

Pharmacokinetics of Paracetamol Glucuronide and Sulphate

Many of the kinetic studies of paracetamol have been extended to include the glucuronide and sulphate conjugates, and some of these merit special attention. The rates of formation of the conjugates in rabbits were much greater than the rates of excretion (Shibasaki *et al.*, 1971). The disposition of intravenous paracetamol sulphate and glucuronide in doses of 56.5–452 and 16.5–264 μmol kg^{-1} respectively in rats was well described by a two-compartment model and the initial rapid distribution phases lasted for 15–30 min. The disposition of both conjugates was similar and essentially linear, and they had much smaller volumes of distribution than paracetamol (Table 10.3) (Watari *et al.*, 1983). In another study, a pharmacokinetic model was developed for the enterohepatic circulation of paracetamol glucuronide following intravenous and intraduodenal administration in rats with and without bile duct cannulation. The model incorporated the lag time between biliary excretion and reabsorption as well as intestinal transit to the site of hydrolysis (Watari *et al.*, 1984). The pharmacokinetic implications of cosubstrate depletion have been investigated in relation to the dose-dependent formation of the glucuronide and sulphate conjugation of paracetamol (Galinsky and Levy, 1981; Levy *et al.*, 1982), and the time course and rate of excretion of paracetamol metabolites was studied in

Table 10.3 Pharmacokinetics of the glucuronide and sulphate conjugates of paracetamol following their intravenous administration in rats.

Conjugate	Total body clearance (ml min kg^{-1})	Renal clearance (ml min kg^{-1})	Elimination half life (min)	Volume of distribution (l kg^{-1})
Glucuronide (16.5–264 μmol kg^{-1})	7.00	6.37	13.38	0.26
Sulphate (56.5–452 μmol kg^{-1})	9.16	7.99	13.64	0.24

From Watari *et al.*, 1983.

man at different dose levels (Slattery *et al.*, 1987). A pharmacokinetic model of paracetamol absorption was proposed with intravenous, oral and intraduodenal administration to establish the relative contributions of glucuronide and sulphate conjugation to intestinal and hepatic first pass metabolism (Tone *et al.*, 1990). There was little or no transplacental transfer of the glucuronide and sulphate conjugates in pregnant sheep and their fetal lambs (Wang *et al.*, 1985, 1986a, 1990).

The volume of distribution of the glucuronide and sulphate conjugates of paracetamol combined was estimated to be 0.24 l kg^{-1} in patients with paracetamol overdosage (Prescott and Wright, 1973), and 14.1 and 19.1 l per 1.73 m^2 in patients with chronic renal failure. In a subsequent study, the volumes of distribution of paracetamol glucuronide and sulphate in patients with chronic renal failure were similar at 0.28 and 0.29 l kg^{-1} respectively. There was marked retention of these conjugates in patients with moderate and severe renal failure (Figure 7.10) (Prescott *et al.*, 1989b).

Saturation Kinetics and Paracetamol Overdosage

Standard biochemical methods have been used for the determination of enzyme kinetics under conditions of saturable paracetamol metabolism such as may occur in studies in isolated hepatocytes and liver microsome and purified enzyme preparations. The Michaelis-Menten constants V_{max} and K_m were usually derived from double reciprocal (Lineweaver Burk) plots and these were also used to elucidate the nature of inhibition of paracetamol metabolism by other interacting drugs (Dybing, 1976; Bolanowska and Gessner, 1978; Carpenter and Mudge, 1981; Watari *et al.*, 1983; Forte *et al.*, 1984; Mitchell *et al.*, 1984b; Emery *et al.*, 1985; Jeffery *et al.*, 1988; Ameer *et al.*, 1992; Bock *et al.*, 1993; Jaw and Jeffery, 1993; McPhail *et al.*, 1993; and others).

The *in vivo* K_m for the sulphate conjugation of paracetamol in rats and man was only about 100 μM (Slattery and Levy, 1979a; Watari *et al.*, 1983; Lin and Levy, 1986), but much greater values of 4.0–40 mM were reported for glucuronide conjugation in rats, mice, pigs and man (Bolanowska and Gessner, 1978; Moldéus, 1978; Slattery and Levy, 1979a; Miners *et al.*, 1990; Monshouwer *et al.*, 1994). In species in which sulphate conjugation was the major route of metabolism, such as the rat and cat, elimination should therefore be saturable and highly dose dependent. Conversely, this effect should be much less obvious in species, such as mouse and man, which depended primarily on glucuronide conjugation for removal. Despite the dependence on saturable sulphate conjugation in the rat, the fall in plasma paracetamol remained linear over a wide range of doses down to low therapeutic concentrations with no sign of a transition from zero to first-order kinetics (Siegers *et al.*, 1978; Price and Jollow, 1982; Watari *et al.*, 1983; Hjelle and Klaassen, 1984; Miller and Jollow, 1986a,b). Failure to observe the expected initial convex (downward) curve of the plasma concentration–time plot was attributed to depletion of inorganic sulphate, and sulphate conjugation kinetics were restored by infusion of sodium sulphate or the sulphate donor N-acetylcysteine. The half life of paracetamol in the rat was highly dose dependent and it ranged from 16.4 min following a dose of 15 mg kg^{-1} to 122 min after 300 mg kg^{-1} (Galinsky and Levy, 1981). A simple physiologically based pharmacokinetic model was proposed to account for the restriction of paracetamol metabolism resulting from sulphate depletion and in the absence of depletion the V_{max} and *in vivo* K_m of the formation of the sulphate conjugate were about 6.5 μmol min kg^{-1} and 100 μM respectively (Lin and Levy, 1986). It was also shown that the sulphate conjugation of paracetamol was maintained in rats with inorganic sulphate retention produced by experimental renal failure (Lin and Levy, 1982). The pharmacokinetic consequences of endogenous cosubstrate depletion for paracetamol have been reviewed (Levy *et al.*, 1982; Levy, 1986).

In man, the plasma paracetamol half life was not obviously dose dependent within the therapeutic range although sulphate conjugation was reduced as the dose was increased within the range of about 350–4000 mg (Davis *et al.*, 1976b; Clements *et al.*, 1984; Slattery *et al.*, 1987). However, the sulphate conjugation of paracetamol was clearly saturated after a large overdose and in some cases less than 10 per cent of the amount excreted in the urine was recovered as the sulphate conjugate (Davis *et al.*, 1976b; Howie *et al.*, 1977; Prescott, 1980; Forrest *et al.*, 1982). The fractional excretion of sulphate conjugate could fall to less than 5 per cent for a time, but subsequently there was a progressive increase up to 40–60 per cent as the total amount of drug in the body decreased (Prescott, 1979b). In patients who developed hepatic necrosis after taking paracetamol in overdosage, the plasma half life was prolonged in relation to the severity of liver damage (Figure 7.4). Some degree of liver damage could be expected if the half life was more than 4 h, while a fatal outcome was likely if it exceeded 10–12 h (Prescott *et al.*, 1971; Prescott and Wright, 1973; Gazzard *et al.*, 1977). It has been claimed that the glucuronide as well as the sulphate conjugation of paracetamol was saturated following overdosage, and that the liver was damaged because a greater fraction was thereby shunted through the route of toxic metabolic activation (Davis *et al.*, 1976b; Slattery and Levy, 1979a; Slattery *et al.*, 1981). A pharmacokinetic model was proposed in which paracetamol was removed via parallel pathways of saturable glucuronide and sulphate conjugation by Michaelis-Menten kinetics and first-order renal excretion and oxidative metabolism to the potentially toxic intermediate (Slattery and Levy, 1979a). The model was said to fit glucuronide (but not sulphate) excretion in one patient who had taken an overdose of paracetamol plus d-propoxyphene (Slattery *et al.*, 1981). Unfortunately this model was based on a very atypical pattern of urinary excretion of paracetamol metabolites in poisoned patients reported by Davis *et al.* (1976b) in which the recovery of cysteine and mercapturic acid conjugates was extraordinarily high while little or no unchanged drug was detected. Their findings differed markedly from those of other investigators using more reliable analytical methods. There appeared to be enormous capacity for glucuronide conjugation in man, and, as shown in Figure 7.4, there was no evidence for a change from zero- to first-order kinetics in poisoned patients as plasma concentrations fell from high toxic to low subtherapeutic levels. The plasma half life was prolonged from the outset in the patients who developed liver damage, and, if anything, the half life increased with time and the concentration–time curve became concave rather than convex downwards. In some patients who subsequently died with liver failure there was virtually complete failure of paracetamol conjugation (Prescott and Wright, 1973). The early prolongation of the paracetamol half life beyond 4 h was probably caused by the liver damage itself rather than saturation of glucuronide conjugation. Notwithstanding the above comments, the glucuronide conjugation of paracetamol could rarely become partially saturated after overdosage with exceptionally high plasma concentrations of the order of 1000 mg l^{-1}, but this was uncommon (Prescott, 1984). The modest prolongation of the plasma paracetamol half life with increasing dose in poisoned patients who did not suffer liver damage could be explained by the effects on sulphate conjugation. In patients treated with cysteamine (which prevented liver damage and probably stimulated sulphate conjugation) the initially prolonged paracetamol half life subsequently shortened towards normal (Prescott *et al.*, 1974).

Extracorporeal Removal of Paracetamol

Techniques such as peritoneal dialysis (MacLean *et al.*, 1968a; Grove, 1971) and haemodialysis (Farid *et al.*, 1972; Kerr, 1973; Winchester *et al.*, 1981; Lieh-Lai *et al.*, 1984) have been recommended for the removal of paracetamol following overdosage but the amounts removed were usually very small and these measures are of no proven benefit. Even with a favourable extraction ratio and dialysis clearance, haemodialysis was not very effective in competing with the liver for removal of paracetamol (Lee *et al.*, 1981a). Charcoal haemoperfusion may be more effective than haemodialysis but the clearance of paracetamol in animals was variable (Willson *et al.*, 1973; Gazzard *et al.*, 1974c; Widdop *et al.*, 1975). Pharmacokinetic models were developed to calculate the *in vivo* clearance of paracetamol by haemoperfusion in dogs (Winchester *et al.*, 1974, 1975). Charcoal haemoperfusion has been advocated for the treatment of paracetamol poisoning (Rigby *et al.*, 1978; Helliwell, 1980; Helliwell and Essex, 1981; Winchester *et al.*, 1981; Zezulka and Wright, 1982) despite failure to demonstrate any benefit in a controlled trial (Gazzard *et al.*, 1974e).

In a study of paracetamol removal by haemodialysis in anephric patients, the extraction ratios for paracetamol and its glucuronide and sulphate conjugates were 0.46–0.78, 0.53–0.57 and 0.13–0.60 respectively. Haemodialysis was the major or sole route of removal of the paracetamol conjugates in these patients (Øie *et al.*, 1975). In another study in patients with chronic renal failure the dialysis clearance of paracetamol and its glucuronide and sulphate conjugates was calculated by arterial-venous difference and simultaneous dialysate measurements. The extraction efficiency of the hollow fibre dialyzer was 47.5 per cent for paracetamol and 43 per cent for the total metabolites. The mean dialysis clearance was 112 ml min^{-1} and 11 per cent of the dose was removed by dialysis for 3 h (Marbury *et al.*, 1980; Lee *et al.*, 1981a). Improved clearance of paracetamol with minimal saturation was claimed for a sorbent suspension reciprocal dialyzer (Shihab-Eldeen *et al.*, 1988). With multiple dosing of paracetamol in patients with chronic renal failure there were good correlations between the observed and expected cumulation of the glucuronide, but not the sulphate conjugate (Martin *et al.*, 1991), and in patients with end-stage renal failure maintained on regular haemodialysis neither conjugate cumulated with repeated dosing as predicted (Martin *et al.*, 1993). The glucuronide conjugate of paracetamol has been proposed as a model molecular mass marker for trans-peritoneal transport (Schoots *et al.*, 1990). As predicted by established phar-macokinetic principles, negligible amounts of paracetamol were removed by exchange transfusion (Fauvelle *et al.*, 1988, 1991). Nevertheless, it has been used without obvious advantage in attempts to treat neonatal paracetamol poisoning (Lederman *et al.*, 1983).

Relationships Between Pharmacokinetics and the Toxicity and Efficacy of Paracetamol

The hepatotoxicity of paracetamol depended on the balance between the rate of formation of toxic N-acetyl-p-benzoquinoneimine, the rate of synthesis of gluta-thione, and the capacity of the parallel safe pathways of elimination. Phar-macokinetic models have been devised to describe the glutathione-dependent threshold dose-toxicity relationships, the production of short-lived reactive metabo-lites and the kinetics of their covalent binding (Gillette, 1974a,b; Jollow *et al.*, 1981; Chen and Gillette, 1988). Although prolongation of the plasma paracetamol half life following overdosage in man was related to liver damage, in animals such as the rat the prolongation with dose was more clearly associated with saturation of sulphate conjugation. In rats the hepatotoxicity of paracetamol was not correlated with pro-longation of the half life, and surprisingly, paracetamol elimination was not impaired by a hepatotoxic dose of carbon tetrachloride (Siegers *et al.*, 1978). It has usually been possible to relate the hepatotoxicity and nephrotoxicity of paracetamol to the kinetics of its metabolic activation but this was not always the case (Tarloff *et al.*, 1989a,b; Adamson *et al.*, 1991).

Pharmacokinetic and Pharmacodynamic Correlations

Little information was available concerning the relationships between the kinetics of paracetamol and its primary therapeutic actions of analgesia and reduction of fever. Nelson and Morioka (1963) drew attention to the more rapid decay in the effects of paracetamol on the pain threshold reported by Flinn and Brodie (1948) than its half life, and concluded that there was a poor correlation between analgesic activity and the body level of the drug. Similarly, no clear relationship was found between pain relief and plasma concentrations of paracetamol in the central or peripheral com-partments following intravenous injection in dental surgery patients (Seymour and Rawlins, 1981). A pharmacokinetic and dynamic analysis of the analgesic effect of paracetamol in man indicated that a second dose taken immediately after cessation of the effect of the first dose produced a greater and more prolonged response than after the first dose (Levy, 1987).

A pharmacokinetic and pharmacodynamic model that incorporated physiologi-cal and thermal properties was developed to relate plasma, central nervous system and urinary concentrations of paracetamol to its temperature-lowering effect in rats following oral dosing. The fall in temperature was delayed and there was reasonable agreement between the observed and predicted time course of the pharmacological effects (Kakemi *et al.*, 1975). A coated bead formulation of paracetamol was produced to provide effective concentrations in a deep tissue compartment using a kinetic model based on population-average pharmacokinetics and pharmacodynamic values combined with dissolution data (Hossain and Ayres, 1992). In children with fever a dose of 5 mg kg^{-1} of paracetamol produced mean plasma concentrations below 5 mg l^{-1} and failed to lower temperature. There was a partial delayed response to 10 mg kg^{-1} with concentrations of about 10 mg l^{-1} and a good response with 20 mg kg^{-1} (Windorfer and Vogel, 1976). In a combined pharmacokinetic and pharmacodynamic study in febrile children, maximum antipyresis was related to the initial temperature and the optimum range of paracetamol concentrations for efficacy was 4–18 mg l^{-1}. This concentration range was said to be lower than for other indications (Wilson *et al.*, 1982b). The maximum plasma concentrations of paracetamol following a dose of 12.5 mg kg^{-1} in febrile children occurred about 2.5 h before the maximum temperature-lowering effect (Brown *et al.*, 1992). There was a mean delay of 106 min in another study in similar children given doses of 10–15 mg kg^{-1} and there was a counterclockwise hysteresis loop with time in the relationship between plasma concentrations of paracetamol and reduction in temperature (Kelley *et al.*, 1992).

11

Pharmacological Actions and Therapeutic Use of Paracetamol

Introduction

Although the introduction of paracetamol into clinical medicine is universally attributed to von Mering (1893), he only referred to it in passing, merely stating that it had antipyretic and 'antineuralgic' properties and advising against its use because it had the same side effects, albeit weaker, as p-aminophenol. No clinical details were given, and doses were not mentioned. Hinsberg and Treupel provided the first substantive report of the properties and clinical use of paracetamol in Munich in 1894. They described acute toxicity studies in two frogs, one guinea pig and several rabbits and dogs, and reported on the antipyretic efficacy of repeated doses of 500 mg of paracetamol in five patients with fever of undisclosed aetiology. Paracetamol produced a prompt fall in temperature of similar magnitude and duration as anti-pyrine, phenacetin and acetanilide (Figure 1.1). At that time the new-found ability to reduce fever with drugs such as acetanilide and phenacetin led to an obsession for their use in the misguided belief that at last a panacea had been found for the 'cure' of all conditions associated with fever. In such circumstances the lack of enthusiasm for paracetamol was surprising, particularly as it was later recognized to be an important urinary constituent following administration of both phenacetin and acetanilide (Sharp, 1915). There was little further interest in paracetamol until it was rediscovered as the major metabolite of acetanilide and phenacetin by Greenberg and Lester (1946), Lester and Greenberg (1947) and Brodie and Axelrod (1948b, 1949) who proposed that the antipyretic and analgesic properties of these drugs depended on their conversion *in vivo* to paracetamol. It was subsequently shown that phenacetin possessed antipyretic activity in its own right without dependence on its metabolism to paracetamol (Burns and Conney, 1965; Conney *et al.*, 1966), but interest in the drug had been rekindled and further studies were soon instigated.

Analgesia

The analgesic efficacy of paracetamol was formally demonstrated by Flinn and Brodie (1948) in a study with pain induced by radiant heat in 12 healthy female subjects. Following administration of a dose of 325 mg there was elevation of the pain threshold that reached a maximum after about 2 h (Figure 11.1). The response was similar to that produced by acetanilide but there was no such effect with placebo. Unlike its precursors, paracetamol was said not to cause meth-aemoglobinaemia (Greenberg and Lester, 1947) and this was confirmed later in studies in medical students given single doses of 3 g (Boréus and Sandberg, 1953). Studies were also carried out in animals and in doses of 45, 91, 106 and 200 mg kg^{-1}, paracetamol increased the pain threshold to radiant heat in rats. The increase with the highest dose was similar to that produced by an equivalent dose of phen-acetin, and paracetamol also had less acute toxicity (Boréus and Sandberg, 1953). In contrast, Frommel *et al.* (1953) were unable to demonstrate significant analgesic activity with 50 mg kg^{-1} of paracetamol in rabbits using electrical stimulation of dental pulp. In another report, paracetamol in doses of 250, 500 and 1000 mg kg^{-1} was generally as effective as phenacetin and amidopyrine in increasing the response time to radiant heat in rats while 1000 mg kg^{-1} of aspirin was ineffective (Renault *et al.*, 1956). Radiant heat was also used to assess the analgesic action of paracetamol combined with other drugs in rats (Boréus *et al.*, 1956). More recent experimental pain models for paracetamol in man have been based on ischaemic pain (López-Fiesco *et al.*, 1992) and electrical stimulation of dental pulp and peripheral nerves (Rohdewald *et al.*, 1982; Bromm *et al.*, 1988; Piguet *et al.*, 1994). It was also neces-sary to take psychological factors into account in the assessment of experimental pain in man (Berntzen *et al.*, 1985).

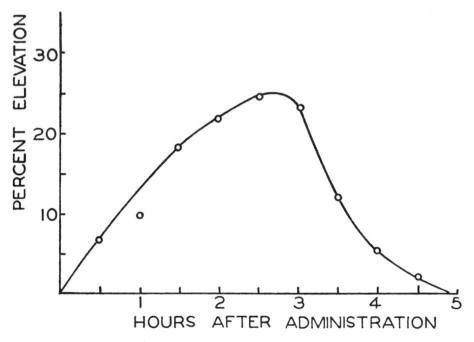

Figure 11.1 The mean elevation of pain threshold to radiant heat in 12 subjects following the oral administration of 325 mg of paracetamol (reproduced with permission from Flinn and Brodie, 1948).

Analgesia in Animals

Standardized tests have been developed in rodents for the screening of paracetamol and related compounds for analgesic activity. Paracetamol was active in many tests including antagonism of: (1) the writhing reaction induced by intraperitoneal injection of phenyl-p-benzoquinone, acetylcholine and acetic acid in mice; (2) hyperalgesia and local oedema after subplantar injection of irritants such as yeast, carrageenan, formalin, trypsin and kaolin, and subcutaneous implantation of cotton thread; (3) withdrawal following electrical, thermal, cold or ultrasound stimulation of the tail; and (4) pain produced by flexion of the tarsotibial joints in the presence of arthritis induced by injection of silver nitrate (Northover and Subramanian, 1961; Vinegar *et al.*, 1976; Glenn *et al.*, 1977; Loux *et al.*, 1977; Ferreira *et al.*, 1978; Pruss *et al.*, 1980; Chipkin *et al.*, 1983; Mohrland *et al.*, 1983; Singh *et al.*, 1983; Okuyama *et al.*, 1984c; Sewell *et al.*, 1984; Behrendt and Cserepes, 1985; Hunskaar *et al.*, 1985b; Luttinger, 1985; Rao and Saifi, 1985; Agudo *et al.*, 1986; Drower *et al.*, 1987; Bhattacharya *et al.*, 1989; Clavelou *et al.*, 1989; Dimova and Stoytchev, 1989; Ferrari *et al.*, 1990; Guasch *et al.*, 1990; Vinegar *et al.*, 1990; Malmberg and Yaksh, 1992; Kanui *et al.*, 1993; Yaksh and Malmberg, 1993). Other experimental pain models that have been used to demonstrate the analgesic efficacy of paracetamol included the mouse hot-plate test; the cold ethanol tail-flick test; ischaemic pain; pleurisy induced by carrageenan; hind paw arthritis induced by subcutaneous injection of *Mycobacterium butyricum* into the tail (adjuvant arthritis); and arthritis produced by intrasynovial injection of urate crystals (Brune *et al.*, 1974; Vinegar *et al.*, 1976; Capetola *et al.*, 1980; Okuyama and Aihara, 1984a; Hunskaar *et al.*, 1986b; Foote *et al.*, 1988; McQueen *et al.*, 1990; Ijølsen *et al.*, 1991b; Castañeda-Hernández *et al.*, 1992; Gelgor *et al.*, 1992a; Perkins and Campbell, 1992; Granados-Soto *et al.*, 1993; López-Muñoz *et al.*, 1993; Wang *et al.*, 1995). With the formalin test, it was said to be possible to dissociate anti-inflammatory and non-anti-inflammatory pain and paracetamol was active against both modalities (Hunskaar and Hole, 1987). Studies of analgesic combinations with and without caffeine usually indicated additive effects or potentiation, although in some reports there was antagonism (Seegers *et al.*, 1981; López-Muñoz *et al.*, 1993). Isobolographic analysis with the combination of paracetamol and buprenorphine in mice suggested synergism (Pircio *et al.*, 1978). Analgesic antagonism was noted with paracetamol and indomethacin in rats, but their antipyretic effects were additive (van Kolfschoten *et al.*, 1983a). The results of studies in animal pain models were not predictable and although paracetamol was usually at least as active as aspirin, it was not always possible to demonstrate analgesic efficacy (Skingle and Tyers, 1979; Pizziketti *et al.*, 1985; Schweizer and Brom, 1985; Vinegar *et al.*, 1989; Rao *et al.*, 1991).

The glucuronide and sulphate conjugates of paracetamol were thought to be pharmacologically inactive (Shibasaki *et al.*, 1979). Paracetamol sulphate had no anti-writhing activity after oral and intraperitoneal administration in mice (Williams *et al.*, 1983) but it markedly potentiated the analgesic effects and acute toxicity of amidopyrine (Ozaki *et al.*, 1972). The thiomethyl and mercapturic acid conjugates had analgesic actions in animals (Hertz and Deghenghi, 1983; Sicardi *et al.*, 1991). The analgesic properties of paracetamol and its 3-monoalkyl and 3,5-dialkyl substituted analogues have been compared (Dearden *et al.*, 1980; Vermeulen *et al.*, 1992) and activity seemed to parallel their oxidation potentials and hepatotoxicity (Harvison *et al.*, 1986b). A thiophene-carboxylate prodrug was said to have greater analgesic activity than paracetamol (Spano and Stacchino, 1979) but efficacy was reduced by fluorine substitution (Barnard *et al.*, 1993c).

Clinical Studies of Analgesia

In a comparison of 600 mg doses of different analgesics in 27 patients with cancer, the pain relief obtained with paracetamol and aspirin was similar and significantly greater in amplitude and duration than with salicylamide or placebo (Wallenstein and Houde, 1954). In another report on 234 patients with musculoskeletal pain, paracetamol in doses of 300 and 600 mg four times daily provided adequate relief in 66 per cent of patients compared with 52 and 53 per cent of groups of 87 and 128 similar patients given aspirin. Paracetamol was better tolerated than aspirin and doses of 3.6 g daily given continuously for as long as 116 days produced no blood, kidney or liver disturbances (Batterman and Grossman, 1955). The analgesic activity of paracetamol was studied in 194 young male and female subjects with pain induced by electrical stimulation of the tooth pulp and radiant heat focused on the forehead, and 166 patients aged 19–70 years with dental pain. Unfortunately the results are difficult to interpret because the paracetamol was given in different combinations with codeine, caffeine, salicylamide and barbiturates (Boréus *et al.*, 1956). Paracetamol 1 g and a combination tablet of aspirin, phenacetin and codeine taken three times daily were compared in a cross-over study in 42 patients with chronic arthritic disorders including rheumatoid arthritis. The combination was considered to be superior by a majority of patients but a significant minority preferred paracetamol (Newton and Tanner, 1956). Further evidence of the efficacy of paracetamol was provided in a comparative study of an aspirin suspension and paracetamol elixir given in doses of 260–520 mg and 130–260 mg respectively for a week in 200 children, aged 4–13 years, following tonsillectomy. Complete and partial pain relief was reported in 88 and 9 per cent respectively of the 100 patients taking paracetamol, and in 67 and 23 per cent of those taking aspirin. There was no difference between the groups in respect of side effects but gross bleeding requiring readmission to hospital occurred in eight patients given aspirin but in none given paracetamol (Reuter and Montgomery, 1964). Reports of the clinical use of paracetamol for analgesia in the 1950s and early 1960s were reviewed by Beaver (1965, 1966) and in general, doses of 600–1000 mg were found to be as effective as aspirin at similar dose levels for pain relief in conditions such as cancer, arthritis and postoperative and postpartum pain. There have since been numerous further reports confirming the analgesic action of paracetamol, including comparisons with new and established drugs in a variety of clinical settings. Details of some of these studies are summarized in Table 11.1.

There have been problems with clinical assessment of the analgesic efficacy of paracetamol. The results of some studies could not be accepted as there were no proper controls or comparisons with established analgesics (Mathieu, 1974; Mugnier, 1978; Messick, 1979; Polity *et al.*, 1993), while in others, the actual drugs given were unknown as the authors referred only to tradenames (Bhounsule *et al.*, 1990; Decousus *et al.*, 1990). Paracetamol was often used as a standard analgesic for comparisons with newer drugs and there was a tendency to use lower, less effective,

Table 11.1 Clinical studies of the analgesic efficacy of paracetamol.

Paracetamol dose	Duration of treatment (days)	Total no. of patients	Age (yr)	Aetiology of pain	Drug comparisons and outcome	Reference
0.25–0.5 g × 1	–	163	not stated	postpartum	P = PL*	Orkin et al., 1957
7.5 g daily	7	75	not stated	rheumatoid arthritis	P < AS	Hajnal et al., 1959
0.6 g × 1	–	373	adult	postpartum	P > PL; P = PH = AS	Lasagna et al., 1967
1 g × 1 or 2	–	103	mean 40	orthopaedic surgery	P > PL; P = AS	Parkhouse and Hallinon, 1967
1 g × 3 daily	14	110	adult	musculoskeletal	P = PBZ + P	McGuinness et al., 1969
0.9 g × 3 daily	7	99	20–70	back pain	P + OP = AS	Hingorani, 1971
1 g × 2	–	350	not stated	dental surgery	P > PL; P = AS = GF	Booy, 1972
0.65 g × 1	–	57	not stated	cancer	P > PL; P = Co; P = AS	Moertel et al., 1972
0.65 g × 1	–	200	17–41	episiotomy	P > PL; P > DP	Hopkinson et al., 1973
0.65–1 g × 1	–	263	16–40	postpartum	P > PL	Hopkinson et al., 1974
0.6 g × 1	–	137	15–38	episiotomy	P + Co > PL; P + Co > P	Levin et al., 1974
1 g × 3 daily	4	67	18–26	dysmenorrhea	P = IBU	Molla and Donald, 1974
1 g × 1	–	225	15–39	episiotomy	P > PL; P > DP	Berry et al., 1975
1 g × 4 daily	14	143	adults	rheumatoid arthritis	P = PL; P < AS; P < IND	Lee et al., 1975
1 g × 1	–	75	13–39	episiotomy	P > PL; P > AS + DP	Smith et al., 1975
0.65 g × 3 daily	–	47	18–35	dental surgery	P + Co > PH; P + Co > AS	Sveen and Gilhuus-Moe, 1975
0.6 g × 1	–	160	16–35	dental surgery	P > PL; P = P + Co	Cooper and Beaver, 1976
0.9 g × 3 daily	3	60	mean 37	fractures	P = P + MX	Eskenazi et al., 1976
0.65 g × 1	–	206	18–65	tension headache	P > PL; P + PT > P	Gilbert et al., 1976
1 g × 1	–	224	15–36	episiotomy	P > PL; P > P + DP	Hopkinson et al., 1976
0.65 g × 1	–	48	adults	postpartum	P > PL; P = DP; P = DP + P	Gruber et al., 1977
0.5 g × 4 daily	3	32	16–29	dental surgery	P = AS; P = AS + P	Skjelbred et al., 1977
0.65 g × 3 daily	3	48	20–70	soft tissue injury	P = DP = MFA	Stableforth, 1977
1 g × 1	–	144	19–85	headache	P > PL; P = AS	Wójcicki et al., 1977b
1 g × 1	–	72	18–91	postoperative	P > PL; P = AS	Wójcicki et al., 1977b
0.325–1 g × 4 daily	3	167	not stated	oral surgery	P + PZ > P + DP	Wright, 1977
0.65 g × 3 daily	–	30	adult	dysmenorrhea	P + DP > FF; P + DP > MFA	Anderson et al., 1978
0.5 g × 1	–	240	18–75	postoperative	P = PL = FP; P + FP > PL	Davie and Gordon, 1978
0.65 g × 2	–	33	not stated	rheumatoid synovitis	P > PL; P > DP	Hardin and Kirk, 1979
0.5 g × 4 daily	3	30	21–27	dysmenorrhea	P = PL = ASA	Janbu et al., 1978, 1979
0.5–1 g × 4 daily	4	24	19–34	dental surgery	P > PL	Skjelbred and Lokken, 1979

(cont.)

Table 11.1 (cont.)

Paracetamol dose	Duration of treatment (days)	Total no. of patients	Age (yr)	Aetiology of pain	Drug comparisons and outcome	Reference
0.65 g × 3 daily	7	98	15–55	soft tissue injury	P + DP < NP	Abbott et al., 1980
0.5–1 g × 1	–	207	mean 23	dental surgery	P500 > PL; P + OX > PL	Cooper et al., 1980
0.5 g × 1	–	299	adult	episiotomy	P > PL; P < DY	Daftary et al., 1980
0.65 g × 4 daily	1	94	adult	postoperative	P = NP = PZ	Filtzer, 1980
1 g × 1	–	113	16–75	dental surgery	P > PL; P = AS	Korberly et al., 1980
1 g × 1	–	689	not stated	migraine	P = AS	Tfelt-Hansen and Olesen, 1980
0.65 g × 1	–	122	>15	postpartum	P > PL; P < AS; P < PP	Bloomfield et al., 1981
1 g × 1	–	119	adult	orthopaedic surgery	P = P = BP	Bullingham et al., 1981
0.5 g × 3 or 4	–	180	not stated	hysterectomy	P > PL; P < DP; P < FQ	Frerich and Krumme, 1981
0.9–1 g × 4 daily	3	100	adult	dental pain	P = P + Co + DX	Ladwa, 1981
0.5 g × 5	–	94	mean 28	dental surgery	P < DP; P = Co	Quiding et al., 1981
1 g (iv) × 1	–	11	not stated	dental surgery	P > PL	Seymour and Rawlins, 1981
0.5 g × 1	–	160	17–77	minor surgery	P = AS = DY = OX	Tigerstedt et al., 1981
1 g × 1	–	80	17–63	orthopaedic surgery	P > PL; TA = PL; P > TA	Winnem et al., 1981
1 g × 4 daily	10	91	not stated	soft tissue injury	P = PL = AN	de Gara et al., 1982
0.65 g × 1	–	127	mean 38–46	orthopaedic surgery	P + DP > PL; P + DP = ZP	Evans et al., 1982
1 g × 4 daily	28	30	21–75	low back pain	P < DF	Hickey, 1982
1 g × 4	1½	51	19–60	dental surgery	P = DF	Irvine et al., 1982
0.65 g × 3 daily	3	39	16–34	dysmenorrhea	P + DP < NP	Langrick and Gunn, 1982
0.65–1 g × 4 daily	3	80	18–45	tonsillectomy	P + Co = P + DP	MacKay and Ananian, 1982
0.5 g × 5	–	93	18–51	dental surgery	P = AP	Quiding et al., 1982a
0.5 g × 5	–	266	not stated	dental surgery	P < P + Co	Quiding et al., 1982b
0.65 g × 3 daily	7–14	184	mean 33	sports injury	P < NP	Simmons et al., 1982
0.8 g × 4 daily	3	24	16–31	dental surgery	P = P + Co	Skjelbred and Lokken, 1982
1 g × 4 daily	3	83	18–65	musculoskeletal	P > PL; P = MZ	Wade and Ward, 1982
1 g × 1	–	86	18–70	dental surgery	P = Co = DF	White and Strunin, 1982
1 g × 4 daily	42	25	adults	osteoarthritis	P > PL	Amadio and Cummings, 1983
0.6 g × 3	–	107	not stated	dental surgery	P > PL; P + Co > PL; P < IBU	Dionne et al., 1983
0.65–1 g × 4 daily	3	83	17–80	dental surgery	P + Co = P + DP	Edmondson and Bradshaw, 1983
1 g × 3 daily	42	39	15–70	arthritis	P < P + MC	Flavell Matts and Boston, 1983
0.6 g × 1	–	132	18–64	postoperative	P > PL; P + Co > P; P = DF	Forbes et al., 1983

(cont.)

Dose		n	Age	Condition	Result	Reference
1 g × 3 daily	?	31	mean 19	dysmenorrhea	P < FL	Frank and Kefford, 1983
1 g × 3 daily	?	25	not stated	dysmenorrhea	P < FL	MacLean, 1983
0.9 g × 3 daily	10	28	18–70	musculoskeletal	P < P + OP	McGuinness, 1983
0.65 g × 1	—	90	18–36	episiotomy	P > PL; P < DF	Melzack et al., 1983
0.9 g × 4 daily	—	27	>18	migraine	P < IBU	Pearce et al., 1983
0.5 g × 3	—	22	18–53	migraine	P = MFA	Peatfield et al., 1983
1 g × 1	—	269	mean 32	headache	P > PL; P = AS	Peters et al., 1983
1 g × 1	—	64	mean 35	meniscectomy	P > PL; P + Co = P	Quiding and Häggquist, 1983
0.5–1 g × 4 daily	2½	80	not stated	dental surgery	P > PL	Seymour, 1983
1 g × 1	—	164	16–75	dental surgery	P > PL; P = P + CF	Winter et al., 1983a
1 g × 1	—	127	16–75	dental surgery	P + PT > PL > AS	Winter et al., 1983b
0.65 g × 1	—	148	15–41	dental surgery	P < PL; P > P + PT	Forbes et al., 1984a
0.65 g × 2	—	129	adult	postoperative	P > PL; P < NB	Forbes et al., 1984b
0.5 g × 2	—	28	18–37	dental surgery	P + DC = DC	Matthews et al., 1984
1 g × 1	—	58	16–78	dental surgery	P > PL; P = AS	Mehlisch and Frakes, 1984
0.5 g × 1	—	12	20–42	dysmenorrhea	P = PL; NP = PL; IBU > PL; IBU > P	Milsom and Andersch, 1984
0.65 g × 4 daily	4	24	not stated	rheumatoid arthritis	P < DP	Mitchell et al., 1984a
1 g × 1	—	89	mean 23	dental surgery	P < NP	Mugnier et al., 1984
0.5 or 1 g × 2	—	92	mean 26	dental surgery	P1000 > P500; P500 = Co	Quiding et al., 1984
0.65 or 1 g × 1	—	476	13–40	episiotomy	P > PL; P < P + AS; P < AS	Rubin and Winter, 1984
0.5 g × 1 (R)	—	91	mean 25	tonsillectomy	P = PZ	Saarnivaara, 1984
0.5–1 g × 4 daily	3	26	18–34	dental surgery	P < P + PMe	Skoglund and Skjelbred, 1984
0.5–1 g × 1 or 2	—	172	adult	dental surgery	P + Co > PL	Ahlström et al., 1985
1 g × 1[a]	—	130	18–65	postoperative	P > PL	Delacroix et al., 1985
0.3 g × 1	—	120	18–65	orthopaedic surgery	P + Co > PL; P + Co < IBU	Heidrich et al., 1985
0.5 g × 4 daily	4	30	18–76	periodontitis	P = FZ	Leguen, 1985
10 mg kg⁻¹ × 1 (R)	—	82	children	tonsillectomy	ineffective	Lindgren and Saarnivaara, 1985
0.5 g × 3 daily	—	90	18–58	dental surgery	P > PL; P = PX	Melzack et al., 1985
0.24 or 0.36 g × 1	—	45	5–12	dental surgery	P > PL; P + Co > PL; P < IBU	Moore et al., 1985b
0.65 g × 4 daily	120	129	18–35	dysmenorrhea	P > PL; P = AS	Pendergrass et al., 1985
0.65 g × 1	—	129	18–40	postoperative	P > PL; P = P + PZ, P + DP, P + Co	Petti, 1985
0.65 g × 4 daily	3	47	16–65	dental surgery	P + DP < SP	Rosen et al., 1985
0.5–1 g × 2 or 3 daily	4	40	18–51	ankle sprain	P = DF	Aghababian, 1986
0.3–0.6 g × 3	—	170	>15	dental surgery	P + Co = GF	Benoit et al., 1986
0.3 × 4 daily	15	40	18–59	back pain	P + Co = DF	Brown et al., 1986
0.12–0.2 g × 3 daily	5	43	5–15	pharyngitis/tonsillitis	P < PX	Caretti, 1986

Table 11.1 (cont.)

Paracetamol dose	Duration of treatment (days)	Total no. of patients	Age (yr)	Aetiology of pain	Drug comparisons and outcome	Reference
1 g × 1	–	99	mean 25	dental surgery	P > PL; P = P + Co	Cooper et al., 1986
0.5 × 1	–	153	adult	oral surgery	P + DH < FL; P + DH = PL	Frame and Rout, 1986
not stated	?	40	>17	arthroscopy	P + Co = DF	Fulkerson and Folcik, 1986
1 g × 1	–	113	mean 33	postoperative	P < P + Co; P > Co	Gertzbein et al., 1986
0.5 g × 3	–	72	18–57	dental surgery	P = FQ	Haanaes et al., 1986
0.4–0.45 g × 3 daily	7	52	18–70	cervical myalgia	P + OP = P + Co	Hoivik et al., 1986
1.3 g × 1	–	100	mean 27	postoperative	P > PL; P < ML	Huang et al., 1986
0.6 g × 4 daily	7	50	18–22	sports injury	P + Co = DF	Indelicato, 1986
0.65 g × 1	–	128	18–70	postoperative	P > PL; P < NB; P < P + NB	Jain et al., 1986
0.5 g × 1	–	80	18–65	postoperative	P + Co > PL	Marhic, 1986
0.5–1 g × 1	–	60	20–70	orthopaedic surgery	P = KR	McQuay et al., 1986
1 g × 4 daily	3	24	18–44	dental surgery	P < ID	Olstad and Skjelbred, 1986a
1 g × 3 or 4 daily	3	24	16–32	dental surgery	P = MP	Olstad and Skjelbred, 1986b
2 g × 2 daily[b]	2½	30	18–34	dental surgery	P > PL	Skoglund, 1986
0.65 g × 1	–	182	adult	dental surgery	P > PL; P + Co = P; ZP > FL > P + Co > P	Sunshine et al., 1986
1 g × 1	–	120	adults	dental surgery	P > PL; P > Co; P + Co > PL	Bentley and Head, 1987
1.5 g daily	15	78	not stated	arthritis	P = GF	Choffray et al., 1987
0.65 g × 2	–	52	16–60	arthroscopy	P + DP < NP	Drez et al., 1987
1 g × 1	–	98	17–38	episiotomy	P + Co > P + DP	Jacobson and Bertilson, 1987
0.65 g × 2	–	45	adult	postoperative	P = PL; P + DP = DP	Liashek et al., 1987
0.24–0.36 g × 1	–	123	7–16	dental surgery	P = PL; P < IBU	McGaw et al., 1987
0.65 g × 1	–	124	18–65	headache	P > PL; P < NP	Miller et al., 1987
1 g × 3 daily	3	97	15–32	episiotomy	P < PX	Ogunbode, 1987
0.3–0.6 g daily	2	100	adult	trauma	P = TENS	Ordog, 1987
0.5 g × 4 daily	3	59	18–40	dental surgery	P = SP	Reijntjes et al., 1987
1.5 g × 2	–	42	21–40	dental surgery	P > PL; P = DF	Rodrigo et al., 1987
0.65 g × 1	–	96	17–62	respiratory infection	P = PL; P < FP	Ryan et al., 1987
0.65–1 g × 3	–	180	mean 29	dental surgery	P + Co > P + DF	Sagne et al., 1987
0.65 g × 4 daily	3	45	adult	dental surgery	P < DP < SP	Shanks et al., 1987
1 g × 2 daily	14	153	not stated	osteoarthritis	P < GF	Amor and Benarrosh, 1988

(cont.)

Dose		n	Age	Condition	Result	Reference
0.6 g × 1	—	143	adult	dental surgery	P = PL; P + Co > PL; P + Co = ML	Cooper et al., 1988
20 mg kg⁻¹ (R)	—	20	1–8	tonsillectomy	P = PE	Gaudreault et al., 1988
0.5–1.0 g × 2	—	150	mean 26	dental surgery	P < DF; P1000 > P500	Nyström et al., 1988
1 g × 1	—	120	mean 41–46	sore throat	P > PL; P < IBU	Schachtel et al., 1988
1 g × 4 daily	14	17	33–68	rheumatoid arthritis	P = IND low = IND high	Seideman and Melander, 1988
0.65 g × 1	—	161	adult	postoperative	P + Co > PL; P + Co = KP	Turek and Baird, 1988
1–4 g daily	3	107	18–64	gynaecological surgery	P + Co = KR	Vangen et al., 1988
0.6 g × 2	—	91	17–74	plastic surgery	P + Co = NP	Vargus Busquets et al., 1988
0.35 g × 1	—	40	18–40	episiotomy	P < AF	Yscla, 1988
1 g × 1	—	59	>16	dental surgery	P > PL; P > IBU	Cooper et al., 1989
0.6 g × 1	—	88	>15	dental surgery	P > PL; P > FL; P > P + Co	Forbes et al., 1989b
not stated	up to 15	14	adults	arthroscopic surgery	P + DP = DF	Jokl and Warman, 1989
4 g × 1c	—	32	18–32	dental pain	P > PL	Moore et al., 1989
1 g × 1	—	116	18–70	migraine	P = TF	Norrelund et al., 1989
1 g × 2	—	32	21–40	dental surgery	P = DF	Rodrigo et al., 1989
1 g × 1	—	37	16–35	postpartum	P > PL; IBU > P	Schachtel et al., 1989
0.65 g × 1	—	200	adult	episiotomy	P > PL; P + PT > P	Sunshine et al., 1989
0.32 g × 3 dailyd	56	43	25–67	fibromyalgia	P > PL	Vaeroy et al., 1989
0.5 g × 1	—	204	not stated	dental pain	P > P + Co	Becker et al., 1990
0.5 g × 1	—	100	not stated	episiotomy	P > PL; P < AL; P < IBU	Bhounsule et al., 1990
0.65 g × 1	—	250	not stated	dental surgery	P > PL; P > TR	Brown et al., 1990
0.6 g × 4 daily	7	75	30–88	cancer	P + Co > PL; P + Co = KR	Carlson et al., 1990
0.6 g × 1 or 2	—	128	16–41	dental surgery	P + Co > PL; P < KR; P + Co > AS	Forbes et al., 1990a
0.6 g × 1	—	206	16–48	dental surgery	P > PL; P < KR; P < IBU	Forbes et al., 1990b
0.5 g × 4	—	21	19–48	dental surgery	P > PL; FL > P	Gallardo and Rossi, 1990
0.325 g	—	31	17–65	headache	P + Co > PL	Gawel et al., 1990
1 g × 4	—	25	adult	dental surgery	P > PL; P = AS; P = IBU; P > DH	Habib et al., 1990
1 g × 3 daily	28	75	42–82	osteoarthritis	P > P + Co	Kjaersgaard-Andersen et al., 1990
0.5–1 g × 1 or 2	—	83	19–65	migraine	P > TF	Larsen et al., 1990
1 g × 1	—	136	17–54	dental surgery	P > PL; P = AS	Lehnert et al., 1990
1 g × 1	—	30	18–70	orthopaedic surgery	P > PL; P = BF	McQuay et al., 1990
1 g × 1	—	760	17–64	dental surgery	P > PL; P < IBU	Mehlisch et al., 1990
30 mg kg⁻¹ × 1e	—	54	adult	postoperative	P = NF	Moreau et al., 1990
0.3 g × 4 daily	4	83	>18	foot surgery	P + Co = FL	Ottinger et al., 1990
0.5–2 g × 1	—	200	adult	dental surgery	P High dose > P low dose	Ström et al., 1990
0.5 g × 3 daily	7	51	40–65	cancer	P < NP, IND, DC	Ventafridda et al., 1990

Table 11.1 (*cont.*)

Paracetamol dose	Duration of treatment (days)	Total no. of patients	Age (yr)	Aetiology of pain	Drug comparisons and outcome	Reference
1 g × 1	–	12	adult	laser pain	P > PL; P > P + Co	Arendt-Nielsen et al., 1991
10 mg kg^{-1} × 3 daily	2	78	6–12	tonsillitis	P > PL; P = IBU	Bertin et al., 1991
0.5 g × 3 daily	7	40	36–79	rheumatoid arthritis	P + Co > PL	Boureau and Boccard, 1991
1 g × 4 daily	28	61	>30	osteoarthritis	P = IBU	Bradley et al., 1991b
0.65 g × 1	–	226	mean 23	dental surgery	P > PL; P + Co > P; P + Co = FL	Cooper and Kupperman, 1991
1 g × 3	7	134	adult	sinusitis	P > PL; P = TP	Frachet et al., 1991
1 g × 4, 2 g × 2	–	15	24–48	laser pain	P > PL	Nielsen et al., 1991
0.5–1 g × 1	–	120	adult	dental surgery	P < MFA	Ragot, 1991
1 g × 1	–	302	18–65	headache	P > PL; P > AS + Co	Schachtel et al., 1991
0.5–1.2 g × 2 daily	5	23	18–34	dental surgery	P2000 > P1000	Skoglund and Pettersen, 1991
1 g × 1	–	139	mean 25	dental surgery	P > PL; P + Co > P; P2000 > P1000	Skoglund et al., 1991
1 g × 1	–	40	21–38	postpartum	P > PL	Skovlund et al., 1991a
1 g × 1	–	36	21–41	postpartum	P = NP	Skovlund et al., 1991b
0.65 g × 1	–	53	20–60	headache	P > PL; P + CF > PL; P = P + CF	Ward et al., 1991
0.125 g × 1 (R)	–	44	children	adenoidectomy	P < DC	Baer et al., 1992
0.8–1 g × 3 daily	7	141	adult	osteoarthritis	P + Co = P + DP	Boissier et al., 1992
1 g × 4 daily	28	182	>30	osteoarthritis	P = IBU	Bradley et al., 1992
1 g × 1	–	22	24–33	hand skin pressure	P = PL; P > IBU; P > DY	Forster et al., 1992
0.65 g × 2	–	86	adult	osteoarthritis	P + DP < DH	Lloyd et al., 1992
0.3 g × 1	–	20	19–30	tourniquet ischaemia	P + NP > PL; P + NP > DY	López-Fiesco et al., 1992
0.5 g × 3 daily	7	120	18–45	dental surgery	P + Co = IBU	Lysell and Anzén, 1992
1 g × 4 daily	6	30	18–40	dental surgery	IBU > P	McQuay et al., 1992
0.5–1.2 g × 1	–	10	25–50	laser pain	P > PL; P slow release > PL	Nielsen et al., 1992
1 g × 1	–	20	adult	cholecystectomy	P = OX	Speranza et al., 1992
0.65 g × 1	–	41	adult	postoperative	P + DP > PL; TR > P	Sunshine et al., 1992
10 mg kg^{-1} × 1	–	31	children	myringotomy	KR > P; P = PL	Watcha et al., 1992
1 g × 4 daily (R)[e]	3	32	adult	cholecystectomy	P = PL; NP = PL	Witjes et al., 1992
0.325–0.65 g × 4	–	262	mean 37	vaccination	P > PL	Aoki et al., 1993
1 g × 1	–	408	adult	termination of pregnancy	P = PL	Cade and Ashley, 1993
0.5–1 g × 4 daily	6	30	39–80	cancer	P500 = P1000	Danninger et al., 1993
0.5 g × 1	–	32	18–53	dental surgery	P > PL; P < PX	Dolci et al., 1993

Dose		n	Age	Condition	Result	Reference
1 g × 1	–	288	18–70	migraine	P > PL; P + DG < P	Hoernecke and Doenicke, 1993
0.5 g × 3 daily	2	200	18–65	dental surgery	P = CX	Marti et al., 1993
1 g × 1	–	59	mean 43	migraine	P + DM = P	MacGregor et al., 1993
1 g × 1	–	40	18–67	postoperative	P < TM	Nappi et al., 1993
0.12–0.29 g × 3 daily	4	35	3–12	adenotonsillectomy	P = NM	Pasquale et al., 1993
0.24–0.4 g × 1	–	60	4–10	dental surgery	P = PL	Primosch et al., 1993
15 mg kg⁻¹ × 1	–	116	2–12	sore throat	P > PL; P = IBU	Schachtel and Thoden, 1993
1 g × 4 daily	14	20	35–73	rheumatoid arthritis	P < NP + P	Seideman, 1993b
1 g × 4 daily	5	20	53–82	coxarthrosis	P < NP + P	Seideman et al., 1993
0.65 g × 1	–	48	adult	postoperative	P = PL; P < KP	Sunshine et al., 1993
0.65 g × 4 daily	42	178	33–85	osteoarthritis	P = NP	Williams et al., 1993
0.5 g × 3 daily	7	40	36–75	rheumatoid arthritis	P + Co > PL	Boureau and Boccard, 1994
0.4 g × 1	–	198	18–65	migraine	P + Co > PL; P + Co = AS	Boureau et al., 1994
0.3–0.5 g × 1	–	232	adult	dental surgery	P + HC > P + Co	Forbes, 1994
15 mg kg⁻¹ × 1	–	44	neonatal	circumcision	P = PL	Howard et al., 1994
1 g × 1	–	226	14–39	dental surgery	P > PL; P < NP	Kiersch et al., 1994
1 g × 1 (R)	–	160	not stated	dental surgery	P = PL; P < AS; P < IBU	Krempien et al., 1994
1 g × 1	–	1915	18–65	headache	P > PL	Migliardi et al., 1994
0.65 g × 1	–	60	13–81	postoperative	P < KR; P = IBU	Morrison and Repka, 1994
0.325–0.4 g × 1	–	160	adult	postoperative	P + DP < KR; KR > P + IBU	Naidu et al., 1994
2.4 g daily	28	390	elderly	chronic pain	P + Co = TR	Rauck et al., 1994
35 mg kg⁻¹ × 1 (R)	–	50	2–15	tonsillectomy	P = KR	Rusy et al., 1995

* PL = placebo, (R) = rectal ± oral administration, ᵃ given as intravenous propacetamol, ᵇ given as paracetamol methionate ester, ᶜ given as benorylate, ᵈ combination with carisoprodol and caffeine, ᵉ taken with sublingual buprenorphine

AF = aceclofenac, AL = 'Analgin' (composition not stated), AN = antrafenine, AP = antipyrine, AS = asprin, BF = bromfenac, BP = buprenorphine, CF = caffeine, Co = codeine, CX = lysine clonixinate, DC = diclofenac, DF = diflunisal, DG = dihydroergotamine, DH = dihydrocodeine, DM = domperidone, DP = d-propoxyphene, DX = doxylamine, DY = dipyrone, FL = flurbiprofen, FP = fenoprofen, FQ = fluproquazone, FZ = fentiazac, GF = glafenine, HC = hydrocodone, IBU = ibuprofen, ID = indoprofen, IND = indomethacin, KP = ketoprofen, KR = ketorolac, MC = metoclopramide, MFA = mefenamic acid, ML = meclofenemate, MP = methylprednisolone, MX = mephenoxalone, MZ = meptazinol, NB = nalbuphine, NF = niflumic acid, NM = nimesulide, NP = naproxen, OP = orphenadrine, OX = oxycodone, PBZ = phenylbutazone, PE = pethidine, PH = phenacetin, PMe = paracetamol methionate ester, PP = pirprofen, PT = phenyltoloxamine, PX = piroxicam, PZ = pentazocine, SP = suprofen, TA = tiaramide, TENS = transcutaneous electrical nerve stimulation, TF = tolfenamic acid, TM = tolmetin derivative, TP = tiaprofenic acid, TR = tramadol, ZP = zomepirac doses. It was also frequently used in combination with other agents, such as codeine and d-propoxyphene, and in such circumstances little could be concluded about the efficacy of paracetamol itself. There were further problems with combinations with drugs such as d-propoxyphene, which had a much longer half life than paracetamol. The consequence of this imbalance was that there would be only a minor contribution to the analgesic effect provided by d-propoxyphene after single doses but a progressively greater effect with repeated administration over several days. The question also arose concerning the equivalence of single and repeated doses of paracetamol, and its efficacy in widely different types of pain ranging for example from tension headache to the pain of episiotomy. Paracetamol was extensively used for the relief of discomfort in the common cold but there was no pharmacological basis for the belief that it could ameliorate symptoms such as sneezing and nasal obstruction. Indeed, it was ineffective against these complaints (Middleton, 1981). Pain has been measured using a variety of methods and efficacy has commonly been assessed by comparisons of pain relief scores or pain intensity differences determined with visual analogue scales (Joyce *et al.*, 1975; Quiding *et al.*, 1981; Quiding and Häggquist, 1983). Variations on this theme included the pain 'thermometer' (White and Strunin, 1982; Schachtel and Thoden, 1993), and particularly for children, the 'faces' scale and objective observations on their behaviour (Tyler *et al.*, 1993). To establish efficacy it was essential to include control groups taking placebo or other standard treatments and an example of the effects of paracetamol with and without codeine on pain relief scores in patients with dental pain is shown in Figure 11.2. As shown in Table 11.1, most studies have been carried out in patients with dental and postoperative pain but the analgesic efficacy of paracetamol has also been demonstrated with experimental pain models based on argon laser stimulation (Arendt-Nielsen *et al.*, 1991; Nielsen *et al.*, 1991), hand pressure (Forster *et al.*, 1992) and electrical and thermal stimulation of cutaneous nerves (Stacher *et al.*, 1979; Bromm and Scharein, 1993). Dental pain was well established as a model for assessment of paracetamol and other analgesics (Bosch *et al.*, 1990; Urquhart, 1994) and a standardized approach was recommended for the evaluation of efficacy in this setting (Saito *et al.*, 1990). Preoperative treatment with paracetamol did not provide additional pain relief in dental surgery (Gustafsson *et al.*, 1983). Self-medication was common in patients suffering from toothache and a survey in 226 patients showed that paracetamol was the most frequently taken drug (Baños *et al.*, 1991). It was also the most popular analgesic to be taken without supervision following dental surgery (Seymour *et al.*, 1983). However, an analysis of the prescribing practices of dentists indicated a switch away from paracetamol to ibuprofen for pain relief (Picozzi and Ross, 1989).

The efficacy of paracetamol and other non-prescription analgesics has also been studied in patients with headache (Schachtel *et al.*, 1991) but there were potential disadvantages with this model because the pain did not always recur when the effect of a single dose of analgesic wore off and there was no true 'peak effect'. In such circumstances the slopes of the straight lines derived as quadratic functions of pain versus time were thought to provide better discrimination between treatments than area under the curve calculations (Gawel *et al.*, 1990). In some studies paracetamol was not effective in the relief of pain associated with inflammation such as in rheumatoid arthritis (Newton and Tanner, 1956; Hajnal *et al.*, 1959; Lee *et al.*, 1975) and it was generally thought to be rather ineffective in these conditions. However, in one report, paracetamol and indomethacin had equianalgesic effects in patients with

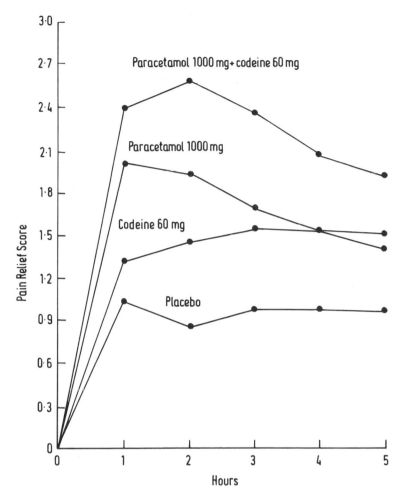

Figure 11.2   Mean pain relief scores in 120 dental surgery patients following administration of paracetamol, codeine and placebo (reproduced with permission from Bentley and Head, 1987).

rheumatoid arthritis (Seideman and Melander, 1988). Other investigators have shown that paracetamol provided pain relief in patients with osteoarthritis and other arthritic conditions (Hardin and Kirk, 1979; Amadio and Cummings, 1983; Choffray *et al.*, 1987; Drez *et al.*, 1987; Kjaersgaard-Andersen *et al.*, 1990; Bradley *et al.*, 1991b; Lloyd *et al.*, 1992) and it was recommended as the first line of analgesic therapy in this condition (Jones and Doherty, 1992). The combination with d-propoxyphene had an effect on well-being that was not seen with paracetamol alone, and this was probably related to the central action of the narcotic analgesic (Mitchell *et al.*, 1984a). The use of paracetamol instead of non-steroidal anti-inflammatory drugs in patients with arthritis was considered to represent cost-conscious prescribing without compromising the quality of care (Greene and Winickoff, 1992). Some paradoxical results have been reported. For example, paracetamol given as suppositories seemed to enhance and prolong pain in both nulli-parous and multiparous women following termination of pregnancy with mifepristone and sulprostone, and this was attributed to a pharmacological interaction between the drugs (Weber and Fontan, 1990; Weber *et al.*, 1990a). Paracetamol has often been combined with a variety of other drugs including antihistamines, hypnotic and sedative drugs, narcotic analgesics and caffeine. In some cases, these combinations seemed difficult to justify and good evidence to support their use was wanting. Although there was evidence that caffeine enhanced analgesic efficacy, there was no obvious mechanistic rationale for this combination (Laska *et al.*, 1983, 1984; Ward *et al.*, 1991; Migliardi *et al.*, 1994). In animals, caffeine decreased paracetamol absorption by slowing gastric emptying and the effect on analgesia depended on the dose (Siegers, 1973). It also enhanced the analgesic efficacy of paracetamol by a pharmacodynamic rather than a pharmacokinetic interaction (Castañeda-Hernández *et al.*, 1992; Granados-Soto *et al.*, 1993) and other agents with enhancing properties included ethylxanthogenate (Dimova and Stoytchev, 1989) and orphenadrine (Hunskaar *et al.*, 1986a). On the other hand, rifampicin decreased the analgesic action of paracetamol, possibly by enhancing its elimination (Dimova and Stoytchev, 1994).

There was continuing debate over the question of whether the analgesic action of paracetamol was mediated by central or peripheral mechanisms and although it was usually effective after systemic absorption, pain could also be relieved by local application. Thus, 12 patients with pain following tooth extraction received in random

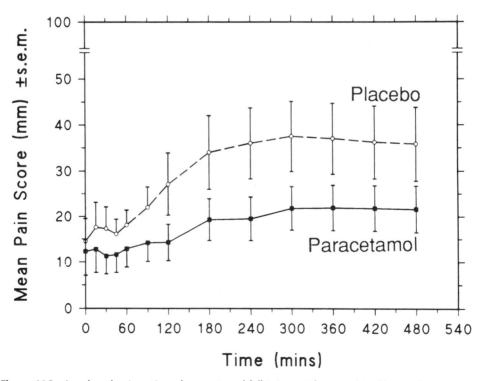

Figure 11.3 Local analgesic action of paracetamol following tooth extraction. Mean pain scores measured on a visual analogue scale in 12 patients receiving paracetamol in their tooth sockets and a systemic placebo or placebo in their tooth sockets and a low systemic dose of paracetamol (50 mg) (reproduced with permission from Moore *et al.*, 1992).

blind order either oral placebo and paracetamol (about 30 mg) in a methylcellulose gel placed in the tooth socket, or gel alone in the socket with 50 mg of oral paracetamol. Similar studies were carried out with aspirin and pain scores were recorded in both groups using visual analogue scales. Significantly less pain was reported with the local paracetamol and aspirin and the response to both drugs was similar (Figure 11.3) (Moore *et al.*, 1992). In an earlier report, the local application of paracetamol to the tongue did not increase the threshold to pain produced by electrical stimulation in healthy subjects and there was no evidence for any local anaesthetic activity (Adriani *et al.*, 1981). The common hypothesis of the mode of action of paracetamol left many questions unanswered and evidence for a central action has been reviewed (Brune *et al.*, 1993).

Anti-inflammatory Activity

Studies of the anti-inflammatory action of paracetamol in animals have yielded rather ambiguous results. Although it did not significantly reduce hyperalgesia and oedema induced by the injection of carrageenan in some reports (Foote *et al.*, 1988), in others it was active in this test and this would usually be interpreted as evidence of anti-inflammatory activity (Vinegar *et al.*, 1976; Glenn *et al.*, 1977; Ferreira *et al.*, 1978; Bhattacharya *et al.*, 1989). Paracetamol had an additive effect with aspirin in reducing carrageenan-induced oedema in rats (Seegers *et al.*, 1979) and it was effective in reducing pleurisy produced by carrageenan as well as adjuvant arthritis in rodents (Vinegar *et al.*, 1976). It also potentiated the analgesic effects of aspirin, indomethacin and flurbiprofen on inflammatory pain in rats (Engelhardt, 1984). In longer-term studies, paracetamol had significant anti-inflammatory and anti-arthritic properties in rats with adjuvant arthritis (Wong and Gardocki, 1983) and it was active in the same pain model following systemic and intracerebroventricular administration (Okuyama and Aihara, 1984b). It also reduced the response to the hyperalgesia produced in rats by adjuvant arthritis and intra-articular injection of uric acid (Davis and Perkins, 1993). In the development of adjuvant arthritis there was an increase in the Fos-like immunoreactive neurones in the rat lumbar spinal cord and this response was not reduced by repeated doses of paracetamol (Abbadie and Besson, 1994). In contrast to these results, paracetamol was inactive in the model of dermal inflammation and erythema produced by ultraviolet radiation in guinea pigs (Adams, 1960; Woodward and Owen, 1979) and there was little or no evidence of anti-inflammatory activity in studies of its effects on leucocyte migration, lysosomal enzyme activity and urate arthritis in pigeons (Brune and Glatt, 1974; Brune *et al.*, 1974, 1994; Brown and Collins, 1977). In doses up to 60 mg kg^{-1}, it did not influence the hyper- and hypoalgesic response to subplantar injection of 5-hydroxytryptamine with pain induced by hind paw pressure in rats (Vinegar *et al.*, 1989). Paracetamol did not antagonize hind paw oedema produced with carrageenan and other irritants (Lewis *et al.*, 1975) and it did not inhibit prostaglandin synthesis in synovial fluid from patients with active rheumatoid arthritis (Crook *et al.*, 1976; Robinson *et al.*, 1978). Paracetamol did not inhibit the activity of cathepsin B_1 obtained from bovine spleen (Kruze *et al.*, 1976) or the enzymes of phospholipase A_2 (Lobo and Hoult, 1994).

It was thought that inflammation involved the formation of free radicals from molecular oxygen and that paracetamol might effectively inhibit prostaglandin synthesis in the presence of cellular peroxides (Hertz and Cloarec, 1984). Depletion of glutathione limited the paw oedema caused by carrageenan, but paracetamol could effectively reduce this response at doses which did not influence glutathione concentrations (Strubelt and Younes, 1984). Previous treatment with large doses of paracetamol protected rats against liver damage following a single toxic dose but did not reduce its anti-inflammatory effects on paw oedema produced by carrageenan (Strubelt *et al.*, 1979). After orthopaedic surgery in dogs, paracetamol in doses of 1.5 g (but not 0.5 g) daily had anti-inflammatory and analgesic effects equivalent at least to those produced by aspirin (Mburu *et al.*, 1988; Mburu, 1991).

The results of clinical studies of the ability of paracetamol to relieve pain associated with inflammation have also been conflicting. Initially, its analgesic efficacy in patients with rheumatoid arthritis appeared to be limited (Newton and Tanner, 1956; Hajnal *et al.*, 1959; Zelvelder, 1961; Boardman and Hart, 1967; Ring *et al.*, 1974; Lee *et al.*, 1975, 1976; Aylward *et al.*, 1976) but there has since been more evidence of efficacy, particularly in comparisons with non-steroidal anti-inflammatory drugs and when used for supplementary analgesia (Hardin and Kirk, 1979; Seideman and Melander, 1988; Boureau and Boccard, 1991, 1994; Seideman, 1993a,b). Paracetamol has been used more extensively for the treatment of other forms of arthritis, particularly osteoarthritis, and analgesic efficacy was usually demonstrated (Amadio and Cummings, 1983; Flavell Matts and Boston, 1983; Choffray *et al.*, 1987; Amor and Benarrosh, 1988; Kjaersgaard-Andersen *et al.*, 1990; Bradley *et al.*, 1991b, 1992; Boissier *et al.*, 1992; Lloyd *et al.*, 1992; Seideman *et al.*, 1993; Williams *et al.*, 1993). In patients with osteoarthritis, treatment with paracetamol for eight weeks had less effect than tiaprofenic acid on the activity of stromelysin, an enzyme which degraded collagen (Vignon *et al.*, 1990). A comparison with diclofenac in 'N of 1' trials in patients with osteoarthritis showed that a significant proportion obtained adequate control of symptoms with paracetamol alone (March *et al.*, 1994). Although the general opinion was that compared with aspirin-like drugs, paracetamol had little anti-inflammatory action, there was increasing support for the view that it was active and that it reduced pain and swelling in inflammatory conditions other than rheumatoid arthritis (Skjelbred and Lokken, 1979, 1993; Skoglund *et al.*, 1989; Mburu *et al.*, 1990). Paracetamol was of particular value for the treatment of osteoarthritis when non-steroidal anti-inflammatory drugs caused gastrointestinal intolerance (Schnitzer, 1993).

Antipyretic Action

With the renewed interest in paracetamol during the 1950s, attention was again directed to its ability to lower the body temperature in the presence of fever. Following oral administration of doses of 91 and 200 mg kg^{-1} in rats with fever induced by subcutaneous injection of yeast, paracetamol and phenacetin had essentially the same temperature-lowering action (Boréus and Sandberg, 1953) while in a similar study in rabbits, 20–150 mg kg^{-1} of paracetamol was more effective than phenacetin and aspirin and had a comparable duration of action (Renault *et al.*, 1956). At doses as low as 2 mg kg^{-1} it was more effective in guinea pigs than larger doses of phenacetin, antipyrine, amidopyrine and quinine and it even lowered the temperature in normothermic animals (Frommel *et al.*, 1953). In another study in mice, rats and guinea pigs, paracetamol and aspirin had similar antipyretic potency and both were more effective than salicylamide (Boxill *et al.*, 1958). When given over a period of five weeks, paracetamol partially reversed the reduction in weight gain caused by heat stress in chickens, but this effect could not be reproduced when the study was repeated under controlled environmental temperature conditions (Subaschandran and Balloun, 1967). In a series of studies, paracetamol was shown to produce a dose-dependent reduction in fever in rats and cats induced by systemic and intracerebral injection of agents such as 5-hydroxytryptamine, endotoxins and pyrogens (Milton and Wendlandt, 1968, 1971; Clark, 1970; Clark and Alderdice, 1972; Clark and Moyer, 1972). Paracetamol also reduced the content of prostaglandin PGE in cerebrospinal fluid collected from the third ventricle in cats with fever induced by bacterial pyrogen (Feldberg *et al.*, 1972, 1973; Feldberg and Gupta, 1973) and when administered centrally, it shifted the log dose-response curve to leucocyte pyrogen to the right (Clark and Coldwell, 1972). Fever associated with increased prostaglandin PGE-like activity in the cerebrospinal fluid was abolished by paracetamol but it had no effect on fever which was not mediated by prostaglandins (Dey *et al.*, 1974, 1975). In one study, paracetamol had a hypothermic action in its own right in rats (Feldberg and Saxena, 1975) but more often it had no effect on normal body temperature (Cranston *et al.*, 1975). Paracetamol abolished or reversed the non-specific febrile response produced in cats by the microinjection of many agents (including saline) into the pre-optic region of the hypothalamus (Dascombe and Milton, 1975). Other investigators confirmed the antipyretic action of paracetamol in different animal models (Dascombe and Milton, 1976; Almeida e Silva and Pela, 1978; Crawford *et al.*, 1979; Dascombe, 1984; Clark *et al.*, 1985; Deeter *et al.*, 1989) and it was also active in crayfish (Casterlin and Reynolds, 1980). In addition to lowering temperature, paracetamol reversed the cardiovascular abnormalities associated with fever caused by contaminating bacterial pyrogens in cats (Rhodes and Waterfall, 1977). It also partially reversed the ruminal stasis associated with fever induced with endotoxin in goats (van Miert *et al.*, 1977) and it had a greater hypothermic action in fasted than fed mice (Walker *et al.*, 1982). Paracetamol prevented the development of cerebral oedema following impact head injury in unanaesthetized rats but gave only partial protection in anaesthetized euthermic animals. These findings were thought to indicate a role for central 5-hydroxytryptamine and prostaglandins in the dynamic process of oedema formation following head injury (Dey and Sharma, 1984). The antipyretic effect of paracetamol in rats was reduced by exposure to hyperbaric helium-oxygen mixtures (Hart, 1978). Efficacy depended on pharmaceutical formulation (Stolar *et al.*, 1973) and it was effective when administered by suppository in rats (Lock *et al.*, 1979). Ascorbic acid had variable effects on the temperature-lowering action of paracetamol in rabbits (Dange *et al.*, 1985) and mice (Mitra *et al.*, 1988) and a circadian rhythm in response was observed in rats (Rachtan and Starek, 1990). Paracetamol was more effective than aspirin in reversing yeast-induced pyrexia in rats (Foote *et al.*, 1988) and this model has stood the test of time as a standard screen for antipyretic activity of paracetamol and related drugs (Guasch *et al.*, 1990).

Clinical Studies of Antipyretic Action

The analgesic and antipyretic efficacy of paracetamol was studied in 121 children with fever and pain associated with a variety of common infectious conditions. Doses ranged from 60 mg every 4 h in patients up to 2 years of age to 240 mg four times daily in children aged more than 3 years. Treatment was considered to be effective in most patients and there were no serious adverse effects. Paracetamol was also given to 20 older children with tuberculosis in doses ranging from 480 to 960 mg daily for five weeks with no untoward haematological events (Cornely and Ritter, 1956). Following administration of paracetamol suppositories to pyrexial infants on 23 occasions, the mean temperature fell from 39.4 to 37.9°C in 4 h (Vest, 1962). In another report paracetamol and aspirin were given alternately to 100 children seen at an outpatient clinic with fever associated with diverse infections. The dose of paracetamol was 60 mg in infants aged less than 1 year, 120 mg for children aged from 1 to 4 years and 240 mg in those more than 4 years old while the dose of aspirin was 65 mg per year of age. Both drugs caused a similar fall in temperature which was maximal at 3 h and lasted for about 6 h. No important adverse effects were noted with either drug (Colgan and Mintz, 1957). In further comparative studies paracetamol was as effective as aspirin and more effective than salicylamide in reducing the temperature in infants and children with fever (Eden and Kaufman, 1967), but it was less active than indomethacin in 123 children aged less than 14 years with fever exceeding 101°F (Brewer, 1968). There have been many subsequent reports of the efficacy of paracetamol in reducing pyrexia, and some of these are summarized in Table 11.2. In one report, a rapid fall in temperature to 35°C in four previously febrile children following the administration of preparations containing paracetamol was actually presented as an adverse hypothermic reaction (van Tittelboom and Govaerts-Lepicard, 1989). Combinations of paracetamol with other drugs have also been used for the treatment of pyrexia (Gramolini and Manini, 1990; Marchioni *et al.*, 1990). Drugs were not often compared with other methods for reducing elevated body temperature but as judged by rectal, epidural and intraventricular temperature monitoring, rectal paracetamol in doses of 1 g was more effective than isolated head cooling, nasopharyngeal cooling and intensive whole body cooling in five pyrexial neurosurgical patients (Mellergård, 1992). Extreme pyrexia could usually be controlled with paracetamol combined with vigorous surface cooling (Simon, 1976) but difficulties were encountered with malignant hyperthermia (Pan *et al.*, 1975) and in patients with hypothalamic lesions (Lipton *et al.*, 1981). The use of paracetamol to reduce fever in children was associated with a fall in respiratory rate and correction factors were calculated to account for this (Gadomski *et al.*, 1994). A new suppository formulation of paracetamol, which was introduced in Tokyo in 1980, became very popular, and a fall in the incidence of febrile convulsions in young children was attributed to its subsequent widespread use (Sunami and Hayashi, 1990). Paracetamol was recommended as emergency treatment for reducing body temperature in patients with febrile convulsions (Odièvre *et al.*, 1990) but in one report it was only partially effective (Schnaiderman *et al.*, 1993).

In children with fever, the antipyretic action was found to depend on the initial temperature, and a highly significant correlation was shown between efficacy as judged by the observed fall relative to the maximum fall in temperature and the plasma concentration of paracetamol. The minimum effective concentration was about 4 mg l^{-1} and as expected on physiological grounds, there was a substantial lag time before the maximum fall in temperature as shown in Figure 11.4 (Wilson *et al.*, 1982b). The delay in pharmacodynamic response to antipyretic drugs reflected the time taken to reduce heat production and increase heat loss after the change in the central set point for temperature regulation and a counterclockwise hysteresis

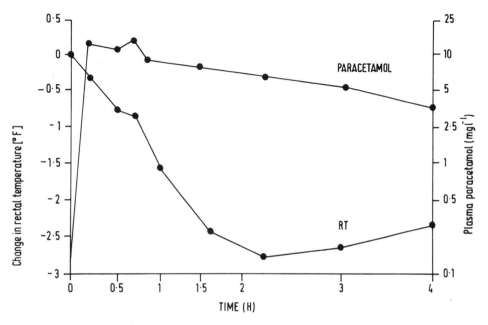

Figure 11.4 The relationship between changes in rectal temperature (RT) and plasma concentrations of paracetamol in eight children with fever following oral administration of a mean dose of 12.4 mg kg^{-1} in a liquid formulation (after Wilson *et al.*, 1982b).

loop was demonstrated by a sequential plot of the fall in temperature against plasma concentrations (Figure 11.5). A well-defined dose-response relationship was established in 26 children between 1.5 and 8 years of age given paracetamol orally in doses of 5, 10 and 20 mg kg^{-1} for acute febrile conditions (Windorfer and Vogel, 1976). There was only a minimal response to 5 mg kg^{-1} but the pyrexia was virtually abolished after 20 mg kg^{-1} (Figure 11.6). The mean maximum plasma concentrations occurred at 30 min at all dose levels and the values were 3.7, 11.9 and 19.7 mg l^{-1} respectively. The correct paediatric dose of paracetamol was a subject for debate, and according to some authorities, underdosing was common (Schechter, 1980; Temple, 1983; Lewis, 1984; Gribetz and Cronley, 1987; Pons *et al.*, 1990; Shann, 1993; Stamm, 1994; Tesler *et al.*, 1994). On the other hand, the *pro re nata* prescribing of paracetamol in hospitals could lead to excessive doses (Penna *et al.*, 1993) and in a survey of its paediatric use in the community in Israel, about 40 per cent of children received an underdose or an overdose (Guberman, 1990).

Although paracetamol is widely used as an antipyretic for relief of a variety of common complaints of presumed bacterial and viral origin, doubts have been expressed concerning the wisdom of this practice (Done, 1959; Rodière and Astruc, 1990; Styrt and Sugarman, 1990; Shann, 1993; Gadomski, 1994). It has been suggested that, by interfering with the natural defence reactions, lowering the body temperature with drugs might adversely influence the course of an infection. Paracetamol was as effective in reducing fever as rimantidine in children with influenza, but it was less effective in reducing the shedding of virus (Thompson *et al.*, 1987). In a study of 56 healthy volunteers with experimental rhinovirus infection, treatment with aspirin or paracetamol in doses of 4 g daily suppressed the production of

215

Table 11.2 Clinical studies of the antipyretic efficacy of paracetamol.

Paracetamol dose	Duration of treatment (days)	Total no. of patients	Age	Cause of fever and complications	Drug comparisons and outcome	Reference
60–360 mg × 4 daily	?	52	2 m–16 y	mixed infection	P effective[1]	Coursin and Kurtz, 1957
150–250 mg × 1 (R)	–	13	1 w–6 m	not stated	P effective[1]	Vest, 1962
80–320 mg × 1	–	130	½–5 y	mixed infection	P > PL; P + TS > P	Steele et al., 1970
80–320 mg × 1	–	120	½–5 y	mixed infection	P < P + AS; P > AS	Steele et al., 1972
60–240 mg × 1	–	39	½–6 y	not stated	P = AS	Tarlin and Landrigan, 1972
5–12 mg kg^{-1} × 1	–	67	½–5 y	not stated	P > PL; P = AS	Hunter, 1973
325–1300 mg (R)	?	79	23–93 y	not stated	P > PL; P oral > P rectal	Maron and Ickes, 1976
12.5 mg kg^{-1} × 1	–	14	1–7 y	mixed infection	P > IBU; P = IBU, AS, AP, IND	Similä et al., 1976
5–20 mg kg^{-1} × 1	–	26	1½–8 y	not stated	20 > 10 > 5 mg kg^{-1}	Windorfer and Vogel, 1976
10 mg kg^{-1} × 1 (R)	–	30	4 m–12 y	mixed infection	P oral = P rectal	Keinänen et al., 1977
10 mg kg^{-1} × 1	–	71	3 m–15 y	various infections	P = AS = AP = MFA	Similä et al., 1977
100–300 mg × 1 (R)	–	105	>3 m^2	mixed infection	P effective[1]	Tomovic and Hagmann, 1977
50–500 mg × 1 (R)^3	–	144	2 w–12 y	mixed infection	oral and rectal P effective	Götte and Liedtke, 1978
10–35 mg kg^{-1} × 1 (R)	–	25	not stated	respiratory infection	P effective[1]	Windorfer, 1978
10 mg kg^{-1} × 1 (R)	–	61	4 m–12 y	mixed infection	P effective[1]	Keinänen-Kiukaanniemi et al. 1979
12–20 mg kg^{-1}	–	37	3 m–6 y	mixed infection	P oral > P rectal[1]	Vernon et al., 1979
300 mg^4	not stated	28	2–8 y	URT	P = IBU	Sheth, 1980
1 g × 1 daily (R)	–	24	19–41 y	gynaecological infection	P = AP	Suma and Lupone, 1980
12 mg kg^{-1} × 1	–	31	<7 y	measles	P effective[1]	Bensaude and Modaï, 1982
12 mg kg^{-1} × 4 daily	?	27	<7 y	mixed infection	P effective[1]	Brusquet et al., 1982
9–12 mg kg^{-1}	–	38	2–7 y	URT, otitis	P = AS; P > CSA	Wilson et al., 1982b
12 mg kg^{-1} × 1 or 2	½	37	<7 y	bacterial/viral infection	P effective[1]	Jean et al., 1983
12 mg kg^{-1} × 4 daily	?	25	<6 y	mixed infection	P effective[1]	Le Fur et al., 1983
12 mg kg^{-1} × 3	–	30	mean 30 m	mixed infection	P effective[1]	Petrus, 1983
10–15, then 3–5 mg kg^{-1}	1	21	4 m–10 y	mixed infection	P effective at both doses[1]	Steru et al., 1983
10–12 mg kg^{-1} × 4 daily	3	25	<14 y	asthma and bronchitis	P effective[1]	Vialatte, 1983
15 mg kg^{-1} × 1	½	69	½–6 y	mixed infection	P = DP	Campos, 1984
12 mg kg^{-1} × 2	½	40	4–38 m	mixed infection	P effective[1]	de Paillerets and Furioli, 1984
12 mg kg^{-1} × 2	½	29	mean 41 m	mixed infection	P effective[1]	Gautry and Bussereau, 1984
125–500 mg × 3 daily (R)	?	30	2 m–10 y	mixed infection	P < IBU	Wilson et al., 1984
8 mg kg^{-1}	–	20	2–12 y	viral and URT	P = IBU	Amdekar and Desai, 1985

Dose		n	Age	Condition	Result	Reference
7.5 mg kg⁻¹ × 4	1	30	3 m–6 y	mixed infection	P effective[1]	Giellen and Bussereau, 1985
62.5–250 mg × 3 daily	5	23	children	URT and measles	P = IBU	Phadke et al., 1985
10 mg kg⁻¹ × 1	—	38	½–16 y	mixed infection	P > TX	Similä and Kylmämaa, 1985
10–15 mg kg⁻¹ × 1	—	46	2–8 y	mixed infection	P = AS	Walker et al., 1986
15 mg kg⁻¹ × 4 daily	?	453	2 m–1½ y	vaccination	P > PL[5]	Ipp et al., 1987
500 mg × 1	—	53	adults	typhoid fever	P < DP	Ajgaonkar et al., 1988
12 mg kg⁻¹ × 2–3 daily	2	12	1–3 y	burn injury	P effective[1]	Childs and Little, 1988
10 mg kg⁻¹ × 4	—	282	2 m–6 y	vaccination	P > PL	Lewis et al., 1988
75 mg × 1	—	263	5 m	vaccination	P = PL	Uhari et al., 1988
6–10 mg kg⁻¹ × 3–4 daily	?	122	4 m–10 y	not stated	P < DC; P = DP	Cedrato et al., 1989
15–20 mg kg⁻¹	—	28	2–8 y	cardiac surgery	P effective[1]	Cullen et al., 1989
10 mg kg⁻¹	—	33	2–11 y	not stated	IBU > P; P > PL	Walson et al., 1989
10–15 mg kg⁻¹	—	54	4 m–4 y	otitis	P + TS > P	Friedman and Barton, 1990
8 mg kg⁻¹ × 1	—	175	4 m–12 y	not stated	P = IBU	Joshi et al., 1990
10 mg kg⁻¹ × 1	—	90	5 m–13 y	not stated	P < IBU	Sidler et al., 1990
10 mg kg⁻¹ × 1	—	118	2–11 y	not stated	P > PL; P < IBU	Walson, 1990
12.5 mg kg⁻¹	—	103	3 m–12 y	non-bacterial infection	P > PL; P = IBU	Wilson et al., 1990
10–15 mg kg⁻¹	variable	225	½–6 y	not stated	P = PL	Kramer et al., 1991
12.5 mg kg⁻¹	—	103	3 m–12 y	acute febrile illness	P > PL; P = IBU	Wilson et al., 1991
10 mg kg⁻¹	—	8	2–12 y	not stated	P < IBU	Kauffman et al., 1992
10–15 mg kg⁻¹		16	1–11 y	not stated	P < IBU	Kelley et al., 1992
15 mg kg⁻¹ × 4 daily	1–2	61	½–11½ y	mixed infection	P = IBU	Walson et al., 1992
10–15 mg kg⁻¹	?	140	2 m–2 y	respiratory infection	P effective[1]	Bonadio et al., 1993
500 mg × 3 daily (R)	2	21	> 65 y	URT	P = NS	Cunietti et al., 1993
100 mg × 1	—	79	8 m–9 y	URT	P = TP	Duhamel et al., 1993
10 mg kg⁻¹ × 4 daily	6	110	3–6 y	febrile convulsions	P = NS	Polidori et al., 1993
44–105 mg kg⁻¹ daily	4	104	½–5 y	mixed infection	P partially effective[1]	Schnaiderman et al., 1993
10 mg kg⁻¹ × 2	—	151	½–5 y	mixed infection	P = IBU	Autret et al., 1994
10–15 mg kg⁻¹	—	75	½–4½ y	viral infection	P + TS > P	Mahar et al., 1994
650 mg × 1	—	150	18–55 y	endotoxin	P > PL; P = KR	Vargas et al., 1994
1 g × 4 daily	?	43	16–58 y	falciparum malaria	P < IND	Wilairatana and Looareesuwan, 1994

[1] no controls or comparison with other drugs; [2] children; [3] repeated doses given over 2–5 days in 40 patients; [4] based on 300 mg adult dose corrected for body weight by Young's formula; [5] ineffective in 70 children aged 1½ years

(R) = rectal ± oral; URT = upper respiratory infection; PL = placebo; AP = amidopyrine; AS = aspirin; CSA = choline salicylate; DC = diclofenac; DP = dipyrone; IBU = ibuprofen; IND = indomethacin; KR = ketorolac; MFA = mefenamic acid; NS = nimesulide; TP = tiaprofenic acid; TS = tepid sponging; TX = tenoxicam

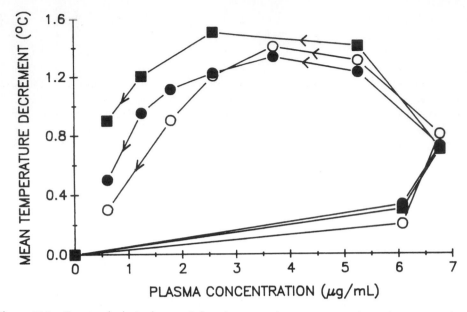

Figure 11.5 Counterclockwise hysteresis loop between plasma concentrations of paracetamol and antipyretic effect plotted in order of increasing time. The three curves were derived from data reported by Windorfer and Vogel 1976, Similä *et al.*, 1977 and Walson and Mortensen, 1989 (reproduced with permission from Hossain and Ayres, 1992).

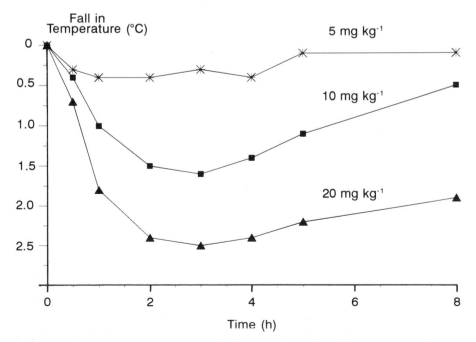

Figure 11.6 The dose-response relationship for the antipyretic effect of paracetamol in children with fever (from Windorfer and Vogel, 1976).

neutralizing antibody and increased nasal symptoms and signs. Compared with placebo, there was a rise in circulating monocytes and a trend towards a longer duration of virus shedding in subjects taking these drugs (Graham *et al.*, 1990). In a placebo-controlled study in 72 children aged 1–12 years with chicken pox, paracetamol 10 mg kg^{-1} taken four times daily for four days did not alleviate symptoms and it may have prolonged the illness (Doran *et al.*, 1989). In another study, 225 children aged 6 months to 6 years with fever of 38°C or more unrelated to bacterial infection received paracetamol 10–15 mg kg^{-1} or placebo every 4 h. There were no significant differences between the groups in the duration of fever or symptoms, and the alleged benefits of lowering temperature with paracetamol were thought to have been exaggerated (Kramer *et al.*, 1991). The temperature response to paracetamol in children with fever gave no useful indication of bacteraemia or the cause of their illness (Baker *et al.*, 1987; Weisse *et al.*, 1987) and its use in such circumstances could interfere with clinical evaluation (Baker *et al.*, 1989). However, in a case control study of 34 febrile children with positive blood cultures and 68 matched controls with negative cultures it was shown that the risk of occult bacteraemia was increased in children who did not respond to paracetamol with a fall in temperature of at least 0.8°C (Mazur *et al.*, 1989). In a subsequent report, the temperature response in children was considered to have a predictive value for occult bacteraemia similar to the white blood cell count but the specificity was low (Mazur and Kozinetz, 1994). Paracetamol did not inhibit the antiviral and antiproliferative action of recombinant human interferon-α_{2a} *in vitro* (Takaoki *et al.*, 1988).

Mechanisms of Analgesic and Antipyretic Action

Although the analgesic actions of aspirin-like drugs were thought to be mediated peripherally by inhibition of prostaglandin synthesis (Vane, 1971) the evidence that paracetamol acted in a similar manner was conflicting, and both central and peripheral mechanisms were probably involved. The antipyretic properties of both drugs were more clearly based on a central action involving prostaglandins (Flower and Vane, 1972).

The mainstay of the evidence for a peripheral analgesic action of paracetamol was provided by Lim *et al.* (1964) in elegant studies with cross-perfused preparations of vaso-isolated but neurally intact spleens in dogs. These investigators showed that the characteristic pain response to injection of bradykinin into the splenic artery of the recipient was blocked by intravenous injection of 178 and 216 mg kg^{-1} of paracetamol in the donor, but not when the same doses were given the same way to the recipient dog. In keeping with the proposed peripheral mechanism of analgesia, the dose of paracetamol required to block the pain response evoked by bradykinin injected into the splenic artery in intact dogs was much smaller when it was injected intra-arterially into the same territory than when it was given intravenously. The ED$_{50}$ values were 14.7 and 108 mg kg^{-1} respectively. Paracetamol also blocked vocalization and the peripheral autonomic responses to pain induced by the intra-arterial injection of bradykinin into the spleen in dogs (Guzman *et al.*, 1964) and it inhibited action potentials in hepatic nerves of the perfused liver arising spontaneously or induced by agents such as acetylcholine, 5-hydroxytryptamine and bradykinin (Andrews and Orbach, 1973). The discovery that many of the actions of aspirin and similar drugs were due to inhibition of biosynthesis of prostaglandins was an important milestone (Vane, 1971) but the position with paracetamol was anomalous because, although it seemed to have little or no anti-inflammatory activity, it clearly possessed analgesic and antipyretic properties. Flower and Vane (1972) showed that paracetamol was inactive against prostaglandin synthetase in dog spleen but that it inhibited prostaglandin synthetase in rabbit brain in a similar manner to aspirin. The concentrations producing 50 per cent inhibition (IC_{50}) were 14 and 11 mg l^{-1} respectively. These findings suggested that the analgesic and antipyretic actions of paracetamol were due to selective central inhibition of prostaglandin synthesis while its lack of anti-inflammatory action was consistent with lack of inhibition peripherally.

Effects of Paracetamol on Prostaglandins

The above hypothesis is not tenable because there is evidence that under certain conditions, paracetamol inhibited the peripheral actions of prostaglandins, including those involved in inflammation. It was shown to suppress the effects of bradykinin, adenosine triphosphate, slow reacting substance C and arachidonic acid in the same way as non-steroidal anti-inflammatory drugs (Vargaftig and Dao Hai, 1973). It also reduced the pain and oedema produced by intraplantar injection of carrageenan (Vinegar *et al.*, 1976; Glenn *et al.*, 1977; Ferreira *et al.*, 1978; Seegers *et al.*, 1979; Bhattacharya *et al.*, 1989) and this was widely accepted as a typical inflammatory response, which was mediated, in part, by peripheral effects of prostaglandins. Inflammation is a complex process that involved migration of polymorphonuclear leucocytes to the site of irritation with subsequent release of arachidonic acid, prostaglandins and chemotactic agents from the phagocytic cells. Isolated rat serosal mast cells released histamine when incubated with paracetamol but only in the presence of liver microsomes obtained from rats induced with polychlorinated biphenyls or phenobarbitone (Mansini *et al.*, 1986). Intraperitoneal injection of prostaglandin PGE_2 enhanced the writhing response to bradykinin in mice, but this effect was only weakly antagonized by oral paracetamol (Walter *et al.*, 1989). In a toxic dose of 600 mg kg^{-1}, oral paracetamol reduced writhing in mice provoked by intraperitoneal injection of zymosan and this was associated with decreased production of prostacyclin (PGI_2) as indicated by the concentrations of its stable metabolite 6-keto-$PGF_{1\alpha}$ in peritoneal fluid (Doherty *et al.*, 1990). At the more realistic dose of 50 mg kg^{-1} intravenously, paracetamol reduced neural activity of joint mechanonociceptors in adjuvant arthritis in rats, and this effect was reversed by local intraarterial injection of cicaprost, a prostacyclin receptor agonist. In this system, prostaglandin PGE_2 was relatively ineffective. These findings indicated that paracetamol had a direct peripheral action on joint capsule pain receptors and that its analgesic action in this model involved inhibition of prostacyclin synthesis (McQueen *et al.*, 1991).

Although paracetamol acted as a reversible inhibitor of platelet cyclooxygenase under certain conditions, the reported effects on prostaglandin production have been variable, and, at times, conflicting. In rabbits, it shared with non-steroidal anti-inflammatory agents the ability to inhibit prostaglandin synthesis (Vargaftig and Dao Hai, 1973) while in another study it had no such effect in rats and did not reduce the production of prostaglandin $PGF_{2\alpha}$ (Glenn *et al.*, 1977). The intravenous administration of arachidonic acid was used as a model for assessment of potential antithrombotic agents but unlike non-steroidal anti-inflammatory drugs, paraceta-mol was ineffective in preventing mortality in this model (DiPasquale and Mellace, 1977). In man, therapeutic doses had no effect on platelet aggregation *in vivo*, but *in vitro* it was almost as active as aspirin in inhibiting aggregation induced by collagen and arachidonic acid (Dupin *et al.*, 1988). Paracetamol did not block the effects of aspirin on cyclooxygenase and platelet function *in vitro* (Rao *et al.*, 1982) and it had a synergistic effect with aspirin in blocking the biosynthesis of prostaglandins by bovine seminal vesicles (Engelhardt, 1984). It inhibited prostaglandin synthesis and the lack of effect on platelet aggregation was thought to be due to its failure to influence thromboxane A_2 production (Drvota *et al.*, 1991). In another report it had no significant effect *in vitro* on platelet aggregation but it inhibited the secretion of 5-hydroxytryptamine by platelets and the vasoconstriction induced by 5-hydroxytryptamine (Verheggen and Schrör, 1987). Paracetamol at concentrations of 150 mg l^{-1} completely inhibited platelet aggregation stimulated by arachidonic acid and collagen, and it also inhibited thromboxane B_2 production and 5-hydroxytryptamine secretion (Shorr *et al.*, 1985). When added to platelet-rich plasma it inhibited aggregation and secretion induced by various agonists, and these effects were attributed to decreased formation of thromboxane B_2 (Lages and Weiss, 1989). In another report, serum thromboxane B_2 concentrations were reversibly reduced in man following a single dose of 18 mg kg^{-1} of paracetamol (Berg *et al.*, 1990).

The non-steroidal anti-inflammatory drugs were thought to inhibit neutrophil function by mechanisms other than those involving prostaglandins, and this could contribute to their anti-inflammatory properties. Unlike these drugs, paracetamol did not inhibit the aggregation of neutrophils in response to a variety of chemo-attractants and it did not alter the viscosity of neutrophil plasma membranes and liposomes (Abramson *et al.*, 1990). It also failed to inhibit the uptake of arachidonic and linoleic acids by cultured human monocytes (Bomalaski *et al.*, 1987). In 53 patients with rheumatoid arthritis, paracetamol in doses of 1 g taken three times a day had no significant effect on leucocyte counts, or on the protein, leukotriene B_4 and prostaglandin PGE_2 content of synovial fluid (Seppälä *et al.*, 1990). Some actions of ethanol were reputed to be caused by the release of prostaglandins, but in studies in volunteers, paracetamol in doses of 325 to 1950 mg did not influence subjective, performance-related and certain physiological effects of ethanol (Pickworth *et al.*, 1992). In mice it did not decrease prostaglandin PGE_2 synthesis in brain *in vivo* but *ex vivo* there was significant dose-related inhibition that correlated with antinociceptive potency as shown by the writhing test (Ferrari *et al.*, 1990). In other studies, paracetamol had no effect, or only a minor effect in reducing the biosynthesis of prostaglandins in rat brain slices and homogenates (Wolfe *et al.*, 1976; Abdel-Halim *et al.*, 1978). Nevertheless, under certain conditions it could inhibit both the constitutive and inducible forms of cyclooxygenase in intact cells (Mitchell *et al.*, 1993).

Paracetamol inhibited the formation of prostaglandins by rabbit kidney micro-somes (Blackwell *et al.*, 1975). It reduced the urinary excretion of prostaglandin PGE_2 and thromboxane B_2 in rats and the effect was proportionately greater in adult than neonatal animals. The renal effects of prostaglandins were age dependent and paracetamol blocked the response of neonatal rats to dehydration but had little effect in weanling and adult animals (Reyes *et al.*, 1989; Meléndez *et al.*, 1990). The renal medullary production of prostaglandins PGE_2 and $PGF_{2\alpha}$ was inhibited in a dose-dependent reversible manner by paracetamol and this represented a direct effect on prostaglandin cyclooxygenase. The concentration for 50 per cent inhibition (IC_{50}) was about 15 mg l^{-1} (Zenser *et al.*, 1978b; Mattammal *et al.*, 1979). In contrast to these findings, paracetamol at concentrations up to 75 mg l^{-1} increased the rate of synthesis of prostaglandins PGE_2 and $F_{2\alpha}$ in rabbit kidney microsomes but as the concentration was increased up to 300 mg l^{-1} there was complete inhibition (Duggin *et al.*, 1982). The inhibitory effect of paracetamol on rat renal medullary cyclooxygenase decreased with increasing incubation time and this was attributed to the cooxidative formation of less inhibitory metabolites (Baumann *et al.*, 1983b). In man, paracetamol has been reported variously as having no effect on the urinary excretion of prostaglandin PGE_2 in healthy female volunteers (Bippi and Frölich, 1990), no effect in healthy young subjects but a reduction in elderly subjects and patients with renal failure (Berg *et al.*, 1990), and a significant reduction in healthy female volunteers (Prescott *et al.*, 1990). In the latter report there was also a lesser reduction in urinary prostaglandin $PGF_{1\alpha}$ and in other studies paracetamol had no effect on the urinary excretion of 2,3-dinorthromboxane B_2 (Vesterqvist and Gréen, 1984). However, a single dose of 500 mg of paracetamol was reported to markedly reduce the urinary excretion of another prostacyclin metabolite, 2,3 dinor-6-keto-$PGF_{1\alpha}$ in healthy subjects (Gréen *et al.*, 1989). Although Bippi and Frölich (1990) found that paracetamol did not reduce urinary prostaglandin PGE_2 excretion significantly in female subjects, the production of its major metabolite was decreased. In another report, paracetamol had no consistent effect on serum concentrations of thromboxane B_2 but it reduced the urinary excretion of prostaglandin PGE_2 in most subjects (Seppälä *et al.*, 1983). P-aminophenol was more active than paracetamol in reducing the synthesis of prostaglandins in the rat renal medulla (Baumann *et al.*, 1983a). Paracetamol did not inhibit the synthesis of prostaglandin PGE_2 and $F_{2\alpha}$ by rat skin (Greaves and McDonald-Gibson, 1972) and it had little or no inhibitory effect on the biotransport of prostaglandins in the rabbit eye and renal cortex (Bito and Salvador, 1976). It had no effect on prostaglandin synthesis by various tissues in the rat except for a minor delayed response in the liver (Fitzpatrick and Wynalda, 1976). It did not potentiate inhibition of the release of prostaglandins PGE_2 and I_2 from mouse peritoneal macrophages by aspirin (Brune and Peskar, 1980) but at high concentrations it produced inhibition itself and at the same time it increased the formation of leukotrienes (Brune *et al.*, 1981, 1984).

There was tissue selectivity in the effect of paracetamol on prostaglandin synthesis and in some studies, it appeared paradoxically to have *increased* the rate synthesis. It increased their production in the rat stomach, and also in rat renal papilla *ex vivo* but not *in vivo* (Danon *et al.*, 1983). It also increased the formation of prostaglandins in the frog heart (Kelemen and Marko, 1988, 1992). Perhaps significantly, paracetamol did not reduce prostaglandin PGE_2 production in preparations of rabbit gastric parietal cells (Levine *et al.*, 1991) and again in contrast to the non-steroidal anti-inflammatory drugs, it did not reduce the binding of prostaglandin $PGF_{2\alpha}$ to human serum proteins (Williams *et al.*, 1991). Unlike non-steroidal anti-inflammatory drugs, paracetamol did not increase the formation of hydroperoxyeicosatetraenoic acid (HPETE) via the lipooxygenase pathway (Siegel *et al.*, 1980). Following oral administration of 100–300 mg kg^{-1} of paracetamol in guinea pigs, prostaglandin production *ex vivo* was stimulated in cell-free preparations from stomach, but not from lung or renal medulla. Similarly, in rats given 50–300 mg kg^{-1}, prostaglandin production was increased in the stomach but decreased in cerebral cortex (Tolman *et al.*, 1983). At concentrations of 3–30 mg l^{-1}, paracetamol stimulated prostaglandin H synthase activity in ram seminal vesicles but at toxic concentrations above 1500 mg l^{-1} the conversion of arachidonic acid to prostaglandin PGG_2 was inhibited (Harvison *et al.*, 1988a). Paracetamol had variable effects on the synthesis of prostaglandin PGE_2 and prostacyclin by the gastric mucosa. In animals and in man it was reported to inhibit (Ali *et al.*, 1977; Konturek *et al.*, 1981; Boughton-Smith and Whittle, 1983), have no effect (Peskar, 1977; Konturek *et al.*, 1984; Tavares *et al.*, 1987), or to stimulate synthesis (Ivey *et al.*, 1978; van Kolfschoten *et al.*, 1982a; Boughton-Smith and Whittle, 1983; Ligumsky *et al.*, 1986). As at other sites, it seemed that in low concentrations paracetamol could enhance the formation of prostaglandins while at high concentrations there was inhibition (Boughton-Smith and Whittle, 1983). Paracetamol inhibited the *ex vivo* formation of leukotriene C_4 by rat gastric mucosa (Trautmann *et al.*, 1991).

The inhibitory actions of paracetamol on the formation of prostaglandins in the central nervous system were less controversial and provided a satisfactory explanation for its antipyretic properties (Flower and Vane, 1972). The prostaglandins, particularly those of the E series, are potent central pyrogens and in animals fever was associated with increased concentrations in cerebrospinal fluid. In cats with fever, paracetamol reduced elevated prostaglandin concentrations in the cerebrospinal fluid in parallel with its temperature-lowering effects (Feldberg and Gupta, 1973; Feldberg *et al.*, 1973; Dey *et al.*, 1974). Arginine vasopressin may be involved in drug-induced antipyresis and while blockade of vasopressin receptors in the ventral septal area of the brain in rats prevented the fall in temperature caused by salicylate in endotoxin fever, it had no effect on the temperature-lowering action of paracetamol (Wilkinson and Kasting, 1990, 1993). It was possible that peripheral anti-inflammatory responses were modulated by central prostaglandin activity. Intracerebroventricular administration of prostaglandin PGD_2 produced a dose-related enhancement of carrageenan-induced oedema in rats which was antagonized by paracetamol (20 and 50 μg) given at the same site. Not surprisingly, these doses had no effect when administered intraperitoneally (Bhattacharya *et al.*, 1989). The intracerebroventricular administration of paracetamol also antagonized the pro-inflammatory action of bradykinin (Bhattacharya *et al.*, 1988). Paracetamol inhibited prostaglandin synthesis in mouse neuroblastoma and rat astrocytoma cell lines and the IC_{50} concentrations were about 100 and 150 mg l^{-1} respectively (Bruchhausen and Baumann, 1982). In these systems, p-aminophenol was more active than paracetamol (Baumann *et al.*, 1983a). The intraperitoneal and intragastric administration of the prostaglandin precursors arachidonic, linolenic and linoleic acids caused anorexia in rats and this effect was inhibited by paracetamol at a dose level of 50 mg kg^{-1} (Doggett and Jawaharlal, 1977).

The picture was further complicated because the effects of paracetamol on prostaglandin synthesis were influenced by a number of factors. Their formation in bull and ram seminal vesicle microsomes could be increased or decreased depending on the concentration of paracetamol and on the presence or absence of cofactors such as hydroquinone and glutathione (Saeed and Cuthbert, 1977; Robak *et al.*, 1978). There were no differences in inhibition of the release of prostaglandins from cultured mouse astrocytes and macrophages, and these findings suggested that there was no specific increased sensitivity of brain cells to account for the analgesic properties of paracetamol (Lanz *et al.*, 1986). Paracetamol slightly diminished carrageenan-induced oedema *in vivo* but it stimulated cyclooxygenase activity *in vitro* in a dose-dependent manner (Robak *et al.*, 1980). Similar concentration-dependent effects have been observed by other investigators. In the absence of cofactors, prostaglandin synthesis by bull seminal vesicle homogenates was increased at low and decreased at high concentrations of paracetamol. In combination with aspirin or indomethacin it strongly potentiated their inhibitory effects on prostaglandin synthesis by the seminal vesicle homogenates but had only a weak effect with rat gastric fundus. It was suggested that paracetamol acted as a phenolic cofactor that stimulated prostaglandin production and also made cyclooxygenase more vulnerable to the effects of aspirin and indomethacin (McDonald-Gibson and Collier, 1979). The antioxidant effect of paracetamol was related to its action on cyclooxygenase (Duniec *et al.*, 1983). The presence of peroxides may be an important factor in the activation of cyclooxygenase and its inhibition by paracetamol was enhanced when peroxide concentrations were lowered by addition of glutathione peroxidase (Hanel and Lands, 1982; Lands and Hanel, 1982). Paracetamol also inhibited the action of manganese protoporphyrin IX in the reconstitution of apoenzyme of prostaglandin H synthase (Thompson and Eling, 1990). In another study in mice with zymosan-induced peritonitis, reduction of superoxide anion by 98 per cent by intraperitoneal administration of superoxide dismutase and catalase did not inhibit the writhing or reduce the antinociceptive potency of paracetamol (Doherty *et al.*, 1990). The activity of cyclooxygenase was thought to be initiated by the formation of peroxidase-related tyrosyl free radical and although paracetamol did not perturb the structure of the radical it caused more rapid decay of the tyrosine radical species (Kulmacz *et al.*, 1991). Befunolol reductase also catalyzed the oxidoreduction of prostaglandins, and this was inhibited by a variety of non-steroidal anti-inflammatory drugs. There were significant correlations between the IC_{50} and the maximum therapeutic doses, and paracetamol was the least active agent (Imamura *et al.*, 1991). Finally, it should be noted that major differences have been reported in the *in vitro* and *in vivo* effects of paracetamol on prostaglandin biosynthesis (Danon *et al.*, 1983). The general conclusion from all of these studies is that paracetamol may either inhibit, stimulate, or have no effect on prostaglandin synthesis depending on tissue selectivity, the source of the enzyme, the drug concentration, the presence or absence of cofactors and experimental conditions. The role of prostaglandins in the peripheral analgesic actions of paracetamol has been a subject for debate (Brune, 1983; Brune and Lanz, 1984; Bannwarth *et al.*, 1993).

Central Versus Peripheral Mechanisms of Action

The central antipyretic action of paracetamol produced by inhibition of prostaglandin synthesis as proposed by Flower and Vane (1972) has been confirmed by other investigators (Feldberg and Gupta, 1973; Feldberg *et al.*, 1973; Dey *et al.*, 1974; Wilkinson and Kasting, 1990). Pretreatment with inducers and inhibitors of oxidative metabolism had variable effects on the hypothermic response to a toxic dose of paracetamol in mice. Intracerebroventricular injection of paracetamol produced a rapid fall in body temperature and brain concentrations correlated with the degree of hypothermia (Massey *et al.*, 1982).

There was also evidence for a central analgesic action of paracetamol. It was effective in reducing the hyperalgesia and oedema produced by carrageenan in rats when given locally and by intraperitoneal or intracerebroventricular injection

(Ferreira *et al.*, 1978). The intra cerebroventricular administration of prostaglandin PGD_2 caused a dose-related enhancement of hind paw oedema induced by injection of carrageenan, and this was antagonized by intracerebroventricular but not by intraperitoneal paracetamol (Bhattacharya *et al.*, 1989). Oral paracetamol antagonized the hyperalgesic effects of intracerebroventricular administration of arachidonic acid and prostaglandins on the vocal response to electrical stimulation in rats (Okuyama and Aihara, 1985) and the intracerebral dose required to abolish the reperfusion hyperalgesia in the rat tail after ischaemia was much smaller than the systemic dose (Gelgor *et al.*, 1992b). The acute responses to pain produced in mice by intrathecal injection of substance P or capsaicin were reduced in a dose-dependent manner by intraperitoneal administration of paracetamol, and these effects were attributed not only to a peripheral action but also to antagonism of nociception at the level of the spinal cord (Hunskaar *et al.*, 1985a; Jurna, 1991). Capsaicin caused the release of prostaglandin PGE_2 from superfused rat spinal cord slices and this effect was inhibited by paracetamol in a dose-dependent manner (Malmberg and Yaksh, 1994). In other studies, intraperitoneal paracetamol produced dose-dependent depression of the nociceptive activity of single neurones of the ventral thalamic nucleus in rats evoked by electrical stimulation of the sural nerve (Figure 11.7). The ED_{50} was 19 mg kg^{-1}. Activity was also recorded in the corresponding ascending axons, but this was not reduced by paracetamol in doses up to 150 mg kg^{-1}. Spontaneous neural activity was not affected (Carlsson and Jurna, 1987; Carlsson *et al.*, 1988; Jurna *et al.*, 1990; Jurna, 1991). The serotoninergic and noradrenergic components of the bulbo-spinal pathways in rats were largely abolished by intrathecal administration of 5,6-dihydroxytryptamine and 6-hydroxydopamine. The pain response to injection of formalin into the hind paws was markedly reduced by intraperitoneal paracetamol in a dose of 400 mg kg^{-1} and this antinociceptive response was reduced in the animals treated with 5,6-dihydroxytryptamine but not in those receiving 6-hydroxydopamine. It was concluded that the spinal serotoninergic system is involved in the analgesic action of paracetamol (Tjølsen *et al.*, 1991a). Further evidence in support of this hypothesis was provided by the reversal of the anti-nociceptive action of paracetamol by the intrathecal administration of tropisetron, a $5\text{-}HT_3$-receptor antagonist (Pélissier *et al.*, 1994).

Paracetamol did not influence spinal reflex potentials in spinal cats (Hara and Murayama, 1992) but it consistently antagonized the nociceptive response to bradykinin in the neonatal rat spinal cord-tail preparation (Dray *et al.*, 1992). Intrathecal paracetamol produced a decrease in the second phase of the response to formalin and it blocked the thermal hyperalgesia induced by spinal injection of N-methyl-D-aspartate and substance P (Malmberg and Yaksh, 1993; Yaksh and Malmberg, 1993). The antagonism of this nociceptive action by L-arginine but not D-arginine suggested a potential central mechanism of action for paracetamol based on inhibition of the L-arginine-nitric oxide pathway (Björkman *et al.*, 1994). Paracetamol inhibited the anti-nociceptive and some of the other actions of morphine in rats (Srivastava *et al.*, 1978; Wallenstein, 1983) and it enhanced the antagonistic action of naloxone (Wong *et al.*, 1980a). Its analgesic effect was reduced by testosterone and by gonadectomy in rats but increased by naloxone (Rao and Saifi, 1985). In rabbits subjected to noxious visceral stimulation caused by distension of the distal colon and somatic pain caused by electrical cervical and lumbar stimulation, paracetamol given intrathecally in doses of 0.5, 2.5, 5 and 10 mg produced dose-dependent antagonism of the visceromotor reflexes and raised the threshold to

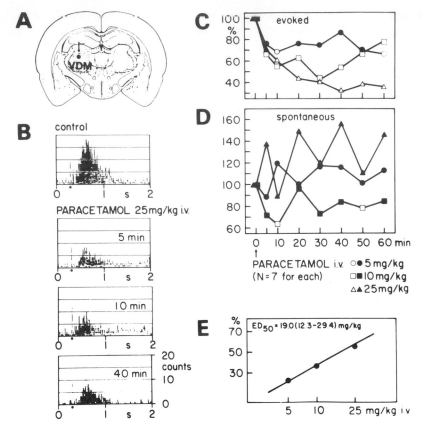

Figure 11.7 Depression by paracetamol of the electrical activity evoked in neurones of the dorsomedial part of the ventral nucleus (VDM) of the thalamus in the rat. A: localization of the neurone in B shown by the dot and arrow; B: peristimulus histograms of activity in a neurone responding to sural nerve stimulation (10 trials each); C and D: time course of depression of evoked and spontaneous activity following administration of different doses of paracetamol; and E: dose-response line for depression of evoked activity in thalamic neurones by paracetamol (reproduced with permission from Carlsson *et al.*, 1988).

lumbar stimulation at the highest dose. Intravenous paracetamol in doses of 10 and 50 mg was inactive. The effects of intrathecal paracetamol were not reversed by naloxone, but were attenuated by the adrenergic antagonist yohimbine. These findings were thought to strongly support a central rather than a peripheral action of paracetamol (Jensen *et al.*, 1992). In healthy volunteers, the threshold to pain as determined subjectively, by visual analogue scores and by the objective nociceptive flexion reflex in response to transcutaneous electrical nerve stimulation was increased by paracetamol 1 g given intravenously as propacetamol, but not by the same dose of aspirin. This indicated a central action because the response involved stimulation of the primary afferent fibres of the sural nerve and not the peripheral pain receptors. The delay in the maximum response to paracetamol was considered to be further evidence in favour of a central action (Piletta *et al.*, 1990, 1991). The overall conclusion from these studies is that the precise mechanism of the analgesic properties of paracetamol remain to be established and that both central and peripheral actions may be involved.

Analgesic and Antipyretic Actions and Plasma Concentrations of Paracetamol

The relationships between plasma concentration and analgesic effects are difficult to determine because of the range of responses to different pain models, different experimental conditions and the variable delay between the time of the maximum plasma concentrations and the maximum pharmacodynamic response. In a study of the effect of subcutaneous and intravenous paracetamol on pain produced by tail pressure in mice there was a convincing linear correlation between analgesic effect and the logarithm of the blood concentration over the range of about 50–350 mg l^{-1} (Figure 11.8). The maximum response was delayed for about 30 min after drug administration by both routes. There was no evidence of a ceiling effect and the rate of decline of analgesic action appeared to be zero order (Shibasaki *et al.*, 1979). In mice with fever induced by yeast, blood concentrations of paracetamol following

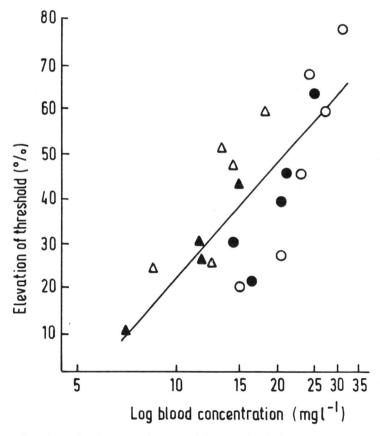

Figure 11.8 The relationship between elevation of the pain threshold to tail pressure and blood concentrations of paracetamol after subcutaneous injection of doses of 149 (▲), 200 (△), 268 (●) and 360 (○) mg kg^{-1} in mice (after Shibasaki *et al.*, 1979).

doscs of 300 and 600 mg kg^{-1} correlated well with the antipyretic response (Mitra *et al.*, 1988). The relationship between plasma concentrations of paracetamol and analgesic effect was also investigated in rats with pain induced by intra-articular injection of uric acid. After oral doses of 100, 178, 316 and 562 mg kg^{-1} of paracetamol with or without caffeine there was a direct relationship between concentration and analgesic response with a sigmoidal model based on the Hill equation (Castañeda-Hernández *et al.*, 1992; Granados-Soto *et al.*, 1992, 1993). In all of these studies the paracetamol concentrations were in the toxic range and greatly exceeded those produced by therapeutic doses in man. According to the time course of drug concentrations following therapeutic doses and changes in pain intensity in clinical studies generally, the range of plasma concentrations for effective analgesia in man was probably about 5–20 mg l^{-1}. However, there have been very few studies in which drug concentrations and analgesic effects have been measured simultaneously in man. As shown in Figure 11.9, peak analgesic effects were delayed relative to peak plasma drug concentrations and this made it difficult to establish direct correlations (Arendt-Nielsen *et al.*, 1991; Nielsen *et al.*, 1991, 1992). It is possible that the rate of rise in drug concentrations was of consequence for the analgesic effect in acute pain (Nielsen *et al.*, 1992). In one report, there was no clear relationship between the analgesic effect of paracetamol in patients with postoperative dental pain and drug concentrations in the central (plasma) or peripheral (brain) compartments (Seymour and Rawlins, 1981). The time course of relief of clinical pain following administration of 1 g of paracetamol was correlated with changes in the

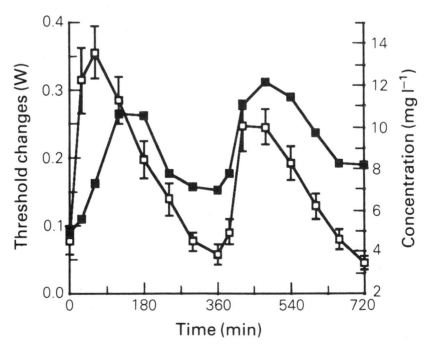

Figure 11.9 Plasma concentrations of paracetamol (□) in relation to changes in threshold (■) to laser-induced pain in 15 subjects following administration of 1 g of paracetamol at 0 and 360 min (reproduced with permission from Nielson *et al.*, 1991).

pain threshold and evoked cortical potential produced by electrical stimulation of the dental pulp in healthy volunteers, and these changes were related to the salivary concentrations of the drug (Derendorf *et al.*, 1982; Rohdewald *et al.*, 1982). A similar relationship was demonstrated with pain produced by intracutaneous electrical stimulation and plasma concentrations of paracetamol (Bromm *et al.*, 1988; Bromm and Scharein, 1993). A dose-dependent analgesic effect was demonstrated in a pain model based on transcutaneous stimulation of the sural nerve in volunteers and the peak effect after intravenous administration of propacetamol was delayed with a counterclockwise hysteresis effect (Piguet *et al.*, 1994). In a pharmacokinetic analysis of the analgesic effect, it was shown that a second dose of paracetamol had a greater and more prolonged effect than the first dose (Levy, 1987).

A complex electrical analogue model of paracetamol-induced antipyresis in the rat was developed by Kakemi *et al.* (1975) in which the delay in onset of effect and physiological functions such as metabolic rate, skin and core temperature, environmental heat transfer coefficient and rate of evaporation of sweat were included. The time course of changes in heat production and body temperature were related to plasma concentrations and the limits for the response were about 16–114 mg l^{-1}. As shown in Figure 11.6, the threshold dose for reduction in temperature in children with fever was about 5 mg kg^{-1} (Windorfer and Vogel, 1976) and the optimum range of plasma concentrations for antipyretic efficacy has been cited as 4–18 mg l^{-1} (Wilson *et al.*, 1982b). Again, the correlations may be obscured by the delay in onset of temperature reduction and sequential time plots of the fall in temperature against plasma concentrations gave a counterclockwise hysteresis loop (Hossain and Ayres, 1992; Kelley *et al.*, 1992). The relationship between concentrations and antipyretic action was influenced by age and initial temperature (Wilson *et al.*, 1982b; Brown *et al.*, 1992) and represented a complex interaction between the processes of drug disposition, heat production and heat loss.

Other Pharmacological Actions of Paracetamol

Paracetamol has other minor pharmacological effects which could usually be related to effects on prostaglandins. In the main these were of little clinical significance.

Effects on Blood and Haemostasis

In usual therapeutic doses, paracetamol had no important effects on platelet function or haemostasis *in vivo* and it was unlikely to cause or aggravate bleeding post-operatively or in patients with coagulation disorders. Rabbit blood or platelet-rich plasma incubated with arachidonic acid caused contraction of superperfused rabbit aorta and rat stomach and colon strips in the same way as prostaglandin PGE_2. This response was attributed to release of prostaglandins from platelets and it was inhibited by prior incubation with paracetamol in concentrations of 0.6–20 mg l^{-1}. There have been several studies of the effects of paracetamol on haemostasis. Mielke and Britten (1970) found that 975 mg of paracetamol had no effect on the bleeding time or platelet aggregation induced by adenosine diphosphate, collagen and adrenaline in 20 normal male subjects and two patients with haemophilia A. Similarly, a single dose of 650 mg had no effect on the bleeding time or platelet function in nine patients with haemophilia, although one developed a haemarthrosis within 24 hours of taking the paracetamol (Kasper and Rapaport, 1972). In a more detailed study, single doses of 975 or 1950 mg of paracetamol again had no effect on the bleeding time or platelet aggregation in healthy volunteers and after repeated doses of 1950 mg daily for one week there was no effect on coagulation factors or fibrinolysis. After treatment for six weeks there was no increase in the bleeding time in three patients with haemophilia and no effect on the bleeding time or platelet aggregation and adhesion in four normal subjects (Mielke *et al.*, 1976). In a double blind crossover study with aspirin and placebo in 23 females, paracetamol in a dose of 0.5 g three times daily had no effect on menstrual blood loss (Petruson *et al.*, 1977). These negative clinical studies have been reviewed (Czapek, 1976; Pearson, 1978). The lack of effect of 1 g of paracetamol on the bleeding time and platelet aggregation induced by collagen and adenosine diphosphate was confirmed in 20 male and 20 female subjects (Seymour *et al.*, 1984). During tonsillectomy in children, intraoperative blood loss was less in those previously given paracetamol than in those receiving ketorolac (Rusy *et al.*, 1995). There was no evidence that the regular use of analgesics including paracetamol in patients with chronic headache was linked to adverse effects on the viscoelastic properties of blood (Oder *et al.*, 1994).

In other studies paracetamol has been shown to have effects on platelet function *in vitro* and this was probably largely a function of concentration. The aggregation of human platelets *in vitro* in response to arachidonic acid and collagen, and to a lesser extent, adenosine diphosphate and ristocetin was reduced to a variable degree by paracetamol in concentrations of 15–150 mg l^{-1}. In addition, there was a marked concentration-dependent decrease in the synthesis of thromboxane B_2 and release of serotonin by platelets after reaction with arachidonic acid (Shorr *et al.*, 1985). In normal subjects paracetamol had no effect on platelet aggregation or secretion induced by adenosine diphosphate, or on thromboxane release at concentrations of 15 mg l^{-1}. However, it inhibited the contraction of bovine coronary arteries mediated by platelet-derived serotonin and thromboxane A_2 (Verheggen and Schrör, 1987). In another report the IC_{50} values for the inhibitory effect of paracetamol on the aggregation of platelets from healthy volunteers *in vitro* in response to collagen, adenosine diphosphate and arachidonic acid were 106, 378 and 106 mg l^{-1} respectively. Paracetamol also reduced serotonin release from platelets and inhibited the synthesis of thromboxane A_2 induced by collagen (Dupin *et al.*, 1988). Similar findings have been reported by other investigators. Paracetamol in doses of 650 mg or 1 g had no effect on platelet aggregation or serotonin release in five of six healthy subjects but in one aggregation in response to arachidonic acid and adrenaline was inhibited *in vivo* at a paracetamol concentration of only 17 mg l^{-1}. Paracetamol inhibited the formation of thromboxane A_2 from arachidonic acid in every subject (Lages and Weiss, 1989). At the toxic concentration of 200 mg l^{-1}, paracetamol inhibited the aggregation of equine platelets *in vitro* in response to arachidonic acid and collagen (Heath *et al.*, 1994).

Although paracetamol had no significant adverse effects on haemostasis, when 650 mg was taken regularly four times a day it produced a mean increase of 3.7 s in the prothrombin time in 62 patients on long-term therapy with a variety of oral anticoagulants (Antlitz *et al.*, 1968). In a subsequent study two doses of 650 mg taken 4 h apart had no effect on the prothrombin time in 10 similar patients (Antlitz and Awalt, 1969). There was no evidence for a clinically important interaction with oral anticoagulants but there has been an anecdotal report of bleeding in a patient on long-term warfarin therapy following the use of paracetamol (Bartle and Blakely, 1991). At toxic concentrations, paracetamol caused dose-dependent inhibition of the migration of human peripheral leucocytes (Brown and Collins, 1977) and it inhibited their adherence to nylon fibre columns (MacGregor, 1976). In doses that inhibited the formation of oedema in the carrageenan pleurisy assay in rats, it reduced neutrophil mobilization by the same magnitude (Vinegar *et al.*, 1978) but it had no adverse effects on leucocyte viability (Austin and Truant, 1978). Paracetamol did not inhibit the phagocytic activity of human peripheral blood monocytes (Klein *et al.*, 1982) and it had no effect on the labelling of leucocytes with indium oxine In^{111} (Augustine *et al.*, 1983). It had no effect on the viscosity of human neutrophil leucocyte plasma membranes (Abramson *et al.*, 1990) but at high concentrations it could limit the microbiocidal action of the myeloperoxidase-peroxide-chloride system of leucocytes (van Zyl *et al.*, 1989). There was no effect on the adherence of *Staphylococcus epidermidis* to medical polymers (Farber and Wolff, 1992). Paracetamol inhibited the oxidative respiratory burst *in vitro* as shown by chemiluminescence and generation of superoxide (Shalabi, 1992) and at the highly toxic concentration of 1000 mg l^{-1} it inhibited interleukin 1 (IL-1) activity and production by human monocytes (Chang *et al.*, 1990). Paracetamol protected red blood cells against various forms of oxidative stress by scavenging free radicals (van der Zee *et al.*, 1988) and therapeutic doses in children produced an increase in the concentration of reduced glutathione in red blood cells (Bernal *et al.*, 1993).

Renal Effects

Most of the reported renal effects of paracetamol can be attributed to its ability to reduce prostaglandin synthesis in the kidney (Zenser *et al.*, 1978b; Mattammal *et al.*, 1979; Haylor, 1980; Abrams *et al.*, 1986; Berg *et al.*, 1990; Prescott *et al.*, 1990; Martin and Prescott, 1994). Except in some patients following acute overdosage, there have been no reports of acute impairment of renal function by paracetamol in predisposed individuals as may occur with aspirin and non-steroidal anti-inflammatory drugs (Plotz and Kimberly, 1981). In short-term studies in healthy young and elderly subjects and in patients with chronic renal failure, paracetamol did not influence the glomerular filtration rate or effective renal blood flow as measured by the inulin, creatinine and p-aminohippurate clearances (Berg *et al.*, 1990; Bippi and Frölich, 1990; Prescott *et al.*, 1990). Similarly, it had no effect on the glomerular filtration rate or other indices of renal function when taken regularly over months or years in patients with rheumatoid arthritis (Edwards *et al.*, 1971) or in elderly subjects (Hale *et al.*, 1989). Paracetamol had no effect on urinary kallikrein excretion but it reduced the activation of plasma kallikrein (Schor *et al.*, 1983).

Paracetamol may have effects on the renal transport of sodium and water and it enhanced the net flow of water across the toad bladder in the presence of vasopressin (Nusynowitz *et al.*, 1966; Bisordi *et al.*, 1980). It also caused a dose-dependent decrease in sodium transport across frog skin and this effect was thought to be mediated by prostaglandins (Hall *et al.*, 1976b). In a dose of 1.2 g, paracetamol increased urine osmolality and reduced urine volume in three patients with diabetes insipidus and in two of these patients taking 2.4–4.8 g daily for several days urine osmolality increased and the volume and free water clearance decreased (Nusynowitz and Forsham, 1966). This modest effect of paracetamol in patients with diabetes insipidus was confirmed in a later report (Cabezas Cerrato *et al.*, 1970). The effects of paracetamol on renal prostaglandins in rats was age dependent. An intraperitoneal dose of 10 mg kg^{-1} blocked the response of newborn rats to dehydration and decreased the urinary excretion of prostaglandin PGE_2 and thromboxane B_2, but it had no such effects in older animals (Reyes *et al.*, 1989; Meléndez *et al.*, 1990; Reyes and Meléndez, 1990). In another study, paracetamol in doses of 15–45 mg kg^{-1} did not antagonize the expected diuresis caused by ethanol in rats (Morato *et al.*, 1992). In toxic concentrations above 2145 mg l^{-1}, paracetamol caused a diuresis and reduced sodium reabsorption in the isolated perfused rat kidney (Emslie *et al.*, 1981b).

In normally hydrated female subjects 1.5 g of paracetamol was said to have reduced sodium and water excretion in successive 3 h collection periods (Haylor, 1980). Unfortunately this cannot be accepted without reservations because there were no proper controls and comparisons were made with the excretion pattern in previous collection periods. Following administration of 40 mg kg day^{-1} of paracetamol for three days in 10 healthy young subjects, nine elderly subjects and nine patients with chronic renal failure, there was a significant decrease in urine sodium excretion in the elderly subjects but no change in the other groups (Berg *et al.*, 1990). In another report there was a decrease in urine sodium output and a delay in the onset of diuresis following an acute water load in 10 healthy young females given paracetamol 1 g four times daily for three days. Unlike indomethacin, paracetamol did not influence plasma renin activity (Prescott *et al.*, 1990). Paracetamol had no effect on the urinary excretion of potassium (Berg *et al.*, 1990; Prescott *et al.*, 1990). The diuresis and natriuresis produced by 20 mg of frusemide was attenuated in 13 healthy volunteers by paracetamol in a dose of 1 g (Abrams *et al.*, 1986). This effect could not be confirmed in a similar study in which 1 g was given four times daily for two days but paracetamol reduced the transient increase in urine prostaglandin excretion and the rise in plasma renin activity caused by frusemide (Martin and Prescott, 1994).

Gastrointestinal Effects

Paracetamol has only minor gastrointestinal effects and these were inconstant and of little practical significance. In rats, it produced some slowing of gastric emptying and delayed the movement of a fluid meal through the gastrointestinal tract. It had little or no effect in antagonizing contraction of the rabbit and guinea-pig ileum induced by histamine and acetylcholine (Weikel and Lish, 1959). There was another report to the effect that paracetamol slowed gastric emptying in rats (Poon *et al.*, 1988b). It had minor effects on antroduodenal motility and gastric emptying in man but no effect on gastric pH (Schurizek *et al.*, 1989a). These effects were of no practical consequence for the use of the absorption kinetics of paracetamol as an indirect measure of gastric emptying rate. Paracetamol inhibited the contraction of rat gastric and colonic strips superperfused with rabbit blood or platelet-rich plasma that had previously been incubated with arachidonic acid, and this effect was attributed to decreased prostaglandin synthesis (Vargaftig and Dao Hai, 1973). It had no significant effect on gastric mucosal blood flow and acid secretion in dogs (Bennett and Curwain, 1977). In concentrations of 1.5–60 mg l^{-1}, paracetamol produced a dose-dependent inhibition of electrically evoked contraction of the myenteric plexus longitudinal muscle preparation of the guinea-pig ileum. The IC_{50} was 14 mg l^{-1} and this effect was readily reversed by washing the drug out of the organ bath or addition of prostaglandin PGE_1 (Miller and Shaw, 1981). The efficacy of naloxone in reversing the inhibitory action of morphine on gastrointestinal propulsion in mice was significantly enhanced by prior treatment with paracetamol (Wong and Wai, 1981). At concentrations of 450–2250 mg l^{-1}, paracetamol increased the absorption of fluid, glucose and sodium by rat isolated duodenal segments but absorption was inhibited at 4500 mg l^{-1} (Diener *et al.*, 1986). The method used for solubilization of the drug at these very high concentrations was not mentioned. Paracetamol seemed to have a variable effect on the gastrointestinal synthesis of prostaglandins. Unlike aspirin, it did not decrease the synthesis of prostaglandin PGE_2 by gastric mucosal and parietal cells (Ota *et al.*, 1988; Romano *et al.*, 1988a; Levine *et al.*, 1991).

Many investigators have shown that in contrast to aspirin and non-steroidal anti-inflammatory drugs, paracetamol does not cause direct gastric mucosal injury in animals (Roth *et al.*, 1963; van Kolfschoten *et al.*, 1982b, 1983b; Manekar and Raul, 1983; Poon *et al.*, 1989; Cho and Ogle, 1990; Bhattacharya *et al.*, 1991) or man (Ivey *et al.*, 1978; Hoftiezer *et al.*, 1982; Stern *et al.*, 1984a; Lanza *et al.*, 1986; Hogan, 1988; Müller *et al.*, 1988, 1990), and when applied locally to the buccal mucosa it did not cause desquamation and ulceration (Roth *et al.*, 1963). As expected in such circumstances, it did not reduce hydrogen and sodium ion flux across the gastric mucosa, or influence the transmucosal potential difference in healthy subjects (Ivey and Settree, 1976; Stern *et al.*, 1984a; Hogan, 1988). Paracetamol largely prevented the fall in gastric transepithelial potential difference produced by aspirin in healthy subjects (de Vos and Barbier, 1985). In rabbits, it did not potentiate pre-stimulated gastric acid secretion (Levine *et al.*, 1991).

Paracetamol actually protected against mucosal damage caused by a variety of gastrotoxic agents. Seegers *et al.* (1978, 1979) showed that in doses of 15–250 mg kg^{-1} paracetamol protected male and female rats against erosive gastric injury produced by aspirin in a dose-dependent manner without influencing the rapid decrease in histamine-stimulated gastric acid output that follows exposure to this drug. Paracetamol displayed a similar dose-dependent protective action against gastric mucosal damage in rats induced by aspirin, indomethacin, ethanol, sodium hydroxide and hydrochloric acid while there was little or no protection against lesions induced by phenylbutazone, glafenine and ibuprofen. With indomethacin, paracetamol protected when given orally or subcutaneously but it was only effective against the toxicity of aspirin when given by the oral route (van Kolfschoten *et al.*, 1982b, 1983b). Other investigators have confirmed that paracetamol can antagonize gastric injury caused by naproxen, indomethacin, aspirin and ethanol in rats (Ivey *et al.*, 1978; Konturek *et al.*, 1982; Ligumsky *et al.*, 1986; Poon *et al.*, 1988b, 1989; Bennett, 1989b; Janjua and Draz, 1991; Trautmann *et al.*, 1991). The protective effect of oral and subcutaneous paracetamol against the toxicity of ethanol in rats was probably not mediated by prostaglandins because it was reduced by vagotomy but not by prior treatment with indomethacin (Poon *et al.*, 1988a, 1989). Paracetamol also inhibited the formation of stress-induced gastric mucosal lesions in rats and this protective effect was abolished by indomethacin (Omura *et al.*, 1994). In contrast to these findings, oral and subcutaneous paracetamol was reported to potentiate gastric ulcers in rats produced by cold restraint stress. There was a decrease in the mast cell counts of the gastric glandular mucosa and the aggravating effects of paracetamol were not antagonized by ranitidine, astemizole, dimethylsulphoxide, sucralfate or verapamil (Cho and Ogle, 1990). In another report, paracetamol, in a dose of 25 mg twice daily for five days, had no effect on total and free gastric acid production in rats and it augmented the gastrotoxicity of ibuprofen 25 mg given in the same dose regimen (Bhattacharya *et al.*, 1991).

At the very high concentration of 750 mg l^{-1}, paracetamol protected rat gastric mucosal cells in culture against the cytotoxic effects of taurocholate. This action was not blocked by indomethacin and it was not associated with changes in the concentrations of prostaglandins PGE_2 and $PGF_{1\alpha}$ in the incubation medium (Ota *et al.*, 1988). Similar findings were observed in human gastric mucosal cell cultures, and again pretreatment with indomethacin did not block this protective action (Romano *et al.*, 1988a,b). In a further report, the protective effect of paracetamol against taurocholate toxicity in gastric mucosal cells was attenuated when non-protein glutathione and cysteine concentrations were reduced by prior treatment with iodoacetamide (Romano *et al.*, 1991). In these two studies, extraordinarily high concentrations of paracetamol (4500 to 6000 mg l^{-1}) were used. In man, 2.6 g of oral paracetamol reduced the gastrotoxicity of aspirin as shown by endoscopic appearances and effects on mucosal hydrogen ion transport and potential difference (Stern *et al.*, 1984b). In contrast, paracetamol given in a dose of 975 mg four times daily for seven days did not protect against endoscopic gastric mucosal injury produced by ibuprofen 600 mg taken four times daily for the same time (Lanza *et al.*, 1986). There have also been negative results in animal studies. Paracetamol did not protect against occult blood loss produced in dogs by aspirin (Leeling *et al.*, 1981) and it failed to protect against gastric mucosal damage caused by ethanol and aspirin with hydrochloric acid in rats (Nakagawa and Okabe, 1987). Unlike aspirin, the use of paracetamol was not associated with a reduced risk of digestive tract cancer (Thun *et al.*, 1993; Peleg *et al.*, 1994).

Effects of Paracetamol on the Central Nervous System

Paracetamol has no obvious effects on central nervous system function even in the case of overdosage. In combination with salicylamide it had no effect on mood, emotions and motivation in normal subjects (Cameron *et al.*, 1967). In doses of 2 g, paracetamol had no discernible effects on mood, mentation and energy in healthy volunteers (Eade and Lasagna, 1967) and it failed to influence the subjective and physiological effects of ethanol in normal subjects (Pickworth *et al.*, 1992). Similarly, in doses of 500 mg and 1 g it had no effect on visuo motor coordination, dynamic visual acuity, critical flicker fusion frequency, digit symbol substitution, complex reaction times and subjective mood in healthy female subjects (Bradley and Nicholson, 1987). The combination of paracetamol and dextropropoxyphene did not influence saccadic eye movements or the ventilatory response to hypercapnia in healthy volunteers (Ali *et al.*, 1985). In another study in 32 volunteers, 1 g of paracetamol had no effect on reaction times and auditory evoked potentials but it caused an increase in spontaneous low frequency electroencephalographic activity (Bromm *et al.*, 1992). Paracetamol had a beneficial effect on sleep in 2931 postoperative patients. This effect was greater in those who had pain and there was at least an additive effect with doxylamine (Smith and Smith, 1985). Not surprisingly, paracetamol had no beneficial effects in patients with acute schizophrenia (Falloon *et al.*, 1978). In a longitudinal prospective study of 1529 women, 41 per cent said that they had taken paracetamol during the first half of pregnancy but this was not related to the intelligence quotient and attention of their children at the age of 4 years (Streissguth *et al.*, 1987).

Paracetamol depressed the compound action potentials of the isolated phrenic nerve in the rat in a reversible dose-dependent fashion (Brodin and Skoglund, 1987). However, this effect was not clinically relevant as it only occurred at supratoxic concentrations up to 8000 mg l^{-1}. Paracetamol antagonized the increase in brain 5-hydroxytryptamine produced in response to bradykinin, cannabis and restraint stress (Bhattacharya and Bhattacharya, 1983; Bhattacharya *et al.*, 1986) and it had little effect on brain concentrations of glutathione in rats (Masukawa *et al.*, 1989; Bien *et al.*, 1992). There was no reinforcing effect of intragastric self-administration of paracetamol in rhesus monkeys. The response rate was lower than with the control solution and there was no evidence of anything resembling a withdrawal syndrome on abstinence (Hoffmeister *et al.*, 1980). Paracetamol increased rapid eye movement (REM) sleep in normal rats but in animals with adjuvant arthritis it decreased wakefulness and increased non-REM sleep irrespective of any effects on the arthritis (Landis *et al.*, 1989). It delayed the onset, and reduced the frequency of audiogenic seizures induced by caffeine in mice, but in doses up to 300 mg kg^{-1} it had no anticonvulsant activity on its own (Deng *et al.*, 1982). Paracetamol also delayed the onset and reduced the severity of convulsions produced by pentylenetetrazole (Wallenstein, 1985, 1991) but it was without effect on convulsions caused by other agents in mice and rats (Steinhauer and Hertting, 1981; Wallenstein and Mauss, 1984). As shown by electroencephalographic changes, paracetamol caused dose-related sedation in rats but in another report it had no effects on the electroencephalogram frequency bands in various cortical areas (Nickel and Zerrahn, 1987).

Cardiovascular and Respiratory Effects

Treatment of rabbits with gram negative bacterial infection with a combination of salicylate and paracetamol did not prevent a fall in blood pressure (Malvin *et al.*, 1979) but the intracerebroventricular administration of paracetamol antagonized the central hypotensive action of clonidine in rats while potentiating the bradycardic effect (Sirén and Karppanen, 1980). Paracetamol had no effect on the gastrointestinal or liver blood flow rate in rabbits (Hierton, 1981) but it depressed the vasoconstrictor response of the mesenteric vasculature to noradrenaline (Stanton *et al.*, 1986). It attenuated the output of prostaglandins from the isolated rat heart in response to arachidonic acid and reduced the duration of coronary vasodilatation (Shaffer *et al.*, 1981). In the voltage clamped frog heart preparation, paracetamol increased the maximum amplitude of the fast inward sodium current in the same way as prostacyclin and this response was abolished by the addition of indomethacin to the perfusion fluid (Kelemen and Marko, 1988). It was also selectively antagonized by lignocaine, quinidine and mexiletine (Marko and Kelemen, 1992). Unlike indomethacin and ibuprofen, paracetamol given to near-term pregnant rats in a dose of 14 mg kg^{-1} produced only minor constriction of the ductus arteriosus of the fetal rats delivered by Caesarean section at different times after dosing. At 24 h there were increases in pericardial fluid, ventricular mass and atrial volume but the significance of these changes is unknown because there was no control group (Momma and Takao, 1990). Paracetamol was said to cause bradycardia without changes in blood pressure in healthy volunteers and anaesthetized dogs (Acharya, 1979).

Paracetamol antagonized the bronchoconstriction induced by adenosine triphosphate, bradykinin and arachidonic acid in anaesthetized guinea pigs and hypotension produced by bradykinin and slow reacting substance C in anaesthetized rabbits and dogs. These effects were dose dependent and were attributed to inhibition of prostaglandin synthesis (Vargaftig and Dao Hai, 1973). Paracetamol partially antagonized the bronchoconstriction produced in anaesthetized guinea pigs by intravenous injection of arachidonic acid (Frey and Dengjel, 1976) and it attenuated the active secretion of chloride ion as shown by the short circuit current in cultured dog tracheal epithelial cells (Mochizuki *et al.*, 1994). In toxic doses it depressed the respiratory rate in rats (Sewell *et al.*, 1984) but in fetal lambs it had an opposite effect which was long lasting (Walker, 1990). Paracetamol did not often aggravate symptoms in patients with aspirin-induced asthma (Szczeklik, 1989) but, if it did, the reaction was usually milder (Fischer *et al.*, 1983). Three aspirin-sensitive asthmatics reacted to 1 g of paracetamol with a fall in the forced expiratory volume of more than 20 per cent and when two of these were desensitized to aspirin they failed to respond to paracetamol (Settipane and Stevenson, 1989). Of 87 patients attending an allergy clinic, 12 experienced increased airways obstruction after taking 1 g of paracetamol (Delaney, 1976). These adverse effects of paracetamol on respiratory function are thought to be mediated by effects on prostaglandins (Fischer *et al.*, 1983; Settipane and Stevenson, 1989; Szczeklik, 1989). Asthma may be provoked in aspirin-sensitive patients by the release of protein-bound prostaglandins, but unlike aspirin and non-steroidal anti-inflammatory drugs, paracetamol did not inhibit the binding of prostaglandin $PGF_{2\alpha}$ to serum proteins (Williams *et al.*, 1991).

Effects on Pregnancy and Reproduction

Despite the wide use of paracetamol, no important adverse or other effects have been recognized following its consumption during pregnancy (Collins, 1981). In rats, paracetamol in a dose of 250 mg kg day^{-1} did not affect fetal length or weight or the incidence of resorptions, and it interfered less with normal fetal growth than aspirin (Lubawy and Garrett, 1977). Paracetamol had little or no effect on ovulation in rabbits (Espey *et al.*, 1982; Espey, 1983) and in clinically realistic doses it had little effect on the ductus arteriosus in fetal and newborn rats (Momma and Takeuchi, 1983; Momma and Takao, 1990). The fetal acid-base balance in febrile women with chorioamnionitis was said to be improved when the temperature was lowered in the mother by rectal administration of paracetamol (Kirshon *et al.*, 1989). Paracetamol did not influence intrauterine pressure in women with dysmenorrhea (Milsom and Andersch, 1984) but it had a paradoxical anti-analgesic effect in women undergoing termination of pregnancy with mifepristone and sulprostone (Weber and Fontan, 1990; Weber *et al.*, 1990a).

Effects on the Eye and Ear

The regular use of paracetamol was associated with a reduced risk of cataracts. In a survey of 300 cataract patients and 609 control subjects in Oxford, the relative risk of developing cataract in those taking paracetamol regularly for at least four months was reduced to 0.42–0.45 (van Heyningen and Harding, 1986; Harding and van Heyningen, 1988). Similar results were reported in a later more detailed study (Harding *et al.*, 1989). Paracetamol also reduced the severity and delayed the onset of cataracts in diabetic rats when given in the drinking water for 160 days (Blakytny and Harding, 1992). There was little binding of radiolabelled paracetamol to bovine soluble lens proteins and an interaction involving metabolic activation was proposed as a mechanism of protection (Shyadehi and Harding, 1991). Protection against cataracts has also been linked to the metal chelating and antioxidant action of paracetamol (Woollard *et al.*, 1990). In contrast to these findings, the acute and subacute administration of paracetamol in toxic doses caused cataracts in susceptible strains of mice and rabbits. This effect was potentiated by prior microsomal enzyme induction with 3-methylcholanthrene and there was a delicate balance between genetic and environmental factors causing ocular toxicity (Shichi *et al.*, 1978, 1980). The metabolic activation of paracetamol seemed to be necessary for cataractogenesis (Lubek *et al.*, 1984, 1988a,b). In toxic doses, paracetamol had no effect on compound action potentials generated by auditory stimulation in guinea pigs, but it potentiated the decrement produced by frusemide (Moorjani *et al.*, 1985).

Miscellaneous Effects

At high and toxic dose levels, paracetamol has multiple adverse effects on intermediary metabolism and these are discussed in Chapters 12 and 13. Paracetamol had radioprotective effects in mice but the mechanism was not established (Allain *et al.*, 1975). It had inhibitory effects on various enzymes including xanthine oxidase (Carlin *et al.*, 1985) and ATPases in human fetal brain (Sarkar *et al.*, 1989) but it did not inhibit serum oxytocinase (Roy *et al.*, 1981, 1982). Paracetamol caused induction of aryl hydrocarbon hydroxylase and cytochrome P450 enzymes in mice (Mostafa *et al.*, 1990), and preincubation of liver slices with high concentrations of paracetamol resulted in increased biosynthesis of lecithin (Lohmann *et al.*, 1984). Paracetamol had no effect on the glycaemic response following a meal in man (Bijlani *et al.*, 1992) and its administration for seven days had no effect on the serum concentrations of thyroid hormones (Faber, 1980). Similarly, it had no effect on serum concentrations of thyroxine, thyroid stimulating hormone or hypothalamic thyreotropin releasing hormone in rats (Tal *et al.*, 1988). Therapeutic doses of paracetamol stimulated the turnover of cysteine and glutathione in man (Lauterburg and Mitchell, 1987), and it blocked the hair follicle stimulating effect of minodoxil by competing with it for sulphate conjugation (Buhl *et al.*, 1990). During chronic administration, paracetamol could aggravate dietary deficiencies of sulphur-containing aminoacids but this did not compromise methylation reactions as shown by folate status and utilization of dietary constituents (Varela-Moreiras *et al.*, 1990, 1993; Prudencio *et al.*, 1994). Paracetamol added to the diet stimulated growth in chickens and rats by an unknown mechanism (Dikstein *et al.*, 1966a,b) and it stimulated hepatic regeneration after two-thirds hepatectomy (White and Gershbein, 1985).

Therapeutic Use of Paracetamol

Paracetamol is used extensively in many countries as a non-prescription analgesic-antipyretic for symptomatic relief in febrile illnesses in children and for the relief of pain and discomfort in a variety of common complaints and disorders. Because it did not have the same potential for adverse effects as aspirin and the non-steroidal anti-inflammatory drugs, paracetamol was considered the treatment of choice for mild-to-moderate pain, and for use during pregnancy (Amadio, 1984). Unreferenced statements were frequently made to the effect that paracetamol had no anti-inflammatory activity but despite these claims it was widely used in patients with rheumatoid arthritis. It could also provide effective relief in osteoarthritis and indeed, it was recommended in full dosage as the first line of analgesic therapy in patients with this condition (Jones and Doherty, 1992). The clinical trials in which paracetamol was compared with non-steroidal anti-inflammatory drugs in patients with osteoarthritis have been critically reviewed. Although the numbers of patients were small, it was more effective than placebo and the frequently repeated assertion that the non-steroidal anti-inflammatory drugs are more effective in relieving pain than paracetamol was not substantiated (Dieppe *et al.*, 1993). In children, paraceta-mol was preferred to aspirin because it was usually as effective and better tolerated (Dalens, 1991; Collet, 1992) and it was indicated particularly for the relief of minor pain (Selbst and Henretig, 1989; Selbst, 1992). Paracetamol was also preferred to aspirin for the relief of pain following surgery for spondylodesis (Koch, 1992) and it was commonly used for postoperative analgesia following a variety of procedures (Baños *et al.*, 1989; Bush *et al.*, 1989; Wiens *et al.*, 1990; Warth *et al.*, 1994). Given postoperatively, it reduced the requirements for morphine (Jespersen *et al.*, 1989; Campbell, 1990) and uncontrolled studies suggested that it was of value in ortho-paedic patients during rehabilitation (Deshayes and Mathieu, 1979). Paracetamol was also used extensively as a 'background' and 'rescue' analgesic (Hutchison *et al.*, 1990; Wong *et al.*, 1993a). The buffering capacity of soluble paracetamol formula-tions provided the further advantage of perioperative acid aspiration prophylaxis (Mills, 1989). The prodrug propacetamol has been used for postoperative analgesia (Delacroix *et al.*, 1985; Moreau *et al.*, 1990; Hans *et al.*, 1993; Beaulieu, 1994) and for the relief of other painful conditions such as otitis (Stipon *et al.*, 1983).

In the United Kingdom, the consumption of paracetamol increased from 1500 million tablets in 1967–1968 to 2854 million tablets in 1973–1974 (Spooner and Harvey, 1976). By 1993, it was the most widely used of all drugs and consumption had risen to about 4000 million tablets annually (Spooner and Harvey, 1993). In 3587 children monitored in hospitals in Boston, USA, between 1974 and 1979, para-cetamol was prescribed for 32 per cent and aspirin for 3 per cent, while during the three months before admission, 23 per cent reported the use of either drug (Mitchell *et al.*, 1982). Following the death of at least seven people caused by the criminal lacing of 'Tylenol' brand of paracetamol in Chicago in 1982, potential users expressed anxiety about the safety of over-the-counter drugs but this did not influ-ence their pattern of consumption (Dershewitz and Levin, 1984). A telephone survey of the use of analgesics by children during an epidemic of influenza revealed that 61 per cent received paracetamol and 14 per cent received aspirin. The declining use of aspirin was attributed to publicity concerning the association with Reye's syndrome (Taylor *et al.*, 1985). In a more recent survey of American pre-school age children, 53.7 per cent had received non-prescription drugs during the preceding month and the most commonly used drug was paracetamol, which was taken by 66.7 per cent (Kogan *et al.*, 1994). Of the drugs prescribed for paediatric inpatients at a teaching hospital, 12.2 per cent were for analgesics and 10.7 per cent of orders were for paracetamol (Summers and Summers, 1986). A prospective study of children aged between 3 months and 3 years in day care with infectious illness in France showed that paracetamol was the most commonly prescribed drug, accounting for 13.5 per cent of prescriptions (Collet *et al.*, 1991). In France, most analgesics were sold on prescription and women were the main consumers. Paracetamol was the most commonly used drug and it was selected for self-medication, prescribed by doctors and recommended by pharmacists on 44.2, 34.5 and 21.2 per cent of occasions respectively (Menard *et al.*, 1993). Over the period 1970–1978, paraceta-mol accounted for less than 5 per cent of analgesic drugs used in Sweden (Gustafsson and Boëthius, 1982) but from 1976 to 1983 there was a rapid increase in sales (Wessling, 1987). In a survey during the last decade in persons born in 1902 in the northern town of Umeå, Sweden, paracetamol was the most frequently used analgesic and the proportion of this population taking it increased from 11 to 28 per cent over the period 1981–1990 (Osterlind and Bucht, 1991). In all the Nordic countries the use of paracetamol increased dramatically from 1978 to 1988. The highest consumption was in Denmark and the lowest in Finland (Ahonen *et al.*, 1991). Headache was an important cause of absence from work in Denmark and paraceta-mol was one of the most commonly taken remedies (Rasmussen *et al.*, 1992). The use of prescribed analgesics increased with age but in Finland few prescriptions were written for paracetamol except for a combination with orphenadrine (Ahonen *et al.*, 1992). Older patients were particularly frequent users of analgesics including parace-tamol (Cupit, 1982) but in Florida from 1978 to 1980 non-prescription aspirin was taken by the elderly more frequently than paracetamol (Stewart *et al.*, 1982). More recent studies have shown a dramatic reversal of this pattern for prescribed analge-sics in the elderly in France (Colomes *et al.*, 1990), Canada (Grymonpre *et al.*, 1991) and Spain (García Domínguez *et al.*, 1992). In an elderly population in Iowa, a substantial proportion of analgesic takers took multiple analgesic drugs. Analgesics were taken more often by females than males, and 9.1 and 6.3 per cent respectively took paracetamol during the preceding week (Chrischilles *et al.*, 1990). As a reflec-tion of the scale of its use in the community, paracetamol was detected in 6.7 per cent of 1176 samples of donor blood (Sharon *et al.*, 1982). It was also a constituent of traditional folk medicines in Southeast Asia (Smith and Nelsen, 1991).

Paracetamol represented 60 per cent of the analgesics prescribed for adult medical and surgical patients in a university affiliated community hospital in New York (Portenoy and Kanner, 1985). It was often prescribed routinely in another American university hospital and its use corresponded more with the hospital service rather than the characteristics and requirements of the patients. The orders were written imprecisely and decisions about administration were generally left to the discretion of the nursing staff (Isaacs *et al.*, 1990). In another survey of paraceta-mol use in hospital, combination analgesics were often used, and in some cases this led to the administration of more than the maximum official dose of the drug (Ward *et al.*, 1992). The successful withdrawal of analgesics including paracetamol after heavy continuous consumption has been described in patients with migraine (Hering and Steiner, 1991). Paracetamol was occasionally taken in excessive doses for prolonged periods and an unusual form of abuse was the intermittent ingestion of 8–30 tablets at once to induce vomiting in patients with bulimia and other eating disorders (Tiller and Treasure, 1992). Other cases have been described where enor-mous doses of paracetamol have been taken over long periods without incident and in one such report, a 58-year-old alcoholic woman apparently took 15–20 g daily for five years without suffering liver damage (Tredger *et al.*, 1995). After more than 100 years, paracetamol itself was said to be in perfect health (Ploin, 1990).

12

General Toxicology

Introduction

Originally, there was no cause for concern about the safety of paracetamol because it was the major metabolite of acetanilide and phenacetin, and apart from a propensity for causing methaemoglobinaemia, these long-established analgesics were generally considered to be very safe. Proper toxicity studies such as would be required today for a new drug were not carried out and the belated discovery that paracetamol could cause hepatic necrosis when administered in toxic doses came somewhat as a surprise (Eder, 1964; Boyd and Bereczky, 1966; Davidson and Eastham, 1966; Thomson and Prescott, 1966). In recent years, the focus of attention has been directed almost exclusively at the liver, and apart from producing methaemoglobinaemia and possibly minor nephrotoxicity in some species, paracetamol is not generally considered to cause significant toxicity in other organ systems.

There was little clinical use of paracetamol during the last century but limited toxicity studies were reported by Hinsberg and Treupel (1894). They gave doses of 50 and 100 mg of paracetamol subcutaneously to two large Hungarian frogs and noted that they became restless and ataxic with irregular respiration. One frog appeared to recover but was found dead the next morning and the other suffered cardiorespiratory arrest 25 min after dosing. A guinea pig, given 1500 mg of oral paracetamol, developed shaking movements and clonic contraction of the jaw muscles with weakness, ataxia and decreased breathing. Although it was kept warm, the animal died during the night. At postmortem examination the organs had a brown-red discolouration with blood-stained peritoneal fluid and pulmonary oedema. The urine gave a positive indophenol reaction. One rabbit, given 6000 mg of paracetamol orally, became lethargic but apparently recovered the next day while another rabbit, given a cumulative dose of 7000 mg intravenously over about 4 h, developed depressed breathing with a progressive fall in pulse rate and blood pressure. Artificial respiration was to no avail. A dose of 100 mg kg^{-1} produced only sleepiness in dogs but there was more marked depression with 200 mg kg^{-1}. Signs of kidney irritation, vomiting and diarrhoea persisted all day after which there was rapid recovery. Doses of 500 and 1000 mg caused cyanosis due to meth-aemoglobinaemia together with sleepiness, ataxia, thirst, lachrimation, vomiting and parotitis. Over the following days there was urgency with the passage of small amounts of brownish-red urine. Hinsberg and Treupel (1894) also gave 500 mg doses of paracetamol to five patients with fever and they remarked on the normal urine chemistry and the absence of any signs of toxicity. Further limited animal toxicity studies indicated that cats were very susceptible to the effects of paraceta-mol while dogs were much more resistant (Heubner, 1913).

Acute Toxicity

Methaemoglobinaemia was the most notorious adverse effect of acetanilide and phenacetin, and when interest in paracetamol was renewed in the middle of the century, it was quickly established that although it shared this toxic effect in some animal species, it did not do so in man (Greenberg and Lester, 1947; Brodie and Axelrod, 1948b, 1949; Boréus and Sandberg, 1953). Paracetamol had a low acute toxicity as judged by the acute lethal dose for 50 per cent of animals (LD_{50}); the results of studies in different species are shown in Table 12.1. The LD_{50} was subject to many variables including the period of assessment in relation to the time of dosing, age, sex, diet, nutritional state and route of administration. Nevertheless, there were important species differences in susceptibility to the lethal toxicity of paracetamol. Mice and hamsters were sensitive species while rats were resistant. The acute LD_{50} of paracetamol was less in fasted than fed mice (Boxill *et al.*, 1958; McLean and Day, 1975; Sonawane *et al.*, 1981; Neuvonen *et al.*, 1985), less in female than male mice (Munoz and Fearon, 1984), less with subcutaneous pellet implantation than oral administration (Munoz and Fearon, 1984), less in mice pretreated with phenobarbitone (McLean and Day, 1975; Neuvonen *et al.*, 1985) and less in mice with dietary deficiencies of vitamin E, methionine or selenium (Peterson *et al.*, 1992). Conversely, the acute oral LD_{50} was increased when L-cysteine and methionine were given with the paracetamol (McLean and Day, 1975; Munoz and Fearon, 1984; Neuvonen *et al.*, 1985). Mice could be made tolerant to a lethal dose of paracetamol (1200 mg kg^{-1}) by pretreatment with sublethal doses of 250 mg kg^{-1} orally twice daily for four days (Piperno *et al.*, 1978). In rats, the mean acute LD_0 and LD_{100} were 900 ± 800 (SE) and 6500 ± 800 mg kg^{-1} respectively and the interval to death varied inversely with dosage (Boyd and Bereczky, 1966). Rabbits survived an oral dose of 3000 mg but died with prostration and convulsions within 24 h of administration of a dose of 5000 mg. In rats given 500 and 800 mg kg day^{-1} for 20 days there were no signs of toxicity, and renal and hepatic histology were said to be normal (Renault *et al.*, 1956). In acute studies in rats and guinea pigs (but not mice), paracetamol was less toxic than aspirin and salicylamide, and signs of toxicity included reduced activity, depression and a decreased respiratory rate. The dose producing neurological toxicity in half the number of animals (TD_{50}) was 144–185 mg kg^{-1} in mice and 268–342 mg kg^{-1} in rats. In anaesthetized dogs, paracetamol produced little change in blood pH, tidal volume, respiratory rate and heart rate, and unlike the other drugs it did not cause myocardial depression. It had no anti-convulsant properties but in toxic doses it increased the pentobarbitone sleeping time in mice (Boxill *et al.*, 1958). No haematological or histological abnor-malities in the liver or kidney were observed in rats given 2 per cent of paracetamol in their chow for 13 weeks (Schnitzer and Smith, 1966).

Table 12.1 The acute LD_{50} of paracetamol in different species.

Species	Route of administration	Mean LD_{50} (mg kg^{-1})	Reference
Rat	oral	> 5000	Boréus and Sandberg, 1953
Rat	oral	4500	Renault *et al.*, 1956
Rat	oral	4450	Boxill *et al.*, 1958
Rat	oral	3710	Boyd and Bereczky, 1966
Rat	ip*	1250–1500	Mitchell *et al.*, 1973b
Rat	oral	5200	McLean and Day, 1974
Rat	oral	5200	McLean and Day, 1975
Rat (age 7 days)	ip	2350	Mancini *et al.*, 1980
Rat (adult)	ip	1580	Mancini *et al.*, 1980
Rat	oral	7000	Poulsen *et al.*, 1981
Rat (age 11 days)	ip	1220	Green *et al.*, 1984b
Rat (age 19 days)	ip	840	Green *et al.*, 1984b
Rat (age 33 days)	ip	1580	Green *et al.*, 1984b
Rat	oral	> 3200	Behrendt and Cserepes, 1985
Rat	oral	> 4000	Guasch *et al.*, 1990
Rat**	ip	400	Hong *et al.*, 1992
Mouse	oral	610	Frommel *et al.*, 1953
Mouse (fasted)	oral	570	Boxill *et al.*, 1958
Mouse (fed)	oral	1020	Boxill *et al.*, 1958
Mouse	oral	875	Rosner *et al.*, 1973
Mouse	oral	449	Whitehouse *et al.*, 1976
Mouse	ip	425	Slattery and Levy, 1977
Mouse (age 7 days)	ip	3850	Mancini *et al.*, 1980
Mouse (adult)	ip	800	Mancini *et al.*, 1980
Mouse	ip	876	McClain *et al.*, 1980
Mouse	ip	340	Nelson *et al.*, 1980a
Mouse	ip	875	Peterson *et al.*, 1980
Mouse (fed)	oral	1500	Sonawane *et al.*, 1981
Mouse (starved)	oral	750	Sonawane *et al.*, 1981
Mouse	ip	480	Abernethy *et al.*, 1983a
Mouse	oral	840	Khairy *et al.*, 1983
Mouse	oral	798–1007	Engelhardt, 1984
Mouse	oral	295	Miners *et al.*, 1984d
Mouse	oral	501–1660	Munoz and Fearon, 1984
Mouse	oral	340	Renton and Dickson, 1984
Mouse	oral	327–610	Neuvonen *et al.*, 1985
Mouse	ip	710	Endo *et al.*, 1988b
Mouse	oral	840	Dimova and Stoytchev, 1989
Mouse	ip	860	Dimova and Stoytchev, 1989
Mouse	oral	925–1212	Guasch *et al.*, 1990
Mouse	ip	820	Ishikawa *et al.*, 1990a
Mouse	ip	460	Juzwiak *et al.*, 1992; Juzwiak, 1993
Mouse	ip	376	Peterson *et al.*, 1992
Mouse	ip	750	Roberts *et al.*, 1992
Mouse	oral	654	Dimova and Stoytchev, 1994
Guinea pig	oral	3500	Boxill *et al.*, 1958
Mosquito (adult)	im***	1920	Richie and Lang, 1985

* intraperitoneal, ** glutamine-free diet, *** intramembranous injection into area between 1st and 2nd thoracic spiracles

The first hint of the hepatotoxicity of paracetamol appeared in 1964 when Eder described severe hepatic necrosis in two of six cats given the relatively low dose of 25 mg kg^{-1} for four weeks followed by 50 mg kg^{-1} for a further 22 weeks. One of these cats had early cirrhosis and two others had moderate and marked fatty degeneration of the liver. In the group as a whole there was anorexia and weight loss by the 23rd week, and by the end of the study four cats had died. In one of these the liver was said to show strong 'marmoration' and the liver pathology was considered severe enough to account for death in two cases. Subsequently, Boyd and Bereczky (1966) observed centrilobular hepatic necrosis in groups of 15–20 rats given single oral doses of 2000–7000 mg kg^{-1} of paracetamol. The liver lesions were only seen in animals dying from one to seven days after dosing and in addition there were degenerative changes in the brain, kidneys, serous salivary glands, thyroid and thymus. The syndrome of acute toxicity was characterized by pallor, hypothermia, decreased food and water intake, tail extension, tremor and a reduced response to stimuli, and premortal signs included stupor and respiratory failure. There was also dose-related weight loss with changes in organ weight and water content (Boyd and Sheppard, 1966). In another study, rats were given 500–4000 mg kg day^{-1} of paracetamol in suspension intragastrically five days a week to determine the lethal doses for 0, 50 and 100 per cent of animals when dosing was continued for 100 days. The mean values for the $LD_{0\ (100\ days)}$, $LD_{50\ (100\ days)}$ and $LD_{100\ (100\ days)}$ were 413, 765 and 1060 mg kg day^{-1} respectively. At the level of the LD_0 the signs of toxicity were hyperreflexia, aciduria, hypertrophy of the cardiac stomach, testicular atrophy, minor hepatic necrosis, nephritis and increased susceptibility to infection. At the highest doses there was also anorexia, hypothermia, prostration, necrosis of salivary glands, thymic atrophy, pneumonitis and marked hepatic necrosis with cirrhosis (Boyd and Hogan, 1968). In 1966 the first cases of liver damage, including two fatalities with fulminant hepatic failure, were reported in man following paracetamol overdosage (Davidson and Eastham, 1966; Thomson and Prescott, 1966).

There have been more recent reports of the acute toxicity of paracetamol and clinical signs in cats and dogs included cyanosis, vomiting, central nervous system depression, hypothermia and facial oedema (Leyland and O'Meara, 1974; Atkins and Johnson, 1975; Duer, 1979; Gaunt *et al.*, 1981; Marcella, 1983; Prasuhn, 1983; Anvik, 1984; St. Omer and Mohammad, 1984; Brown, 1985; Judson, 1985; Savides *et al.*, 1985; Hjelle and Grauer, 1986; Jones *et al.*, 1992b). At doses up to 300 mg kg^{-1} intraperitoneally, paracetamol produced no discernible changes in activity or consciousness in mice but they were less active and appeared to be sedated at higher doses. Rats were often prostrated by large doses and appeared moribund with doses above 750 mg kg^{-1}. Death usually occurred within 12 h and the cause was not apparent (Mitchell *et al.*, 1973b; McMurtry *et al.*, 1978). Rats given 400 mg kg^{-1} intraperitoneally became lethargic and tachypnoeic with piloerection. Postmortem examination revealed large quantities of fluid in the peritoneal and thoracic cavities suggestive of a diffuse capillary leak (Hong *et al.*, 1992). Following an oral dose of 1500 mg kg^{-1} in mice there was decreased activity, tremor, an exaggerated response to noise and loss of the righting reflex together with anaemia, leucopenia and thrombocytopenia. Histological examination of the liver showed moderate to marked centrilobular congestion at 3 h with necrosis at 9 h after dosing (Piperno *et al.*, 1978). In another study, standard and germ-free mice were examined at intervals up to 48 h after oral administration of 300 and 600 mg kg^{-1} of paracetamol. In addition to the expected necrosis of the liver, there were degenerative and necrotic changes in the kidney, bronchiolar epithelium, testis and lymphoid follicles of the spleen and small intestine (Placke *et al.*, 1987b). In dogs, an oral dose of 600 mg kg^{-1} caused cyanosis due to methaemoglobinaemia, facial and paw oedema, lachrimation, pruritus, bloody vomiting and melaena usually without impairment of the sensorium. Biochemical and haematological abnormalities included leucocytosis, increased prothrombin time, alkalosis, hypokalaemia, and elevation of blood aspartate aminotransferase, creatine phosphokinase, bilirubin and ammonia concentrations. There were no remarkable changes in blood amylase, urea, creatinine, glucose and cholesterol. No definite histological abnormalities were observed in dogs killed 2–3 h after dosing, but after 24–48 h there was palpebral oedema, centrilobular hepatic necrosis, renal tubular dilatation and haemorrhage into the bladder, stomach and small intestine (Piperno *et al.*, 1978). An oral dose of 100 mg did not produce clinical effects in dogs but after 200 mg kg^{-1} three of four animals had methaemoglobinaemia and one developed haematuria. After 500 mg kg^{-1} there was vomiting, methaemoglobinaemia, haematuria, depression, oedema of the face, paws and forelegs lasting 1–3 days. These signs were associated with decreased blood concentrations of glutathione and increased alanine aminotransferase and alkaline phosphatase activity. One dog died 18–24 h after dosing and was found to have haemorrhagic congestion of the liver and kidney. No gross lesions were seen at postmortem examination of the other three dogs but the histological findings included centrilobular hepatic necrosis, biliary stasis, 'nephrosis', atrophy and depletion of splenic follicles and pulmonary congestion and oedema (Savides *et al.*, 1984).

Cats were very susceptible to the toxicity of paracetamol (Leyland and O'Meara, 1974; Duer, 1979; Prasuhn, 1983; Sundlof, 1990). They readily developed methaemoglobinaemia but they did so to a lesser extent than with phenacetin and acetanilide (Renault *et al.*, 1956). Two of five cats given 325 mg of paracetamol orally at 0 and 4 h died and manifestations of toxicity included cyanosis, depression, anorexia and facial and submandibular oedema. Doubling the dose of paracetamol in another four cats was uniformly fatal. There were minor elevations of serum alanine aminotransferase activity but at postmortem examination there was no histological evidence of hepatic necrosis (St. Omer and McKnight, 1980). In another study, six cats received 20, 60 and 120 mg kg^{-1} on separate occasions. After the middle dose some cats had haematuria and haemoglobinuria, and after the high dose they all developed methaemoglobinaemia, salivation, vomiting, depression and facial oedema. These signs persisted for 12–48 h and were associated with a fall in the whole blood concentration of glutathione and variable elevation of alanine aminotransferase activity and prothrombin time (Savides *et al.*, 1984). The marked susceptibility of cats to the effects of paracetamol was confirmed by numerous other reports of severe toxicity following accidental poisoning with the drug (Steele, 1974; Finco *et al.*, 1975; St. Omer and McKnight, 1980; Nash and Oehme, 1984; Ilkiw and Ratcliffe, 1987). N-acetylcysteine has been used with limited success for the treatment of paracetamol poisoning in cats and dogs (Gaunt *et al.*, 1981; St. Omer and Mohammad, 1984; Judson, 1985; Savides *et al.*, 1985).

Nephrotoxicity and Hepatotoxicity

The nephrotoxicity and hepatotoxicity of paracetamol are discussed in Chapters 13 and 14 respectively.

Toxic Effects on the Blood

Methaemoglobinaemia

Methaemoglobinaemia was the major toxic effect of paracetamol on the blood but there were striking species differences in susceptibility in this respect. Despite frequent claims in many learned reviews and reference works that paracetamol caused methaemoglobinaemia in man, this was not the case (Greenberg and Lester, 1947; Boréus and Sandberg, 1953; Vest, 1962; Thomas *et al.*, 1966; Windorfer and Vogel, 1976) while conversely, it could produce such severe methaemoglobinaemia in cats, dogs and pigs as to threaten life (Gazzard *et al.*, 1975b; St. Omer and McKnight, 1980; Hjelle and Grauer, 1986; Henne-Bruns *et al.*, 1988b; Kelly *et al.*, 1992). These differences were not simply a function of dose because significant methaemoglobinaemia was not seen in man even following gross overdosage. Methaemoglobinaemia following the administration of paracetamol has been reported in cats (Renault *et al.*, 1956; Eder, 1964; Finco *et al.*, 1975; Nash and Oehme, 1984; Nash *et al.*, 1984b; Savides *et al.*, 1984; Ilkiw and Ratcliffe, 1987; Weiss *et al.*, 1990; Hornfeldt, 1992), dogs (Gazzard *et al.*, 1975b; Piperno *et al.*, 1978; Savides *et al.*, 1984; Kelly *et al.*, 1992), pigs (Henne-Bruns *et al.*, 1988a,b) and rats (Peters *et al.*, 1972; Udosen *et al.*, 1989; Udosen and Ebong, 1991). In contrast to these findings, methaemoglobinaemia was not observed in mice (Piperno *et al.*, 1978), or in other studies in pigs (Miller *et al.*, 1976a) and dogs (Francavilla *et al.*, 1989). One possible explanation for the latter negative result was that the paracetamol was injected subcutaneously in solution in dimethylsulphoxide, a compound which is known to protect against its toxicity (Siegers, 1978a; Jeffery and Haschek, 1988; Park *et al.*, 1988). However, dimethylsulphoxide was also used as the solvent for paracetamol in another study in dogs in which there was said to be uncontrollable methaemoglobinaemia (Kelly *et al.*, 1992). Methaemoglobin was produced by the oxidation of ferrous to ferric iron in haemoglobin, and this process could be reversed by administration of reducing agents such as ascorbic acid, methylene blue and N-acetylcysteine (Gazzard *et al.*, 1975b; St. Omer and McKnight, 1980; Ilkiw and Ratcliffe, 1987; Hornfeldt, 1992). It was seen in the most dramatic form in acute high dose toxicity studies and was usually present in only minor degree during chronic administration (Eder, 1964; Peters *et al.*, 1972). The dose-dependent formation of methaemoglobinaemia following single administration of paracetamol in cats is shown in Figure 12.1. Glutathione status was important for prevention of the oxidation of haemoglobin, and paracetamol-induced methaemoglobinaemia was associated with decreased blood concentrations of glutathione (Nash and Oehme, 1984; Nash *et al.*, 1984b). The inhibition of hepatic glutathione synthesis in dogs by prior treatment with buthionine sulphoximine resulted in gross methaemoglobinaemia following intravenous infusion of paracetamol (Kelly *et al.*, 1992).

Anaemia

Anaemia has been observed in some acute toxicity studies of paracetamol in cats (Finco *et al.*, 1975; Ilkiw and Ratcliffe, 1987), dogs (Francavilla *et al.*, 1989), pigs (Henne-Bruns *et al.*, 1988a,b) and mice (Piperno *et al.*, 1978). In some cases the anaemia was caused by oxidative haemolysis with the appearance of Heinz bodies

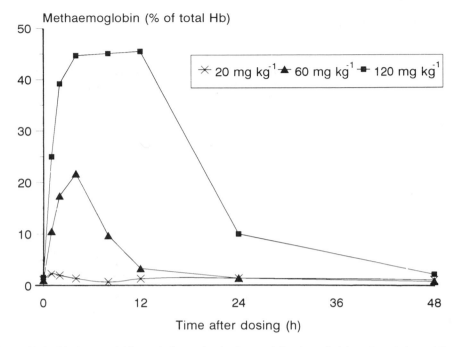

Figure 12.1 Methaemoglobinaemia formation in six cats following administration of three different doses of paracetamol on three occasions three weeks apart (from Nash *et al.*, 1984a).

in the peripheral blood (Finco *et al.*, 1975; Miller *et al.*, 1976a; Gaunt *et al.*, 1981; Goldenthal, 1982; Harvey *et al.*, 1986; Ilkiw and Ratcliffe, 1987) and it has also been attributed to gastrointestinal bleeding in the setting of acute hepatic failure (Francavilla *et al.*, 1989). In a case of paracetamol poisoning in a cat, the haemato-crit fell to 7 per cent in seven days (Malley, 1987) and chronic poisoning in a dachs-hund was associated with Heinz bodies, reticulocytosis and abnormal red blood cell morphology with abundant eccentrocytes (Harvey *et al.*, 1986). In chronic toxicity studies there was a mild hyperchromic anaemia in rats (Peters *et al.*, 1972) and a minor decrease in the life span of erythrocytes in rabbits and dogs (Pletscher *et al.*, 1958). In other reports there was no evidence of anaemia or haemolysis (Eder, 1964; Schnitzer and Smith, 1966). Paracetamol reduced the glutathione content of red blood cells and increased their osmotic fragility in rats (Raheja *et al.*, 1984). It also reduced the glutathione concentration in red blood cells in cats (Gaunt *et al.*, 1981; Nash *et al.*, 1984b) and at grossly toxic concentrations it had a similar effect on human red blood cells and caused haemolysis *in vitro* (Altorjay *et al.*, 1993). In contrast, treatment of children with therapeutic doses for several days resulted in an increase in the glutathione content of erythrocytes (Bernal *et al.*, 1993). Incubation of human red blood cell membranes ('white ghosts') with N-acetyl-p-benzoquinoneimine resulted in the inhibition of membrane transport systems and modification of the cytoskeletal proteins (Nicotera *et al.*, 1990).

Haemostasis

Prolongation of the prothrombin time (Piperno *et al.*, 1978; Savides *et al.*, 1984; Kelly *et al.*, 1992) and reduced concentrations of fibrinogen (Miller *et al.*, 1976a) have been observed in animals with severe paracetamol intoxication. Such findings are to be expected in the presence of severe liver damage and hepatic failure. In therapeutic doses paracetamol had no adverse effects on haemostasis in healthy subjects or patients with haemophilia (Mielke, 1981) and it did not influence platelet aggregation in healthy volunteers (Cronberg *et al.*, 1984).

Effects on White Blood Cells and Platelets

Leucocytosis and thrombocytopenia have been described in dogs, cats and pigs with severe paracetamol-induced liver necrosis (Finco *et al.*, 1975; Miller *et al.*, 1976a; Piperno *et al.*, 1978) while leucopenia was reported in mice (Piperno *et al.*, 1978). In two similar reports of the same acute toxicity study in pigs, there was a decrease in the peripheral blood lymphocyte count (Henne-Bruns *et al.*, 1988a,b). Paracetamol had no effect on the white blood cell count in a chronic toxicity study in rats (Peters *et al.*, 1972), but in man it inhibited the function of polymorphonuclear leucocytes (Shalabi, 1992) and could possibly interfere with their antimicrobial action (van Zyl *et al.*, 1989). At toxic concentrations, paracetamol inhibited the migration of human leucocytes (Brown and Collins, 1977), but in another study it did not inhibit human neutrophil chemotaxis (Matzner *et al.*, 1984). Glutathione synthetase deficiency in man (5-oxoprolinuria) was associated with an increased sensitivity of circulating lymphocytes to the cytotoxicity of paracetamol in the presence of an activating mouse liver microsomal drug metabolizing system, and a model was developed on this basis for the assessment of toxicity caused by drug metabolites (Spielberg, 1980; Spielberg and Gordon, 1981; Leeder *et al.*, 1988). Toxicity in lymphocytes was marked at paracetamol concentrations that caused more than 80 per cent depletion of glutathione (Spielberg, 1980) and the cytotoxicity of paracetamol in this model was reversed by the addition of N-acetylcysteine (Spielberg, 1983, 1984, 1985).

Reticulo-endothelial System, Thyroid and Salivary Glands

Necrotic and atrophic changes were noted in lymphoid tissue, mesenteric lymph nodes, intestinal Peyer's patches, splenic follicles and thymus in acute toxicity studies in cats, dogs, mice and rats (Boyd and Bereczky, 1966; Boyd and Hogan, 1968; Piperno *et al.*, 1978; Duer, 1979; Savides *et al.*, 1984; Placke *et al.*, 1987b). Degenerative changes were also seen in the salivary glands in rats and cats (Boyd and Bereczky, 1966; Boyd and Hogan, 1968; St. Omer and McKnight, 1980) and the thyroid gland in rats (Boyd and Bereczky, 1966). The depletion of hepatic glutathione following administration of paracetamol was associated with impairment of the clearance of microparticles from the circulation by phagocytes (Hennighausen and Engel, 1989).

Pulmonary and Cardiovascular Toxicity

Pulmonary lesions have been described occasionally in acute toxicity studies with paracetamol in mice, rats, dogs and pigs. In mice, acute necrosis of the bronchiolar epithelium was seen and exfoliation of the necrotic mucosa caused partial obstruction of the smaller airways (Placke *et al.*, 1987b; Bartolone *et al.*, 1989a). Following

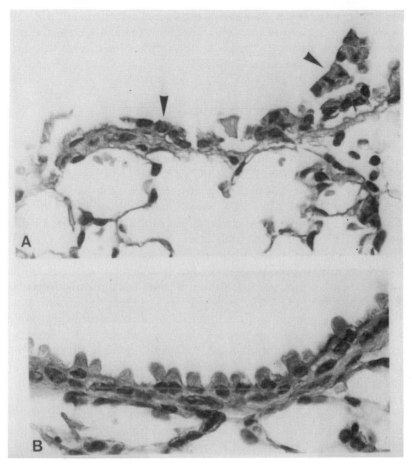

Figure 12.2 Necrosis of Clara cells (arrows) in bronchial epithelium in a mouse 6 h after intraperitoneal administration of 800 mg kg^{-1} of paracetamol (A). The normal appearance in a control mouse is shown in (B). Original magnification × 1000 (reproduced with permission from Jeffery and Haschek, 1988).

doses of 800 mg kg^{-1} there was similar necrosis of the non-ciliated bronchiolar epithelial (Clara) cells (Figure 12.2) together with nasal epithelial necrosis, which was not prevented by administration of dimethylsulphoxide (Jeffery and Haschek, 1988). Pulmonary oedema with inflammatory cell infiltrates was observed in pigs, cats and dogs (Miller *et al.*, 1976a; Duer, 1979; Anvik, 1984; Kelly *et al.*, 1992) but it was difficult to relate this to paracetamol toxicity *per se* in the presence of acute hepatic failure. Pulmonary oedema and pneumonitis was present in rats given doses of paracetamol exceeding the LD$_{50}$ for 100 days (Boyd and Hogan, 1968), but again these were probably preterminal events. Toxic doses of paracetamol caused depletion of pulmonary glutathione in rats (Micheli *et al.*, 1994).

Oral paracetamol had no significant adverse cardiopulmonary effects in anaesthetized dogs (Boxill *et al.*, 1958) and a 'therapeutic' dose of 14 mg kg^{-1} of paracetamol given orally to pregnant rats, just before delivery by Caesarean section at term, had only minor cardiovascular effects on the fetal circulation compared with those produced by aspirin, ibuprofen and indomethacin (Momma and Takao, 1990).

There was little change in the diameter of the ductus arteriosus but over 24 h there was some increase in atrial and ventricular volume, ventricular mass and pericardial fluid. The significance of these changes is uncertain because there was no control group for comparison.

Central Nervous System Toxicity

Central nervous system effects such as depression, listlessness, hypo-reactivity, lethargy, weakness, loss of righting reflex, tail extension, ataxia, over-reaction to noise, tremor, and somnolence progressing to stupor and coma, sometimes with convulsions, have been described in high dose acute toxicity studies in mice, rats, cats, dogs and pigs (Boxill *et al.*, 1958; Boyd and Bereczky, 1966; Mitchell *et al.*, 1973b; Finco *et al.*, 1975; Gazzard *et al.*, 1975b; Miller *et al.*, 1976a; Piperno *et al.*, 1978; Savides *et al.*, 1984; Francavilla *et al.*, 1989; Kelly *et al.*, 1992). In some studies attempts had been made to develop animal models of fulminant hepatic failure and the picture was complicated further by general anaesthesia and adminis-tration of other agents such as dimethylsulphoxide, buthionine sulphoximine and methylene blue (Gazzard *et al.*, 1975b; Miller *et al.*, 1976a; Francavilla *et al.*, 1989; Kelly *et al.*, 1992). Assessment of the central effects of paracetamol was not possible in the presence of hepatic encephalopathy, severe acidosis, hypoglycaemia, severe methaemoglobinaemia or pulmonary oedema, although abnormalities related to liver failure would tend to be of late onset. In chronic toxicity studies in rats given paracetamol in doses corresponding to the LD_{50} over 100 days, behavioural changes included: listlessness; reduced reflexes; an augmented response to stimuli such as prodding; jarring the cage or blowing against the grain of the fur; and tremor and convulsions were additional premortal signs (Boyd and Hogan, 1968). Hypothermia, which was presumably of central origin, has been mentioned in both acute (Miller *et al.*, 1976a; Alhava *et al.*, 1978; St. Omer and McKnight, 1980; Massey *et al.*, 1982) and chronic toxicity studies (Boyd and Hogan, 1968). It seems unlikely that there are major species differences in the central nervous system tox-icity of paracetamol. Piperno *et al.* (1978) remarked on the lack of effect of paraceta-mol on the sensorium of dogs given single oral doses of 600 mg kg^{-1} in contrast to a marked depressant effect in mice given 1500 mg kg^{-1} but this probably reflected the differences in dose and severity of intoxication. Very large doses of paracetamol, up to 4000 and 6000 mg kg^{-1}, have been given to rats by many investigators without any comment about central nervous system effects, but in one report they were said to be rendered moribund by a dose of 750 mg kg^{-1} (Mitchell *et al.*, 1973b). On balance, it seems likely that the depressant effects noted above were secondary to metabolic effects and toxicity in other systems. In the absence of very high plasma paracetamol concentrations above about 1000 mg l^{-1}, severe metabolic acidosis, hypoglycaemia or hepatic encephalopathy, overdosage of paracetamol alone did not cause impairment of consciousness in man (Zezulka and Wright, 1982; Prescott, 1983; Flanagan and Mant, 1986). A single oral dose of 2 g had no effect on mood, energy and mentation in a placebo-controlled study in healthy volunteers (Eade and Lasagna, 1967). Paracetamol inhibited $Na^+K^+ATPase$ and $Mg^{2+}ATPase$ in the cerebrum and cerebellum of 10–32-week human fetuses in a dose-dependent fashion (Sarkar *et al.*, 1989). Very large doses of paracetamol caused minor depletion of glutathione in rat brain, primarily affecting the thalamus, medulla and cerebral cortex (Masukawa *et al.*, 1989; Micheli *et al.*, 1993; Cerretani *et al.*, 1994) but in another study it had no such effect (Bien *et al.*, 1992).

Gastrointestinal System

Gastrointestinal mucosal inflammation, haemorrhage and oedema have been observed in rats and dogs following single high toxic doses of paracetamol (Boyd and Bereczky, 1966; Piperno *et al.*, 1978) and there was gastroenteritis in rats given oral doses equivalent to the LD_{50} over 100 days (Boyd and Hogan, 1968). Unlike aspirin and non-steroidal anti-inflammatory drugs, paracetamol in smaller doses did not cause gastrointestinal ulceration in guinea pigs (Manekar and Raul, 1983), rats (Mann and Sachdev, 1977; Seegers *et al.*, 1978; Wong and Gardocki, 1983; Engelhardt, 1984; Foote *et al.*, 1988) or, as shown by endoscopy and biopsy, in man (Vickers, 1967; Ivey *et al.*, 1978; Konturek *et al.*, 1981, 1984; Hoftiezer *et al.*, 1982; Ivey, 1983; Stern *et al.*, 1984a; Graham and Smith, 1985; Lanza *et al.*, 1986; Müller *et al.*, 1988, 1990; Bennett, 1989a). Again, unlike aspirin, direct application of paracetamol to the human buccal mucosa did not cause local desquamation and necrosis (Roth *et al.*, 1963), nor did it cause exfoliation of gastric mucosal cells in healthy subjects as shown by DNA loss in gastric washings (Corinaldesi *et al.*, 1978). The lack of significant gastric mucosal toxicity in man was confirmed by studies of its effects on the transmucosal potential difference (Stern *et al.*, 1984a; Hogan, 1988). Paracetamol also failed to augment histamine-stimulated acid secretion as indicated by the aminopyrine uptake ratio in isolated rabbit gastric parietal cells (Levine *et al.*, 1991). In rats and in man, paracetamol actually protected against gastric mucosal injury produced by aspirin, non-steroidal anti-inflammatory drugs, ethanol and other irritants (Seegers *et al.*, 1978, 1979, 1980a; van Kolfschoten *et al.*, 1982b, 1983b; Stern *et al.*, 1984b; de Vos and Barbier, 1985; Poon *et al.*, 1988b, 1989; Trautmann *et al.*, 1991; Kohút *et al.*, 1992). It also protected against taurocholate-induced damage to cultured gastric epithelial cells (Ota *et al.*, 1988; Romano *et al.*, 1988a).

In contrast to these findings, intraperitoneal and oral paracetamol caused dose-dependent gastric ulceration in rats (Daas *et al.*, 1978; Strubelt and Hoppenkamps, 1983). It potentiated gastric lesions produced by aspirin and ibuprofen in rats (Engelhardt, 1984; Bhattacharya *et al.*, 1991) and it worsened stress-induced gastric ulceration (Cho and Ogle, 1990). In addition, paracetamol did not prevent gastric mucosal injury caused by ibuprofen in man (Lanza *et al.*, 1986). Paracetamol had variable effects on the production of prostaglandins by rat gastric mucosa and it did not consistently reverse the inhibition of synthesis produced by aspirin (van Kolfschoten *et al.*, 1981). In another report, the protective effect of paracetamol against ethanol-induced gastric mucosal injury was associated with reduced formation of leukotriene C_4 but not prostaglandin 6-keto-$PGF_{1\alpha}$ (Trautmann *et al.*, 1991). While there was some evidence that the gastro-protective effect of paracetamol was mediated by the activity of thiols rather than prostaglandins (Romano *et al.*, 1991), oral paracetamol depleted glutathione in rat stomach and proximal small intestine but not in the jejunal and ileal segments (Siegers *et al.*, 1989). N-acetyl-p-benzoquinone-imine and p-benzoquinone were potentially toxic arylating metabolites of paracetamol that could be formed in the stomach by its reaction with nitrite (Ohta *et al.*, 1988a). Paracetamol did not increase occult gastrointestinal blood loss in healthy subjects (Johnson and Driscoll, 1981; Konturek *et al.*, 1984). At very high concentrations, paracetamol inhibited the absorption of fluid, glucose and sodium by isolated rat duodenal segments (Diener *et al.*, 1986).

Pancreatic Toxicity

In mice given 300 and 400 mg kg^{-1} of paracetamol intraperitoneally, electron microscopy showed pancreatic damage with cytoplasmic vacuolation, damaged cytoplasmic membranes and secretory granules and pyknotic nuclei. Paracetamol cysteine protein adducts were not detected in pancreatic cytosol suggesting that this form of toxicity was not mediated by metabolic activation (Ferguson *et al.*, 1990).

Oculotoxicity

Toxic doses of paracetamol produced irreversible anterior cataracts associated with the Ah locus in susceptible strains of mice (Shichi *et al.*, 1978). Further studies indicated a strong correlation between the Ah^b allele and cataract formation following administration of a very large dose of paracetamol (1000 mg kg^{-1}) in four inbred strains of mice previously induced with 3-methylcholanthrene. Cataracts developed without depletion of lenticular glutathione but there were differences between susceptible and resistant strains in the delivery of paracetamol metabolites to the lens (Shichi *et al.*, 1980). Similar dose-related cataract formation was reported in another study, and cataracts were also produced within one week following chronic administration of large doses of paracetamol in rabbits previously induced with phenobarbitone, β-naphthoflavone and 3-methylcholanthrene. Cataracts did not occur in the absence of induction (Lubek *et al.*, 1984, 1988a). The formation of cataracts in susceptible strains of mice was associated with increased metabolic activation of paracetamol as shown by production of the cysteine conjugate (Lubek *et al.*, 1988b). Unlike aspirin, paracetamol did not protect against cataracts formed by the binding of malondialdehyde to soluble lens proteins (Riley and Harding, 1993).

Reproductive Toxicity

Testicular atrophy was noted in rats given toxic doses of paracetamol over a period of 100 days (Boyd and Hogan, 1968; Boyd, 1970) and testis weight was reduced following daily administration of toxic doses of paracetamol to rats for 70 days (Jacqueson *et al.*, 1984). A single toxic dose produced testicular atrophy and spermatidic degeneration in mice (Placke *et al.*, 1987b) and it reduced epididymal (but not testicular) glutathione concentrations in rats (Gandy *et al.*, 1990). In another study in rats a toxic dose of 3000 mg kg^{-1} of paracetamol had little or no effect on testicular glutathione concentrations (Micheli *et al.*, 1994). In mice given 1 per cent of the drug chronically in their diet, a continuous breeding protocol showed cumulative effects on reproduction and abnormal sperm with reduced birthweight and retarded growth (Reel *et al.*, 1992). In another report, paracetamol interfered with the normal growth of the rat fetus and placenta to a lesser extent than aspirin (Lubawy and Garrett, 1977). The glutathione concentration in fetal mouse liver was less than adult liver but doses of 100 and 250 mg kg^{-1} of paracetamol given between days 6 and 13 of gestation had no teratogenic effect (Lambert and Thorgeirsson, 1976). Paracetamol caused low level morphological transformations of mouse embryo cells (Patierno *et al.*, 1989), but had no adverse effect on the development of cultured salivary glands from fetal mice (Lyng, 1989). At concentrations as low as 50 mg l^{-1}, it caused abnormalities in cultured rat embryos. Embryotoxicity appeared to be enhanced when glutathione synthesis was inhibited with buthionine sulphoximine and decreased when glutathione synthesis was stimulated with N-acetylcysteine (Stark *et al.*, 1989a; Weeks *et al.*, 1990). The incidence of neural defects, such as abnormal closure of the anterior neuropores in cultured rat embryos, was increased when paracetamol and its 3-hydroxy metabolite were added to the medium but not when paracetamol was administered by intra-amniotic injection (Harris *et al.*, 1989; Stark *et al.*, 1990). p-Aminophenol produced a greater incidence of abnormalities and the morphological changes were distinct from those produced by paracetamol. Deacetylation of paracetamol increased its embryotoxicity (Harris *et al.*, 1988; Stark *et al.*, 1989b). The administration of large doses of paracetamol before and during pregnancy induced mosaic aneuploidy (Tsuruzaki *et al.*, 1982) and it increased the frequency of micronuclei, major malformations and embryotoxicity in pregnant rats (Ying and Lou, 1993). Exposure of the embryos of the South African clawed frog (*Xenopus laevis*) to paracetamol caused mortality and malformations that were aggravated by the presence of an exogenous metabolic activation system (Fort *et al.*, 1992). The teratogenicity of diphenylhydantoin in mice was related to glutathione status and was potentiated by previous administration of paracetamol (Wells, 1983). This potentiation also depended on poor and extensive metabolizer status of diphenylhydantoin (Lum and Wells, 1986). Paracetamol suppressed the synthesis of progesterone by porcine granulosa cells and was thought to have the potential for causing reproductive toxicity in man (Haney *et al.*, 1988).

Many of these studies were carried out with toxic doses of paracetamol and there was no good evidence that in therapeutic doses it had similar effects on reproduction in man. Paracetamol had a favourable teratogenicity risk rating (Friedman *et al.*, 1990) but there have been occasional anecdotal accounts of malformations following its use during pregnancy and these included polyhydramnios with neonatal renal failure (Char *et al.*, 1975), bilateral anophthalmia (Golden and Perman, 1980) and cranio-facial and digital malformation (Golden *et al.*, 1982). In a case control study, the relative risk of gastroschisis was increased in women who had taken paracetamol during the first trimester of pregnancy (Werler *et al.*, 1992). Paracetamol reduced the production of prostacyclin by cultured endothelial cells and it reduced the formation of prostacyclin, but not thromboxane, in pregnant women (O'Brien *et al.*, 1993). Unlike aspirin, paracetamol has not been shown to have prostaglandin-dependent adverse effects on the duration of pregnancy or the course of labour (Collins, 1981; Rudolph, 1981). Most pregnant women knew that the risk of drug-induced damage in the unborn child was greatest during the first three months of pregnancy and most would restrict their use of analgesics to paracetamol (Butters and Howie, 1990).

Genotoxicity and Mutagenicity

The toxic effects of paracetamol on the liver raised the possibility that it might also have genotoxic and mutagenic effects, and interest in this subject was sharpened further by a report indicating that it caused liver tumours in mice (Flaks and Flaks, 1983). There was little evidence that paracetamol was mutagenic and studies of its ability to induce mutations in different strains of *Salmonella typhimurium* and *Escherichia coli* with and without metabolic activation have been largely negative (King *et al.*, 1979; Ishidate and Yoshikawa, 1980; Wirth *et al.*, 1980; Dybing *et al.*, 1984; Oldham *et al.*, 1986; Jasiewicz and Richardson, 1987; Burke *et al.*, 1994). A dose-related increase in revertant colonies was observed with paracetamol in the presence of metabolic activation in one of five strains of *Salmonella* (Oldham *et al.*, 1986), and in another study, negative findings could have been related to the use of dimethylsulphoxide as the solvent (Jasiewicz and Richardson, 1987). Although N-acetyl-p-benzoquinoneimine, the reactive metabolite of paracetamol, produced severe bacterial cytotoxicity, it did not induce mutations (Dybing *et al.*, 1984). There was evidence of a mutagenic effect of paracetamol in two strains of *Salmonella* in the presence of nitrous acid. The mutagen was identified as 4-acetyl-amino-6-diazo-2,4-cyclohexadienone, but its formation in the digestive tract in man was considered to be negligible (Ohta *et al.*, 1988b). Paracetamol did not cause important mutagenicity in other test systems including sex-linked recessive lethality in *Drosophila* (King *et al.*, 1979) and the development of ouabain resistance in cultured mouse embryo cells (Patierno *et al.*, 1989). It also reduced the mutagenicity of N-nitrosodimethylamine in the higher plant *Arabidopsis thalania* (Gichner *et al.*, 1993).

At cytotoxic concentrations, paracetamol caused single strand breaks in DNA and increased DNA repair synthesis in cultured rat hepatocytes while N-acetyl-p-benzoquinoneimine caused extensive single strand breaks in DNA in hepatoma cells (Dybing *et al.*, 1984). N-hydroxyparacetamol decreased DNA synthesis in rat kidney cells and interfered with normal cell cycle progression (Djordjevic *et al.*, 1986). However, paracetamol did not cause DNA strand breaks in cultured human skin fibroblasts incubated with ram seminal vesicle microsomes (Nordenskjöld and Moldéus, 1983). The metabolic activation of paracetamol during the respiratory burst in human granulocytes and neutrophils derived from a leukaemic cell line resulted in binding to both DNA and RNA (Corbett *et al.*, 1989, 1992). Significant species differences have been observed in susceptibility to the genotoxic effects of paracetamol. It increased unscheduled DNA synthesis in hepatocytes from mice but not in hepatocytes from hamsters and guinea pigs. There was a minor increase with rat hepatocytes and the response was increased in mice by induction with Arochlor 1254 or 3-methylcholanthrene. The narrow range of doses required to produce cytotoxicity and genotoxicity made it difficult to predict whether initial damage to DNA would result in a mutation, or whether the cells would die before a mutation could be expressed (Holme and Søderlund, 1986). In another study, paracetamol had no effect on DNA repair assays in rat hepatocytes (Milam and Byard, 1985). Paracetamol inhibited DNA synthesis and caused a small increase in single strand DNA breaks in V79 Chinese hamster cells. At concentrations of 450 and 2500 mg l^{-1}, it decreased unscheduled DNA synthesis and DNA repair synthesis induced by ultraviolet light (Hongslo *et al.*, 1988). Paracetamol also had a synergistic effect with ultraviolet light on cell death and DNA repair in peripheral blood lymphocytes and proliferating leukaemic cells (Brunborg *et al.*, 1994). It inhibited replicative DNA synthesis in a concentration-dependent manner above 15 mg l^{-1}, and the concentration for 50 per cent inhibition was about 25 mg l^{-1}. The effect was inhibited by ascorbate, indicating that it was caused by an oxidation product (Holme *et al.*, 1988; Hongslo *et al.*, 1989, 1990b). Paracetamol induced a low frequency of non-neoplastic morphological transformations in mouse embryo cells, and the effect was dependent on metabolic activation (Patierno *et al.*, 1989). The structure-activity relationships of paracetamol analogues for inhibition of replicative DNA synthesis in V79 Chinese hamster cells showed that the relevant factors were the partial atomic charge on the ring carbon attached to the phenolic oxygen, the partial charge on the phenoxy radical oxygen and the energy difference between the parent phenolic paracetamol analogue and the corresponding radical dissociation products (Richard *et al.*, 1991). The structure-activity relationships for the DNA repair test were investigated for more than 300 chemicals, including paracetamol (Williams *et al.*, 1989b).

Cytogenetic assays have clearly indicated a clastogenic action of paracetamol on mammalian cells *in vitro* but studies *in vivo* have been limited and the findings inconsistent. Paracetamol did not cause micronucleus formation in mice (King *et al.*, 1979) and in a normal rat kidney cell line, the fraction of micronucleated cells was only increased at concentrations above 1500 mg l^{-1} (Dunn *et al.*, 1987). Chromosomal abnormalities in meiotic cells after single and repeated doses in male mice were minor and probably not significant (Laxminarayana *et al.*, 1980) but paracetamol increased the frequency of micronuclei in rat blastocysts collected on the 4th day of pregnancy (Lou *et al.*, 1993). In another report, paracetamol induced a small but statistically significant increase in micronuclei in mice that was not dose related (Sicardi *et al.*, 1991). Paracetamol could cause damage to DNA as shown by chromosomal aberrations and sister chromatid exchanges, and such effects have been observed with cell cultures *in vitro* and also in studies *in vivo* (Ishidate *et al.*, 1978; Anantha Reddy, 1984; Shimame, 1985; Sasaki, 1986; Holme *et al.*, 1988; Hongslo *et al.*, 1988, 1990b; Müller *et al.*, 1991; Giri *et al.*, 1992). In another study, the aberrations were rare and statistically insignificant (Anantha Reddy and Subramanyam, 1985). Mitotic indices for human lymphocytes *in vitro* decreased with increasing paracetamol concentrations and there were significant increases in chromatid and isochromatid gaps and breaks (Watanabe, 1982). In other reports, the adverse effects of paracetamol on chromosomes were also dose dependent (Hongslo *et al.*, 1988; Müller *et al.*, 1991; Giri *et al.*, 1992). It was proposed that the genotoxicity of paracetamol was caused by inhibition of ribonucleotide reductase (Hongslo *et al.*, 1990b) and although the effects on sister chromatid exchange parallelled the inhibition of DNA synthesis, these two actions were probably unrelated as they did not occur at comparable concentrations (Holme *et al.*, 1988). Subsequent studies showed that paracetamol destroyed the tyrosyl ribonucleotide reductase ribosyl free radical (Hongslo *et al.*, 1990a). Paracetamol could induce single strand breaks in DNA at low concentrations even in organs that had a low capacity for its metabolic activation and these effects were probably due to its inhibiting effect on ribonucleotide reductase (Hongslo *et al.*, 1994).

Some investigators have claimed to show that paracetamol has genotoxic effects in man at normal therapeutic dose levels. It did not cause DNA strand breaks in cultures of human skin fibroblasts incubated with sheep seminal vesicle microsomes (Andersson *et al.*, 1982) but in another study with cultured human fibroblasts there was an increase in sister chromatid exchange (Wilmer *et al.*, 1981). Others have reported chromosomal aberrations induced by paracetamol in cultured human lymphocytes (Kawachi *et al.*, 1980; Watanabe, 1982). In 11 healthy subjects given 1 g of paracetamol on three occasions over a period of 8 h, the incidence of aberrant lymphocytes in peripheral blood increased transiently from 1.7 to 2.8 per cent, and this effect was reduced by ascorbic acid taken at the same time (Kocisová *et al.*,

1988). In a similar study there was a minor decrease in unscheduled DNA synthesis in lymphocytes from peripheral blood and the frequency of micronucleated buccal cells increased from a control value of 0.19 to 0.38 per cent at 72 h after dosing (Topinka *et al.*, 1989). In further similar studies in healthy subjects given the same dose of paracetamol there was no increase in micronucleus formation in peripheral lymphocytes (Kocisová and Srám, 1990a,b). However, there was an increase in micronuclei in buccal cells associated with an increase in the frequency of aberrant cells as shown by cytogenetic analysis (Srám *et al.*, 1989, 1990). A small but statistically significant increase in the frequency of sister chromatid exchange and chromatid breaks in lymphocytes from healthy subjects was observed following administration of 3 g of paracetamol over 8 h. With an *in vitro* lymphocyte system, paracetamol at concentrations of 150–1500 mg l^{-1} increased sister chromatid exchange and inhibited replicative DNA synthesis (Hongslo *et al.*, 1991). In another report, however, there was no consistent or dose-related change in unscheduled DNA synthesis in human lymphocytes incubated with paracetamol at the same high concentration (Binková *et al.*, 1990). Paracetamol delayed the repair of damage to DNA induced by ultraviolet light and increased single strand DNA breaks in human blood mononuclear cells in culture (Hongslo *et al.*, 1993). In contrast to these reports, paracetamol in a dose of 1 g taken three times over 8 h had no effect on the frequency of structural chromosome aberrations in peripheral blood lymphocytes in a placebo-controlled study in groups of six male and six female subjects matched according to their cell cycle kinetics (Kirkland *et al.*, 1992). In a 37-year-old man with immune deficiency, tonsillar carcinoma and myelodysplasia, a (1;7) (p11;p11) translocation was attributed (without evidence) to abuse of paracetamol and codeine for seven years (Fyfe and Wright, 1990).

The genotoxicity and mutagenicity of paracetamol has been reviewed (Hayashi, 1992; Giri, 1993; Hongslo and Holme, 1994) and the overall conclusions are that while it is clearly not active in bacterial tests for mutagenicity, clastogenic effects have been demonstrated in mammalian cell systems *in vitro*. Many of the latter studies have been conducted with the drug at very high concentrations. The results of studies *in vivo* have been conflicting and some reports that apparently showed effects with therapeutic doses in man have been criticized (Kirkland *et al.*, 1992). Attention was also drawn to statistical problems and the close similarity of the reported effects of paracetamol and the dye Green S on the induction of chromosome aberrations and sister chromatid exchange in different studies. The remarkable coincidence in the apparent clastogenicity of these unrelated compounds was finally attributed to a methodological artefact rather than a biological response (Chételat *et al.*, 1992).

Carcinogenicity

The recognition of uroepithelial neoplasia as a long-term complication of analgesic nephropathy and the observation of liver tumours in chronic toxicity studies in mice has caused concern in some quarters about the potential carcinogenicity of paracetamol. It has not been possible to induce tumours consistently with paracetamol in carcinogenicity studies in animals. Paracetamol did not increase the frequency of bladder tumours induced by the carcinogen N-2-fluorenylacetamide in male and female mice, and, if anything, it reduced the incidence in males (Weisburger *et al.*,

1973). Renal tumours did not develop in rats given 0.535 per cent of paracetamol in their diet for up to 117 weeks. Four animals had bladder tumours or papillomas, but the incidence was not significantly different in controls or rats given other analgesics (Johansson, 1981). In another study, groups of 40 male and female rats received 0.5 and 1.0 per cent of paracetamol in their diet for up to 18 months. Bladder carcinomas developed in three rats, and bladder hyperplasia or papillomas occurred in 6–13 per cent of animals. There were no such lesions in control rats (Flaks *et al.*, 1985). Paracetamol did not induce renal or bladder tumours in groups of 50 rats given 0.45 and 0.9 per cent of paracetamol in the diet for up to two years (Hiraga and Fujii, 1985). The chronic administration of phenacetin and antipyrine produced uroepithelial hyperplasia in rats, and similar but less marked changes were observed in rats treated with 0.5, 1.0 and 1.5 per cent of paracetamol in the diet for 12 weeks (Johansson *et al.*, 1989). Analgesics and other agents which cause renal papillary damage may also cause uroepithelial hyperplasia but it was not possible to show progression to invasive carcinoma (Bach and Gregg, 1988). It was proposed that analgesics caused urothelial carcinoma by peroxidase-mediated activation but no direct evidence was put forward to support this theory (Bach and Bridges, 1984).

In early studies, the co-administration of paracetamol reduced the incidence of liver tumours induced by N-2-fluorenylacetamide and its N-hydroxy derivative in mice and hamsters (Weisburger *et al.*, 1973) and it did not produce liver tumours in rats when fed at 0.535 per cent in the diet for up to 117 weeks (Johansson, 1981). In contrast, Flaks and Flaks (1983) reported a very high incidence of liver cancer and cellular abnormalities in mice fed paracetamol 0.5 and 1.0 per cent in the diet for 18 months. The total incidence of liver cell tumours in the high dose male mice was 87 per cent and hepatocellular carcinoma developed in 21.7 per cent of animals. The corresponding values in females were 19.2 and 4.3 per cent respectively. In a similar study carried out in rats there was hepatic enlargement and 20 per cent of animals of both sexes developed neoplastic liver nodules (Flaks *et al.*, 1985). These findings have not been confirmed by other investigators. Paracetamol did not induce tumours in any system in male rats given 0.45 and 0.9 per cent, or females given 0.65 and 1.3 per cent in the diets for 104 weeks (Hiraga and Fujii, 1985), and in mice receiving 6000 and 12 000 parts per million in their diet for 40 weeks there was no evidence of carcinogenicity despite hepatic necrosis and hyperplasia (Ward *et al.*, 1988). Maruyama and Williams (1988) reviewed the findings in two previously reported carcinogenicity studies in which mice received 0.3, 0.6 or 1.25, and 1.1 or 1.25 per cent of paracetamol in the diet for 41 and 48 weeks respectively (Weisburger *et al.*, 1973; Amo and Matsuyama, 1985). Despite extensive centrilobular hepatic necrosis at the higher dose levels, no neoplastic lesions were found. In rats with liver damage and cirrhosis produced by a diet devoid of choline, short- and longer-term administration of paracetamol did not induce liver tumours (Maruyama *et al.*, 1990). Paracetamol had no hepatic tumour-initiating activity in rats given 10 doses of 1000 mg kg^{-1} orally over five weeks, or a single dose of 500 mg kg^{-1} 24 h after two-thirds hepatectomy. These treatments were followed by administration of 0.1 per cent of phenobarbitone in the drinking water as a promoting agent for 12 weeks (Hasegawa *et al.*, 1988). Paracetamol did not cause any significant hepatic changes in a two-year carcinogenicity study in rats (Harada *et al.*, 1989). In another study, rats aged 6, 26 and 46 weeks were given single doses of diethylnitrosamine followed by feeding 1.3 per cent of paracetamol in the diet for six weeks. Two-thirds hepatectomy was performed three weeks after administration of the diethylnitrosamine. Paracetamol inhibited the formation of abnormal foci in the liver in all age groups (Hasegawa *et al.*, 1991). In other studies it did not act as a promoter of pre-neoplastic and focal γ-glutamyltransferase-positive proliferative hepatic lesions (Tsuda *et al.*, 1984b; Edwards and Lucas, 1985; Maronpot *et al.*, 1989; Ward *et al.*, 1989) and, indeed, it inhibited the formation of these and neoplastic lesions produced by a variety of agents (Yamamoto *et al.*, 1973; Tsuda *et al.*, 1984a,c, 1988; Kurata *et al.*, 1985; Masui *et al.*, 1986). Paracetamol had no effect on hepatocyte intercellular communication at non-toxic levels in mice and this was consistent with the absence of tumour promotion activity (Ruch and Klaunig, 1986). It did not cause tumour progression in a rat leukaemia transplant model (Dieter *et al.*, 1992) and it increased the efficacy of anti-tumour alkylating agents against a mouse mammary carcinoma in culture (Teicher *et al.*, 1993). The possibility was raised that paracetamol could react in the stomach with nitrite in drinking water to produce carcinogenic nitrosamines (Lykkesfeldt and Poulsen, 1993; Nielsen and Lings, 1993) but in a previous report the main products of this reaction were N-acetyl-p-benzoquinoneimine and p-benzoquinone (Ohta *et al.*, 1988a). Unlike aspirin and other non-steroidal anti-inflammatory drugs, the regular use of paracetamol was not consistently related to a decreased risk of colonic and other gastrointestinal cancers (Thun *et al.*, 1993). In a follow-up survey of 143 574 outpatients in the Kaiser-Permanente Medical Care Program over the period 1969–1972, positive associations were found for the use of paracetamol and cancer of the pharynx and melanoma, while negative associations were noted for cancer of the colon and uterus (Friedman and Ury, 1980). Although the possibility could not be entirely excluded, paracetamol was probably not a carcinogen in man (Rane and Orrenius, 1985). Animal carcinogenicity studies with paracetamol have been reviewed and the potential risks to humans were evaluated (IARC Monograph, 1990).

Cytotoxicity

Extensive toxicity studies have been carried out with paracetamol in isolated hepatocytes, and these are discussed in Chapter 14. The cytotoxic effects of paracetamol have also been studied in other cell lines. At very high concentrations it inhibited mitosis in human peripheral blood lymphocytes that had been stimulated by exposure to phytohaemagglutinin (Timson, 1968). Acute and chronic cytotoxicity was demonstrated in cultures of human hepatoma HepG2 cells at concentrations of 1057 and 150 mg l^{-1} respectively (Hall *et al.*, 1993) and the cytotoxicity of N-acetyl-p-benzoquinoneimine against Hepa 1c1c-9 cells was increased when glutathione was depleted by prior exposure to buthionine sulphoximine (Riley *et al.*, 1993). In experiments with cultures of V79 Chinese hamster lung fibroblasts, paracetamol cytotoxicity was not increased as expected by the addition of a rat or hamster S9 microsomal metabolic activating fraction (Horner *et al.*, 1987). On the other hand, in cultures of human BCL-D1 embryonic lung cells, cytotoxicity was enhanced by inclusion of an S9 fraction obtained from rats induced by pretreatment with Arochlor 1254 but the susceptibility of V79 Chinese hamster cells, murine fibroblasts and MRC-5 human embryo lung fibroblasts was not increased to the same extent (Benford *et al.*, 1990). The cytotoxicity of paracetamol was greater in cultures of V79 Chinese hamster cells than HeLa cells (Fortunati *et al.*, 1993). The cytotoxic effects of paracetamol have been demonstrated in other studies in cultures of HeLa cells (Ekwall and Acosta, 1982), L929 mouse fibroblasts (Kemp *et al.*, 1988; Nordin *et al.*, 1991), mouse 3T3 cells (Jover *et al.*, 1992; Wakuri *et al.*, 1993), chick embryo neurones (Weiss and Sawyer, 1993), human HL-60 promyelocytic leukacmia cells (Wakuri *et al.*, 1993) and rat skeletal muscle cells (Gülden *et al.*, 1994). Cytotoxicity was also shown in cultures of toad kidney epithelial A6 cells by changes in the transepithelial potential difference and transepithelial electrical resistance (Bjerregaard, 1993).

Metabolic Effects

The effects of high toxic doses of paracetamol on intermediary metabolism and other processes have been studied *in vivo* and in isolated perfused liver and kidney, tissue slices, cell cultures and mitochondrial preparations. It had little effect on renal glucose synthesis in rats *in vivo* but at concentrations of 75–600 mg l^{-1} it inhibited the synthesis of glucose from lactate in isolated hepatocytes and decreased the availability of adenosine triphosphate (Tange *et al.*, 1977). Inhibition of mitochondrial energy metabolism by paracetamol *in vitro* was reported with concentrations of 1500 to 6000 mg l^{-1} and this was associated with reduced oxygen consumption, decreased glucose synthesis, reduced hepatic adenosine triphosphate, impaired coupled and uncoupled respiration and changes in mitochondrial potential (Porter and Dawson, 1979; Meyers *et al.*, 1988; Itinose *et al.*, 1989; Ramsay *et al.*, 1989; Burcham and Harman, 1990; Nazareth *et al.*, 1991; Strubelt and Younes, 1992). Under certain conditions the effects were reversible (Itinose *et al.*, 1989; Ramsay *et al.*, 1989) and they appeared to be dependent on the metabolic activation of paracetamol as judged by their prevention with piperonyl butoxide (Meyers *et al.*, 1988) and N-acetylcysteine (Burcham and Harman, 1990). Paracetamol inhibited NADH-linked respiration and N-acetyl-p-benzoquinoneimine inhibited all phases of mitochondrial respiration (Ramsay *et al.*, 1989). The site-specific inhibition of cellular respiration and dramatic depletion of adenosine triphosphate caused by paracetamol was also produced by N-acetyl-p-benzoquinoneimine, and it preceded the loss of glutathione and the loss of cell membrane integrity (Andersson *et al.*, 1990; Burcham and Harman, 1990, 1991). Paracetamol and its reactive metabolite had independent effects on hepatic respiration and these differed in respect of reversibility (Esterline *et al.*, 1989). Paracetamol and 3-hydroxyparacetamol had similar inhibitory effects on mitochondrial respiration and it was proposed that this might explain the acidosis and depression of consciousness sometimes seen in poisoned patients with very high plasma paracetamol concentrations (Esterline and Ji, 1989). In rats given doses of 375 and 750 mg kg^{-1}, there were differential effects on mitochondrial coupled energy metabolism in the liver and dehydrogenase activities were reduced even at the lower dose. Changes in phase transition temperatures and activation energies were thought to be related to effects on membrane fluidity (Katyare and Satav, 1989, 1991). The inhibition of mitochondrial respiration was an early event in the course of paracetamol hepatotoxicity (Donnelly *et al.*, 1994). At toxic concentrations paracetamol inhibited growth and suppressed the uptake of [^{14}C]-thymidine, [^{14}C]-uridine and [^{14}C]-acetate by the protozoan *Tetrahymena pyriformis* (Okano *et al.*, 1984). It also increased the sensitivity of *Escherichia coli* to radiation damage and it inhibited post-irradiation synthesis of DNA and protein (Shenoy and Gopalakrishna, 1977).

The hepatotoxicity of paracetamol in weanling mice previously induced with 3-methylcholanthrene was potentiated by prior infection with influenza B virus. There was a significant incidence of atypical fatty liver pathology and this was said to resemble the microvesicular steatosis seen in human Reye's syndrome, a condition associated with mitochondrial swelling and impaired energy metabolism (MacDonald *et al.*, 1984). Unlike aspirin, paracetamol did not increase mitochondrial membrane conductance or the proton transport of phospholipids across the membrane, and this was considered to be relevant to the lack of association between the use of paracetamol and Reye's syndrome (Gutknecht, 1992). A causal relationship between Reye's syndrome and aspirin was now accepted but no such relationship has been demonstrated with paracetamol. Indeed, there was an inverse relationship between the previous use of paracetamol and Reye's syndrome, and as the use of aspirin in children has declined with a fall in the incidence of the condition, the use of paracetamol has increased (Halpin *et al.*, 1982; Waldman *et al.*, 1982; Hurwitz *et al.*, 1987; Hall *et al.*, 1988; Forsyth *et al.*, 1989; Orlowski *et al.*, 1990; Porter *et al.*, 1990). There was one anomalous report of seven children with Reye's syndrome seen over the period 1982–1987. None had been exposed to salicylate but three had been treated with paracetamol (Rinaldi *et al.*, 1989). Paracetamol was reported to cause hypoglycaemia and seizures in a child (Ruvalcaba *et al.*, 1966), and hypoglycaemia caused by impaired gluconeogenesis has been observed following overdosage (Record *et al.*, 1975a). Hypoglycaemia has also been associated with the use of paracetamol in combination with d-propoxyphene (Leuzinger *et al.*, 1978; Blaison *et al.*, 1991). Paracetamol interfered with blood glucose estimation based on enzymic or electrochemical oxidation (Farrance and Aldons, 1981; Fleetwood and Robinson, 1981; Saeger *et al.*, 1992). In the case of paracetamol overdosage, spuriously high glucose concentrations could lead to inappropriate action with potentially disastrous consequences (Copland *et al.*, 1992; Farah *et al.*, 1982). In contrast to these findings, hyperglycaemia with a diminished response to insulin and impaired glucose tolerance has been reported in patients with mild-to-moderate paracetamol poisoning (Thomson and Prescott, 1966; Record *et al.*, 1975a). In mice, toxic doses of paracetamol caused hyperglycaemia and hepatic glycogen was depleted to a similar extent and with the same time course as depletion of glutathione. Both effects could be prevented with N-acetylcysteine (Hinson *et al.*, 1983) and the hyperglycaemia was associated with increased concentrations of immuno-precipitable insulin (Hinson *et al.*, 1984). The depletion of hepatic glycogen caused by toxic doses of paracetamol in mice was associated with plasma membrane damage and activation of glycogen phosphorylase *a*. Although N-acetylcysteine reduced plasma membrane damage, it did not prevent activation of phosphorylase *a* or glycogen depletion (Burcham and Harman, 1989). The formation of paracetamol cysteine protein adducts was correlated with hepatotoxicity, but not with paracetamol-induced pancreatic damage and elevation of serum insulin concentrations (Ferguson *et al.*, 1990).

In concentrations up to 6000 mg l^{-1}, paracetamol rapidly inhibited the incorporation of [^{14}C]-leucine into protein in isolated rat hepatocytes (Gwynn *et al.*, 1979) and following treatment with 750 mg kg day^{-1} of paracetamol for six weeks there was decreased metabolic utilization of nitrogen in rats fed with protein-sufficient, but not protein-deficient diets (Varela-Moreiras *et al.*, 1991). After a delay, rats given a diet containing 1 per cent of paracetamol for up to 10 weeks excreted large amounts of 5-oxoproline (pyroglutamate) in the urine and this could be prevented by the addition of methionine to the diet. The 5-oxoprolinuria reflected depletion of sulphur containing amino acids with consequent disruption of the glutathione cycle (Ghauri et al., 1993) and atypical pyroglutamate acidaemia and aciduria have also been observed in patients taking paracetamol (Creer et al., 1989; Pitt, 1990; Pitt et al., 1990). Paracetamol taken for a 'cold' was proposed as the trigger for type II citrullinaemia in a 19-year-old man (Shiohama et al., 1993). The chronic ingestion of paracetamol in high doses in rats caused growth retardation which was attributed to depletion of sulphur-containing amino acids (McLean et al., 1989). Chronic administration of paracetamol in the diet of mice decreased their growth rate and reduced the hepatic content of cysteine and glutathione. These effects were reversed by supplementation of the diet with methionine. Although methionine requirements were increased, the susceptibility to hepatic lipid peroxidation was not enhanced and the availability of methyl groups for methylation reactions was not compromised (Reicks et al., 1988, 1992; Reicks and Hathcock, 1989). Chronic treatment with paracetamol did not impair the metabolic utilization of dietary fat in rats (Varela-Moreiras et al., 1990) and again, it did not reduce the availability of methyl groups as shown by a normal hepatic folate content and distribution (Varela-Moreiras et al., 1993). However, it was proposed that the weight loss observed in chronic toxicity studies in rats was due to methionine and cysteine deficiencies (Poulsen and Thomsen, 1988). It should be noted that deficiencies of these amino acids would be most likely to occur in rats as they can tolerate enormous doses of paracetamol over long periods, and there would be heavy demands because sulphate conjugation was the dominant route for its elimination in this species. Glycine and glutamate were also necessary for glutathione synthesis and their concentrations in the liver were reduced by toxic doses of paracetamol (Endo et al., 1988b). The metabolic consequences of methionine deficiency induced by chronic administration of paracetamol have been reviewed (Hathcock, 1990).

The short-term consumption of therapeutic doses of paracetamol reduced plasma concentrations of inorganic sulphate, but contrary to expectations, concentrations were elevated in patients taking the drug chronically in doses of up to 12 g daily (Hendrix-Treacy et al., 1986). Similar elevation of plasma inorganic sulphate was noted during prolonged intake of paracetamol (Blackledge et al., 1991). The rate of turnover of the pool of cysteine available for the synthesis of glutathione was markedly increased in healthy volunteers following doses of 600 and 1200 mg (Lauterburg and Mitchell, 1987), and in another report it was claimed that regular takers of paracetamol with chronic headache had lower plasma concentrations of glutathione than unspecified control subjects (Trenti et al., 1992). In mice, a single dose of 190 mg kg^{-1} of paracetamol had little effect on blood sulphate concentrations (de Vries et al., 1990) but in rats as little as 15 mg kg^{-1} produced a significant fall and a dose of 200 mg kg^{-1} also decreased the synthesis of glycosaminoglycan in patellar cartilage (van der Kraan et al., 1988). With chronic administration of 200 mg kg^{-1} of paracetamol twice daily, serum inorganic sulphate and glycosaminoglycan content of cartilage were reduced during the first four weeks, but the changes were insignificant from the fourth to the ninth week (van der Kraan et al., 1990). Paracetamol caused a significant reduction in the concentration of inorganic sulphate in the cerebrospinal fluid in rats (Morris et al., 1984) but doses of 1.5 g had little or no effect on concentrations in the cerebrospinal fluid in man (Morris et al.,

1986). Thyroid function was reduced in rats given 473 mg kg^{-1} of paracetamol daily for eight weeks, and increased lipofuchsin pigment was observed in the thyroid follicular epithelium (Pataki *et al.*, 1974). Paracetamol had no effect on the anti-viral and anti-proliferative properties of recombinant human interferon-α_{2a}, and it could therefore be used for symptomatic treatment of the influenza-like adverse reactions produced by the interferon (Takaoki *et al.*, 1988).

13

Nephrotoxicity

Introduction

As phenacetin was removed from the non-prescription market in most countries in the belief that it was the primary cause of analgesic nephropathy, it was not surprising that as its major metabolite, paracetamol came under intense scrutiny. Although there was no good evidence that paracetamol was an important cause of chronic renal disease in man, it remained a prime suspect and some investigators have gone to great lengths in attempts to prove its guilt. In man, paracetamol could cause acute renal failure following overdosage, and prolonged abuse of analgesic combinations caused analgesic nephropathy characterized by renal papillary necrosis. Attempts have been made, therefore, to reproduce these two distinct types of renal lesion in animal models.

Acute Nephrotoxicity

Boyd and Bereczky (1966) described tubular, papillary and interstitial oedema and degeneration in rats given 2000–7000 mg kg^{-1} of paracetamol but other investigators were unable to demonstrate renal lesions or impairment of tubular function in this species following oral, intraperitoneal or intravenous doses of 300–2250 mg kg^{-1} (Calder et al., 1971; Arnold et al., 1973; Mitchell et al., 1973b; Arnold et al., 1976; Tange et al., 1977; Smail et al., 1981). Similar negative findings were reported in mice given doses of 150–750 mg kg^{-1} (Mitchell et al., 1973b; Smail et al., 1981; Endo et al., 1988a). McMurtry et al. (1978) were able to produce moderate dose-related proximal tubular necrosis with subcutaneous paracetamol in Fischer 344 rats, and nephrotoxicity was increased by prior induction with 3-methylcholanthrene and phenobarbitone, and decreased by inhibition of metabolic activation with cobaltous chloride. N-hydroxyparacetamol also caused proximal tubular necrosis in rats (Healey et al., 1978). Other acute nephrotoxicity studies with paracetamol in rats, mice, hamsters, dogs and pigs are summarized in Table 13.1. In general it has not proved easy to produce acute renal lesions in animals with paracetamol even with heroic doses causing major toxicity and death. It was necessary

Table 13.1 Acute nephrotoxicity studies of paracetamol in animals.

Species	Dose (mg kg^{-1})	Route of administration	Age (months)	Nephrotoxicity	Reference
Rat	2000–7000	oral	Y[1]	renal tubular degeneration and oedema	Boyd and Bereczky, 1966
Rat	300	iv	NS[2]	no renal lesions	Calder et al., 1971
Rat	3710	oral	NS	no tubular necrosis	Arnold et al., 1973
Rat	500–1500	ip	NS	no renal lesions	Mitchell et al., 1973b
Rat[3]	450	iv	NS	no effects on renal tubular synthesis of glucose	Tange et al., 1977
Rat (F-344)	250	sc	NS	minimal tubular necrosis	McMurtry et al., 1978
Rat (F-344)	500	sc	NS	mild tubular necrosis	McMurtry et al., 1978
Rat (F-344)	750	sc	NS	moderate tubular necrosis	McMurtry et al., 1978
Rat[4] (F-344)	250	sc	NS	severe tubular necrosis	McMurtry et al., 1978
Rat[5] (F-344)	750	sc	NS	moderate tubular necrosis	McMurtry et al., 1978
Rat[6] (F-344)	750	sc	NS	no renal lesions	McMurtry et al., 1978
Rat (Gunn)	148–966	oral	NS	papillary necrosis in 5 of 30 animals	Axelsen, 1980
Rat (Gunn)	900	iv	NS	papillary and tubular necrosis, especially in homozygotes	Briggs et al., 1982
Rat	900	iv	NS	minor tubular necrosis	Briggs et al., 1982
Rat (SD,f)	450	iv	NS	no renal lesions	Hart et al., 1982a
Rat (SD,f)	300	ip	NS	no renal lesions	Hart et al., 1982a
Rat (SD,f)	3000	oral	NS	no renal lesions	Hart et al., 1982a
Rat (SD,f)[4]	450	iv	NS	no renal lesions	Hart et al., 1982a
Rat (SD,f)[4]	1500	oral	NS	isolated tubular cell necrosis	Hart et al., 1982a
Rat (SD,f)[4]	2250	oral	NS	no renal lesions	Hart et al., 1982a
Rat (SD,f)	2250	oral	1	no renal lesions	Hart et al., 1982a
Rat (SD,m)	300	iv	NS	isolated tubular cell necrosis	Hart et al., 1982a
Rat (SD,m)	1500	oral	NS	no renal lesions	Hart et al., 1982a
Rat (W,f)	300	iv	NS	no renal lesions	Hart et al., 1982a
Rat (W,f)	1500	oral	NS	no renal lesions	Hart et al., 1982a
Rat[7] (F-344)	250	ip	NS	mild cortical tubular necrosis, no increase in plasma urea	Newton et al., 1983b
Rat[7] (F-344)	750	ip	NS	mild cortical tubular necrosis, blood urea increased	Newton et al., 1983b
Rat[7] (F-344)	900	ip	NS	moderate cortical tubular necrosis, blood urea increased	Newton et al., 1983b
Rat[7] (SD)	250	ip	NS	no renal lesions, no increase in blood urea	Newton et al., 1983b
Rat[7] (SD)	750	ip	NS	no renal lesions, no increase in blood urea	Newton et al., 1983a
Rat[7] (SD)	900	ip	NS	no renal lesions, no increase in blood urea	Newton et al., 1983a
Rat	1000	ip	11 days	no renal lesions	Green et al., 1984b

(cont.)

Species (strain)	Dose	Route	Duration	Effect	Reference
Rat	1250	ip	11 days	no renal lesions	Green et al., 1984b
Rat	750	ip	19 days	no renal lesions	Green et al., 1984b
Rat	1250	ip	33 days	no renal lesions	Green et al., 1984b
Rat (F-344)	750	ip	NS	cortical tubular necrosis, blood urea increased, no effect on tubular function[8]	Newton et al., 1985a
Rat (F-344)	600	ip	2–4	blood urea not increased, no renal lesions	Beierschmitt et al., 1986b
Rat (F-344)	600	ip	12–15	blood urea increased, tubular necrosis	Beierschmitt et al., 1986b
Rat (F-344)	600	ip	22–25	blood urea increased, tubular necrosis	Beierschmitt et al., 1986b
Rat[9] (F-344)	600	ip	2–4	blood urea not increased, minimal tubular necrosis	Beierschmitt et al., 1986b
Rat[9] (F-344)	600	ip	12–15	blood urea increased, tubular necrosis	Beierschmitt et al., 1986b
Rat (F-344)	300	ip	2–4	blood urea not increased, no tubular necrosis	Beierschmitt et al., 1986c
Rat (F-344)	300	ip	12–14	blood urea not increased, no tubular necrosis	Beierschmitt et al., 1986c
Rat (F-344)	300	ip	22–25	blood urea not increased, no tubular necrosis	Beierschmitt et al., 1986c
Rat (F-344)	600	ip	2–4	blood urea not increased, no tubular necrosis	Beierschmitt et al., 1986c
Rat (F-344)	600	ip	12–14	blood urea not increased, no tubular necrosis	Beierschmitt et al., 1986c
Rat (F-344)	600	ip	22–25	blood urea increased, mild tubular necrosis	Beierschmitt et al., 1986c
Rat (F-344)	800	ip	2–4	blood urea not increased, no tubular necrosis	Beierschmitt et al., 1986c
Rat (F-344)	800	ip	12–14	blood urea increased, moderate tubular necrosis	Beierschmitt et al., 1986c
Rat (F-344)	800	ip	22–25	blood urea increased, severe tubular necrosis	Beierschmitt et al., 1986c
Rat[9] (Gunn)	1800[10]	iv	NS	renal papillary necrosis, distal tubular necrosis	Henry and Tange, 1987
Rat[9] (Albino)	1800[10]	iv	NS	no renal lesions	Henry and Tange, 1987
Rat (W)	1000	oral	$1\frac{1}{2}$	no functional or histological changes	de Morais and Wells, 1988
Rat (Gunn)[t]	1000	oral	$1\frac{1}{2}$	variable papillary and cortical tubular necrosis	de Morais and Wells, 1988
Rat (Gunn)[m]	1000	oral	$1\frac{1}{2}$	variable papillary and cortical tubular necrosis	de Morais and Wells, 1988
Rat (W)	1000	oral	3	no functional or histological changes	de Morais and Wells, 1988
Rat (Gunn)[t]	1000	oral	3	increased blood urea, variable papillary and tubular necrosis	de Morais and Wells, 1988
Rat (Gunn)[m]	1000	oral	3	increased blood urea, variable papillary and tubular necrosis	de Morais and Wells, 1988
Rat (W)	500	ip	3	no increase in blood urea	de Morais and Wells, 1989
Rat (Gunn)[t]	500	ip	3	increased blood urea	de Morais and Wells, 1989
Rat (Gunn)[m]	500	ip	3	increased blood urea	de Morais and Wells, 1989
Rat	500–1000	NS	NS	proximal tubular necrosis	Furuhama et al., 1989a
Rat	750–1000	NS	NS	plasma urea and creatinine increased	McCrae et al., 1989
Rat	1500	oral	NS	plasma urea and creatinine increased	Siegers and Möller-Hartmann, 1989
Rat (F-344)	250–750	ip	2	no increase in blood urea	Tarloff et al., 1989a
Rat (F-344)	1000	ip	2	blood urea increased	Tarloff et al., 1989a
Rat (SD)	250–1000	ip	2	no increase in blood urea	Tarloff et al., 1989a

Table 13.1 (cont.)

Species	Dose (mg kg^{-1})	Route of administration	Age (months)	Nephrotoxicity	Reference
Rat (F-344)	250–750	iv	2	no increase in blood urea	Tarloff et al., 1989a
Rat (SD)	250–750	iv	2	no increase in blood urea	Tarloff et al., 1989a
Rat (SD)	750	ip	2–3	no increase in blood urea	Tarloff et al., 1989b
Rat (SD)	750	ip	9–12	blood urea increased	Tarloff et al., 1989b
Rat (SD)	750	iv	3	no increase in blood urea	Tarloff et al., 1989b
Rat (SD)	500	iv	12	blood urea increased	Tarloff et al., 1989b
Rat (F-344)	250	ip	2	no increase in blood urea	Tarloff et al., 1989c
Rat (F-344)	250	ip	3	no increase in blood urea	Tarloff et al., 1989c
Rat (F-344)	250	ip	9–12	no increase in blood urea	Tarloff et al., 1989c
Rat (F-344)	500	ip	2	no increase in blood urea	Tarloff et al., 1989c
Rat (F-344)	500	ip	3	no increase in blood urea	Tarloff et al., 1989c
Rat (F-344)	500	ip	9–12	no increase in blood urea	Tarloff et al., 1989c
Rat (F-344)	750	ip	2	no increase in blood urea	Tarloff et al., 1989c
Rat (F-344)	750	ip	3	no increase in blood urea	Tarloff et al., 1989c
Rat (F-344)	750	ip	9–12	blood urea increased, severe tubular necrosis	Tarloff et al., 1989c
Rat (F-344)	1000	ip	2	blood urea increased, moderate tubular necrosis	Tarloff et al., 1989c
Rat (F-344)	1000	ip	3	blood urea increased, mild tubular necrosis	Tarloff et al., 1989c
Rat (F-344)	1000	ip	9–12	animals died	Tarloff et al., 1989c
Rat (SD)	250	ip	2	no increase in blood urea	Tarloff et al., 1989c
Rat (SD)	250	ip	3	no increase in blood urea	Tarloff et al., 1989c
Rat (SD)	250	ip	9–12	no increase in blood urea	Tarloff et al., 1989c
Rat (SD)	500	ip	2	no increase in blood urea	Tarloff et al., 1989c
Rat (SD)	500	ip	3	no increase in blood urea	Tarloff et al., 1989c
Rat (SD)	500	ip	9–12	no increase in blood urea	Tarloff et al., 1989c
Rat (SD)	750	ip	2	no increase in blood urea	Tarloff et al., 1989c
Rat (SD)	750	ip	3	no increase in blood urea	Tarloff et al., 1989c
Rat (SD)	750	ip	9–12	blood urea increased, moderate tubular necrosis	Tarloff et al., 1989c
Rat (SD)	1000	ip	2	no increase in blood urea, no tubular necrosis	Tarloff et al., 1989c
Rat (SD)	1000	ip	3	blood urea increased, mild tubular necrosis	Tarloff et al., 1989c
Rat (SD)	1000	ip	9–12	animals died	Tarloff et al., 1989c
Rat (F-344)	140	ip	NS	no histological or functional changes	Fowler et al., 1991
Rat	500–1500	oral	NS	increased plasma creatinine, enzymuria	Möller-Hartmann and Siegers, 1991

	dose	route	age	effect	reference
Rat (RHA)	750	ip	4	no functional change	de Morais et al., 1992a
Rat (Gunn)[1]	750	ip	4	increased blood urea	de Morais et al., 1992a
Rat (Gunn)[m]	750	ip	4	increased blood urea	de Morais et al., 1992a
Rat	200–1000	ip	3	GFR and PAH clearance decreased, not glucose reabsorption	Trumper et al., 1992
Rat	600	oral	2	enzymuria	Casadevall et al., 1993
Mouse	150–750	oral	NS	no renal lesions	Mitchell et al., 1973b
Mouse	600	oral	2	'nephrosis', cortical and outer medullary tubular dilatation	Placke et al., 1987b
Mouse	400, 800	oral	>20 days	no definite kidney damage	Skoglund et al., 1987
Mouse[11]	300	oral	NS	no renal lesions but increased serum creatinine	Younes et al., 1988
Mouse	600	oral	3	proximal tubular necrosis	Bartolone et al., 1989a
Mouse	600	oral	3	proximal tubular necrosis, increased blood urea	Emeigh Hart et al., 1991a
Mouse	900–1200	oral	2½	increased serum creatinine	Hu et al., 1993a
Mouse	600	ip	2½	tubular necrosis, increased blood urea	Emeigh Hart et al., 1994
Mouse	600	ip	3–4	mild tubular necrosis, increased blood urea	Hoivik et al., 1995
Hamster	300	ip	NS	no renal lesions	El-Hage et al., 1983
Hamster	200–400[12]	ip	W[13]	no papillary necrosis or other renal lesions	Carlton and Engelhardt, 1989
Hamster	200[14]	ip	W	no papillary necrosis or other renal lesions	Carlton and Engelhardt, 1989
Dog	600	oral	NS	renal tubular dilatation	Piperno et al., 1978
Dog	500	oral	NS	'nephrosis'	Savides et al., 1984
Dog	1150	sc	NS	no histological renal damage	Panella et al., 1990
Cat	120	oral	mature	no renal lesions	Savides et al., 1985
Pig	1000–4000	oral	Y	early tubular degeneration	Miller et al., 1976a

[1] young; [2] not stated; [3] isolated renal tubular cells *ex vivo*; [4] pretreated with 3-methylcholanthrene; [5] pretreated with phenobarbitone; [6] pretreated with cobaltous chloride; [7] also given frusemide; [8] as shown by uptake of PAH and tetraethylammonium by kidney slices; [9] unilateral nephrectomy; [10] two doses of 900 mg kg⁻¹ 48 hours apart; [11] pretreated with phorone to deplete glutathione; [12] given with potentially protective dimethylsulphoxide; [13] weanlings; [14] 200 mg kg⁻¹ daily for 2–5 days

W = Wistar; SD = Sprague Dawley; F-344 = Fischer F-344; f = female; m = male; t = heterozygous; m = homozygous

267

to use susceptible strains such as Fischer 344 (McMurtry *et al.*, 1978; Newton *et al.*, 1985a; Beierschmitt *et al.*, 1986c; Tarloff *et al.*, 1989c) and homozygous Gunn rats (Briggs *et al.*, 1982; Henry and Tange, 1984, 1987), while in some studies unilateral nephrectomy was performed in order to potentiate toxicity (Henry *et al.*, 1983; Henry and Tange, 1984, 1987; Beierschmitt *et al.*, 1986b). As shown in Table 13.1, the typical renal lesion in susceptible animals was proximal tubular necrosis and an example is shown in Figure 13.1. Primary cultures of postnatal rat kidney epithelial cells showed only minimal morphological changes and leakage of lactic dehydrogenase after exposure to 150 mg l^{-1} of paracetamol for 24 h (Smith *et al.*, 1986c). A modest increase in the urinary excretion of N-acetyl-β-D-glucosamidinase (NAG) and alanine aminopeptidase in rats given an oral dose of 600 mg kg^{-1} of paracetamol was further evidence that it could cause acute tubular injury (Casadevall *et al.*, 1993). A similar increase in urinary N-acetyl-β-D-glucosamidinase and γ-glutamyl transferase was reported in rats given 1000 and 1500 mg kg^{-1} of paracetamol (Möller-Hartmann and Siegers, 1991). In some studies paracetamol caused functional renal impairment as shown by elevation of the blood urea or creatinine (Newton *et al.*, 1983b; Younes *et al.*, 1988; McCrae *et al.*, 1989; Siegers and Möller-Hartmann, 1989; Tarloff *et al.*, 1989a,b; Emeigh Hart *et al.*, 1991a; Möller-Hartmann and Siegers, 1991), but it had little or no effect on the tubular synthesis and transport of glucose (Tange *et al.*, 1977; Tarloff *et al.*, 1989c; Trumper *et al.*, 1992), or p-aminohippurate and tetraethylammonium uptake by kidney slices (Newton *et al.*, 1985a; Tarloff *et al.*, 1989a, 1990). Paracetamol had only a minor

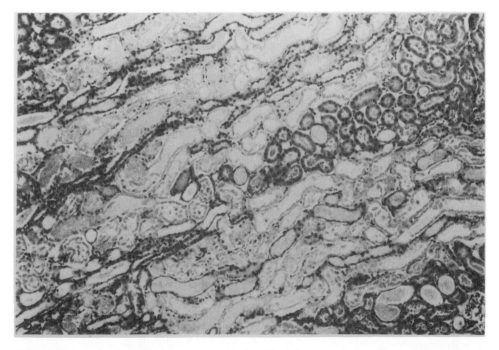

Figure 13.1 Acute renal tubular necrosis in Fischer rats following subcutaneous injection of 750 mg kg^{-1} of paracetamol. There is extensive cortical necrosis involving the distal proximal tubules (reproduced with permission from McMurtry *et al.*, 1978).

inhibitory effect on protein synthesis, glucose utilization and lactate production in the dog kidney (Davidson *et al.*, 1973a,b). Basal and nystatin-stimulated oxygen consumption was reduced and lactic dehydrogenase release increased when proximal tubular cells from mice were incubated with very high concentrations of 1500 and 3750 mg l^{-1} of paracetamol. Isolated proximal tubular cells from rats and baboons were much less responsive and there was only a small effect at the higher concentration (Tyson *et al.*, 1991). In another report, 'nephrotoxicity' was shown by effects on the uptake of p-aminohippurate and leakage of lactic dehydrogenase in rat renal slices incubated with paracetamol in supratoxic concentrations up to 7550 mg l^{-1} (Tarloff *et al.*, 1990). Contrary to the intentions of the authors of the latter reports, these findings only demonstrated the remarkable lack of renal toxicity of paracetamol at realistic dose levels.

The uptake of α-methylglucose by isolated proximal tubular cells from rat kidney was proposed as an *in vitro* model for nephrotoxicity but paracetamol had little effect in this system, even at concentrations as high as 750 mg l^{-1} (Boogaard *et al.*, 1989). Trumper *et al.* (1992) reported a dose-dependent fall in glomerular filtration rate and renal blood flow as shown by decreased inulin and p-aminohippurate clearances in rats given 200, 500 and 1000 mg kg^{-1} of paracetamol intraperitoneally (Figure 13.2). The urine to plasma osmolality ratio was reduced but there were no changes in water and electrolyte excretion or glucose reabsorption and the renal glutathione content was only reduced with the highest dose. The maximum decrease in glomerular filtration rate and p-aminohippurate clearance was delayed until 16 h after dosing and it was concluded that proximal tubular function was preserved but that distal tubular function was depressed, probably as a result of renal haemodynamic changes. The increase in serum creatinine produced by paracetamol in another study was attributed to glomerular damage in the absence of signs of tubular dysfunction but there was no histological evidence of glomerular or other renal lesions (Younes *et al.*, 1988). In Gunn rats given 900 mg kg^{-1} of paracetamol intravenously, papillary necrosis was observed in three of 12 homozygotes, but not in heterozygotes or albino rats (Briggs *et al.*, 1982). The same dose produced minor patchy necrosis of the tip of the papilla with damage to the collecting ducts and loops of Henle in 18 unilaterally nephrectomized homozygous Gunn rats. There was also patchy necrosis of single tubular cells in the distal third of the proximal tubules. Unfortunately, the frequency and severity of the papillary lesions were not stated but similar damage was not observed in albino rats (Henry and Tange, 1987). Renal papillary necrosis and minor tubular lesions were also noted in other studies with Gunn rats (de Morais *et al.*, 1992a). Chronic renal lesions were observed in uninephrectomized homozygous Gunn rats following single intravenous doses of paracetamol combined with aspirin and antipyrine (Henry and Tange, 1984). In this model, paracetamol in a dose of 900 mg kg^{-1} tended to produce tubular necrosis while aspirin (450 mg kg^{-1}) and antipyrine (940 mg kg^{-1}) uniformly produced papillary necrosis (Henry *et al.*, 1983).

The pretreatment of rats with 150 mg kg^{-1} of paracetamol was said to exacerbate papillary necrosis and tubular toxicity induced with 2-bromoethanamine (Bach and Gregg, 1988) but in another study it did not produce papillary necrosis in hamsters or potentiate the lesions induced by 2-bromoethylene (Carlton and Engelhardt, 1989). In the latter report, the paracetamol was given dissolved in dimethylsulphoxide and this might have protected against toxicity (Siegers, 1978a; Jeffery and Haschek, 1988). The acute tubular toxicity of paracetamol was enhanced by

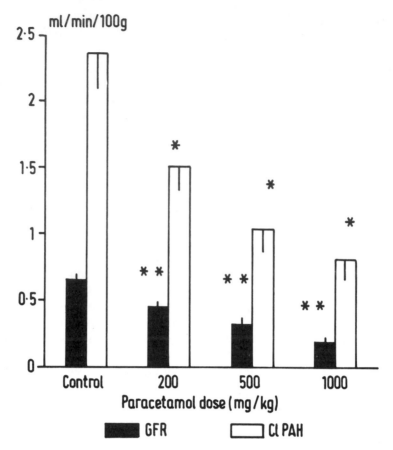

Figure 13.2 Dose-related decrease in glomerular filtration rate (GFR) and renal blood flow (p-aminohippurate clearance) (Cl PAH), in male Wistar rats treated with 200, 500 and 1000 mg kg^{-1} of paracetamol by intraperitoneal injection (after Trumper *et al.*, 1992).

stimulation of its metabolism by prior induction with 3-methylcholanthrene and phenobarbitone, and decreased by inhibition with cobalt chloride (McMurtry *et al.*, 1978). Paracetamol caused acute impairment of renal function in mice previously depleted of glutathione by administration of phorone (Younes *et al.*, 1988). The acute nephrotoxicity of paracetamol was dose dependent and age dependent with increased resistance in young animals (Table 13.1). Male mice were more susceptible than females to the acute nephrotoxicity of paracetamol in one study (Hu *et al.*, 1993a), but in another, the position was reversed (Mugford and Tarloff, 1995). Castration protected male mice against paracetamol nephrotoxicity (Emeigh Hart *et al.*, 1994) and in CD-1 mice only males exhibited cytochrome P450-dependent selective covalent binding to protein and renal tubular toxicity (Hoivik *et al.*, 1995). The greater susceptibility of female than male rats to nephrotoxicity in one study could not be attributed to sex differences in the bioactivation of paracetamol by oxidation and deacetylation (Mugford and Tarloff, 1995).

Chronic Nephrotoxicity

Early studies with paracetamol were prompted by increasing concern about its possible role in the aetiology of analgesic nephropathy. This condition was originally described as a chronic interstitial nephritis (Spühler and Zollinger, 1953) and it was not until later that renal papillary necrosis was recognized as the primary lesion (Lindeneg *et al.*, 1959; Kincaid-Smith, 1967). At first, chronic pyelonephritis was thought to play a central role and chronic toxicity studies were carried out in animals with experimental urinary tract infections induced by techniques such as intracardiac, intravenous or intravesical injection of bacteria with or without 'massage' of the kidneys (Miescher and Studer, 1961; Angervall *et al.*, 1962a,b,c) and the surgical introduction of glass beads into the bladder (Vivaldi, 1968). It was conceivable that paracetamol might have aggravated infection in some of these studies, but in others it had no such effect (Hedwall and Heeg, 1961; Vivaldi, 1968). Chronic nephrotoxicity studies with paracetamol are listed in Table 13.2. Various abnormalities were described but there was no consistent picture and in a number of studies paracetamol did not produce any histological or functional abnormalities, even when given in very large doses. It was soon obvious that papillary necrosis could not be produced easily with any reasonable dose of paracetamol, and even with 3000 mg kg^{-1} daily the lesions were minor and the incidence was low (Boyd and Hogan, 1968; Nanra *et al.*, 1973b, 1978). Other analgesics such as aspirin produced renal papillary necrosis more readily than paracetamol and the incidence with these drugs in combination was similar to that observed with aspirin alone (Nanra and Kincaid-Smith, 1970, 1973; Nanra *et al.*, 1973b, 1980; Molland, 1978; Qamar and Alam, 1988; Burrell *et al.*, 1990, 1991). The severity of paracetamol-induced papillary necrosis was increased by water deprivation (Nanra and Kincaid-Smith, 1973; Nanra *et al.*, 1978) and urinary tract infection (Furman *et al.*, 1981). The lesions occurred spontaneously in the Gunn rat, but were aggravated by paracetamol and could be produced with a single dose of about 240 mg kg^{-1} (Axelsen, 1975, 1980). The incidence of papillary necrosis in Gunn rats given single oral doses of aspirin, phenacetin and paracetamol is compared in Figure 13.3. Other workers have confirmed the susceptibility of Gunn rats to renal impairment and papillary and cortical necrosis induced by paracetamol (Briggs *et al.*, 1982; de Morais and Wells, 1988, 1989; de Morais *et al.*, 1992a). Paracetamol did not enhance renal papillary necrosis previously induced in pigs by the administration of 2-bromoethanamine (Gregg *et al.*, 1990).

The papillary lesions produced by paracetamol in animals were similar to those produced by other analgesics and they undoubtedly represented the same process that caused analgesic nephropathy in man. The earliest lesion consisted of patchy necrosis of the structures adjacent to of the tip of the papilla (papillary necrobiosis), and this progressed to a bland acellular necrosis extending into the medulla and involving the matrix, collecting ducts, thin loops of Henle, interstitial cells and the endothelium of the medullary microvasculature. There was usually a sharp line of demarcation between the necrotic and viable tissue. The basement membranes of the blood vessels and tubules were thickened, and secondary changes of cortical fibrosis with tubular atrophy only developed after papillary necrosis was established (Burrell *et al.*, 1990, 1991; Burrell and Yong, 1991). Papillary damage produced by paracetamol and other analgesics was associated with uroepithelial hyperplasia

Table 13.2 Chronic nephrotoxicity studies of paracetamol in animals.

Species	Dose (mg kg day^{-1})	Duration (weeks)	Outcome	Reference
Rat	350	4	focal cortical infiltrates and tubular degeneration, loss of enzyme activity	Eisalo and Talanti, 1961
Rat[1]	290–340	21	variable focal interstitial nephritis (also present in controls)	Angervall et al., 1962a
Rat[1]	100, 400	21	'nephritis' in all 'massaged' kidneys including controls	Angervall et al., 1962b
Rat[1]	300	21	'nephritis'	Angervall et al., 1962b
Rat[1]	100, 410	22	'nephritis' in all 'massaged' kidneys including controls	Angervall et al., 1962c
Rat	400	42	reduced urinary concentrating capacity	Angervall et al., 1964
Rat	2% of diet	13	no histological renal damage	Schnitzer and Smith, 1966
Rat	500–4000	14	congestion, fatty degeneration, tubular necrosis	Boyd and Hogan, 1968
Rat[2]	200	26–52	no histological changes or increased frequency of urinary infection	Vivaldi, 1968
Rat	not stated[3]	20	papillary necrosis in 2 of 9 rats, water diuresis	Nanra and Kincaid-Smith, 1970
Rat	1500–3000	5–9	no papillary necrosis or interstitial nephritis, some tubular degeneration	Peters et al., 1972
Rat[4]	3000	19	no histological or functional abnormality	Nanra et al., 1973b
Rat[4]	?450[5]	21	necrobiosis of papillary tip	Nanra et al., 1973b
Rat	380[3]	12–30	papillary necrosis in 3 of 8 rats, water deprivation	Nanra and Kincaid-Smith, 1973
Rat	380[3]	12–30	papillary necrosis in 2 of 9 rats, water diuresis	Nanra and Kincaid-Smith, 1973
Rat (Gunn)	268	4	renal papillary necrosis in 1 of 10 rats	Axelsen, 1975
Rat (Gunn)	420	4	renal papillary necrosis in 1 of 5 rats	Axelsen, 1975
Rat	200	29	no renal lesions	Thomas et al., 1977a

Rat	894	48	intermediate renal papillary necrosis in 3 of 5 rats	Molland, 1978
Rat	360[6]	48	renal papillary necrosis in 5 of 5 rats (cortical lesions in 4)	Molland, 1978
Rat	3000	8–20	papillary necrosis in 3 of 7 rats, water deprivation	Nanra et al., 1978
Rat	250[3]	72	renal papillary necrosis in 6 of 8 rats	Nanra et al., 1980
Rat	300	12–32	no renal lesions	Furman et al., 1981
Rat[7]	300	12–32	papillary necrosis in 4 of 12 rats, cortical scars and abscesses	Furman et al., 1981
Rat	900	8	reversibly increased urine microglobulin, albumin and NAG[8]	Bernard et al., 1988
Rat	6–12 000[9]	40	no renal lesions	Ward et al., 1988
Rat	310–1610	6–12	papillary necrosis in 40% at highest dose, urothelial hyperplasia	Johansson et al., 1989
Rat	380[6]	65	papillary necrosis in 5 of 10 rats, decreased urine concentration	Burrell et al., 1990
Rat	140–210	40–83	no histological renal lesions	Burrell and Yong, 1991
Rat	190–360[6]	20–63	variable papillary necrosis, decreased urine concentration	Burrell et al., 1991
Rabbit	85–340	30	variable inflammatory infiltrates, no rise in blood urea	Miescher and Studer, 1961
Rabbit[10]	85–340	30	no renal lesions, no rise in blood urea	Miescher and Studer, 1961
Rabbit	300	4	'pyelitis' in 4 of 7 rabbits	Qamar and Alam, 1988
Rabbit	150[6]	4	interstitial nephritis or 'pyelitis' in 2 of 7 rabbits	Qamar and Alam, 1988
Cat	25–50	26	no histological or functional changes	Eder, 1964
Pig	100	4	no renal pathology or impairment of function	Gregg et al., 1990

[1] intracardiac/intravenous *E. coli* + massage of kidney 10 days before end of study; [2] glass bead inserted in bladder, *E. coli* injection; [3] given with aspirin and caffeine; [4] one or two rats only; [5] presumed dose, given with aspirin and caffeine; [6] given with aspirin; [7] with induced pyelonephritis; [8] potentiation of cadmium nephrotoxicity, NAG = N-acetyl-β-D-glucosaminidase; [9] parts per million; [10] with repeated intravenous injections of *Proteus* bacilli during last 10 weeks

273

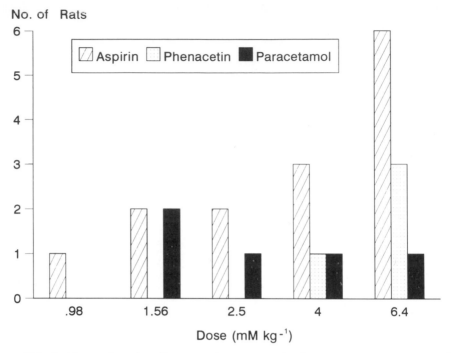

Figure 13.3 Incidence of renal papillary necrosis in groups of six homozygous Gunn rats treated with different single doses of oral aspirin, phenacetin and paracetamol (from Axelsen, 1980).

(Johansson *et al.*, 1989). With minor lesions such as those shown in Figure 13.4, there could be re-epithelialization and attempts at healing of the papillary stump (Furman *et al.*, 1981) but more advanced lesions were irreversible with no evidence of repair (Burrell *et al.*, 1991). Apart from a reduced urinary concentration capacity in some studies (Angervall *et al.*, 1964) and reduced fractional excretion of urea (Peters *et al.*, 1972), chronic toxicity studies with paracetamol showed no consistent impairment of renal function (Miescher and Studer, 1961; Bernard *et al.*, 1988; Gregg *et al.*, 1990). Paracetamol, given for two months, increased subsequent chronic nephrotoxicity of cadmium in rats (Bernard *et al.*, 1988).

The main conclusion to be drawn from these studies is that it was difficult to produce acute tubular necrosis or renal papillary necrosis in animals with paracetamol and that the latter lesion could be produced more readily with aspirin and other analgesics. The relevance of chronic toxicity studies of paracetamol in animals subjected to intracardiac, intravenous and intravesical injections of bacteria, sometimes with kidney massage, was questionable, as was the administration of doses as high as 3000 mg kg^{-1}. Acute papillary necrosis produced in animals by single doses of compounds such as ethyleneimine has been proposed as a model for chronic analgesic nephropathy in man (Bach and Hardy, 1985), but this hardly seems realistic. In practice, acute impairment of renal function following consumption of paracetamol in man was very rare unless it was taken in overdosage, and there was no evidence of nephrotoxicity when it was taken in full dosage for long periods (Edwards *et al.*, 1971). Until recently there have been very few reports of analgesic nephropathy in patients taking paracetamol alone (Nanra *et al.*, 1978; Prescott,

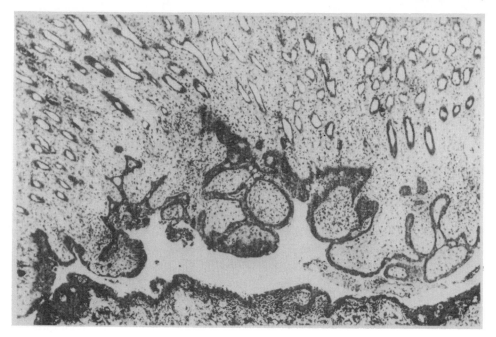

Figure 13.4 Minor renal papillary necrosis in the rat showing an increase in fibrous tissue and re-epithelialization of the necrotic stump of the papilla. The rat was treated with 300 mg kg^{-1} of oral paracetamol daily for 28 weeks and received twice weekly intravesical injections of *Escherichia coli* to induce pyelonephritis (reproduced with permission from Furman *et al.*, 1981).

1982a) but several cases have now been reported from Malaysia (Segasothy *et al.*, 1984, 1986a, 1988).

Mechanisms of Nephrotoxicity

The ways in which paracetamol causes nephrotoxicity have not been clearly established but at least two different mechanisms presumably would have to be invoked to account for acute proximal tubular necrosis and chronic renal papillary necrosis. Possible mechanisms include metabolic activation of paracetamol to produce an arylating cytotoxic intermediate, inhibition of synthesis of vasodilator prostaglandins resulting in renal medullary ischaemia and direct cytotoxicity. Mechanisms involving the metabolic activation of paracetamol were favoured by most investigators and these included: (1) cytochrome P450- and NADPH-dependent oxidation to produce toxic N-acetyl-p-benzoquinoneimine in the kidney in the same way as in the liver; (2) NADPH-independent cooxidation of paracetamol to N-acetyl-p-benzoquinoneimine by renal prostaglandin synthetase; (3) deacetylation of paracetamol to the more nephrotoxic p-aminophenol, which may also be subject to further metabolic activation; and (4) conjugation with glutathione and conversion of the resulting cysteine conjugate by renal cysteine conjugate β-lyase to a reactive cytotoxic intermediate. Models of acute papillary necrosis such as that induced by 2-bromethanamine have been proposed as a means of gaining a better understanding of the mechanisms involved (Bach and Hardy, 1985; Bach and Gregg, 1988; Bach *et al.*, 1988; Gregg *et al.*, 1989). Although the relevance of these models of acute papillary necrosis in animals has been defended, the circumstances can hardly be considered representative of chronic renal papillary necrosis in man caused by the long-term abuse of analgesics over periods of many years. From a mechanistic point of view it is necessary to consider the localization in the nephron of paracetamol-induced renal lesions, regional differences in drug concentrations and the effects of predisposing factors.

The Renal Distribution of Paracetamol

Bluemle and Goldberg (1968) reported that, unlike salicylate, paracetamol was concentrated up to 10-fold in the inner renal medulla compared with the cortex in hydropenic dogs, and proposed that the renal papillary necrosis allegedly produced by phenacetin was caused by high local concentrations of paracetamol. The urine-to-plasma concentration ratio of paracetamol (but not phenacetin) was increased in healthy subjects during vasopressin antidiuresis indicating that paracetamol reabsorption was enhanced under these conditions (Barraclough, 1972; Barraclough and Nilam, 1973). Paracetamol was shown to be filtered at the glomerulus in dogs and subsequently reabsorbed in the tubules by simple diffusion. Under conditions of oliguria, it was concentrated maximally in the distal nephron and collecting ducts and toxicity was thought to be related to high concentrations locally. The cortico-medullary concentration gradient was inversely related to the urine flow rate. Paracetamol glucuronide and sulphate conjugates were not reabsorbed and also became concentrated in the tubular fluid of the distal nephron (Duggin and Mudge, 1975, 1976). It was widely hypothesized that the paracetamol formed from phenacetin taken by analgesic abusers caused renal papillary necrosis because it was concentrated by the countercurrent mechanism in the inner medulla and papilla (Duggin, 1977, 1980; Shelley, 1978; Mudge, 1982; Bach and Hardy, 1985; Walker, 1991). The extent of the covalent binding of paracetamol to renal proteins was said to correspond to its concentration in the inner medulla (Walker and Duggin, 1988) and the effect of hydropenia in concentrating paracetamol in the distal nephron was consistent with clinical and experimental evidence that the incidence of analgesic-induced renal papillary necrosis was increased by dehydration (Nanra and Kincaid-Smith, 1970, 1973; Nanra *et al.*, 1970a,b, 1973b; Rosner, 1974).

Although these arguments were persuasive, it must be pointed out that the concentration of a drug at a particular site was not in itself a basis for toxicity. There was no similar cortico-medullary concentration gradient for salicylate (Bluemle and Goldberg, 1968), yet this agent produced renal papillary necrosis much more readily than paracetamol. In addition, loss of urinary concentration capacity was the earliest functional defect in analgesic nephropathy and if the concentration of paracetamol in the inner medulla was an essential factor in its genesis, analgesic-induced renal papillary necrosis would be a minor self-limiting condition.

Cytochrome P450-dependent Metabolic Activation of Paracetamol

Following the discovery of the mechanisms of paracetamol hepatotoxicity it was proposed that it caused acute renal tubular injury in the same way through conversion to the reactive arylating intermediate N-acetyl-p-benzoquinoneimine, and that as in the liver, glutathione played a crucial protective role. In keeping with this hypothesis, the covalent binding of paracetamol to renal proteins and the severity of proximal tubular necrosis in susceptible male Fischer rats was reduced when its metabolic activation was decreased by treatment with cobaltous chloride. As in the liver, there was an inverse relationship between depletion of renal glutathione and covalent binding, and the nephrotoxicity of paracetamol was potentiated when glutathione was depleted by prior administration of diethylmaleate and decreased when its synthesis was stimulated with cysteine. The covalent binding of paracetamol to renal microsomes was enzyme dependent, and required NADPH and oxygen. Pretreatment with 3-methylcholanthrene increased the toxicity and covalent binding of paracetamol in the liver, but had little or no effect in the kidney. Tubular necrosis was most extensive at the sites of greatest cytochrome P450 activity (Mitchell *et al.*, 1977; McMurtry *et al.*, 1978). The oxidation and glutathione conjugation of paracetamol occurred primarily in rat liver while conversion of the glutathione to the mercapturic acid conjugate was catalyzed primarily by kidney cells (Moldéus *et al.*, 1978).

Subsequent studies confirmed that paracetamol undergoes metabolic activation in the kidney (but to a lesser extent than in the liver) with covalent binding to renal proteins, depletion of renal glutathione and production of the cysteine and mercapturic acid conjugates (Joshi *et al.*, 1978; Mudge *et al.*, 1978; Jones *et al.*, 1979; Hart *et al.*, 1980; Ross *et al.*, 1980; Emslie *et al.*, 1981a,b, 1982; Newton *et al.*, 1982a, 1983a,b, 1985b; Emeigh Hart *et al.*, 1991a, 1994; Hoivik *et al.*, 1995). The covalent binding of paracetamol in the kidney after a toxic dose was about one-fifth of that observed in the liver (Fischer *et al.*, 1981). It was emphasized that the acute nephrotoxicity of paracetamol depended on its metabolic activation (Duggin, 1980; Bach and Bridges, 1984; Bach and Hardy, 1985; Dybing, 1985; Walker and Duggin, 1988; Walker, 1991) and again it was shown that renal toxicity could be prevented by inhibition of its oxidation and covalent binding with agents such as piperonyl butoxide and diethyldithiocarbamate (Younes *et al.*, 1988; Bartolone *et al.*, 1989a; Emeigh Hart *et al.*, 1991a; Möller-Hartmann and Siegers, 1991). Large doses of paracetamol reduced renal concentrations of glutathione, and toxicity did not occur unless it was depleted (Mitchell *et al.*, 1977; McMurtry *et al.*, 1978; Mudge *et al.*, 1978; Duggin, 1980; Duggin *et al.*, 1980; Newton *et al.*, 1982a; Younes *et al.*, 1988; Tarloff *et al.*, 1990; Emeigh Hart *et al.*, 1991a; Hu *et al.*, 1993a; Walker and Fawcett, 1993). The covalent binding of paracetamol in kidney slices and the isolated perfused rat kidney was reduced by the addition of glutathione (Joshi *et al.*, 1978; Emslie *et al.*, 1981a) while prior depletion of glutathione with phorone increased the severity of renal impairment produced by paracetamol (Younes *et al.*, 1988). Inducing agents had variable effects on paracetamol metabolism and nephrotoxicity. 3-Methylcholanthrene enhanced the renal metabolic activation of paracetamol (Emslie *et al.*, 1981a) but had less effect on its covalent binding in kidney than in liver (Mudge *et al.*, 1978). Renal depletion of glutathione was enhanced by pretreatment with polybrominated biphenyls and decreased by piperonyl butoxide (Newton *et al.*, 1982a). Prior depletion of renal glutathione with diethylmaleate decreased the formation of the mercapturic acid conjugate of paracetamol in the isolated perfused kidney, presumably because of its reduced availability (Emslie *et al.*, 1981a). The depletion of glutathione in the kidney by paracetamol was time dependent and greater in male than female mice (Hu *et al.*, 1993a), and as in the

277

liver, it was dose dependent within limits (McMurtry *et al.*, 1978; Mudge *et al.*, 1978; Tarloff *et al.*, 1990). The depletion of renal glutathione and cysteine by paracetamol was less, and recovery was more complete in young than in mature and elderly mice (Richie *et al.*, 1992). Species differences in glutathione depletion corresponded with differences in covalent binding and nephrotoxicity (Mudge *et al.*, 1978; Emeigh Hart *et al.*, 1991a).

Significant strain, age and sex differences in susceptibility to acute paracetamol nephrotoxicity have been observed in rats, and in some cases these differences could be related to variation in renal cytochrome P450 content (Newton *et al.*, 1983b; Beierschmitt and Weiner, 1986; Beierschmitt *et al.*, 1986b; Tarloff *et al.*, 1989a,b,c; 1990; Kaloyanides, 1991; Hu *et al.*, 1993a). In one report, the activities of renal glucuronyl transferase and sulphotransferase were not reduced in young compared with older rats and it was considered unlikely that susceptibility to nephrotoxicity was related to the renal metabolism of paracetamol (Tarloff *et al.*, 1991). Studies with monoclonal antibodies directed against cytochrome CYP2E1 showed that this isoform accounted for about half of the oxidation of paracetamol in mouse liver and kidney. Its activity corresponded with sex differences in susceptibility to nephrotoxicity and renal damage was most severe in the proximal tubules where cytochrome CYP2E1 was localized (Hu *et al.*, 1993a; Hoivik *et al.*, 1995). In another report, renal cytochrome P450 in rats was shown to be increased by treadmill exercise (Piatkowski *et al.*, 1993). When mouse proximal tubular cells were incubated with paracetamol there was selective arylation of 33, 44, 58 and 130 kD proteins and a similar pattern was found *in vivo* (Bartolone *et al.*, 1989a; Emeigh Hart *et al.*, 1991b; Tyson *et al.*, 1991). In rats, the covalent binding of paracetamol to kidney proteins was unaffected by hepatectomy indicating that the nephrotoxic metabolite was formed *in situ* rather than formed in the liver and subsequently transported to the kidney (Breen *et al.*, 1982a). As in the liver, lipid peroxidation was probably not a primary mechanism of toxicity as its inhibition with desferrioxamine did not influence paracetamol nephrotoxicity (Younes *et al.*, 1988).

Taken together, these findings support the existence of cytochrome P450 and NADPH-dependent metabolic activation and covalent binding of paracetamol with glutathione protection as a mechanism of the acute proximal tubular necrosis produced by large doses in susceptible animals and for the acute renal failure that may rarely occur in man following overdosage. Some inconsistencies have been reported, however. In one study paracetamol-induced glutathione depletion in rat kidney slices did not precede cytotoxicity (Tarloff *et al.*, 1990). In another, paracetamol caused marked depletion of glutathione in the liver, but not in the kidney. Administration of the glutathione precursors methionine and N-acetylcysteine prevented hepatic but not renal toxicity suggesting different mechanisms of toxicity (Möller-Hartmann and Siegers, 1991). In the isolated perfused kidney of the Gunn rat the glucuronide conjugation of paracetamol was reduced but there was no corresponding increase in oxidative metabolism. This suggested that the enhanced nephrotoxicity of paracetamol in this strain was not caused by increased renal formation of a reactive metabolite (Emslie *et al.*, 1982). It is also necessary to question the relevance of some of these findings because of the enormous doses of paracetamol used. For example, in one report rat renal slices were incubated with paracetamol at a concentration of 7550 mg l^{-1} in attempts to produce toxicity (Tarloff *et al.*, 1990).

Metabolic Activation of Paracetamol by Prostaglandin Endoperoxide Synthetase

The cytochrome P450 and NADPH-dependent metabolic activation of paracetamol could account for the proximal tubular necrosis. However, it could not account for the papillary necrosis of analgesic nephropathy because cytochrome P450 was restricted largely to the renal cortex and outer medulla while there was negligible activity in the inner medulla and papilla (Zenser *et al.*, 1978a, 1979; Mohandas *et al.*, 1981a; Zenser and Davis, 1984). The more extensive and persistent covalent binding of paracetamol to the renal inner medulla than to the cortex also pointed to a different mechanism of paracetamol activation (Joshi *et al.*, 1978; Mudge *et al.*, 1978; Mohandas *et al.*, 1981a). The renal metabolism and covalent binding of paracetamol in the mouse was largely dependent on NADPH but in the rabbit there appeared to be a different system altogether that was independent of NADPH and inhibited by fluoride (Mohandas *et al.*, 1977, 1979). It was subsequently found that paracetamol rapidly formed a glutathione conjugate when it was incubated with microsomes from sheep seminal vesicles in the presence of arachidonic acid and glutathione, and the reaction was catalyzed by prostaglandin synthetase as it was inhibited by indomethacin (Moldéus and Rahimtula, 1980; Harvison *et al.*, 1988a). The inner renal medulla was rich in this enzyme complex, which consisted of a cyclooxygenase component which converted arachidonic acid to prostaglandin PGG_2 and a hydroperoxidase component which could oxidize other compounds while reducing the latter to prostaglandin H_2. The same prostaglandin endoperoxide synthetase-dependent cooxidation of paracetamol was shown to take place in the kidney where it occurred primarily in the inner medulla (Boyd and Eling, 1981; Mohandas 1981a,b; Duggin *et al.*, 1982; Moldéus *et al.*, 1982a; Zenser and Davis, 1984; Larsson *et al.*, 1985) and the glutathione conjugate was the same as that formed by the oxidation of paracetamol by cortical mixed function oxidase (Moldéus *et al.*, 1982a). The metabolic activation of paracetamol by NADPH-dependent cytochrome P450 was greatest in rabbit renal cortex and least in the inner medulla while the order was opposite for oxidation by prostaglandin endoperoxide synthetase (Mohandas *et al.*, 1981a,b). The inner renal medulla and papilla might appear to be particularly vulnerable to damage from the covalent binding of paracetamol because the concentration of reduced glutathione was lowest at these sites and increased progressively in the outer medulla and cortex. In addition, the activity of glutathione peroxidase and reductase was very low in the renal medulla (Mohandas *et al.*, 1984). Microsomal prostaglandin H synthase prepared from rabbit renal medulla activated paracetamol, which was then bound covalently to protein. The binding was inhibited by glutathione, which combined with the activated paracetamol to form the glutathione conjugate (Moldéus and Rahimtula, 1980; Boyd and Eling, 1981; Eling *et al.*, 1990).

As might be expected, the prostaglandin-dependent cooxidation and covalent binding of paracetamol to rabbit renal proteins was inhibited by aspirin and indomethacin (Mohandas *et al.*, 1981a,b; Duggin *et al.*, 1982). In other studies aspirin inhibited cyclooxygenase but it apparently had little effect on hydroperoxidase in the presence of peroxide substrates and it did not prevent the renal cooxidation of paracetamol (Zenser *et al.*, 1983; Zenser and Davis, 1984). This was an important point because by inhibiting cyclooxygenase, aspirin and other non-steroidal anti-inflammatory drugs would be expected to protect against paracetamol-induced papillary necrosis. In practice, the opposite seemed to apply because there was clinical and experimental evidence that analgesic combinations were more nephrotoxic than the individual drugs administered alone. Aspirin can cause depletion of renal glutathione and could thus have a synergistic effect on the nephrotoxicity of paracetamol (Duggin *et al.*, 1980; Walker and Duggin, 1988; Walker, 1991).

The renal medullary prostaglandin-dependent cooxidation of paracetamol to a cytotoxic metabolite has been widely accepted as definitive proof that paracetamol played a fundamental role in the aetiology of papillary necrosis and analgesic nephropathy (Bach and Bridges, 1984; Bach and Hardy, 1985; Walker and Duggin, 1988; Gregg *et al.*, 1989; Kaloyanides, 1991; Walker, 1991; Walker and Fawcett, 1993). However compelling and plausible this mechanism may be, the fact remained that it was very difficult to produce experimental renal papillary necrosis with paracetamol (or phenacetin), and analgesic nephropathy associated with the use of paracetamol alone was very rare.

Nephrotoxicity Mediated by p-Aminophenol

The possibility that the renal toxicity of paracetamol might be related to its conversion to p-aminophenol has recently attracted attention. Intravenous p-aminophenol produced proximal renal tubular necrosis in rats while paracetamol had no such effect (Calder *et al.*, 1971), and in subsequent studies the acute nephrotoxicity of a series of quinols and catechols was related to their oxidation-reduction potential (Calder *et al.*, 1975). Further studies showed that p-aminophenol caused depletion of renal glutathione and was bound covalently in the kidney to a greater extent than in the liver (Crowe *et al.*, 1979). On the basis that p-aminophenol was a minor metabolite of paracetamol in hamsters (Gemborys and Mudge, 1981) and that it was formed from paracetamol in the mouse kidney, it was proposed as a mediator of analgesic nephropathy in man (Carpenter and Mudge, 1981). The presumed metabolic activation of p-aminophenol seemed to be independent of cytochrome P450 and some other mechanism appeared to be involved as inducers and inhibitors of mixed function oxidase had no consistent effect on its nephrotoxicity (Calder *et al.*, 1979). The rank order of deacetylation activity in rat tissue homogenates incubated with paracetamol at the high concentration of 1660 mg l^{-1} was liver > renal cortex > renal medulla and the reaction was highly pH dependent. Although the renal lesions produced by p-aminophenol were confined to the cortex, a strong case was made for its primary involvement in the pathogenesis of analgesic nephropathy (Mudge, 1982). In another study, the *in vitro* deacetylation of paracetamol was greater in rat liver than in kidney, and there was least conversion in brain (Baumann *et al.*, 1984). Only a very small fraction of a dose of paracetamol was excreted in the urine as p-aminophenol in the Fischer F344 rat but the proportion increased with the dose of paracetamol. p-Aminophenol was also formed from paracetamol in the isolated perfused kidney and induction with β-naphthoflavone and polybrominated biphenyls protected against its nephrotoxicity. The renal lesions produced by p-aminophenol and paracetamol were similar and it was proposed that the nephrotoxicity of paracetamol depended on its deacetylation to p-aminophenol, which was then subject to metabolism in the kidney to an electrophilic intermediate (Newton *et al.*, 1982b). Strain differences in susceptibility to the renal toxicity of paracetamol could not be attributed to differences in its deacetylation to p-aminophenol as the covalent binding of ring-[^{14}C] paracetamol to renal microsomal protein and the excretion of p-aminophenol were similar in susceptible Fischer F344 rats and resistant Sprague Dawley rats (Newton *et al.*, 1983b). On the other hand, p-aminophenol produced lesions in both strains that were similar to, but more severe than, those produced by paracetamol in Fischer F344 rats. At concentrations above 750 mg l^{-1}, the covalent binding of p-aminophenol to renal microsomes was greater in Fischer F344 than Sprague Dawley rats (Newton *et al.*, 1983c). Studies with ring- and acetyl-$[^{14}C]$ paracetamol revealed that the compound binding to renal subcellular fractions was derived from p-aminophenol. Thus, paracetamol could apparently cause renal cortical damage as a consequence of its metabolic activation by two mechanisms, i.e. directly through NADPH-dependent cytochrome P450, and after deacetylation to p-aminophenol (Newton *et al.*, 1983a). The covalent binding of ring-$[^{14}C]$ paracetamol to renal cortical protein was four-fold greater than the binding of acetyl-$[^{14}C]$ drug in Fischer F344 rats but the binding of the two forms in Sprague Dawley rats was not different. As the renal binding of ring-$[^{14}C]$ paracetamol was four-fold greater in the former than the latter strain, it was proposed that the differences in susceptibility to renal toxicity were dependent on the formation of p-aminophenol (Newton *et al.*, 1985b). Inhibition of the deacetylation of paracetamol with bis(p-nitrophenyl) phosphate reduced its covalent binding to rat renal cortical homogenates and pretreatment with this agent reduced the renal toxicity of paracetamol but not that of p-aminophenol. It was concluded that the nephrotoxicity of paracetamol was diminished by reducing its conversion to p-aminophenol (Newton *et al.*, 1985a). In some reports, there was no marked effect of age on the formation of p-aminophenol, and unlike paracetamol, its nephrotoxicity in rats was apparently not related to strain or age (Tarloff *et al.*, 1989b,c). However, the deacetylation of paracetamol was proportionally greater in old than young rats because microsomal formation of the reactive metabolite was reduced to the extent of 50 per cent in aged rats (Beierschmitt and Weiner, 1986). Treadmill exercise enhanced the renal deacetylation of paracetamol and this effect was more marked in young than middle-aged rats (Piatkowski *et al.*, 1993). There were major species differences in the presumed role of p-aminophenol in the renal toxicity of paracetamol. In mice, tubular necrosis produced by paracetamol was associated with arylation of proteins by metabolites retaining the acetyl group (i.e. not p-aminophenol) and renal toxicity was not influenced by inhibition of its deacetylation. On the other hand, the nephrotoxicity of paracetamol (but not p-aminophenol) was reduced when microsomal oxidation was inhibited with pipero-piperonyl butoxide. Immunochemical analysis revealed covalent binding with a nephrotoxic dose of paracetamol but not with p-aminophenol. The antibody was directed primarily against the N-acetyl group of the bound metabolite of paracetamol, and as it did not react with the renal protein from mice given a nephrotoxic dose of p-aminophenol, it was unlikely that deacetylation preceded binding or that there was acetylation of bound p-aminophenol. Thus, the acute renal toxicity of paracetamol in mice did not involve p-aminophenol and was probably dependent on activation by cytochrome P450 (Emeigh Hart *et al.*, 1991a,b). Sex differences in susceptibility to the acute nephrotoxicity of paracetamol in rats were not related to differences in bioactivation by deacetylation or microsomal oxidation (Mugford and Tarloff, 1995).

The hypothesis that p-aminophenol was the primary cause of acute tubular necrosis produced by paracetamol was hardly tenable and its involvement in the pathogenesis of chronic analgesic nephropathy was even less likely. The inconsistencies and species differences in the formation of p-aminophenol cannot easily be reconciled and although it was claimed to be a urinary metabolite of paracetamol in man (Clark *et al.*, 1986) it has never been identified as such by other investigators. In studies with deuterium-labelled paracetamol, there was much less exchange of the acetyl group in man than in rats (Baty *et al.*, 1988). Some investigators have gone to great lengths in attempts to prove that p-aminophenol was involved in analgesic nephropathy caused by paracetamol. In one report, the polymerization of p-aminophenol in blood *in vitro* was described and its alleged further conversion to melanin and lipofuchsin was presented in support of unreferenced claims that paracetamol caused chronic renal disease, haemolytic anaemia and the deposition of lipofuchsin in tissues in man (Hegedus and Nayak, 1991).

Paracetamol Cysteine Conjugate

Some halogenated hydrocarbons caused renal toxicity through their conjugation with glutathione. The glutathione conjugates were hydrolyzed by renal γ-glutamyl transferase to the cysteinylglycine conjugates, which in turn were converted by dipeptidases to 3-cysteine conjugates. The cysteine conjugates could then be converted by cysteine conjugate β-lyase in renal tubular cells to reactive sulphur-containing species, which caused nephrotoxicity (Elfarra and Anders, 1984; Kaloyanides, 1991; Finkelstein *et al.*, 1992). It has been suggested that the glutathione conjugate of paracetamol was exported from the liver to the kidney where it might cause renal toxicity through the β-lyase mechanism (Möller-Hartmann and Siegers, 1991). Fowler *et al.* (1991) showed that 4-amino-3-S-glutathionylphenol (the glutathione conjugate of p-aminophenol) produced dose-dependent proximal tubular necrosis in Fischer F344 rats. The renal necrosis was very similar histologically and functionally to that produced by p-aminophenol, but occurred at lower doses. In another report, incubation of renal tubular cells with p-aminophenol glutathione conjugate caused dose- and time-dependent loss of cell viability. Cytotoxicity was decreased if γ-glutamyl transferase was inhibited with avicin and nephrotoxicity was also reduced when the organic cation transport system was inhibited with tetraethylammonium. Biliary diversion of metabolites and glutathione depletion reduced the nephrotoxicity of p-aminophenol and this was in keeping with a causative role for the glutathione conjugate (Klos *et al.*, 1992).

Paracetamol nephrotoxicity was probably not mediated by cysteine conjugate β-lyase. Inhibition of renal γ-glutamyl transferase with avicin or inhibition of cysteine conjugate β-lyase with amino oxyacetic acid did not reduce the nephrotoxicity of paracetamol or p-aminophenol in rats, and the cysteine conjugate of paracetamol was not nephrotoxic in doses up to 810 mg kg^{-1} (Furuhama *et al.*, 1989b; McRae *et al.*, 1990). A positive dose-response for paracetamol nephrotoxicity in the absence of a dose-response relationship for the formation of the paracetamol cysteine protein adduct also suggested that toxicity was not related to this conjugate (Furuhama *et al.*, 1989a). Further evidence against this mechanism was provided by the absence of renal toxicity in Fischer F344 rats following intravenous administration of up to 810 mg kg^{-1} of the cysteine conjugate of paracetamol while the parent drug produced nephrotoxicity at doses of 750 and 1000 mg kg^{-1} (McCrae *et al.*, 1989). Similarly, p-aminophenol in a dose of 110 mg kg^{-1} produced a significant increase in blood urea nitrogen in rats while the equivalent dose given as the glutathione conjugate had no effect (Eyanagi *et al.*, 1991).

Renal Medullary Ischaemia

Microvascular degeneration and vasoconstriction leading to medullary ischaemia have long been favoured as the primary mechanism of analgesic nephropathy. However, it was not certain how this might apply to the pathogenesis of renal papillary necrosis produced by paracetamol as distinct from other analgesics, and it has not been possible to establish whether the vascular lesions precede or follow other degenerative changes (Kincaid-Smith *et al.*, 1968; Nanra and Kincaid-Smith, 1970; Molland, 1978; Shelley, 1978; Prescott, 1979b, 1982a; Duggin, 1980; Bach and Bridges, 1984; Bach and Hardy, 1985). The renal medulla was thought to be particularly vulnerable to ischaemic damage because the blood flow was very sluggish and the tissue oxygenation is low. Medullary perfusion was reduced in rats treated with analgesics for up to 20 weeks and it was reduced further by hypovolaemic shock but not by dehydration (Nanra *et al.*, 1973a,b). It was widely accepted that analgesic nephropathy produced by aspirin and non-steroidal anti-inflammatory drugs was caused by inhibition of the renal synthesis of vasodilator prostaglandins leading to medullary ischaemia and papillary necrosis (Nanra and Kincaid-Smith, 1973; Molland, 1978; Shelley, 1978; Nanra, 1980; Prescott, 1982a; Bach and Hardy, 1985). In normal doses these drugs could also cause acute prostaglandin-dependent impairment of renal function in patients with compromised renal perfusion but this effect did not seem to be shared by paracetamol (Plotz and Kimberly, 1981; Nanra, 1983).

Paracetamol has been reported to have variable effects on renal prostaglandins. It inhibited the formation of prostaglandins PGE_2, PGD_2 and $PGF_{2\alpha}$ by rabbit renal medulla (Blackwell *et al.*, 1975). There was no reduction in the whole kidney concentrations of prostaglandins PGE_2 and $PGF_{2\alpha}$ in rats given a realistic oral dose of 12 mg kg^{-1} of paracetamol (Bannwarth and Netter, 1994) but in concentrations up to 750 mg l^{-1} it caused a dose-dependent reversible decrease in these prostaglandins associated with a decrease in cyclic adenosine monophosphate (AMP). The inhibition was overcome by adding arachidonic acid but it was not influenced by glutathione. A similar effect was observed *in vivo* following administration of an intraperitoneal dose of 375 mg kg^{-1} (Zenser *et al.*, 1978b). Paracetamol reversibly inhibited the conversion of arachidonic acid to prostaglandin PGE_2 by cyclo-oxygenase in the rat inner medulla and the concentration required for half maximum inhibition was about 15 mg l^{-1} (Mattammal *et al.*, 1979). In another report, however, the corresponding inhibitory concentration for prostaglandin synthetase in rat medulla was 150 mg l^{-1} and p-aminophenol was four to five times more active (Bruchhausen and Baumann, 1982). The greater inhibitory effect of p-aminophenol was noted in other reports (Baumann *et al.*, 1983a,b). Paracetamol could produce either inhibition, stimulation or have no effect on prostaglandin synthesis *in vitro*, depending on the source of the enzyme, drug concentration and experimental conditions. It has been reported to increase the formation of prostaglandin PGE_2 in the rat renal papilla *ex vitro* (Danon *et al.*, 1983) and it was suggested that the stimulation of prostaglandin synthesis in such circumstance made tissues more vulnerable to the effects of aspirin (McDonald-Gibson and Collier,

1979). The effect of paracetamol on renal prostaglandins was shown to be age dependent in rats. The renal production of prostaglandin PGE_2 was greater in neonatal than adult rats, and it was more resistant to inhibition by paracetamol (Reyes *et al.*, 1989; Meléndez *et al.*, 1990). In unanaesthetized newborn rats, paracetamol blocked, rather than enhanced, the increase in urine osmolality caused by water deprivation and this effect was not seen in weanling and adult animals (Reyes and Meléndez, 1990). In man, paracetamol reduced water and sodium excretion in healthy females (Haylor, 1980; Prescott *et al.*, 1990) but in another study it produced a similar effect in elderly subjects but not in young subjects or patients with chronic renal failure (Berg *et al.*, 1990). The reported effects on renal prostaglandins have also been variable. The urinary excretion of prostaglandin PGE_2 was reduced in healthy females in one study (Prescott *et al.*, 1990) but not in another (Bippi and Frölich, 1990), while a significant decrease was reported in elderly subjects and patients with chronic renal failure but not in young healthy subjects of both sexes (Berg *et al.*, 1990). In another report it reduced the urinary excretion of prostaglandins in female subjects and blunted the increase induced by frusemide (Martin and Prescott, 1994). The overall conclusion is that paracetamol had less effect on renal prostaglandins than aspirin and non-steroidal anti-inflammatory drugs, and its actions were variable and inconsistent. If the ischaemia hypothesis for the pathogenesis of renal papillary necrosis was correct, this could account for the difficulty in producing this condition with paracetamol in animals and for the rarity of analgesic nephropathy associated with the use of paracetamol alone in man.

Other Mechanisms

It was possible that paracetamol caused renal tubular and papillary necrosis by a direct cytotoxic action although there was no evidence to support such a mechanism apart from the concentration of the drug in the distal nephron (Bluemle and Goldberg, 1968; Duggin and Mudge, 1975, 1976). The proximal tubules have great powers of regeneration and injury at this site was usually rapidly reversible. In contrast, the regenerative capacity of cells of the lower nephron seemed to be very limited and they could eventually 'die out' with chronic exposure to paracetamol or toxic metabolites to give papillary necrosis (Prescott, 1982a). Verapamil prevented the changes in glomerular filtration rate and tubular function produced by high concentrations of paracetamol in the isolated perfused rat kidney but it was not known whether this effect had a haemodynamic or metabolic basis (Trumper *et al.*, 1993). In toxic doses paracetamol had effects on intermediary metabolism in the kidney. It inhibited glucose synthesis from lactate in rat kidney *in vitro* (Tange *et al.*, 1977) and in another report it inhibited respiration, gluconeogenesis and reduced adenosine triphosphate levels in rat kidney cells (Porter and Dawson, 1979). These effects were proposed as mechanisms of cytotoxicity but their relevance is uncertain as very high concentrations of paracetamol were used (1500 and 600 mg l^{-1} respectively).

14

Hepatotoxicity

Introduction

Although the hepatotoxicity of paracetamol was discovered relatively recently, it rapidly became a cause for concern and attracted much adverse publicity because the drug was used increasingly for self-poisoning and this was frequently complicated by some degree of acute liver damage. There had been no hint of liver damage in the limited toxicity studies carried out before paracetamol was reintroduced into clinical medicine in the 1950s, and hepatotoxicity had not been recognized during the long and widespread medical use of its prodrugs acetanilide and phenacetin. Eder (1964) first reported hepatic necrosis and early cirrhosis in six cats given 25 mg kg^{-1} of paracetamol for four weeks followed by 50 mg kg^{-1} for a further 22 weeks. Four cats died during the study and in two the liver pathology was considered to be sufficient to account for death. Boyd and Bereczky (1966) then described extensive centrilobular hepatic necrosis with sinusoidal congestion in male Wistar rats given paracetamol orally in doses of 2000–7000 mg kg^{-1}, and hepatic necrosis was the main finding in animals dying within 1–7 days. Dose-related hepatic necrosis and cirrhosis were subsequently reported in rats given oral paracetamol for 100 days in doses up to 4000 mg kg^{-1} (Boyd and Hogan, 1968). Davidson and Eastham (1966) reported fatal liver necrosis in two patients who had taken paracetamol in overdosage, and at the same time, Thomson and Prescott (1966) described another patient with liver damage following an overdose. Over the next few years there was a steady increase in the number of cases of paracetamol poisoning with liver damage in the United Kingdom (MacLean *et al.*, 1968a; Proudfoot and Wright, 1970; Prescott *et al.*, 1971; Clark *et al.*, 1973b) and subsequently there have been many hundreds of reports worldwide. The biochemical mechanisms of paracetamol hepatotoxicity involving metabolic activation and covalent binding with a crucial protective role for glutathione were elucidated in a classic series of studies by Mitchell and his colleagues (Jollow *et al.*, 1973; Mitchell *et al.*, 1973b,c; Potter *et al.*, 1973) and this resulted in the rational development of effective antidotal therapy of overdosage (Mitchell *et al.*, 1974; Prescott *et al.*, 1974, 1977b; Crome *et al.*, 1976b; Rumack and Peterson, 1978). Paracetamol has since become a popular model agent for the study of experimental chemically induced hepatic necrosis.

Pathology

The pathological changes in the liver produced by toxic doses of paracetamol have been studied extensively by conventional light microscopy (including histochemical and immunohistological techniques), and by scanning and transmission electron microscopy. The lesions of acute hepatic necrosis developed and evolved with time, so the extent and nature of the abnormalities observed depended on the time interval between dosing and examination. Most studies have been carried out in rats, mice and hamsters and the histological appearances were essentially the same in these species. Similar histological changes have been observed following the administration of paracetamol in cats (Eder, 1964; St. Omer and McKnight, 1980; Savides *et al.*, 1984; Granados-Soto *et al.*, 1993) and dogs (Piperno *et al.*, 1978; Savides *et al.*, 1984; Granados-Soto *et al.*, 1993). Hepatic necrosis and degeneration have also been observed in broiler birds following repeated intramuscular administration of paracetamol (Mohapatra *et al.*, 1993). More detailed studies, sometimes involving very large numbers of animals, have been performed in attempts to produce models of acute hepatic failure with paracetamol in dogs (Gazzard *et al.*, 1975b; Landa Garcia *et al.*, 1984; Ortega *et al.*, 1985; Francavilla *et al.*, 1988, 1989; Panella *et al.*, 1990; Kelly *et al.*, 1992) and pigs (Miller *et al.*, 1976a; Henne-Bruns *et al.*, 1988a,b). Both species developed severe methaemoglobinaemia and haemolysis, and dogs in particular were not suitable for this purpose (Terblanche and Hickman, 1991). Claims have also been made for a 'low dose' (2500 mg kg^{-1}) intravenous infusion model for paracetamol liver injury (Funatsu *et al.*, 1987).

Light Microscopy

The first detailed histopathological study of experimental hepatic necrosis produced by paracetamol was reported by Dixon *et al.* (1971) in rats given single oral doses of 2500 and 3500 mg kg^{-1}. Some rats died within four days and survivors were examined on days 5, 7, 14, 21 and 28. In three of five rats dying within 24 h there was loss of basophilic granules in the cytoplasm of centrilobular hepatocytes with fine hydropic vacuolation and mild-to-moderate sinusoidal congestion. When death occurred between 24 and 48 h there was marked hepatic congestion with dilatation of the central vein and disruption of the surrounding sinusoids, which were packed with red blood cells. Necrosis of centrilobular cells was advanced with nuclear disintegration, pyknosis, karyorrhexis and cytoplasmic eosinophilia. The structure of the liver was largely preserved but in some areas the eosinophilic anuclear cells coalesced to form amorphous masses. The extent of necrosis varied from small foci surrounding the central vein to confluent areas involving the centrilobular and midzonal regions (Figure 14.1). In more severely affected animals, hydropic vacuolation spread into the periportal hepatocytes, and bridging necrosis extended to the remaining areas so that only the portal tracts were preserved amidst an amorphous mass of necrotic hepatocytes and red blood cells (Figure 14.2). At 3–5 days the centrilobular zones were infiltrated with macrophages and occasional polymorphonuclear cells, and there was little evidence of continuing necrosis (Figure 14.3). A further feature at this time was active regeneration of hepatocytes with mitotic figures, cytoplasmic basophilia and hyperchromatic nuclei (Figure 14.4). The reticulin framework was preserved but there was widespread loss of hepatocytes. On

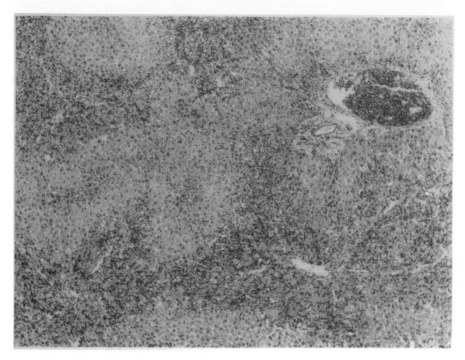

Figure 14.1 Acute hepatic necrosis involving centrilobular and mid-zonal hepatocytes 36–48 h after administration of a hepatotoxic dose of paracetamol in the rat (magnification × 40) (reproduced with permission from Dixon *et al.*, 1971).

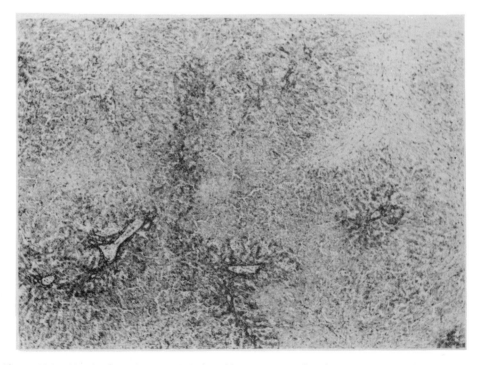

Figure 14.2 Massive hepatic necrosis induced by paracetamol in the rat at 36–48 h showing a narrow rim of surviving hepatocytes around the portal tracts (reticulin stain, magnification × 40) (reproduced with permission from Dixon *et al.*, 1971).

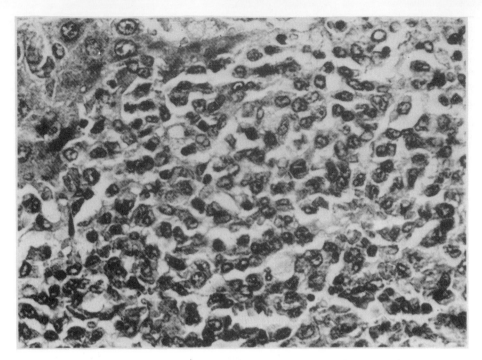

Figure 14.3 Paracetamol-induced hepatic necrosis in the rat after five days showing cellular infiltrate of macrophages and polymorphonuclear leucocytes (magnification × 360) (reproduced with permission from Dixon *et al.*, 1971).

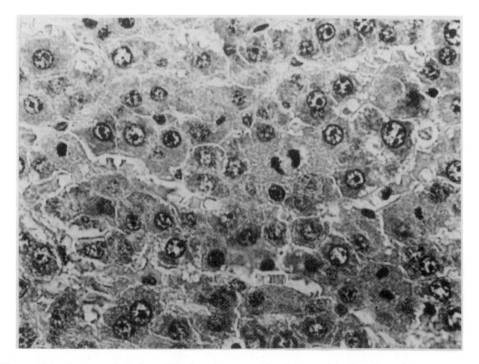

Figure 14.4 Regeneration of surviving hepatocytes with mitotic activity five days after administration of a toxic dose of paracetamol in the rat (magnification × 360) (reproduced with permission from Bartolone *et al.*, 1989b).

the 7th day restoration was advanced and by the 14th, 21st and 28th days the appearances were normal apart from scattered residual foci of collapsed reticulin. The sequence of events could be summarized as centrilobular necrosis followed by macrophage infiltration, regeneration and rapid complete recovery. Similar findings were reported in mice and rats by Mitchell *et al.* (1973b), who also noted early loss of hepatic glycogen and sparing of the Kupffer cells. The changes occurred more rapidly in mice than in rats and the extent of necrosis at various times after administration was dose dependent within species. In mice, glycogen loss and vacuolization of centrilobular hepatocytes resulted in clear demarcation of the affected centrilobular areas from the rest of the liver by 2 h and gross necrosis was evident by 6 h reaching a maximum by 24–48 h. Necrosis was established by 12 h in hamsters with the maximum damage at 24–48 h and regeneration was evident at 48–72 h (Potter *et al.*, 1974). In mice given 500 mg kg^{-1} of paracetamol orally, the earliest detectable abnormality was vacuolation along the sinusoidal margins of centrilobular cells at 1 h after dosing. Centrilobular congestion was conspicuous by 3 h and at this time there was necrosis of single cells as evidenced by swollen 'balloon' cells. By 6 h, centrilobular necrosis was established in many animals (Walker *et al.*, 1980). A similar sequence of events was observed in another study in mice treated with 600 mg kg^{-1} of oral paracetamol. Glycogen was depleted in centrilobular areas by 2 h and staining with oil-Red-O revealed intracellular lipid droplets by 4 h after doses of 600 mg kg^{-1} and 8 h after doses of 300 mg kg^{-1}. Following the smaller dose, the histological appearances had nearly returned to normal by 18–24 h (Placke *et al.*, 1987a).

Many other investigators have described the histological changes in the liver following toxic doses of paracetamol. The early depletion of glycogen was confirmed (Dixon *et al.*, 1975a; Chiu and Bhakthan, 1978; Linscheer *et al.*, 1980; Klugmann *et al.*, 1984; MacDonald *et al.*, 1984; Price *et al.*, 1987; Skoglund *et al.*, 1987; Bhatia *et al.*, 1988; McLean *et al.*, 1989; Ansari *et al.*, 1991; Juzwiak *et al.*, 1992; Rainska *et al.*, 1992; Muriel *et al.*, 1993) and there were frequent references to initial vacuolation of affected hepatocytes, which was often attributed to hydropic change (Dixon *et al.*, 1975a; Buttar *et al.*, 1976; Piperno *et al.*, 1978; Strubelt *et al.*, 1979; Linscheer *et al.*, 1980; Sato *et al.*, 1981b; Walker *et al.*, 1981, 1985; Raheja *et al.*, 1983b; Savides *et al.*, 1984; Ortega *et al.*, 1985; Gale *et al.*, 1987; Henne-Bruns *et al.*, 1988a; Francavilla *et al.*, 1989; Roberts *et al.*, 1991b; Muriel *et al.*, 1993; Sakr, 1993; Yamada *et al.*, 1993). The later appearance of lipid droplets (steatosis) was also noted in the necrotic hepatocytes (Dixon *et al.*, 1971; Gazzard *et al.*, 1975b; Walker *et al.*, 1980; Poulsen *et al.*, 1981; Rosenbaum *et al.*, 1984; Helliwell *et al.*, 1985; Placke *et al.*, 1987a; Davies *et al.*, 1991; Rainska *et al.*, 1992). The liver was congested with red blood cells at an early stage and the necrotic lesions were frequently haemorrhagic in nature (Dixon *et al.*, 1971; Miller *et al.*, 1976a; Chiu and Bhakthan, 1978; Walker *et al.*, 1981, 1983b,c; Ginsberg *et al.*, 1982; Sharma *et al.*, 1983; Savides *et al.*, 1984; Ortega *et al.*, 1985; Hazelton *et al.*, 1986a; Placke *et al.*, 1987a; Guarner *et al.*, 1988; Jeffery and Haschek, 1988; Francavilla *et al.*, 1989; McLean *et al.*, 1989; Panella *et al.*, 1990; Devictor *et al.*, 1992; Madhu *et al.*, 1992b). The hepatic sequestration of erythrocytes contributed to acute anaemia in pigs (Miller *et al.*, 1977) and in mice, the congestion resulted in a rapid increase in liver weight with striking enlargement and engorgement of the liver (Figure 14.5) (Corcoran *et al.*, 1985a). Following oral administration of 750 mg kg^{-1} of paracetamol in mice, extensive confluent necrosis was always associated with massive congestion. As a

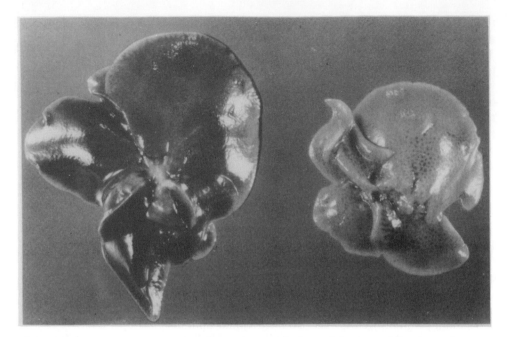

Figure 14.5 Massive engorgement and congestion in the liver of the mouse following oral administration of 1200 mg kg^{-1} of paracetamol (left). The liver on the right was from a control mouse, which had also been treated with N-acetylcysteine to prevent hepatotoxicity (reproduced with permission from Corcoran *et al.*, 1985a).

consequence of the sequestration of red blood cells in the liver there was a significant decrease in the haematocrit of peripheral blood, and an increase in liver size, weight, content of water and haemoglobin, and an increase in the ^{125}I-albumin space. These changes reached a maximum at 4 h after which time they regressed (Figure 14.6) (Walker *et al.*, 1985). Congestion of the liver with blood following a toxic dose of paracetamol was responsible for the increase in liver weight and could be so extreme as to cause early hypovolaemic shock (Wright and Moore, 1991). The congestion observed with severe necrosis was also associated with reduced liver blood flow (Funatsu *et al.*, 1987) and it was referred to as intrahepatic bleeding (Murase *et al.*, 1986). It was suggested that neutrophil accumulation in the hepatic microcirculation might aggravate toxicity by impeding blood flow. However, hepatotoxic doses of paracetamol did not upregulate the messenger RNA for intercellular adhesion molecule-1 (ICAM-1), a critical determinant of neutrophil adhesion and activation, and ultimately, of neutrophil-mediated tissue injury (Welty *et al.*, 1993).

When necrosis of hepatocytes became established, macrophages and inflammatory cells were seen to infiltrate the zone of injury to clear away the cellular debris and allow regeneration and repair (Figure 14.7). The extent of this inflammatory reaction varied according to the severity of the necrosis, and within species it was time dependent. In rats, for example, the maximum macrophage response occurred 3–5 days after administration of a hepatotoxic dose of paracetamol (Dixon *et al.*, 1971; Zieve *et al.*, 1985a), and in mice there was an intense inflammatory reaction at the junction of necrotic and surviving hepatocytes after three days (Roberts *et al.*,

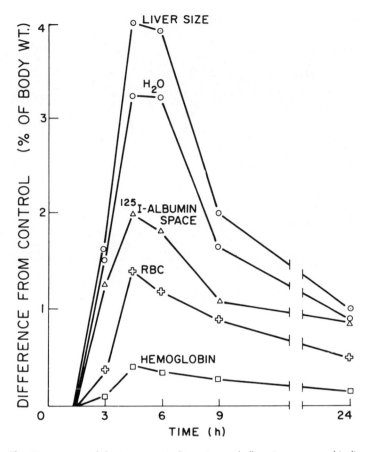

Figure 14.6 The time course of the increases in liver size and albumin space, and in liver water, red blood cell and haemoglobin content resulting from hepatic congestion following oral administration of a hepatotoxic dose of 750 mg kg^{-1} of paracetamol in mice (reproduced with permission from Walker *et al.*, 1985).

1991b). The cellular response was described variously as inflammatory, polymorphonuclear, granulocytic, neutrocytic, neutrophilic and leucocytic with or without a greater or lesser macrophage response (Mitchell *et al.*, 1973b; Dixon *et al.*, 1975a; Linscheer *et al.*, 1980; Calder *et al.*, 1981b; Sato *et al.*, 1981b; Raheja *et al.*, 1982; Ghosh and De, 1983; Klugmann *et al.*, 1984; Hazelton *et al.*, 1986a; Bhatia *et al.*, 1988; Endo *et al.*, 1988a; Younes *et al.*, 1988; Francavilla *et al.*, 1989; Roberts *et al.*, 1991b; Juzwiak *et al.*, 1992; Madhu *et al.*, 1992b; Muriel *et al.*, 1993). In other reports the infiltration was referred to as lymphocytic (Buttar *et al.*, 1976; Sakr, 1993) or even eosinophilic (Handa and Sharma, 1990). Other investigators have observed a predominately macrocytic or histiocytic response (Strubelt *et al.*, 1979; Zieve *et al.*, 1985a) and the cells were described as plump, with bulky cytoplasm and indented 'monocytoid' nuclei. Acidophil or Councilman-like bodies have been noted occasionally (Dixon *et al.*, 1975a; Linscheer *et al.*, 1980; Mehrotra *et al.*, 1983; Ortega *et al.*, 1985).

Even with doses of paracetamol that did not produce frank necrosis, there was centrilobular accumulation of activated macrophages. Compared with the resident

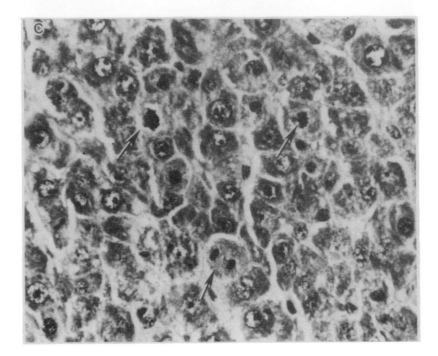

Figure 14.7   Prominent mitotic activity in hepatocytes 54 h after acute paracetamol-induced hepatic necrosis in the rat (magnification × 400) (reproduced with permission from Zieve *et al.*, 1985a).

Kupffer cells, these cells were highly vacuolated, generally larger, more actively phagocytic and had greater levels of migration. Macrophage accumulation and activation appeared to be mediated by factors released from the hepatocytes, and were time and dose dependent (Laskin and Pilaro, 1986; Laskin *et al.*, 1986). In turn, the macrophages appeared to release substances that activated endothelial cells and both cell types produced reactive mediators which were cytotoxic to injured hepatocytes (Laskin, 1991). Potentiation of the hepatotoxicity of allyl alcohol and 1,1-dichloroethylene by previous exposure to paracetamol was attributed to the formation of these mediators (Wright and Moore, 1991). However, other studies have suggested that infiltrating polymorphs do not contribute to parenchymal hepatic cell injury (Jaeschke *et al.*, 1991).

In severe acute paracetamol-induced hepatic necrosis, the reticulin framework of the liver lobule was largely preserved and regeneration occurred after the infiltration of macrophages. Three to five days after administration of a toxic dose of paracetamol in rats many cells showed evidence of regeneration with increased cytoplasmic basophilia, double nuclei and mitotic figures but these changes were less obvious by the seventh day. The first signs of regeneration could be observed at 48 h in rats (Mitchell *et al.*, 1973b; Dixon *et al.*, 1975a) and at 24 h in mice (Juzwiak *et al.*, 1992). Mitotic activity in hepatocytes became a prominent feature in rats given repeated daily doses of paracetamol over periods of 4–7 days (Strubelt *et al.*, 1979; Juzwiak *et al.*, 1992; Rainska *et al.*, 1992). Protection against paracetamol hepatotoxicity with diltiazem was associated with increased mitotic activity (Deakin *et al.*, 1991). Following acute paracetamol-induced hepatic injury in rats there was a biphasic rise in the activity of liver ornithine decarboxylase, an enzyme that reflected the earliest phases of cell multiplication. The early peak preceded the peak occurrence of histological necrosis that was followed in turn by the maximal response of liver thymidine kinase activity (which reflected DNA synthesis), histological regeneration as shown by mitoses, and repair (Zieve *et al.*, 1985a, 1986). There was no evidence of continuing necrosis seven days after a toxic dose of paracetamol in rats but the hepatocytes showed increased basophilia, hyperchromatic nuclei and few mitotic figures. After 14–28 days the appearances had returned essentially to normal (Dixon *et al.*, 1971). Similar sequences of morphological and biochemical abnormalities were seen in rat and hamster liver slices incubated with toxic concentrations of paracetamol. The toxicity observed in liver slices was an excellent predictor of hepatotoxicity *in vivo* (Miller *et al.*, 1993a).

Histochemical and Immunohistochemical Changes

Following the administration of hepatotoxic doses of paracetamol, many investigators noted the early loss of liver glycogen as shown by periodic acid-Schiff (PAS) staining, and as necrosis developed there was progressive loss of activity of other liver enzymes including ethanol, lactic, malic, isocitric and succinic dehydrogenases, glucose-6-phosphatase, γ-glutamyltransferase, acid phosphatase, NADPH-cytochrome *c* reductase, cytochrome oxidase and aniline hydroxylase (Dixon *et al.*, 1975a; Chiu and Bhakthan, 1978; Smail *et al.*, 1981; Sharma *et al.*, 1983; Bhatia *et al.*, 1988). With long-term administration of paracetamol there were no histochemical abnormalities in one study (Bhatia and Bhatia, 1990), but in another there was slight enhancement of focal lesions that were positive for γ-glutamyl transferase but no promotion of glutathione S-transferase positive nodules (Maruyama *et al.*, 1990). Glycogen phosphorylase *a* activity was assayed histochemically in rats as an indication of free cytosolic Ca^{2+} concentrations. It increased progressively, starting in the perivenous zone and spreading to midzonal and periportal areas 9–24 h after administration of a toxic dose of paracetamol. The increase in glycogen phosphorylase *a* activity preceded the major loss of membrane integrity as shown by increasing serum aminotransferase activity and the uptake of trypan blue by perfused hepatocytes (Behrendt and Cserepes, 1985; Jepson *et al.*, 1987; Horton and Wood, 1989).

The 3-(cystein-S-yl)-paracetamol-protein adduct was considered to be the definitive end-product of the critical covalent binding of paracetamol that caused the injury and necrosis of hepatocytes. Accordingly, anti-serum specific for this adduct was used to demonstrate its formation, distribution and concentration in the livers of treated mice, and the correlation with cell injury as a function of dose and time. The adduct could be shown immunohistochemically within the liver lobule, and it appeared in a progressive central-to-peripheral pattern. There was a good correlation between the intensity of the immunohistochemical response and the amount of adduct in hepatic supernatant as shown by particle concentration fluorescence immunoassay. The immunochemically detectable adduct appeared before the onset of centrilobular necrosis and was localized in distinctive lobular zones in a dose-dependent manner (Figure 14.8). The binding of paracetamol to liver proteins occurred before depletion of total hepatic glutathione, and at doses that did not produce hepatic necrosis. There was immunohistochemical evidence of the binding

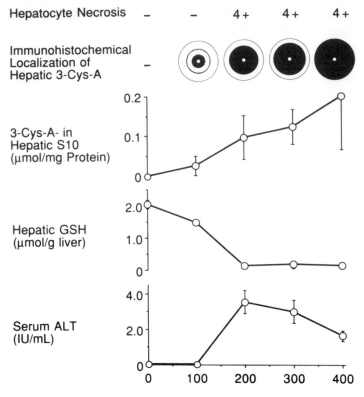

Hepatocyte Necrosis — — 4+ 4+ 4+

Immunohistochemical Localization of Hepatic 3-Cys-A

3-Cys-A- in Hepatic S10 (μmol/mg Protein)

Hepatic GSH (μmol/g liver)

Serum ALT (IU/mL)

Dose Response: mg/kg Acetaminophen

Figure 14.8 The dose–response relationship between paracetamol (acetaminophen)-induced hepatotoxicity at 2 h in mice and the liver content and immunohistochemical localization of the 3-(cystein-S-yl) paracetamol protein adduct (3-Cys-A). Histological hepatic necrosis was graded in severity from 1 + to 4 + and the relative density of the immunohistochemically localized 3-(cystein-S-yl paracetamol protein adduct is represented as circular symbols in which diameter and darkness of shading symbolically represent relative differences in the area and intensity of binding around representative centrilobular regions (reproduced with permission from Roberts *et al.*, 1991b).

of paracetamol to the hepatocyte nucleus. The paracetamol-protein adduct was also found in metabolically active and dividing hepatocytes and in the macrophages in the regenerating liver (Roberts *et al.*, 1991b). The effects of paracetamol-induced liver damage on α-fetoprotein and the antigens of liver cell plasma membranes in regenerating mouse liver have been studied using immunohistochemical methods (Gleiberman *et al.*, 1983).

Individual Variation

Considerable individual variation was noted in the susceptibility to paracetamol-induced hepatic necrosis but the severity always parallelled the extent of covalent binding of the drug (Jollow *et al.*, 1973). The survival of pigs given toxic doses of paracetamol as a model for experimental fulminant hepatic failure was unpredictable, and the mean survival time was not inversely related to dose as would normally be expected (Miller *et al.*, 1976a). Not only was there individual variation in the histological extent of damage between animals, but there was also variation in the distribution of necrosis within the different lobes of the liver in a particular animal (Kelleher *et al.*, 1977; Calder *et al.*, 1981b; Leonard *et al.*, 1985a; Guarner *et al.*, 1988; Martinelli *et al.*, 1989). In some cases there were large areas of confluent necrosis in the same lobe of the liver as central veins about which there was comparatively little damage (Walker *et al.*, 1985; Francavilla *et al.*, 1989).

Histological Scores

Arbitrary scores have been developed according to the proportion of necrotic cells within representative areas as observed by light microscopy in attempts to quantitate the extent of paracetamol-induced acute hepatic damage (Mitchell *et al.*, 1973b; Linscheer *et al.*, 1980; El-Hage *et al.*, 1983; Leonard *et al.*, 1985a; Zieve *et al.*, 1985a; Jaszewski and Sheridan, 1987; Panella *et al.*, 1990; and many others). Automated techniques based on the differential staining properties of viable and necrotic cells with correction for the non-parenchymal cells have also been described (Dixon *et al.*, 1975b).

Electron Microscopy

There have been several reports of the ultrastructural changes produced in the liver by toxic doses of paracetamol. In rats, 6 h after a dose of 3000 mg kg^{-1}, there was disorganization and matrix swelling of the mitochondria followed at 12 h by disintegration of the canalicular system and breakdown of the plasma membrane. Further changes at 24 and 48 h included condensation of the nucleus and vacuolation of the cytoplasm of the necrotic cells with mitochondrial degeneration. After phagocytosis by macrophages, the collections of cellular debris aggregated to form large, generally spherical electron-dense inclusions. These spherical acidophil bodies were observed within macrophages, or lying free in the sinusoids, and were composed of compacted mitochondrial endoplasmic reticulun and small clear vesicles. In the hepatocytes adjacent to the zone of necrosis the cells were dense and contained vacuoles loosely packed with amorphous electron-dense material. The cytoplasm contained well-formed regular endoplasmic reticulum surrounding mitochondria of normal size but with dense matrices and irregular cristae. The microvilli were reduced in size and number (Dixon *et al.*, 1975b). In the hepatocytes of hamsters there was progressive loss of structural integrity of the endoplasmic reticulum, swelling of the cisternae into vesicles with fatty infiltration and vacuolation, and sinusoidal congestion. Subsequent changes included collapse and denaturation of the plasma membrane and the appearance of lamellated myeloid figures. Parasinusoidal Kupffer cells were seen to phagocytose the cellular debris and there was extensive accumulation of membrane-bound aggregates of the myeloid figures (Chiu and Bhakthan, 1978). In a time course study in mice given doses of 300 and 600 mg kg^{-1} of paracetamol, vesiculation, vacuolation and mitochondrial and plasma membrane degeneration culminated in widespread centrilobular necrosis by 8 h after the higher dose. With 300 mg kg^{-1} the lesions were restricted and developed more slowly (Placke *et al.*, 1987a). In dogs, vesiculation of the smooth endoplasmic reticulum was associated with lamellar and myelin-like structures (Ortega *et al.*, 1985). These electron microscopic findings, and in particular, the early and extensive mitochondrial disorganization were confirmed by other investigators (Linscheer *et al.*, 1980; Sato *et al.*, 1981a; Marzella *et al.*, 1986; Funatsu *et al.*, 1987; Henne-Bruns *et al.*, 1988a,b; González *et al.*, 1992; Kelly *et al.*, 1992; Harris and Hamrick, 1993).

In detailed scanning and transmission electron microscopic studies of paracetamol-induced hepatic necrosis in mice, the sequence of events was observed in relation to the development of hepatic congestion. There was early endocytic vacuolation and loss of microvilli with enlargement of the Disse space. The vacuoles were largely membrane-bound and sometimes contained remnants of the microvillae. Hepatic congestion developed as red blood cells entered the enlarged Disse space and endocytic vacuoles through enlarged pores in the sinusoidal lining cells (Walker *et al.*, 1980, 1983c). During the first seven days of chronic administration of paracetamol in rats, there was loss of the microvilli at the sinusoidal and biliary surfaces of the hepatocytes together with swelling and vacuolation of the mitochondria. By the 12th–14th week of dosing, lipid vacuoles in the hepatocytes were associated with granular mitochondria showing loss of the cristae and containing electron-dense bodies. There was also fragmentation of the rough endoplasmic reticulum (Mehrotra *et al.*, 1983).

Cytotoxicity

The cytotoxic properties of paracetamol and N-acetyl-p-benzoquinoneimine have been demonstrated in hepatocytes isolated from rats (Hayes *et al.*, 1984, 1986; Hill and Burk, 1984; van de Straat *et al.*, 1986; Koo *et al.*, 1987; Kyle *et al.*, 1987, 1988; 1990; Tee *et al.*, 1987; Andersson *et al.*, 1990; Lawrence and Benford, 1990; Smolarek *et al.*, 1990; O'Brien *et al.*, 1991; and others), mice (Acosta *et al.*, 1980; Holme *et al.*, 1984, 1991; Harman, 1985; Harman and McCamish, 1986; Birge *et al.*, 1989; Bruno *et al.*, 1992; Harman *et al.*, 1992b; Grewal and Racz, 1993), hamsters (Harman and Fischer, 1983; Boobis *et al.*, 1986, 1990; Tee *et al.*, 1986b, 1987; Lupo *et al.*, 1987; Hardwick *et al.*, 1992a,b), rabbits, dogs and monkeys (Smolarek *et al.*, 1990), and man (Boobis *et al.*, 1986; Tee *et al.*, 1987; Larrauri *et al.*, 1989; Lawrence and Benford, 1990). In most studies, the hepatocytes were isolated by treatment with collagenase and prepared as hepatocyte suspensions or primary monolayer cultures where the growing cells adhered to a collagen-coated glass surface. The viability of hepatocytes was assessed by their ability to exclude trypan blue and adhere to glass, and toxicity was shown by the appearance of characteristic 'blebbing' of the cell membrane (Walker *et al.*, 1983a; Tee *et al.*, 1986b, 1987; Koo *et al.*, 1987; Harman *et al.*, 1992b; Nasseri-Sina *et al.*, 1992). Toxicity was assessed quantitatively by the fraction of cells unable to exclude trypan blue (Tee *et al.*, 1986b, 1987; Andersson *et al.*, 1990) and leakage of substances such as lactic dehydrogenase from the damaged hepatocytes (Moldéus, 1978). Cytotoxicity was also shown by necrosis of cells and disintegration of the monolayer with detachment of large areas (Milam and Byard, 1985). Other methods used to determine the viability of hepatocytes after exposure to paracetamol included the intracellular fluorescence of 2,'7'-bis-(2-carboxyethyl)-5-(6)-carboxyfluorescein (Riley *et al.*, 1993), protein staining with sulphorhodamine B

(Hall *et al.*, 1993), kenacid blue R binding to protein (Benford *et al.*, 1990) and the uptake and metabolism of p-iodonitrotetrazolium violet (Bruschi and Priestly, 1990).

The cytotoxicity of paracetamol varied considerably between species and this variation was related to differences in the extent of metabolic activation (Boobis *et al.*, 1986; Tee *et al.*, 1987; Smolarek *et al.*, 1990). Hepatocytes isolated from rats, rabbits, monkeys and man were relatively resistant while those from mouse, hamster and dog were more sensitive (Boobis *et al.*, 1986; Tee *et al.*, 1987; Gómez-Lechón *et al.*, 1988; Smolarek *et al.*, 1990; O'Brien *et al.*, 1991). Paracetamol cytotoxicity was concentration and time dependent (Acosta *et al.*, 1980; Harman and Fischer, 1983; Beales *et al.*, 1985; Boobis *et al.*, 1986; Harman and McCamish, 1986; Tee *et al.*, 1986b, 1987; Gómez-Lechón *et al.*, 1988; Birge *et al.*, 1989; Bruschi and Priestly, 1990; Smolarek *et al.*, 1990; Bruno *et al.*, 1992; Hardwick *et al.*, 1992b; Harman *et al.*, 1992b; Grewal and Racz, 1993; and others), and was always associated with intracellular glutathione depletion (Harman and Fischer, 1983; Harman, 1985; Boobis *et al.*, 1986; Farber *et al.*, 1988; Donatus *et al.*, 1990; Burcham and Harman, 1991; Grewal and Racz, 1993). In comparative cytotoxicity studies with the human hepatoma cell line HepG2, acute exposure to paracetamol at a concentration of 1057 mg l^{-1} produced 50 per cent hepatotoxicity and chronic exposure at 151 mg l^{-1} caused significant morphological changes (Hall *et al.*, 1993). The cytotoxicity of paracetamol was greater in hepatocytes than in non-hepatic cell lines (Ekwall and Acosta, 1982; Jover *et al.*, 1992; Shrivastava *et al.*, 1992).

The most obvious morphological sign of pre-lethal paracetamol toxicity in isolated hepatocytes was blebbing of the cell membrane (Figure 14.9). This preceded the increase in permeability to trypan blue and leakage of lactic dehydrogenase from damaged cells, and was attributed to decreased plasma membrane stability caused by the effects of calcium on the cell cytoskeleton (Moore *et al.*, 1985a; Tee *et al.*, 1986b; Koo *et al.*, 1987; Nasseri-Sina *et al.*, 1992). Bleb formation did not correlate with, but preceded, the rise in intracellular calcium associated with lethal cytotoxicity produced by paracetamol (Harman *et al.*, 1992b). By means of rhodamine-phalloidin fluorescence microscopy it was shown that rat hepatocytes cultured in monolayers developed a characteristic pattern of prominent polar aggregates of short F-actin microfilament bundles when exposed to toxic concentrations of paracetamol. These changes occurred before blebbing, loss of trypan blue exclusion and release of lactic dehydrogenase into the medium (Koo *et al.*, 1987). In one report, incubation of rat monolayer hepatocyte cultures with 600 and 2400 mg l^{-1} of paracetamol did not result in blebbing despite damage as shown by trypan blue exclusion and release of lactic dehydrogenase. However, dimethylsulphoxide had been used as the solvent (Hayes and Pickering, 1985). Paracetamol had little effect on enzyme release or DNA content in isolated trout hepatocytes but it interfered with cell-to-cell aggregation (Blair *et al.*, 1989).

The morphological abnormalities of paracetamol toxicity in isolated hepatocytes as shown by scanning and transmission electron microscopy were similar to those observed *in vivo*. The changes included surface blebbing, progressive loss of microvilli, gross distortion of the cell membrane, mitochondrial abnormalities and loss of microvilli in the bile canaliculi (Tee *et al.*, 1986b). In another report, bleb formation was again a prominent feature. The process was considered to be analogous to the endocytic vacuolation observed at the cell margins due to intravascular pressure from the sinusoids, and caused by dysfunction of the microfilament component of

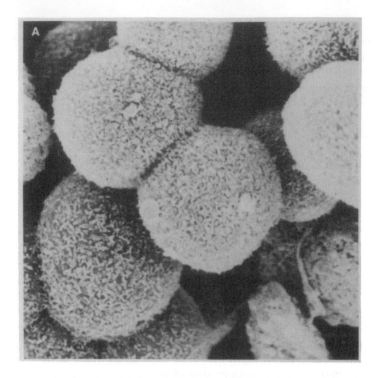

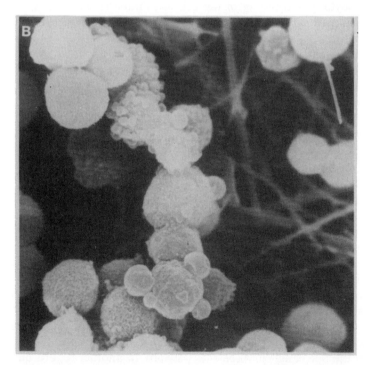

Figure 14.9 Scanning electron micrographs of isolated hamster hepatocyes showing (A) normal appearances following incubation in buffer alone (× 2250) and (B) cytotoxicity with blebbing after incubation with 2.5 mM paracetamol for 90 min (× 900) (reproduced with permission from Tee *et al.*, 1986b).

the cytoskeleton (Walker *et al.*, 1983a). Paracetamol-induced changes in the smooth endoplasmic reticulum and the distribution of glycogen in hepatocytes have also been noted (Gómez-Lechón *et al.*, 1988). Hepatotoxicity was associated with fragmentation of DNA (Shen *et al.*, 1991, 1992) and early loss of large genomic DNA (Ray *et al.*, 1990, 1991, 1993b).

Chronic Administration and Tolerance

Histological liver damage was greater in rats given single doses of 500 and 1000 mg kg^{-1} than it was after the same doses had been given twice daily for seven days (Buttar *et al.*, 1976). There was severe hepatic necrosis initially in rats given 1000 mg kg^{-1} of paracetamol daily for four days, but tolerance appeared to develop rapidly and only minor changes were evident after the fourth day (Strubelt *et al.*, 1979). Following the administration of 330 mg kg^{-1} of paracetamol in the diet for eight weeks there was initial moderate damage after which there was evidence of subacute hepatitis (Mehrotra *et al.*, 1982). Tolerance to the acute hepatotoxicity of paracetamol was also seen in rats given the relatively small dose of 200 mg kg^{-1} orally six days a week for up to 14 weeks. Centrilobular necrosis increased in severity up to the fifth day after which the changes regressed. By 12–14 weeks the only abnormalities were diffusely scattered ballooned hepatocytes, congested sinusoids and prominent Kupffer cells (Mehrotra *et al.*, 1983). Similarly, hepatic necrosis induced by a single dose of 400 mg kg^{-1} of paracetamol in mice greatly reduced the mortality produced by a second dose of 750 mg kg^{-1} given 24 h later (Jaszewski and Sheridan, 1987), and previous repeated administration of small daily doses of paracetamol reduced the severity of liver necrosis produced by a large hepatotoxic dose (Bhatia *et al.*, 1988). In contrast to these findings, other investigators have noted continuing hepatic necrosis and degeneration in cats and rats dosed daily with paracetamol for periods of weeks or months (Eder, 1964; Boyd and Hogan, 1968). In rats given 4250 mg kg^{-1} of paracetamol daily for 18 weeks, hepatic function as shown by the protrhombin index was depressed to a lesser extent than in rats given a single dose although, not surprisingly, histological examination of the chronically treated rats showed varying degrees of hepatic necrosis (Poulsen and Thomsen, 1988). In mice given diets containing 5000 and 10 000 parts per million of paracetamol for up to 70 weeks, more than half of the high-dose group died before 24 weeks and only 16 per cent survived the experiment. Histological abnormalities included hepatocytomegaly with bizarre nuclei, variable hepatic necrosis, cirrhosis and lipofuchsin deposition (Hagiwara and Ward, 1986). In another study in mice maintained on diets containing the same amounts of paracetamol for 24 weeks, there was some continuing hepatic necrosis with post-necrotic changes and prominent hepatocytomegaly (Waalkes and Ward, 1989). Mice examined after treatment with 300 mg kg^{-1} daily for 4, 8, 12, 16, 20 and 24 weeks showed minor histological abnormalities but no evidence of hepatic necrosis or fibrosis (Bhatia and Bhatia, 1990). Further evidence that repeated administration of large doses of paracetamol could cause continuing severe liver injury was shown by centrilobular necrosis and fibrosis with little inflammatory cell or macrophage response in rats given a diet containing up to 1.25 per cent of paracetamol for 41 and 48 weeks (Maruyama and Williams, 1988). In mice given 1 per cent of paracetamol in the diet for three months, the livers became shrunken and nodular with the appearances of chronic active hepatitis (Ham *et al.*, 1981) and in another report, fibrosis was observed in rats given a diet containing 1.25 per cent paracetamol for 41 weeks (Amo and Matsuyama, 1985). Liver function tests were abnormal in a dachshund which had been given 325 mg of paracetamol daily by its owner for six weeks (Harvey *et al.*, 1986). Progressive hepatic damage with coagulation necrosis, occasional fibrosis and an increasing lymphofollicular reaction was also reported in broiler birds given daily intramuscular paracetamol for eight weeks (Mohapatra *et al.*, 1993). In rats given approximately 300 mg kg^{-1} of paracetamol daily in the diet for up to 24 weeks, there was no evidence of hepatic necrosis but there was fatty change and focal 'ballooning' of hepatocytes associated with swelling of mitochondria and distension of the rough endoplasmic reticulum (Bhatia and Bhatia, 1990). There was no evidence of hepatic pathology in rats given 200 mg kg^{-1} of paracetamol daily with and without the same dose of aspirin for 200 days (Thomas *et al.*, 1977a) and following the administration of 20 mg kg^{-1} of paracetamol daily for 90 days in rats the histological findings were limited to minor macro- and microvesicular fatty change (Khedun *et al.*, 1993).

Biochemical Abnormalities

The acute hepatic injury produced by paracetamol was associated with a variety of biochemical abnormalities and these could usually be attributed to release of intracellular constituents into the circulation following loss of integrity of the cell membrane, or interference with normal hepatocyte metabolism and function. One of the most sensitive and dramatic indicators of acute hepatocyte injury was the release of intracellular enzymes such as lactic dehydrogenase and aminotransferases into the circulation, or, in the case of *in vitro* studies, into the suspending solvent or culture medium. Walker *et al.* (1974) observed dramatic increases in the plasma activity of aspartate and alanine aminotransferases (AST, SGOT and ALT, SGPT respectively) in rats 24 h after administration of 4000 mg kg^{-1} of paracetamol and there was a close correlation between histological evidence of hepatic necrosis and plasma enzyme activities. In a similar, more detailed study, Dixon *et al.* (1975b) also found a good correlation between histological liver damage and plasma transaminase activity at 24 h after dosing (Figure 14.10) but the relationship was less certain during recovery after 36 and 72 h. The increase in serum aspartate and alanine aminotransferase was time and dose dependent as shown in hamsters in Figure 14.11. There was a similar pattern in rats following an oral dose of 1000 mg kg^{-1} of paracetamol with a delay before the aspartate and alanine transaminase activities began to increase at 12 h and maximum elevation to 56–100 times the respective control values at 18 h. The enzyme activities then declined rapidly and were approaching control values by 72 h (Buttar *et al.*, 1976). In most acute toxicity studies with paracetamol *in vivo*, activity of plasma aminotransaminases has been measured routinely as the primary index of liver damage, and the same dose and time dependence of the response was observed (Strubelt *et al.*, 1979; Linscheer *et al.*, 1980; Green *et al.*, 1984b; Corcoran *et al.*, 1985a; Fouse and Hodgson, 1987; Lee *et al.*, 1987; Brzeznicka and Piotrowski, 1989; Panella *et al.*, 1990; Roberts *et al.*, 1991b; and others). Other intracellular enzymes released into the circulation following acute paracetamol-induced hepatic necrosis that have been monitored for this purpose include sorbitol dehydrogenase (Strubelt *et al.*, 1974, 1978, 1979; Buttar *et*

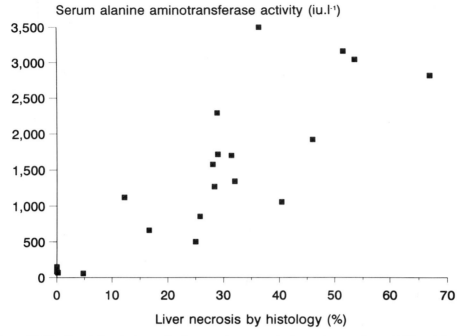

Figure 14.10 Correlation between the increase in serum alanine aminotransferase (ALT) activity and extent of histological hepatic necrosis 24 h after oral administration of 4000 mg kg^{-1} of paracetamol in rats (data from Dixon *et al.*, 1975b).

al., 1976; Siegers and Younes, 1979; Strubelt and Breining, 1980; Younes and Siegers, 1980b, 1985a,b; Ginsberg *et al.*, 1982; Zieve *et al.*, 1986; Lupo *et al.*, 1987; Placke *et al.*, 1987a; Burcham and Harman, 1988; Pakuts *et al.*, 1988; Rikans and Moore, 1988; Brzeznicka and Piotrowski, 1989; Siegers and Möller-Hartmann, 1989; Werner and Wendel, 1990; Davies *et al.*, 1991; Dwivedi *et al.*, 1991; Madhu and Klaassen, 1991; Szymanska *et al.*, 1991; Liu *et al.*, 1992c; Nicholls-Grzemski *et al.*, 1992; Harvey *et al.*, 1993); alkaline phosphatase (Miller *et al.*, 1976a; El-Hage *et al.*, 1983; Ghosh and De, 1983; Ortega *et al.*, 1985; Corcoran and Wong, 1987; Fouse and Hodgson, 1987; Henne-Bruns *et al.*, 1988a,b; Udosen *et al.*, 1989; Handa and Sharma, 1990; Nakae *et al.*, 1990a; Raje and Bhattacharya, 1990; Ansari *et al.*, 1991; Udosen and Ebong, 1991; Chattopadhyay *et al.*, 1992; Gilani and Janbaz, 1992; Juzwiak *et al.*, 1992; Muriel *et al.*, 1992; Shukla *et al.*, 1992a,b; Singh *et al.*, 1992; Visen *et al.*, 1993); lactic dehydrogenase (Green *et al.*, 1984b; Ortega *et al.*, 1985; Fouse and Hodgson, 1987; Nicholls-Grzemski *et al.*, 1992; Strubelt and Younes, 1992); γ-glutamyltranspeptidase (Dwivedi *et al.*, 1991; Muriel *et al.*, 1992, 1993); glutamic dehydrogenase (Strubelt *et al.*, 1974; Siegers *et al.*, 1978; Sato *et al.*, 1981a,b; Ansari *et al.*, 1991; Shukla *et al.*, 1992b); acid phosphatase (Acosta *et al.*, 1980; Ansari *et al.*, 1991; Chattopadhyay *et al.*, 1992; Shukla *et al.*, 1992b); gluta-thione S-transferase (Davies *et al.*, 1991; Wang and Peng, 1993); isocitric dehydroge-nase (Kapetanovic and Mieyal, 1979; Mitra *et al.*, 1991); malic dehydrogenase (Zieve *et al.*, 1985a, 1986); argininosuccinate lyase (Acosta *et al.*, 1980); ornithine carbamyltransferase (Hirayama *et al.*, 1983); carboxylesterase (Huang *et al.*, 1993); and N-acetyl-β-D-glucosamidinase (Deakin *et al.*, 1991). In general, changes in the

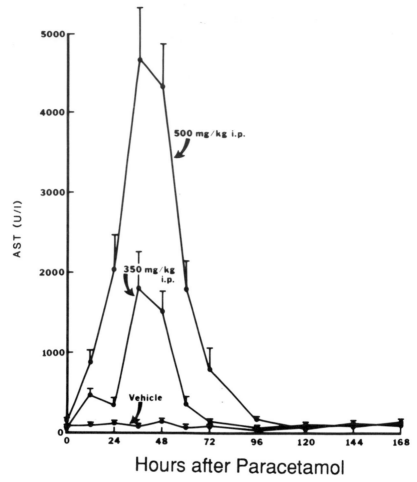

Figure 14.11   Dose- and time-dependent increases in plasma aspartate aminotransferase activity in hamsters following intraperitoneal administration of 350 and 500 mg kg^{-1} of paracetamol (reproduced with permission from Lee *et al.*, 1987).

activity of these enzymes parallelled those of the aminotransferases but with differences in the relative magnitude of the response. During recovery from massive hepatic necrosis caused by paracetamol, the processes of regeneration and repair were preceded by increased liver thymidine kinase and ornithine decarboxylase activity (Zieve *et al.*, 1985b, 1986, 1988; Zieve, 1989).

In studies with perfused liver preparations, liver slices, cultured hepatocytes and suspensions of isolated hepatocytes, the cytotoxicity of paracetamol was usually demonstrated by the release of intracellular lactic dehydrogenase into the perfusate or medium using the oxidation of NADH as described by Moldéus (1978). Again, the release of lactic dehydrogenase from hepatocytes damaged by exposure to toxic concentrations of paracetamol was dose and time dependent (Figure 14.12) (Mitchell *et al.*, 1985; Harman and McCamish, 1986; Horton and Wood, 1989; Shen *et al.*, 1991; Harman *et al.*, 1992b; Strubelt and Younes, 1992). Similar results were reported with exposure to N-acetyl-p-benzoquinoneimine, the presumed toxic

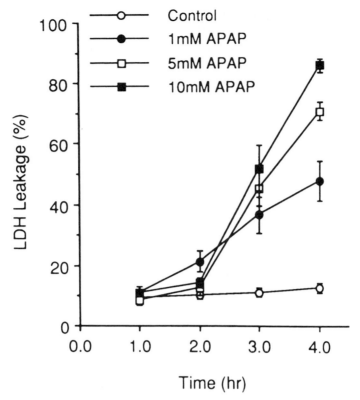

Figure 14.12 The dose- and time-dependent release of lactic dehydrogenase from isolated mouse hepatocyes incubated with toxic concentrations of paracetamol (APAP) (reproduced with permission from Harman *et al.*, 1992b).

metabolite of paracetamol (Holme *et al.*, 1984; Harman *et al.*, 1991; Nasseri-Sina *et al.*, 1992). The cytotoxicity of paracetamol has also been shown by the leakage from damaged hepatocytes of aspartate and alanine aminotransferases (Acosta *et al.*, 1980; Tyson *et al.*, 1980; Fouse and Hodgson, 1987; Lauterburg, 1987; Gómez-Lechón *et al.*, 1988; Leng-Peschlow, 1988; Farghali *et al.*, 1992; Strubelt and Younes, 1992; Visen *et al.*, 1993); alkaline phosphatase (Visen *et al.*, 1993); isocitric dehydrogenase (McLean and Nuttall, 1978; Devalia *et al.*, 1982; Beales *et al.*, 1985); argininosuccinate lyase (Acosta *et al.*, 1980); [14C]-5'-adenosine monophosphate (Shirhatti and Krishna, 1985); potassium (McLean and Nuttall, 1978; Harman and Fischer, 1983; Leng-Peschlow, 1988; Bruschi and Priestly, 1990); and protein (Larrauri *et al.*, 1989). The changes in enzyme activity usually followed the same pattern as with lactic dehydrogenase but the relative magnitude of the responses differed (Acosta *et al.*, 1980). There was a reciprocal relationship between the activity of the enzymes in hepatocytes and the perfusate or culture medium. With damage to the cell membrane, the initially high intracellular activity decreased as the enzymes leaked out into the extracellular fluids and cytotoxicity could be assessed by a decrease in liver enzyme content (Shukla *et al.*, 1992a; Singh *et al.*, 1992). Intracellular lactic dehydrogenase was considered a better indicator than released lactic dehydrogenase of the number of viable hepatocytes following exposure to paracetamol

(Chao *et al.*, 1988). In this study the extrapolated concentration of paracetamol required to release 50 per cent of the enzyme was extraordinarily high at 9211 mg l^{-1} and the results must be interpreted with caution because dimethyl sulphoxide (concentration unstated) was used as the solvent.

Impairment of Hepatic Function and Metabolism

The impairment of hepatic function and metabolism produced by toxic doses of paracetamol has been studied in whole animals as well as in the perfused liver and in isolated and cultured hepatocytes. Mitochondrial damage was an early and consistent histological finding in hepatic necrosis induced by paracetamol (Walker *et al.*, 1980; Placke *et al.*, 1987a), and it was associated with major depression of mitochondrial function as shown by inhibition of mitochondrial respiration and energy metabolism with reduced oxygen consumption and reduced ATP content (Hirayama *et al.*, 1983; Bates *et al.*, 1988; Burcham and Harman, 1988, 1990, 1991; Meyers *et al.*, 1988; Esterline and Ji, 1989; Katyare and Satav, 1989, 1991; Ramsay *et al.*, 1989; Tirmenstein and Nelson, 1989, 1990; Harman *et al.*, 1991; Shukla *et al.*, 1992a,b; Strubelt and Younes, 1992; Visen *et al.*, 1993; Donnelly *et al.*, 1994). There was similar depression of mitochondrial energy metabolism with N-acetyl-p-benzoquinoneimine (Andersson *et al.*, 1989, 1990; Esterline *et al.*, 1989; Burcham and Harman, 1991; Harman *et al.*, 1991). This early inhibition of mitochondrial energy metabolism by paracetamol and N-acetyl-p-benzoquinoneimine was associated with damage to the plasma membrane and disruption of intracellular calcium homeostasis. The resulting increase in cytosolic concentrations of free calcium was formerly considered to be the primary step in the sequence of events leading to irreversible injury and cell death (Jepson *et al.*, 1987; Lauterburg, 1987; Burcham and Harman, 1988; Long and Moore, 1988; Horton and Wood, 1989, 1991; Nicotera *et al.*, 1989; Bruschi and Priestly, 1990; Hardwick *et al.*, 1992a,b; Harman *et al.*, 1992b; Strubelt and Younes, 1992; Vu *et al.*, 1992; Grewal and Racz, 1993; Harris and Hamrick, 1993). Toxic doses of paracetamol also produced an increase in nuclear calcium concentrations with DNA fragmentation, which was characteristic of calcium-mediated endonuclease activation (Shen *et al.*, 1991, 1992). Similar findings were reported in other studies in which there was also substantial loss of large genomic DNA (Ray *et al.*, 1990, 1991, 1993b). Paracetamol inhibited the plasma membrane Na^+/K^+-ATPase pump (Negro *et al.*, 1981; Ginsberg and Cohen, 1985; Corcoran *et al.*, 1987a) and it induced changes in mitochondrial and plasma membrane potentials (Nazareth *et al.*, 1991). It also caused reversible changes in the fluorescence polarization of lipid soluble probes indicating an action on the lipids of microsomal membranes (Araya *et al.*, 1987a,b). The effects of paracetamol-induced hepatic failure on intermediary metabolism have been investigated *in vivo* using ^{31}P nuclear magnetic resonance (Bates *et al.*, 1988) and this technique was also used in metabolic studies with perfused isolated hepatocytes immobilized on agarose threads (Farghali *et al.*, 1992).

Hepatotoxic doses of paracetamol impaired the conjugation and biliary excretion of bilirubin (Davis *et al.*, 1975b) and there have been many reports of hyperbilirubinaemia in such circumstances (Gazzard *et al.*, 1975b; Miller *et al.*, 1976a; Ghosh and De, 1983; Poulsen *et al.*, 1985c; Henne-Bruns *et al.*, 1988a,b; Francavilla *et al.*, 1989, 1993; Udosen *et al.*, 1989; Ansari *et al.*, 1991; Dwivedi *et al.*, 1991;

Udosen and Ebong, 1991; Hong *et al.*, 1992; Kelly *et al.*, 1992; Rainska *et al.*, 1992; Shukla *et al.*, 1992a,b; Strubelt and Younes, 1992). In some of these studies, paracetamol-induced haemolysis could have contributed to the increased bilirubin concentrations. Toxic doses of paracetamol reduced the choleretic response to bromsulphthalein in rats with bile fistulae (Buttar, 1976) and greatly reduced its clearance by competing for its hepatic uptake and conjugation with glutathione (Davis *et al.*, 1975a; Buttar, 1976; Strubelt *et al.*, 1979; Mitra *et al.*, 1991). There was inhibition of bile secretion with reduced excretion of cholesterol and bile acids (Skakun and Shmanko, 1984), and a decrease in biliary efflux of iron (Benzick *et al.*, 1994). After administration of a therapeutic dose of 20 mg kg^{-1} of paracetamol daily for 90 days in rats, there was a reduction in the clearance of bromsulphthalein by isolated perfused liver preparations (Khedun *et al.*, 1993). Toxic doses of paracetamol reduced the hepatic clearance of kallikrein (de Toledo and Borges, 1993) and inhibited the hepatic uptake of microparticles such as colloidal carbon and albumin microspheres (Buhring *et al.*, 1991). However, even in high dosage, paracetamol did not reduce the galactose elimination capacity in rats (Poulsen *et al.*, 1981, 1985c). Other biochemical consequences of paracetamol toxicity were impaired hepatic synthesis of protein as shown by a reduced liver uptake and incorporation of [^{14}C]- and [^{3}H]-leucine (Thorgeirsson *et al.*, 1976; Beales *et al.*, 1985; Lawrence and Benford, 1990; Lindenthal *et al.*, 1993), and [^{14}C]-valine (Vonen and Morland, 1984), and decreased serum albumin concentrations (Murase *et al.*, 1986; Francavilla *et al.*, 1988, 1993; de Toledo and Borges, 1993; Rao *et al.*, 1993). In one report the reduction in protein synthesis was not dependent on depletion of glutathione (Bruno *et al.*, 1986) but in another, protein synthesis by hepatocytes declined in association with covalent binding and glutathione depletion and was reversible following exposure for up to 4 h, but not after 12 h. There was decreased synthesis of a protein with an apparent molecular weight of 56–58 kD, which coincided with increased production of another protein of 32 kD (Bruno *et al.*, 1991). There was also accumulation of triglycerides (Buttar *et al.*, 1976; Thorgeirsson *et al.*, 1976; Curzio *et al.*, 1980; Handa and Sharma, 1990) and increased blood concentrations of ammonia (Gazzard *et al.*, 1975b; Miller *et al.*, 1976a; Francavilla *et al.*, 1988, 1989, 1993) and insulin (Ferguson *et al.*, 1990). Paracetamol inhibited glycogen synthesis in isolated rat hepatocytes (Krack *et al.*, 1980) and gluconeogenesis was said to be impaired in rats given the relatively low dose of 20 mg kg^{-1} daily for 90 days (Khedun *et al.*, 1993).

The reduced synthetic capacity of the liver produced by paracetamol toxicity also caused impairment of haemostasis as shown by prolongation of the prothrombin time as a result of decreased production of hepatic clotting factors (Miller *et al.*, 1976a; Poulsen *et al.*, 1981, 1985b; Raheja *et al.*, 1983b; Francavilla *et al.*, 1989, 1993; Deakin *et al.*, 1991; Hughes *et al.*, 1991; Kelly *et al.*, 1992). Paracetamol hepatotoxicity has also been associated with an increased acute phase inflammatory response with elevation of serum α_2-macroglobulin (de Toledo and Borges, 1993), increased plasma concentrations of α_1-glycoprotein (Sugihara *et al.*, 1992) and decreased plasma concentrations of Gc (vitamin D-binding protein) with increased Gc : G-actin complexes (Lee *et al.*, 1987). Increased complexing of circulating group-specific component (Gc, vitamin D-binding protein) in hamsters was closely related to the extent of liver damage produced by paracetamol (Young *et al.*, 1987). In other reports, changes were observed in the binding of low density lipoprotein to hepatocytes (Singh *et al.*, 1992), and liver histone messenger RNA was decreased

(Smith *et al.*, 1992). Paracetamol increased the liver content of metallothionein in a dose-dependent fashion (Wormser and Calp, 1988; Waalkes and Ward, 1989) and it caused a redistribution of previously administered cadmium from the liver to the kidney while increasing its urinary and faecal excretion (Gale *et al.*, 1986b). Contrary to expectations, concentrations of tumour necrosis factor (TNF-α) were not increased in paracetamol-induced hepatic failure (Devictor *et al.*, 1992), but liver erythropoeitin content was increased in liver that was regenerating after paracetamol-induced necrosis (Liu *et al.*, 1981).

Many investigators have reported reduced activity of drug metabolizing enzymes with acute hepatic injury produced by paracetamol. The liver content of cytochrome P450 was reduced in some reports (Thorgeirsson *et al.*, 1976; Willson and Hart, 1977; Strubelt *et al.*, 1979; Sato *et al.*, 1981b; Gumbrecht and Franklin, 1983; Leng-Peschlow, 1988; Dwivedi *et al.*, 1991; Juzwiak *et al.*, 1992), but in others there was either little or no decrease (Chiu and Bhakthan, 1978; Rikans and Moore, 1988), or its activity was only reduced in animals previously induced by treatment with 3-methylcholanthrene or phenobarbitone (Poulsen *et al.*, 1985b; Murase *et al.*, 1986). These differences were probably related to differences in the severity of liver damage. Toxic doses of paracetamol also reduced the activity of aminopyrine demethylase (Willson and Hart, 1977; Strubelt *et al.*, 1979; Murase *et al.*, 1986; Speck and Lauterburg, 1991), aniline hydroxylase (Thorgeirsson *et al.*, 1976; Willson and Hart, 1977; Chiu and Bhakthan, 1978; Strubelt *et al.*, 1979), ethylmorphine N-demethylase (Aikawa *et al.*, 1978a), p-N-anisole demethylase (Poulsen *et al.*, 1985b) and bilirubin glucuronyl transferase (Willson and Hart, 1977). Aminopyrine demethylation was a sensitive indicator of paracetamol-induced liver damage, and it was decreased even after minimal injury (Sultatos *et al.*, 1978). The extent of impairment of the elimination of ^{99m}Tc-mebrofenin was also proposed as a sensitive early measure of the severity of paracetamol-induced liver damage (Sawas-Dimopoulou and Soulpi, 1987). Paracetamol had relatively little effect on the pattern of rat microsomal cytochrome P450 fractions as determined by anion exchange chromatography (Iversen and Franklin, 1985). The effects of acute liver damage on hepatic drug metabolizing enzymes were usually modest and there were poor correlations with histological appearances and standard biochemical tests of liver function (Willson and Hart, 1977). In other studies, hepatic necrosis produced by paracetamol resulted in marked impairment of the elimination of antipyrine (Kelleher *et al.*, 1977; Knights *et al.*, 1983) but not of levonorgestrel (Gommaa and Osman, 1983). Tolerance to the hepatotoxicity of paracetamol caused by the previous administration of toxic doses was attributed to inhibitory effects on its toxic metabolic activation (Poulsen *et al.*, 1985b; Jaszewski and Sheridan, 1987; Bhatia *et al.*, 1988). Similarly, liver damage caused by previous treatment with carbon tetrachloride protected against paracetamol hepatotoxicity (Curzio *et al.*, 1980) and toxicity following administration of both agents was less than predicted (Shelton and Weber, 1981). There was dissociation of the effects of paracetamol on subcellular function in rats as shown by the galactose elimination capacity, prothrombin index and drug metabolizing enzyme activity (Poulsen and Andreasen, 1980).

Correlations Between Histological and Biochemical Liver Injury

Close correlations have been reported between the histological severity of acute hepatic necrosis produced by paracetamol and standard biochemical tests of liver function, such as elevation of plasma aminotransferase activity and prolongation of the prothrombin time (Walker *et al.*, 1974; Dixon *et al.*, 1975b; Buttar *et al.*, 1976; Willson and Hart, 1977; Strubelt *et al.*, 1979; Linscheer *et al.*, 1980; Poulsen *et al.*, 1981; Raheja *et al.*, 1982, 1983b; Leonard and Dent, 1984; Munoz and Fearon, 1984; Corcoran *et al.*, 1985a; Leonard *et al.*, 1985a; Hazelton *et al.*, 1986a; Lee *et al.*, 1987; van de Straat *et al.*, 1987c; Young *et al.*, 1987; Wormser *et al.*, 1990; Deakin *et al.*, 1991; Roberts *et al.*, 1991b; Szymanska *et al.*, 1992; Speck *et al.*, 1993). The hepatotoxicity of paracetamol also correlated with the formation of covalently bound 3-(cystein-*S*-yl)paracetamol protein adduct in the liver (Pumford *et al.*, 1989; Ferguson *et al.*, 1990). This adduct was considered to be the ultimate index of paracetamol hepatotoxicity, and a specific particle concentration fluorescence immunoassay was developed for its immunohistological localization. The formation, distribution and concentration of the adduct was correlated with histological and biochemical liver cell injury as a function of dose and time (Figure 14.8) (Roberts *et al.*, 1991a,b).

Mechanisms of Paracetamol Hepatotoxicity

The essential mechanisms of paracetamol hepatotoxicity were first described by Mitchell and his colleagues more than 20 years ago in an elegant series of studies (Jollow *et al.*, 1973; Mitchell *et al.*, 1973b,c; Potter *et al.*, 1973). It was shown that toxicity was dependent on the formation of a reactive metabolite of paracetamol by hepatic mixed function oxidase. Thus, hepatic necrosis in mice and rats was potentiated when the elimination of paracetamol was enhanced by prior induction of drug-metabolizing enzymes with phenobarbitone, while inhibition of its metabolism and disappearance with piperonyl butoxide dramatically protected against hepatotoxicity. Pretreatment with 3-methylcholanthrene also potentiated paracetamol-induced hepatic necrosis whereas inhibition of the synthesis of cytochrome P450 with cobaltous chloride prevented liver damage (Mitchell *et al.*, 1973b). There was further development of the central role of the metabolic activation of paracetamol in the production of liver injury (Mitchell *et al.*, 1973a, 1974; Mitchell, 1975a,b). Hepatic necrosis was associated with extensive covalent binding of radiolabelled paracetamol to mouse liver proteins, and maximum binding preceded the development of recognizable histological injury. Both necrosis and covalent binding were dose dependent, and the extent of binding in individual animals was always directly proportional to the severity of the necrosis. The pretreatment of mice with phenobarbitone, piperonyl butoxide and cobalt chloride changed the rate of metabolism of paracetamol and the severity of the hepatic lesions, and affected the extent of hepatic binding of the radiolabelled metabolite similarly. It was proposed that paracetamol hepatotoxicity was caused by the covalent binding of a chemically reactive metabolite to vital liver macromolecules (Jollow *et al.*, 1973). In studies *in vitro*, the binding of [^{3}H]-paracetamol to the aminoacids of microsomal proteins was linear in respect to time and protein concentration. As binding depended on the availability of reduced nicotinamide adenine dinucleotide phosphate and oxygen, and was inhibited by carbon monoxide or cobaltous chloride pretreatment, it was considered to be mediated by cytochrome P450-dependent mixed function oxidase. The extent of binding *in vitro* correlated with treatments that altered the severity of hepatic necrosis and binding *in vivo* (Potter *et al.*, 1973).

The administration of hepatotoxic doses of paracetamol caused dose-dependent depletion of liver glutathione and its fundamental protective role was established. The prior depletion of hepatic glutathione with diethylmaleate potentiated paracetamol-induced liver damage and increased the covalent binding while pretreatment with cysteine, a precursor of glutathione, prevented liver damage and reduced the degree of covalent binding. Most importantly, it was shown that the covalent binding of the toxic metabolite of paracetamol to hepatic macromolecules did not occur until the availability of glutathione was exhausted through conjugation with the metabolite (Figure 14.13) Thus, glutathione protected against electrophilic attack by the toxic arylating metabolite of paracetamol (Mitchell *et al.,* 1973c). Species differences in susceptibility to the hepatotoxicity of paracetamol were correlated with the fraction excreted as mercapturic acid conjugates derived from the conjugation of the toxic metabolite of paracetamol with glutathione. The formation of the mercapturic acid conjugate was highest in susceptible mice and hamsters and lowest in resistant rats. Again, the formation of mercapturic acid conjugate was increased by treatments that augmented hepatotoxicity and decreased by treatments that protected against hepatotoxicity. The activity of the pathway of mercapturic acid formation *in vivo* reflected the activity of the hepatotoxic pathway of metabolism. The metabolic intermediate, which was normally conjugated with glutathione in the mercapturic acid pathway, was considered to be the same as the electrophilic metabolite which depleted glutathione after toxic doses and arylated

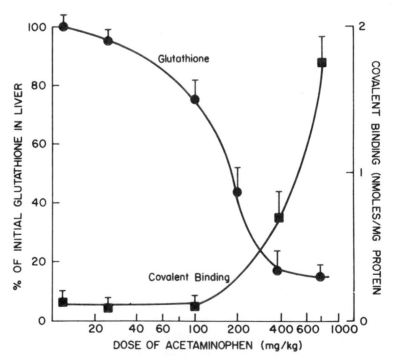

Figure 14.13   Relationship between depletion of hepatic glutathione and covalent binding of [³H]-paracetamol (acetaminophen) 2 h after intraperitoneal injection of increasing doses of paracetamol in mice (reproduced with permission from Mitchell *et al.,* 1973c).

hepatic macromolecules causing cell death (Jollow *et al.*, 1974). The mercapturic acid conjugate of paracetamol derived from the conjugate with glutathione was identified in the urine of volunteers given the drug and the recovery was dose dependent. Thus, paracetamol was shown to be converted to an electrophilic metabolite that reacted with glutathione in man in the same way as in animals. Glutathione-like nucleophiles such as cysteamine protected mice against the arylation of hepatic macromolecules and death caused by the toxic metabolite of paracetamol (Mitchell *et al.*, 1974). At the same time, early administration of cysteamine was shown to effectively prevent liver damage in patients who had taken hepatotoxic overdoses of paracetamol (Prescott *et al.*, 1974). Subsequent investigation has centred largely on the identity and formation of the toxic metabolite, the nature of covalent binding, specific target proteins and the role of specific mechanisms of cell injury such as 'oxidative stress' and disturbances of calcium homeostasis.

The Toxic Metabolite of Paracetamol

The essential requirement of metabolic activation for the toxicity of paracetamol, and the modulation of hepatotoxicity by treatments that increased or decreased the activity of cytochrome P450-dependent mixed function oxidases have been confirmed repeatedly over the years by countless investigators. Initially, it was proposed that the toxic metabolite might be N-hydroxyparacetamol, which would dehydrate immediately to form the highly reactive N-acetyl-p-benzoquinoneimine (Mitchell *et al.*, 1973a, 1974; Potter *et al.*, 1973; Davis *et al.*, 1974a; Jollow *et al.*, 1974; Mitchell, 1975a). This hypothesis was investigated further (Hinson *et al.*, 1977; Gemborys *et al.*, 1978, 1980; Healey *et al.*, 1978; Healey and Calder, 1979; Calder *et al.*, 1981a; Holme *et al.*, 1982a,b) but it became obvious that N-hydroxyparacetamol could not be the primary hepatotoxic metabolite. It was synthesized but was found to be relatively stable at physiological pH and it did not dehydrate immediately as supposed (Gemborys *et al.*, 1978; Healey *et al.*, 1978). In addition, it was not much more toxic than paracetamol itself as it would be expected to be if it were a minor metabolite (Healey *et al.*, 1978). N-hydroxyparacetamol could not be identified as a microsomal metabolite of paracetamol, although, paradoxically, it could be formed from phenacetin (Hinson *et al.*, 1979b; Calder *et al.*, 1981a), and it did not increase the covalent binding of paracetamol to microsomal protein (Nelson *et al.*, 1980b). Since there was no evidence of incorporation of ^{18}O in the metabolism of paracetamol and no loss of label during the metabolism of $[^{18}O]$-paracetamol, the possibility of an epoxide precursor of N-acetyl-p-benzoquinoneimine was excluded (Hinson *et al.*, 1979a, 1981; Hoffmann *et al.*, 1990). The failure of added epoxide hydrolase to block the covalent binding of the reactive metabolite of paracetamol was interpreted as further evidence against the formation of an epoxide intermediate (Hinson *et al.*, 1980b; Steele *et al.*, 1983).

There was considerable biochemical evidence that N-acetyl-p-benzoquinoneimine was the reactive metabolite of paracetamol (Miner and Kissinger, 1979b; Corcoran *et al.*, 1980; Corcoran and Mitchell, 1981; Hinson *et al.*, 1981; Huggett and Blair, 1982, 1983a; Nelson, 1982, 1990; Hinson, 1983; Dahlin *et al.*, 1984; Potter and Hinson, 1986a, 1987a; Harvison *et al.*, 1988b; Hoffmann *et al.*, 1990), and its properties were consistent with this hypothesis (Blair *et al.*, 1980; Dahlin and Nelson, 1982; Holme *et al.*, 1984; Albano *et al.*, 1985). Miner and Kissinger (1979b) generated N-acetyl-p-benzoquinoneimine electrochemically and found that the synthetic form reacted with a range of nucleophiles to produce sulphydryl adducts that were indistinguishable from those formed during the microsomal metabolism of paracetamol. Paracetamol and N-hydroxyparacetamol both formed the quinoneimine as a common arylating intermediate (Corcoran *et al.*, 1980) and its production by direct oxidation of paracetamol via the cytochrome P450-dependent mixed function oxidase system was proposed as the mechanism of hepatotoxicity (Calder *et al.*, 1981a). N-acetyl-p-benzoquinoneimine was considerably more toxic than the parent drug in mice and its decomposition kinetics were complex (Dahlin and Nelson, 1982). It was subsequently identified as an oxidation product of the microsomal metabolism of paracetamol and was rapidly reduced back to the parent drug by a variety of reductants. It also was bound covalently to microsomal proteins, and this binding was inhibited by glutathione and ascorbic acid. N-acetyl-p-benzoquinoneimine reacted readily with nucleophiles such as glutathione to form paracetamol and its glutathione conjugate (Dahlin *et al.*, 1984). The covalent binding characteristics of synthetic N-acetyl-p-benzoquinoneimine parallelled closely those of the reactive species generated metabolically from paracetamol (Streeter *et al.*, 1984b).

The precise mechanism of the formation of N-acetyl-p-benzoquinoneimine by microsomal enzymes has not been established but the possibilities included a direct one electron transfer to give a phenoxy radical and N-acetyl-p-benzosemiquinoneimine, a direct two electron transfer to yield N-acetyl-p-benzoquinoneimine or an indirect reaction involving active oxygen (van de Straat *et al.*, 1988b). The evidence favoured a two electron rather than a one electron transfer (Dahlin *et al.*, 1984; Potter and Hinson, 1987a, 1989; Harvison *et al.*, 1988b; van de Straat *et al.*, 1988b; Hoffmann *et al.*, 1990; Nelson, 1990; Vermeulen *et al.*, 1992) and proton nuclear magnetic resonance relaxation measurements indicated the phenolic function of paracetamol as the site of its oxidative bioactivation (van de Straat *et al.*, 1987a). Theoretical considerations supported a two electron transfer mechanism (Loew and Goldblum, 1985) but also a role for phenoxy radicals (Koymans *et al.*, 1989). The production of phenoxy radicals by one electron transfer had been proposed previously by de Vries (1981) but N-acetyl-p-benzosemiquinoneimine formed in this process would generate superoxide or some other form of active oxygen (Nelson *et al.*, 1981a; Rosen *et al.*, 1983). Several reports have raised the possibility that paracetamol could initiate oxidation or free radical reactions (Gerson *et al.*, 1985; Harman, 1985; Moore *et al.*, 1985a; Tee *et al.*, 1986b). Phenoxy free radicals were detected during the microsomal metabolism of paracetamol (Fischer *et al.*, 1985c) and the properties of the radicals formed by its one electron oxidation were studied by pulse radiolysis (Bisby *et al.*, 1985). Free radical reactions could result from the enzymic redox cycling of N-acetyl-p-benzoquinoneimine (Rosen *et al.*, 1983) or from the one electron oxidation of paracetamol to form a semiquinone radical (Potter and Hinson, 1987a). It was also possible that the quinoneimine could be converted to the semiquinoneimine by a one electron reduction (van de Straat *et al.*, 1987d; Potter and Hinson, 1989). The protective effects of antioxidants (Harman, 1985) and thiol reducing agents (Tee *et al.*, 1986b) against paracetamol liver damage supported an oxidative mechanism of toxicity, as did the potentiation by agents that enhanced oxidative stress such as 1,3-bis(chloroethyl)-N-nitrosourea and ferric ions (Gerson *et al.*, 1985; Younes *et al.*, 1986). Horseradish peroxidase and prostaglandin H synthetase probably catalyzed primarily the one electron oxidation of paracetamol (Rosen *et al.*, 1983; Ross *et al.*, 1984; West *et al.*, 1984; Fischer *et al.*, 1985b; Potter *et al.*, 1985, 1986; Mason and Fischer, 1986; Potter and Hinson, 1987b, 1989; Keller and Hinson, 1991). In a recent study involving labelled analogues of paracetamol with analysis of the thioether metabolites, it was concluded that paracetamol was converted to N-acetyl-p-benzoquinoneimine not by the generation of a free oxygenated intermediate, but by sequential removal of two electrons from the substrate. A scheme was proposed that appeared to account for all the known oxidative metabolites of paracetamol (Hoffmann *et al.*, 1990). The different isoenzymes of cytochrome P450 have different specificities for the different pathways of paracetamol metabolism including the formation of N-acetyl-p-benzoquinoneimine (Morgan *et al.*, 1982, 1983; Ioannides *et al.*, 1983b; Steele *et al.*, 1983; Potter and Hinson, 1987a; van de Straat *et al.*, 1987a; Harvison *et al.*, 1988b; Raucy *et al.*, 1989, 1991; Prasad *et al.*, 1990; Jeffery *et al.*, 1991; Thummel *et al.*, 1993), and the effects of structural modification of paracetamol on its toxicity and metabolism have been investigated (Nelson *et al.*, 1978; Fernando *et al.*, 1980; Fischer and Mason, 1984; Rosen *et al.*, 1984; Fischer *et al.*, 1985b,c; Mason and Fischer, 1986; Streeter *et al.*, 1986; van de Straat *et al.*, 1986, 1987c,d; Andersson *et al.*, 1989; Donatus *et al.*, 1990; Barnard *et al.*, 1993a).

Depending on the conditions, N-acetyl-p-benzoquinoneimine could act both as an electrophile and an oxidant (Calder *et al.*, 1974; Miner and Kissinger, 1979b; Blair *et al.*, 1980; Corcoran *et al.*, 1980; Hinson *et al.*, 1981; Albano *et al.*, 1983, 1985; Rosen *et al.*, 1983; Dahlin *et al.*, 1984; Powis *et al.*, 1984; Streeter *et al.*, 1984b; Andersson *et al.*, 1989). It reacted with nucleophiles to form the corresponding conjugates (Miner and Kissinger, 1979b) and in particular it reacted with glutathione to yield the glutathione conjugate of paracetamol at the same time regenerating the parent drug and forming oxidized glutathione (Corcoran *et al.*, 1980; Hinson *et al.*, 1982; Huggett and Blair, 1982; Dahlin *et al.*, 1984; Powis *et al.*, 1984; Rosen *et al.*, 1984; Albano *et al.*, 1985; Potter and Hinson, 1986a,b, 1989; van de Straat *et al.*, 1986, 1987b, 1988b; Coles *et al.*, 1988; Nelson *et al.*, 1991). The glutathione conjugate was identified as an important biliary metabolite of paracetamol (Hinson *et al.*, 1982) and the amount appearing in the bile was a reliable index of the toxic activation of paracetamol (Madhu *et al.*, 1989). Toxic doses of paracetamol did not increase the biliary excretion of oxidized glutathione indicating that N-acetyl-p-benzoquinoneimine produced *in vivo* was not acting as an oxidant (Smith and Mitchell, 1985; Smith and Jaeschke, 1989). N-acetyl-p-benzoquinoneimine also reacted with thiol groups on proteins to give paracetamol-protein adducts. Cysteine residues were identified as the major sites of arylation and the primary adduct formed *in vitro* and *in vivo* was 3-(cystein-S-yl)paracetamol (Streeter *et al.*, 1984b; Hoffmann *et al.*, 1985a). N-acetyl-p-benzoquinoneimine could also cause oxidation of protein thiols (Birge *et al.*, 1988). In general, it had the same cytotoxic effects as paracetamol and similar effects on covalent binding, glutathione depletion, calcium homeostasis and intermediary metabolism (Holme *et al.*, 1984; Albano *et al.*, 1985; Moore *et al.*, 1985a; Potter and Hinson, 1986a; Rundgren *et al.*, 1988; Andersson *et al.*, 1989, 1990; Esterline *et al.*, 1989; Burcham and Harman, 1991; Harman *et al.*, 1991; Nasseri-Sina *et al.*, 1992).

Covalent Binding

The essential role of the covalent binding of paracetamol to hepatic macromolecules and microsomal protein in the causation of liver damage as described originally by

Mitchell and his colleagues (Jollow *et al.*, 1973; Mitchell *et al.*, 1973c; Potter *et al.*, 1973) has since been confirmed by many other investigators. The binding was dose dependent and only occurred after critical depletion of hepatic reduced glutathione to 20–30 per cent of the initial values (Figure 14.13). It was dependent on cytochrome P450, and was similar *in vitro* and *in vivo*; in the latter case binding was linear in respect of time and protein concentration (Potter *et al.*, 1973, 1974; Lake *et al.*, 1981). Treatments that increased and decreased hepatotoxicity also increased and decreased the covalent binding of paracetamol in the same way (Jollow *et al.*, 1973; Mitchell *et al.*, 1973c; Potter *et al.*, 1973, 1974; Davis *et al.*, 1974a, 1976a; Pessayre *et al.*, 1980; Hinson *et al.*, 1981; Lake *et al.*, 1981; Walker *et al.*, 1983b; Corcoran *et al.*, 1985a; Kyle *et al.*, 1990; McDanell *et al.*, 1992). Marked species differences in susceptibility to paracetamol hepatotoxicity in mice, hamsters, rats, guinea pigs, rabbits and man also corresponded with differences in the extent of covalent binding (Davis *et al.*, 1974a; Aikawa *et al.*, 1978b; Tee *et al.*, 1987). The covalent binding of paracetamol was correlated with the extent of metabolic activation in rats as shown by the urinary recovery of the cysteine and mercapturic acid conjugates (Davis *et al.*, 1976a). Covalent binding was greatest in the liver with relatively little binding in other tissues such as kidney, muscle and brain (Jollow *et al.*, 1973; Potter *et al.*, 1974; Fischer *et al.*, 1981; Nakae *et al.*, 1990a). Although paracetamol was bound mostly to proteins there was minor binding to microsomal phospholipids (Wendel and Hallbach, 1986). In mouse liver homogenates, radiolabelled paracetamol was bound to cytosolic protein and microsomes with preferential binding to glutathione S-transferase (Wendel and Cikryt, 1981). As shown by autoradiographic studies, the intrahepatic localization of covalently bound paracetamol in the liver and the extent of binding were correlated with the centrilobular distribution and the severity of the hepatic necrosis (Jollow *et al.*, 1973; Potter *et al.*, 1974). More recently, a similar centrilobular distribution of the paracetamol protein adduct was demonstrated in animals and man by specific immunohistochemical techniques (Figure 14.14) (Bartolone *et al.*, 1987, 1989b; Birge *et al.*, 1990; Roberts *et al.*, 1991b). [³H]-Paracetamol was bound to human liver microsomal proteins in a non-specific manner (Lecoeur *et al.*, 1994). The covalent binding of N-acetyl-p-benzoquinoneimine to cellular protein also correlated with cytotoxicity, and was similar to the binding of paracetamol (Streeter *et al.*, 1984b; Albano *et al.*, 1985; Tee *et al.*, 1987).

In addition to glutathione itself, other sulphydryl nucleophiles such as cysteamine, cysteine, N-acetylcysteine, α-mercaptopropionylglycine and dithiothreitol reduced the covalent binding of the reactive metabolite of paracetamol to liver proteins (Potter *et al.*, 1973; Mitchell *et al.*, 1974; Buckpitt *et al.*, 1979; Stramentinoli *et al.*, 1979; Lake *et al.*, 1981; Massey and Racz, 1981; Mitchell *et al.*, 1981b; Corcoran *et al.*, 1985a; Speeg *et al.*, 1985; Corcoran and Wong, 1986; Harman and Self, 1986; Hjelle *et al.*, 1986; Kitteringham *et al.*, 1988). Conversely, the binding and toxicity of paracetamol were increased when glutathione was depleted by prior exposure to agents such as diethyl maleate (Mitchell *et al.*, 1973c) and doxorubicin (Wells *et al.*, 1980), while the circadian rhythm in liver non-protein sulphydryl content was associated with corresponding changes in the extent of covalent binding (Schnell *et al.*, 1983). The covalent binding of paracetamol *in vitro* (but not *in vivo*) was reduced by ascorbic acid (Lake *et al.*, 1981; Miller and Jollow, 1984; Peterson and Knodell, 1984; Jonker *et al.*, 1988; Kitteringham *et al.*, 1988), and a similar discrepancy between the effects on paracetamol binding *in vitro* and *in vivo* was observed with

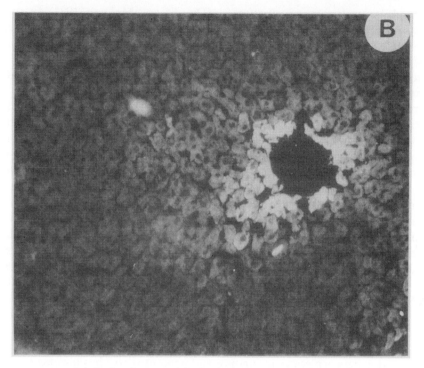

Figure 14.14 Centrilobular localization of the binding of paracetamol to mouse hepatocytes as shown by indirect immunohistochemical staining 2 h after oral administration of a dose of 600 mg kg^{-1} (× 122) (reproduced with permission from Bartolone *et al.*, 1989b).

fish oil (Speck and Lauterburg, 1991). Enhancement and reduction in the extent of covalent binding were reported with a variety of treatments that increased or decreased the formation of the reactive metabolite of paracetamol (Jollow *et al.*, 1973; Potter *et al.*, 1973, 1974; Pessayre *et al.*, 1980; Hinson *et al.*, 1981; Mitchell *et al.*, 1981b; Harman and Fischer, 1983; Renton and Dickson, 1984; Speeg *et al.*, 1985; Letteron *et al.*, 1986; Wells and To, 1986b; Ishikawa *et al.*, 1990a; Speck *et al.*, 1993). Although phenobarbitone was considered to be a classical inducer of cyto-chrome P450-dependent mixed function oxidase, in some reports it had relatively little effect on the isoenzymes involved in the metabolic activation of paracetamol and it did not increase the covalent binding or hepatotoxicity of paracetamol as might have been expected (Potter *et al.*, 1974; Ioannides *et al.*, 1983b; Steele *et al.*, 1983; Poulsen *et al.*, 1985b; van de Straat *et al.*, 1986; Kyle *et al.*, 1988; Larrauri *et al.*, 1989).

Although covalent binding seemed to be essential for the development of parace-tamol hepatotoxicity, there have been some discordant findings and a direct cause and effect relationship has been questioned. In mice, peak covalent binding (and presumably maximum injury) had occurred by 2 h yet N-acetylcysteine was still able to protect against liver damage when given as late as $4\frac{1}{2}$ h after the paracetamol (Piperno *et al.*, 1978). In another report the extent of covalent binding of parace-tamol was considered insufficient to account for toxicity. There was less binding to hepatocytes that were damaged by incubation with paracetamol for 1 h than in cells which had survived after exposure for 4 h (Devalia and McLean, 1983). In addition, N-acetylcysteine (Gerber *et al.*, 1977), α-mercaptopropionylglycine (Labadarios *et al.*, 1977), 3-O-methyl(+)catechin (Devalia *et al.*, 1982), α-tocopherol and diphenylphenylenediamine (Albano *et al.*, 1983), calcium EDTA (Beales *et al.*, 1985), cimetidine (Peterson *et al.*, 1983), dithiodithreitol (Tee *et al.*, 1986b), disulfiram (Poulsen *et al.*, 1987; Jørgensen *et al.*, 1988), chlorpromazine (Saville *et al.*, 1988), desferrioxamine (Gerson *et al.*, 1985) and liposome-encapsulated superoxide dismutase (Nakae *et al.*, 1990a) were all said to protect against paracetamol hepatotoxicity without significantly reducing the extent of covalent binding. Furthermore, although susceptibility to the hepatotoxicity of paracetamol was increased by chronic intake of ethanol (Walker *et al.*, 1983b) and 1,3-bis(chloroethyl)-1-nitrosourea (Gerson *et al.*, 1985) there was no increase in the extent of covalent binding. In mice given a toxic dose of paracetamol, late treatment with piperonyl butoxide produced changes in the pattern of selective protein arylation but not in total covalent binding (Brady *et al.*, 1991). Similarly, differences in susceptibility to paracetamol hepatotoxicity with age were associated with differences in selective protein arylation but not with total covalent binding (Beierschmitt *et al.*, 1989). In another report, the toxicity of paracetamol was comparable in hepatocytes isolated from mice of different ages but covalent binding was much greater in the young (Harman and McCamish, 1986). Fasting increased the susceptibility of mice to paracetamol hepatotoxicity but did not increase the extent of covalent binding (Strubelt *et al.*, 1981).

Dissociation between covalent binding and hepatotoxicity has also been reported in studies with paracetamol analogues. Thus, N-methylparacetamol produced more covalent binding than paracetamol but it was not hepatotoxic and had no useful analgesic activity (Forte and Nelson, 1980; Harvison *et al.*, 1986b). Similarly, large doses of 3-hydroxyacetanilide (the meta- isomer of paracetamol) produced at least as much if not more covalent binding than equivalent toxic doses of paracetamol but with less depletion of glutathione and no hepatotoxicity (Nelson, 1980; Streeter *et al.*, 1984a; Garle *et al.*, 1988; Tirmenstein and Nelson, 1989; Roberts *et al.*, 1990; Holme *et al.*, 1991). Indeed, it was not possible to cause liver damage with 3-hydroxyacetanilide, even in hamsters and mice sensitized by prior induction with 3-methylcholanthrene and phenobarbitone or depletion of glutathione with borneol or diethyl maleate (Roberts *et al.*, 1990; Tirmenstein and Nelson, 1991). Compared with paracetamol, 3-hydroxyacetanilide was bound less to mitochondrial proteins and unlike paracetamol it did not inhibit plasma membrane ATPase or cause oxidation of protein thiols (Tirmenstein and Nelson, 1989, 1990). Only by depleting mitochondrial glutathione to less than 20 per cent of control values with combined treatment with diethyl maleate and buthionine sulphoximine was it possible to produce liver toxicity in mice with 3-hydroxyacetanilide (Tirmenstein and Nelson, 1991). Further discrepancies between covalent binding and toxicity have been noted with 3,5-dimethylparacetamol and 2,6-dimethylparacetamol. The former analogue was hepatotoxic with little covalent binding while the latter was not hepatotoxic even though it was bound to a much greater extent (Porubek *et al.*, 1987; Birge *et al.*, 1988, 1989; Rossi *et al.*, 1988; Bruno *et al.*, 1991, 1992). Despite the lack of covalent binding of 3,5-dimethylparacetamol, it caused cytotoxicity with depletion of glutathione and oxidation of protein thiols. Conversely, although 2,6-dimethylparacetamol was bound covalently and depleted glutathione, it did not cause loss of protein thiols or hepatotoxicity (Birge *et al.*, 1988). In keeping with these findings,

N-acetyl-p-benzoquinoneimine and the corresponding reactive metabolite of 3,5-dimethylparacetamol (but not that of 3-hydroxyacetanilide or 2,6-dimethyl-paracetamol) caused cross-linking of bovine serum albumin molecules *in vitro* (Streeter *et al.*, 1986). The cytotoxicity of 3,5-dimethylparacetamol appeared to be dependent on deacetylation and the product could be trapped by conjugation with glutathione (Rossi *et al.*, 1988). However, p-aminophenol did not cause liver injury although it was bound covalently to a much greater extent than paracetamol (McLean *et al.*, 1980). Although the covalent binding hypothesis has stood the test of time (Yamada, 1983), these discordant observations must raise doubts about the presumed direct causal relationship between the covalent binding and toxicity of paracetamol. The most likely explanation for these anomalous results was that the critical determinant of hepatotoxicity was the covalent binding of paracetamol to specific protein targets, which accounted for only a small proportion of the total amount of protein that was arylated.

The Role of Glutathione

As with covalent binding, depletion of hepatic glutathione appeared to be an essential factor for paracetamol-induced liver damage and arylation by the toxic metabolite of paracetamol *in vitro* was prevented by the addition of glutathione or its precursor cysteine (Potter *et al.*, 1973). Conversely, prior depletion of hepatic glutathione with diethyl maleate potentiated the hepatotoxicity of paracetamol in mice while treatment with cysteine prevented liver damage. Paracetamol caused a dose- and time-dependent decrease in hepatic glutathione (Figures 14.13 and 14.15) and covalent binding to hepatic macromolecules did not occur until the availability of glutathione was exhausted through conjugation with the reactive metabolite. Changes in the availability of glutathione caused by diethyl maleate or cysteine increased or decreased respectively the covalent binding to hepatic macromolecules (Mitchell *et al.*, 1973c). Other treatments that increased or decreased the formation of the toxic metabolite of paracetamol caused greater or lesser depletion of hepatic glutathione and the decrease was not due to its oxidation to the disulphide dimer. Covalent binding and toxicity only occurred after depletion of glutathione to less than about 30 per cent of normal (Potter *et al.*, 1974). The toxic metabolite of paracetamol was preferentially detoxified by conjugation with glutathione, and the severity of hepatic necrosis in rats, mice, hamsters, guinea pigs and rabbits correlated directly with the rate and extent of hepatic glutathione depletion (Davis *et al.*, 1974a). These early observations were developed further by other investigators. Paracetamol was shown to cause a dose- and time-dependent decrease in intracellular glutathione in isolated hepatocyte suspensions and cultures, which correlated with cytotoxicity as manifested by blebbing, leakage into the medium of potassium and enzymes such as lactic dehydrogenase, and failure to exclude trypan blue (Moldéus, 1978; Harman and Fischer, 1983; Dawson *et al.*, 1984; Holme *et al.*, 1984; Bruno *et al.*, 1985; Harman, 1985; Hue *et al.*, 1985; Milam and Byard, 1985; Mitchell *et al.*, 1985; Harman and Self, 1986; Hayes *et al.*, 1986; Tee *et al.*, 1986b, 1987; van de Straat *et al.*, 1986; Leng-Peschlow, 1988; Larrauri *et al.*, 1989; Willson *et al.*, 1991; Nasseri-Sina *et al.*, 1992; and others). Glutathione played an important role in maintaining calcium homeostasis and hepatocyte integrity (Moore *et al.*, 1985a) and again the increase in phosphorylase *a* and rise in plasma aminotransferase activity produced by toxic doses of paracetamol only occurred after

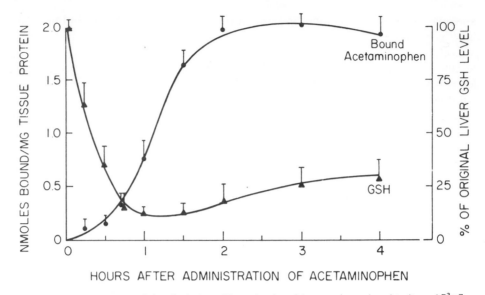

Figure 14.15 Time course of the depletion of hepatic glutathione and covalent binding of [^{3}H]-paracetamol (acetaminophen) following the intraperitoneal administration of a dose of 750 mg kg^{-1} in mice (reproduced with permission from Mitchell *et al.*, 1973c).

hepatic glutathione had fallen to 20 per cent of normal (Corcoran *et al.*, 1988). The reduction in hepatic glutathione persisted with the chronic administration of paracetamol (Strubelt *et al.*, 1979; Reicks *et al.*, 1988; Reicks and Hathcock, 1989; Reicks and Crankshaw, 1993), but in one study there was no depletion in rats given 500 mg kg^{-1} twice daily for seven days (Buttar *et al.*, 1977).

N-acetyl-p-benzoquinoneimine itself reacted directly with glutathione under different conditions to yield paracetamol, its glutathione conjugate and oxidized glutathione (Huggett and Blair, 1982; Rosen *et al.*, 1983, 1984; Albano *et al.*, 1985; Davies *et al.*, 1986; van de Straat *et al.*, 1988b) and depending on the conditions, the same products could be formed from one and two electron oxidation of paracetamol by peroxidases (Potter and Hinson, 1986a,b, 1987a,b, 1989). When incubated with mouse liver microsomes, N-acetyl-p-benzoquinoneimine formed the glutathione conjugate of paracetamol with regeneration of the parent drug (Dahlin *et al.*, 1984). The rapid depletion of intracellular glutathione in isolated hepatocytes by N-acetyl-p-benzoquinoneimine was correlated with its cytotoxicity (Holme *et al.*, 1984; Moore *et al.*, 1985a; Tee *et al.*, 1987; van de Straat *et al.*, 1987b; Harman *et al.*, 1991) and prior depletion of glutathione in mouse hepatoma cultures by exposure to buthionine sulphoximine potentiated its cytotoxicity (Riley *et al.*, 1993). The oxidative metabolism of paracetamol consumed hepatic glutathione and its depletion depended, therefore, on drug metabolizing enzyme activity (Aikawa *et al.*, 1978b). In another study the loss of liver glutathione was proposed as a marker for the generation of reactive metabolites of paracetamol and other agents (Garle *et al.*, 1988). The formation of the glutathione conjugate of paracetamol correlated directly with the loss of intracellular glutathione (Moldéus, 1978; Farber *et al.*, 1988; Harman *et al.*, 1991) and the viability of hepatocytes (Dawson *et al.*, 1984). Adduct formation with hepatic macromolecules was inversely related to the glutathione content

(Szymanska *et al.*, 1992). The decrease in plasma concentrations of glutathione induced by paracetamol was considered to reflect reduced hepatic glutathione in rats (Adams *et al.*, 1983) and in man (Lauterburg *et al.*, 1984c), but in another report paracetamol depleted liver glutathione in rats without lowering plasma concentrations (Di Simplicio *et al.*, 1984). Paracetamol has been used as a probe for the study of glutathione turnover (Lauterburg *et al.*, 1980; Lauterburg and Smith, 1986).

Other investigators confirmed that the effect of large doses of paracetamol on lowering hepatic glutathione was dose dependent (Buttar *et al.*, 1977; Wendel *et al.*, 1982; Mitchell *et al.*, 1985; Brzeznicka and Piotrowski, 1989; Larrauri *et al.*, 1989; Madhu *et al.*, 1989; Chen *et al.*, 1990) and that toxicity did not occur until the concentrations fell to less than about 20 per cent of control values (Strubelt *et al.*, 1974; Kapetanovic and Mieyal, 1979; Williamson *et al.*, 1982; Hirayama *et al.*, 1983; Bruno *et al.*, 1985; Klaassen *et al.*, 1985; Mitchell *et al.*, 1985; van de Straat *et al.*, 1986; Placke *et al.*, 1987a; Corcoran *et al.*, 1988; Kitamura *et al.*, 1989; and others). Because the availability of glutathione for inactivation of the toxic metabolite of paracetamol was a critical determinant of toxicity, there was a dose threshold for toxicity. This threshold dose varied greatly between species, and as it was exceeded there was a rapid and disproportionate increase in hepatotoxicity (Figure 14.16) (Jollow *et al.*, 1974, 1981; Potter *et al.*, 1974; Mitchell, 1975b; Jollow, 1980; Wendel *et al.*, 1982; Corcoran *et al.*, 1985a; van de Straat *et al.*, 1987c; Nakae *et al.*, 1988; Brzeznicka and Piotrowski, 1989; Pumford *et al.*, 1989). A similar phenomenon was observed in patients taking paracetamol in overdosage and the average threshold dose for severe liver damage in man was 250–300 mg kg^{-1} (Prescott,

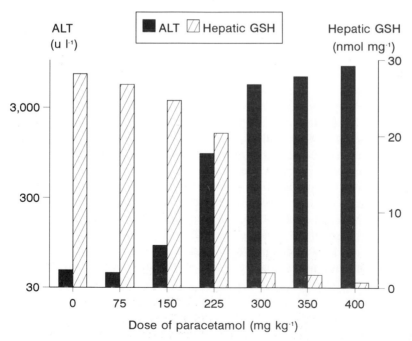

Figure 14.16   Dose-threshold effect for depletion of hepatic glutathione and hepatic necrosis as shown by plasma alanine aminotransferase activity (ALT) in mice treated with increasing doses of intraperitoneal paracetamol (data from Wendel *et al.*, 1982).

1983). The time course of changes in hepatic glutathione following exposure to toxic doses of paracetamol depended on experimental conditions, dose, species and whether the studies were carried out *in vivo* or *in vitro*. *In vivo* there was usually an initial rapid fall followed by a slow recovery, often with a degree of overshoot (Strubelt *et al.*, 1974; Buttar *et al.*, 1977; Moldéus, 1978; Hassing *et al.*, 1979; Viña *et al.*, 1980; Price and Jollow, 1982; Williamson *et al.*, 1982; Hirayama *et al.*, 1983; Raheja *et al.*, 1983b; Siegers *et al.*, 1983a; Peterson and Knodell, 1984; Mitchell *et al.*, 1985; Poulsen *et al.*, 1985b; Price *et al.*, 1987; Skoglund *et al.*, 1987; Micheli and Giorgi, 1988; Kaneo *et al.*, 1989a,b; Kitamura *et al.*, 1989; Larrauri *et al.*, 1989; Lawrence and Benford, 1990; Lew and Quintanilha, 1991; Hong *et al.*, 1992). Species and strain differences in susceptibility to paracetamol toxicity were associated with corresponding differences in the extent of glutathione depletion (Davis *et al.*, 1974a; Aikawa *et al.*, 1978b; Tsui and Madsen, 1979; Willson *et al.*, 1991), and there were similar correlations in respect of sex (Raheja *et al.*, 1983b) and age differences (Mitchell *et al.*, 1985; Harman and McCamish, 1986; Rikans and Moore, 1988; Chen *et al.*, 1990). Other factors that simultaneously influenced hepatic glutathione and susceptibility to toxicity included: fasting (Buttar *et al.*, 1977; Pessayre *et al.*, 1980; Lauterburg and Mitchell, 1982; Adams *et al.*, 1983; Schnell *et al.*, 1984; Joyave *et al.*, 1985; Price *et al.*, 1987; Raheja *et al.*, 1987; Saville *et al.*, 1988); dietary deficiency of riboflavin (Raheja *et al.*, 1983c, 1987), methionine (Reicks and Hathcock, 1984, 1989); and α-tocopherol and selenium (Hill and Burk, 1984); chronic ethanol consumption (Walker *et al.*, 1983b); diabetes (Price and Jollow, 1982); decreased body temperature (Kalhorn *et al.*, 1990); exercise (Lew and Quintanilha, 1991); circadian rhythms (Hassing *et al.*, 1979; Schnell *et al.*, 1983, 1984; Miller *et al.*, 1986); and exposure to light (Schnell *et al.*, 1984). In one study, fasting caused a paradoxical increase in hepatic glutathione (Miller *et al.*, 1986). Many agents that increased or decreased the hepatotoxicity of paracetamol were shown to have corresponding effects on the depletion of hepatic glutathione (Fossa *et al.*, 1979; Kapetanovic and Mieyal, 1979; Linscheer *et al.*, 1980; Pessayre *et al.*, 1980; Albano *et al.*, 1981; Raheja *et al.*, 1982, 1983a, 1984; Rosen *et al.*, 1983; Klugmann *et al.*, 1984; Renton and Dickson, 1984; Joyave *et al.*, 1985; Speeg *et al.*, 1985; Younes and Siegers, 1985b; Letteron *et al.*, 1986; Jeffery and Haschek, 1988; Mitra *et al.*, 1988; Saville *et al.*, 1988; Bertelli *et al.*, 1990; Kalhorn *et al.*, 1990; Szymanska *et al.*, 1991, 1992; Juzwiak *et al.*, 1992; Madhu *et al.*, 1992b; Rainska *et al.*, 1992; Speck *et al.*, 1993; Farag and Abdel-Meguid, 1994; and others). In many cases the changes in glutathione status were probably secondary.

Treatment with agents such as diethyl maleate, buthionine sulphoximine and phorone markedly reduced hepatic glutathione, but this in itself did not normally cause toxicity (Mitchell *et al.*, 1973c; Högberg and Kristoferson, 1977; Raheja *et al.*, 1983a; Hill and Burk, 1984; Hue *et al.*, 1985; Mitchell *et al.*, 1985; Corcoran *et al.*, 1988; Kyle *et al.*, 1988; Yeung, 1988; Speck *et al.*, 1993). However, pretreatment with these agents augmented the depletion of glutathione induced by paracetamol and enhanced its hepatotoxicity (Högberg and Kristoferson, 1977; Raheja *et al.*, 1983a; Hue *et al.*, 1985; Mitchell *et al.*, 1985; Hayes *et al.*, 1986; Younes *et al.*, 1986; Porubek *et al.*, 1987; Szymanska *et al.*, 1992). They antagonized to a variable extent the effects of agents such as cysteine, N-acetylcysteine, methionine, dimethyl sulphoxide, ascorbic acid, propylthiouracil and captopril on hepatic glutathione and paracetamol toxicity (Raheja *et al.*, 1983a; Miners *et al.*, 1984d; Jeffery and Haschek, 1988; Yeung, 1988; Mitra *et al.*, 1991). Like buthionine sulphoximine, methionine sulphoximine inhibited glutathione synthesis and reversed the protective effect of N-acetylcysteine on paracetamol hepatotoxicity (Dawson *et al.*, 1984). Oxidative injury to hepatocytes has been proposed as a mechanism of paracetamol toxicity and this was supposed to occur as a result of the production of active oxygen species during its metabolic activation. These reactive species might form damaging peroxides that could be neutralized by reaction with glutathione peroxidase to produce oxidized glutathione, which in turn would be reduced by glutathione reductase. A marked increase in the output of oxidized glutathione, therefore, could be interpreted as evidence of oxidative damage, but this did not normally occur with the microsomal metabolism of paracetamol (Adams *et al.*, 1983; Lauterburg *et al.*, 1984b; Miller and Jollow, 1984; Smith and Mitchell, 1985; van de Straat *et al.*, 1986; Porubek *et al.*, 1987; Farber *et al.*, 1988; Andersson *et al.*, 1989; Smith and Jaeschke, 1989; Benzick *et al.*, 1994). Inhibition of glutathione reductase with 1,3-bis(chloroethyl)-1-nitrosourea (BCNU) increased the glutathione depletion and toxicity of paracetamol and N-acetyl-p-benzoquinoneimine, and also increased modestly the efflux of oxidized glutathione (Albano *et al.*, 1985; Hayes *et al.*, 1986; Kyle *et al.*, 1988; Harman *et al.*, 1991; Adamson and Harman, 1993). 1,3-Bis(chloroethyl)-1-nitrosourea and diethyl maleate had differential effects on the toxicity of paracetamol and its 3,5-dimethyl- and 2,6-dimethyl- analogues (Porubek *et al.*, 1987), and as judged by the effects of the reductase inhibitor, paracetamol and N-acetyl-p-benzoquinoneimine had different mechanisms of cytotoxicity (Harman *et al.*, 1991). Potentiation of the toxicity of paracetamol by 1,3-bis(chloroethyl)-1-nitrosourea was prevented by liposome-encapsulated superoxide dismutase without influencing hepatic glutathione, and this was interpreted as evidence for a role of superoxide in paracetamol hepatotoxicity (Nakae *et al.*, 1990a).

The formation of glutathione was limited by the availability of cysteine, and treatment with cysteine and its prodrugs facilitated its synthesis. Toxicity and the depleting effect of paracetamol on hepatic glutathione were effectively antagonized by a variety of thiols and potential sulphydryl donors, including cysteine itself (Strubelt *et al.*, 1974; Estrela *et al.*, 1983; Miners *et al.*, 1984d; Yeung, 1988; Larrauri *et al.*, 1989; Dalhoff and Poulsen, 1993c); cystathione (Kitamura *et al.*, 1989); methionine (Viña *et al.*, 1980, 1989; Miners *et al.*, 1984d); cysteamine (Strubelt *et al.*, 1974; Miners *et al.*, 1984d); N-acetylcysteine (Viña *et al.*, 1980, 1989; Massey and Racz, 1981; Bonanomi *et al.*, 1982; Estrela *et al.*, 1983; Lauterburg *et al.*, 1983; Dawson *et al.*, 1984; Miners *et al.*, 1984d; Corcoran *et al.*, 1985b; Klaassen *et al.*, 1985; Speeg *et al.*, 1985; Davies *et al.*, 1986; Harman and Self, 1986; Hazelton *et al.*, 1986a; Hjelle *et al.*, 1986; Yeung, 1988; Larrauri *et al.*, 1989; Fiaschi *et al.*, 1990); α-mercaptopropionylglycine (Harman and Self, 1986); dimethyl sulphoxide (Jeffery and Haschek, 1988); dithiothreitol (Davies *et al.*, 1986; Harman and Self, 1986; Tee *et al.*, 1986b; Porubek *et al.*, 1987); dithiocarb (Strubelt *et al.*, 1974); thioproline (Larrauri *et al.*, 1989); L-2-oxo- and L-2-methylthiazolidine-4-carboxylic acids (Strubelt *et al.*, 1974; Klaassen *et al.*, 1985; Hazelton *et al.*, 1986a; Fiaschi *et al.*, 1990), captopril and penicillamine (Yeung, 1988); and propylthiouracil (Raheja *et al.*, 1982, 1983a, 1987). The D- isomers of 2-methylthiazolidine-4-carboxylic acid and N-acetylcysteine were ineffective in reversing the effects of paracetamol on toxicity and hepatic glutathione, presumably because they did not stimulate glutathione synthesis (Klaassen *et al.*, 1985; Corcoran and Wong, 1986), while methionine and 2-oxothiazolidine-4-carboxylic acid did not increase glutathione or prevent the toxicity of paracetamol in human hepatocytes (Larrauri *et al.*, 1989). Methionine was ineffective in preventing toxicity in hepatocytes that had been exposed previously to a toxic concentration of paracetamol (Davies *et al.*, 1986), and N-acetylcysteine did not prevent glutathione depletion and liver damage in mice when given intravenously 2 h before a toxic dose of paracetamol (Wendel *et al.*, 1982). N-acetylcysteine, glutathione and ascorbic acid antagonized the effects of N-acetyl-p-benzoquinoneimine in reducing the glutathione content of hepatocytes and prevented cytotoxicity (Holme *et al.*, 1984; Nasseri-Sina *et al.*, 1992). Glutathione itself had only a modest effect on paracetamol-induced toxicity and depletion of hepatic glutathione *in vivo* when given intraperitoneally (Strubelt *et al.*, 1974) and orally (Viña *et al.*, 1989), but greater efficacy was claimed with the intravenous administration of glutathione incorporated into liposomes (Wendel *et al.*, 1982) or conjugated with dextran (Kaneo *et al.*, 1989a,b). Although, in general, changes in glutathione status have corresponded well with changes in susceptibility to paracetamol toxicity, there have been exceptions and anomalies. There was a poor correlation between cytotoxicity and the glutathione content in cultured human hepatocytes (Larrauri *et al.*, 1989), and in other studies protection against toxicity without prevention of glutathione depletion was reported for α-mercaptopropionylglycine (Labadarios *et al.*, 1977), dimethylaminoethanol (Siegers and Younes, 1979), cimetidine (Mitchell *et al.*, 1981b; Peterson *et al.*, 1983), ascorbic acid (Peterson and Knodell, 1984), dithiothreitol (Tee *et al.*, 1986b), chlorpromazine (Saville *et al.*, 1988), anethol dithiolthione (Warnet *et al.*, 1989a,b) and iloprost (Nasseri-Sina *et al.*, 1992). Tienilic acid inhibited glutathione S-transferase, and would be expected to deplete glutathione, but it did not potentiate paracetamol hepatotoxicity (Ahokas *et al.*, 1984).

Oxidative Stress and Lipid Peroxidation

Lipid peroxidation was a well-established mechanism of toxicity for agents such as carbon tetrachloride and the question of a similar mechanism for paracetamol arose following reports of protection against its hepatotoxicity by free radical scavengers and antioxidants such as vitamin E (α-tocopherol) and propylgallate (Kelleher *et al.*, 1976a,b). In subsequent studies, toxic doses of paracetamol were found to produce some degree of lipid peroxidation that was correlated *in vivo* and *in vitro* and increased by fasting. It was absolutely dependent on depletion of glutathione but depletion in itself did not necessarily result in lipid peroxidation (Chiu and Bhakthan, 1978; Wendel *et al.*, 1979, 1982; Flaccavento *et al.*, 1980b; Sonawane *et al.*, 1980; Wendel and Feuerstein, 1981; Fairhurst *et al.*, 1982; Albano *et al.*, 1983; Barber *et al.*, 1983; Thelen and Wendel, 1983; Wendel, 1983). Lipid peroxidation involved the generation of reactive oxygen species, such as superoxide anions, hydroxyl radicals and hydrogen peroxide, which could cause peroxidation of unsaturated membrane lipids resulting in loss of cellular integrity and viability. The toxicity of peroxides could be prevented by their reaction with glutathione peroxidase to form oxidized glutathione, which in turn would be converted back to reduced glutathione by glutathione reductase. Increased formation of oxidized glutathione following exposure to paracetamol was therefore taken as a sensitive indicator of oxidative stress (Adams *et al.*, 1983; Harman *et al.*, 1992a; Adamson and Harman, 1993). Lipid peroxidation was usually assessed *in vivo* by measurement of expired ethane and pentane as scission products of peroxidized fatty acids, and *in vitro* by the formation of malondialdehyde. It was proposed that the metabolism of paracetamol involved one electron oxidation, which generated a phenoxy radical and hydrogen peroxide. The former would donate an electron to molecular oxygen thereby forming superoxide anion and reactive N-acetyl-p-benzoquinoneimine. The superoxide and hydrogen peroxide would then give rise to lipid peroxidation (de Vries, 1981; Rosen *et al.*, 1983; Farber and Gerson, 1984; Fischer and Mason, 1984). The protection against paracetamol hepatotoxicity shown by a variety of free radical scavengers and antioxidants was widely accepted as evidence for an oxidative mechanism of toxicity (Kelleher *et al.*, 1976a; McLean and Nuttall, 1976; Albano *et al.*, 1983; Mansuy *et al.*, 1986; Farber *et al.*, 1988; Jeffery *et al.*, 1988; Kyle *et al.*, 1988, 1990; Donatus *et al.*, 1990).

Other investigators have described increased lipid peroxidation following exposure to toxic doses of paracetamol under different conditions, but prior induction of mixed function oxidase by pretreatment with 3-methylcholanthrene or phenobarbitone was usually necessary in resistant species such as the rat (Gutteridge and Wardle, 1981; Harman and Fischer, 1983; Beales *et al.*, 1985; Mitchell *et al.*, 1985; Younes and Siegers, 1985; Mansuy *et al.*, 1986; Kyle *et al.*, 1987; Farber *et al.*, 1988; van de Straat *et al.*, 1988a,b; Younes *et al.*, 1988; Nakae *et al.*, 1990a; Dwivedi *et al.*, 1991; Muriel *et al.*, 1992, 1993; Singh *et al.*, 1992; Szymanska *et al.*, 1992; Li *et al.*, 1994b; Özdemirler *et al.*, 1994). Lipid peroxidation produced by paracetamol was correlated with reduced excretion of bile and increased plasma aminotransferase activity (Skakun and Shmanko, 1984). Paracetamol potentiated lipid peroxidation induced by carbon tetrachloride (Flaccavento *et al.*, 1980a) and when it was given in combination with theophylline and caffeine there was a greater loss of glutathione and more lipid peroxidation than with paracetamol alone (Farag and Abdel-Meguid, 1994). There were also reports of reduction of lipid peroxidation, often with corresponding protection against hepatotoxicity, following treatment with a variety of agents including: α-tocopherol (Fairhurst *et al.*, 1982; Albano *et al.*, 1983; Mansuy *et al.*, 1986); diphenyl-p-phenylenediamine (Albano *et al.*, 1983; Farber *et al.*, 1988; Kyle *et al.*, 1988, 1990); calcium ethylenediaminetetraacetic acid (EDTA) (Beales *et al.*, 1985); curcumin (Donatus *et al.*, 1990); picroliv (Dwivedi *et al.*, 1991; Singh *et al.*, 1992); glutathione (Wendel *et al.*, 1982; Wendel, 1983); N-acetylcysteine, cysteamine and butylated hydroxytoluene (Fairhurst *et al.*, 1982); anisyldithiolthione, propylgallate and levamisole (Mansuy *et al.*, 1986); silymarin and related compounds (Campos *et al.*, 1988; Muriel *et al.*, 1992; Singh *et al.*, 1992); superoxide dismutase in liposomes (Nakae *et al.*, 1990a,b); diethyldithiocarbamate, SKF 525A, metyrapone, pyrazole and α-naphthoflavone (Wendel and Feuerstein, 1981); colchicine (Muriel *et al.*, 1993); and ebselen (Li *et al.*, 1994b).

There was indirect evidence to support the theory that paracetamol toxicity was mediated by oxidative stress. The protective effect of allopurinol against paracetamol hepatotoxicity was thought to be related to its antioxidant action rather than inhibition of the formation of reactive oxygen (Jaeschke, 1990); and the formation of high molecular weight protein aggregates in the livers of rats following the administration of toxic doses of paracetamol was interpreted as evidence for a contribution by lipid peroxidation to liver damage (Minamide *et al.*, 1992). In some reports, paracetamol appeared to increase the efflux of oxidized glutathione (Kyle *et al.*, 1990; Adamson and Harman, 1993) and its toxicity was increased by inhibition of glutathione reductase with 1,3-bis(chloroethyl)-1-nitrosourea (Gerson *et al.*, 1985; Kyle *et al.*, 1987, 1988, 1990; Farber *et al.*, 1988; Nakae *et al.*, 1988, 1990a; Harman *et al.*, 1991; Adamson and Harman, 1993; Ito *et al.*, 1994). In other studies, lipid peroxidation could not be demonstrated without inhibition of glutathione reductase (Farber *et al.*, 1988; Ellouk-Achard *et al.*, 1994) and the potentiating effect of 1,3-bis(chloroethyl)-1-nitrosourea was reversed by diphenyl-p-phenylenediamine and desferrioxamine (Nakae *et al.*, 1988). In contrast to these findings, others reported that treatment with 1,3-bis(chloroethyl)-1-nitrosourea had no effect on paracetamol hepatotoxicity (Smith and Mitchell, 1985), mortality (Smith *et al.*, 1985) and the time course or degree of cytotoxicity (Porubek *et al.*, 1987; Andersson *et al.*, 1989). As might be expected in a mechanism involving oxidative stress, toxicity was reduced if superoxide was removed by the addition of superoxide dismutase (Kyle *et al.*, 1987; Nakae *et al.*, 1990a,b) and if hydrogen peroxide was removed by adding catalase (Kyle *et al.*, 1987). Copper (II) (3,5-diisopropylsalicylate)$_2$, a synthetic superoxide dismutase, had an insignificant effect on paracetamol toxicity (Joyave *et al.*, 1985), but other copper compounds depressed lipid peroxidation (Wendel and Heidinger, 1980). In some reports, superoxide dismutase did not inhibit paracetamol-induced lipid peroxidation in rat liver postmitochondrial supernatant fractions (Wendel and Heidinger, 1980; Fairhurst *et al.*, 1982). The activities of glutathione peroxidase and glutathione reductase were higher in hepatocytes from young than from adult mice, and the resistance of cells from the young mice to the cytotoxicity of paracetamol was put forward as evidence for a mechanistic role of peroxides (Adamson and Harman, 1989). Glutathione peroxidase activity was reduced by a selenium-deficient diet and this was associated with protection against paracetamol hepatotoxicity (Burk and Lane, 1983). The oxidative component of paracetamol hepatotoxicity was associated with the later stages of injury, and it could be reduced by ebselen, a selenium-containing compound with glutathione peroxidase activity (Harman *et al.*, 1992a).

Perioxidative damage to cell membranes was iron dependent and the initiation of lipid peroxidation required the presence of active iron. The finding that desferrioxamine (deferoxamine) could reduce paracetamol hepatotoxicity and mortality was consistent with an oxidative mechanism of toxicity (Gerson *et al.*, 1985; Kyle *et al.*, 1988, 1990; Harman *et al.*, 1991, 1992a; Sakaida *et al.*, 1992; Adamson and Harman, 1993; Benzick *et al.*, 1994; Ito *et al.*, 1994). Desferrioxamine depressed the formation of malondialdehyde without preventing hepatic glutathione depletion or reducing the covalent binding of [^{3}H]-paracetamol to liver proteins (Sakaida *et al.*, 1995). Desferrioxamine reduced the output of oxidized glutathione (Adamson and Harman, 1993), and paracetamol reduced the biliary efflux of iron (Benzick *et al.*, 1994; Gupta, 1994). Resistance to the hepatotoxicity of paracetamol induced by desferrioxamine was restored by the addition of ferrous and ferric ions. Superoxide dismutase and catalase prevented injury in the presence of ferric iron, and catalase (but not superoxide dismutase) protected with ferrous iron (Kyle *et al.*, 1987). Treatment of rats with ferrous fumarate for three weeks increased lipid peroxidation produced by paracetamol (Younes *et al.*, 1989). Again, there were contradictory findings and desferrioxamine completely or partially inhibited lipid peroxidation without protecting against paracetamol toxicity (Younes and Siegers, 1985a; Porubek *et al.*, 1987; Siegers *et al.*, 1988; Younes *et al.*, 1988).

There were other examples of dissociation of lipid peroxidation from toxicity (Fairhurst and Horton, 1984; Beales *et al.*, 1985; Tee *et al.*, 1986b; Donatus *et al.*, 1990), and this was also shown in studies with 3-mono- and 3,5-dimethyl substituted derivatives of paracetamol (van de Straat *et al.*, 1987b, 1988a). It was also possible that the demonstration of lipid peroxidation was method dependent (Gutteridge and Wardle, 1981). These and other discrepancies have made it difficult to accept oxidative stress and lipid peroxidation as primary mechanisms of paracetamol toxicity (Badr, 1994). Some investigators were unable to demonstrate that paracetamol caused lipid peroxidation, and under certain conditions (notably with liver microsomal incubations) it appeared to act as an antioxidant and a scavenger of superoxide and other radicals so that it actually protected against lipid peroxidation (Högberg and Kristoferson, 1977; Aikawa *et al.*, 1978a; Anundi *et al.*, 1979; Hughes *et al.*, 1981; Negro *et al.*, 1981; Albano *et al.*, 1983; DuBois *et al.*, 1983; Muller, 1983; Reiter and Wendel, 1983; Wendel and Hallbach, 1986; Porubek *et al.*, 1987; Farber *et al.*, 1988; Tsokos-Kuhn *et al.*, 1988a; van de Straat *et al.*, 1988a,b; van Steveninck *et al.*, 1989; Garrido *et al.*, 1991; Pavlovich *et al.*, 1991; Reicks *et al.*, 1992; Kamiyama *et al.*, 1993). Paracetamol was less active than 5-aminosalicylic acid as an inhibitor of membrane lipid peroxidation and a scavenger of peroxyl radicals (Dinis *et al.*, 1994). The inhibition of lipid peroxidation by paracetamol and its analogues was related to their lipophilicity (van de Straat *et al.*, 1988) and their half-wave oxidation potentials (Porubek *et al.*, 1987). Paracetamol also inhibited the spontaneous formation of hydrogen peroxide by rat liver microsomes (van de Straat *et al.*, 1988b) and its antioxidant action was concentration dependent (Farber *et al.*, 1988; Pavlovich *et al.*, 1991). In addition to these findings, most investigators have shown that contrary to expectations in the event of oxidative stress, paracetamol did not significantly increase the production of oxidized glutathione (Adams *et al.*, 1983; Lauterburg *et al.*, 1984b; Miller and Jollow, 1984; Smith and Mitchell, 1985; van de Straat *et al.*, 1986; Porubek *et al.*, 1987; Farber *et al.*, 1988; Andersson *et al.*, 1989; Smith and Jaeschke, 1989; Benzick *et al.*, 1994). There have also been contradictory reports concerning the effects of vitamin E. Initially, dietary deficiency potentiated paracetamol hepatotoxicity, and the addition of vitamin E conferred some protection (Kelleher *et al.*, 1976b). Similarly, α-tocopherol reduced lipid peroxidation and toxicity produced in isolated hepatocytes by paracetamol (Albano *et al.*, 1983). On the other hand, at a concentration of 1887 mg l^{-1}, paracetamol reduced lipid peroxidation and increased the viability of hepatocytes from vitamin E-deficient rats (DuBois *et al.*, 1983), and in another report, vitamin E-deficient rats were resistant to paracetamol toxicity while susceptibility was restored by correcting the deficiency (Mitchell *et al.*, 1981a). Lipid peroxidation could not proceed without the generation of active oxygen by the one electron oxidation of paracetamol and there was no evidence that this occurred during its microsomal metabolism (Powis *et al.*, 1984; van de Straat *et al.*, 1988b) as distinct from metabolism by a peroxidase and hydrogen peroxide system (Keller and Hinson, 1991). In addition, there was no evidence that paracetamol was bound covalently to alkyl residues of hepatic lipids (Smith *et al.*, 1984). In some cases the confusing results of these studies of oxidative stress and lipid peroxidation could have been due to the use of dimethyl sulphoxide as the solvent for paracetamol by some investigators (Wendel and Feuerstein, 1981; Wendel *et al.*, 1982; Mitchell *et al.*, 1985; Kyle *et al.*, 1987, 1988, 1990; Nakae *et al.*, 1988, 1990a,b; Garrido *et al.*, 1991; Harman *et al.*, 1991). Nitric oxide appeared to have a role as liver damage induced by paracetamol was increased when its cytokine-mediated formation was inhibited with N^G-monomethyl-L-arginine. These findings were thought to indicate protection by nitric oxide against oxidative damage as a result of regulation of hepatic glutathione status (Kuo and Slivka, 1994). The overall conclusion was that oxidative stress was unlikely to be an important mechanism in paracetamol toxicity (Smith and Mitchell, 1985; Porubek *et al.*, 1987; Brent and Rumack, 1993) and the lipid peroxidation observed in animals receiving paracetamol was probably the result, rather than the cause of toxicity (Mitchell *et al.*, 1981a).

Calcium Homeostasis

Disruption of intracellular calcium homeostasis has been considered as a primary event in paracetamol hepatotoxicity. Moore *et al.* (1985a) found that paracetamol and N-acetyl-p-benzoquinoneimine increased cytosolic free Ca^{2+} as shown by increased glycogen phosphorylase *a* activity, and that this was accompanied by blebbing of hepatocytes and loss of mitochondrial Ca^{2+}. The disturbance of Ca^{2+} balance always preceded cell death and the loss of mitochondrial Ca^{2+} preceded membrane damage. It was concluded that loss of protein-bound thiols was responsible for inhibition of high affinity Ca^{2+}-ATPase activity in the plasma membrane and that this ultimately resulted in cytotoxicity and cell death. Tsokos-Kuhn and her colleagues (1985) reported inhibition by paracetamol of ATP-dependent Ca^{2+} uptake by plasma membrane vesicles and proposed that inhibition of plasma membrane Ca^{2+} regulation was a connecting link between the alkylation hypothesis and the perturbed Ca^{2+} homeostasis hypothesis of lethal cell injury. Other investigators subsequently showed that toxic doses of paracetamol caused an increase in phosphorylase *a* activity, and hence, by inference, an increase in cytosolic Ca^{2+}, and that this was an early event which seemed to precede, or coincide with morphological and biochemical signs of toxicity (Corcoran *et al.*, 1987b, 1988; Long and Moore, 1988; Saville *et al.*, 1988; Burcham and Harman, 1989; Horton and Wood, 1989; Tsokos-Kuhn, 1989; Yamamoto, 1990; Vu *et al.*, 1992). The increase in phosphorylase *a* occurred at the same time as glutathione was depleted, and disruption of Ca^{2+} homeostasis appeared to be a consequence of arylation and covalent binding (Corcoran *et al.*, 1987b, 1988). The changes in cytosolic Ca^{2+} were dose and time dependent, and were associated with an increase in mitochondrial Ca^{2+} concentration (Burcham and Harman, 1988). Investigation of the translocation of Ca^{2+} across liver cell plasma membranes following toxic doses of paracetamol revealed an increase in the calcium space with early influx of Ca^{2+} before the onset of irreversible cellular injury (Lauterburg, 1987). The increase in hepatocyte Ca^{2+} content correlated with the extent of histological liver damage (Landon *et al.*, 1986) and histochemical changes in the activity of perivenous phosphorylase *a* preceded major loss of cell membrane integrity (Jepson *et al.*, 1987). Paracetamol-induced accumulation of Ca^{2+} in the isolated perfused rat liver was associated with metabolic and biochemical indices of hepatotoxicity (Strubelt and Younes, 1992), and depletion of glutathione was related to the increase in glycogen phosphorylase *a* (Vu *et al.*, 1992). Cytotoxicity depended on prolonged elevation of cytosolic Ca^{2+}, and increased activity of phosphorylase *a* was associated with inhibition of the Ca^{2+} pump of the plasma membrane, but not that of the endoplasmic reticulum (Long and Moore, 1988). The time sequence of the changes in free Ca^{2+} and phosphorylase *a* activity was studied using freeze-clamped liver samples and paracetamol toxicity was thought to be caused by direct arylation of susceptible thiols of liver plasma membranes, and in particular, the ATP-dependent Ca^{2+} pump (Tsokos-Kuhn *et al.*, 1988a,b, 1989).

The paracetamol-induced increase in cytosolic Ca^{2+} caused activation of several enzymes including phospholipase A_2 and this resulted in the release of arachidonic acid and the formation of cytodestructive prostaglandins. Some protection against hepatotoxicity was observed with inhibitors of phospholipase A_2, such as quinine, corticosteroids, aspirin and non-steroidal anti-inflammatory drugs (Horton and Wood, 1989) and also with sulotroban, a thromboxane receptor antagonist (Horton and Wood, 1991). Early (0–2 h) and late (6–12 h) phases were recognized in the loss of Ca^{2+} homeostasis caused by paracetamol in mouse hepatocytes. The late changes corresponded with loss of nuclear sequestration of calcium and this could have involved phospholipase A_2 since toxicity was reduced by inhibitors such as chlorpromazine and diltiazem (Harris and Hamrick, 1993). The disturbances of calcium balance induced by paracetamol were associated with an increase in nuclear Ca^{2+}, which was parallelled by an increase in fragmented DNA with substantial loss of large genomic DNA. The DNA fragments accumulated in a ladder-like pattern that was characteristic of Ca^{2+}-mediated activation of endonuclease. These early changes were correlated with subsequent cytotoxicity and were thought to play a significant role in cell necrosis produced by paracetamol (Ray *et al.*, 1990, 1991, 1993b; Shen *et al.*, 1991, 1992). DNA fragmentation and cytotoxicity were virtually abolished by aurintricarboxylic acid, a Ca^{2+} endonuclease inhibitor, and ethyleneglycol-bis-(β-aminoethylether)-N,N,N′,N′,-tetraacetic acid (EGTA), a chelator of calcium required for endonuclease activation (Shen *et al.*, 1992). Pretreatment with chlorpromazine, and to a lesser extent verapamil, prevented both the increase in nuclear Ca^{2+} and biochemical signs of paracetamol hepatotoxicity (Ray *et al.*, 1993b). Chlorpromazine also inhibited the paracetamol-induced increase in phosphorylase *a* and hepatotoxicity in fed and fasted mice in a dose-dependent fashion and this was attributed to 'negative sensitivity modulation to calcium in hepatocytes' (Saville *et al.*, 1988). In keeping with the postulated role of calcium in paracetamol toxicity, other investigators reported protection and decreased accumulation of Ca^{2+} following treatment with Ca EDTA (Beales *et al.*, 1985; Hue *et al.*, 1985), chlorpromazine (Landon *et al.*, 1986; Kamiyama *et al.*, 1993), diltiazem (Deakin *et al.*, 1991; Thibault *et al.*, 1991; Kamiyama *et al.*, 1993), nifedipine (Landon *et al.*, 1986) and verapamil, gallopamil and ethyleneglycol-bis-(β-aminoethylether)-N,N,N′,N′,-tetraacetic acid (Thibault *et al.*, 1991). Trifluoperazine prevented the increase in phosphorylase *a* and Ca^{2+}, and protected against paracetamol liver damage in mice, but it also caused hypothermia and all protection was lost if normothermia was maintained (Yamamoto, 1990). The increase in cytosolic calcium concentration was antagonized by prior loading of hamster hepatocytes with the chelator Quin 2-AM, and there was also protection when after initial exposure, paracetamol was removed from the incubation medium. The Quin 2-AM had less effect on blebbing than on cell viability, and the increase in Ca^{2+} was thought to be the cause of cell death (Boobis *et al.*, 1990). In another study with Quin 2, the effect of paracetamol on cytosolic Ca^{2+} was studied over five days. Concentrations increased before cytotoxicity was apparent and were correlated with biochemical evidence of toxicity. The changes in Ca^{2+} and cytotoxicity were reversed by promethazine and ethyleneglycol-bis-(β-aminoethyl ether)-N,N,N′,N′,-tetraacetic acid (Bruschi and Priestly, 1990). Paracetamol had no effect on intracellular Ca^{2+} in hamster V79 and HeLa cells in culture (Fortunati *et al.*, 1993).

N-acetyl-p-benzoquinoneimine and its 3,5-dimethyl- and 2,6-dimethyl- derivatives caused arylation and/or oxidation of plasma membrane ATPase in isolated hepatocytes (Andersson *et al.*, 1989). 2,6-Dimethyl N-acetyl-p-benzoquinoneimine produced greater loss of protein thiols, greater accumulation of cytosolic Ca^{2+}, and greater inhibition of plasma membrane ATPase than 3,5-dimethyl N-acetyl-p-benzoquinoneimine. The cytotoxic effects of these analogues and of N-acetyl-p-benzoquinoneimine itself were preceded by a sustained rise in cytosolic free Ca^{2+}. Both arylation and oxidation of protein thiols were thought to cause the increase in Ca^{2+} and cytotoxicity, and arylation of critical thiols appeared to be the more lethal reaction (Nicotera *et al.*, 1989). Paracetamol decreased plasma membrane calcium ATPase and reduced the ability of isolated mitochondria to sequester calcium, but 3-hydroxyacetanilide had no such effects (Tirmenstein and Nelson, 1989). Studies with radiolabelled paracetamol and mouse liver proteins suggested inactivation of the microsomal Ca^{2+} pump by adduct formation as there was binding to proteins with N-terminal sequences identical to calreticulum, an intraluminal Ca^{2+} sequestration protein and thiol:protein disulphide oxidoreductase (Zhou *et al.*, 1993).

Recent studies suggested that the rise in free cytosolic Ca^{2+} was not the primary trigger for paracetamol toxicity. Concentrations of paracetamol that caused plasma membrane damage in mouse hepatocytes also activated phosphorylase *a* and caused loss of glycogen. The latter effect could be dissociated from cytotoxicity since N-acetylcysteine and 2,4-dichloro-6-phenylphenoxyethylamine reduced plasma membrane damage but had no effect on phosphorylase *a* or loss of glycogen (Burcham and Harman, 1989). The increase in cytosolic Ca^{2+} produced by paracetamol in isolated hepatocytes accompanied, but did not precede loss of viability, and chelation of cytosolic Ca^{2+} with fura-2 did not prevent cytotoxicity (Davies *et al.*, 1992; Hardwick *et al.*, 1992b; Grewal and Racz, 1993). It was possible to produce a greater increase in Ca^{2+} with the ionophore 4-bromo-A23187 without causing cell death than with a toxic dose of paracetamol, and paracetamol had no effect on the increase in calcium concentrations produced by vasopressin (Hardwick *et al.*, 1992a,b). In another study, the increase in cytosolic free Ca^{2+} in hepatocytes incubated with paracetamol was delayed for more than 2 h and it occurred shortly before the decrease in viability, but well before the appearance of blebbing. There was no sustained increase in Ca^{2+} concentrations before or during the time when irreversible toxic events occurred in the hepatocytes (Harman *et al.*, 1992b).

Thiol Oxidation and Arylation

The consensus of recent opinion has favoured oxidation and arylation of critical protein thiols as the cause of paracetamol hepatotoxicity and oxidation in particular was a plausible alternative hypothesis to covalent binding as a mechanism of toxicity. N-acetyl-p-benzoquinoneimine has both electrophilic and oxidative properties, and thiols and antioxidants can protect against liver damage. The development of this hypothesis was facilitated by a model first described by Mclean and Nuttall (1978) in which rat liver slices were exposed to paracetamol for 2 h as a first phase during which damage was sustained as a result of its metabolic activation and covalent binding to cell structures. This damage only became manifest during a second post-exposure phase of incubation for 4 h in paracetamol-free medium. In this way it was possible to separate the initial covalent binding of paracetamol from the subsequent events leading to cell injury and death. McLean and Nuttall (1978) found that antioxidants such as methylene blue, promethazine and (+)catechin prevented injury when added after the exposure to paracetamol had ended, indicating the existence of a reversible process subsequent to the covalent binding of paracetamol metabolites to sensitive cell sites. This two-phase model was used extensively to study the initiation of cell damage and the mechanisms of reversal of the post-arylation events leading to hepatocyte injury and death (Devalia *et al.*, 1982; Harman and Fischer, 1983; Holme *et al.*, 1984; Beales *et al.*, 1985; Harman, 1985; Boobis *et al.*, 1986, 1990; Davies *et al.*, 1986, 1992; Harman and Self, 1986; Tee *et al.*, 1986b, 1987; Grewal and Racz, 1993; and others).

The toxicity of paracetamol and N-acetyl-p-benzoquinoneimine was associated with loss of cellular protein thiols (Albano *et al.*, 1985; Moore *et al.*, 1985a; Porubek *et al.*, 1987; Andersson *et al.*, 1989; Nicotera *et al.*, 1989; Tirmenstein and Nelson, 1990) and their effects on mitochondrial thiols were considered particularly relevant (Nelson *et al.*, 1991). The loss of protein thiols seemed to be due largely to oxidation since hepatotoxicity could be reduced or prevented by antioxidants such as methylene blue, (+)catechin, 3-O-methyl(+)catechin and promethazine (McLean and Nuttall, 1978), and diphenylphenylenediamine and α-tocopherol (Harman, 1985). The thiol reductant dithiothreitol was even more effective in reversing hepatotoxicity after exposure to paracetamol and restoring protein thiols (Boobis *et al.*, 1986, 1990; Harman and Self, 1986; Tee *et al.*, 1986b; Nelson *et al.*, 1991; Grewal and Racz, 1993), and when added to the incubation medium shortly after exposure to N-acetyl-p-benzoquinoneimine it also reversed toxicity caused by this agent (Albano *et al.*, 1985; Davies *et al.*, 1986; Lauriault and O'Brien, 1991). The timing was critical and in another report dithiothreitol only partially restored the loss of protein thiols induced by N-acetyl-p-benzoquinoneimine (Nicotera *et al.*, 1989). N-acetyl-p-benzoquinoneimine seemed to cause largely oxidative damage to sulphydryl groups of key enzymes, which was lethal in cells that had been depleted of glutathione, and this oxidation could be reversed by thiol reductants (Davies *et al.*, 1986). Dithiothreitol probably acted by reducing N-acetyl-p-benzoquinoneimine back to paracetamol, converting oxidized glutathione back to the reduced form and regenerating protein thiols by reducing mixed protein disulphides (Lauriault and O'Brien, 1991). N-acetylcysteine and glutathione (but not methionine) also reduced cytotoxicity in hepatocytes after exposure to paracetamol and N-acetyl-p-benzoquinoneimine (Green and Fischer, 1984; Boobis *et al.*, 1986; Davies *et al.*, 1986; Holme and Jacobsen, 1986; Grewal and Racz, 1993).

It was possible to dissociate the oxidative and arylating properties of paracetamol and its 3,5-dimethyl- and 2,6-dimethyl- analogues. Like N-acetyl-p-benzoquinoneimine, 3,5-dimethyl-N-acetyl-p-benzoquinoneimine depleted protein thiols in isolated hepatocytes and oxidation appeared to be the primary mechanism of toxicity as judged by ready reversal with dithiothreitol (Andersson *et al.*, 1989; Nicotera *et al.*, 1989). In another report, 3,5-dimethyl-N-acetyl-p-benzoquinoneimine did not deplete protein thiols or cause toxicity unless glutathione had been reduced artificially by treatment with 1,3-bis(chloroethyl)-1-nitrosourea or diethyl maleate. Toxicity was again reversed by dithiothreitol and it was concluded that damage could be produced by protein thiol oxidation without lipid peroxidation (van de Straat *et al.*, 1987a). 2,6-Dimethyl-N-acetyl-p-benzoquinoneimine was found to bind more extensively to protein thiols than the 3,5-dimethyl analogue and it caused irreversible arylation. It was more cytotoxic, and it was more difficult to reverse toxicity with dithiothreitol (Nicotera *et al.*, 1989; Lauriault and O'Brien, 1991). The loss of protein thiols produced by these paracetamol analogues was greater than could be accounted for by the degree of covalent binding. Paracetamol and 3,5-dimethylparacetamol caused the formation of protein aggregates of high molecular weight which were not linked by disulphide bonds (Birge *et al.*, 1988). A significant fraction of the protein thiol loss produced by paracetamol was attributed to oxidation but 3-hydroxyacetanilide had no such effects. It was proposed that the associated conversion of xanthine oxidase to the oxidized form caused a transient increase in activated oxygen which, together with reduced activities of glutathione peroxidase and thioltransferase, contributed to protein thiol oxidation (Tirmenstein and Nelson, 1990). Collectively, these findings indicate an important role for oxidation and arylation of thiols in paracetamol hepatotoxicity but anomalous results have been reported. Dithiocarb protected against the toxicity of N-acetyl-p-benzoquinoneimine and its 2,6-dimethyl derivative in isolated rat hepatocytes and it appeared to form conjugates (Lauriault and O'Brien, 1991). In another study, dithiocarb and metyrapone had some protective effect against toxicity in hamster hepatocytes when added after exposure to paracetamol and these agents clearly had a protective action separate from their ability to inhibit the metabolic activation of the drug. Contrary to expectations, N-acetylcysteine and α-mercaptopropionylglycine failed to protect mouse hepatocytes from plasma membrane damage when added after exposure to paracetamol (Harman and Self, 1986).

Target Proteins for Paracetamol Arylation

Early characterization of the thioether metabolites of paracetamol was consistent with the possibility of arylation of cysteinyl thiol groups and the corresponding conjugates were subsequently found to represent the major protein-bound residues of paracetamol. Studies with bovine serum albumin indicated that the reactive metabolite of paracetamol became covalently bound to protein cysteinyl thiols (Streeter *et al.*, 1984b). Similar results were obtained with N-acetyl-p-benzoquinoneimine and this caused cross-linking of the albumin molecules that could not be reversed with dithiothreitol (Streeter *et al.*, 1986). The [^{14}C]-paracetamol adduct with bovine serum albumin was shown to contain only one major radiolabelled amino-acid adduct that was identified as the 3-cysteinyl conjugate, and the site of the binding was probably at cysteine residue 34 (Hoffmann *et al.*, 1985b). Cysteine residues were the primary targets for arylation by the reactive metabolite of paracetamol and the major adduct formed with mouse liver protein was shown to be the 3-cysteinyl conjugate (Hoffmann *et al.*, 1985a).

A competitive enzyme-linked immunosorbent assay was developed for the paracetamol cysteine protein adduct and this could be detected in mice following administration of toxic doses of the drug (Roberts *et al.*, 1987a, 1989; Potter *et al.*, 1989). Peak concentrations in liver proteins were observed at 2 h after a dose of 400 mg kg^{-1} after which time the concentrations declined. In contrast, the appearance of the paracetamol cysteine protein adduct in the circulation was delayed with a sustained peak after 6–12 h. In patients with liver damage following paracetamol poisoning there was a good correlation between plasma concentrations of the paracetamol cysteine protein adduct and the severity of hepatotoxicity as shown by increased plasma alanine aminotransferase activity (Hinson *et al.*, 1990). The adduct appeared first in mouse liver cytosol and as concentrations declined, the adducts were detected in serum in parallel with increasing aminotransferase activity. The highest concentrations of the paracetamol cysteine protein adduct were found in plasma membranes and mitochondria (Pumford *et al.*, 1990b). Polyacrylamide gel electrophoresis revealed more than 15 proteins containing the paracetamol cysteine adducts, and the pattern of their distribution of molecular weights was similar in liver supernatant and serum. The temporal relationship between the appearance of the adducts in serum and their disappearance from the liver suggested that the adducts were released from the liver into the circulation following lysis of the hepatocytes (Pumford *et al.*, 1990a). A similar time sequence of the formation and distribution of the specific paracetamol cysteine protein adduct in mice was correlated with cell injury (Roberts *et al.*, 1991b). Changes in serum insulin and injury to pancreatic β-cells in mice given toxic doses of paracetamol were not associated with the appearance of the paracetamol cysteine protein adduct in the pancreas (Ferguson *et al.*, 1990). Both enzyme-linked immunosorbent assays and particle concentration fluorescent immunoassays were developed for the demonstration of the paracetamol cysteine protein adduct (Benson *et al.*, 1989; Roberts *et al.*, 1991a; Pohl, 1993).

With the use of specific affinity purified antisera against paracetamol-bound liver proteins it was possible to localize binding to centrilobular hepatocytes, and resolution of the proteins showed predominant bands at about 44 and 58 kD (Bartolone *et al.*, 1987, 1988, 1989b). With antibodies directed specifically towards 2,6-dimethylparacetamol there was similar binding to a 58 kD protein but only minimal binding to the 44 kD protein (Birge *et al.*, 1989). Immunochemical analysis of proteins from activated human liver cytosol revealed selective binding of paracetamol to proteins of 38, 58 and 130 kD. In mouse liver, most binding of paracetamol occurred with 44 and 58 kD proteins. However, the pattern of binding to proteins in the liver of a patient who died after taking paracetamol in overdosage was similar to those observed *in vitro* in mouse and human liver (Birge *et al.*, 1990, 1991b). In another report, there was a similar pattern of binding of paracetamol to hepatic and renal proteins *in vitro* and *in vivo* in mice and in man (Tyson *et al.*, 1991). Following exposure to toxic doses of paracetamol, hepatocytes from mice were able to resynthesize the 56–58 kD proteins (Bruno *et al.*, 1991). The post-exposure protection against paracetamol-induced liver damage by piperonyl butoxide was associated with changes in the selective arylation of proteins, and the critical target appeared to be in the 58 kD protein band (Brady *et al.*, 1991). The earliest detectable target for the binding of paracetamol was a 44 kD protein and this behaved as a peripheral membrane protein associated with the endoplasmic reticulum (Birge *et al.*, 1991c). In another study, it was shown that the major cytosolic protein of 58 kD that bound paracetamol could also be modified by glutathiolation under oxidative conditions (Birge *et al.*, 1991a). The *de novo* hepatic synthesis of the 58 kD paracetamol-binding protein diminished progressively after exposure of mouse hepatocytes to paracetamol and 3,5-dimethylparacetamol (but not 2,6-dimethyl-paracetamol), and after incubation for more than 8 h the protein was not detectable during recovery. In contrast, the synthesis of a 32 kD protein was stimulated by paracetamol and its 3,5-dimethyl, but not the 2,6-dimethyl derivative (Bruno *et al.*, 1992). Determination of the amino-acid sequences of the 58 kD target protein for paracetamol binding indicated the presence of only eight cysteine residues and this low content raised the possibility of binding to non-thiol sites (Bartolone *et al.*,

1992). The major immunologically detectable cytosolic target protein for paracetamol was homologous with a specific selenium-binding protein (Bartolone *et al.*, 1992) and similar identity with a selenium-binding protein was reported for a paracetamol-binding protein of molecular weight 55 kD (Pumford *et al.*, 1992). An autoantibody to protein disulphide isomerase was detected in rats with liver damage following treatment with diethylmaleate and paracetamol (Nagayama *et al.*, 1994), but its formation was presumably the result, rather than the cause, of toxicity.

The molecular mechanisms of paracetamol hepatotoxicity have been extensively reviewed (Hinson, 1980; Monks and Lau, 1988; Nelson, 1990; Nelson and Pearson, 1990; Vermeulen *et al.*, 1992; Boelsterli, 1993). Overall, the probable mechanism was depletion of cellular glutathione by N-acetyl-p-benzoquinoneimine followed by covalent binding to, and oxidative depletion of, protein thiol groups causing disturbances of intermediary metabolism and calcium homeostasis. Lipid peroxidation was more likely to be the result than the cause of hepatotoxicity.

Factors Influencing the Hepatotoxicity of Paracetamol

The hepatotoxicity of paracetamol depended primarily on the balance between the rate of formation of its toxic reactive metabolite and the rate of synthesis of hepatic glutathione. Consequently, many factors and treatments have been shown to increase or decrease the hepatotoxicity of paracetamol, and these were usually related to effects on its toxic metabolic activation or hepatic glutathione status.

Drugs and Chemicals

Toxicity was usually potentiated by classic inducers of cytochrome P450 enzymes such as phenobarbitone (Jollow *et al.*, 1973; Mitchell *et al.*, 1973b; Walker *et al.*, 1973; McLean and Day, 1974, 1975; Miller *et al.*, 1976a; Streeter and Timbrell, 1979; Younes and Siegers, 1980b; Massey *et al.*, 1982; Sharma *et al.*, 1983; Blouin *et al.*, 1987; Kyle *et al.*, 1988; Birge *et al.*, 1989; Burk *et al.*, 1990) and 3-methylcholanthrene (Mitchell *et al.*, 1973b; Potter *et al.*, 1974; Thorgeirsson *et al.*, 1975; Jollow, 1980; Pessayre *et al.*, 1980; Gemborys and Mudge, 1981; Hart *et al.*, 1982a; Albano *et al.*, 1983; Lazarte *et al.*, 1984; van de Straat *et al.*, 1986; Lupo *et al.*, 1987; Kyle *et al.*, 1988; Lubek *et al.*, 1988b; Nakae *et al.*, 1988; Larrauri *et al.*, 1989; Kalhorn *et al.*, 1990; Roberts *et al.*, 1990; Willson *et al.*, 1991; Szymanska *et al.*, 1992). Indeed, many investigators found that it was necessary to pretreat resistant species, such as the rat, with these inducers in order to produce liver injury with any reasonable dose of paracetamol. 3-Methylcholanthrene was invariably more effective in potentiating toxicity than phenobarbitone, and several investigators reported paradoxical results with phenobarbitone that could even protect against liver damage (Potter *et al.*, 1974; Pessayre *et al.*, 1980; Gemborys and Mudge, 1981; Poulsen *et al.*, 1985b; Younes and Siegers, 1985a; Lupo *et al.*, 1987; Larrauri *et al.*, 1989; Kalhorn *et al.*, 1990). In one report, the potentiation of toxicity by phenobarbitone was due to inhibition of glucuronide conjugation rather than increased metabolic activation (Douidar and Ahmed, 1987). The distribution of covalently bound paracetamol shifted from centrilobular to periportal areas following induction with 3-methylcholanthrene (Satoh *et al.*, 1979). As expected, there was protection against paracetamol hepatotoxicity with inhibitors of microsomal oxidation such as cobaltous chloride (Jollow *et al.*, 1973; Mitchell *et al.*, 1973b; Jollow, 1980; Roberts *et al.*, 1986), SKF 525A (Massey *et al.*, 1982; Kyle *et al.*, 1988) and piperonyl butoxide (Jollow *et al.*, 1973; Mitchell *et al.*, 1973b; Potter *et al.*, 1974; Jollow, 1980; Massey *et al.*, 1982; Harman and Fischer, 1983). Susceptibility to the toxicity of paracetamol was greatly increased if glutathione was depleted with diethylmaleate (Mitchell *et al.*, 1973c, 1985; Potter *et al.*, 1974; Raheja *et al.*, 1983a; Albano *et al.*, 1985; Tsokos-Kuhn *et al.*, 1985; Hayes *et al.*, 1986; Porubek *et al.*, 1987; Roberts *et al.*, 1990; Willson *et al.*, 1991; Szymanska *et al.*, 1992; James *et al.*, 1993), or its synthesis inhibited with buthionine sulphoximine (Miners *et al.*, 1984d; Hue *et al.*, 1985; Hayes *et al.*, 1986; Wong and Corcoran, 1987; Yeung, 1988; Davies *et al.*, 1991; Bray *et al.*, 1992b; Kelly *et al.*, 1992; James *et al.*, 1993). Glutathione itself was not very effective in reversing paracetamol liver toxicity and its systemic availability after oral administration was negligible (Witschi *et al.*, 1992). It did not enter hepatocytes readily but protection could be enhanced by its administration in liposomes and as esters and glutathione-dextran macromolecular conjugates (Gazzard *et al.*, 1974b; Strubelt *et al.*, 1974; Benedetti *et al.*, 1975; Malnoë *et al.*, 1975; Negro *et al.*, 1981; Wendel *et al.*, 1982; Hirayama *et al.*, 1983; Wendel, 1983; Kaneo *et al.*, 1989a,b, 1994; Viña *et al.*, 1989; Uhlig and Wendel, 1990). There was good protection against liver necrosis with glutathione precursors such as cysteine (Mitchell *et al.*, 1973b; Strubelt *et al.*, 1974; Negro *et al.*, 1981; Miners *et al.*, 1984d; Munoz and Fearon, 1984; Yeung, 1988) and methionine and its analogues (McLean and Day, 1975; Stramentinoli *et al.*, 1979; Miners *et al.*, 1984d; Picciòla *et al.*, 1986; Skoglund *et al.*, 1986; Viña *et al.*, 1986, 1989; McLean *et al.*, 1989; Bray *et al.*, 1992b). N-acetylcysteine was proposed as an antidote for paracetamol poisoning in man (Prescott and Matthew, 1974) and it was subsequently shown to be very effective (Prescott *et al.*, 1977, 1979; Rumack and Peterson, 1978). There has since been great interest in N-acetylcysteine and the mechanism of its protective action against experimental paracetamol hepatotoxicity (Piperno and Berssenbruegge, 1976; Gerber *et al.*, 1977; Piperno *et al.*, 1978; Aliverti and Zaninelli, 1980; St. Omer and McKnight, 1980; Massey and Racz, 1981; Mitchell *et al.*, 1981b; Walker *et al.*, 1981, 1982, 1983a, 1985; Whitehouse *et al.*, 1981; Bonanomi *et al.*, 1982; Jackson, 1982; Ioannides *et al.*, 1983a; Khairy *et al.*, 1983; Lauterburg *et al.*, 1983; Banda and Quart, 1984a; Dawson *et al.*, 1984; Miners *et al.*, 1984d; Corcoran *et al.*, 1985a,b, 1987b; Klaassen *et al.*, 1985; Savides *et al.*, 1985; Speeg *et al.*, 1985; Boobis *et al.*, 1986; Corcoran and Wong, 1986; Davies *et al.*, 1986; Harman and Self, 1986; Hayes *et al.*, 1986; Hazelton *et al.*, 1986a; Hjelle *et al.*, 1986; Letteron *et al.*, 1986; Wong *et al.*, 1986; Banda and Quart, 1987; Bruno *et al.*, 1988; Yeung, 1988; Burcham and Harman, 1989, 1990; Viña *et al.*, 1989; Wormser and Ben-Zakine, 1990; Butterworth *et al.*, 1992; Nasseri-Sina *et al.*, 1992; Peterson and Brown, 1992; Shen *et al.*, 1992; Donnelly *et al.*, 1994; Gomez *et al.*, 1994).

N-acetylcysteine inhibited the covalent binding of paracetamol by about 70 per cent when it protected against liver necrosis and the time interval between its administration after dosing with paracetamol was critical for efficacy. Efficacy also depended on the route of administration (Piperno *et al.*, 1978; Corcoran *et al.*, 1985a). In mouse liver microsomal incubations, N-acetylcysteine and other thiols decreased the covalent binding of paracetamol and formed the corresponding adducts (Buckpitt *et al.*, 1979; Tredger *et al.*, 1981), and depending on the conditions, N-acetylcysteine could react directly with N-acetyl-p-benzoquinoneimine *in vitro* to form paracetamol and its mercapturic acid conjugate (Huggett and Blair, 1983a). In one report, N-acetylcysteine apparently protected against liver damage without reducing the covalent binding of paracetamol (Gerber *et al.*, 1977). N-acetylcysteine was thought to protect primarily through pre-arylation mechanisms to decrease the amount of reactive metabolite available for initiation of hepatic injury (Corcoran *et al.*, 1985a). It had no major effect on the overall disposition and metabolism of paracetamol, but it greatly increased the biliary excretion of the glutathione conjugate and it appeared to act by increasing glutathione synthesis to provide more glutathione for detoxification of the reactive metabolite (Corcoran *et al.*, 1985b). Similar conclusions were reached by other investigators (Lauterburg *et al.*, 1983; Pratt and Ioannides, 1985; Whitehouse *et al.*, 1985; Hjelle *et al.*, 1986). N-acetylcysteine could also protect against post-arylation toxicity under certain conditions, and in this context it appeared to restore the functional capacity of the proteolytic system to facilitate the removal of arylated proteins from cells (Bruno *et al.*, 1988). It also increased glycogen deposition in rat liver independently of any action on paracetamol (Itinose *et al.*, 1994). A kinetic analysis suggested that in the doses used as an antidote for paracetamol poisoning, N-acetylcysteine would substantially increase the mobilization and excretion of zinc (Brumas *et al.*, 1992). Given alone, N-acetylcysteine was reported to paradoxically reduce hepatic glutathione content (Viña *et al.*, 1980). Dithiothreitol was able to reverse post-arylation toxicity in isolated hepatocytes, but unlike N-acetylcysteine, it had an additional effect which probably involved regeneration of critical protein thiols (Rafeiro *et al.*, 1994).

A toxic dose of paracetamol caused depletion of inorganic sulphate and this was reversed by N-acetylcysteine acting as a sulphate donor (Lin and Levy, 1981). In this way the protective L-isomer produced a modest increase in the excretion of sulphate in mice but it did not increase the sulphate conjugation of paracetamol. Conversely, the D-isomer did not protect against toxicity yet it significantly increased the sulphate conjugation of paracetamol (Wong *et al.*, 1986). Thus N-acetylcysteine protected against the hepatotoxicity of paracetamol by stimulating glutathione synthesis and not by enhancing its sulphate conjugation (Hjelle *et al.*, 1986). Inhibition of gastric emptying with impaired absorption of paracetamol was proposed as a mechanism whereby N-acetylcysteine afforded protection (Whitehouse *et al.*, 1981). Methionine also protected against paracetamol toxicity and it acted as a glutathione precursor after enzymic conversion to cysteine. S-adenosylmethionine, the product of the first stage of this process, protected against liver damage (Stramentinoli *et al.*, 1979; Bray *et al.*, 1992b) and maintained the glutathione content of human hepatocytes incubated with toxic concentrations of paracetamol (Ponsoda *et al.*, 1991). Other prodrugs of cysteine that were effective in preventing paracetamol liver damage included cystathione (Kitamura *et al.*, 1989); D-glucose-cysteine (Gomez *et al.*, 1994); thiazolidine-4-carboxylate and its derivatives (Strubelt *et al.*, 1974; Nagasawa *et al.*, 1982, 1984; Williamson *et al.*, 1982; Klaassen *et al.*, 1985; Hazelton *et al.*, 1986a; Roberts *et al.*, 1987b); and ribose-cysteine (Roberts *et al.*, 1992). The oral administration of L-2-oxothiazolidine-4-carboxylate greatly increased plasma concentrations of cysteine in man (Porta *et al.*, 1991). In one study, the rank order of protection by metabolic precursors against paracetamol toxicity in human hepatocytes was N-acetylcysteine > thioproline > cysteine > 2-oxo-4-thiazolidine carboxylate > methionine (Larrauri *et al.*, 1989). The protective agent oltipraz (5-[pyrazinyl]-4-methyl-1,2-dithiol-3-thione) increased hepatic glutathione in hamsters but its efficacy seemed to be related more to increasing the rate of elimination of paracetamol by stimulating its glucuronide conjugation (Davies and Schnell, 1991). Propylthiouracil appeared to protect against paracetamol toxicity by forming an adduct directly with the reactive metabolite (Yamada *et al.*, 1981).

Many other agents have been reported to modify paracetamol-induced liver damage (Table 14.1). In some cases it was possible to establish mechanisms with reasonable certainty but in many reports mechanisms were assumed without any supporting evidence. As shown in the table, the findings in different studies have not always been consistent and in some cases the results have been diametrically opposite. Some toxic interactions were complex with the outcome depending on species, relative effects on toxic and non-toxic metabolic pathways, cytochrome P450 isoenzyme specificity, induction state and dose as reported, for example, with caffeine (Nouchi *et al.*, 1986; Sato and Izumi, 1989; Lee *et al.*, 1991a,b; Liu *et al.*, 1992b), aspirin (Thomas *et al.*, 1977a; de Vries *et al.*, 1981, 1984; Engelhardt, 1984; Douidar *et al.*, 1985; van Bree *et al.*, 1989) and H_2-receptor antagonists (Miners *et al.*, 1984b; Mitchell *et al.*, 1984b; Speeg *et al.*, 1984; Emery *et al.*, 1985; Black, 1987; Rogers *et al.*, 1988; Sachs and Kowalsky, 1988). Prostanoids such as iloprost were effective in protecting against paracetamol hepatotoxicity at remarkably low concentrations (Stachura *et al.*, 1981; Nasseri-Sina *et al.*, 1987, 1988, 1992; Guarner *et al.*, 1988; Davies *et al.*, 1992; Monto *et al.*, 1994) and this depended on protein synthesis as protection was abolished by cycloheximide (Fawthrop *et al.*, 1992). Protection by cholestyramine was attributed to interference with the absorption and enterohepatic circulation of paracetamol (Dordoni *et al.*, 1973; Siegers and Möller-Hartmann, 1989) but a mechanism involving lithocholate production was also proposed (Rosa *et al.*, 1984). A pharmacokinetic model was developed to describe the dose-response relationships following induction and inhibition of the microsomal enzymes involved in paracetamol hepatotoxicity (Jollow *et al.*, 1981). Several investigators have shown that dimethylsulphoxide protected against liver damage produced by paracetamol and possible mechanisms included scavenging of free radicals and inhibition of its metabolic activation (Siegers, 1978a; Younes and Siegers, 1980b; El-Hage *et al.*, 1983; Jeffery and Haschek, 1988; Jeffery *et al.*, 1988, 1991; Park *et al.*, 1988; Arndt *et al.*, 1989). This must be a matter of concern because many investigators used dimethylsulphoxide as the solvent for paracetamol in their toxicity studies (Wendel and Feuerstein, 1981; Wendel *et al.*, 1982; Estrela *et al.*, 1983; Costa and Murphy, 1984; Holme *et al.*, 1984, 1991; Gerson *et al.*, 1985; Harman, 1985; Harman *et al.*, 1991; Mitchell *et al.*, 1985; Streeter *et al.*, 1986; Koo *et al.*, 1987; Kyle *et al.*, 1987, 1988, 1990; Francavilla *et al.*, 1989; Madhu *et al.*, 1989; Nakae *et al.*, 1990a,b; Panella *et al.*, 1990; Garrido *et al.*, 1991; Lauriault and O'Brien, 1991; Thibault *et al.*, 1991; Kelly *et al.*, 1992; Fortunati *et al.*, 1993; Riley *et al.*, 1993). Other protective agents such as ethanol and propylene glycol have also been used as solvents for paracetamol in toxicity studies. The results of such studies must therefore be interpreted with caution. Many of these complex toxicological interactions depended not only on effects on paracetamol metabolism, but also on effects on glutathione status, and data from studies in animals obviously cannot be extrapolated directly to man.

Ethanol

There has been concern that chronic excessive consumption of ethanol might

Table 14.1 Some agents reported to increase or decrease the hepatotoxicity of paracetamol in animals.

Agent	Species	Hepatotoxicity	Suggested mechanism	Reference
Acetone	rat	increased	enhanced toxic metabolic activation	Moldéus and Gergely, 1980b
Acetone	rat	decreased	reduced toxic metabolic activation	Price and Jollow, 1983
Acetone	rat	increased	not stated	Kyle et al., 1988
Acetone	mouse	increased	enhanced toxic metabolic activation	Jeffery et al., 1991
Acetylcorynoline	mouse	decreased	reduced metabolic activation, increased glutathione	Lu et al., 1994
N-Acetyl-DL-penicillamine	mouse	no change		Zera and Nagasawa, 1980
Allopurinol	mouse	decreased	not known	Gale and Smith, 1988
Allopurinol	mouse	decreased	inhibition of xanthine oxidase	Tirmenstein and Nelson, 1990
Allyl alcohol	rat	increased	prevention of compensatory hyperfunction	Poulsen et al., 1985a
3-Aminobenzamide	mouse	increased	inhibition of DNA repair	Shen et al., 1992
Andrographolide	rat	decreased	not known	Handa and Sharma, 1990
Andrographolide	rat[1]	decreased	action on plasma membrane	Visen et al., 1993
Anethole dithiolthione	mouse	decreased	elevation of hepatic glutathione	Ansher et al., 1983
Anethole trithione	mouse	decreased	prevented depletion of glutathione	Warnet et al., 1989a
Anethole dithiolthione	mouse	decreased	acted as glutathione substitute	Warnet et al., 1989b
Arginine thiazolidine carboxylate	mouse	decreased	prodrug of cysteine	Pagella et al., 1980
Artemisia scoparia	rat	decreased	not known	Gilani and Janbaz, 1993
Ascorbic acid	mouse	no change		Hargreaves et al., 1982
Ascorbic acid	mouse	no change		Romero-Ferret et al., 1983
Ascorbic acid	hamster	no change		Miller and Jollow, 1984
Ascorbic acid	mouse	decreased	antioxidant	Peterson and Knodell, 1984
Ascorbic acid	mouse	decreased	scavenger of reactive metabolite	Jonker et al., 1988
Ascorbic acid esters	mouse	decreased	antioxidant	Mitra et al., 1988
Ascorbic acid esters	mouse	decreased	elevation of hepatic glutathione	Mitra et al., 1991
Ascorbyl palmitate	mouse	decreased	antioxidant	Hargreaves et al., 1982
Aspirin	mouse	decreased	reduced absorption rate	Whitehouse et al., 1976
Aspirin	rat	no change		Thomas et al., 1977a
Aspirin	rat	decreased	not known	Lock et al., 1982
Aspirin	mouse	decreased	not known	de Vries et al., 1984
Aspirin	mouse	decreased	increased glutathione conjugation	Engelhardt, 1984
Aspirin	mouse	decreased	inhibition of prostaglandin synthesis	Ben-Zvi et al., 1990
Aspirin	hamster	increased	inhibition of prostaglandin synthesis	Nasseri-Sina et al., 1992

(cont.)

Aurintricarboxylic acid	mouse[1]	decreased	inhibition of Ca^{2+} endonuclease	Shen et al., 1992
Azadirachta indica	rat	decreased	none	Chattopadhyay et al., 1992
Ban-zhi-lian	mouse	decreased	stabilization of hepatocellular membrane	Lin et al., 1994a
Benzylimidazole	mouse	decreased	inhibition of thromboxane synthesis	Guarner et al., 1988
Berberis aristata	rat	decreased	not known	Gilani and Janbaz, 1992
1,3-Bis(chloroethyl)-1-nitrosourea	rat[1]	increased	inhibition of glutathione reductase	Albano et al., 1985
1,3-Bis(chloroethyl)-1-nitrosourea	rat[1]	increased	inhibition of glutathione reductase	Gerson et al., 1985
1,3-Bis(chloroethyl)-1-nitrosourea	rat	decreased	none	Smith and Mitchell, 1985
1,3-Bis(chloroethyl)-1-nitrosourea	rat[1]	increased	inhibition of glutathione reductase	Hayes et al., 1986
1,3-Bis(chloroethyl)-1-nitrosourea	rat[1]	increased	inhibition of glutathione reductase	Koo et al., 1987
1,3-Bis(chloroethyl)-1-nitrosourea	rat[1]	increased	inhibition of glutathione reductase	Kyle et al., 1987
1,3-Bis(chloroethyl)-1-nitrosourea	mouse[1]	increased	inhibition of glutathione reductase	Farber et al., 1988
1,3-Bis(chloroethyl)-1-nitrosourea	rat[1]	increased	inhibition of glutathione reductase	Kyle et al., 1988
1,3-Bis(chloroethyl)-1-nitrosourea	rat[1]	increased	inhibition of glutathione reductase	Nakae et al., 1988
1,3-Bis(chloroethyl)-1-nitrosourea	rat[1]	increased	inhibition of glutathione reductase	Adamson and Harman, 1989
1,3-Bis(chloroethyl)-1-nitrosourea	mouse[1]	increased	inhibition of glutathione reductase	Kyle et al., 1990
1,3-Bis(chloroethyl)-1-nitrosourea	rat[1]	increased	inhibition of glutathione reductase	Nakae et al., 1990a
1,3-Bis(chloroethyl)-1-nitrosourea	rat	increased	inhibition of glutathione reductase	Nakae et al., 1990b
1,3-Bis(chloroethyl)-1-nitrosourea	rat[1]	increased	inhibition of glutathione reductase	Harman et al., 1991
1,3-Bis(chloroethyl)-1-nitrosourea	mouse[1]	increased	inhibition of glutathione reductase	Adamson and Harman, 1993
1,3-Bis(chloroethyl)-1-nitrosourea	rat[1]	increased	inhibition of glutathione reductase	Ito et al., 1994
Bis-(p-nitrophenyl)-phosphate	mouse	decreased	esterase inhibition	Wong and Corcoran, 1987
Borneol	hamster	increased	enhanced toxic metabolic activation	Smith and Jollow, 1977
Butanediol	rat	decreased	reduced toxic metabolic activation	Price and Jollow, 1983
p-Butoxyacetanilide	mouse[1]	decreased	reduced toxic metabolic activation	Kapetanovic and Mieyal, 1979
Butylhydroxyanisole	mouse[1]	no change		Moldéus et al., 1982b
Butylhydroxyanisole	mouse	decreased	increased hepatic glutathione	Ansher et al., 1983
Butylhydroxyanisole	mouse	decreased	increased hepatic glutathione	Miranda et al., 1983
Butylhydroxyanisole	mouse	decreased	reduced toxic metabolic activation	Rosenbaum et al., 1984
Butylhydroxyanisole	mouse	decreased	increased glucuronide conjugation	Hazelton et al., 1986b
Butylhydroxyanisole	mouse	decreased	reduced conjugation	Wang and Peng, 1993
CaEDTA	rat[1]	decreased	not known	Beales et al., 1985
Caffeine	rat	increased	not known	Sato et al., 1985
Caffeine	mouse	decreased	reduced toxic metabolic activation	Gale et al., 1986a
Caffeine[2]	mouse	increased	enhanced toxic metabolic activation	Gale et al., 1986a
Caffeine	mouse	decreased	?reduced toxic metabolic activation	Gale et al., 1987

335

Table 14.1 *(cont.)*

Agent	Species	Hepatotoxicity	Suggested mechanism	Reference
Caffeine	mouse	decreased	reduced toxic metabolic activation	Gale and Smith, 1988
Caffeine	rat	increased	increased depletion of glutathione	Kalhorn et al., 1990
Caffeine	mouse	decreased	prevention of glutathione depletion	Rainska et al., 1992
Captopril	mouse	decreased	acted as alternative nucleophile	Yeung, 1988
Captopril	rat	no change		Habior, 1992
Carbon disulphide	mouse	decreased	reduced toxic metabolic activation	Masuda and Nakayama, 1982
Carbon tetrachloride	rat	decreased	reduced toxic metabolic activation	Curzio, 1980
Carboxymethylcellulose	mouse	increased	increased depletion of glutathione	Klugmann et al., 1984
S-Carboxymethylcysteine	hamster	no change		Ioannides et al., 1983a
(+)Catechin	rat[3]	decreased	antioxidant	McLean and Nuttall, 1976
(+)Catechin	rat[3]	decreased	antioxidant	McLean and Nuttall, 1978
(+)Catechin	rat[3]	decreased	not known	Devalia et al., 1982
Cernitins	mouse	decreased	prevention of glutathione depletion	Juzwiak et al., 1992
Chlordecone	mouse	increased	enhanced toxic metabolic activation	Fouse and Hodgson, 1987
Chlorpromazine	rat	decreased	calcium channel blockade	Landon et al., 1986
Chlorpromazine	mouse	decreased	reduced calcium effect	Saville et al., 1988
Chlorpromazine	mouse	decreased	inhibition of phospholipase A_2	Harris and Hamrick, 1993
Chlorpromazine	mouse	decreased	decreased calcium accumulation	Ray et al., 1993b
Cholestyramine	rat	decreased	reduced lithocholate production	Rosa et al., 1984
Cholestyramine	rat	decreased	interruption of paracetamol enterohepatic cycling	Siegers and Möller-Hartmann, 1989
Cichorium intybus	rat	decreased	not known	Gilani et al., 1993
Cimetidine	rat	decreased	reduced toxic metabolic activation	Mitchell et al., 1981b
Cimetidine	mouse	decreased	reduced toxic metabolic activation	Rudd et al., 1981
Cimetidine	mouse	decreased	none	Donn et al., 1982
Cimetidine	rat	decreased	reduced toxic metabolic activation	Drew et al., 1982
Cimetidine	mouse	decreased	reduced toxic metabolic activation	Jackson, 1982
Cimetidine	mouse	decreased[4]	reduced toxic metabolic activation	Abernethy et al., 1983a
Cimetidine	mouse	decreased	reduced toxic metabolic activation	Peterson et al., 1983
Cimetidine	mouse	decreased	reduced toxic metabolic activation	Lazarte et al., 1984
Cimetidine	rat	no change		Leonard and Dent, 1984
Cimetidine	rat	decreased	reduced toxic metabolic activation	Speeg et al., 1985
Cimetidine	mouse	decreased	reduced toxic metabolic activation	Yurdakök et al., 1985

Cimetidine	rat	decreased	reduced toxic metabolic activation	Murase et al., 1986
Cimetidine	rat	decreased	reduced toxic metabolic activation	Okuno et al., 1987
Clofibrate	mouse	decreased	not known	Nicholls-Grzemski et al., 1992
Clofibrate	mouse	decreased	peroxisome proliferation	Priestly et al., 1993
Clofibrate	mouse	decreased	reduced metabolic activation and covalent binding	Manautou et al., 1994
Coenzyme A	mouse	decreased[4]	prevention of glutathione depletion	Bertelli et al., 1990
Colchicine	rat	decreased	antioxidant	Muriel et al., 1993
Copper (II)(3,5-diisopropylsalicylate)	mouse	decreased	acted as synthetic superoxide dismutase	Joyave et al., 1985
Corticosteroids	rat	decreased	inhibition of phospholipase A_2	Horton and Wood, 1989
Corticosterone	rat	no change		Harvey et al., 1993
Cortisol	rat	no change		Harvey et al., 1993
Corynebacterium parvum	rat[1]	decreased	reduced metabolic activation, Kupffer cell activation	Raiford and Thigpen, 1994
Curcumin	rat[1]	no change		Donatus et al., 1990
(+)-Cyanidanol	rat	decreased	reduced toxic metabolic activation	Younes and Siegers, 1980a,b
Cystathionine	mouse	decreased	cysteine precursor	Kitamura et al., 1989
Cysteamine	rat	decreased	stimulation of glutathione synthesis	Gazzard et al., 1974b
Cysteamine	mouse	decreased	not known	Mitchell et al., 1974
Cysteamine	mouse	decreased	repletion of glutathione	Strubelt et al., 1974
Cysteamine	mouse	decreased	reduced toxic metabolic activation	Miners et al., 1984d
Cysteamine	hamster	decreased	not known	Miller and Jollow, 1986a
Cysteamine	rat	decreased	reduced toxic metabolic activation	Peterson et al., 1989
Cysteamine	mouse	decreased	reduced toxic metabolic activation	Peterson and Brown, 1992
Cysteine isopropyl ester	mouse	decreased	stimulation of hepatic glutathione synthesis	Butterworth et al., 1992
N-Demethylricinine	rat	decreased	stabilization of plasma membrane	Shukla et al., 1992a
N-Demethylricinine	rat[1]	decreased	stabilization of plasma membrane	Visen et al., 1992
Desferrioxamine	rat	decreased	reduced oxidative stress	Gerson et al., 1985
Desferrioxamine	mouse	no change		Younes and Siegers, 1985a
Desferrioxamine	rat	decreased	reduced oxidative stress	Nakae et al., 1988
Desferrioxamine	mouse	no change		Siegers et al., 1988
Desferrioxamine	mouse	no change		Younes et al., 1988
Desferrioxamine	rat	decreased	chelation of iron	Harman et al., 1991
Desferrioxamine	rat	decreased	prevention of lipid peroxidation	Sakaida et al., 1992
Desferrioxamine	mouse[1]	decreased	reduced oxidative stress	Adamson and Harman, 1993
Desferrioxamine	rat[1]	decreased	reduced lipid peroxidation	Ito et al., 1994
Desferrioxamine	rat	decreased	chelation of iron, reduced active oxygen	Sakaida et al., 1995
Dexamethasone	mouse	increased	decreased hepatic glutathione	Madhu et al., 1992b

Table 14.1 (cont.)

Agent	Species	Hepatotoxicity	Suggested mechanism	Reference
DPPPE[5]	mouse	decreased	reduced toxic metabolic activation	Burcham and Harman, 1989
Dichloralphenazone	mouse	increased	enhanced toxic metabolic activation	Streeter and Timbrell, 1979
2,4-Dichloro-4-phenol	hamster	increased	inhibition of sulphate conjugation	Miller and Jollow, 1986b
Dichlorophenolindophenol	rat[3]	decreased	antioxidant	Mourelle and McLean, 1989
Dichlorophenolindophenol	rat[3]	decreased	antioxidant	Mourelle et al., 1990
Diethyl ether	mouse	increased	enhanced toxic metabolic activation	To and Wells, 1986
Diethyl ether	mouse	increased	enhanced toxic metabolic activation	Wells and To, 1986a
Diethyl ether	mouse	increased	none	Wells and To, 1986b
Diethyl ether	mouse	increased	enhanced toxic metabolic activation	Gale and Smith, 1988
Diethylhexylphthalate	mouse	decreased	not known	Nicholls-Grzemski et al., 1992
Dihydroxydibutyl ether	rat	decreased	not known	Fregnan et al., 1982
Diisopropylfluorophosphate	mouse	decreased	esterase inhibition	Wong and Corcoran, 1987
Diltiazem	mouse	decreased	calcium channel blockade	Kobusch and du Souich, 1990
Diltiazem	mouse	decreased	calcium antagonist	Deakin et al., 1991
Diltiazem	rat[1]	decreased	calcium antagonist	Thibault et al., 1991
Diltiazem	mouse	decreased	phospholipase A_2 inhibition	Harris and Hamrick, 1993
Dimercaprol	mouse	no change		Mitchell et al., 1974
Dimercaprol	mouse	no change		Strubelt et al., 1974
Dimethylaminoethanol	mouse	decreased	reduced toxic metabolic activation	Siegers and Younes, 1979
Dimethyl prostaglandin E_2	rat	decreased	none	Stachura et al., 1981
Dimethyl prostaglandin E_2	rat	decreased	not known	Raheja et al., 1985
Dimethyl prostaglandin E_2	hamster[1]	decreased	not known	Nasseri-Sina et al., 1988
Dimethyl prostaglandin E_2	mouse	decreased	not known	Renic et al., 1992
Dimethyl prostaglandin E_2	rat	decreased	stabilization of microsomal membrane	Monto et al., 1994
Dimethylsulphoxide	mouse	decreased	reduced toxic metabolic activation	Siegers, 1978a
Dimethylsulphoxide	hamster	decreased	free radical scavenger	El-Hage et al., 1983
Dimethylsulphoxide	mouse	decreased	free radical scavenger	Jeffery and Haschek, 1988
Dimethylsulphoxide	mouse	decreased	reduced toxic metabolic activation	Park et al., 1988
Dimethylsulphoxide	rat[1]	decreased	prevention of glutathione depletion	Ren and Cong, 1994
2,4-Dinitrophenol	rat	increased	not known	Strubelt, 1981
Diphenylphenylenediamine	rat	increased	not known	Kelleher et al., 1976a
Diphenylphenylenediamine	mouse	decreased	antioxidant	Albano et al., 1983

Compound	Species	Mechanism	Effect	Reference
Diphenylphenylenediamine	mouse[1]	antioxidant	decreased	Harman, 1985
Diphenylphenylenediamine	rat[1]	antioxidant	decreased	Farber et al., 1988
Diphenylphenylenediamine	rat[1]	antioxidant	decreased	Nakae et al., 1988
Diphenylphenylenediamine	rat[3]	antioxidant	decreased	Mourelle and McLean, 1989
Diphenylphenylenediamine	rat[1]	antioxidant	decreased	Kyle et al., 1990
Diphenylphenylenediamine	rat[1]	antioxidant	decreased	Harman et al., 1991
Disulfiram	rat	reduced toxic metabolic activation	decreased	Poulsen et al., 1987
Disulfiram	rat	reduced toxic metabolic activation	decreased	Jorgensen et al., 1988
Dithiocarb	mouse	repletion of hepatic glutathione	decreased	Strubelt et al., 1974
Dithiocarb	rat	none	decreased	Siegers et al., 1978
Dithiocarb	rat	reduced toxic metabolic activation	decreased	Younes and Siegers, 1980a
Dithiocarb	rat	reduced toxic metabolic activation	decreased	Younes and Siegers, 1980b
Dithiocarb	mouse	reduced toxic metabolic activation	decreased	Masuda and Nakayama, 1982
Dithiocarb	hamster[1]	?antioxidant	decreased	Harman and Fischer, 1983
Dithiocarb	mouse	reduced toxic metabolic activation	decreased	Younes et al., 1988
Dithiocarb	rat[1]	conjugation with reactive metabolite	decreased	Lauriault and O'Brien, 1991
Dithiocarb	rat[6]	radical scavenger	decreased	Strubelt and Younes, 1992
Dithiothreitol	hamster[1]	thiol reduction	decreased	Boobis et al., 1986
Dithiothreitol	hamster[1]	thiol reduction	decreased	Davies et al., 1986
Dithiothreitol	mouse[1]	thiol reduction	decreased	Harman and Self, 1986
Dithiothreitol	hamster[1]	thiol reduction	decreased	Tee et al., 1986b
Dithiothreitol	rat[1]	thiol reduction	decreased	Porubek et al., 1987
Dithiothreitol	hamster[1]	thiol reduction	decreased	Boobis et al., 1990
Dithiothreitol	rat[1]	thiol reduction	decreased	Lauriault and O'Brien, 1991
Dithiothreitol	mouse[1]	thiol reduction	decreased	Grewal and Racz, 1993
Doxorubicin	mouse	depletion of glutathione	increased	Wells et al., 1980
Ebselen	mouse[1]	reduced oxidative stress	decreased	Harman et al., 1992a
Ebselen	rat[1]	synthetic glutathione peroxidase activity	decreased	Li et al., 1994b
EGTA[7]	mouse[1]	depletion of intracellular Ca^{2+}	decreased	Bruschi and Priestly, 1990
EGTA[7]	rat[1]	depletion of intracellular Ca^{2+}	decreased	Thibault et al., 1991
EGTA[7]	mouse[1]	chelation of Ca^{2+}	decreased	Shen et al., 1992
Endotoxin	mouse	not known	decreased	Ishikawa et al., 1990b
Enoxacin	rat	reduced toxic metabolic activation	decreased	Nakanishi and Okuno, 1990
Epidermal growth factor	mouse[1]	effects on glutathione metabolism	decreased	Wang and Zhang, 1994
Ethylxanthogenate	mouse	reduced toxic metabolic activation	decreased	Dimova and Stoytchev, 1990
Famotidine	rat		no change	Murase et al., 1986

(cont.)

Table 14.1 (cont.)

Agent	Species	Hepatotoxicity	Suggested mechanism	Reference
Fenitrothion	mouse	decreased	reduced toxic metabolic activation	Ginsberg et al., 1982
Ferulate	mouse	decreased	reduced conjugation	Wang and Peng, 1993
Ferulate	mouse	decreased	not known	Wang and Peng, 1994
Fructose	rat[3]	decreased	increased intracellular ATP	Mourelle et al., 1991
Fructose	rat[6]	decreased	anaerobic synthesis of ATP	Strubelt and Younes, 1992
Fructus schizandrae	mouse	decreased	reduced toxic metabolic activation	Liu and Wei, 1987
Fulvotomentosides	mouse	decreased	reduced toxic metabolic activation	Liu et al., 1992c, 1994a
Galactosamine	hamster	increased	decreased glucuronide conjugation	Smith and Jollow, 1976
Gallopamil	rat[1]	decreased	calcium antagonist	Thibault et al., 1991
Garcinia kola	rat	decreased	reduced toxic metabolic activation	Akintonwa and Essien, 1990
D-Glucose-L-cysteine	mouse	decreased	cysteine precursor	Gomez et al., 1994
Glutathione-dextran	mouse	decreased	maintenance of hepatic glutathione	Kaneo et al., 1994
Goldthioglucose	mouse[1]	increased	inhibition of glutathione peroxidase	Adamson and Harman, 1989
Gomisin A	rat	decreased	suppression of lipid peroxidation	Yamada et al., 1993
Hepatogard	rat	decreased	none	Rao et al., 1993
Hydrocortisone	rat	no change		Nimmo et al., 1973a
Halothane	mouse	increased	enhanced toxic metabolic activation	Wells et al., 1986
Hippophae rhamnoides	mouse	decreased	prevention of glutathione depletion	Cheng et al., 1990; Cheng, 1992b
ICRF-187	hamster	decreased	chelation of divalent cations	El-Hage et al., 1983
Ibuprofen	hamster[1]	increased	inhibition of prostaglandin synthesis	Nasseri-Sina et al., 1992
Iloprost	hamster[1]	decreased	not known	Nasseri-Sina et al., 1987
Iloprost	hamster[1]	decreased	not known	Davies et al., 1992
Iloprost	not stated[1]	decreased	not known	Fawthrop et al., 1992
Iloprost	hamster[1]	decreased	not known	Nasseri-Sina et al., 1992
Imidazole	rat	decreased	inhibition of thromboxane synthesis	Horton and Wood, 1989
Imidazole	mouse	decreased	inhibition of thromboxane synthesis	Ben-Zvi et al., 1990
Indomethacin	mouse	decreased	inhibition of prostaglandin synthesis	Ben-Zvi et al., 1990
Insulin + growth factors	dog	no change		Francavilla et al., 1993
Interleukin 1α	mouse	decreased	increased cyclic AMP	Renic et al., 1993
Isaxonine	rat[1]	increased	glutathione depletion	Shrivastava et al., 1994
Isoniazid	rat	increased	enhanced toxic metabolic activation	Burk et al., 1990
Jigrine	rat	decreased	antioxidant effect	Kapur et al., 1994

Compound	Species	Effect	Mechanism	Reference
Ketoconazole	mouse	increased	none	Walker et al., 1989
Kopsinine	mouse	decreased	facilitated regeneration	Huang and Liu, 1989
Kopsinine F	mouse	decreased	reduced toxic metabolic activation	Zhang and Liu, 1989
Lipopeptides	mouse	decreased	reduced toxic metabolic activation	Migliore-Samour et al., 1989
Lipopolysaccharides	mouse	decreased	reduced toxic metabolic activation	Ishikawa et al., 1990a
Lobenzarit	mouse	decreased	unspecified action on glutathione	González et al., 1992
Lovastatin	mouse	increased	none	Raje and Bhattacharya, 1990
Malotilate	mouse	decreased	unspecified interaction with bioactivation	Younes and Siegers, 1985b
Mepyramine	rat	no change		Nimmo et al., 1973a
α-Mercaptopropionylglycine	mouse	decreased	acted as nucleophile	Labadarios et al., 1977
α-Mercaptopropionylglycine	rat	decreased	none	Negro et al., 1981
α-Mercaptopropionylglycine	rat	decreased	conjugation with reactive metabolite	Hirayama et al., 1983
α-Mercaptopropionylglycine	mouse[1]	decreased	none	Walker et al., 1983a
α-Mercaptopropionylglycine	mouse[1]	decreased	maintenance of hepatic glutathione	Harman and Self, 1986
α-Mercaptopropionylglycine	mouse	decreased	acted as nucleophile	Sakr, 1993
Methotrexate	chick[1]	increased	depletion of glutathione	Sinclair et al., 1987
Methotrexate	chick[1]	increased	depletion of glutathione	Lindenthal et al., 1993
Methoxsalen	rat	decreased	reduced toxic metabolic activation	Letteron et al., 1986
p-Methoxyacetanilide	mouse	decreased	reduced toxic metabolic activation	Kapetanovic and Mieyal, 1979
3-O-Methyl(+)catechin	rat[1]	decreased	not known	Devalia et al., 1982
Methylene blue	rat[3]	decreased	?antioxidant	McLean and Nuttall, 1976
Methylene blue	rat[3]	decreased	?antioxidant	McLean and Nuttall, 1978
4-Methylpyrazole	rat	decreased	reduced toxic metabolic activation	Burk et al., 1990
4-Methylpyrazole	rat	decreased	reduced toxic metabolic activation	Brennan et al., 1994
Methylthiazolidine-4-carboxylate	mouse	decreased	cysteine prodrug	Nagasawa et al., 1982
Methylthiazolidine-4-carboxylate	mouse	decreased	cysteine prodrug	Klaassen et al., 1985
Methylthiazolidine-4-carboxylate	mouse	decreased	cysteine prodrug	Hazelton et al., 1986a
Metyrapone	mouse	decreased	reduced metabolic activation	Fossa et al., 1979
Metyrapone	mouse	decreased[4]	reduced metabolic activation	Goldstein and Nelson, 1979
Metyrapone	mouse	decreased	reduced metabolic activation	Nelson et al., 1980a
Metyrapone	mouse	decreased	reduced metabolic activation	Massey et al., 1982
Metyrapone	hamster[1]	decreased	?antioxidant	Harman and Fischer, 1983
Mirex	mouse	increased	enhanced toxic metabolic activation	Fouse and Hodgson, 1987
Misoprostol	rat	decreased	stabilization of plasma or lysosomal membranes	Lim et al., 1994
Morphine	mouse	increased	depletion of glutathione	Skoulis et al., 1989
MSF[8]	rat/mouse	decreased	reduced lipid peroxidation	Zanoli, 1981

Table 14.1 (*cont.*)

Agent	Species	Hepatotoxicity	Suggested mechanism	Reference
β-Naphthoflavone	rat[1]	decreased	reduced toxic metabolic activation	Kyle et al., 1987
β-Naphthoflavone	rat[1]	decreased	reduced toxic metabolic activation	Kyle et al., 1988
β-Naphthoflavone	rat	increased	increased toxic metabolic activation	Tuntaterdtum et al., 1993
Neurotensin	mouse[1]	decreased	increased glutathione synthesis	Li et al., 1994a
N[G]-Monomethyl-L-arginine	rat[1]	increased	inhibition of synthesis of protective nitric oxide	Kuo and Slivka, 1994
Nifedipine	rat	decreased	calcium channel blockade	Landon et al., 1986
Non-steroidal anti-inflammatory drugs	rat	decreased	inhibition of cyclooxygenase	Horton and Wood, 1989
Norfloxacin	rat	decreased	reduced toxic metabolic activation	Nakanishi and Okuno, 1990
Ofloxacin	rat	no change		Nakanishi and Okuno, 1990
OKY 1581	mouse	decreased	inhibition of thromboxane synthesis	Guarner et al., 1988
Oleanolic acid	mouse	decreased	decreased toxic activation, increased glucuronidation	Liu et al., 1993, 1994a
Oltipraz	mouse	decreased	increased hepatic glutathione	Ansher et al., 1983
Oltipraz	hamster	decreased	increased hepatic glutathione	Davies et al., 1991
Oxmetidine	rat	no change		Leonard and Dent, 1984
Oxothiazolidine-4-carboxylate	mouse	decreased	cysteine prodrug	Williamson et al., 1982
Oxothiazolidine-4-carboxylate	mouse	decreased	cysteine prodrug	Klaassen et al., 1985
Oxothiazolidine-4-carboxylate	mouse	decreased	cysteine prodrug	Hazelton et al., 1986a
Penicillamine	mouse	no change		Strubelt et al., 1974
Penicillamine	mouse	decreased	acted as nucleophile	Yeung, 1988
Pentoxiphylline	mouse	increased	not known	Welty et al., 1993
Phenacetin	mouse	decreased	reduced toxic metabolic activation	Kapetanovic and Mieyal, 1979
Phenanthroline	mouse	decreased	chelation of ferric iron	Ito et al., 1994
Phenazine methosulphate	rat[1]	increased	not known	Mourelle and McLean, 1989
Phenylephrine	rat[3]	increased	depletion of glutathione	Harbison et al., 1991
Phenylmethylsulphonylfluoride	mouse	decreased	esterase inhibition	Wong and Corcoran, 1987
Phenylpropanolamine	mouse	increased	depletion of glutathione	James et al., 1993
Phorone	mouse	increased	depletion of glutathione	van Doorn et al., 1978
Phosphatidylcholine	mouse	decreased	not known	Jaeschke et al., 1987
Phosphonothioates	rat	decreased	reduced toxic metabolic activation	Furukawa et al., 1986
Picroliv	rat	decreased	reduced toxic metabolic activation	Ansari et al., 1991
Picroliv	rat	decreased	not known	Dwivedi et al., 1991
Picroliv	rat[1]	decreased	blockade of hepatic receptors	Visen et al., 1991

(cont.)

Compound	Species	Effect	Mechanism	Reference
Picroliv	rat[1]	decreased	antioxidant	Singh et al., 1992
Pollen extract	mouse	decreased	related to glutathione	Juzwiak, 1993
Polychlorinated biphenyls	rat[1]	increased	enhanced toxic metabolic activation	Hayes et al., 1984
Poly (rI.rC)	mouse	decreased	reduced toxic metabolic activation	Renton and Dickson, 1984
Polyinosinic-polycytidylic acid	mouse	decreased[9]	reduced toxic metabolic activation	Kalabis and Wells, 1990
Polysaccharide peptide	rat	decreased	reduced oxidative stress, reduced covalent binding	Yeung et al., 1994
Pregnenolone-16α-carbonitrile	hamster	decreased	reduced toxic metabolic activation	Madhu and Klaassen, 1991
Pregnenolone-16α-carbonitrile	mouse	decreased		Madhu et al., 1992b
Pregnenolone-16α-carbonitrile	rat	no change	not known	Harvey et al., 1993
Prednisolone	mouse	decreased	stimulation of glutathione synthesis	Speck et al., 1993
Promethazine	rat	no change		Nimmo et al., 1973a
Promethazine	rat[3]	decreased	antioxidant	McLean and Nuttall, 1976
Promethazine	rat[3]	decreased	antioxidant	McLean and Nuttall, 1978
Promethazine	rat[1]	decreased	not known	Devalia et al., 1982
Promethazine	mouse[1]	decreased	antioxidant	Harman, 1985
Promethazine	mouse[1]	decreased	depletion of extracellular Ca^{2+}	Bruschi and Priestly, 1990
Propargyline	mouse	increased	inhibition of cystathionase	Kitamura et al., 1989
Propolis extract	mouse	decreased	increased hepatic glutathione	González et al., 1994
Propranolol	mouse	decreased[4]	reduced hypoxia	Rosner et al., 1973
Propranolol	rat	no change		Gazzard et al., 1974b
Propylene glycol	mouse	decreased	reduced toxic metabolic activation	Hughes et al., 1991
Propylene glycol	mouse	decreased	reduced toxic metabolic activation	Snawder et al., 1993
Propylgallate	rat	decreased	antioxidant	Kelleher et al., 1976a
Propylthiouracil	rat	decreased	prevention of glutathione depletion	Cho et al., 1980
Propylthiouracil	rat	decreased	increased hepatic glutathione	Linscheer et al., 1980
Propylthiouracil	rat	decreased	multifactorial	Raheja et al., 1982
Propylthiouracil	rat	decreased	none	Raheja et al., 1983a
Propylthiouracil	rat	decreased	reduced toxic metabolic activation	Raheja et al., 1987
Prostaglandin E_1	mouse	no change		Renic et al., 1992
Prostaglandin E_2	mouse	decreased	not known	Renic et al., 1992
Quin-2	hamster[1]	decreased	chelation of Ca^{2+}	Boobis et al., 1990
Quinacrine	rat	decreased	inhibition of phospholipase A_2	Horton and Wood, 1989
Ranitidine	rat	increased	inhibition of glucuronide conjugation	Leonard and Dent, 1984
Ranitidine (50 mg kg^{-1})	rat	increased	inhibition of glucuronide conjugation	Leonard et al., 1985a
Ranitidine (> 100 mg kg^{-1})	rat	decreased		Leonard et al., 1985a
Ranitidine	rat	increased	inhibition of paracetamol conjugation	Leonard et al., 1985b

Table 14.1 (cont.)

Agent	Species	Hepatotoxicity	Suggested mechanism	Reference
Ranitidine	rat	increased	altered paracetamol metabolism	Rogers et al., 1985
Ranitidine	rat	no change		Murase et al., 1986
Ranitidine	dog	decreased	reduced toxic metabolic activation	Francavilla et al., 1989
Ranitidine	mouse	increased	none	Yurdakök et al., 1989
Ranididine	dog	decreased	reduced toxic metabolic activation	Panella et al., 1990
Ribose-cysteine	mouse	decreased	cysteine prodrug	Roberts et al., 1992
Ricinin	rat	no change		Shukla et al., 1992a
Ricinus communis	rat[1]	decreased	stabilization of plasma membrane	Visen et al., 1992
SA 3443	mouse	decreased	reduced glutathione depletion	Tanaka et al., 1991
Saikosaponins	mouse	decreased	increased glutathione conjugation	Lee et al., 1993
Salicylate	mouse	increased	competition for glucuronide conjugation	Douidar et al., 1985
Saponins	mouse	decreased	none	Liu et al., 1994a
Selenium	rat	decreased	stimulation of glutathione peroxidase	McLean and Day, 1974
Selenium	rat	decreased	increased glutathione conjugation	Schnell et al., 1988
Selenium	hamster	decreased	reduced toxic metabolic activation	Madhu et al., 1992a
Silipide	mouse	decreased	antioxidant	Conti et al., 1992
Silvex	mouse	decreased	not known	Nicholls-Grzemski et al., 1992
Silybin	rat	decreased	prevention of glutathione depletion	Campos et al., 1988
Silybin	rat	decreased	prevention of glutathione depletion	Campos et al., 1989
Silybin	mouse	no change		Conti et al., 1992
Silybinin	rat[6]	decreased	reduced toxic metabolic activation	Leng-Peschlow, 1988
Silybinin	rat	decreased	reduced toxic metabolic activation	Garrido et al., 1989
Silymarin	mouse	no change		Strubelt et al., 1974
Silymarin	rat	decreased	not known	Fregnan et al., 1982
Silymarin	rat[1]	decreased	blockade of hepatic receptors	Visen et al., 1991
Silymarin	rat	decreased	antioxidant	Muriel et al., 1992
Silymarin	rat	decreased	stabilization of plasma membrane	Shukla et al., 1992a
Silymarin	rat	decreased	stabilization of plasma membrane	Shukla et al., 1992b
Silymarin	rat[1]	decreased	none	Visen et al., 1993
Sodium sulphate	mouse	decreased	increased sulphate conjugation	Slattery and Levy, 1977
Sodium sulphate	cat	decreased	increased sulphate conjugation	Savides et al., 1985
Sodium sulphate	hamster	no change		Miller and Jollow, 1986b

Compound	Species	Effect	Mechanism	Reference
Substituted thiazolidine carboxylates	mouse	decreased	cysteine prodrugs	Nagasawa et al., 1984
Sucrose	rat	decreased	not known	Martinelli et al., 1989
Sulotroban	rat	decreased	thromboxane receptor antagonist	Horton and Wood, 1991
Superoxide dismutase	rat	decreased	prevention of lipid peroxidation	Nakae et al., 1990a
Superoxide dismutase	rat	decreased	prevention of lipid peroxidation	Nakae et al., 1990b
Theobromine	rat	no change		Kalhorn et al., 1990
Theophylline	rat	increased	increased glutathione depletion	Kalhorn et al., 1990
Thiazolidine-4-carboxylate	mouse	decreased	none	Strubelt et al., 1974
Thiazolidine-4-carboxylate	mouse	decreased	cysteine prodrug	Nagasawa et al., 1982
Thiazolidine-4-carboxylates	rat[1]	decreased	cysteine prodrugs	Roberts et al., 1987b
Thioacetamide	rat	decreased	stimulation of hepatic tissue repair	Chanda et al., 1995
Thioctic acid	rat	no change		Gazzard et al., 1974b
Thioctic acid	mouse	no change		Strubelt et al., 1974
Tienilic acid	mouse	no change		Ahokas et al., 1984
α-Tocopherol	rat	decreased		Gazzard et al., 1974b
α-Tocopherol	rat	decreased	antioxidant	Walker et al., 1974
α-Tocopherol	rat	decreased	not known	Kelleher et al., 1976b
α-Tocopherol	mouse[1]	decreased	antioxidant	Albano et al., 1983
α-Tocopherol (liposomes)	mouse	decreased	not known	Werner and Wendel, 1990
Trifluoperazine	mouse	decreased	inhibition of calmodulin	Yamamoto, 1990
Triterpenoids	mouse	decreased	not known	Liu et al., 1994b
Ursolic acid	rat	decreased	stabilization of plasma membrane	Shukla et al., 1992b
Verapamil	rat[1]	decreased	calcium antagonist	Thibault et al., 1991
Verapamil	mouse	decreased	reduced calcium accumulation	Ray et al., 1993b
Wedelia chinensis	mouse	decreased	reduced activation or increased glucuronidation	Lin et al., 1994b
Xylitol pentanicotinate	mouse	decreased[4]	reduced hypoxia	Rosner et al., 1973
Zinc	rat	decreased	reduced toxic metabolic activation	Pour et al., 1985
Zinc	mouse	decreased	not known	Chengelis et al., 1986
Zinc	mouse	decreased	increased hepatic glutathione	Szymanska et al., 1991
Zinc	hamster	decreased	reduced toxic metabolic activation	Madhu et al., 1992a

[1] isolated hepatocytes; [2] pretreatment for three days; [3] liver slices; [4] decreased mortality; [5] 2,4-dichloro-6-phenylphenoxyethylenediamine; [6] isolated perfused liver; [7] ethyleneglycol-bis(β-aminoethylether)-N,N,N',N'-tetraacetic acid; [8] 2,4-monofurfurylidene-tetra-O-methylsorbitol; [9] biphasic response with increased toxicity 32 days after administration

enhance the hepatotoxicity of paracetamol in man, and this potentially toxic interaction has been studied in animals. The situation was complicated because acute and chronic consumption of ethanol have opposite effects on paracetamol toxicity, and with acute ingestion, the timing in relation to the taking of paracetamol could be critical. Unfortunately, the findings in animals have often been uncritically extrapolated to man but this was not justified because of different experimental conditions and species differences. The acute administration of ethanol protected against paracetamol hepatotoxicity and increased survival in mice and rats (Wong *et al.*, 1980b; Sato and Lieber, 1981; Sato *et al.*, 1981b; Altomare *et al.*, 1984a; Banda and Quart, 1984a,b; Tredger *et al.*, 1985; Lieber *et al.*, 1987; Serrar and Thevenin, 1987; Thummel *et al.*, 1988, 1989; Garrido *et al.*, 1989). This protective effect was species dependent, and maximum protection in the mouse was observed when the ethanol was given early before the paracetamol (Thummel *et al.*, 1989). Ethanol protected even when given 3–4 h, or even 6 h, after a toxic dose of paracetamol (Banda and Quart, 1984a; Serrar and Thevenin, 1987), but toxicity was increased when it was given 16–18 h beforehand (Strubelt *et al.*, 1978; Carter, 1987). It also reduced the toxicity of paracetamol in rat liver slices (Mourelle and McLean, 1989; Mourelle *et al.*, 1990). Ethanol given with paracetamol did not cause lipid peroxidation and it did not influence the inhibiting effect of paracetamol on lipid peroxidation *in vitro* (Kamiyama *et al.*, 1993). The reduced hepatotoxicity of paracetamol produced by acute administration of ethanol was widely attributed to inhibition of its metabolic activation as shown in some studies by decreased glutathione conjugation (Wong *et al.*, 1980b; Sato *et al.*, 1981b, 1991; Sato and Lieber, 1981; Altomare *et al.*, 1984b; Tredger *et al.*, 1985b, 1986; Lieber *et al.*, 1987). Ethanol reduced the glucuronide conjugation of paracetamol in rats (Minnigh and Zemaitis, 1980) and it decreased both glucuronide and glutathione conjugation by the isolated perfused rat liver (Schlager *et al.*, 1987). It also inhibited the glutathione conjugation of paracetamol by rat liver microsomes (Sato *et al.*, 1991). In human liver microsomes, ethanol seemed to inhibit the metabolic activation of paracetamol by an indirect process (Thummel *et al.*, 1989). It was proposed that the protection by ethanol was mediated by acetaldehyde as this effect was blocked by pyrazole (Mourelle *et al.*, 1990) while acetaldehyde reduced paracetamol liver toxicity in rats (Liu *et al.*, 1992a) and decreased the formation of its glutathione conjugate by rat liver microsomes (Sato *et al.*, 1991). Other investigators have raised the possibility of protection by a mechanism involving NADPH (Thummel *et al.*, 1988; Mourelle and McLean, 1989; Mourelle *et al.*, 1990). The acute administration of ethanol in rats did not cause oxidative stress but it reduced the rate of glutathione synthesis (Lauterburg *et al.*, 1984a).

In contrast to the effects of acute intake of ethanol, chronic administration for periods of weeks or months enhanced the hepatotoxicity of paracetamol and increased mortality in hamsters, mice, rats and baboons. This increased susceptibility was usually associated with stimulation of the metabolic activation of paracetamol and increased production of glutathione-derived conjugates (Teschke *et al.*, 1979; Moldéus *et al.*, 1980a; Peterson *et al.*, 1980; Sato *et al.*, 1981a; Lieber, 1983; Rosen *et al.*, 1983; Walker *et al.*, 1983b; Altomare *et al.*, 1984a,b; Tredger *et al.*, 1985; Carter, 1987; Lieber *et al.*, 1987). A methionine-deficient diet greatly increased the potentiating effect of ethanol on liver damage induced by paracetamol (Reicks and Hathcock, 1984). In some studies, chronic consumption of ethanol was found to increase the glucuronide conjugation of paracetamol without inducing its metabolic activation (Tredger *et al.*, 1985, 1986b). It also enhanced the depletion of glutathione (Rosen *et al.*, 1983; Vendemiale *et al.*, 1984) and reduced the biliary excretion of the glutathione conjugate of paracetamol (Vendemiale *et al.*, 1984; Madhu *et al.*, 1989). When the chronic ingestion of ethanol was discontinued 24 h before administration of paracetamol in hamsters there was marked resistance to hepatotoxicity compared with animals continuing with ethanol and control hamsters not given any ethanol at all (Singletary *et al.*, 1980; Rosen *et al.*, 1983). In other circumstances, the effects of acute and chronic intake of ethanol on paracetamol hepatotoxicity tended to cancel out (Altomare *et al.*, 1984b).

In rats, the binding of paracetamol to proteins and its cysteine conjugation seemed to be catalyzed by different isozymes of cytochrome P450, and the enhanced toxicity caused by chronic ingestion of ethanol more closely parallelled the changes in protein binding than cysteine conjugation (Prasad *et al.*, 1990). The major ethanol-inducible isoform of cytochrome P450 in rabbits was P450 3a (now referred to as CYP2E1), and together with P450 4 and 6 it had a high capacity for the oxidation of paracetamol (Morgan *et al.*, 1983; Coon *et al.*, 1984; Coon and Koop, 1987). Monospecific antibodies were used to identify a cDNA for the isozyme P450 3a in rabbit liver and the entire sequence of 492 amino acids was determined (Khani *et al.*, 1987). Similarities were noted in the N-terminal sequences with those of human cytochrome P450j (Lieber, 1988). In the rat, nine isoforms of cytochrome P450 were found to catalyze the formation of N-acetyl-p-benzoquinoneimine from paracetamol (Harvison *et al.*, 1988b) and the most efficient was CYP3A1 (Lee *et al.*, 1991a). A molecular mechanism for the alleged enhanced susceptibility of chronic ethanol abusers to liver damage promoted by paracetamol was proposed on the basis that the isoforms CYP2E1 and CYP1A2 were largely responsible for the generation of N-acetyl-p-benzoquinoneimine by human liver microsomes, and that ethanol caused induction of CYP2E1 in animals (Raucy *et al.*, 1989). However, at more realistic therapeutically relevant concentrations of paracetamol, the major isoform of cytochrome P450 involved in the formation of N-acetyl-p-benzoquinoneimine by human liver was shown to be CYP3A4 (Thummel *et al.*, 1993). It is not known to what extent this isozyme is inducible by ethanol in man. Studies of the *in vitro* binding of paracetamol to human liver microsomes revealed that there was no specific binding to CYP2E1 (Lecoeur *et al.*, 1994). In induced mice, CYP2E1 was important in the bioactivation of paracetamol at low doses while CYP1A2 contributed more to bioactivation and toxicity at higher doses (Snawder *et al.*, 1994b).

Species, Strain and Other Genetic Differences

In early studies of paracetamol hepatotoxicity it soon became obvious that there were major species differences in susceptibility. Hamsters and mice were sensitive while guinea pigs, rabbits and rats were resistant. The severity of hepatic damage in the different species correlated directly with the rate of metabolic activation of paracetamol and rate of depletion of glutathione (Davis *et al.*, 1974a; Aikawa *et al.*, 1978b). These species differences were confirmed by other investigators using liver slices (Wormser *et al.*, 1990), liver microsomal preparations (Liu *et al.*, 1991) and isolated hepatocytes (Moldéus, 1978; Green *et al.*, 1984a), and the rank order of decreasing sensitivity to paracetamol toxicity in cultured hepatocytes was dog, rabbit, rat and monkey (Smolarek *et al.*, 1990). Paracetamol was more toxic to hepatocytes obtained from hamsters and mice than those from rats and man, and these species differences were related to differences in the rates of its conversion to the toxic metabolite N-acetyl-p-benzoquinoneimine (Boobis *et al.*, 1986; Seddon *et al.*, 1987; Tee *et al.*, 1987). Organ cultures from urodele amphibians deacetylated paracetamol and in liver cell cultures it depleted glycogen and released lactic dehydrogenase. In contrast, organ cultures from anuran amphibians did not metabolize paracetamol and were not susceptible to toxicity (Clothier *et al.*, 1982). Paracetamol produced cytotoxicity in cultured trout liver cells and the morphological changes included re-arrangement of the mitochondria so that they became clustered adjacent to the nucleus (Miller *et al.*, 1993c). At cytotoxic concentrations, paracetamol maintained the activity of cytochrome CYP1A1 in previously induced trout hepatocytes in culture (Miller *et al.*, 1993b). Strain differences in the resistance of rats to paracetamol liver toxicity were also related to differences in the extent of metabolic activation (Hart *et al.*, 1982a; Price and Jollow, 1986) but not to differences in glutathione depletion (Willson *et al.*, 1991). With inbred strains of mice, there was a correlation between *in vivo* and *in vitro* susceptibility (Whitehouse *et al.*, 1990). Genetically determined differences in the inducibility of aryl hydrocarbon hydroxylase by 3-methylcholanthrene, β-naphthoflavone, 2,3,7,8-tetrachlorodibenzo-p-dioxin and phenobarbitone in two inbred strains of mice were reflected in corresponding differences in sensitivity to paracetamol toxicity (Thorgeirsson *et al.*, 1975) and in another report, both toxicity and inducibility of cytochrome P450 were controlled by the Ah locus (Nebert *et al.*, 1976). Paracetamol was more toxic to the liver in Gunn rats with homozygous and heterozygous glucuronyl transferase deficiency than Wistar rats, and this was attributed to enhanced metabolic activation as a result of reduced glucuronide conjugation in the former (Calder *et al.*, 1981b; de Morais and Wells, 1988, 1989, 1992a). The major species differences in susceptibility to paracetamol between rats and hamsters was also observed in a liver slice model of toxicity (Miller *et al.*, 1993a).

Age

The acute toxicity of paracetamol as shown by mortality and the LD_{50} was less in young than adult mice and rats (Mancini *et al.*, 1980; Sonawane *et al.*, 1980; Adamson *et al.*, 1991). However, in other reports, the seven-day mortality was greater in young mice aged 7–9 and 16–19 days than in adults (Alhava *et al.*, 1978), and mortality was greater in 19-day-old rats than in those aged 11 and 33 days (Green *et al.*, 1984b). Otherwise, there was a rather consistent picture of resistance to paracetamol hepatotoxicity in neonatal and young mice and rats compared with adults (Nebert *et al.*, 1976; Hart and Timbrell, 1979; Hart *et al.*, 1982a; Beierschmitt *et al.*, 1986a, 1989; Adamson and Harman, 1988; Adamson *et al.*, 1991). Similar resistance in the young has been reported in studies with mouse liver slices (Wormser and Ben-Zakine, 1990) and hepatocytes (Adamson and Harman, 1989). In contrast to these findings, cultured hepatocytes from 1-, 2- and 3-week-old mice were as susceptible to paracetamol toxicity as those from adults despite greater covalent binding in the young mice (Harman and McCamish, 1986). In one study, paracetamol was not more toxic in old rats (Rikans and Moore, 1988; Rikans, 1989, 1991) but, in another, it caused more liver necrosis and lethality in old than in middle-aged and young mice (Adamson *et al.*, 1991). Paracetamol was much more toxic in older than in younger Gunn rats, but there was no such difference with Wistar rats (de Morais and Wells, 1988). Young mosquitoes were more resistant to

paracetamol toxicity while very old mosquitoes were more sensitive and these differences were related to glutathione status (Richie and Lang, 1985). These age-related
differences in susceptibility to paracetamol toxicity have been related variously to
differences in metabolic activation (Hart and Timbrell, 1979; Al-Turk and Stohs,
1981; Beierschmitt *et al.*, 1986a; de Morais and Wells, 1988), glutathione availability
(Al-Turk and Stohs, 1981; Richie and Lang, 1985), selective protein arylation
(Beierschmitt *et al.*, 1989) and the activity of glutathione peroxidase, glutathione
reductase, and superoxide dismutase (Adamson and Harman, 1988, 1989). Paradoxically, young animals may have less hepatic glutathione than older animals (Lambert
and Thorgeirsson, 1976; Hart and Timbrell, 1979), and as assessed by paracetamol
probe analysis, glutathione turnover and synthesis in rats decreased with age
(Lauterburg *et al.*, 1980). The recovery of hepatic glutathione content following a
toxic dose of paracetamol was much slower in aged than in young and mature mice
(Chen *et al.*, 1990).

Sex

Female Sprague Dawley rats were more resistant than males to paracetamol hepatotoxicity, and this may have been due to more extensive metabolic activation in the
latter (Hart *et al.*, 1982a). Similar results were obtained in another study in the same
strain of rat although hepatic glutathione was depleted earlier in the females. Castration of male rats decreased, and ovariectomy of female rats tended to increase
susceptibility to hepatotoxicity (Raheja *et al.*, 1983b). In contrast to these reports,
susceptibility to paracetamol-induced liver damage was greater, and the LD_{50} was
less in female than in male mice (Munoz and Fearon, 1984).

Route of Administration

The toxicity of paracetamol in rats appeared to be greater after intraperitoneal than
oral administration (Colin *et al.*, 1986a) while an opposite result was observed in
mice (Corcoran *et al.*, 1985a). In a study in which paracetamol was given intravenously, intraperitoneally and orally, no useful conclusion could be drawn as there
was little or no toxicity with any route (Hart *et al.*, 1982a). Plasma concentrations
were higher, and hepatotoxicity was greater in mice given paracetamol by intraperitoneal injection compared with oral administration (Esteban *et al.*, 1993a,b).

Diet and Nutrition

The hepatotoxicity of paracetamol was increased in mice and rats with dietary deficiencies of protein (McLean and Day, 1974, 1975), vitamin E (Walker *et al.*, 1974;
McLean *et al.*, 1980; Peterson *et al.*, 1992) and the sulphur amino acids cysteine
and methionine (Reicks and Hathcock, 1984; McLean *et al.*, 1989; Price and
Jollow, 1989b; Peterson *et al.*, 1992). Selenium deficiency reduced the activity of
glutathione peroxidase, reduced lipid peroxidation and protected against paracetamol hepatotoxicity (Burk and Lane, 1983). However, in other studies, selenium deficiency aggravated toxicity (Raheja *et al.*, 1987; Peterson *et al.*, 1992). Prolonged

treatment with paracetamol caused deficiencies of methionine and cysteine, and reduced hepatic glutathione (Reicks *et al.*, 1988). A diet deficient in riboflavin protected against the toxicity of paracetamol (Raheja *et al.*, 1983c) and paracetamol did not cause hepatic tumours in rats maintained on a choline deficient diet (Maruyama *et al.*, 1990). A diet containing fish oil had a protective effect against paracetamol-induced liver toxicity in mice (Speck and Lauterburg, 1991) but D-limonene did not prevent depletion of hepatic glutathione by paracetamol as anticipated (Reicks and Crankshaw, 1993). The addition of 0.75 per cent butyl hydroxyanisole to the diet reduced the covalent binding of paracetamol to mouse hepatic and renal protein, and this was attributed to increased liver glutathione content (Miranda *et al.*, 1985). An exclusive diet of sucrose for 42 h protected against paracetamol hepatotoxicity and this was thought to be due to reduced activity of liver cytochrome P450 (Martinelli *et al.*, 1993). In rats receiving total parenteral nutrition, the addition of glutamine supplements decreased the hepatotoxicity of paracetamol and produced less depletion of hepatic glutathione (Hong *et al.*, 1992). Susceptibility to paracetamol-induced liver toxicity was increased in obese overfed Sprague Dawley rats (Corcoran and Wong, 1987) but reduced in obese Zucker rats, particularly when they were pretreated with phenobarbitone (Blouin *et al.*, 1987).

Fasting

There was a uniformly increased susceptibility to the hepatotoxicity of paracetamol in fasted mice, hamsters and rats, and this was usually associated with reduced

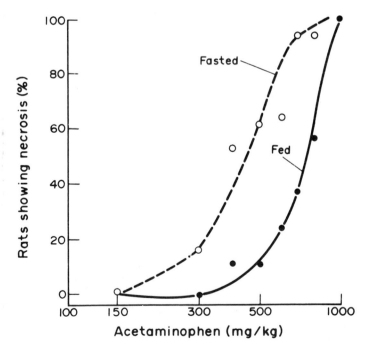

Figure 14.17   The effect of fasting on the dose-toxicity response curve following intraperitoneal administration of paracetamol (acetaminophen) in rats (reproduced with kind permission from Elsevier Science Ltd, from Price *et al.*, 1987).

hepatic glutathione content (Pessayre *et al.*, 1979, 1980; Strubelt *et al.*, 1981; Lauterburg and Mitchell, 1982; Walker *et al.*, 1982; Joyave *et al.*, 1985; Furukawa *et al.*, 1986; Miller *et al.*, 1986; Price *et al.*, 1987; Saville *et al.*, 1988). The effect of fasting was to move the dose-response curve for toxicity to the left (Figure 14.17). The acute LD_{50} of paracetamol in rats was almost halved by fasting for 18 h (McLean and Day, 1974) and starvation caused a marked fall in hepatic glutathione in mice with increased lipid peroxidation following a toxic dose of paracetamol (Wendel *et al.*, 1979). Paracetamol hepatotoxicity was greatly reduced in isolated perfused livers taken from fed compared with fasted rats (Strubelt and Younes, 1992). Pharmacokinetic factors could contribute to the potentiation of toxicity caused by fasting (Price *et al.*, 1987) and fasting could reduce hepatic glutathione (Pessayre *et al.*, 1979) and interfere with the proper utilization of glutathione for detoxification of the reactive metabolite of paracetamol (Miller *et al.*, 1986).

Other Factors

Many other factors have been reported to influence the toxic effects of paracetamol on the liver and these include: viral infection (MacDonald *et al.*, 1984; Renton and Dickson, 1984); immunological incompetence (Svendsen *et al.*, 1989); leukaemia (Lavigne *et al.*, 1982); diabetes and ketosis (Price and Jollow, 1982, 1983, 1986; Jeffery *et al.*, 1991); thyroid status (Raheja *et al.*, 1982); pregnancy (Larrey *et al.*, 1986); hyperoxia and hypoxia (Strubelt and Breining, 1980; Strubelt, 1981; Marzella *et al.*, 1986); exercise and endurance training (Lew and Quintanilha, 1991); circadian rhythms (Schnell *et al.*, 1983, 1984); and individual variation (Wells and To, 1986b; Young *et al.*, 1987). Active liver regeneration produced by partial hepatectomy protected against paracetamol hepatotoxicity in mice (Uryvaeva and Faktor, 1976).

15

Adverse Reactions and Interactions

Introduction

Paracetamol was re-introduced into clinical medicine as a combination with aspirin and caffeine ('Triogesic') in the USA in 1950. Soon after, three cases of agranulocytosis following its use were notified to the company and although the product was hastily withdrawn, subsequent investigation cast doubt on a causative role for paracetamol and it was put back onto the market in 1956 (Spooner and Harvey, 1976). Batterman and Grossman (1955) gave paracetamol in doses of 300 and 600 mg four times daily to 234 patients with musculoskeletal pain for up to 25 weeks. Untoward events were insignificant and occurred at the same rate (11 per cent) as with placebo. Chronic toxicity studies with a dose of 3.6 g daily for 116 weeks failed to reveal any haematological, renal or hepatic disturbances. Other clinical studies soon confirmed that paracetamol was well tolerated and that it produced few side effects of any consequence (Beaver, 1965). In most clinical reports paracetamol either did not cause side effects worthy of mention, or if it did, the incidence was similar to that observed in patients receiving placebo (Colgan and Mintz, 1957; Tarlin and Landrigan, 1972; Berry et al., 1975; Smith et al., 1975; Maron and Ickes, 1976; Keinänen et al., 1977; Skjelbred et al., 1977; Amadio and Cummings, 1983; Matthews et al., 1984; Mehlisch and Frakes, 1984; Milsom and Andersch, 1984; Amdekar and Desai, 1985; Jain et al., 1986; Gaudreault et al., 1988; Schachtel et al., 1988, 1989, 1991; Cooper et al., 1989; Gawel et al., 1990; Habib et al., 1990; Lehnert et al., 1990; McQuay et al., 1990; Nielsen et al., 1991, 1992; Wilson et al., 1991; Kauffman et al., 1992; Watcha et al., 1992; van Kraaij et al., 1994; and others). The most common complaints were nausea, vomiting, tiredness, headache, drowsiness and dizziness (Bloomfield et al., 1981; Frank and Kefford, 1983; Forbes et al., 1983, 1989b; McQuay et al., 1986; Olstad and Skjelbred, 1986b; Bentley and Head, 1987; Walson et al., 1989, 1992; Mehlisch et al., 1990; Ström et al., 1990; Arendt-Nielsen et al., 1991; Bertin et al., 1991; Skovlund et al., 1991a,b; Witjes et al., 1992; and others). In many reports of the clinical efficacy of paracetamol there was simply no mention of adverse effects, while in others the interpretation of the incidence of specific symptoms was difficult because no details were given of the methods of assessment and there was often no proper control data. In addition, paracetamol was frequently given in combination with other drugs, making it difficult if not impossible to establish any cause and effect relationship. Adverse effects have often been attributed to paracetamol without any supporting evidence as for example in the (erroneous) statement that in usual dosage it produced drowsiness, meth-aemoglobinaemia and impaired mentation (Henriques, 1970). In 60 patients with chronic knee pain, treated with 4 g of paracetamol daily for four weeks, there was a minor but statistically significant increase in plasma aspartate aminotransferase activity (Bradley *et al.*, 1991b) but no abnormalities were observed in most other studies where haematological and biochemical safety monitoring was performed (Cornely and Ritter, 1956; Keinänen *et al.*, 1977; Seideman and Melander, 1988; Walson *et al.*, 1989; Kauffman *et al.*, 1992; Cunietti *et al.*, 1993). Detailed monitoring of laboratory tests in 119 children receiving single doses of placebo, paracetamol or one of two doses of ibuprofen for fever revealed no significant abnormalities except that the blood urea nitrogen was said be increased in the active treatment groups. The mean blood urea nitrogen concentrations were 10.8 and 11.7 mg dl^{-1} after treatment with placebo and paracetamol respectively but the number of children given paracetamol was not stated and there was no validation of a statistically significant difference (Kelley *et al.*, 1993). As judged by published records and adverse reports to the Drug Abuse Warning Network in relation to estimated use, the incidence of adverse effects was much lower with paracetamol than with aspirin (Winick, 1989) and in general, paracetamol was preferred to aspirin and other non-narcotic analgesics because it was tolerated better (Ivey, 1983; Selbst, 1992; Aarbakke, 1994; Strom, 1994). Paracetamol has been taken continuously in doses ranging from 7.5 to as much as 20 g daily without apparent toxicity (Hajnal *et al.*, 1959; Boardman and Hart, 1967; Fyfe and Wright, 1990; Tredger *et al.*, 1995).

Allergy

Allergic reactions to drugs have been classified as: (1) anaphylactic shock, anaphylactoid reactions and acute dyspnoea; (2) urticaria, bronchial asthma and drug fever; (3) skin rashes, special exanthemas, conjunctivitis and vascular purpura; (4) serum sickness and allergic vasculitis; (5) thrombocytopenia, agranulocytosis and neutropenia, and pulmonary infiltration with eosinophilia; and (6) hepatic and renal reactions. These reactions have a more or less typical time pattern in relation to exposure to the drug (Hoigné *et al.*, 1990).

Anaphylaxis

Severe anaphylactic reactions to paracetamol were rare and few properly documented cases have been reported. There were also problems with definitions and some patients reported as such seem only to have had urticaria. Sharma *et al.* (1979) described a one-month-old Indian boy who developed extreme flushing of the skin with bronchospasm and severe respiratory distress an hour after being given 42 mg of paracetamol. He had recovered by the next day but was then given 50 mg of paracetamol, which produced an identical reaction. Stricker *et al.* (1985) gave brief details of five cases of acute hypersensitivity to paracetamol that had been reported to The Netherlands Centre for Monitoring of Adverse Reactions to Drugs over an unspecified period. Most had developed urticaria and other manifestations included bronchospasm, hypotension and collapse. Of five patients reported as reacting to paracetamol with anaphylaxis, four had urticaria, two had bronchospasm and two were hypotensive. The Australian Adverse Drug Reaction Registry had records of 60 systemic reactions to paracetamol in 43 patients, most of which were urticarial. Hypotensive collapse and airways obstruction were noted in three and two patients respectively (Leung *et al.*, 1992). There have been single case reports of severe reactions characterized by the rapid onset of urticaria and angioneurotic oedema with hypotension, bronchospasm and sometimes collapse and loss of consciousness (Roblot *et al.*, 1987; Simon *et al.*, 1988; Stempel *et al.*, 1991; Doan and Greenberger, 1993; Ispano *et al.*, 1993). In one case which was reported twice, an additional feature was the sudden onset of vomiting and diarrhoea (Le Van *et al.*, 1989; Le Van and Grilliat, 1990). Challenge tests with paracetamol (performed unwittingly in some patients) were positive. Seven of 38 patients with allergy to analgesics also had reactions to paracetamol when challenged and in one case there was life-threatening anaphylaxis (Kalyoncu, 1994).

Urticarial Reactions

Quincke's oedema has been described (Stricker *et al.*, 1985; Roblot *et al.*, 1987; Kennedy, 1989) and there have been reports of urticaria, pruritic reactions and angioneurotic oedema without major systemic upset following the use of paracetamol (Michelson, 1975; Sharma *et al.*, 1979; Cole, 1985; Idoko *et al.*, 1986; Leung *et al.*, 1992; Martin *et al.*, 1993; Kalyoncu, 1994). Attempts have been made to determine the incidence of allergic reactions to analgesics including paracetamol in hospital patients (Oberholzer *et al.*, 1993) and paracetamol was well tolerated in 25 patients who reacted to aspirin with urticaria or angioedema (Grzelewska-Rzymowska *et al.*, 1992).

Isolated rat serosal mast cells incubated with paracetamol liberated histamine only when S10 liver microsomal fractions were included and this indicated the involvement of an intermediate metabolite (Mansini *et al.*, 1986). Further evidence for the role of metabolic activation in the immunogenicity of paracetamol was shown by the ability to immunize mice with highly substituted conjugates of paracetamol with keyhole limpet haemocyanin and bovine serum albumin produced by its reaction with horseradish peroxidase (Chesham and Davies, 1985).

Asthma

Bronchospasm was an important manifestation in acute allergic reactions to paracetamol and the question of cross-tolerance in patients with aspirin sensitivity has been a cause for concern. From early reports it seemed that patients with urticaria and asthma induced by aspirin could take paracetamol without risk of serious consequences (Feinberg and Feinberg, 1955; Fisherman and Cohen, 1973; Szczeklik *et al.*, 1975; Delaney, 1976). However, other investigators found that patients with sensitivity to aspirin and non-steroidal anti-inflammatory drugs could also develop bronchospasm after taking paracetamol and the reported incidence varied from 0 to 60 per cent (Table 15.1). Patients who reacted to paracetamol invariably reacted

Table 15.1 The incidence of cross-tolerance to paracetamol in patients with aspirin-induced bronchial asthma

No. of patients with aspirin sensitivity	No. (%) reacting to paracetamol with asthma	Reference
3	5 (60)	Smith, 1971
11	0	Szczeklik *et al.*, 1975
50	0	Delaney, 1976
49	3 (6)	Szczeklik *et al.*, 1977
69	2 (3)	Spector *et al.*, 1979
10	3 (30)	Delaney, 1983
15	0	Falliers, 1983
9	0	Díez Gómez *et al.*, 1984
32	6 (18.8)	Barles *et al.*, 1988
38*	7 (18.4)	Kalyoncu, 1994
34	13 (38.2)	Settipane *et al.*, 1994

* Unspecified allergic reactions to aspirin

similarly to aspirin (Spector *et al.*, 1979; Settipane and Stevenson, 1989). Case reports of paracetamol-induced asthma indicated that as with aspirin, it could be severe and associated with rhinitis, urticaria and angioedema (Chafee and Settipane, 1967; Assem, 1976; Schmid, 1977; Henochowicz, 1986; Ellis *et al.*, 1989). Because of uncertainty about the frequency of cross-reaction, a controlled challenge with paracetamol was recommended in children with aspirin-induced asthma (Weinberger, 1978). Paracetamol was less likely than aspirin to produce adverse pulmonary reactions in young asthmatics. Of 25 such patients, four reacted to aspirin and two to paracetamol (Fischer *et al.*, 1983) and 15 asthmatics who were not sensitive to aspirin failed to react to paracetamol (Falliers, 1983). Three patients with hypertrophic rhinitis who were intolerant of aspirin and a variety of non-steroidal anti-inflammatory drugs were not sensitive to paracetamol (Prieto *et al.*, 1986). In another report, two of three patients who were intolerant of both aspirin and paracetamol did not react to paracetamol after desensitization to aspirin. Two patients were also desensitized to increasing doses of paracetamol and were refractory to doses of 1.5 but not 2 g (Settipane and Stevenson, 1989). It was estimated that the incidence of sensitivity to paracetamol in Polish patients with aspirin-induced asthma was about 4 per cent, and although paracetamol could usually be taken with impunity, it was recommended that an initial test dose of half a tablet should be given (Szczeklik, 1986, 1989). Of 112 patients with intolerance of various non-steroidal anti-inflammatory drugs manifest mostly by urticaria or angioedema, only three reacted to paracetamol (Ispano *et al.*, 1993).

The mechanism of paracetamol-induced asthma was not known but in one case, the adverse reaction might have been caused by use of the yellow dye tartrazine (Chafee and Settipane, 1967). Skin testing and measurement of histamine release *in vitro* were not helpful indicators of sensitivity to paracetamol (Assem, 1976; Ellis *et al.*, 1989). Unlike non-steroidal anti-inflammatory agents, paracetamol did not cause the release of prostaglandin $PGF_{2\alpha}$ *in vitro* or inhibit its binding to plasma proteins (Williams *et al.*, 1991). Paradoxically, paracetamol and several non-steroidal anti-inflammatory drugs relieved bronchospasm in one patient with asthma (Resta *et al.*, 1984).

Dermatological Reactions

Cutaneous reactions to paracetamol were uncommon. In a survey of eruptions seen by 202 Italian dermatologists between 1988 and 1991, 354 were considered to be definitely or possibly caused by antipyretic analgesics and non-steroidal anti-inflammatory drugs. Fixed eruptions, non-specific exanthema and urticaria or angio-oedema due to paracetamol were recorded on three, four and two occasions respectively. Skin reactions were observed in a further 59 cases following the use of paracetamol with multiple other drugs (Gruppo Italiano Studi Epidemiologici in Dermatologia (GISED), 1993). The most commonly reported dermatological reactions to paracetamol were fixed eruptions characterized by recurrent, discrete and often dusky blue-brown lesions occurring at the same sites over a period of time (Henriques, 1970; Wilson, 1975; Verbov, 1985; Meyrick Thomas and Munro, 1986; Bharija and Kanwar, 1987; Valsecchi, 1989; Duhra and Porter, 1990; Cohen *et al.*, 1992; Zemtsov *et al.*, 1992; Rademaker and Salmon, 1994). In other reports of fixed eruptions attributed to paracetamol, multiple other drugs had been taken (Olumide, 1979; Guin *et al.*, 1987; Guin and Baker, 1988). Skin testing with paracetamol was uniformly negative (Meyrick Thomas and Munro, 1986; Guin and Baker, 1988; Valsecchi, 1989) but challenge tests with oral administration resulted in the reappearance of the typical rash (Wilson, 1975; Shukla, 1982; Bharija and Kanwar, 1987; Valsecchi, 1989; Duhra and Porter, 1990; Cohen *et al.*, 1992). Of 113 patients with proven fixed drug eruptions, nine (7.9 per cent) were caused by paracetamol (Thankappan and Zachariah, 1991). Other less commonly reported dermatological reactions attributed to paracetamol were generalized urticaria (Michelson, 1975), acute generalized pustulosis (Mensing, 1993), progressive pigmentary purpura or Schamberg's disease (Abeck *et al.*, 1992), familial pemphigus (Brenner *et al.*, 1990), vascular purpura (Dussarat *et al.*, 1988) and cutaneous vasculitis (Shiohara *et al.*, 1992).

Paracetamol has rarely been involved in severe, life-threatening and fatal skin reactions. A 44-year-old woman died after developing fatal Stevens Johnson syndrome with haemolysis following the use of mefenamic acid, frusemide and paracetamol (Chan *et al.*, 1991). There have been reports of toxic epidermal necrolysis (Lyell's syndrome) in patients taking paracetamol alone (Kamanabroo and Schmitz-Landgraf, 1988; Sakellariou *et al.*, 1991) and in combination with other drugs (Gérard *et al.*, 1982; Roupe *et al.*, 1986; Sakellariou *et al.*, 1991). Generalized sensitivity reactions with multisystem involvement have also been reported. A 43-year-old woman became unwell with fever, diffuse erythematous rash, cervical and axillary lymphadenopathy, eosinophilia and hepatitis. She had been given numerous other drugs including bromazepam, allopurinol, aspirin, penicillin, erythromycin and oxomemazine, and it is not clear why this reaction was attributed to paracetamol (Guérin *et al.*, 1984). In another report, a 15-month-old girl developed unexplained fever, conjunctivitis, oedema, cervical lymphadenopathy, a maculopapular then erythematous rash with abnormal liver function tests and jaundice. A year later there was a similar reaction following administration of paracetamol and a subsequent challenge test was positive (Hurvitz *et al.*, 1984). A maculopapular rash in a breast-fed infant was attributed to consumption of paracetamol by the mother (Matheson *et al.*, 1985).

Respiratory and Cardiovascular Systems

Paracetamol alone had no significant effect on respiratory function in 19 patients with severe chronic obstructive lung disease (Munck *et al.*, 1990). Reversible pneumonitis with respiratory symptoms and diffuse radiographic shadowing was attributed to paracetamol in two cases (Kitaguchi *et al.*, 1992; Kudeken *et al.*, 1993) and in another similar case involving polypharmacy there was a skin rash and peripheral eosinophilia (Kondo *et al.*, 1993). Radiation pneumonitis occurred in a 63-year-old woman being treated for breast cancer following the withdrawal of a combination of paracetamol and dextropropoxyphene (Halpern *et al.*, 1985).

Paracetamol had no obvious cardiovascular effects but it was said to cause bradycardia in healthy subjects (Acharya, 1979) and to potentiate bradycardia induced by sotalol (Tongia, 1982). Repeated febrile illnesses in a 7-year-old boy with immunodeficiency were associated with reversible prolongation of the P-R interval on electrocardiography and a similar transient conduction defect was noted in a previously healthy 4-week-old infant. Both children had been given paracetamol and for some reason this was thought to have caused the electrocardiographic abnormalities (Entacher *et al.*, 1993). A case of Torsades de pointes ventricular tachycardia was reported in a patient taking terfenadine and paracetamol. It was suggested without evidence that the paracetamol inhibited the metabolism of terfenadine causing cumulation and cardiotoxicity (Matsis and Easthope, 1994).

Adverse Haematological Effects

Adverse effects on the blood have been reported infrequently following the normal therapeutic use of paracetamol.

Methaemoglobinaemia

Unlike its precursors acetanilide and phenacetin, paracetamol did not cause significant methaemoglobinaemia even in susceptible young children (Greenberg and Lester, 1947; Brodie and Axelrod, 1949; Boréus and Sandberg, 1953; Vest, 1962, 1963; Friederiszick and Toussaint, 1966; Thomas *et al.*, 1966; Windorfer and Vogel, 1976; Götte and Liedtke, 1978). Kiese and Menzel (1962) observed a statistically significant but otherwise quite trivial increase in methaemoglobin in 22 subjects given two doses of 843 mg of paracetamol, and a methaemoglobin concentration of 1.64 per cent was noted in a 10-week-old infant with minor paracetamol poisoning (Horwitz *et al.*, 1977). MacLean *et al.* (1968b) reported the presence of methaemoglobin (concentration not stated) in a 20-year-old woman who apparently became cyanosed after taking paracetamol (dose not mentioned). This latter report was unique as significant methaemoglobinaemia has never been reported otherwise in man, even after gross overdosage.

Thrombocytopenia

There have been isolated case reports of thrombocytopenia associated with the use of paracetamol. Heading (1968) described reversible acute thrombocytopenic purpura in a 63-year-old woman in whom challenge tests with paracetamol were positive, and thrombocytopenia, which developed in a 61-year-old man soon after he started to take paracetamol, was complicated by gastrointestinal bleeding (Skokan *et al.*, 1973). In another case of thrombocytopenia associated with consumption of paracetamol, a migration inhibitory factor test with the drug was positive (Shoenfeld *et al.*, 1980). Circulating antibodies to the sulphate conjugate of paracetamol were demonstrated in a 22-year-old man who presented with gross purpura and a platelet count of 4000 cu mm^{-1} following the ingestion of aspirin, paracetamol, salicylamide and caffeine (Eisner and Shahidi, 1972). A patient with known aspirin-induced thrombocytopenia apparently developed thrombocytopenia after taking paracetamol on one occasion despite having used it for years previously without incident (Scheinberg, 1979). No challenge test was performed and a causative role for paracetamol in this case seems doubtful. In another report, there was thrombocytopenic purpura with absence of megakaryocytes in an 80-year-old man who took oxyphenbutazone and paracetamol (Font *et al.*, 1981). Oxyphenbutazone was the more likely culprit. Purpura fulminans developed in a 32-year-old alcoholic woman who took alcohol to excess with paracetamol for three days following a serious car accident in which she killed two of her seven children. However, grossly abnormal liver function tests on admission with a rapid recovery were typical of acute hepatic necrosis caused by paracetamol overdose, a possibility not mentioned by the authors (Guccione *et al.*, 1993). Two types of antiplatelet antibodies were demonstrated in the presence of toxic concentrations of paracetamol in a patient with thrombocytopenia that was thought to be caused by the drug (Lerner *et al.*, 1985). In a case control study, the annual incidence of drug-induced thrombocytopenic purpura was estimated at 18 cases per million population. There was no increased risk associated with the use of paracetamol (Kaufman *et al.*, 1993).

Aplastic Anaemia and Agranulocytosis

After its reintroduction into medicine in 1950 as 'Triogesic', the marketing of paracetamol was suspended following reports of three cases of agranulocytosis to the American manufacturer E. R. Squibb. However, a causal relationship was considered unlikely (Lloyd, 1961; Spooner and Harvey, 1976). Ten years later, there was another report of agranulocytosis in a 78-year-old woman who had been taking paracetamol in doses up to 2 g daily for many weeks. No other drugs were involved. The clinical picture was typical with a minimum neutrophil count of 240 cu mm^{-1} and recovery was rapid when the drug was discontinued (Lloyd, 1961). There were subsequent reports of pancytopenia after the use of paracetamol in combination with pentazocine (Datta, 1973) and dextropropoxyphene (Webster, 1973). These were followed by case reports of agranulocytosis (with fatalities) attributed to the use of paracetamol (MacKinnon and Menon, 1974; Maraninchi *et al.*, 1981; Hirsch *et al.*, 1982; Benkirane-Agoumi *et al.*, 1986; Chichmanian *et al.*, 1989; Lacotte *et al.*, 1990). In another report, paracetamol was considered to be the cause of agranulocytosis in five patients although few details were provided, and as in many other reports, other drugs had also been taken (Jouet *et al.*, 1980). In most cases, bone marrow examination revealed a picture of maturation arrest of myelocytes. In one patient, agranulocytosis occurred after ingestion of a single dose of 600 mg and although paracetamol was implicated on the basis of the effects of high concentrations on cultured bone marrow cells, there was a further episode of agranulocytosis without exposure to paracetamol (Maraninchi *et al.*, 1981). In another patient, paracetamol was supposed to have caused agranulocytosis after it had been taken regularly for three years (Hirsch *et al.*, 1982). It was usually difficult to implicate a drug as a cause of agranulocytosis with any degree of certainty and deliberate challenge was too dangerous to contemplate. No single agent could be identified as a cause of agranulocytosis in a 67-year-old woman taking multiple drugs until a recurrence was clearly associated with renewed ingestion of paracetamol (Chichmanian *et al.*, 1989). In another report, agranulocytosis in a 20-year-old woman with pharyngitis was attributed to paracetamol or penicillin, and it was rapidly reversed by stopping these drugs and administration of granulocyte colony stimulating factor (Ramos Fernandez de Soria *et al.*, 1994).

The incidence of agranulocytosis caused by paracetamol must be very low considering its extensive worldwide use. In a survey of 15 patients with agranulocytosis, paracetamol was said to be the cause in three but no details were given (Duhamel *et al.*, 1977) while in another study of 63 patients seen between 1968 and 1978 it was thought to be responsible in five cases (Heit and Heimpel, 1982). An international study of the relationship between drug usage and blood dyscrasias was carried out in Israel, Spain, Germany, Italy, Hungary, Bulgaria and Sweden. There was no association between consumption of paracetamol and agranulocytosis or aplastic anaemia (International Agranulocytosis and Aplastic Anemia Study, 1986).

Effects on White Blood Cell Function and Infection

Following the administration of 1.3 g of paracetamol in healthy volunteers there was significant inhibition of the ability of granulocytes to adhere to nylon fibre columns (MacGregor, 1976), but paracetamol did not adversely affect the viability of polymorphonuclear leucocytes (Austin and Truant, 1978). The phagocytic activity of monocytes was not decreased in subjects who took 500 mg of paracetamol four times daily for five days (Klein *et al.*, 1982) and it also had no inhibitory effect on the chemotaxis of neutrophils obtained from healthy subjects (Matzner *et al.*, 1984). In contrast to these findings, paracetamol inhibited human polymorphonuclear cell function *in vitro* as shown by decreased luminochemiluminescence produced by the oxidative respiratory burst and reduced phagocytic activity (Shalabi, 1992). It also competed with chloride ions as a substrate for human leucocyte myeloperoxidase and, therefore, could interfere with its microbiocidal action (van Zyl *et al.*, 1989). In a study of the effects of anti-rheumatic drugs on the *in vitro* immunological responses of human peripheral blood lymphocytes, paracetamol in low therapeutic and high toxic concentrations enhanced, then inhibited, phytomitogen-induced blastogenesis (Panush, 1976; Panush and Ossakow, 1979).

In a 15-year-old girl with acute Epstein-Barr viral infection and psychosis, the ingestion of paracetamol was considered to have masked the symptoms and signs of infection and delayed the making of the proper diagnosis (Jarvis *et al.*, 1990). A 37-year-old man abused paracetamol and codeine tablets for seven years, taking as much as 18 g of paracetamol a day. He presented with weight loss, anorexia, fever, jaundice and candidiasis. Investigation revealed immunodeficiency with T-cell defects and myelodysplasia but a negative test for human immunodeficiency virus. Karyotyping of the bone marrow showed a (1;7) (p11;p11) translocation leaving trisomy 1p and 7p and monosomy 7q. He received radiotherapy for a squamous cell tonsillar carcinoma and died with disseminated aspergillosis. For some reason, the chromosomal translocations and their consequences were attributed to the use of paracetamol (Fyfe and Wright, 1990). There was no objective evidence to support this claim. The local application of paracetamol to third molar sockets after surgical extraction did not interfere with wound healing (Moore *et al.*, 1992). Paracetamol had no effect on the clinical resolution of influenza in children (Thompson *et al.*, 1987), but in another report it was thought to have worsened the illness in children with fever (Sugimura *et al.*, 1994). It also had no adverse effect on the biological responses to interferon and the immune responses to vaccination (Uhari *et al.*, 1988; Witter *et al.*, 1988; Gross *et al.*, 1994).

Anaemia

The use of paracetamol was not associated with aplastic anaemia in a major international study (International Agranulocytosis and Aplastic Anemia Study, 1986) but a case control study in France indicated a moderate risk with an odds ratio of 1.8 to 2.0 for intake during the previous five years or during the last year. There was no significant association with the therapeutic use of paracetamol (Baumelou *et al.*, 1993). There have been occasional reports of haemolytic anaemia. A 28-year-old man was found to be icteric and anaemic (haemoglobin concentration 4 g 100 ml^{-1}) after taking paracetamol in unstated doses for two weeks on account of malaise and fever. A direct Coombe's test was positive and the patient recovered after withdrawal of the drug. Paracetamol was 'proved' to be the cause because a few drops of the patient's blood haemolyzed when mixed with a paracetamol solution of unstated strength (Mehrotra and Gupta, 1973). Another patient developed a haemolytic anaemia with thrombocytopenia on two occasions after taking paracetamol. A Coombe's test was positive and a haemolyzing drug-dependent factor was demonstrated (Manor *et al.*, 1976). There have been other reports of haemolytic anaemia and thrombocytopenia (Kornberg and Polliack, 1978) and a chronic haemolytic anaemia responsive to corticosteroids was eventually traced to excessive and inappropriate use of a combination of paracetamol with dextropropoxyphene (Fulton and McGonigal, 1989). Patients with glucose-6-phosphate dehydrogenase deficiency may be at increased risk of drug-induced haemolysis and, although paracetamol was generally considered to be safe in this condition, several cases have been reported following its use (Bartsocas *et al.*, 1982; Heintz *et al.*, 1989). In one case, severe haemolysis and renal failure complicated an overdose of paracetamol in a 28-year-old man with the Hillbrow enzyme variant (Cayanis *et al.*, 1975). Paracetamol also caused asymptomatic shortening of the red cell survival time in a patient with the Mahidol variant of glucose-6-phosphate dehydrogenase (Pootrakul and Panich, 1983). Paracetamol did not cause haemolysis in a comparison with placebo in 17 young patients with glucose-6-phosphate dehydrogenase deficiency, but unfortunately the dose was not specified (Cottafava *et al.*, 1990). It did not decrease the red blood cell glutathione content, but it had a variable effect on the time of acid haemolysis (Altorjay *et al.*, 1993). Paracetamol was included in long lists of drugs said to cause haemolytic anaemia (Valbonesi *et al.*, 1979; Durán-Suárez, 1984), but it was not considered to pose a great risk for patients with glucose-6-phosphate dehydrogenase deficiency (Beutler, 1984).

Effects on Haemostasis

With increasing awareness of the adverse effects of aspirin on platelet function there was considerable interest in the effects that paracetamol might have on haemostasis. It was immediately obvious that patients with bleeding disorders such as haemophilia might be at increased risk of haemorrhage after taking aspirin. Mielke and Britten (1970) first showed that 975 mg of paracetamol had no effect on the bleeding time in healthy subjects or in two patients with haemophilia. It also had no effect on platelet aggregation. A similar lack of effect of therapeutic doses of paracetamol on platelet aggregation, platelet factor 3, blood loss from skin puncture and the bleeding time was confirmed in subsequent reports (Sutor *et al.*, 1971; Kasper and Rapaport, 1972; Mielke *et al.*, 1976; Waltman *et al.*, 1976; Pearson, 1978; Mielke, 1981; Cronberg *et al.*, 1984; Seymour *et al.*, 1984). A six-week course of 1950 mg of paracetamol daily had no effect on the bleeding time in three haemophiliacs and no effect on platelet aggregation or platelet adhesion in four normal subjects (Mielke *et al.*, 1976). In addition, it did not influence the coagulation proteins or fibrinolytic system (Mielke, 1981).

In more detailed studies of the effects of paracetamol on haemostatic mechanisms, it was found that preincubation with toxic concentrations of paracetamol (150 mg l^{-1}) completely inhibited the aggregation of human platelets induced by arachidonic acid and collagen, and the secretion of $[^{14}C]$-serotonin and production of thromboxane B_2 in response to arachidonic acid was also inhibited. At the same high concentrations, N-acetyl-p-benzoquinoneimine had similar effects but it did not alter the formation of thromboxane B_2 or collagen-induced platelet aggregation (Shorr *et al.*, 1985). Similar effects of toxic concentrations of paracetamol were described on platelet aggregation, and inhibition of release of serotonin and thromboxane synthesis in platelets stimulated with collagen (Dupin *et al.*, 1988). Paracetamol had no effect on platelet aggregation *in vitro* but it inhibited the release of adenosine triphosphate (ATP) and platelets exposed to paracetamol inhibited the serotonin-mediated constriction of bovine coronary artery strips (Verheggen and Schrör, 1987). In another study, paracetamol added *in vitro* to human platelets inhibited aggegation, secretion and thromboxane B_2 formation in response to collagen, adrenaline and arachidonic acid. Following ingestion of 650 and 1000 mg of paracetamol, platelet aggregation and secretion were not altered in four healthy subjects but were inhibited in one other subject who also had the highest plasma concentrations of the drug (Lages and Weiss, 1989).

Therapeutic doses of paracetamol had no effect on menstrual blood loss in normal subjects (Petruson *et al.*, 1977; Janbu *et al.*, 1978, 1979; Pendergrass *et al.*, 1984, 1985) or in women with intrauterine contraceptive devices (Hahn and Petruson, 1979). In studies of blood loss after surgery, paracetamol caused a minor increase in bleeding time after tooth extraction but it was less than that caused by aspirin and there was no correlation between the bleeding time and postoperative blood loss (Pawlak *et al.*, 1978). In 409 patients given paracetamol after tonsillectomy there was less bleeding than in 423 given aspirin (Stage *et al.*, 1988) and there was less bleeding during and after hip replacement in patients who took paracetamol preoperatively than in those who had taken aspirin and non-steroidal anti-inflammatory drugs (Faunø *et al.*, 1993). Overall, it seems that paracetamol could cause minor dose-related changes in platelet function but in therapeutic doses it had no adverse effects on haemostasis, even in patients with bleeding disorders such as haemophilia (Czapek, 1976; Mielke, 1981). Abnormal viscoelastic properties of whole blood in patients with chronic headache could not be attributed to the use of analgesics, including paracetamol (Oder *et al.*, 1994).

Paracetamol in Donor Blood

Paracetamol was detected in 72 (6.12 per cent) of 1176 samples of donor blood in Jerusalem (Sharon *et al.*, 1982). In another survey in Halifax, Nova Scotia, paracetamol was present in 10 of 400 blood samples but none of the donors had admitted taking the drug during the previous 24 h (MacIntyre *et al.*, 1986).

Adverse Gastrointestinal Effects

Gastrointestinal Function

In therapeutic doses, paracetamol had no important effects on gastrointestinal function and it did not influence xylose absorption and excretion (Markiewicz, 1975). Following administration of 20 mg kg^{-1} as tablets with 40 ml of water in healthy volunteers, there was a minor decrease in the frequency and duration of antral propagation activity as measured by manometry, but no change in gastric pH (Schurizek *et al.*, 1989a). Diarrhoea and faecal incontinence in a patient given paracetamol syrup regularly was attributed to the sorbitol content of the formulation (James *et al.*, 1992).

Peptic Ulcer

A strong association between the consumption of analgesics containing aspirin and chronic gastroduodenal ulceration was established in a series of epidemiological studies originating in Australia (Duggan, 1980; Ivey, 1983). Paracetamol did not cause direct gastroduodenal mucosal ulceration or injury. Roth *et al.* (1963) showed that in contrast to aspirin, it did not produce acute gastric mucosal damage in cats, and it did not cause gross buccal mucosal lesions in man when a fragment of tablet was placed between the cheek and gum. In a survey of 127 patients with gastric and duodenal ulcer in Sydney, there was a strong association with heavy analgesic use in comparison with matched control patients. The relative risks for gastric ulcer were similar for all aspirin-containing and paracetamol-containing preparations (17 and 24 respectively). For paracetamol alone the relative risk was also 24 but there were only 12 patients in this group. There was no link between analgesic use and duodenal ulcer (Piper *et al.*, 1981). Analgesic use was then compared in 99 gastric ulcer patients and 199 control subjects. Again there was a strong association with heavy analgesic use and a dominant effect of combinations containing paracetamol (Piper *et al.*, 1982). In a later report by the same authors, aetiological factors were studied in 104 patients with gastric ulcer and 208 control subjects in relation to smoking, and exposure to alcohol and lifetime, five-year and one-year use of analgesics. There was a significant association between gastric ulcer and the use of aspirin and non-steroidal anti-inflammatory drugs but not paracetamol (McIntosh *et al.*, 1985). The previously reported association of gastric ulcer with paracetamol could have been due to a tendency of patients with dyspepsia to replace aspirin and non-steroidal anti-inflammatory drugs with paracetamol, which was perceived as safer (Piper and McIntosh, 1988). In another similar study, too few peptic ulcer patients used paracetamol for any conclusion to be drawn concerning a causative role (Duggan *et al.*, 1986). A different approach was taken in a survey of the use of analgesics by 1327 new users of cimetidine over the age of 65 years compared with 5308 similar subjects not prescribed cimetidine. Analgesics were consumed more commonly by the patients receiving cimetidine and again the positive association with aspirin and non-steroidal anti-inflammatory drugs extended to paracetamol (Avila *et al.*, 1988). In 113 patients with dyspeptic symptoms in whom there was no endoscopic evidence of peptic ulcer, oesophagitis or cancer, there was a significant association with paracetamol consumption but it was not stated how many of these patients had also taken aspirin. Twenty-two patients had macroscopic duodenitis and 17 had a previous history of peptic ulcer (Talley *et al.*, 1988). In later reports, there was no significant association between dyspepsia and the use of paracetamol in a community (Talley *et al.*, 1994b) or in outpatients referred for endoscopy (Talley *et al.*, 1994a). The prior use of analgesics was investigated in 192 patients with previously diagnosed gastric and duodenal ulcer and 225 new cases in comparison with 411 matched community control subjects. More recurrent than new cases used paracetamol daily while fewer recurrent than new cases used aspirin or non-steroidal anti-inflammatory drugs. Thus, a diagnosis of gastric or duodenal ulcer caused a decrease in the use of aspirin and an increase in the use of paracetamol (McIntosh *et al.*, 1988). In patients with duodenal ulcer, the periods of dyspepsia were lengthened with increasing use of paracetamol (McIntosh *et al.*, 1991). Another case control study was carried out in an urban black population in South Africa and again there was a strong association between heavy use of analgesics and gastric ulcer. There were no differences between users of aspirin and paracetamol alone and in combination, and users of non-steroidal anti-inflammatory drugs. Only 50 patients were studied and it was not stated how many took paracetamol alone and in combination with other drugs (Mohamed *et al.*, 1990). In another report, of 541 gastric ulcer patients, 30 per cent were taking aspirin, 20 per cent non-steroidal anti-inflammatory drugs, and 8 per cent paracetamol, and patients presenting with gastric ulcer who had a previous history of the disease were more likely to use paracetamol, presumably on medical advice (Brazer *et al.*, 1990). Finally, there was an increased risk of perforation or haemorrhage in peptic ulcer patients who regularly took 1 g or more of paracetamol daily but not in those who took less (Savage *et al.*, 1993).

Although most of these studies indicated a strong association between the use of paracetamol and peptic ulcer disease, this association was generally considered to be an artefact caused by the preferential use of paracetamol rather than aspirin and non-steroidal anti-inflammatory drugs by patients with dyspeptic symptoms.

Gastrointestinal Haemorrhage

There was no evidence that paracetamol caused occult or overt gastrointestinal haemorrhage. Goulston and Skyring (1964) measured the faecal excretion of ^{51}Cr after isotope labelling of red blood cells in 27 hospital patients, given 4 g of paracetamol daily for five days. The mean daily blood loss was 0.8 ml compared with 0.6 ml during the control period. In 10 of these patients given aspirin, the mean daily loss increased from 0.7 to 3.3 ml daily. Paracetamol did not increase bleeding in 18 patients who had pre-existing gastrointestinal blood loss. In a similar study in eight patients, the mean daily faecal blood losses were 4.6, 1.3 and 1.2 ml with daily intake of 2.25 g of aspirin, 4 g of paracetamol and 600 mg of flufenamic acid respectively (Tudhope, 1966). In other studies with ^{51}Cr-labelled red blood cells in patients with osteoarthritis and rheumatoid arthritis, administration of 2.6–5.2 g of paracetamol daily did not increase occult gastrointestinal blood loss (Loebl *et al.*, 1977; Tringham *et al.*, 1980; Johnson and Driscoll, 1981).

The association between the use of aspirin and non-steroidal anti-inflammatory drugs and acute upper gastrointestinal haemorrhage was well established. In a study of 346 patients admitted to hospital with haematemesis or melaena, previous intake of paracetamol was more common than in matched controls but there was no association between bleeding and habitual use of paracetamol. It was concluded that paracetamol was taken in part, for the symptoms of bleeding but it did not necessarily cause bleeding (Coggon *et al.*, 1982). The same conclusions were drawn in another report of the same data (Langman *et al.*, 1983). In another case control study of 230 patients with bleeding peptic ulcer there was no significant association with previous or regular consumption of paracetamol (Faulkner *et al.*, 1988). In other similar studies in Israel, Belgium, Spain and France there was no evidence that paracetamol increased the risk of major upper gastrointestinal haemorrhage (Levy *et al.*, 1988; Holvoet *et al.*, 1991; Laporte *et al.*, 1991; Begaud *et al.*, 1993). In a survey of drug use by 71 patients with bleeding peptic ulcer 17 (24 per cent) took paracetamol regularly but the significance of this finding could not be assessed as no information was given about its use by controls (Marriott *et al.*, 1993). There was no association between paracetamol use and gastrointestinal bleeding in a report from the Boston Collaborative Drug Surveillance Program (Jick, 1981) or with complications of bleeding peptic ulcer in 1144 patients in a more recent multicentre study in the United Kingdom (Langman *et al.*, 1994). A switch from non-steroidal anti-inflammatory drugs to paracetamol was recommended as a means of reducing the number of patients admitted to hospital with gastrointestinal bleeding (Walt, 1995).

Endoscopic Studies

The effects of paracetamol on the gastric mucosa have been observed directly by endoscopic examination in a number of studies. The administration of 650 mg of paracetamol intragastrically did not cause endoscopic mucosal damage in 33 males and 37 females attending a gastroenterology service whereas under the same conditions aspirin produced gastric lesions in 17 patients (Vickers, 1967). A similar failure to produce endoscopic gastroduodenal lesions was reported following single and repeated therapeutic doses of paracetamol for periods of 1–14 days (Loebl *et al.*,

1977; Ivey *et al.*, 1978; Hoftiezer *et al.*, 1982; Stern *et al.*, 1984a; Lanza *et al.*, 1986; Hogan, 1988; Müller *et al.*, 1988, 1990). Endoscopic biopsy examination of the gastric mucosa in patients with osteoarthritis who had been switched to a combination of paracetamol and dextropropoxyphene for one week showed varying degrees of acute and chronic gastritis. After continued treatment with the combination for four weeks in 12 patients, similar changes were observed on repeat endoscopy (McIntyre *et al.*, 1981). In one report, paracetamol was said to cause clinical signs in two of eight patients and three had mucosal hyperaemia on endoscopy. However, no information was provided on dose, the reasons for taking paracetamol, underlying pathology and the previous or concurrent use of other drugs (Misra *et al.*, 1990). Paracetamol provided some protection against endoscopic gastric mucosal injury caused by aspirin and ethanol in five healthy subjects with occlusion of the pylorus with a balloon catheter (Stern *et al.*, 1984b). In other studies, paracetamol did not prevent gastric injury as assessed by endoscopy in healthy volunteers given aspirin (Graham and Smith, 1985) or ibuprofen (Lanza *et al.*, 1986).

Experimental Studies

Gastric mucosal injury caused changes in the permeability to ions and hence the potential difference across the gastric mucosal barrier. Paracetamol did not increase gastric mucosal permeability as measured directly in healthy subjects (Gordon *et al.*, 1974) and unlike aspirin it had no effect on H^+ and Na^+ ion transport and did not reduce the transmucosal potential difference (Ivey and Settree, 1976). Changes in the potential difference across the gastric mucosa were closely related to the severity of injury caused by a variety of agents and the lack of effect of paracetamol was confirmed by other investigators (Ivey *et al.*, 1978; Massarrat and Strutwolf, 1979; Stern *et al.*, 1984a; Hogan, 1988). Paracetamol gave some protection against gastric mucosal injury induced by aspirin as shown by attenuation of the fall in potential difference (de Vos and Barbier, 1985).

Unlike aspirin, paracetamol did not increase the exfoliation of gastric mucosal cells as shown by DNA loss (Corinaldesi *et al.*, 1978). It inhibited glucosamine synthesis by human gastric mucosal cell homogenates but this effect was considered to be unrelated to the genesis of peptic ulcer (Goodman *et al.*, 1977). Prostaglandins were thought to be involved in the gastric mucosal damage produced by aspirin and related drugs. In some circumstances paracetamol seemed to stimulate rather than inhibit prostaglandin synthesis and this could explain not only its lack of gastric toxicity but also protection against gastric injury produced by aspirin and non-steroidal anti-inflammatory drugs (Seegers *et al.*, 1979, 1980a, 1982; van Kolfschoten *et al.*, 1981; Trautmann *et al.*, 1991). Prostaglandins were probably not involved in any gastroprotective effects of paracetamol in man. It did not influence the synthesis of prostaglandins PGE_2 and $PGF_{2\alpha}$ by human gastric mucosa (Peskar, 1977; Konturek *et al.*, 1984; Bennett, 1989b) and although it protected human gastric epithelial cells against injury induced by taurocholate this effect appeared to be unrelated to stimulation of prostaglandin synthesis (Romano *et al.*, 1988a). On the other hand, indomethacin blocked the protective action of paracetamol against gastric injury produced by aspirin and ethanol (Stern *et al.*, 1984b).

The overall conclusion from these studies is that therapeutic doses of paracetamol do not cause gastric mucosal injury, peptic ulcer or gastrointestinal bleeding. It was recommended as the analgesic of choice in patients with gastrointestinal disease (Caradoc-Davies, 1984; Ivey, 1986; Elliott, 1990).

Oesophageal Ulceration

Dysphagia in a 35-year-old woman following the ingestion of a combination of paracetamol and dextropropoxyphene was shown by endoscopy to be due to linear oesophageal ulceration. The ulcer healed on withdrawal of the drugs (Finet *et al.*, 1990).

Acute Biliary Pain with Cholestasis

A patient had recurrent attacks of abdominal pain followed by transiently abnormal liver function tests after taking aspirin, naproxen and paracetamol. Another patient with aspirin intolerance also had recurrent abdominal pain with abnormal liver function tests after taking paracetamol and codeine. No further episodes occurred after the patients were told to avoid analgesics including paracetamol. In the absence of other causes, it was proposed that paracetamol caused cholestasis and biliary pain (Waldum *et al.*, 1992). Another case was reported in a 25-year-old woman who became unwell with abdominal pain several days after taking unstated doses of paracetamol for three or four days for toothache. Investigations were normal but the liver function tests were consistent with biliary obstruction and did not return to normal for five months (Wong *et al.*, 1993b). In these cases, a cause and effect relationship seemed most unlikely.

Rectal Ulceration and Stenosis

There have been numerous reports of proctitis, rectal ulceration and stenosis in patients using suppositories containing paracetamol in combination with dextropropoxyphene (Vincens *et al.*, 1982; Blanchi *et al.*, 1984; Laplanche *et al.*, 1984; Hemet *et al.*, 1986; Fenzy and Bogomoletz, 1987; Rotenberg *et al.*, 1988; Marteau *et al.*, 1990; Raclot and Minazzi, 1993) and aspirin (Lanthier *et al.*, 1987; Ozoux *et al.*, 1987; Ramboer and Verhamme, 1987; Gainant *et al.*, 1989; Baekelandt *et al.*, 1990; Puy Montbrun *et al.*, 1990; Legallicier *et al.*, 1991; D'Haens *et al.*, 1993; van Gossum *et al.*, 1993; Yousfi *et al.*, 1993). Many patients were middle-aged females with a neurotic or psychiatric background (D'Haens *et al.*, 1993) and dependence on the preparations containing the narcotic analgesic dextropropoxyphene was sometimes such that abuse continued despite clear warnings of the consequences and recurrence of the rectal lesions (Vincens *et al.*, 1982). The rectal ulceration was severe in some reports with associated vaginal ulceration and even the formation of a rectovaginal fistula (Laplanche *et al.*, 1984; Raclot and Minazzi, 1993). In some cases major reconstructive surgery was necessary for the relief of intractable stenosis (Hemet *et al.*, 1986; Lanthier *et al.*, 1987; Gainant *et al.*, 1989; Legallicier *et al.*, 1991; Raclot and Minazzi, 1993; van Gossum *et al.*, 1993). It does not seem reasonable to attribute severe local mucosal damage solely to the paracetamol content of the suppositories, at least not in the patients who took it in combination with aspirin. The use of suppositories containing paracetamol only were well tolerated with no significant local adverse effects (Gustafsson *et al.*, 1979).

Ulcerative Colitis

The use of paracetamol during the previous four weeks was associated with relapse of ulcerative colitis but a direct causal relationship was not implied (Rampton *et al.*, 1983).

Colorectal Cancer

There was no significant reduction in the risk for colorectal cancer in patients taking paracetamol frequently as was the case for aspirin and non-steroidal anti-inflammatory drugs (Thun *et al.*, 1991, 1993; Logan *et al.*, 1993; Muscat *et al.*, 1994).

Hepatotoxicity

Acute hepatic necrosis was a common complication of paracetamol overdosage and it was inevitable that sooner or later liver damage would be suspected during its normal therapeutic use. In the numerous clinical studies of the comparative clinical efficacy of paracetamol there were no consistent findings to suggest hepatotoxicity. There were no changes in liver function tests in 20 normal subjects given 3 g daily for 10 days (Khalil *et al.*, 1978) or in 11 patients who took total doses of 200–700 g of paracetamol with dextropropoxyphene over periods of 5–39 months (Hutchinson *et al.*, 1986). In a case control study of drug-induced liver disease in a population of 280 000 individuals over a period of five years, there were 12 instances requiring hospitalization. None were attributed to the use of paracetamol despite the esti-mated exposure of more than 60 000 persons to the drug (Beard *et al.*, 1986). Simi-larly, in a survey of 3959 liver biopsies in 1981 and 1983, there were 301 cases of suspected drug-induced liver toxicity but in the final analysis paracetamol was not implicated in any (Koch *et al.*, 1985). Minor abnormalities have been noted in some studies (Shufman and Machtey, 1979). Sporadic minor elevation in plasma amino-transferase activity occurred in 15 healthy subjects taking 3.9 g of paracetamol daily for one week (Lanza *et al.*, 1986) and a statistically significant but clinically insignifi-cant increase was observed in 61 patients with osteoarthritis given 4 g daily for four weeks (Bradley *et al.*, 1991b). The previous use of paracetamol was determined in 45 patients with chronic active hepatitis but there was no evidence to suggest that it had been an initiating factor (Neuberger *et al.*, 1980). In a survey of hepatic injury in 53 chronic haemodialysis patients, episodes were linked twice to the use of paraceta-mol and aspirin, and once to paracetamol taken with oxomemazine. No details were given and most of the patients had active viral hepatitis (Simon and Meyrier, 1982). In another report, 56 per cent of 118 young adults had some disturbance of liver function during an epidemic of measles in Israel. More than half of the patients given paracetamol had raised plasma aminotransferase activity compared with 15 per cent of those given dipyrone. The mean cumulative dose of paracetamol was higher in the patients with abnormal liver function tests (11.6 g) than in those without (7.6 g) (Ackerman *et al.*, 1989). An unusual outbreak of fulminant hepatitis was reported in eight previously healthy children. A viral aetiology was likely, but there was an unusual pattern of zonal necrosis and all the children had been given therapeutic doses of paracetamol (Alonso *et al.*, 1994).

The safety of paracetamol in patients with pre-existing liver disease has also been questioned. Liver function tests were monitored in 30 patients with hepatosplenic bilharziasis before, during and after administration of 3 g of paracetamol daily for 10 days. The mean serum aspartate and alanine aminotransferase activities and bilirubin concentration increased from 20.6 to 31.4 units, 17.3 to 29.9 units and 0.92 to 1.25 mg 100 ml^{-1} respectively. Two patients were said to have developed hepatic precoma during treatment, which improved rapidly after the drug was discontinued. However, no details were given, it is not known what other drugs they received and there was no proper control group of similar patients not given paracetamol (Khalil *et al.*, 1978). No adverse effects on hepatic function were observed in 11 patients with cirrhosis and 12 patients without liver disease given 3 g of paracetamol daily for five days (Andreasen and Hutters, 1979). In six patients with chronic stable liver disease who took 4 g of paracetamol daily for five days there was no evidence of toxicity or drug accumulation, but in a crossover comparison with placebo in a further 20 similar patients treated for 13 days, liver function tests deteriorated in one patient taking paracetamol. However, subsequent challenges with 4 g a day of paracetamol taken for 10 and 14 days failed to produce a similar response and it was concluded that there was no contraindication to the use of paracetamol in patients with stable chronic liver disease (Benson, 1983). Similar conclusions were reached in another study in which it was shown that the glutathione conjugation of paracetamol was not impaired in 15 patients with chronic liver disease as evidenced by the production of normal amounts of the cysteine and mercapturic acid conjugates (Forrest *et al.*, 1979).

Acute and Chronic Liver Damage with Therapeutic Use

In the late 1970s, case reports of chronic liver disease began to appear in patients who had been taking therapeutic doses of paracetamol on a regular basis. A 59-year-old woman who had also been exposed to cleaning solvents developed abnormal liver function tests with histological appearances on liver biopsy of chronic active hepatitis after taking 2.925 g of paracetamol daily for a year. The liver function tests returned to normal when the drug was discontinued and deteriorated again on rechallenge with the same dose (Johnson and Tolman, 1977). There was a rather similar report concerning a 53-year-old man who had taken 4 g of paracetamol daily for about a year. Although there was a minor deterioration in liver function tests on challenge, repeat liver biopsies a long time after the drug had been stopped showed continuing and progressive liver damage. Paracetamol metabolism and hepatic glutathione content were normal (Bonkowsky *et al.*, 1978). Three other cases of toxic hepatitis were attributed to paracetamol but one alcoholic patient had clearly taken a major overdose and the others had taken excessive doses (Barker *et al.*, 1977). Another ex-alcoholic patient, who had taken paracetamol in combination with chlormezanone, had abnormal liver function tests and atypical liver biopsy appearances of cholestasis, steatosis and fibrosis (Olsson, 1978). There was also a

Table 15.2 Some case reports of atypical liver damage following the therapeutic use of paracetamol.

Age and sex	Max. stated daily dose	Max. amino-transferase $(\mu\,l^{-1})$	Histology[1]	Predisposing or associated factors	Reference
59F	2.9 g for 1 year	1150	CAH;CH	unidentified cleaning solvents	Johnson and Tolman, 1977
40M	3.6 g ? period	188	–	infectious mononucleosis, tetracycline	Rosenberg et al., 1977
37F	3.6 g for 2 weeks	410	–	infectious mononucleosis	Rosenberg et al., 1977
53M	3.9 g for 1 year	200	CAH		Bonkowsky et al., 1978
55M	2.7 g for 1 week	43[2]	CF;CS	ex-alcoholic, chlormezanone	Olsson, 1978
66M	4.0 g for 10 years	155	PCB		Arthurs and Fielding, 1980
53M	1.16 g for 12 years	120	MCH		Itoh et al., 1983
48F	4–5 g for 5 months	739	AHN;CH		Bravo-Fernández et al., 1988
33F	5.3 g for 5 years	6540	AHN;CF	taken intermittently, ?overdose	Koga et al., 1991

[1] AHN = acute hepatic necrosis, CAH = chronic active hepatitis, CH = cirrhosis, CF = chronic fibrosis, CS = cholestasis, MCH = micronodular cirrhosis, PCB = primary biliary cirrhosis; [2] μkat/l

report of hepatic dysfunction following the normal use of paracetamol in two patients with infectious mononucleosis (Rosenberg *et al.*, 1977; Rosenberg and Neelon, 1978). Challenge tests in a 53-year-old man with micronodular cirrhosis allegedly caused by consumption of 1.16 g of paracetamol daily for 12 years were quite unconvincing (Itoh *et al.*, 1983), and primary biliary cirrhosis in a 66-year-old man was attributed to the taking of 4 g daily for ten years (Arthurs and Fielding, 1980). These were anecdotal reports and no evidence was provided in support of the claims. Two patients who had taken paracetamol for one year were included in a series of 26 cases of drug-induced hepatotoxicity. Apart from the mention of 'hydropic degeneration' as the finding on liver biopsies, no other details were given (Lozano Gutierrez *et al.*, 1984). Another patient presented with a three-week history of hepatitis following the stated intake of 4–5 g of paracetamol daily for five months. A liver biopsy showed centrilobular necrosis and cirrhosis (Bravo-Fernández *et al.*, 1988). A 33-year-old Japanese woman took excessive doses of paracetamol (up to 5.3 g daily) intermittently for five years because of 'headache, fret and fume' and presented with an apparent overdose. A liver biopsy showed a picture of centrilobular necrosis and chronic liver damage with-fibrosis (Koga *et al.*, 1991). Apart from the case of overdosage referred to above by Barker *et al.* (1977), these patients do not conform to any clear pattern and the histological appearances of liver biopsies differed from those observed with acute liver injury following overdosage. The details of these atypical cases are summarized in Table 15.2. Other atypical reactions included an isolated increase in serum γ-glutamyltranspeptidase (Weber and Dölle, 1992) and toxic hepatitis following the chronic use of benorylate and penicillamine (Sacher and Thaler, 1977).

Soon after the first descriptions of chronic hepatitis in patients taking paracetamol over prolonged periods, there appeared dozens of reports of acute liver damage caused by paracetamol allegedly taken with 'therapeutic intent' in normal or near normal doses. At first sight, it seemed that many of these patients had taken little more than the maximum recommended daily dose for short periods because of acute pain, and there were no warning symptoms of toxicity before liver damage occurred. Details of these cases are summarized in Table 15.3. The clinical picture on presentation was usually typical of acute overdosage with nausea and vomiting, hepatic tenderness, gross elevation of plasma aminotransferase activity, impaired haemostasis and mild jaundice. Many of the patients were chronic alcoholics. Histological examination of the liver invariably showed the typical appearances of acute centrilobular hepatic necrosis, although in chronic alcoholics this was sometimes superimposed on a degree of fibrosis or cirrhosis (Goldfinger *et al.*, 1978; Levinson, 1983; Leist *et al.*, 1985; Lesser *et al.*, 1986; O'Dell *et al.*, 1986; Bidault *et al.*, 1987; Luquel *et al.*, 1988; Foust *et al.*, 1989). In keeping with a preceding episode of acute poisoning, the maximum elevation of aminotransferases was usually observed on the day of admission after which there was a rapid return to normal. Some adult patients were said to have suffered acute liver damage after taking single doses of paracetamol as low as 1 g (Grinblat *et al.*, 1980), 1.2 g (Luquel *et al.*, 1988), 1.35 g (Pomiersky and Blaich, 1985), 1.5 g (Rustgi *et al.*, 1993) and 2.6 g (Lesser *et al.*, 1986), or repeated doses of as little as 1–2 g daily (Florén *et al.*, 1987; Luquel *et al.*, 1988; Hartleb, 1994). As would be consistent with an acute overdose, some patients died with fulminant hepatic failure (McClain *et al.*, 1980; Kaysen *et al.*, 1985; Leist *et al.*, 1985; Lesser *et al.*, 1986; Bell *et al.*, 1987a; Shimizu *et al.*, 1989; Wootton and Lee, 1990; Patel, 1992), and again it was remarkable that some patients died after

Table 15.3 Cases reported as liver damage following the alleged therapeutic use of paracetamol.

Age and sex	Max. stated dose	Histology[1]	Max. amino-transferase (μ l^{-1})	Predisposing or associated factors	Reference
59F	30 g in 4 days	AHN	6200	alcoholic, overdose	Barker et al., 1977
67F	6.5 g/day, 1 week	AHN	1040	cachexia, overdose[2]	Barker et al., 1977
50F	6.5 g/day, 3 weeks	AHN	400	overdose[2]	Barker et al., 1977
3½F	unknown	–	73	also dextropropoxyphene	Horwitz et al., 1977
46F	5.4 g, 2 days	AHN	9400	alcoholic, died	Vilstrup et al., 1977
1¾F	19 g, 7 days	–	2750	overdose	Calvert and Linder, 1978
36F	9.7 g	CH[3]	1960	alcoholic, overdose	Goldfinger et al., 1978
3½F	>5 g, 1 day	AHN	22 000	overdose	Nogen and Bremner, 1978
55M	2.7 g/day, 1 week	CF,CS	43[4]	previous alcoholic, ?overdose	Olsson, 1978
30M	8 g/day, 1 week	AHN;CF	1321	overdose, narcotic and analgesic abuse	Ware et al., 1978
5½F	unknown	–	2230	salicylate intoxication, hyperpyrexia	Bickers and Roberts, 1979
31F	1 g,[5] 2 yr + overdose	CAH;CH[6]	10 860	overdose[2]	Arthurs and Fielding, 1980
5wkM	unknown	AHN	1920	presumed overdose, child died	Atwood, 1980
36F	>6.4 g	AHN;CAH	8460	alcoholic, overdose	Gerber et al., 1980
27F	4 g/day, 10 days + overdose	AHN;?CAH	4590	alcoholic, overdose, pancreatitis	Gerber et al., 1980
40F	1 g over 2 days	–	85	previous halothane anaesthesia	Grinblat et al., 1980
36M	4.5 g/day, ?duration	AHN	>3300	alcoholic, overdose[2]	LaBrecque and Mitros, 1980
29F	3 g/day, ?duration	AHN	3300	alcoholic	LaBrecque and Mitros, 1980
46F	6–10 g/day, 10 days	–	2180	abuse of glutethimide and other drugs	Leibowitz and Kuhn, 1980
53M	3.9 g/day, unspecified	–	19 710	alcoholic	Licht et al., 1980
48M	10 g, 2 days	–	6960	alcoholic, overdose	McClain et al., 1980
53M	10 g	AHN	9940	alcoholic, overdose	McClain et al., 1980
43M	50 g, 3 days	AHN	7720	alcoholic, overdose	McClain et al., 1980
1?	1.5 g, 14 h	–	810	gross overdose, child died	Mühlendahl and Krienke, 1980
3½F	5.4 g, 36 h	AHN	16 000	overdose[2]	Mühlendahl and Krienke, 1980
1F	unknown	AHN	4320	alcoholic, died	Weber and Cutz, 1980
23F	6 g	–		alcoholic, died	Johnson et al., 1981
37F	10 g/day, several weeks	AHN	14 500	alcoholic, died	Black et al., 1982
2mthM	4.2 g, 28 h	AHN		gross overdose, child died	Montoya Cabrera et al., 1982
3M	8 g/day, several weeks	AHN		given as benorylate, overdose,[2] child died	Symon et al., 1982
1¼M	>2 g, 4 days	AHN	10 230	overdose, use of more than one product	Agran et al., 1983

(cont.)

Age/Sex	Dose	Value	Code	Comments	Reference
2F	>11 g, 70 h	30000	AHN	overdose[2]	Clark et al., 1983
63M	10 g, 2 days	15390	AHN	alcoholic, overdose,[2] psittacosis	Davis et al., 1983
7wkF	not stated	1180	—	overdose[2]	Greene et al., 1983
6wkM	not stated	2350	—	overdose[2,7]	Greene et al., 1983
60F	7 g/day, 'fairly long time'	not stated	AHN;CF	use o` more than one product	Laake et al., 1983
41M	10 g/day, 1 week	6500	AHN	alcoholic, overdose[2]	Levinson, 1983
65M	3 g/day, 20 days	1080	AHN	alcoholic	Saenz de Santa Maria et al, 1983
1?	3–5.3 g	195	—	overdose,[2] probably poisoned by parents	Taylor and Betts, 1983
??	$16\frac{1}{4}$ g, $2\frac{1}{2}$ days	9310	—	alcoholic, overdose	Erickson and Runyon, 1984
??	13–18 g, 2 days	5130	—	alcoholic, overdose	Erickson and Runyon, 1984
??	<90 g in 8 days	9400	—	alcoholic, overdose	Erickson and Runyon, 1984
24F	29.5 g, 1 day	6226	—	28 weeks pregnant, fetal death	Haibach et al., 1984
42M	unknown	848	—	alcoholic, overdose[2]	Himmelstein et al., 1984
27F	12.5 g, 1 day	750	—		Jakobsen et al., 1984
48F	1 g for 3 months	465	—	phenobarbitone	Pirotte, 1984
53M	10 'Lobac'[8] tablets, 2 days	126[4]	—	alcoholic	Sköld and Rönnborg, 1984
50M	3 'Lobac'[8] tablets/day, 14 days	66[4]	—	alcoholic	Sköld and Rönnborg, 1984
49M	3 'Lobac'[8] tablets, ?period	6.2[4]	—	alcoholic	Stolt and Johnsen, 1984
$1\frac{1}{2}$F	120 mg/2h, 2 days	2160	—	overdose[2]	Swetnam and Florman, 1984
48F	3.25 g/day, 3 weeks	>1800	AHN	alcoholic, abuse of other drugs	Zabrodski and Schnurr, 1984
41F	19.5 g in 3 days	23000	AHN	alcoholic, overdose	Kaysen et al., 1985
27M	10 g in 4 days	1663	—	alcoholic, overdose[2]	Kaysen et al., 1985
54F	?23.9 g in 1 day	17500	AHN	alcoholic	Kaysen et al., 1985
33M	unknown	>3000	FM;HS[6]	alcoholic, ?overdose[2]	Kaysen et al., 1985
30M	40 g in 4 days	16504	—	alcoholic, ?overdose, use of more than one product	Kaysen et al., 1985
28M	6–7 g in 1 day	29700	FM;CF	alcoholic, overdose[2]	Kaysen et al., 1985
28M	5–6 g in 1 day	19750	—	alcoholic, overdose[2]	Leist et al., 1985
40M	?15 g in 2 days	2396	AHN;CF	alcoholic, overdose[2]	Leist et al., 1985
46F	1.35 g	283	—	chlormezanone	Leist et al., 1985
38M	3.7g	6600	FN		Pomiersky and Blaich, 1985
31F	6.4 g	1308	AHN	overdose	Yasunaga et al., 1985
34M	4.5 g	>100[4]	—	alcoholic, took 'Lobac' tablets	Yasunaga et al., 1985
39M	5 g/day, ?6 days	8270	—	alcoholic	Frisinette-Fich et al., 1986
38M	4.4 g/day, 2 days	13496	—	alcoholic, overdose[2]	Kartsonis et al., 1986
47M	2.6 g, 2 days	9072	AHN;FM;CH	alcoholic, overdose[2]	Kartsonis et al., 1986
38F	6 g/day, ?duration	5260	CF[6]	alcoholic, previous episode	Lesser et al., 1986; O'Dell et al., 1986

Table 15.3 (cont.)

Age and sex	Max. stated dose	Predisposing or associated factors	Histology[1]	Max. aminotransferase (μ l⁻¹)	Reference
53M	2.6–3.9 g/day, ?duration	alcoholic	—	19 700	Seeff et al., 1986
30M	12.5 g, 3 days	alcoholic	—	>10000	Seeff et al., 1986
39M	21 g, 1 week	alcoholic	—	3160	Seeff et al., 1986
58M	4–6 g/day, ?duration	alcoholic	—	2870	Seeff et al., 1986
34F	'not excessive'	alcoholic	—	26 900	Seeff et al., 1986
49F	3.7 g/day, 3 days	alcoholic	—	6888	Seeff et al., 1986
7mthM	456 mg kg⁻¹, 3 days	overdose[2]	—	7120	Smith et al., 1986a
18F	3.2 g/day	alcoholic, overdose	—	4795	Bell et al., 1987a
34M	8 g/day	alcoholic, 'Lobac'	—	1074	Bell et al., 1987a
32F	3.4 g/day	alcoholic	—	13 420	Bell et al., 1987a
57F	2.4–3.2 g/day	alcoholic	AHN	16 180	Bell et al., 1987a
56F	2.4–3.2 g/day	alcoholic, overdose[2]	—	22 940	Bell et al., 1987a
36F	5–6 g/day, 6 weeks	other drugs, overdose	?AHN	unknown	Bidault et al., 1987
37F	5 g/day, 3 weeks	alcoholic, overdose	AHN;CF;FM	unknown	Bidault et al., 1987
30F	3 g/day, 3 months	niflumic acid	AHN	unknown	Bidault et al., 1987
77F	not stated	alcoholic	—	5.2[4]	Denison et al., 1987
29M	not stated	alcoholic		490[4]	Denison et al., 1987
39M	not stated	alcoholic	—	400[4]	Denison et al., 1987
59M	not stated	alcoholic	—	240[4]	Denison et al., 1987
73M	not stated	alcoholic	—	110[4]	Denison et al., 1987
58F	1–1.5 g/day, ?duration	alcoholic, 'slight intoxication', ?with paracetamol	AHN	49[4]	Florén et al., 1987
46F	3–4 g/day, ?duration	alcoholic, ?overdose, dextropropoxyphene	AHN	88.4[4]	Florén et al., 1987
25M	not known	?overdose		9140	Litovitz et al., 1987
48F	10 g, 12 h	overdose, cholelithiasis	AHN	>5000	Baeg et al., 1988
39M	8 g, 1 day	alcoholic, other drugs, salicylate, naproxen etc	—	1.9[4]	Björck et al., 1988
54M	20 g, 7 days	alcoholic, other drugs	—	1.0[4]	Björck et al., 1988
18M	88 g, 47 days	many other drugs including salicylate	—	1.2[4]	Björck et al., 1988
51M	45 g, 7 days	alcoholic, chlormezanone	—	75[4]	Björck et al., 1988
6F	7 g, 3 days	overdose,[2] measles	AHN	10450	Blake et al., 1988
3F	not stated	febrile illness, other drugs	—	17000	de Nardo et al., 1988
47M	6 g, 12 h	alcoholic, overdose	—	17 220	Keaton, 1988

Patient	Dose	Amount	Type	Comment	Reference
65M	1.5 g/day, 2 days	3200	MCH	alcoholic	Luquel et al., 1988
49M	1.2 g	1870	AHN	alcoholic	Luquel et al., 1988
45M	5 g/day, ?duration	7180	—	alcoholic, diphenylhydantoin	McClain et al., 1988
60F	6 g/day ?duration	16 700	—	alcoholic, ?overdose, also took phenobarbitone	McClain et al., 1988
25F	7.4 g/day, ?duration	7740	—	also took primidone and phenobarbitone	McClain et al., 1988
44F	unknown	1560	AHN	overdose,[2] multiple drugs	McClain et al., 1988
43M	17 g/day	7720	—	alcoholic, renal failure	McClain et al., 1988
48M	5 g/day	6920	—	alcoholic	McClain et al., 1988
24M	9 g, 1 day	6456	AHN	alcoholic, overdose, viral hepatitis, heroin abuse	Pezzano et al., 1988
37F	29 g, 3 days	17 670	—	alcoholic, overdose	Foust et al., 1989
7M	5 g, 2 days	1762	—	multiple organ failure	Fudin et al., 1989
1F	580 mg kg^{-1}, 32 h	13 640	—	overdose,[2] other unspecified drugs	Henretig et al., 1989
2F	520 mg kg^{-1}, 3 days	7360	—	overdose,[2] diphenhydramine, varicella	Henretig et al., 1989
5F	excessive, several days	4000	AHN	overdose[2]	Litovitz et al., 1989
8F	excessive, several days	>15 000	AHN	overdose[2]	Litovitz et al., 1989
>17F	15 tablets/day, 1 month	9500	—	?overdose	Litovitz et al., 1989
33M	9 g, 2 days	49 × N[9]	AHN	epileptic, induction by phenobarbitone assumed	Marsepoil et al., 1989
48M	5.4 g, 3 days	136	—	overdose,[2] other drugs	Sánchez-Guisande et al., 1989
28F	44 g, 4 days	7401	—	alcoholic, overdose	Wootton and Lee, 1990
28F	6 g/day, 5 days	11 380	—	alcoholic, overdose	Wootton and Lee, 1990
47M	5–6 g/day, 4 days	4472	—	alcoholic, overdose	Wootton and Lee, 1990
49M	6.5 g/day, 5 days	21 660	—	alcoholic, overdose	Wootton and Lee, 1990
37F	6 g/day, 2 days	4736	—	alcoholic, overdose	Wootton and Lee, 1990
37M	4 g/day, 3 days	10 941	—	alcoholic	Wootton and Lee, 1990
40M	not stated	11 050	—	alcoholic	Wootton and Lee, 1990
½F	500 mg	3516	—	overdose[2]	Augustin and Schmoldt 1991a,b
4½F	500 mg/day, 3 days	5060	—	barbiturate, fever, ceftriaxone, poor nutrition	Chiossi et al., 1991
66M	20 g/day, 4 weeks	9240	—	alcoholic, overdose[2]	Kumar and Rex, 1991
65F	6 g/day, ?duration	3199	—	alcoholic, overdose	Kumar and Rex, 1991
43F	5 g/day, ?duration	14 920	—	alcoholic, overdose	Kumar and Rex, 1991
55M	6 g/day, ?duration	7225	—	alcoholic, overdose	Kumar and Rex, 1991
59M	5 g/day, 1 month	3000	—	alcoholic, overdose	Kumar and Rex, 1991
34M	10 g/day, ?duration	4052	—	alcoholic, overdose	Kumar and Rex, 1991
??	7 g, 3 days	6955	—	alcoholic, overdose	Cheng, 1992a
3½F	7.8 g, 2 days	9158	—	overdose[2]	Douidar et al., 1992
46M	3 g/day, 1 week	30 000	—	alcoholic	Edwards and Oliphant, 1992

(cont.)

375

Table 15.3 (cont.)

Age and sex	Max. stated dose	Max. amino-transferase (μ l^{-1})	Histology[1]	Predisposing or associated factors	Reference
25M	5–6 g, 2–3 days	174[4]	–	previous gastroenteritis, overdose	Eriksson et al., 1992
46F	3–4 g/day, ?duration	250[4]	–	alcoholic	Eriksson et al., 1992
30F	not known	25 127	AHN	overdose[2]	Litovitz et al., 1992
1½F	not known	13 617	–	overdose,[2] opiates, child died	Litovitz et al., 1992
13½F	2.5 g	4470	AHN		Patel, 1992
31M	3.3 g, 1½ days	5724	–	previous alcoholic, zidovudine, HIV[10]	Shriner and Goetz, 1992
3M	>2.2 g, 50 h	unknown	–	overdose[2]	Chao, 1993
2mth?	1.6 g, 60 h	1320	–	overdose[2]	Claass et al., 1993
21F	3.25 g	21 294	–	alleged potentiation by isoniazid	Crippin, 1993
7M	194 mg kg^{-1}, 3 days	368	–		Entacher et al., 1993
32F	6 g/day, 3 days	4471		alcoholic, overdose	Guccione et al., 1993
61M	not known	7700	–	alcoholic, overdose[2]	Hanson, 1993
29M	20 g, 1 day	2200	–	overdose, other drugs	Pedersen et al., 1993
38M	1.5 g	11 250[11]	–	fasting	Rustgi 1993
21M	36.5 g, 4 days	5000	–	use of more than one product	Sivaloganathan et al., 1993
13mthM	1 g/day, 4 days	14 100	–	overdose[2]	Day and Abbott, 1994
3½F	3.8 g, 2 days	11 282	–	overdose[2]	Douidar et al., 1994
43M	6 g/day, 'weeks'	4063	–	alcoholic	Drenth et al., 1994
10F	not known	14 150	AHN	overdose,[2] child died	Nadir et al., 1994
43F	6 g/day, 4 days	>600	–	anti-tuberculous and other drugs taken, overdose	Nolan et al., 1994
32F	2.4 g/day, ?duration	920	–	isoniazid, rifampicin, pyrazinamide	Nolan et al., 1994
9F	1.3 g+more in hospital	5027	AHN	subacute mercury poisoning	Zwiener et al., 1994

[1] histology key: AHN = acute hepatic necrosis, CAH = chronic active hepatitis, CF = chronic fibrosis, CH = cirrhosis, CS = cholestasis, FM = fatty metamorphosis, MCH = micronodular cirrhosis, FN = focal necrosis, HS = hyaline sclerosis; [2] overdose confirmed by drug concentration measurement; [3] biopsy performed several months later; [4] μkat/l; [5] per week; [6] no acute necrosis; [7] possibly intentional; [8] composition not stated; [9] × normal values; [10] also taking trimethoprim and sulphamethoxazole; [11] liver transplant

apparently taking as little as 2.5 g (Patel, 1992), 3–3.9 g (Kaysen *et al.*, 1985), 2.4–3.2 g daily (Bell *et al.*, 1987a) and 4.8 g (Shimizu *et al.*, 1989). Acute renal failure developed in a number of patients and some required treatment with haemodialysis (Gerber *et al.*, 1980; Grinblat *et al.*, 1980; McClain *et al.*, 1980, 1988; Johnson *et al.*, 1981; Clark *et al.*, 1983; Jakobsen *et al.*, 1984; Stolt and Johnsen, 1984; Kaysen *et al.*, 1985; Yasunaga *et al.*, 1985; Frisinette-Fich *et al.*, 1986; Bell *et al.*, 1987a; Björck *et al.*, 1988; Blake *et al.*, 1988; de Nardo *et al.*, 1988; Keaton, 1988; Luquel *et al.*, 1988; Pezzano *et al.*, 1988; Henretig *et al.*, 1989; Marsepoil *et al.*, 1989; Sánchez-Guisande *et al.*, 1989; Wootton and Lee, 1990; Denison *et al.*, 1991; Cheng, 1992a; Eriksson *et al.*, 1992; Claass *et al.*, 1993; Pedersen *et al.*, 1993; Sivaloganathan *et al.*, 1993; Bonkovsky *et al.*, 1994; Douidar *et al.*, 1994).

Many reports of toxicity involved young children who had been given excessive doses of paracetamol by parents and doctors (Calvert and Linder, 1978; Nogen and Bremner, 1978; Agran *et al.*, 1983; Greene *et al.*, 1983; Swetnam and Florman, 1984; Smith *et al.*, 1986a; Henretig *et al.*, 1989; Claass *et al.*, 1993; Kurt *et al.*, 1993; Douidar *et al.*, 1994; Ferenc *et al.*, 1994) and regrettably in some the outcome was fatal (Weber and Cutz, 1980; Montoya Cabrera *et al.*, 1982; Clark *et al.*, 1983; Blake *et al.*, 1988; de Nardo *et al.*, 1988; Chao, 1993). Attention has been drawn to the dangers of errors of dosing of paracetamol in children (Velásquez-Jones, 1983; Litovitz, 1992), but in one case poisoning was probably intentional (Hickson *et al.*, 1983). Liver damage in a 17-year-old girl, who allegedly took only 1.5–2 g of paracetamol daily, was attributed without evidence to 'chemical hypoxia' and a synergistic effect of thyroxine on mitochondrial respiration (Hartleb, 1994) and in another case, toxicity following the claimed ingestion of 1–3 g daily was said to be related to increasing age with chronic renal and cardiorespiratory insufficiency (Bonkovsky *et al.*, 1994). In a retrospective survey of patients admitted to one hospital from January 1987 to July 1993, 49 were identified with paracetamol hepatotoxicity. Twenty-one (43 per cent) were said to have taken the paracetamol for therapeutic purposes but all had taken more than the recommended maximum daily dose. Recent fasting was thought to be a more important risk factor than chronic alcoholism. Ten patients (20.4 per cent) admitted to taking more than 10 g of paracetamol daily and this 'unintentional hepatic toxicity' was clearly the result of major overdosage. It was claimed that fasting predisposed to toxicity by causing induction of the oxidative metabolism of paracetamol but no evidence was provided to support such a mechanism in man (Whitcomb and Block, 1994). The simultaneous use of several different products, each of which contained paracetamol, contributed to toxicity in some patients (Agran *et al.*, 1983; Laake *et al.*, 1983; Kaysen *et al.*, 1985; Sivaloganathan *et al.*, 1993). It was not always easy to differentiate paracetamol-induced liver damage from other pathology such as viral hepatitis (Roschlau, 1986), and, in some reports, other potentially hepatotoxic drugs may have been responsible (Powers *et al.*, 1986; Raabe *et al.*, 1987; Hatamori *et al.*, 1993). Unintentional overdosage with paracetamol was considered to be a constant phenomenon. In a retrospective survey of enquiries to the Stockholm Poisons Information Centre during 1988–1990, about 7 per cent concerned repeated or subacute 'therapeutic' overdosage. An analysis of the outcome in 50 such cases showed that liver damage was mild or moderate in 35, but 10 developed severe toxicity and there was one death. As the admitted doses varied from 6 g a day for a week to 40 g over two days, these cases clearly come into the category of overdosage and in such circumstances toxicity would be expected (Persson, 1991). The Danish Committee on Adverse Drug Reactions had also received reports of acute liver damage and cholestatic reactions following the use of paracetamol in therapeutic doses (Friis and Andreasen, 1992). In contrast to these numerous reports claiming that paracetamol could be dangerously hepatotoxic when taken for therapeutic purposes, particularly by chronic alcoholics, a 58-year-old woman who drank excessively did not suffer liver damage despite consumption of 15–20 g daily for five years. Studies showed that she had abnormally slow clearance and reduced toxic metabolic bioactivation of paracetamol (Tredger *et al.*, 1995).

Chronic Intake of Alcohol and Inducing Drugs

It was assumed without question that chronic alcoholics and patients taking inducing drugs were at increased risk from the hepatotoxicity of paracetamol as a result of increased metabolic activation and this was a convenient explanation for the severe liver damage that appeared to follow the consumption of modest, otherwise non-toxic doses of paracetamol. This belief has no secure foundation. The original report that suggested potentiation of paracetamol hepatotoxicity following over-dosage in chronic alcoholics and patients taking inducing drugs was based on a comparison of only eight non-induced and eight potentially induced patients, of whom only three were alcoholics (Wright and Prescott, 1973). In contrast to the findings in animals, the chronic use of potentially inducing drugs, such as anti-convulsants and rifampicin, and the chronic excessive consumption of ethanol had little or no effect on the extent of the toxic metabolic activation of paracetamol in man as shown by the production of its glutathione-derived conjugates. Pretreatment of healthy subjects with phenobarbitone increased the recovery of the mercapturic acid conjugate of paracetamol in one study (Mitchell *et al.*, 1974) but in another, the excretion of the cysteine and mercapturic acid conjugates was not increased in patients with proven induction resulting from the chronic use of anticonvulsants and rifampicin (Prescott *et al.*, 1981). Conflicting results have also been obtained with ethanol. The urinary recovery of the cysteine and mercapturic acid conjugates of paracetamol was increased (but still remained within normal limits) in nine alco-holics without liver damage compared with six control subjects and nine patients with alcoholic cirrhosis (Villeneuve *et al.*, 1983) and 11 chronic alcoholics produced more potentially hepatotoxic metabolites of paracetamol than healthy subjects although the difference was only just statistically significant (Chern *et al.*, 1993). In contrast, the toxic metabolic activation of paracetamol was not enhanced in heavy drinkers (Critchley *et al.*, 1982; Prescott and Critchley, 1983a) although its clearance was increased (Dietz *et al.*, 1984). In other studies, the urinary excretion of the cys-teine and mercapturic acid conjugates of paracetamol was not higher in chronic alcoholics, arguing against substantially increased metabolic activation (Lauterburg and Velez, 1988; Tredger *et al.*, 1995). There was no evidence of induction of drug-metabolizing enzymes in liver biopsies from chronic alcoholics except in the pres-ence of active alcoholic liver damage and enzyme activity returned to normal levels rapidly when alcohol was discontinued (Hoensch, 1984). In another study there was no decrease in the formation of the mercapturic acid conjugate of paracetamol in chronic alcoholics as expected when they abstained from alcohol for two weeks (Skinner *et al.*, 1990). The rate of elimination of paracetamol was reduced in alco-holics with liver disease, but there was little difference between drinking and abstinent alcoholics without cirrhosis (Shamszad *et al.*, 1975). It was claimed that the production of the hepatotoxic metabolite of paracetamol was enhanced in chronic alcoholics because it was eliminated more rapidly than in healthy controls. Unfortunately, there was no information about the metabolism of paracetamol in this study (Girre *et al.*, 1993). Chronic alcoholics taking paracetamol in overdosage were not at increased risk of hepatotoxicity in one study (Rumack, 1983), but in another the opposite conclusion was reached, possibly because the alcoholic patients had taken larger doses (Bray *et al.*, 1991). If chronic alcoholics are at increased risk of paracetamol-induced liver damage (as they may be), the most likely mechanism seems to be glutathione deficiency. Even so, they had sufficient glutathione to easily detoxify a single dose of at least 2 g (Lauterburg, 1985; Lauterburg and Velez, 1988). The belief that therapeutic doses of paracetamol can cause severe hepatotoxicity in human chronic alcoholics and patients who have taken potentially inducing drugs has been perpetuated from one report to another without any clear proof or justification.

Therapeutic Use Versus a Therapeutic Dose

Mitchell *et al.* (1974) calculated that a single dose of at least 15 g of paracetamol would be required to deplete hepatic glutathione in an adult to the point where liver injury could occur, and this agrees remarkably well with the threshold dose for toxicity observed in overdose patients (Prescott, 1983). It is inconceivable that as little as 1–2.5 g of paracetamol could cause fatal liver damage or severe injury requiring transplantation as claimed (Lesser *et al.*, 1986; Patel, 1992; Rustgi *et al.*, 1993). It was often stated that the paracetamol was taken for 'therapeutic purposes' and some authors referred to the unhappy circumstances of severe toxicity following grossly excessive doses as 'therapeutic misadventure' (Seeff *et al.*, 1986; McClain *et al.*, 1988; Kumar and Rex, 1991). In addition, there was frequently a lack of clarity about the distribution of doses over the periods of time cited. In most of the reports in Table 15.3 it was obvious from the typical clinical course and from drug concentration measurements when available, that substantial acute overdoses had been taken just before admission. This will be no surprise to those who have experience in dealing with poisoned patients because they know that overdoses are often denied and the amounts minimized, while chronic alcoholics are notoriously unreliable historians. In this context, some reports have been severely criticized (Hall *et al.*, 1986a,b, 1987; Brandon, 1993; Goulding, 1993). It was irresponsible to describe the consumption of 20, 30 or even 40 g of paracetamol over two or three days as normal therapeutic use as implied by some authors, and by the same token the consequences of taking 20 g of paracetamol daily for four weeks can hardly be blamed on 'therapeutic misadventure' (Kumar and Rex, 1991). If ethanol potentiated paracetamol hepatotoxicity to such a dangerous degree as claimed, and if as supposed, normal therapeutic doses could cause severe and even fatal liver damage, it was surprising that there has been no experimental verification of this or reports of positive challenge tests in such patients. In addition, many reports of chronic liver toxicity would be expected considering the enormous use of paracetamol. The safety of paracetamol taken in recommended doses and the question of potentiation of toxicity in man by ethanol and inducing drugs has been a subject of continuing comment and debate (Craig, 1980; Black, 1984; Black and Raucy, 1986; Prescott,

1986a,b; Regal, 1986; Maddrey, 1987; Ackerman and Levy, 1988; Mitchell, 1988; Lieber, 1990b; Schenker and Maddrey, 1991; Rex and Kumar, 1992; Lee, 1994; Tredger *et al.*, 1995; and others). Even in alcoholics, the use of paracetamol was thought to be associated with a lower risk of toxicity than other non-prescription analgesics (Aarbakke, 1994; Strom, 1994).

Nephrotoxicity

In the past, phenacetin was almost universally condemned as the cause of analgesic nephropathy, a form of renal disease characterized by papillary necrosis progressing to chronic renal failure. As paracetamol was the major metabolite of phenacetin, it is not surprising that it too came to be regarded with the utmost suspicion. Phenacetin has been banned, or its availability greatly restricted for some time in most countries and the focus of attention has rightfully shifted to aspirin and the non-steroidal anti-inflammatory drugs as the analgesics most likely to cause renal toxicity in clinical practice. Indeed, the weight of objective evidence indicates that taken alone, phenacetin and paracetamol are probably the safest non-narcotic analgesics as far as the kidney is concerned (Prescott, 1982a). Phenacetin was never taken alone, but always in combination with other potentially nephrotoxic drugs and on this point it is salutary to recall the comments made by Alfred Gilman (1964). He aptly compared the situation with the scientist who came to the conclusion that it was possible to get drunk by drinking soda as he had become inebriated on three successive occasions after drinking scotch and soda, bourbon and soda, and rye and soda! There was very little evidence that paracetamol played anything other than a very minor role as a causal agent in analgesic nephropathy, but in common with other non-narcotic analgesics it could cause acute renal failure following overdosage. The aetiology and pathogenesis of analgesic nephropathy, and the roles of phenacetin, paracetamol and other analgesics have been subjects of long and vigorous debate for decades (Gsell *et al.*, 1957; Nordenfeldt and Ringertz, 1961; Prescott, 1966b, 1982a; Kincaid-Smith, 1967; Dubach *et al.*, 1968, 1991; Gault *et al.*, 1968; Calder *et al.*, 1971; Stewart and Gallery, 1976; Nanra *et al.*, 1978; Shelley, 1978; McCredie *et al.*, 1982; Mihatsch *et al.*, 1982a; Schwarz, 1987; Elseviers and de Broe, 1988; Pommer *et al.*, 1989; Nanra, 1993; Lornoy, 1994; and many others). Paracetamol suffered unjust guilt by association and, despite an almost complete lack of evidence, it was widely assumed to be the nephrotoxic metabolite of phenacetin. Indeed, some investigators remain convinced that paracetamol is dangerously nephrotoxic and have gone to extraordinary lengths in attempts to force proof of its guilt in this respect. Analgesic nephropathy remained a serious problem in countries such as Belgium, Germany and Switzerland (Drukker *et al.*, 1986; Pommer *et al.*, 1986; Elseviers and de Broe, 1988; Wing *et al.*, 1989), and the late complication of uroepithelial malignancy was a further cause for concern (Hultengren *et al.*, 1965; Bengtsson *et al.*, 1968; Johansson *et al.*, 1974; Porpaczy and Schramek, 1981; Mihatsch and Knüsli, 1982b; McCredie *et al.*, 1983b; and others).

The adverse renal effects of drugs such as aspirin, paracetamol and non-steroidal anti-inflammatory agents seemed to involve at least two different and apparently unrelated forms of toxicity. The first was acute renal failure due to proximal tubular necrosis or reduced renal perfusion and it occurred in predisposed individuals in whom the renal circulation was compromised, and following acute overdosage. Possible mechanisms included cytotoxicity and ischaemia resulting from reduced renal synthesis of vasodilator prostaglandins. The other form was renal papillary necrosis, which progressed insidiously to end-stage renal failure with continued consumption of analgesics over the course of many months or years. Although the same mechanisms of cytotoxicity and ischaemia could be operating as in acute tubular damage this seemed unlikely, and in analgesic nephropathy the primary site of injury was the renal papilla and inner medulla. It was necessary, therefore, to distinguish between the acute and chronic nephrotoxicity of paracetamol.

Experimental Studies in Man

There have been few studies of the acute renal effects of paracetamol in man but unlike aspirin, it was not thought to have toxic effects unless it was taken in overdose (Plotz and Kimberly, 1981). In a dose of 3.6 g daily for five days it produced an appreciable increase in urinary renal tubular cell excretion in only a small minority of healthy subjects (Prescott, 1965, 1966a), and this effect was not related to individual differences in paracetamol metabolism and excretion (Prescott *et al.*, 1968). Renal tubular damage may be associated with increased urinary excretion of tubular enzymes but in six subjects given 650 mg of paracetamol four times a day for four days there was no increase in the urinary output of N-acetyl-D-β-glucosaminidase (Proctor and Kunin, 1978). A single dose of 2 g caused an increase in urinary lactic dehydrogenase in all of five subjects during water diuresis and in three during antidiuresis. Similar results were obtained with γ-glutamyltransferase but there was no increase with N-acetyl-β-D-glucosaminidase, β-galactosidase or leucine aminopeptidase (Metz *et al.*, 1986). Given for three days in doses of 3 g daily, paracetamol had no effect on urinary β_2-microglobulin excretion in 10 healthy subjects (Weise *et al.*, 1981). In other studies there were no changes in the glomerular filtration rate as shown by the renal clearance of creatinine in healthy subjects taking 3 g daily for two days (Bippi and Frölich, 1990) and in young and elderly healthy volunteers and patients with chronic impairment of renal function given 40 mg kg day^{-1} for three days (Berg *et al.*, 1990). Paracetamol 4 g daily for three days had no effect on the renal clearances of inulin and p-aminohippurate in healthy young females but it reduced the total body clearance of p-aminohippurate by inhibiting its acetylation (Prescott *et al.*, 1990). In these and other studies paracetamol had variable effects on the renal production of prostaglandins, and on sodium and water excretion (Haylor, 1980; Berg *et al.*, 1990; Bippi and Frölich, 1990; Martin and Prescott, 1994). In healthy female volunteers given 4 g of paracetamol daily for three days there was a marked reduction in the urinary excretion of prostaglandins and sodium, and impaired ability to excrete a water load. The reduction in sodium output was similar to that produced by indomethacin (Prescott *et al.*, 1990).

Acute Renal Failure

Acute renal failure was a well-recognized complication of acute paracetamol poisoning, and it usually occurred in patients with severe liver damage (Proudfoot and Wright, 1970; Prescott and Wright, 1973; Wilkinson *et al.*, 1977; Cobden *et al.*, 1982; Prescott *et al.*, 1982; Björck *et al.*, 1988; Jones and Vale, 1993). The overall

Table 15.4 Reported cases of acute renal failure following the alleged therapeutic use of paracetamol.

Age and sex	Max. stated daily dose	Max. plasma creatinine (μmol l^{-1})	Max. amino-transferase (μ l^{-1})	Renal histology[1]	Comments	Reference
20mthF	19 g, 7 days	258	1960	–	creatinine clearance 7.25 ml min 1.73 m^2	Calvert and Linder, 1978
36F	9.75 g	1290	1960	–	alcoholic, meprobamate, peritoneal dialysis	Goldfinger et al., 1978
5wkM	not known	–	1920	TN	fatal hepatorenal failure	Atwood, 1980
36F	6.4 g	56[2]	6300	–	alcoholic, overdose, peritoneal dialysis	Gerber et al., 1980
27F	4 g/day, 10 days	418	4590	–	alcoholic, overdose, other drugs, oliguria	Gerber et al., 1980
40F	1 g	1513	175	TN	previous halothane anaesthesia, other drugs, UTI[3]	Grinblat et al., 1980
46F	6–10 g/day, 10 days	160	2180	–	multiple drug abuse	Leibowitz and Kuhn, 1980
58M	10 g	–	9940	TN	alcoholic, overdose, fatal hepatorenal failure	McClain et al., 1980
43M	50 g, 3 days	66[2]	7720	TN	alcoholic, overdose, peritoneal dialysis	McClain et al., 1980
1F	not known	345	16000	TN	fatal hepatorenal failure	Weber and Cutz, 1980
23F	6 g	668	4320	–	alcoholic, drug abuse, haemodialysis	Johnson et al., 1981
20M	0.75 g	330	–	TN	other drug, oliguria	Gabriel et al., 1982
27M	0.65 g	518	–	TN	anuria for 48 h	Gabriel et al., 1982
2mthM	4.2 g, 28 h	–	–	TN	overdose, given rectally, fatal hepatorenal failure	Montoya Cabrera et al., 1982
2F	11 g, 70 h	–	30000	TN	overdose,[4] given rectally, fatal hepatorenal failure	Clark et al., 1983
63M	10 g, 2 days	436	15390	–	psittacosis	Davis et al., 1983
27M	3.9 g	730	5178	–	alcoholic, overdose,[4] haemodialysis	Himmelstein et al., 1984
27F	12.5 g, 1 day	302	750	TN		Jakobsen et al., 1984
49M	not stated	690	6.2[5]	–	alcoholic, apparently took 6 'Lobac' daily	Stolt and Johnsen, 1984
45M	8.4 g	240	10100	–	alcoholic, oliguria	Fleckenstein, 1985
41F	19.5 g, 3 days	356	23000	TN	alcoholic, overdose,[4] fatal hepatorenal failure	Kaysen et al., 1985
27M	10 g, 4 days	721	1663	–	alcoholic, overdose,[4] haemodialysis	Kaysen et al., 1985
54F	?3.9 g	561	6520	TN	alcoholic, overdose,[4] fatal hepatorenal failure	Kaysen et al., 1985
30M	40 g, 3 days	240	16504	–	alcoholic, overdose[4]	Kaysen et al., 1985
33M	unknown	739	>3000	–	alcoholic, ?overdose, ?iatrogenic renal failure	Kaysen et al., 1985
28M	7 g, 1 day	365	29700	–	alcoholic, overdose[4]	Leist et al., 1985
28M	6 g, 1 day	641	19750	–	alcoholic, overdose,[4] drug abuse, peritoneal dialysis	Leist et al., 1985
38M	3.7 g	409	6600	–	alcoholic	Yasunaga et al., 1985
34M	4.5 g	>1700	>100[5]	–	oliguria, haemodialysis, took 'Lobac'	Frisinette-Fich et al., 1986
47M	2.6 g, 2 days	400	9072	–	alcoholic, overdose,[4] died from sepsis 4 wk later	Lesser et al., 1986
32M	3.4 g/day	>700	13420	–	alcoholic, took 'Lobac'	Bell et al., 1987a
29M	not stated	625	490[5]	–	alcoholic, 'chronic' intoxication	Denison et al., 1987, 1991
39M	not stated	1380	400[5]	–	alcoholic, 'chronic' intoxication	Denison et al., 1987, 1991

Age/Sex	Dose			Renal histology	Comments	Reference
59M	not stated	264	240[5]	–	alcoholic, 'chronic' intoxication	Denison et al., 1987, 1991
40M	0.8 g	907	normal	TN	intermittent alcoholic, other drugs	Björck et al., 1988
25M	8 g	350	normal	TN	'practical joke'	Björck et al., 1988
39M	8 g	1294	1.9[5]	–	alcoholic, also took naproxen and salicylate	Björck et al., 1988
54M	20 g, 7 days	1264	1.0[5]	–	alcoholic, took other drugs including salicylate	Björck et al., 1988
18M	88 g, 47 days	442	1.2[5]	TN	took many other drugs including salicylate	Björck et al., 1988
51M	45 g, 7 days	1190	75[5]	–	alcoholic, overdose, also took salicylate	Björck et al., 1988
6F	>7 g, 3 days	–	10400	TN	overdose, fatal hepatic failure, haemodialysis, sepsis	Blake et al., 1988
3F	not stated	–	17000	–	fatal hepatorenal failure	de Nardo et al., 1988
47M	6 g, 12 h	1531	17220	–	alcoholic, ?overdose, haemodialysis	Keaton, 1988
65M	3 g, 2 days	520	3200	–	alcoholic, hepatic failure, haemodialysis	Luquel et al., 1988
49M	1.2 g	1431	1879	–	alcoholic, GI haemorrhage, haemodialysis	Luquel et al., 1988
60F	6 g/day	383	16700	–	alcoholic, also taking phenobarbitone	McClain et al., 1988
25F	7.4 g/day	934	7740	–	alcoholic, also taking primidone and phenobarbitone	McClain et al., 1988
44F	not stated	249	1560	–	overdose, obesity, multiple drugs	McClain et al., 1988
24M	9 g, 1 day	767	6456	–	alcoholic, overdose,[4] drug abuse, HIV, haemodialysis	Pezzano et al., 1988
7M	5 g, 2 days	407	1764	–	pneumonia, haemofiltration, haemodialysis	Fudin et al., 1989
22mthF	6.5 g, 3 days	208	7360	–	overdose,[4] oliguria, varicella	Henretig et al., 1989
33M	9 g, 2 days	1190	49[6]	TN	taking phenobarbitone	Marsepoil et al., 1989
48M	5.4 g, 3 days	1059	136	–	overdose[4]	Sánchez-Guisande et al., 1989
40M	not stated	–	11050	–	alcoholic, fatal hepatorenal failure	Wootton and Lee, 1990
59M	5 g/day, 1 month	–	3000	–	alcoholic, fatal hepatic failure	Kumar and Rex, 1991
34M	10 g/day	–	4052	–	alcoholic, testicular cancer, fatal	Kumar and Rex, 1991
??	7 g, 3 days	472	6955	–		Cheng, 1992a
25M	6 g/day, 3 days	228	174[5]	–	gastroenteritis	Eriksson et al., 1992
46F	6 g, 1 day	636	250[5]	–	alcoholic	Eriksson et al., 1992
8 wk?	1.6 g, 60 h	338	1320	–	after surgery for ureter stenosis, candidiasis	Claass et al., 1993
14M	not stated	203	–	–	other drugs including flurbiprofen	McIntire et al., 1993
12F	not stated	460	–	–	ibuprofen also taken for several days	McIntire et al., 1993
29M	20 g	1479	2200	–	overdose, haemodialysis	Pedersen et al., 1993
21M	36.5 g, 4 days	275	>5000	–	alcoholic, haemodialysis	Sivaloganathan et al., 1993
39M	1.5 g, 4 days	694	38	TN	alcoholic	Brevet et al., 1994
3½F	7.68 g, 2 days	481	11282	–	overdose,[4] peritoneal dialysis	Douidar et al., 1994
43M	6 g/day, 'weeks'	1727	4063	–	alcoholic, haemodialysis	Drenth et al., 1994
10F	not known	303	14150	TN	overdose,[4] haemodialysis, died	Nadir et al., 1994

[1] Renal histology: TN = tubular necrosis; [2] blood urea nitrogen, mg 100 ml^{-1}; [3] urinary tract infection; [4] overdose according to measured paracetamol concentration; [5] μkat/l; [6] × normal

incidence was low, and it was reduced further by the availability of specific antidotal therapy with N-acetylcysteine and methionine. In a series of 2060 unselected patients admitted to hospital in Edinburgh with paracetamol overdosage over the period 1969–1980, 33 (1.6 per cent) developed acute renal failure (Prescott *et al.*, 1982) and in other reports on similar unselected patients the incidence was about 1 per cent (Hamlyn *et al.*, 1978; Cobden *et al.*, 1982). Renal failure occurred in 7 per cent of 90 highly selected patients with liver damage from paracetamol poisoning but the incidence was much higher with fulminant hepatic failure where the risk was similar to that with hepatic failure from other causes (Wilkinson *et al.*, 1977). Most patients who developed renal failure following declared overdose of paracetamol also had hepatic necrosis but biochemical liver damage was occasionally absent (Prescott *et al.*, 1982; Pillans and Hall, 1985; Kher and Makker, 1987; Björck *et al.*, 1988; Campbell and Baylis, 1992) or minimal (Grinblat *et al.*, 1980; Kleinman *et al.*, 1980; Cobden *et al.*, 1982; Sánchez-Guisande *et al.*, 1989). Renal failure as a complication of paracetamol overdose is described in Chapter 16, but there was a large grey area of overlap with so-called therapeutic overdose. Acute renal failure has been described following accidental overdosage of paracetamol in children and also in many patients following its alleged use with therapeutic intent, often in apparently normal, or near normal, doses. Details of these patients are summarized in Table 15.4. Many were chronic alcoholics. Most patients who were presented as taking paracetamol for therapeutic purposes had clearly taken an overdose two or three days previously, as shown by the typical pattern of grossly abnormal but rapidly improving liver function tests following admission together with plasma drug concentrations when measured. Some patients had also taken other potentially nephrotoxic analgesics (Baños Gallardo *et al.*, 1987). Others apparently suffered renal damage after allegedly taking very small doses of the order of 1 g or less (Grinblat *et al.*, 1980; Gabriel *et al.*, 1982; Baños Gallardo *et al.*, 1987; Luquel *et al.*, 1988). These reports were difficult to accept for overdosage was not excluded and challenge tests were not performed after recovery. One patient had apparently taken the suspected preparation (a combination of paracetamol with dextropropoxyphene) in the same low dose many times previously without incident (Gabriel *et al.*, 1982). In another case, cardiac failure and pre-existing renal disease were thought to be precipitating factors and subsequent studies showed a decrease rather than the expected increase in the metabolic activation of paracetamol (Bonkovsky *et al.*, 1994). Despite numerous dramatic case reports, there has not been one properly authenticated case of acute renal failure produced by normal therapeutic doses of paracetamol.

Acute renal failure induced by paracetamol was usually heralded by back pain and oliguria with proteinuria and microscopic haematuria. As shown by renal biopsies, the underlying pathology was acute tubular necrosis and this was confirmed by electron microscopy (Kleinman *et al.*, 1980; Björck *et al.*, 1988). Distal tubular damage was observed in one report (Cobden *et al.*, 1982) and in another the appearances were described as acute interstitial nephritis (Pusey *et al.*, 1983). Focal microvascular changes have also been noted (Björck *et al.*, 1988). Acute renal failure induced by paracetamol was usually of rapid onset and possible predisposing factors included ingestion of other drugs, dehydration caused by vomiting and lack of food intake as a result of anorexia. The impairment of renal function was reversible but some patients required treatment with peritoneal or haemodialysis.

Several other reports require comment. Drugs were considered to be the cause in

147 of 398 cases of acute renal failure seen in 58 French nephrology units over a period of one year. Paracetamol was mentioned in five cases and in four of these it was said to have been taken in therapeutic doses without major liver involvement. Acute tubular necrosis was observed in two patients, one of whom had taken an overdose (Kleinknecht *et al.*, 1986a,b). In another study, 18 patients with acute renal failure associated with the use of antipyretic analgesics were seen in 12 months. Paracetamol had been taken by five patients including two who had also taken other analgesics (Heidbreder *et al.*, 1986). A 7-year-old boy had recurrent episodes of acute renal failure and macroscopic haematuria associated with respiratory infections. Renal biopsies showed mesangial glomerulonephritis with acute interstitial nephritis and the lesions were attributed to therapeutic doses of paracetamol, which were presumably taken for the respiratory infections (Gallego *et al.*, 1991). Although a basophil degranulation test with paracetamol was positive, no details were given and otherwise it is difficult to see why it was implicated in this case. Paracetamol had no additional adverse effects on renal function in patients with malignant disease treated with cisplatin (de Gislain *et al.*, 1990).

Analgesic Nephropathy

Paracetamol has been unjustifiably indicted as a cause of analgesic nephropathy on the illogical grounds that it was the major metabolite of phenacetin and therefore had the same effects. It has been said that: 'we did not need to regard paracetamol as a flagship now that its parent substance (i.e. phenacetin) has been wrecked' (Bengtsson and Lindholm, 1977); 'at present paracetamol remains more than suspect as a major aetiological factor in analgesic nephropathy in this country' (South Africa) (Furman, 1982); 'paracetamol as a metabolite of phenacetin must also be classified as nephrotoxic' (Schulz, 1990); and 'since paracetamol is an important metabolite of phenacetin, there is reason to regard bad news about phenacetin as having possibly distressing implications for paracetamol as well' (Stolley, 1991). There have been calls to control the availability of paracetamol and to restrict it to prescription-only use (Mihatsch *et al.*, 1980b, 1982a). The mistaken belief that paracetamol and phenacetin shared the same renal toxicity has been reinforced by the use of non-specific methods for urine screening for covert analgesic use that gave positive results following the ingestion of both phenacetin and paracetamol (Dubach, 1967a; Baumeler *et al.*, 1975; Schulz, 1990). Thus, many authors referred to phenacetin and paracetamol together as though they could be equated one with the other (Mihatsch *et al.*, 1980b, 1982a; Hangartner *et al.*, 1987; Schwarz *et al.*, 1989; Ballé and Schollmeyer, 1990; Paller, 1990; Schulz, 1990; Steenland *et al.*, 1990; Hauser *et al.*, 1991; Stolley, 1991). The manner in which assumptions about paracetamol could be made without evidence and subsequently enshrined in the folklore of analgesic nephropathy was illustrated by the story of capillarosclerosis of the renal pelvis. This was proposed as a specific indicator of the abuse of phenacetin on the basis of extensive autopsy studies in patients with analgesic nephropathy who had taken mixed analgesics including phenacetin (Mihatsch *et al.*, 1983). It was then extended to include paracetamol despite the total lack of any supporting evidence and it was then even stated that capillarosclerosis was proved to be pathognomonic of paracetamol abuse (Bethke and Schubert, 1985; Schubert and Bethke, 1986). A subsequent report of capillarosclerosis in one of 98 hospital autopsies was attributed to the consumption of 1.35 g of paracetamol daily for three months in a patient with diabetes, severe atherosclerosis, metastatic thyroid carcinoma, bilateral lower limb amputations and fatal sepsis (Karttunen *et al.*, 1982). The other drugs taken by this patient were not even mentioned. Some authors still failed to record the analgesic drugs taken by patients with analgesic nephropathy and referred only to the amount of phenacetin consumed without mentioning the other (more nephrotoxic) analgesics taken with it (Gonwa *et al.*, 1980; Mihatsch *et al.*, 1980a; Porpaczy and Schramek, 1981; Mihatsch and Knüsli, 1982; Thieler *et al.*, 1990; and others).

There have been few chronic studies of the renal effects of paracetamol in man. Comprehensive tests of renal function were performed in 18 patients who had taken 2–30 kg of paracetamol over periods of years for arthritic conditions. There was no correlation between paracetamol intake and any aspect of renal function and there was no worsening of renal function in 13 patients followed up 13 months later after they had taken a further mean dose of 2 kg of the drug (Edwards *et al.*, 1971). In a survey of 109 outpatients, consumption of aspirin and paracetamol alone and in combination was related to minor increases in serum urea concentrations, although these were still within the normal range. The use of paracetamol was determined by urine screening but this would also have included phenacetin (Joubert *et al.*, 1977). Of 4058 patients, 181 were identified as regular users of single analgesics and non-steroidal anti-inflammatory drugs. At follow-up one year later, there was no change in the estimated creatinine clearance in 147 patients who had been taking paracetamol (Hale *et al.*, 1989). Following the withdrawal of phenacetin in Canada the incidence of papillary necrosis decreased by 50 per cent despite the increasing use of paracetamol as a single agent (Wilson and Gault, 1982). In Belgium, phenacetin disappeared from the market over the period 1983–1991, but analgesic nephropathy still accounted for about 15 per cent of patients requiring dialysis. There was a strong geographical correlation between the distribution of analgesic mixtures and analgesic nephropathy, but not with the use of single drugs (Elseviers and de Broe, 1994b). A multinational survey of 359 patients with analgesic nephropathy in 15 European countries showed that all but 11 had abused analgesic mixtures containing two analgesics and caffeine or codeine (Elseviers and de Broe, 1994a).

There have been few adequately documented reports of analgesic nephropathy in patients taking paracetamol alone or in combination with other analgesics. The first cases to be described were a 45-year-old man, who was found to have unilateral renal papillary necrosis with mild impairment of renal function seven months after excessive consumption of paracetamol and chlormezanone (Krikler, 1967), and a 53-year-old woman, who had taken three tablets of paracetamol daily for 10 years together with other analgesics including aspirin and phenacetin, (Master, 1973). Two other possible cases (Koutsaimanis and De Wardener, 1970) were subsequently shown to have taken aspirin and phenacetin, which could have been responsible (Kerr, 1970). Paracetamol was apparently taken by one patient with papillary necrosis in one report (Parker and Shaw, 1975) and by five in another, but no details were given (Nanra, 1979). In three series of patients with analgesic nephropathy, paracetamol had been taken by 2 of 190 patients (Nanra *et al.*, 1978), 2 of 91 patients (McCredie *et al.*, 1982) and 1 of 48 patients (Schwarz *et al.*, 1985), but, again, no details were provided. Of perhaps greater significance was a series of reports from Malaysia of analgesic nephropathy associated with paracetamol as the sole analgesic taken. Following a review of 1011 intravenous urograms, Segasothy *et al.* (1984) found seven cases of renal papillary necrosis due to the excessive consumption of paracetamol alone. In a later study, the number of patients with papillary necrosis had risen to 28 and these included a further five patients who had taken paracetamol in combination with local remedies that contained aspirin and phenacetin (*Chap Kaki Tiga* and *Chap Harimau*) (Segasothy *et al.*, 1986a). In a subsequent survey of 180 patients with end-stage renal disease, 14 patients gave a history of analgesic abuse and 11 of these had taken paracetamol and one paracetamol with aspirin and phenacetin. Seven of these patients had renal papillary necrosis and in five it was attributed to the excessive consumption of paracetamol. Altogether, 15 patients had papillary necrosis associated with the use of paracetamol, but this included previously published cases (Segasothy *et al.*, 1988). The other drugs taken were not mentioned. In a further report on the use of computed tomography and ultrasound in the diagnosis of analgesic nephropathy, there was mention of three patients who had taken paracetamol alone and two who had taken it with other analgesics (Segasothy *et al.*, 1994b). Of 69 patients with analgesic nephropathy, 38 had taken large amounts of non-steroidal anti-inflammatory drugs and 31 had taken other drugs including paracetamol alone (11 cases) or with aspirin and phenacetin (6) (Segasothy *et al.*, 1994a). These reports are unique and analgesic nephropathy apparently due to the use of paracetamol alone has not been described elsewhere on this scale.

Over the years there have been a few reports of individual patients with analgesic nephritis who apparently took paracetamol in combination with aspirin and other non-steroidal anti-inflammatory drugs (Prescott, 1966b; Davies *et al.*, 1970; New Zealand Rheumatism Association Study, 1974; Goldberger and Talner, 1975; Nanra and Kincaid-Smith, 1975; Cove-Smith and Knapp, 1978; Nanra *et al.*, 1978; Wortmann *et al.*, 1980; Knapp and Avioli, 1982; McCredie *et al.*, 1982; Schwarz *et al.*, 1985; Allen *et al.*, 1986). In addition, the use of paracetamol by patients with established analgesic nephropathy could result in deterioration in renal function (Nanra *et al.*, 1978) and in a later study this was associated with positive urine tests for paracetamol (Schwarz *et al.*, 1989). Continuing covert analgesic abuse has always been a problem. Patients with analgesic nephropathy were found to have paracetamol in their blood more frequently than those with other renal disease (Schwarz *et al.*, 1988) and of 22 transplanted patients with analgesic nephropathy, 41 per cent had paracetamol in more than half the urine samples tested over one year compared with only 7 per cent in other renal transplant patients (Furman *et al.*, 1976). In another study, patients with analgesic nephropathy who had received renal transplants did not have a higher frequency of positive urine tests for paracetamol (Schwarz *et al.*, 1992). Blood tests for paracetamol and salicylate were positive more often in patients with analgesic nephropathy in whom renal function continued to deteriorate than in those with stable renal function (Hauser *et al.*, 1991). Although the positive urine tests in these studies indicated the intake of phenacetin or paracetamol, the emphasis seems to have shifted to paracetamol. As judged by urine screening for the use of phenacetin or paracetamol, urinary tract infection was an important factor in patients with analgesic nephropathy (Dubach, 1981, 1984) and chronic pancreatitis was identified as an associated complication (Hangartner *et al.*, 1987).

There were anecdotal reports of neonatal renal failure following the maternal use of paracetamol and other drugs during pregnancy (Char *et al.*, 1975) and retroperitoneal fibrosis with hydronephrosis following consumption of paracetamol with dextropropoxyphene for 10 months (Critchley *et al.*, 1985). In another report, hypomagnesaemia and mild renal impairment were noted in a 71-year-old woman, with a hysterectomy for carcinoma of the uterus, who had taken increasing doses of paracetamol up to 3.9 g daily for seven years. The patient had received radiotherapy and a renal biopsy showed chronic interstitial nephritis with glomerular lesions (Tuso and Nortman, 1992). It is not clear why these changes were attributed to paracetamol or why its use in normal doses should be referred to as 'abuse'. Apart from slower excretion of total drug, the metabolism of radiolabelled paracetamol was not abnormal in patients with analgesic nephropathy (Thomas *et al.*, 1980), and aspirin and caffeine did not affect the metabolism of paracetamol formed from phenacetin in healthy subjects (Mineshita *et al.*, 1989).

Epidemiological Studies

Epidemiological studies have been carried out in attempts to define the role of analgesics in the aetiology of chronic renal disease. There were major difficulties with establishing reliably the use of these drugs over periods of many years, especially as different agents were often taken at different times. Another potentially confusing factor was the determination of paracetamol in the urine of analgesic takers as a marker for the consumption of phenacetin. Although urine testing could be valuable for verification of drug use, major discrepancies were observed between the claimed and actual intake of analgesics (Schwarz *et al.*, 1984). A longitudinal study of analgesic use in relation to renal function was performed in female workers in Swiss watch factories on the basis of initial urine tests that were positive for paracetamol (for intake of phenacetin) or salicylate. The study group consisted of 623 women with objective evidence of regular intake of phenacetin-containing analgesics and a matched control group of women who did not use these drugs regularly. Renal function was monitored for 20 years and the final analysis showed excess mortality in the analgesic takers with positive urine tests with increased relative risks for renal and cardiovascular disease and cancer (Dubach *et al.*, 1968, 1971, 1975, 1983, 1991). There was no such association with the use of salicylate and it was not possible to differentiate between the use of phenacetin and paracetamol. Paracetamol was detected in the urine of 47 of 515 outpatients (4.1 per cent) and a significant proportion had hypertension and increased plasma creatinine concentrations (Heilmann *et al.*, 1976). Again, it was not possible to distinguish between consumption of phenacetin and paracetamol. Belgium had the second highest world incidence of analgesic nephropathy and the geographical distribution of such patients with terminal renal failure correlated with the presence of analgesic factories in the neighbourhood of Antwerp. Three of the five most popular brands were made in this area, but only one contained paracetamol in which it was combined with aspirin and caffeine (Vanherweghem and Even-Adin, 1982). A case control study of analgesic use was carried out in 527 patients with end-stage renal disease and 1047 matched controls. The risk of terminal renal disease was not associated with the use of any analgesic, including paracetamol (Murray *et al.*, 1983). Capillarosclerosis in the renal pelvis as a sign of the abuse of analgesics containing phenacetin was found in 1.5 per cent of men and 3.9 per cent of women in a study of 500 unselected autopsy examinations. These figures were considered to reflect the extent of the abuse of phenacetin and paracetamol in the community. There was evidence that three patients had taken paracetamol in combination with other analgesics (Bethke and Schubert, 1985). Analgesic abuse was a major problem in some parts of what was formerly the Federal Republic of Germany but paracetamol (usually taken in combination with other analgesics) made only a modest contribution to the total consumption of analgesics. The European Dialysis and Transplant Association data probably underestimated the real extent of analgesic nephropathy (Pommer *et al.*, 1986).

Patients with leprosy used analgesics extensively and paracetamol was taken most commonly. However the average intake was only 1.3 g daily and of 28 patients who consented to intravenous urographic examination, none had renal papillary necrosis (Segasothy *et al.*, 1986b). In Sydney, the use of analgesics was compared in 91 of 675 renal outpatients who had renal papillary necrosis and 120 matched renal control patients. The consumption of paracetamol was not associated with an increased risk of papillary necrosis (McCredie and Stewart, 1988). In another case control study of regular intake of analgesics in 921 patients receiving renal replacement therapy there was a significant relationship between renal disease and analgesic use, and the risk increased with dose. No similar relationship could be shown with single analgesics including paracetamol but the numbers involved were very small (Pommer *et al.*, 1989). In south-west Germany, paracetamol was found in the urine of 4.1 per cent of 169 factory workers, 3.5 per cent of 198 general practice patients and 2 per cent of renal patients, and renal pelvic capillarosclerosis was observed in one of 258 autopsies. These findings were considered to indicate the habitual use of 'paracetamol-type' analgesics in that area (Mohr *et al.*, 1990). At the Group Health Co-operative at Puget Sound, 17 new cases of undiagnosed renal disease were identified between 1984 and 1989 among 378 769 users of non-prescription analgesics. Four were heavy users of analgesics and had taken paracetamol in combination with aspirin, ibuprofen and other drugs. Paracetamol was exonerated in two patients as renal function did not deteriorate further with its continued use, and in the other patients the intake of paracetamol was minimal (Derby and Jick, 1991). In a comparative study, the elderly and patients with coronary artery disease were at increased risk of impairment of renal function following the use of ibuprofen but not paracetamol (Murray *et al.*, 1990). Of 79 patients with headache, 68 had migraine and most (81 per cent) had taken combination rather than single analgesics. Non-steroidal anti-inflammatory drugs were taken most often (96.2 per cent of patients) followed by paracetamol (70.9 per cent). Sixty-five patients were said to abuse analgesics but only one of 45 of these was shown to have renal papillary necrosis associated with the consumption of paracetamol and mefenamic acid for 20 years (Rahman *et al.*, 1993b).

A survey by telephone interview was conducted in 554 adults with newly diagnosed renal disease and 516 matched control subjects in North Carolina. The risk of renal disease was increased in daily users of paracetamol after adjustment for the intake of aspirin and phenacetin and the odds ratio was 3.21 (confidence interval 1.05–9.80). The authors concluded that the long-term daily use of paracetamol was associated with an increased risk of chronic renal disease (Sandler *et al.*, 1989). This report was criticized because more than 55 per cent of the 554 patients were not available for interview and the analgesic history had to be obtained by proxy. Only 10 per cent of the controls were similarly unavailable. The number of daily users of paracetamol was very small (30 patients and five controls) and the differences between the groups only just reached statistical significance. The reclassification of just one individual would have rendered the findings insignificant. Only 19 per cent of the whole group of patients were classified as having interstitial nephritis and this was the only category of renal disease that could reasonably be attributed to the use of analgesics (Gates and Temple, 1989). In another similar survey by telephone interview of 716 patients with end-stage renal failure and 361 control subjects in Maryland, Virginia, West Virginia and Washington DC, there was a positive association between the cumulative use of paracetamol and terminal renal disease. Consumption of more than one tablet a day was classed as heavy use, and this was associated with a doubling of the risk of renal failure (Perneger *et al.*, 1994). However, the patients and controls differed significantly in respect of age and sex and the renal diagnoses were not specified. Despite these shortcomings, it was confidently stated that the use of paracetamol increased the odds of end-stage renal disease in patients with a variety of underlying renal diseases (including diabetic nephropathy), and that reduced consumption of paracetamol would reduce the overall incidence of end-stage renal disease by 8–10 per cent. The authors claimed that a cause and effect relationship was 'biologically plausible since paracetamol is a metabolite of phenacetin'. There was no mention of analgesic nephropathy in any of the 716 renal patients and the reasons for the use of analgesics were not given. As the authors admitted, it was possible that paracetamol was preferred to aspirin and non-steroidal anti-inflammatory drugs on the grounds of safety in patients with advanced renal failure.

Urinary Tract Cancer

Urinary tract cancer was a well-recognized long-term complication of analgesic nephropathy that could occur in up to 10 per cent of patients. The most common tumour was transitional cell carcinoma of the renal pelvis (Hultengren *et al.*, 1965; Bengtsson *et al.*, 1968; Johansson *et al.*, 1974; Blohmé and Johansson, 1981; Porpaczy and Schramek, 1981; Mihatsch and Knüsli, 1982; Prescott, 1982a; McLaughlin *et al.*, 1983; McCredie *et al.*, 1983a, 1989, 1990, 1993; and others), and a clear association between heavy analgesic use and tumours of the bladder and ureter has also been reported (Porpaczy and Schramek, 1981; Mihatsch and Knüsli, 1982b; Piper *et al.*, 1985, 1986; McCredie and Stewart, 1988; McCredie *et al.*, 1988, 1989, 1993; Hauser *et al.*, 1990; Nørgaard and Jensen, 1990; and others). Uroepithelial hyperplasia has been regarded as a premalignant condition and there was a high incidence of atypical urothelial changes in patients with end-stage analgesic nephropathy (Blohmé and Johansson, 1981). It has been produced with a variety of analgesic drugs in animals and it was probably a non-specific response to chronic injury (Prescott, 1982a; Bach *et al.*, 1988). More recently, malignancy, particularly uroepithelial cancer, has emerged as a major complication of renal transplantation in patients with analgesic nephropathy (Hauser *et al.*, 1990). Because of the long induction period of these cancers there have been real difficulties in attributing risk to any single analgesic drug. As with analgesic nephropathy itself, most workers have uncritically attributed these uroepithelial and renal tumours to abuse of phenacetin despite the fact that it was always taken with other analgesics, and unfortunately, paracetamol has again attracted guilt by association. Indeed, in some studies phenacetin and paracetamol have been considered together as though their actions were the same (McLaughlin *et al.*, 1983), and in others it was not possible to differentiate between the consequences of consumption of these drugs because both had usually been taken (McLaughlin *et al.*, 1985). Some 25 years ago it was recommended (illogically) that the sale of paracetamol should be restricted in Switzerland because of the long-term risk of urinary tract tumours in patients who had abused phenacetin containing analgesics (Brunner *et al.*, 1978; Mihatsch *et al.*, 1980a; Mihatsch and Knüsli, 1982). An increase in the incidence of transitional cell carcinoma of the lower urinary tract was recorded in Vienna in 300 urological patients with a history of long-term use of analgesic combinations containing phenacetin. In addition, 26 patients had bladder cancer and one had ureteric cancer. In some patients the tumours were multifocal. Although the patients apparently took only analgesics containing phenacetin, it was stated that as phenacetin was metabolized to paracetamol, the harmful effect of both on the kidneys was identical (Porpaczy and Schramek, 1981).

The relationship between regular use of paracetamol and tumours of the renal tract has been investigated in case control studies and these are summarized in Table 15.5. In all reports but two, there was no statistically significant association between the use of paracetamol and renal cell carcinoma or tumours of the renal pelvis, ureter or bladder. A population-based case control interview study of 74 patients with renal pelvic cancer and 679 controls indicated a four-fold risk in individuals who used phenacetin or paracetamol regularly for three or more years. There were only seven long-term users of these drugs. Two used phenacetin compounds only, one used paracetamol compounds and four took phenacetin and paracetamol together (McLaughlin *et al.*, 1983). Similar inconclusive results in respect of paracetamol were noted in a later report, also based on 74 patients (McLaughlin *et*

Table 15.5 Case control studies of the regular use of paracetamol and malignant tumours of the renal tract.

Site of tumour	No. of cases	No. of controls	Significant association	Reference
Renal pelvis	36	307	No[1]	McCredie *et al.*, 1983a
Renal pelvis	31	440	No	McCredie *et al.*, 1983b
Bladder	154	440	No	McCredie *et al.*, 1983b
Renal pelvis	74	697	No	McLaughlin *et al.*, 1983
Renal adenoma	548	624	No	MacLure and MacMahon, 1985
Renal cell	495	697	No	McLaughlin *et al.*, 1985
Renal pelvis	74	697	Yes[2]	McLaughlin *et al.*, 1985
Bladder	173	173	No	Piper *et al.*, 1985
Renal pelvis, ureter and bladder	381	808	No	McCredie and Stewart, 1988
Renal cell	360	985	No	McCredie *et al.*, 1988
Renal pelvis	121	187	No[2]	Ross *et al.*, 1989
Ureter	66	187	No[2]	Ross *et al.*, 1989
Bladder	143	120	No[2]	Berleur and Cordier, 1992
Renal cell	518	1351	No	Kreiger *et al.*, 1993
Renal cell	489	523	Yes	McCredie *et al.*, 1993
Renal pelvis	147	523	No	McCredie *et al.*, 1993
Renal cell	440	691	No	Chow *et al.*, 1994
Renal cell	1774	2359	No	McCredie *et al.*, 1995

[1] analgesics not containing phenacetin, [2] including analgesics containing phenacetin

al., 1985). In a similar study of 154 women with cancer and 440 controls in Sydney there was no association between cancer of the bladder or renal pelvis (31 patients) and the use of analgesics not containing phenacetin (McCredie *et al.*, 1983b). Likewise, there was a negative result for cancer of the ureter in 36 men (McCredie *et al.*, 1983a). In both of these studies there was a significant link with intake of analgesic mixtures containing phenacetin. In further reports it was not possible to substantiate an increased risk of cancer of the renal pelvis, ureter or bladder with the intake of paracetamol (McCredie *et al.*, 1986; McCredie and Stewart, 1988). A minor decrease in the incidence of end-stage renal failure following restriction of the sale of phenacetin in Australia was not followed by a parallel decrease in renal or uroepithelial cancer. Other investigators confirmed a positive association between the incidence of bladder cancer and the use of phenacetin containing analgesics in 173 young women but again there was no relationship to the consumption of paracetamol (Piper *et al.*, 1985, 1986). Another case control study of patients with carcinoma of the renal pelvis and ureter revealed a significant increase in risk in individuals with a history of continuous use of non-prescription analgesics for more than 30 days, but this risk did not extend to paracetamol unless the phenacetin and paracetamol data were combined (Ross *et al.*, 1989). In a study of 147 cases of renal pelvic cancer, the risks were increased by the use of aspirin and phenacetin mixtures to a far greater extent than with paracetamol where the difference between cases and controls was not significant. These findings were interpreted as showing a weak link between paracetamol and renal pelvic cancer (McCredie *et al.*, 1993) but the excess risk could also have been due to the previous use of other analgesics including phenacetin (Vanchieri, 1993). Hypercalaemia was reported as a manifestation of transitional cell carcinoma of the renal pelvis in a 45-year-old woman who had taken unspecified large amounts of aspirin, phenacetin, paracetamol and codeine for 10 years (Derbyshire *et al.*, 1989). Renal function had remained normal in a 42-year-old woman during 17 years use of paracetamol for headache. However, there was a deterioration after she took a Chinese herbal remedy for two-and-a-half years and she was found to have a transitional cell carcinoma of the renal pelvis. This was attributed to the herbal remedy rather than paracetamol (Vanherweghem *et al.*, 1995). There was concern in Denmark and Norway about analgesic-induced bladder cancer, particularly in women, and although it was recognized that there was insufficient evidence to incriminate paracetamol as a cause, excessive use was discouraged (Nørgaard and Jensen, 1990; Berg, 1994).

It had also been suspected that paracetamol might be a cause of renal parenchymal cancer. An association with the long-term use of phenacetin-containing products was shown in women but this did not extend to the duration of use of aspirin or paracetamol (McLaughlin *et al.*, 1984). In a subsequent case control study of 495 cases of renal cell cancer the use of phenacetin containing analgesics for more than 36 months was associated with a two-fold increase in risk. There was no significant link with products containing paracetamol but the numbers were small (McLaughlin *et al.*, 1985). Similar negative findings in respect of paracetamol were reported in two other surveys of patients with renal adenocarcinoma (MacLure and MacMahon, 1985; McCredie *et al.*, 1988). The risk of renal cell cancer was found to be increased somewhat in a survey of 155 554 patients with diagnoses of rheumatoid arthritis, osteoarthritis and back pain who were more or less regular users of analgesics. It was not possible to determine the risks for individual drugs but about half of the patients with osteoarthritis were constant users of non-steroidal anti-inflammatory drugs or paracetamol (Mellemgaard *et al.*, 1992). In a further case control study involving the whole of the Danish population there was no association between renal cell carcinoma and the use of paracetamol (Mellemgaard *et al.*, 1994). A case control study of patients with renal cell cancer showed that there was no increased risk with the use of paracetamol (Kreiger *et al.*, 1993), but, in another report, the risk was apparently increased similarly by the use of aspirin and phenacetin mixtures and paracetamol taken in any form (McCredie *et al.*, 1993). The possibility that the increased risk observed with paracetamol was related to previous use of phenacetin-containing combinations could not be excluded. In an international study involving 1774 cases of renal cell cancer and 2359 controls in Minnesota, USA, Australia, Denmark, Sweden and Germany, there was no association with the use of paracetamol although the number of regular users was too small to entirely exclude the possibility (McCredie *et al.*, 1995).

The overall conclusion must be that despite intensive efforts to prove the nephrotoxicity of paracetamol and despite the development of plausible mechanisms whereby it could cause tubular and papillary necrosis, it is most unlikely to cause serious renal damage in man unless it is taken in substantial overdosage. There have been rare reports of unexplained acute renal failure in young adults following the alleged consumption of small therapeutic doses and the risk of renal papillary necrosis or cancer of the urinary tract as a complication of long-term use must be very low considering the scale on which the drug is used. There was no reliable evidence that paracetamol caused chronic renal damage in man (Aarbakke, 1994).

Central Nervous System Effects

A single dose of 2 g of paracetamol had no significant effect on mood or mentation in 20 healthy young men (Eade and Lasagna, 1967) and a combination of 468 mg each of paracetamol and salicylamide had no influence on mood, emotion and motivation in 78 male and 78 female volunteers (Cameron *et al.*, 1967). In a more recent study, doses of 500 and 1000 mg had no adverse effects on visuomotor coordination, dynamic visual acuity, critical flicker fusion frequency, digit symbol substitution, complex reaction time or subjective assessment of mood in seven healthy females (Bradley and Nicholson, 1987). Paracetamol produced minor non-specific changes in the spontaneously recorded electroencephalograms in healthy medical students (Bromm and Scharein, 1993) but it had no effect on polygraphically recorded sleep in 37 subjects (Murphy *et al.*, 1994). After taking a combination of chlorzoxazone and paracetamol, a 21-year-old man experienced headaches, disorientation and a dream-like state that disappeared when the medication was discontinued (Liederman and Boldus, 1967). Paracetamol was unlikely to have caused these symptoms. The question was raised as to the possibility that chronic ingestion of paracetamol might cause headache (Cantwell-Simmons *et al.*, 1993) and withdrawal of analgesics (including paracetamol) in patients with chronic headache resulted in improvement (Diener *et al.*, 1989). Paracetamol was one of the drugs detected most frequently at post-mortem examinations of Federal Aviation Authority civilian aviation fatalities in 1989 (13 of 377 cases), but no particular significance was attached to this finding (Kuhlman *et al.*, 1991). Paracetamol could cause a reduction in the concentration of inorganic sulphate in the cerebrospinal fluid, but this was probably of no practical significance (Morris *et al.*, 1984, 1986).

Abuse

In self-administration studies with paracetamol in rhesus monkeys, there was no reinforcing effect and there was lower dosing rate than with the solvent alone (Hoffmeister *et al.*, 1980). There have been occasional reports of the abuse of paracetamol but there was no widespread habitual excessive consumption as occurred in the past with phenacetin-containing analgesics. In the few cases of abuse that have been reported, combination preparations, which included habit forming drugs such as caffeine, sedatives and narcotic analgesics, were usually taken (Nakra *et al.*, 1973; Vincens *et al.*, 1982; Rotenberg *et al.*, 1988; Fyfe and Wright, 1990). In one unusual report, paracetamol was taken in large doses (up to 30 tablets) by four young women with eating disorders to induce vomiting. In one patient, the associated nausea and anorexia reduced the risk of her binging the next day (Tiller and Treasure, 1992). Two of 64 alcoholic patients were classed as abusers of paracetamol and claimed to take 12–14 and 30 tablets daily (Seifert *et al.*, 1993) and another such patient apparently took as much as 25 g daily (Tredger *et al.*, 1995). As shown in Tables 15.3 and 15.4, abuse of paracetamol (particularly by chronic alcoholics) resulted in hepatic and renal toxicity (Denison *et al.*, 1991).

In some areas it was common practice to screen the urine of patients with analgesic nephropathy for p-aminophenol as a guide to analgesic abuse. Unfortunately, this test could not distinguish between the use of phenacetin and paracetamol as both drugs were hydrolyzed to p-aminophenol. Urine tests showed that continuing analgesic abuse was frequent in patients with analgesic nephropathy despite denial of the habit (Furman *et al.*, 1976; Hauser *et al.*, 1991), and distinctive personality traits were demonstrated in female industrial workers in whom urine tests were regularly positive for p-aminophenol (Hobi *et al.*, 1976). Using a specific assay, paracetamol was found in the urine in 7 of 169 (4.1 per cent) factory workers in Heidelberg, and it was concluded that habitual use of 'paracetamol-type' analgesics continued in the general population (Mohr *et al.*, 1990). In none of these reports could it be determined whether phenacetin or paracetamol had been taken. Paracetamol was said to be abused most by patients with headache, but no supporting data were provided (Elkind, 1991). In South Australia, sustained abuse of paracetamol was not believed to be common (Mathew, 1992). The definition of abuse is problematical and patients taking less than the maximum recommended daily dose of paracetamol for conditions such as hip pain have been accused unreasonably of abusing the drug (Tuso and Nortman, 1992). Patients with chronic headache and migraine frequently took paracetamol but it was not properly established whether this represented true abuse (Rahman *et al.*, 1993a). Patients with chronic tension-type headache were at particular risk of becoming drug-dependent and acquiring analgesic-induced headache (Schnider *et al.*, 1994).

Effects on Pregnancy and the Newborn

Paracetamol was used increasingly as an analgesic during pregnancy but adverse effects including an increased risk of congenital abnormalities have not been noted following its normal therapeutic use (Crombie *et al.*, 1970; Nelson and Forfar, 1971; Collins, 1981; Heymann, 1986). There was an isolated unconfirmed reference stating that paracetamol exhibited an activity indistinguishable from other prostaglandin inhibitors in closing the ductus arteriosus in the sheep fetus (Peterson, 1985). No untoward effects were observed in 13 women given paracetamol at different times during pregnancy (Lasfargues and Brehon, 1979). A survey of drugs prescribed for 6837 women during the first trimester of pregnancy showed that 493 were given paracetamol and 328 paracetamol with codeine. The prevalence of congenital disorders was not remarkable (6 and 15 per 1000 respectively) (Jick *et al.*, 1981). In a similar study of 6509 mothers, 2 of 350 women who had been prescribed paracetamol, and 9 of 347 who had been prescribed paracetamol with codeine, delivered children with congenital disorders (Aselton *et al.*, 1985). The findings in these studies were similar to those expected for the background incidence of congenital disorders. In another report, 735 of 1371 women took drugs (mostly prescribed) during the first trimester of pregnancy but only 60 had been given paracetamol (Grupo de Trabajo DUP España, 1991b). Throughout the whole of pregnancy, drugs were taken by 93 per cent of the women but paracetamol was only taken by 138 (1.1 per cent) (Grupo de Trabajo DUP España, 1991a). However, in an international study of drug use during pregnancy in 14 778 women, analgesics (mostly paracetamol) had been taken by 2193 (17 per cent) (Bonati, 1991). The total consumption of paracetamol during pregnancy would undoubtedly be substantial when non-prescription use was also taken into account. A survey of pregnant women in Glasgow showed that most would only take an analgesic preparation containing paracetamol for minor complaints, and very few would opt for aspirin (Butters and Howie, 1990). According to an analysis of current information on teratogenicity in man, there was negligible risk from paracetamol (Friedman *et al.*, 1990).

As might be expected from the frequency of use of paracetamol and the natural incidence of congenital malformations, anecdotal cases involving paracetamol have been reported. An infant with neonatal renal failure was born after her mother had experienced severe polyhydramnios during the pregnancy. The child died at the age of eight weeks and at post-mortem examination the renal pathology included multiple dilated distal tubules containing granular eosinophilic casts. The mother had taken paracetamol daily and 'Benedictin' intermittently during pregnancy and for some reason the renal lesions were attributed to the paracetamol (Char *et al.*, 1975). A 20-year-old woman delivered a male infant with anophthalmia at 37 weeks of gestation. During early pregnancy she had been given dicyclomine, phenobarbitone, amitriptyline, dextropropoxyphene and paracetamol (Golden and Perman, 1980). Another woman who was prescribed phenobarbitone, dextropropoxyphene and paracetamol during pregnancy gave birth to an infant with cranio-facial and digital malformations (Golden *et al.*, 1982). In these reports it was clearly impossible to establish the cause of these disorders. In another study, there was no relationship between the taking of paracetamol during pregnancy and subsequent measures of intelligence quotient and attention decrements in the offspring (Streissguth *et al.*, 1987).

Adverse Metabolic Effects

Metabolic abnormalities have occasionally been attributed to paracetamol. Hypoglycaemia was documented following the administration of 30 mg of paracetamol in a 43-month-old child whose mother had toxaemia of pregnancy and whose delivery was complicated by respiratory distress, hypoglycaemia and convulsions. He had previously reacted to aspirin with hypoglycaemia (Ruvalcaba *et al.*, 1966). Hypoglycaemia was also reported in three patients following the use of a combination analgesic containing dextropropoxyphene and paracetamol (Leuzinger *et al.*, 1978; Blaison *et al.*, 1991). Doses of 1 g of paracetamol eight hourly for seven days had no effect on serum concentrations of thyroxine, triiodothyronine, reverse triiodothyronine, 3,3'-diiodothyronine and 3,5'-diiodothyronine in healthy subjects (Faber, 1980). Hypothermia was reported as a side effect in four children with fever given therapeutic doses of paracetamol. However, the fall in temperature was mild (35°C) and transient (van Tittelboom and Govaerts-Lepicard, 1989). 5-Oxoprolinuria (pyroglutamic aciduria) was described in patients taking paracetamol (Creer *et al.*, 1989; Pitt, 1990; Pitt *et al.*, 1990) and was thought to have been related to effects on glutathione and glycine metabolism (Persaud and Jackson, 1991). Type II citrullinaemia in a 19-year-old man was thought to have been triggered by paracetamol taken for a 'cold' but no objective information was provided in support of this theory (Shiohama *et al.*, 1993).

Reye's Syndrome

A causal relationship between the use of aspirin and Reye's syndrome in children and young adults has finally been accepted but no such relationship has been demonstrated with paracetamol. Indeed, there was an inverse relationship between the previous use of paracetamol and Reye's syndrome, and as the use of aspirin in children has declined with a fall in the incidence of the condition, the use of paracetamol has increased (Halpin *et al.*, 1982; Waldman *et al.*, 1982; Hurwitz *et al.*, 1987; Hall *et al.*, 1988; Forsyth *et al.*, 1989; Orlowski *et al.*, 1990; Porter *et al.*, 1990). Despite the marked decrease in the incidence of Reye's syndrome following curtailment of the use of aspirin, cases were still being reported, and in some there was a history of the use of aspirin and/or paracetamol (Rinaldi *et al.*, 1989; Poss *et al.*, 1994).

Interference with Laboratory Tests

There have been reports of interference by paracetamol with laboratory tests including those for uric acid (Smith and Payne, 1979) and aminoacids (Shih *et al.*, 1985). Interference would be method dependent and there were particular problems with the analysis of glucose using glucose oxidase (Kaufmann-Raab *et al.*, 1976; Wright and Foster, 1980; Farrance and Aldons, 1981; Fleetwood and Robinson, 1981; Roddis, 1981; Farah *et al.*, 1982; Townsend, 1983). Paracetamol was one of the most serious sources of interference with glucose assays based on peroxidase-linked reactions with electrochemical detection (Cowell and Ford, 1987; Bindra *et al.*, 1991; Moatti-Sirat *et al.*, 1992) and it was necessary to develop special membranes to avoid interference with implantable glucose sensors (Groom and Luong, 1993; Jaffari and Pickup, 1994; Moatti-Sirat *et al.*, 1994; Zhang *et al.*, 1994). Paracetamol caused minimal interference with an electrocatalytic glucose sensor employing direct electrochemical oxidation (Saeger *et al.*, 1992) and in another approach, surface-bound tyrosinase was used to remove paracetamol biocatalytically and thus reduce interference (Wang *et al.*, 1993). Paracetamol could also interfere with the estimation of urinary metanephrine and catecholamines (Wilson *et al.*, 1985).

Drug Interactions

Apart from possible potentiation of the hepatotoxicity of paracetamol by ethanol and drugs that cause induction of drug metabolizing enzymes, no serious adverse drug reactions involving paracetamol have been confirmed in man. As described in Chapter 14, many compounds were shown to modify the hepatotoxicity of paraceta-mol in animals by altering its metabolic activation or influencing glutathione status, but such interactions are unlikely to be relevant to its normal clinical use. Multiple interactions have also been described in man between paracetamol and drugs which increased or decreased its rate of absorption through effects on gastric emptying. These are summarized in Chapter 4 and will not be discussed further here. Absorp-tion interactions involving paracetamol seem to be of little clinical significance, although in one report the absorption of aluminium was greatly increased in a patient maintained on haemodialysis. This was attributed to the citrate content of an effervescent formulation of paracetamol (Main and Ward, 1992). Known phar-macokinetic and pharmacodynamic interactions of paracetamol in man are sum-marized in Table 15.6 and the subject has been reviewed (Hayes, 1981; Prescott and Critchley, 1983a; Lacroix *et al.*, 1985; Sachs and Kowalsky, 1988). Additional studies of some interactions have been carried out *in vitro* and in animals. Dose-dependent competition for sulphate conjugation was demonstrated between parace-tamol and ethinyloestradiol in human intestinal mucosa obtained from surgical specimens (Rogers *et al.*, 1987a). It was noted that the incidence of neutropenia as an adverse effect of zidovudine (azidothymidine, AZT) was increased in patients who also took paracetamol and an interaction based on competition for glucuronide conjugation was proposed (Richman *et al.*, 1987). It was later shown that paraceta-mol did not impair the metabolism of zidovudine in patients infected with human immunodeficiency virus (HIV), and, if anything, paracetamol increased its clearance (Steffe *et al.*, 1990; Sattler *et al.*, 1991; Burger *et al.*, 1994a,b). Similar negative results were demonstrated in studies with human liver microsomes (Sim *et al.*, 1991; Rajaonarison *et al.*, 1991, 1992; Kamali and Rawlins, 1992) and there was little or no effect in studies with isolated rat hepatocytes and rat liver microsomes (Cretton and Sommadossi, 1991; Ameer *et al.*, 1992; Ameer, 1993). In other studies of poten-tial clinical significance, paracetamol increased the biliary excretion of metabolites of trimetrexate by the perfused rat liver (Webster *et al.*, 1987) and it inhibited alcohol dehydrogenase and reduced the first pass metabolism of ethanol by rat gastric mucosa (Palmer *et al.*, 1991). In rats, paracetamol depressed the metabolism of phenylbutazone, but not oxyphenbutazone or ketophenylbutazone (Niwa and Nakayama, 1968), yet it had no effect on the metabolism of indomethacin (van Kolfschoten *et al.*, 1985) or antipyrine (Vial *et al.*, 1990).

Some reports of interactions have been inconsistent and, in the case of chloram-phenicol, completely opposite results have been reported by different investigators (Table 15.6). These discrepancies may have been related to auto-induction of chlor-amphenicol metabolism and differences in dose, patient selection, experimental design and analytical methodology (Choonara, 1987; Spika and Aranda, 1987). On

Table 15.6 Drug interactions involving therapeutic doses of paracetamol in man.

Pharmacokinetic interactions

Interacting drug	Result of interaction	Proposed mechanism	Reference
p-Aminohippurate	reduced acetylation of PAH	inhibition of acetylation	Prescott et al., 1990
Amylobarbitone	no effect on amylobarbitone elimination		Kinsella et al., 1979
Anticonvulsants	no effect on anticonvulsant metabolism		Neuvonen et al, 1979
Anticonvulsants	enhanced elimination, reduced bioavailability of paracetamol	induction	Perucca and Richens, 1979
Anticonvulsants	enhanced elimination of paracetamol	induction, increased glucuronide conjugation	Prescott et al., 1981
Anticonvulsants	increased clearance of paracetamol	increased glucuronide conjugation and oxidation	Miners et al., 1984c
Antipyrine	no effect on antipyrine elimination		Awni et al., 1990
Anti-TB drugs[1]	enhanced elimination of paracetamol	induction	Madhusudanarao et al., 1988a
Aspirin	increased blood aspirin concentration	?esterase inhibition	Cotty et al., 1977
Butyl hydroxyanisole	no effect		Verhagen et al., 1989
Caffeine	minor changes of no significance	possibly due to formulation differences	Wójcicki et al., 1994
Chloramphenicol	greatly increased chloramphenicol half life	competition for glucuronide conjugation	Buchanan and Moodley, 1979
Chloramphenicol	no effect on chloramphenicol disposition		Rajpurohit and Krishnaswamy, 1984
Chloramphenicol	no effect on chloramphenicol kinetics		Kearns et al., 1985
Chloramphenicol	decreased half life of chloramphenicol		Spika et al., 1986
Chloramphenicol	reduced steady-state chloramphenicol concentrations		Bravo et al., 1987
Chloramphenicol	no effect on chloramphenicol kinetics		Stein et al., 1989
Chloroquine	increased rate of paracetamol absorption	increased gastric emptying rate	Adjepon-Yamoah et al., 1986
Chloroquine	no effect on chloroquine absorption or disposition		Essien et al., 1988
Cimetidine	no effect on paracetamol kinetics[2]		Abernethy et al., 1983a
Cimetidine	no effect on paracetamol kinetics or disposition		Critchley et al., 1983
Cimetidine	no effect on paracetamol disposition		Miners et al., 1984c
Cimetidine	decreased oxidation of paracetamol	inhibition of metabolic activation	Mitchell et al., 1984b
Cimetidine	no effect on paracetamol kinetics		Chen and Lee, 1985
Cimetidine	no effect on paracetamol disposition		Vendemiale et al., 1987
Cimetidine	no effect on paracetamol disposition and kinetics		Slattery et al., 1989
Codeine	no effect on codeine metabolism		Somogyi et al., 1991
Diazepam	no effect on diazepam elimination		Mulley et al., 1978
Diftalone	no effect on diftalone elimination		Buniva et al., 1977
Fenoldopam	increased fenoldopam concentrations	competition for sulphate conjugation	Ziemniak et al., 1987
Ibuprofen	no effect on elimination of either drug		Wright et al., 1983

Drug	Effect	Mechanism	Reference
Indomethacin	no effect on indomethacin elimination		Seideman, 1991
Isoniazid	reduced clearance of paracetamol	reduced metabolic activation	Epstein et al., 1991
Lamotrigine	decreased half life of lamotrigine	not known	Depot et al., 1990
Methotrexate	increased volume of paracetamol distribution	high fluid intake	Kamali et al., 1988
Omeprazole	no effect on paracetamol disposition[3]		Xiaodong et al., 1994
Oral contraceptives	reduced paracetamol half life	increased rate of metabolism	Abernethy et al., 1982b
Oral contraceptives	increased paracetamol clearance	increased glucuronidation and oxidation	Miners et al., 1983
Oral contraceptives	increased paracetamol clearance	increased glucuronidation and oxidation	Mitchell et al., 1983
Oral contraceptives	increased ethinyloestradiol concentrations	competition for sulphate conjugation	Rogers et al., 1987b
Oral contraceptives	no effect on levonorgestrel kinetics		Rogers et al., 1987b
Oral contraceptives	increased ethinyloestradiol concentrations	competition for sulphate conjugation	Back et al., 1990
Oxaprozin	no effect on oxaprozin elimination		Scavone et al., 1986
Primaquine	no effect on paracetamol disposition		Back and Tjia, 1987
Probenecid	decreased clearance of paracetamol	competition for glucuronide conjugation and excretion	Kamali, 1993
Ranitidine	no effect on paracetamol disposition		Jack et al., 1985
Ranitidine	no effect on paracetamol disposition		Thomas et al., 1988
Rifampicin	increased rate of paracetamol elimination	increased glucuronide conjugation	Prescott et al., 1981
Terfenadine	cardiac arrhythmia[4]	presumed accumulation of terfenadine	Matsis and Easthope, 1994
Toluene	increased blood toluene concentrations	inhibition of metabolism	Löf et al., 1990
Zidovudine	no effect on zidovudine conjugation		Steffe et al., 1990
Zidovudine	no effect on zidovudine clearance		Sattler et al., 1991
Zidovudine	no effect on kinetics or disposition of either drug		Burger et al., 1994a,b

Pharmacodynamic interactions

Drug	Effect	Mechanism	Reference
Antihypertensives	no significant effect of paracetamol on blood pressure		Chalmers et al., 1984
Antihypertensives	no effect of paracetamol on blood pressure	not known	Radack et al., 1987
Anticoagulants[5]	increased prothrombin time[6]		Antlitz et al., 1968
Anticoagulants[5]	no effect on prothrombin time		Antlitz and Awalt, 1969
Coumarins	increased prothrombin time	reduced synthesis of clotting factors	Boeijinga et al., 1982, 1983
Frusemide	antagonism of diuretic and natriuretic effect of frusemide	not stated	Abrams et al., 1986
Frusemide	no effect on diuretic and natriuretic effect of frusemide		Martin and Prescott, 1994
Sotalol	increased bradycardia produced by sotalol	not stated	Tongia, 1982
Warfarin	increased prothrombin time (case report)	overdose, other drugs	Justice and Kline, 1988
Warfarin	bleeding (case report)	not known	Bartle and Blakely, 1991
Warfarin	increased prothrombin time (brief case report)	not known	Kaye, 1991

[1] Rifampicin + isoniazid + pyrazinamide + ethambutol; [2] minor reduction in mercapturic acid production on prolonged therapy with cimetidine; [3] paracetamol formed by metabolism of phenacetin; [4] unconfirmed anecdotal report; [5] including warfarin, dicoumarol, anisinidone and phenprocoumon; [6] mean increase 3.5 sec

the basis of an anecdotal case report, isoniazid was said to potentiate the hepato-toxicity of paracetamol by inducing its metabolism and increasing the formation of toxic metabolite (Crippin, 1993). The circumstances strongly suggested that, as expected, dose of paracetamol had been taken and other investigators showed that in fact, isoniazid was a potent inhibitor of the metabolic activation of paracetamol in man (Epstein *et al.*, 1991; Zand *et al.*, 1993). Omeprazole was proposed as an aryl hydrocarbon-type inducer of human cytochrome P450, and as such it would be expected to enhance paracetamol metabolism and toxicity (Diaz *et al.*, 1990; Peter-sen, 1993). However, it was subsequently shown in man to have no effect on the kinetics of paracetamol formed from phenacetin (Xiaodong *et al.*, 1994). Other inter-actions have been assumed to occur without any supporting evidence. Severe hepa-totoxicity was reported in an alcoholic patient receiving long-term zidovudine therapy following the alleged ingestion of 3.3 g of paracetamol over 36 h. The clini-cal course was typical of paracetamol overdosage but it was assumed without evi-dence that zidovudine had potentiated toxicity by inhibiting the glucuronide conjugation of paracetamol (Shriner and Goetz, 1992). Subsequent studies refuted this possibility (Steffe *et al.*, 1990; Sattler *et al.*, 1991; Burger *et al.*, 1994a,b). In other reports it was suggested that liver toxicity could have resulted from interactions between paracetamol and ranitidine (Bredfeldt and von Huene, 1984) and interferon plus vinblastine (Kellokumpu-lehtinen *et al.*, 1989), but this seemed unlikely. The only dramatic and potentially lethal interaction attributed to the normal use of paracetamol was ventricular tachycardia (Torsades de pointe) in one patient also taking terfenadine. The interaction was not confirmed and no mechanism was estab-lished (Matsis and Easthope, 1994). It might appear that paracetamol could interact with oral anticoagulants but the findings were inconsistent and when potentiation occurred in formal studies, it was minor (Wells *et al.*, 1994). Paracetamol did not interfere with the glucuronide conjugation of 7-hydroxy-4-methylcoumarin by human liver microsomes (Irshaid *et al.*, 1990).

16

Paracetamol Overdose

Introduction

In 1966, Davidson and Eastham reported acute liver damage in a 30-year-old woman and a 28-year-old man following overdosage with paracetamol in Edinburgh. Both patients died 3–4 days later with fulminant hepatic failure and post-mortem examination revealed acute centrilobular hepatic necrosis affecting all areas. At the same time Thomson and Prescott (1966) reported another patient who suffered liver damage after taking an overdose and they mentioned two other cases including toxic necrosis of the liver with a fatal outcome in a 13-year-old girl. Over the next few years there were increasing numbers of reports of patients with severe and fatal liver damage following overdosage with paracetamol in the United Kingdom (Brown, 1968; MacLean et al., 1968a; Rose, 1969; Toghill et al., 1969; Proudfoot and Wright, 1970; Prescott et al., 1971; Sanerkin, 1971; Will and Tomkins, 1971; Farid et al., 1972; Clark et al., 1973b). The incidence of self-poisoning was increasing rapidly at that time in most Western countries, and with the increasing availability of paracetamol it was inevitable that it would be used more and more for this purpose. An early report from South Africa (Pimstone and Uys, 1968) was followed three years later by the first case report from the USA (Boyer and Rouff, 1971). These reports of paracetamol poisoning were soon followed by others from many countries including Australia (Benson and Boleyn, 1974; Rigby et al., 1978; Oh and Shenfield, 1980; Breen et al., 1982b; Ho and Beilin, 1983; Hardwicke et al., 1986; Kritharides et al., 1988; McGrath, 1989; Brotodihardjo et al., 1992; Campbell and Oates, 1992; Henderson et al., 1993), Belgium (Melis and Bochner, 1990; van Vyve et al., 1993; Buylaert et al., 1994), Canada (Antaki et al., 1978; Holzbecher et al., 1981; Sutherland et al., 1981; Zabrodski and Schnurr, 1984; Lacroix et al., 1989; Campbell and Baylis, 1992; Chow et al., 1992), Chile (Brahm et al., 1992), Denmark (Vilstrup et al., 1977; Jorgensen, 1985; Jensen, 1986; Sørensen et al., 1986; Strøm et al., 1986; Jensen et al., 1987; Ott et al., 1990a; Fisker et al., 1991; Kondrup et al., 1992; Nielsen and Nielsen, 1992; Pedersen et al., 1993), Finland (Haapanen, 1982), France (Commandre et al., 1976; Garnier et al., 1982; Bismuth et al., 1983; Belin et al., 1988; Harry et al., 1989; Navelet et al., 1990; Weber et al., 1990b; Duchene et al., 1991; Coirault et al., 1993; Brevet et al., 1994),

Germany (Horwitz *et al.*, 1977; Mühlendahl and Krienke, 1980; Baumgarten *et al.*, 1983; Mühlendahl, 1987; Homann *et al.*, 1990; Augustin and Schmoldt, 1991a,b; Michaelis *et al.*, 1991; Claass *et al.*, 1993; Rump and Keller, 1994), Holland (van Heijst *et al.*, 1976; Stegeman-Castelen *et al.*, 1983; van Berge Henegouwen and Savelkoul, 1994), Hong Kong (Chan *et al.*, 1993), Ireland (Fitzgerald and Drury, 1977; Arthurs and Fielding, 1980; Malone *et al.*, 1992), Israel (Shnaps *et al.*, 1980, 1981; Levy and Oren, 1985; Oren and Levy, 1992, 1993; Winkler and Halkin, 1992, 1993), Italy (de Nardo *et al.*, 1988; Chiossi *et al.*, 1991), Japan (Ikejiri *et al.*, 1979; Yasunaga *et al.*, 1985; Sakai *et al.*, 1987; Ohtani *et al.*, 1989; Shimazaki *et al.*, 1989; Shimizu *et al.* 1989; Koga *et al.*, 1991; Yamakawa, 1992), Mexico (Montoya Cabrera *et al.*, 1982), New Zealand (Cairns *et al.*, 1983; Buchanan, 1991; Edwards and Oliphant, 1992), Norway (Reikvam and Skjoto, 1978; Skjoto and Reikvam, 1979; Laake *et al.*, 1983; Jacobsen *et al.*, 1984; Bodd *et al.*, 1985; Bell *et al.*, 1987a,b; Jakobsen *et al.*, 1987; Rygnestad, 1989; Boberg *et al.*, 1994), Singapore (Chao, 1993), South Africa (Müller *et al.*, 1983; Pillans and Hall, 1985; Monteagudo and Folb, 1987), Spain (Frati *et al.*, 1983; Manrique Larralde *et al.*, 1988; Marruecos *et al.*, 1988; Sánchez-Guisande *et al.*, 1989), Sweden (Alván *et al.*, 1976; Andersson *et al.*, 1976; Bæhrendtz *et al.*, 1976; Olsson, 1978; Frisinette-Fich *et al.*, 1986; Denison *et al.*, 1987, 1991; Florén *et al.*, 1987; Weiss *et al.*, 1987; Björck *et al.*, 1988; Eriksson *et al.*, 1992; Alsén *et al.*, 1994) and Switzerland (Enrico and Buchser, 1983). Intentional self-poisoning with paracetamol became a matter of concern in many countries and in some it attracted much adverse publicity. There were particular problems with paracetamol poisoning. An overdose did not produce any early characteristic or specific symptoms and signs, and it did not normally cause impairment of consciousness unless taken in combination with central nervous system depressants. As a result, the gravity of the situation was often not appreciated when the patient was first seen yet fulminant hepatic failure could develop within three or four days with an unpleasant and rapidly fatal outcome. In addition, early recognition and treatment was essential to prevent liver damage and death in severely poisoned patients. Paracetamol poisoning was almost always intentional in older children and adults, but accidental in infants and young children. A sensational outbreak of poisoning referred to as 'the paracetamol tragedy' in Nigeria in 1990 resulted in the deaths of 109 children. However, the poisoning was caused not by paracetamol but by ethylene glycol, which had been used instead of propylene glycol in a locally produced paediatric elixir formulation (Alubo, 1994).

Epidemiology

Simple analgesics, including paracetamol, tended to be taken in overdose more often by young adults (especially females) who had not been prescribed drugs, than by the middle-aged or elderly (National Poisons Information Service Monitoring Group, 1981; Prescott and Highley, 1985; Muscari, 1987; Wynne *et al.*, 1987; Hawton and Fagg, 1992a; Malone *et al.*, 1992; Chan *et al.*, 1993; Alsén *et al.*, 1994). The reasons for intentional self-poisoning with paracetamol were similar to those for self-poisoning generally and the motives are often manipulative. Unfortunately, many authors still referred to self-poisoning incorrectly as 'attempted suicide' or a 'suicidal gesture'. This was simply not true as most young adults who take an overdose of paracetamol have no intention of killing themselves. They usually take it on impulse because of failure to cope with personal problems and at the time they do not seriously consider the possibility that their actions might result in their death. Major overdoses could be taken for apparently trivial reasons in what appeared to be an irresponsible game of toxicological Russian roulette. The level of knowledge about paracetamol and its potential toxicity in patients who had taken it in overdose was poor (McNicholl, 1992; Myers *et al.*, 1992), and initially there was no obvious reason for a preference for paracetamol apart from its ready availability (Gazzard *et al.*, 1976a,b). In a more recent survey of 80 patients in Oxford who had taken an overdose of paracetamol, it was chosen because it was available and the dangers seemed to be recognized. However, there was a lack of knowledge of the specific effects and the timing of these effects (Hawton *et al.*, 1995). 'Copycat' self-poisoning with paracetamol might have been encouraged by media publicity and television (Davis and Williams, 1975; Volans, 1976; Collins, 1993; Waldron, 1993), but on the other hand, better information might have prompted some patients to seek help early when they would not have done so otherwise (O'Connell and Feeley, 1993). The most common age group for self-poisoning with paracetamol was 18–25 years and females outnumbered males in a ratio of about 2 : 1 (Gazzard *et al.*, 1976a; Hamlyn *et al.*, 1978; Breen *et al.*, 1982b; Prescott, 1983; Bodd *et al.*, 1985; Levy and Oren, 1985; Monteagudo and Folb, 1987; Augustin and Schmoldt, 1991a,b; Oren and Levy, 1992). In one report, paracetamol was taken in five of 23 episodes of self-poisoning by adolescents and young adults with anorexia nervosa who may have been at particular risk of toxicity (Woolf and Gren, 1990). Paracetamol was used by the elderly less frequently for self-poisoning (Schernitski *et al.*, 1980; Wynne *et al.*, 1987). In one report of 737 cases of self-poisoning, paracetamol was taken by 41 per cent of patients aged less than 35 years, 25 per cent of those aged 35–64 years and by only 11 per cent of patients aged 65 years or more (Wynne *et al.*, 1987). Paracetamol was usually taken in a domestic environment but overdosage in motor vehicles has been reported (Bauman *et al.*, 1989).

Incidence

The frequency of use of paracetamol for poisoning has increased greatly in many countries in recent years and this has been largely due to increased availability as sales have risen and overtaken those of other analgesics. Paracetamol has been used more often than aspirin for self-poisoning in Edinburgh since 1976 (Proudfoot and Park, 1978). In addition to availability, its use for this purpose was influenced by cultural factors and local fashions of analgesic use. The use of paracetamol for self-poisoning in hospital patients over the years in different countries is summarized in Table 16.1. These reports cannot be compared directly because of geographical and temporal differences in incidence, and variation in the criteria for referral and admission. Thus, paracetamol does not feature prominently among the drugs taken by poisoned patients in intensive care units because most patients who took it in overdosage were managed in medical wards. As shown in Table 16.1, paracetamol was used increasingly for self-poisoning over the years and this was particularly obvious when studies were repeated at intervals in the same area (Prescott *et al.*, 1971; Prescott, 1978, 1983; Platt *et al.*, 1988; Rygnestad, 1989; Fisker *et al.*, 1991; Hawton and Fagg, 1992b; Kelly and Galloway, 1992; McGoldrick *et al.*, 1992; Nielsen and Nielsen, 1992; Buylaert *et al.*, 1994). Other investigators have drawn

Table 16.1 Incidence of paracetamol poisoning in hospital overdose patients.

Country	Period	Setting	Age	Total no. of cases	No. (%) taking paracetamol	Reference
Australia	1977–79	Hospital admissions	adult	963	(8.1)	Myers et al., 1981
Australia	1980–82	Hospital admissions	adult	747	59 (7.9)	Hardwicke et al., 1986
Australia	1983–88	Hospital admissions	child	407	27 (6.6)	Campbell and Oates, 1992
Australia	1985–86	Hospital admissions	adult	325	35 (10.8)	McGrath, 1989
Australia	1986–91	Intensive Care Unit	adult	732	66 (9.0)	Henderson et al., 1993
Australia	1986–91	Emergency Department	adult	1000	150 (15.0)	Henderson et al., 1993
Australia	1989	Emergency Department	adult	323	48 (14.9)	Hodgkinson et al., 1991
Australia	1993	Hospital admissions	adult	26	5 (19.2)	Stanton et al., 1994
Belgium	1980–88	Intensive Care Unit	child	470	12 (2.6)	Melis and Bochner, 1990
Canada	1983–86	Emergency Department	child	1666	77 (4.6)	Lacroix et al., 1989
Canada	1983–86	Hospital admissions	child	687	24 (3.5)	Lacroix et al., 1989
Canada	1983–86	Intensive Care Unit	child	137	1 (0.7)	Lacroix et al., 1989
Canada	1986–88	Emergency Department	adult	1001	196 (19.6)	Chow et al., 1992
Denmark	1979–83	Intensive Care Unit	adult	1011	10 (1.0)	Fisker et al., 1991
Denmark	1984–88	Intensive Care Unit	adult	922	74 (8.0)	Fisker et al., 1991
England	1954–75	Hospital admissions	adult	5866	270 (4.6)	Jones, 1977
England	1971–72	Hospital admissions	adult	100	3 (3.0)	Lockhart and Baron, 1987
England	1974–81	Hospital admissions	<5 yr	1100	41 (3.7)	Lawson et al., 1983
England	1976	Hospital admissions	adult	873	125 (14.3)	Hawton and Fagg, 1992b
England	1978–79	Hospital admissions	adult	296	52 (17.4)	Platt et al., 1988
England	1982–86	Hospital admissions	adult	737	241 (32.7)	Wynne et al., 1987
England	1983–84	Hospital admissions	adult	94	16 (17.0)	Lockhart and Baron, 1987
England	1983–84	Hospital admissions	adult	246	69 (28.1)	Platt et al., 1988
England	1988	Emergency Department	adult	843	(43.0)	Underhill et al., 1990
England	1990	Hospital admissions	adult	869	365 (42.5)	Hawton and Fagg, 1992b

Country	Year	Type	Age	Number	Number (%)	Reference
Ireland	1986–90	Hospital admissions	adult	467	60 (8.6)	Coakley et al., 1994
New Zealand	1989	Emergency Department	adult	531	56 (10.6)	Buchanan, 1991
New Zealand	1992	Emergency Department	all	622	105 (16.9)	Hall and Curry, 1994
N. Ireland	1976	Emergency Department	not stated	265	2 (0.8)	Kelly and Galloway, 1992
N. Ireland	1980–82	Hospital admissions	adult	1055	107 (10.1)	Murphy et al., 1984b
N. Ireland	1986	Emergency Department	not stated	228	21 (9.2)	Kelly and Galloway, 1992
N. Ireland	not stated	Hospital admissions	adult	100	39 (39.0)	McNicholl, 1992
Norway	1978	Hospital admissions	adult	303	17 (5.6)	Rygnestad, 1989
Norway	1980	Hospital admissions	adult	1125	34 (3.0)	Jacobsen et al., 1984
Norway	1987	Hospital admissions	not stated	425	52 (12.2)	Rygnestad, 1989
Scotland	1970–79	Hospital admissions	adult	2204	214 (9.7)	Sangster et al., 1981
Scotland	1971–85	Hospital admissions	adult	3516	160 (4.6)	McMurray et al., 1987
Scotland	1972–77	Hospital admissions	adult	1318	119 (9.0)	Lawson and McCallum, 1979
Scotland	1978–79	Hospital admissions	adult	1738	299 (17.2)	Platt et al., 1988
Scotland	1980–81	Hospital admissions	adult	4232	606 (14.3)	Prescott, 1982b
Scotland	1983	Emergency Department	adult	73	11 (15.1)	Willcox, 1985
Scotland	1983–84	Hospital admissions	adult	1598	289 (18.1)	Platt et al., 1988
Scotland	1994	Hospital admissions	adult	2432	885 (36.4)	Prescott, 1995
Spain	1974–80	Intensive Care Unit	adult	91	2 (2.2)	Frati et al., 1983
Spain	1975–85	Intensive Care Unit	not stated	183	5 (2.7)	Manrique Larralde et al., 1988
Switzerland	1981–82	Intensive Care Unit	adult	103	1 (1.0)	Enrico and Buchser, 1983
USA	1975–78	Emergency Department	> 55 yr	61	1 (1.6)	Schernitski et al., 1980
USA	1978	Hospital admissions	not stated	94	4 (4.3)	McGoldrick et al., 1992
USA	1978–79	Emergency Department	all	82	9 (11.0)	Soslow, 1981
USA	1979	Hospital admissions	> 18 yr	92	15 (16.3)	Stein et al., 1993
USA	1986–88	Hospital admissions	adult	133	27 (20.0)	Kerr, 1989
USA	1988	Hospital admissions	not stated	146	9 (6.2)	McGoldrick et al., 1992
USA	1989	Hospital admissions	> 18 yr	91	12 (13.2)	Stein et al., 1993
Wales	1989	Hospital admissions	not stated	1000	(29.0)	Janes and Routledge, 1992

attention to the increasing popularity of paracetamol for poisoning and the increasing occurrence of fatal overdosage (Prescott *et al.*, 1976c; Volans, 1976; Meredith and Goulding, 1980; Whittington and Barclay, 1981; Breen *et al.*, 1982b; Thomas *et al.*, 1983; Osselton *et al.*, 1984; Adams, 1986; McCoy and Trestrail, 1988; Crowe, 1989; Kumar *et al.*, 1990; Ott *et al.*, 1990a; Augustin and Schmoldt, 1991a; Persson, 1991; Farmer, 1994). In Boston, Massachusetts, only 7 per cent of samples from 164 overdose patients seen from 1984 to 1985 were positive for paracetamol (Mahoney *et al.*, 1990) but in a survey of samples submitted for drug screening in Michigan, the detection rate for paracetamol increased from 6.5 per cent in 1977 to 11 per cent in 1986 (McCoy and Trestrail, 1988) and similar results were found in a comparable study in Norway (Rygnestad *et al.*, 1990). Toxicology screening of 177 patients admitted to a trauma service gave a positive result in 72 per cent but only 3 (1.7 per cent) had taken paracetamol (Clark and Harchelroad, 1991). Over a period of five months in 1986, 486 patients were seen with suspected drug overdose including 114 who were thought to have taken paracetamol (23.5 per cent). It was found that 71 (62.3 per cent) of these had insignificant drug concentrations, while of 365 patients who were thought not to have taken paracetamol, significant serum concentrations were detected in seven (1.9 per cent) (Ashbourne *et al.*, 1989). Paracetamol or salicylate were detected in 18.4 per cent of 949 consecutive toxicology requests in 1987 in San Antonio, and again, there was very poor agreement between the drugs found and the drugs expected according to the history from the patients (Schwartz *et al.*, 1990). Other investigators have long been aware of the unreliability of the history given by self-poisoners and attention has been drawn to the lack of correlation between the dose claimed to have been taken and the measured drug concentrations in plasma (Ambre and Alexander, 1977; Prescott, 1978; Shnaps *et al.*, 1980; Read *et al.*, 1986). Paracetamol has become the most popular single agent for self-poisoning in the United Kingdom and in recent reports it was used by 30–40 per cent of patients (Wynne *et al.*, 1987; Platt *et al.*, 1988; Hawton and Fagg, 1992b; Janes and Routledge, 1992; McNicholl, 1992). Of 2432 adult overdose admissions to the Royal Infirmary of Edinburgh during 1994, paracetamol was taken alone or in combination with other drugs in 885 cases (36.4 per cent) (Prescott, 1995). Paracetamol was also the drug taken most frequently by child and adolescent self-poisoners (51 per cent of ingestions) in Tasmania (Tulloch *et al.*, 1994).

Paracetamol accounted for a smaller proportion of telephone enquiries to Poisons Information Services (Table 16.2). Again, the numbers were higher for recent years and as expected, the percentages of calls involving paracetamol were greater when considering enquiries that were confined to drugs. In 1993, there were 4577 calls about drugs to the Scottish Poisons Information Bureau and of these, 609 (13.3 per cent) concerned paracetamol (Prescott, 1995). Paracetamol was frequently taken in combination with other drugs and alcohol, and these often dominated the symptomatology (National Poisons Information Service Monitoring Group, 1981; Breen *et al.*, 1982b; Garnier *et al.*, 1982; Thomas *et al.*, 1983; Bodd *et al.*, 1985; Monteagudo and Folb, 1987; Brotodihardjo *et al.*, 1992; Kelly and Galloway, 1992; Malone *et al.*, 1992). Drug combinations containing paracetamol with barbiturates and narcotic analgesics were also taken by drug abusers (Dawson and Whyte, 1990). There was particular concern about overdosage with combinations of paracetamol plus dextropropoxyphene (e.g. coproxamol) because the latter could cause rapidly fatal cardiorespiratory depression (Carson and Carson, 1976; Sengupta and Peat, 1977; Whittington, 1977; Harvey and Spooner, 1978; Spooner and Harvey, 1978,

Table 16.2 Frequency of enquiries relating to paracetamol poisoning in calls to Poisons Information Services.

Country	Period	Total no. of calls	No. (%) involving paracetamol	Reference
USA	1977–78	1956	230 (11.8)[1]	Saracino *et al.*, 1980
Canada	1980	43 008	661 (1.5)	Freeman and Manoguerra, 1982
France	1974–81	230 000	115 (0.05)	Garnier *et al.*, 1982
France	1974–83	350 000	1600 (0.5)	Bismuth *et al.*, 1983
USA	1981–82	3381	66 (1.9)	Paulozzi, 1983
South Africa	1986–91	1877	265 (14.1)[1]	Müller *et al.*, 1993
Hong Kong	1988–92	255[2]	(7.1)	Chan *et al.*, 1994b
Scotland	1993	4577	609 (13.3)[1]	Prescott, 1995

[1] Enquiries about drugs only; [2] children only

1993; Sangster *et al.*, 1981; Whittington and Barclay, 1981; Dwyer and Jones, 1984; Vale *et al.*, 1984; Hardwicke *et al.*, 1986; Crowe, 1989; Crome, 1993; Farmer, 1994).

Severity of Poisoning and Incidence of Complications

The severity of poisoning with paracetamol as shown by plasma concentration measurements and the incidence of complications and mortality in different reports are summarized in Table 16.3. There was considerable variation, and unfortunately, the results of different studies cannot be compared directly because the selection criteria varied enormously and there were major differences between some investigators in the criteria used to define liver damage and renal failure. In addition, the prognosis was poorer and the incidence of complications higher in early reports when treatment was less effective and specific antidotal therapy was not available. A further complicating factor was associated overdosage with other drugs and this applied particularly to poisoning with the combination of paracetamol and dextropropoxyphene in the United Kingdom. In some series, patients were selected on the basis of high and potentially toxic plasma paracetamol concentrations (Douglas *et al.*, 1976; Vale *et al.*, 1981) while others included seriously poisoned patients who had been referred to specialist units (Clark *et al.*, 1973b; Portmann *et al.*, 1975; Helliwell and Essex, 1981; Harrison *et al.*, 1990b). Not surprisingly, in these reports the incidence of severe liver damage, renal failure and death was high. In contrast, only some 5–20 per cent of unselected hospital patients were at risk of severe liver damage according to the plasma paracetamol concentrations, and in most recent reports a substantially smaller proportion actually suffered this complication (Table 16.3). From 1988–1991, only 15 of 655 overdose admissions to the Prince of Wales Hospital, Hong Kong, required specific antidotal therapy for paracetamol poisoning (Chan *et al.*, 1994c). Similarly, the overall incidence of renal failure was very low. The reports of largely unselected patients give a balanced picture of the outcome of paracetamol poisoning in general, which contrasts sharply with the impression of inevitably disastrous hepatic and renal toxicity implied by numerous dramatic case

Table 16.3 Severity and complications of poisoning in patients admitted to hospital with paracetamol overdose.

Country	Period	Age	Total no. of patients	No. (%) at risk of liver damage[1]	No. (%) with liver damage[2]	No. of deaths	No. (%) with renal failure	Reference
Scotland	1968–70	adult	41	–	10 (24.4)	1	1 (2.4)	Proudfoot and Wright, 1970
England	1971–72	adult	60	–	49 (81.7)	12	6 (10.0)	Clark et al., 1973b
England	1974–75	adult	155	20 (12.9)	8 (5.2)	3	–	James et al., 1975
England	1966–74	adult	220	–	200 (90.1)	29	–	Portmann et al., 1975
England	not stated	not stated	38	38 (100)	12 (31.6)	2	4 (10.5)	Douglas et al., 1976
England	1975	not stated	775[3]	50 (6.5)	–	10	–	Goulding et al., 1976
USA	1976–77	not stated	45	–	5 (11.1)	1	3 (6.7)	Cohen and Burk, 1978
England	1974–75	adult	201	16 (8.0)	14 (7.9)[4]	7	2 (1.1)	Hamlyn et al., 1978
USA	1973–76	<5 yr	16	2 (12.5)	0	0	–	Rumack and Peterson, 1978
Israel	1977–79	adult	22	0	0	0	0	Shnaps et al., 1980
England	not stated	not stated	73	–	47 (64.4)	14	–	Helliwell and Essex, 1981
England	1978–79	all	173	20 (11.6)	–	1[5]	–	NPIS,[6] 1981
England	1974–79	adult	132	132 (100)[7]	24 (18.2)	2	3 (0.8)	Vale et al., 1981
Australia	1977–81	adult	103	–	4 (3.9)	1[5]	1 (1.0)	Breen et al., 1982b
France	1974–81	all	75	–	0	0	0	Garnier et al., 1982
Scotland	1969–72	adult	360	57 (15.8)	28 (7.8)	3	3 (0.8)	Prescott, 1983
Norway	1980	not stated	34	–	0	0	–	Jacobsen et al., 1984
USA	1976–84	1–6 yr	417	55 (13.2)	3 (0.7)	0	0	Rumack, 1984
Norway	1981–82	adult	130	7 (5.4)	0	0	0	Bodd et al., 1985

Israel	1978–83	all	49	2 (10.0)[8]	0	0	Levy and Oren, 1985
Denmark	1980–84	adult	95	26 (27.4)	13 (13.7)	0	Jensen, 1986
England	1982	not stated	100	16 (16.0)	6 (6.0)	–	Read et al., 1986
England	1982–83	not stated	147[9]	–	–	83	Read et al., 1986
Scotland	1971–85	adult	116	15 (12.9)	–	–	McMurray et al., 1987
South Africa	1981–85	adult	91	39 (42.9)	14 (15.4)	4 (4.4)	Monteagudo and Folb, 1987
USA	1976–85	all	11195	1462 (13.1)	395 (3.5)	28	Smilkstein et al., 1988
France	1985–88	not stated	114	5 (4.4)	2	2	Harry et al., 1989
England	1987–88	adult	273	62 (50.4)[10]	148 (54.2)[11]	–	Jones et al., 1989
England	1986–89	adult	150[9]	–	–	72	Harrison et al., 1990b
Scotland	1974–86	child	140	1 (0.8)	0	0	Kumar et al., 1990
France	1982–88	not stated	61	3 (4.9)	2 (3.3)	1[12]	Weber et al., 1990b
Australia	1985–90	all	306	–	21 (6.9)	5 (1.6)	Brotodihardjo et al., 1992
Israel	1984–89	all	89[13]	6 (6.7)	0	0	Oren and Levy, 1992
Hong Kong	1989–91	adult	104	11 (10.6)	6 (5.8)	0	Chan et al., 1993
England	not stated	all	333	75 (22.5)	13 (3.9)	3	Spooner and Harvey, 1993
USA	1982	adult	28	10 (35.7)	0	0	Ros and Conrad, 1994
USA	1986–87	child	866	3 (0.3)	–	–	Bond et al., 1994

[1] As defined by plasma aminotransferase activity exceeding 1000 units l^{-1} but defined differently by different authors – see original text; [2] usually with plasma paracetamol concentrations; [3] enquiries to National Poisons Information Service; [4] 14 of 178 patients; [5] multiple drugs; [6] National Poisons Information Service Monitoring Group; [7] all severely poisoned and treated with methionine; [8] two of 20 patients in whom measurements were made; [9] selected patients referred with liver damage; [10] 62 of 125 patients; [11] plasma aspartate aminotransferase >45 u l^{-1}; [12] other nephrotoxic analgesics taken; [13] only 34 patients admitted

reports. In overdose, paracetamol could undoubtedly cause serious and fatal toxicity but this was uncommon and was now essentially confined to patients who did not receive early treatment with N-acetylcysteine or methionine.

Mortality

The primary cause of death from poisoning with paracetamol was hepatic failure and the risk depended on many factors including other drugs taken, and the availability of effective treatment. Cysteamine was introduced in 1974 (Prescott *et al.*, 1974), and methionine and N-acetylcysteine had come into general use by the end of the decade. In England and Wales, the official number of hospital admissions for paracetamol overdose rose from 150 in 1968 to 7000 in 1973, and deaths attributed to the taking of paracetamol alone rose over this period from 6 to 77 annually (Volans, 1976). The number of deaths thought to be caused by paracetamol alone increased to 144 in 1977 (Meredith *et al.*, 1981), 152 in 1980 (Meredith and Vale, 1984) and 176 in 1984 (Meredith *et al.*, 1986). Other data from the Office of Population Censuses and Surveys concerning the numbers of deaths in England and Wales caused by paracetamol poisoning indicated higher rates rising from 111 in 1973 to 559 in 1980 (Osselton *et al.*, 1984). From 1976 to 1980, the total number of deaths involving paracetamol in England and Wales was put at 959, and of these 641 (66.8 per cent) were attributed to paracetamol as a single substance. From 1986 to 1990 the corresponding figures were 1515 and 839 (55.4 per cent) (Farmer, 1994).

Fatalities from paracetamol overdose in the USA seemed to be uncommon. Only three deaths in 2410 cases were recorded from 1973 to 1975 (0.12 per cent) (Rumack and Peterson, 1978), and according to the American Association of Poison Control Centers Data Collection System reports for 1988–1991, in a total of 396 505 exposures to paracetamol there were only 253 deaths (0.06 per cent) (Litovitz *et al.*, 1989, 1990, 1991, 1992). In a survey of exposure to paracetamol from the same source in 1984, there were 10 deaths in reports on 2637 adults (0.4 per cent) but no deaths in 2231 children (Veltri and Rollins, 1988). Young children rarely ingested large doses themselves and this probably explains the low incidence of severe and fatal liver damage in this age group (Meredith *et al.*, 1978b; Rumack and Peterson, 1978; Meredith and Goulding, 1980; Peterson and Rumack, 1981; Volans, 1991). Up to 1977 there was only one recorded childhood death from paracetamol in the United Kingdom (Fraser, 1980). In Denmark, greatly increased sales of paracetamol over the period 1978–1986 were accompanied by an increase in the number of hospital admissions for overdosage from 26 to 202 with a corresponding increase in mortality (Ott *et al.*, 1990a,b). From 1982 to 1984, there were 19 deaths attributed wholly or partly to paracetamol poisoning (Jensen *et al.*, 1987). There was a marked increase in the number of deaths in which paracetamol was detected at legal examinations in south Florida over the period 1972–1981. Of a total of 95 such deaths, a fatal outcome was attributed to a variety of drugs in 40 cases, but to paracetamol in only four cases (Thomas *et al.*, 1983). In a similar analysis of 142 deaths in New Zealand from 1975 to 1987, only two were caused by an overdose of paracetamol (Cairns *et al.*, 1983). The number of deaths in Leeds, UK, attributed to paracetamol from 1977 to 1987 fluctuated from year to year and the total numbers for paracetamol and aspirin over this period were 27 and 35 respectively (Crowe, 1989). From

1983 to 1992, non-narcotic analgesics accounted for 10.8 per cent of 352 fatal overdoses in Edinburgh and paracetamol was responsible for 73.5 per cent of these (Obafunwa and Busuttil, 1994). A toxicological survey of 73 suicides in southern Sweden in 1989 revealed paracetamol in 15 cases but it was not known to what extent it contributed to the outcome (Alsén *et al.*, 1994).

The official mortality data for paracetamol have been exaggerated by the inclusion of deaths caused by dextropropoxyphene taken with it in combined preparations despite evidence that the dextropropoxyphene had a far more immediate and dangerous effect than paracetamol (Sengupta and Peat, 1977). It was pointed out that hepatic necrosis was present in only a minority of deaths officially attributed to paracetamol, and that a significant proportion of deaths occurred suddenly outside hospital (Dixon, 1976). In contrast, death from paracetamol-induced hepatic failure was delayed and almost always occurred in hospital. Dextropropoxyphene was a prime suspect in these early deaths and it was clear that the official numbers of deaths attributed to paracetamol were overestimated by a substantial margin (Harvey and Spooner, 1978). Subsequent analyses of the deaths recorded as caused by paracetamol confirmed that many deaths had been wrongly attributed and had in fact been caused by dextropropoxyphene (Lesna, 1978; Meredith and Goulding, 1980; Dwyer and Jones, 1984; Meredith and Vale, 1984; Vale *et al.*, 1984; Spooner and Harvey, 1993). Half of the deaths recorded as being due to paracetamol and a quarter of the deaths attributed to paracetamol with dextropropoxyphene could not be substantiated when subjected to independent scrutiny. In 1979 and 1983, 41 per cent of 317 patients who were thought to have died from paracetamol alone did so either outside hospital or on arrival there. In 119 of 130 such patients who died outside hospital there was no evidence of hepatic necrosis at necropsy (Meredith *et al.*, 1986). The official returns for deaths alleged to be caused by paracetamol from 1975 to 1990 in England and Wales were reassessed according to whether or not there was hepatic necrosis and whether death occurred outside hospital or immediately on arrival. The results of this analysis are shown in Figure 16.1. It was calculated that over the period 1975–1990, a total of 1514 deaths might properly have been attributed to paracetamol whereas the official total of 7671 represented about a five-fold overestimate (Spooner and Harvey, 1993). In 1987, of 957 deaths from drug overdosage in England and Wales, 124 (12.9 per cent) were caused by the combination of paracetamol and dextropropoxyphene while 101 (10.6 per cent) were attributed to paracetamol alone (Crome, 1993). The picture was somewhat different with deaths occurring in unselected hospital overdose patients where the mortality, although variable, was now considerably less than 1 per cent (Table 16.3). Before effective treatment became available in 1974, the mortality from liver failure in unselected hospital patients in Scotland and England was 1–3 per cent and less than 10 per cent of patients suffered severe liver damage with plasma aminotransferase activity exceeding 1000 units l^{-1} (Table 16.4) (Hamlyn *et al.*, 1978; Prescott, 1983). Avoidable factors often contributed to mortality in patients with paracetamol overdose, and the most important were delays in starting specific treatment and in referral to specialist centres (Canalese *et al.*, 1981a). Current figures suggested that paracetamol was involved in about 500 overdose deaths per annum in England and Wales, but that in only about 150 was death due to paracetamol-induced hepatic failure (Bray, 1993; Makin and Williams, 1994). Paracetamol poisoning was the commonest cause of acute liver failure in the UK and it accounted for 250 of 342

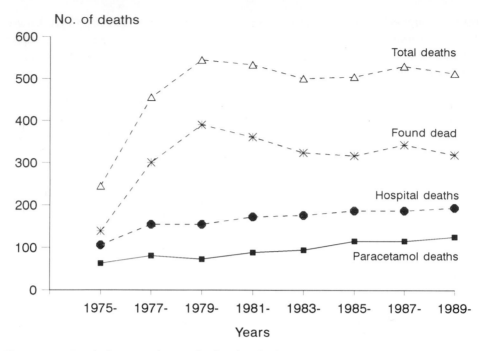

Figure 16.1 Deaths from suicide in England and Wales from 1975 to 1990 attributed to paracetamol and classified according to whether the victims were found dead, or whether they died in hospital from paracetamol toxicity or other causes. Only the cases classified as paracetamol deaths had hepatic necrosis at post-mortem examination (data from Spooner and Harvey, 1993).

cases (73 per cent) admitted to the Liver Failure Unit at King's College Hospital London during 1992–1994 (Williams, 1994). Once fulminant hepatic failure developed, the prognosis was very poor. Over the period 1973–1988, 396 such patients were referred to King's College Hospital and the overall mortality rate was 61 per cent. Of 99 patients admitted during 1986–1988, 60 per cent developed acute renal failure requiring dialysis (Bray *et al.*, 1992a). There have been important advances in

Table 16.4 Complications and mortality in patients with paracetamol overdosage in Newcastle upon Tyne and Edinburgh not receiving specific antidotal therapy.[1]

No. of patients	No. severely poisoned[2]	No. with severe liver damage	No. of deaths in hepatic failure	No. with renal failure[3]
Newcastle upon Tyne, 1974–1975				
180	29 (16%)	14 (7.8%)[4]	7 (3.9%)	2 (1.1%)
Edinburgh, 1969–1972				
360	57 (16%)	28 (7.8%)[5]	3 (0.8%)	3 (0.8%)

[1] From Prescott, 1983; [2] plasma paracetamol concentrations above line joining plots of 200 mg l^{-1} at 4 h and 30 mg l^{-1} at 15 h on a semilogarithmic graph; [3] requiring dialysis; [4] plasma aspartate aminotransferase >600 u l^{-1}; [5] plasma asparate aminotransferase >1000 u l^{-1}

the treatment of fulminant hepatic failure, and the survival rate in patients with grade III–IV encephalopathy caused by paracetamol overdose has now increased to 64 per cent (Williams, 1994).

Preventive Measures

In attempts to reduce the problems caused by children taking paracetamol, child resistant containers were introduced in the UK in 1976 (Ferguson *et al.*, 1992). In some countries the number of tablets that could be purchased in a single pack was restricted as a preventative measure (Bismuth *et al.*, 1983; Bodd *et al.*, 1985; Garnier and Bismuth, 1993) and another factor that limited intake in France was the popularity of an effervescent formulation, which was physically difficult to take in a large dose (Garnier *et al.*, 1982; Garnier and Bismuth, 1993). Perhaps as a result of these measures, paracetamol poisoning was much less of a problem in France than in the UK. This was illustrated by the lack of reports of fatal overdoses in children in France, but three deaths had occurred in young foreigners all of whom had bought their tablets in other countries (Bismuth *et al.*, 1983). Paracetamol was used extensively as a single analgesic in the UK and as a result large doses could be ingested by self-poisoners. In contrast, in countries such as Germany, serious toxicity was said to be much less of a problem because paracetamol was marketed largely in combination with other analgesics and this limited the dose in each tablet and hence the amount taken in overdose (Forth, 1993). The use of paracetamol lozenges that were difficult to swallow was also proposed as a means of limiting the amount that could be taken (Mahadeva *et al.*, 1986).

Children

The causes of paracetamol poisoning in children differed according to age. Up to about 1 year, poisoning was usually the consequence of the misguided administration of excessive doses, often repeated, by parents and doctors while from 1 to 5 years, it was usually accidental when paracetamol was left within reach and found and eaten by an inquisitive child. With increasing age above 5 years, paracetamol was taken deliberately more and more for manipulative purposes in the same way as adults (Levy and Oren, 1985; Jonville *et al.*, 1988, 1990; Veltri and Rollins, 1988; Kumar *et al.*, 1990; Melis and Bochner, 1990). Accidental poisoning was commonest in the 2–3-year-old age group (Rumack, 1984). Although paracetamol poisoning in older children generally did not result in serious toxicity, the administration of excessive doses by parents to young children has caused severe and fatal liver damage especially when doses were repeated (Calvert and Linder, 1978; Nogen and Bremner, 1978; Weber and Cutz, 1980; Montoya Cabrera *et al.*, 1982; Agran *et al.*, 1983; Clark *et al.*, 1983; Greene *et al.*, 1983; Swetnam and Florman, 1984; Smith *et al.*, 1986a; Blake *et al.*, 1988; de Nardo *et al.*, 1988; Henretig *et al.*, 1989; Litovitz *et al.*, 1989; Augustin and Schmoldt, 1991a; Chiossi *et al.*, 1991; Campbell and Oates, 1992; Chao, 1993; Douidar *et al.*, 1994; Zwiener *et al.*, 1994). In the light of these reports, it was suggested that the margin of safety of paracetamol in this age group might be lower than appreciated (Penna and Buchanan, 1991). However, as discussed in Chapter 14, in most cases the amounts administered represented gross overdosage. Dosing errors with liquid formulations were common, but they did not often result in toxicity (Litovitz, 1992). Over the period 1958–1977, 598 deaths from accidental poisoning in children were recorded in the UK but only one was caused by paracetamol (Fraser, 1980).

From 1975 to 1977, the National Poisons Information Service in London received 3139 calls about paracetamol and 580 of these referred to children aged less than 13 years. Further information was available on 116 children and only 3 of 56 had potentially toxic plasma paracetamol concentrations. Two children, aged 11 and 13 years, suffered severe liver damage (Meredith *et al.*, 1978b, 1979). Thirteen cases of accidental poisoning in children with paracetamol and four due to dosing errors were reported among 230 000 calls made to the Centre Anti-Poisons de Paris from 1974 to 1981. There were no complications (Garnier *et al.*, 1982). Of 101 enquiries about children taking paracetamol in Tours from 1983 to 1986, 15 per cent were less than 1 year old, 70 per cent were between 1 and 5 years of age and 15 per cent were more than 5 years old. The amounts ingested were small and there was no toxicity (Jonville *et al.*, 1988, 1990). In the UK in 1978 and 1979, poisoning was confirmed by toxicological analysis in 95 of 287 children aged between 10 days and 14 years, and salicylate or paracetamol were encountered in 15 per cent of cases (Flanagan *et al.*, 1981a). Analgesics were taken by 28.1 per cent of 6562 children under the age of 6 years admitted to hospital for poisoning from 1975 to 1986. Aspirin was taken most often at the beginning of this period and paracetamol at the end (Ferguson *et al.*, 1992). Children accounted for 13 of 49 patients (26.5 per cent) admitted to hospital in Jerusalem with paracetamol poisoning from 1973 to 1983 (Levy and Oren, 1985), but in a later study from Australia, paracetamol was only involved in 7 of 306 admissions of children to hospital for drug overdose (Brotodihardjo *et al.*, 1992). Of 130 hospital overdose patients in Norway with blood samples found to contain paracetamol, only two were children aged less than 2 years (Bodd *et al.*, 1985). In Antwerp, 896 children were admitted to hospital for poisoning from 1980 to 1988 but only 12 had taken paracetamol (Melis and Bochner, 1990), while in an Australian report covering the period 1983–1988, only 27 of 407 similar paediatric admissions (7 per cent) involved paracetamol (Campbell and Oates, 1992). Of 417 children under the age of 6 years, 55 (13.2 per cent) were at risk of hepatotoxicity with plasma paracetamol concentrations above a 'treatment line' on a semilogarithmic graph joining the points of 200 mg l^{-1} at 4 h and 50 mg l^{-1} at 12 h after ingestion. Three of these children had severe liver damage with plasma aminotransferase activity exceeding 1000 units l^{-1} but, in all, treatment with N-acetylcysteine had been delayed for more than 16 h (Rumack, 1984). In other studies paediatric poisoning with paracetamol was relatively benign (Kumar *et al.*, 1990) and, of 77 cases seen over three years in Montreal, 24 were admitted to hospital and one was treated in an intensive care unit (Lacroix *et al.*, 1989). Analgesics topped the list of drugs in reports of poisoning in children under the age of 6 years made to American Poison Control Centres during 1990–1992 (Woolf and Lovejoy, 1993) but there were only six instances of major toxicity in a total of 2171 exposures to paracetamol in children (Litovitz and Manoguerra, 1992). In another report on an estimated 19 000 children exposed to paracetamol in 1986 and 1987, only 2091 were referred to hospital. Of these, the records of only 866 could be assessed and according to timed measurements of the plasma paracetamol concentrations, only three were at risk of toxicity (Bond *et al.*, 1994).

Clinical Features

During the first few hours after ingestion of a hepatotoxic dose of paracetamol there were no specific early symptoms or signs to indicate the severity of intoxication. Anorexia, nausea and vomiting usually developed within a few hours followed by right upper quadrant abdominal pain and hepatic tenderness. The vomiting usually subsided within 24–48 h but it could be protracted and compromise oral treatment with N-acetylcysteine (Maurer and Zeisler, 1978; Melethil *et al.*, 1981; Sutherland *et al.*, 1981; Smith, 1986; Robertson *et al.*, 1986; Foust *et al.*, 1989; Price *et al.*, 1991; Bonfiglio *et al.*, 1992; Reed and Marx, 1994). Hepatic tenderness could persist for 36–72 h, by which time mild jaundice was often apparent. In most patients there were no further complications and recovery was rapid and complete (Rose, 1969; Proudfoot and Wright, 1970; Matthew, 1973; Ferguson *et al.*, 1977; Williams and Davis, 1977; Cohen and Burk, 1978; Prescott, 1978, 1983; Leen and Welsby, 1984; Weber *et al.*, 1990b; van Vyve *et al.*, 1993; and many others). Drowsiness was often mentioned as a presenting feature, but this was probably more a reflection of the expectations of the patient and the medical attendants than any effect of the drug. There was no early impairment of consciousness unless alcohol or other central nervous system depressants were taken except in rare cases of very severe poisoning with acidosis and exceptionally high plasma paracetamol concentrations above 800–1000 mg l^{-1} (Zezulka and Wright, 1982; Flanagan and Mant, 1986). In the latter circumstances impaired consciousness and coma were usually of short duration and there were no characteristic neurological findings. In one isolated case coma was associated with hypotension and respiratory depression requiring endotracheal intubation and mechanical ventilation suggesting intake of other drugs while in others there was hyperventilation (Zezulka and Wright, 1982; Flanagan and Mant, 1986). Depression of consciousness with very high plasma paracetamol concentrations was associated with hypothermia in a 1-year-old child (Lieh-Lai *et al.*, 1984), but in other cases, hypothermia with coma and respiratory acidosis were more likely to have been caused by dextropropoxyphene, codeine, ethanol, nitrazepam and other depressant drugs that had been taken with the paracetamol (van Heijst *et al.*, 1976; Pond *et al.*, 1982b; Hartnell *et al.*, 1983; Kritharides *et al.*, 1988; Block *et al.*, 1992).

In a minority of severely poisoned patients (now essentially those who present too late for effective treatment with N-acetylcysteine or methionine), acute liver failure supervened after 3–6 days with deepening jaundice, and drowsiness, asterixis, tremor, confusion and delirium progressing to coma. Associated findings included hypoglycaemia, metabolic acidosis, hyperventilation, cerebral oedema, renal failure, sepsis, disseminated intravascular coagulation, haemorrhage and terminal cardiac arrhythmias (Davidson and Eastham, 1966; MacLean *et al.*, 1968a; Pimstone and Uys, 1968; Rose, 1969; Toghill *et al.*, 1969; Clark *et al.*, 1973b; Davis and Williams, 1975; Williams and Davis, 1977; Canalese *et al.*, 1981a; Sutherland *et al.*, 1981; Wakeel *et al.*, 1987; Thornton and Losowsky, 1989; Navelet *et al.*, 1990; and others). Convulsions were probably related to hypoglycaemia (Sørensen *et al.*, 1986; Olson *et al.*, 1994), and in one case pre-existing cerebral atrophy was an additional factor (Sakai *et al.*, 1987). Even in specialist liver units, the prognosis of paracetamol-induced fulminant hepatic failure was poor, but it has improved steadily over the years (Williams and Davis, 1977; Canalese *et al.*, 1981a; Gimson *et al.*, 1983; O'Grady *et al.*, 1988, 1989, 1991; Harrison *et al.*, 1990a,b; Bray *et al.*, 1991,

Table 16.5 Some reported cases of liver damage following paracetamol overdosage.

Age and sex	Alleged dose (g)	Plasma paracetamol (mg l⁻¹)	Time after ingestion (h)	Max. plasma amino-transferase (units l⁻¹)	Max. plasma bilirubin (μmol l⁻¹)	Max. prothrombin time ratio	Histology[1]	Treatment[2]	Comments	Reference
54M	35	760	?	216	75	–	–	–	impaired glucose tolerance	Thomson and Prescott, 1966
40F	30	–	–	7000	100	2.3	AHN	HF	fatal hepatorenal failure	MacLean et al., 1968a
41M	12.5	–	–	>8000	100	1.6	AHN	–	cardiac abnormalities	MacLean et al., 1968a
26F	?	–	–	2320	177	76%[3]	AHN	HF	fatal hepatic failure	Pimstone and Uys, 1968
46M	37	–	–	–	95	–	AHN	–	diuresis, fatal	Rose, 1969
37M	25	–	–	>2000	21	12%[3]	–	–		Rose, 1969
33F	35	–	–	–	120	2.4	AHN	HF	fatal hepatic failure	Toghill et al., 1969
29F	?	–	–	4000	93	5%[3]	AHN		renal failure	Boyer and Rouff, 1971
19F	20	18	10	1350	27	2.9	–	–	ECG changes	Will and Tomkins, 1971
34M	75	–	–	>4000	78	11%[3]	–	–	given prednisone	Chakrabarti and Lloyd, 1973
26F	25	–	–	1190	83	–	–	–		Benson and Boleyn, 1974
25F	45	30	48	10000	365	3.2	AHN	HF[4]	recovered hepatic failure	Benson and Boleyn, 1974
22F	20	40	8	normal	–	–	–	D,P	no liver damage	Benson and Boleyn, 1974
59M	90	152	36	>2000	88	2.5	AHN	HF,D	fatal hepatic failure	Benson and Boleyn, 1974
30F	?	–	–	1250	612	–	AHN	–	fatal hepatorenal failure	Alván et al., 1976
16M	51	9	?	3200	58	20%[3]	CF[5]	MET		Andersson et al., 1976
88F	?	–	–	5000	?	30%[3]	–	–	dextropropoxyphene	Commandre et al., 1976
24F	13	–	–	8795	202	5.0	AHN	HF	fatal hepatic failure	McJunkin et al., 1976
32F	25	220	?	2920	37	–	AHN	CYS	fatal hepatic failure	van Heijst et al., 1976
41F	25	15000[6]	?	4137	140	1.5	–	–	pancreatitis	Coward, 1977
21F	23	–	–	3302	22	1.4	–	–		Ferguson et al., 1977
16F	5.9	–	–	4750	26	40%[3]	–	–		Fernandez and Fernandez-Brito, 1977
26M	30	160	5.5	??	32	1.4	–	MET		Fitzgerald and Drury, 1977
31F	60	–	–	300	102	5.2	–	–	renal failure, pancreatitis	Gilmore and Tourvas, 1977
18F	?	–	–	12000	43	–	–	–	other drugs	Groarke et al., 1977
25F	?	–	–	60	–	–	–	–		Groarke et al., 1977
18F	?	1082[7]	12	644	–	20%[3]	–	CYS	coma, other drugs	Jones and Thomas, 1977
24M	32.5	9.5	20	3900	27	1.3	–	AR		Krenzelok et al., 1977
54F	36	–	–	2800	450	2.5	–	HF	renal failure	Merritt and Joyner, 1977
26F	16	–	–	350	–	–	–	NAC		Peterson and Rumack, 1977
31M	55	–	–	2814	38	32%[3]	AHN	MET		Vilstrup et al., 1977
16M	18.2	–	–	9248	–	–	–	–		Antaki et al., 1978
3½F	11.3	94	24	20376	22	1.6	–	–		Arena et al., 1978
30F	24	–	–	160	3	1.3	–	NAC		Carloss et al., 1978

Patient	Age					Ratio	Histology	Treatment	Comments	Reference
27F	25	–	–	140	3	1.9	–	NAC		Carloss et al., 1978
24F	?	–	–	240	2	1.2	–	NAC		Carloss et al., 1978
19F	?	?	–	8540	–	5.4	AHN	HF	fatal hepatic failure	Carloss et al., 1978
20F	33	?	71	>5000	560	4.2	CF	–	recovered hepatic failure	Cohen and Burk, 1978
17F	15	–	–	>2750	21	3.2	AHN	–		Cohen and Burk, 1978
21F	30	18	–	9760	44	2.5	AHN	–	renal failure	Cohen and Burk, 1978
45F	?	–	145	>500	70	4.5	AHN	–	fatal hepatorenal failure	Cohen and Burk, 1978
63F	24	7	–	460	190	3.5	AHN	–	fatal hepatic failure	Kim and Dillman, 1978
19M	23	21	170	281	12	53%[3]	–	NAC		Maurer and Zeisler, 1978
26M	?	?	145	10000	252	>3.4	CF, CS	NAC[8]	31 paracetamol overdoses	Prescott et al., 1978a
53M	?	?	50	2800	92	5%[3]	AHN	–	fatal	Reikvam and Skjoto, 1978
47F	25	20	223	3195	–	–	AHN	CYS	fatal, dextropropoxyphene	Reikvam and Skjoto, 1978
21F	60	2	100	2682	–	–	–	NAC[8]	hyperpyrexia, salicylate	Reikvam and Skjoto, 1978
53	27	18	460[7]	148	77	1.6	–	NAC	unnecessary haemodialysis	Rigby et al., 1978
34F	?	?	214	4360	77	1.3	AHN	MET		Scalley and Conner, 1978
20F	15	–	–	9550	–	–	–	–	therapeutic abortion	Silverman and Carithers, 1978
20M	55	17	–	45	–	?	AHN	HP	anorexia nervosa	Newman and Bargman, 1979
31M	25	?	–	2800	98	–	AHN	–		Petersen and Vilstrup, 1979
21F	?	?	100	2682	55	2.9	–	NAC	hyperpyrexia, salicylate	Skjoto and Reikvam, 1979
31F	?	12	75	10860	146	3.3	–	NAC	histology inexplicable	Arthurs and Fielding, 1980
69F	?	?	150	393	51	5	CAH, CH	–	hypothermia, barbiturates	Helliwell, 1980
50F	?	?	290	>8000	21	1	–	NAC	fatal, other drugs	Hutchinson et al., 1980
26M	16	?	1860[6]	146	54	4.2	–	NAC	renal failure	Kleinman et al., 1980
22F	25	70	760[6]	>1500	83	1.9	–	–		Golden et al., 1981
21M	11.7	19	3	9040	80	3.9	–	NAC		Golden et al., 1981
19F	50	7.5	32	11720	92	?	–	NAC	renal failure	Jeffery and Lafferty, 1981
19F	15	?	–	4040	–	?	–	NAC[8]	renal failure	Jeffery and Lafferty, 1981
26M	26	?	260000[6]	3660	–	?	–	NAC[8]		Melethil et al., 1981
15F	30	?	165	8280	–	4.8	AHN	CYS[8]	fatal hepatic failure	Sutherland et al., 1981
45?	25	–	48	732	–	17%[3]	–	–	renal failure	Cobden et al., 1982
18?	50	?	124	>1000	–	41%[3]	–	–	renal failure	Cobden et al., 1982
23F	17	?	34	>2000	–	29%[3]	–	–	renal failure	Cobden et al., 1982
20?	25	?	–	8440	–	27%[3]	–	–	renal failure	Cobden et al., 1982
41?	29	–	–	260	–	21%[3]	–	–	renal failure	Cobden et al., 1982
26?	10	?	390	3980	–	70%[3]	–	–	renal failure	Cobden et al., 1982
38?	50	?	226	>5000	–	28%[3]	–	–	renal failure	Cobden et al., 1982
17?	11	–	–	4200	–	33%[3]	–	–	renal failure	Cobden et al., 1982
19?	30	–	328	2150	–	24%[3]	–	NAC[8]	renal failure	Cobden et al., 1982
25?	50	?	–	–	–	12%[3]	–	–	renal failure	Cobden et al., 1982
36F	30	?	60	2284	14	1.3	–	–	renal failure	Curry et al., 1982

Table 16.5 (cont.)

Age and sex	Alleged dose (g)	Plasma paracetamol (mg l⁻¹)	Time after ingestion (h)	Max. plasma amino-transferase (units l⁻¹)	Max. plasma bilirubin (μmol l⁻¹)	Max prothrombin time ratio	Histology[1]	Treatment[2]	Comments	Reference
3M	3	112	4	16 280	34	–	–	NAC[8]	accidental overdose	Czajka and Whitington, 1982
47F	?	680	?	5760	–	–	–	NAC	coma, other drugs	Farah et al., 1982
21F	25	316	8	16 400	–	–	–	CYS	renal failure	Harris, 1982
28F	58	485	22	>7000	94	40%[3]	–	NAC[8]	hypothermia, many drugs	Pond et al., 1982b
43F	?	1150	?	312	–	4.1	–	NAC	died, brain haemorrhage	Raper et al., 1982
28M	16	18	21	1296	–	–	FN	–	fatal paraquat overdose	Siefkin, 1982
56F	75	959	11.5	258	44	1.6	–	NAC	acidosis	Zezulka and Wright, 1982
38F	10	–	–	–		48%[3]	AHN	–	renal failure	Baumgarten et al., 1983
53M	50	260	14	44	normal	1.5	–	–	hypothermia, other drugs	Hartnell et al., 1983
22F	32.5	159	?	4300	30	1.7	–	MET	delivered normal infant	Lederman et al., 1983
26F	15	58	20	3000	–	11%[3]	–	–	renal failure	Stegeman-Castelen et al., 1983
22F	4.8	–	–	>10 000	37	1.5	AHN	GSH	also haemodialysis	Wakushima et al., 1983
1M	10	863	5	5520	130	–	–	NAC		Lieh-Lai et al., 1984
17F	25	236	8	4572	64	41%[3]	–	NAC		Stokes, 1984
19F	10	16	18	16 336	66	2.8	–	NAC[8]	renal failure	Dabbagh and Chesney, 1985
50F	80	476	?	119	–	–	–	NAC	also MET, other drugs	Jorgensen, 1985
19M	25	62	21	>2000	–	–	–	NAC[8]	laparotomy, pancreatitis	Caldarola et al., 1986
51F	75	725	20	776	–	–	–	–	other drugs, died, ?cause	Clark et al., 1986
54M	50	302	48	7870	–	–	–	–		Clark et al., 1986
26F	40	45	36	<6000	–	–	–	–	hepatorenal failure	Clark et al., 1986
45F	?	1100	34	123	30	–	–	–	coma, acidosis	Flanagan and Mant, 1986
59F	?	950	4	243	–	2.3	–	MET	acidosis, coma	Flanagan and Mant, 1986
50F	?	900	?	–	–	–	–	–	hepatorenal failure	Flanagan and Mant, 1986
80F	?	1140	?	–	–	1.3	–	NAC	fatal hepatic failure	Flanagan and Mant, 1986
17M	100	950	5	normal	–	1.8	–	NAC	acidosis, coma	Flanagan and Mant, 1986
32F	64	198	10	5720	206	3.3	–	NAC[8]	15-week pregnancy	Ludmir et al., 1986
19M	42	230	9	1160	–	normal	–	NAC		Smith, 1986
16F	15	79	?	11 700	–	2.2	–	–	taking anticonvulsants	Smith et al., 1986b
60F	25	60	34	>800	–	14%[3]	AHN	HF	fatal hepatic failure	Sorensen et al., 1986
17F	29	–	–	9950	39	30%[3]	–	–		Bell et al., 1987b
39M	36	–	–	11 520	110	17%[3]	–	–	renal failure	Bell et al., 1987b
56F	20	24	24	10 670	55	40%[3]	–	–		Bell et al., 1987b
44F	30	–	–	4695	26	24%[3]	–	–	renal failure, fatal	Bell et al., 1987b
25F	20	–	–	5076	23	30%[3]	–	–		Bell et al., 1987b

Age/sex									Clinical features	Reference
36M	25	—	—	23 660	128	7%[3]	—	—	fatal	Bell et al., 1987b
27F	?	12	?	11 439	29	—	—	—		Jakobsen et al., 1987
8F	?	408	17	16 000	137	5%[3]	AHN	NAC	fatal hepatic failure	Jakobsen et al., 1987
30F	?	385	?	2529	88	—	AHN	NAC	drug abuse, fatal	Jakobsen et al., 1987
39F	?	—	—	3360	56	2.7	AHN	HF	drug abuse, renal failure	Sakai et al., 1987
15F	?	41	55	1075	188	15%[3]	AHN	HF	fatal hepatic failure	Wakeel et al., 1987
27F	24	—	—			—	—	NAC[8]		Belin et al., 1988
37M	23	—	—	88[9]		—	—	—	renal failure	Björck et al., 1988
35F	12.5	130	14	15 456	48	3.9	—	NAC[8]	renal failure	Davenport and Finn, 1988
33M	75	361	8	16 000	69	5.3	—	NAC	renal failure	Davenport and Finn, 1988
30F	?	190	?	4240	725	4.2	—	NAC	hypothermia, renal failure	Kritharides et al., 1988
24M	15.5	—	—	8030	61	23%[3]	—	NAC[8]		Manrique Larralde et al., 1988
26F	30	—	—	3000	26	1.4	—	NAC		McClain et al., 1988
24F	30	235	7	7120	51	—	AHN	NAC		McClain et al., 1988
28F	30	—	—	685	34	1.3	—	NAC		McClain et al., 1988
15F	7.5	—	—	3390		1	—	NAC	renal failure	McClain et al., 1988
16F	10	94	5.5	>5000	48	2.2	—	NAC[8]		McClain et al., 1988
20M	?	37	11	637	103	6.2	AHN	GSH	fatal hepatorenal failure	Minton et al., 1988
84F	?	47	8	119 200	148	—	AHN	NAC[8]		Bartle et al., 1989
24F	4.8	448	12	5269		3.5	AHN	NAC	renal and myocardial failure	Ohtani et al., 1989
22F	50	310	?	217		<10%[3]	—	HF	normal infant delivered	Rosevear and Hope, 1989
19M	39	—	—	5530	114	29%[3]	—	HF	dextropropoxyphene	Ruane et al., 1989
27M	6.4	—	—	6980	60	7.5	—	HF	hepatorenal failure	Shimazaki et al., 1989
36F	3.2	67	18	13 600		10%[3]	—	HF	hepatorenal failure	Shimazaki et al., 1989
43M	25	12	28	9990	126	5.4	—	NAC	fatal bleeding varices	Thornton and Losowsky, 1989
35M	14	2	11	12 230	130	1.8	—	NAC	recovered hepatic failure	Homann et al., 1990
14M	45	250	10	209[9]	106	—	—	—	recovered hepatic failure	McClements et al., 1990
19F	11.5	—	—	12 500	256	10	AHN	NAC[8]	renal failure	Murphy et al., 1990
48M	50	6	21	10 780	546	6.1	—	—	thrombocytopenia	Thornton and Losowsky, 1990
19M	35	5.5	72	7040	44	37%[3]	AHN	—	recovered hepatic failure	Thornton and Losowsky, 1990
21F	16	78	36	5990	189	8%[3]	AHN	—		Weber et al., 1990b
18F	10.5	410	4	8140		3.0	—	LTP	rejection, 'myocarditis'	Hoffmann et al., 1991
34F	11	154	11.5	91	10	—	AHN	NAC	renal failure, 'pancreatitis'	Mofenson et al., 1991
31F	?	253	16	9700		—	—	NAC		Rolband and Marcuard, 1991
16F	15	13	72	54	22	1	—	NAC	fatal hepatic failure	Price et al., 1991
20F	13	131	24	6660		—	—	NAC[8]	other drugs	Bonfiglio et al., 1992
18F	30	—	—	10 571		—	—	LTP	survived liver transplant	Mrvos et al., 1992
16F	?	—	—	18 375	320	2.5	—	LTP	survived liver transplant	Mrvos et al., 1992
32?	85	—	—	3070		3.8	—	GSH	hepatic failure	Yamakawa, 1992
24?	8.6	—	—			—	AHN	—		Yamakawa, 1992

Table 16.5 (cont.)

Age and sex	Alleged dose (g)	Plasma paracetamol (mg l⁻¹)	Time after ingestion (h)	Max. plasma amino-transferase (units l⁻¹)	Max. plasma bilirubin (µmol l⁻¹)	Max prothrombin time ratio	Histology[1]	Treatment[2]	Comments	Reference
29M	50	32	23	6080	38	2.1	–	–	flupenthixol, ECG changes	Armour and Slater, 1993
25F	15	–	–	6623	148	1.8	–	–	Caesarian section	Friedman et al., 1993
17M	31	134	12	11660	29	2.1	–	NAC[8]	renal failure	Knoop et al., 1993
18F	60	10	48	8430	80	4.7	–	LTP	bioartificial liver support	Rozga et al., 1993
24F	12.5	84	15	11000	–	3.3	–	NAC[8]	hypoglycaemia	van Vyve et al., 1993
28M	25	56	24	13480	68	2.9	–	NAC[8]		van Vyve et al., 1993
16F	10	114	?	3270	20	–	–	NAC[8]		Walson and Groth, 1993
18F	20	–	–	11400	140	–	–	NAC[8]	hepatorenal failure	Boberg et al., 1994
18F	14	–	–	8146	–	<10%[3]	–	LTP	rejection, fatal	Boberg et al., 1994
32F	29	106	–	14100	–	17%[3]	–	NAC[8]	renal failure	Boberg et al., 1994
37M	25	146	8	12474	44	3.0	–	–		Fischereder and Jaffe, 1994
41F	142	136	12	7800	–	<8%[3]	–	NAC[8]	fatal hepatic failure	Rump and Keller, 1994
46F	8	3	72	7780	100	5.5	AHN	NAC[8]	recovered hepatic failure	Viallon et al., 1994
37F	17.5	328	7	48	–	–	–	NAC	chronic abuse	Wylie and Fraser, 1994

[1] Histology: AHN = acute hepatic necrosis, CAH = chronic active hepatitis, CF = chronic fibrosis, CH = cirrhosis, CS = cholestasis, FN = focal necrosis; [2] treatment: HF = hepatic failure regime, D = dimercaprol, P = penicillamine, CYS = cysteamine, MET = methionine, AR = arginine, NAC = N-acetylcysteine, GSH = gluthione, LTP = liver transplant; [3] quick, or thrombotest %; [4] also cholestasis and micronodular cirrhosis; [5] no mention of hepatic necrosis; [6] as stated, but incorrect units given; [7] inappropriate method of analysis which also included metabolites; [8] late treatment; [9] µkat l⁻¹

1992a; Keays *et al.*, 1991; Makin and Williams, 1994; Mutimer *et al.*, 1994). Acute renal failure (hepatorenal syndrome) occurred in more than 50 per cent of patients and the incidence in fulminant hepatic failure due to paracetamol poisoning was the same as with other causes (Wilkinson *et al.*, 1977; O'Grady *et al.*, 1988; Makin and Williams, 1994). Acute renal failure could also occur within 24–48 h after ingestion of an overdose of paracetamol and it was not always associated with hepatic failure, or indeed with any biochemical evidence of hepatotoxicity (Proudfoot and Wright, 1970; Clark *et al.*, 1973b; Prescott and Wright, 1973; Prescott, 1978; Kleinman *et al.*, 1980; Cobden *et al.*, 1982; Prescott *et al.*, 1982; Pillans and Hall, 1985; Kher and Makker, 1987; Björck *et al.*, 1988; McClain *et al.*, 1988; Duchene *et al.*, 1991; Jones and Vale, 1993; and others). The delayed onset of acidosis and hypoglycaemia with increasing lethargy, confusion and coma was the normal course of events in paracetamol-induced fulminant hepatic failure but it has been reported as though it were an unusual occurrence (Zabrodski and Schnurr, 1984). This picture of late presentation was typical of patients who arrived in hospital with incipient hepatic failure several days after taking an overdose of paracetamol (Black *et al.*, 1982; McClain *et al.*, 1988; Thornton and Losowsky, 1989). Most patients who presented late were dehydrated and already had severe liver damage and renal failure. A mistaken diagnosis of viral hepatitis could easily be made in less severely poisoned patients who presented with anorexia, vomiting, hepatic tenderness and jaundice (Leen and Welsby, 1984; Roschlau, 1986), and in other cases the possibility of Reye's syndrome was raised on occasion (Little, 1976; Weber and Cutz, 1980; Agran *et al.*, 1983; Smith *et al.*, 1986a; Nesbitt and Minuk, 1988; Augustin and Schmoldt, 1991a,b). Regrettably, some patients with abdominal pain following paracetamol overdosage were referred for surgical opinion and subjected to needless laparotomy or laparoscopy before the correct diagnosis was recognized (Gilmore and Tourvas, 1977; Baumgarten *et al.*, 1983; Caldarola *et al.*, 1986; Baeg *et al.*, 1988) and in one such case the outcome was fatal (Canalese *et al.*, 1981a). Unfortunately, myths and misconceptions about the clinical features of paracetamol poisoning in man have been perpetuated as, for example, in the incorrect statements that paracetamol in overdose caused methaemoglobinaemia, cyanosis, haemolysis, hypoxia, skin lesions, chills, bone marrow depression, drowsiness, excitement, delirium, convulsions, coma and death from respiratory failure (Henriques, 1970; Chakrabarti and Lloyd, 1973; Golden *et al.*, 1981). Unsupported statements have also been made about fatal doses (Smith, 1981). Thousands of patients with paracetamol poisoning have now been reported in the world literature and the topic has been the subject of countless comments, editorials and reviews. Some case reports are summarized in Table 16.5. Paracetamol hepatotoxicity following overdosage has even been reported where there was no liver damage (Ambre and Alexander, 1977; Rumack and Peterson, 1978; Shnaps *et al.*, 1980; Jackson, 1981, 1982; Byer *et al.*, 1982; Garnier *et al.*, 1982; Jacobsen *et al.*, 1984; Bodd *et al.*, 1985; Levy and Oren, 1985; Robertson *et al.*, 1986; Kadri *et al.*, 1988; Mathis *et al.*, 1988; Kumar *et al.*, 1990; Block *et al.*, 1992; Brahm *et al.*, 1992; Oren and Levy, 1992; Ros and Conrad, 1994).

Biochemical Abnormalities

The most dramatic biochemical consequence of acute hepatic necrosis produced by paracetamol overdosage was the rapid release into the circulation of large amounts of intracellular enzymes such as the aspartate and alanine aminotransferases (AST or SGOT and ALT or SGPT respectively). Other abnormalities reflected impairment of the synthetic and excretory functions of the liver, compensatory mechanisms and the process of regeneration. Paracetamol-induced liver damage was usually assessed by measurement of plasma alanine or aspartate aminotransferase activity, bilirubin concentration and the prothrombin time (as an index of the hepatic synthesis of clotting factors). Notwithstanding the importance of detecting liver damage, it was suggested that baseline liver function tests were unnecessary in patients suspected of taking an overdose of paracetamol during the preceding 18 h (Ros and Conrad, 1994).

Plasma Enzyme Activity

Following an overdose of paracetamol there was a lag period of 8–36 h before the rise in plasma aminotransferase activity and the delay was inversely related to the severity of the liver injury. The aminotransferase activity then increased dramatically to reach a maximum of as much as 20 000 or 30 000 units l^{-1} on the third or fourth day after which, in patients who survived, there was a slower decrease with a return to normal values over a period of 1–3 weeks (Figure 16.2) (Rose, 1969; Proudfoot and Wright, 1970; Prescott *et al.*, 1971; Clark *et al.*, 1973b; Stewart and Simpson, 1973; Davis and Williams, 1975; Cohen and Burk, 1978; Wilson *et al.*, 1978; Petersen and Vilstrup, 1979; Saunders *et al.*, 1980; Black *et al.*, 1982; Lieh-Lai *et al.*,1984; Beckett *et al.*, 1985a; Mann *et al.*, 1989; Ohtani *et al.*, 1989). The record elevation so far seems to be 119 200 units l^{-1} for alanine aminotransferase in a 24-year-old Japanese woman (Ohtani *et al.*, 1989). The initial increase in plasma aminotransferase activity was related to the histological severity of hepatic necrosis as shown by liver biopsies, and increases above 400–600 units l^{-1} were always associated with severe histological damage (James *et al.*, 1975; Eastham *et al.*, 1976; Gazzard *et al.*, 1977; Hamlyn *et al.*, 1978). In another report, aminotransferase activity varied greatly and no significant correlation could be demonstrated with the extent of liver damage as assessed by the hepatocyte volume fraction (Portmann *et al.*, 1975). An unusually high aspartate to alanine aminotransferase ratio was observed in two alcoholic patients with paracetamol hepatotoxicity and this was considered to be of diagnostic significance (Himmelstein *et al.*, 1984). Similar dramatic increases in plasma enzyme activity in paracetamol poisoning have been reported for lactic dehydrogenase (Prescott *et al.*, 1971; Stewart and Simpson, 1973; Wright and Prescott, 1973; Emby and Fraser, 1977; Hamlyn *et al.*, 1978; Reikvam and Skjoto, 1978; Wilson *et al.*, 1978; Bickers and Roberts, 1979; Greene *et al.*, 1983; Erickson and Runyon, 1984; Zabrodski and Schnurr, 1984; Jakobsen *et al.*, 1987; Blake *et al.*, 1988; de Nardo *et al.*, 1988; Mann *et al.*, 1989; Ohtani *et al.*, 1989; van Vyve *et al.*, 1993; and others), and hydroxybutyrate dehydrogenase (Prescott *et al.*, 1971; Stewart and Simpson, 1973; Wright and Prescott, 1973; Commandre *et al.*, 1976). It was claimed that the ratio of the plasma alanine aminotransferase to lactic dehydrogenase activities had some diagnostic value in differentiating between viral hepatitis and ischaemic and paracetamol-induced hepatic injury (Cassidy and Reynolds, 1994). Paracetamol-induced hepatic necrosis also caused a dramatic increase in the activity of plasma glutathione S-transferases, a group of cytosolic proteins of low molecular weight present in high concentration

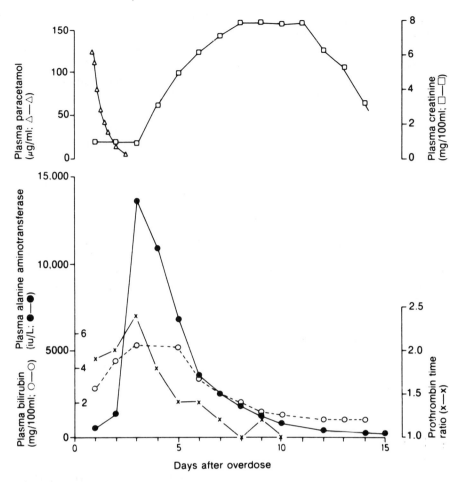

Figure 16.2 Increases in plasma alanine aminotransferase, bilirubin and creatinine, and the prothrombin time ratio in a 53-year-old man admitted too late for effective treatment with N-acetylcysteine following paracetamol overdosage. The rapid fall in plasma concentrations of paracetamol is also shown (reproduced with permission from Prescott, 1983).

in hepatocytes. The increase preceded the rise in aminotransferases and provided a much more sensitive index of hepatocellular integrity (Hayes *et al.*, 1983; Beckett *et al.*, 1985a,b, 1989). The plasma concentration of F-protein, another cytosolic protein, was also a sensitive indicator of paracetamol-induced hepatic injury (Beckett *et al.*, 1989).

In contrast to the striking elevation of the aminotransferases, dehydrogenases and glutathione S-transferases, there was no great increase in the plasma activity of other enzymes. There was little or no rise in plasma alkaline phosphatase activity in most patients with paracetamol poisoning (Thomson and Prescott, 1966; Toghill *et al.*, 1969; Proudfoot and Wright, 1970; Prescott *et al.*, 1971; Clark *et al.*, 1973b; Stewart and Simpson, 1973; Cohen and Burk, 1978; Hamlyn *et al.*, 1978; Petersen and Vilstrup, 1979; Jakobsen *et al.*, 1987; Mann *et al.*, 1989), but in some with very severe liver damage there was a slow persistent rise associated with hyper-bilirubinaemia that coincided with a delayed cholestatic phase of recovery (Benson and Boleyn, 1974; Merritt and Joyner, 1977; Cohen and Burk, 1978; Hutchinson *et al.*, 1980; Kritharides *et al.*, 1988; Shimazaki *et al.*, 1989; Thornton and Losowsky, 1990). Minor increases in plasma γ-glutamyltransferase activity have been observed (Stewart and Simpson, 1973; Coward, 1977; Krenzelok *et al.*, 1977; Rigby *et al.*, 1978; Stokes, 1984; Pillans and Hall, 1985; Jakobsen *et al.*, 1987; Sakai *et al.*, 1987; Manrique Larralde *et al.*, 1988; Shimazaki *et al.*, 1989; McClements *et al.*, 1990; Mrvos *et al.*, 1992; Friedman *et al.*, 1993; Wylie and Fraser, 1994) and this appeared to involve mostly the hydrophilic form of the enzyme (Huseby, 1981). Increased plasma amylase has been observed in some patients with paracetamol poisoning but the changes were usually modest and variable without clinical evidence of pancreatitis (Douglas *et al.*, 1976; Cohen and Burk, 1978; Hamlyn *et al.*, 1978; Nogen and Bremner, 1978; Black *et al.*, 1982; Clark *et al.*, 1983; Erickson and Runyon, 1984; Kaysen *et al.*, 1985; Sakai *et al.*, 1987; Hoffmann *et al.*, 1991; Yamakawa, 1992; Rump and Keller, 1994). These changes could represent impaired removal of amylase by the damaged liver, but except in patients with pancreatitis other investigators have not noted consistently increased plasma amylase activity. In some cases, increased plasma amylase and lipase may have been related to chronic alcoholism (Erickson and Runyon, 1984). Variable increases in plasma creatine phosphokinase activity have been noted in some patients with paracetamol poisoning. A cause and effect relationship could not be established as other drugs had been taken, some patients were alcoholics, and others had hyperpyrexia associated with salicylate intoxication (Hamlyn *et al.*, 1978; Reikvam and Skjoto, 1978; Bickers and Roberts, 1979; Kaysen *et al.*, 1985; Blake *et al.*, 1988; Mann *et al.*, 1989). Minor changes have been observed in plasma cholinesterase activity (Stewart and Simpson, 1973; Sakai *et al.*, 1987).

Bilirubin

The increase in plasma bilirubin concentration following paracetamol overdosage is much less pronounced than the rise in aminotransferases, and in some patients with mild-to-moderate hepatic necrosis the bilirubin concentration could remain within normal limits. Indeed, death in liver failure after paracetamol overdosage has been reported without clinical jaundice (Emby and Fraser, 1977). As with aminotransferases, the increase in bilirubin concentrations was delayed with maximum abnormalities usually occurring on the third or fourth days (Figure 16.2) (Clark *et al.*, 1973b; Lieh-Lai *et al.*, 1984). In some severely poisoned patients the maximum increase was delayed further and bilirubin concentrations continued to rise until the end in patients who died with hepatic failure (Benson and Boleyn, 1974; Davidson *et al.*, 1976; Cohen and Burk, 1978; Hutchinson *et al.*, 1980; Black *et al.*, 1982; Kritharides *et al.*, 1988; Mann *et al.*, 1989; McClements *et al.*, 1990). The plasma bilirubin had prognostic significance and concentrations above about 70 μmol l^{-1} (4 mg 100 ml^{-1}) on the third to the fifth day indicated impending hepatic encephalopathy, especially when the prothrombin time ratio exceeded 2.2 at the same time (Clark *et al.*, 1973b; Gazzard *et al.*, 1977). In chronic alcoholics and very severely poisoned patients, there could be a delayed cholestatic phase during recovery when the plasma bilirubin concentrations and alkaline phosphatase activity remained elevated for a considerable time (Benson and Boleyn, 1974; Merritt and Joyner, 1977; Cohen and Burk, 1978; Kritharides *et al.*, 1988; Shimazaki *et al.*, 1989; Thornton and Losowsky, 1990). During the first few days after an overdose the bilirubin in plasma was largely unconjugated as a result of impaired hepatic glucuronide conjugation (Clark *et al.*, 1973b; Davidson *et al.*, 1976; Emby and Fraser, 1977; Wilson *et al.*, 1978) and studies in rats confirmed that paracetamol liver damage greatly reduced the activities of bilirubin glucuronyl transferase and cytochrome P450 (Davidson *et al.*, 1976). Hepatic biliverdin reductase activity was also reduced after an overdose of paracetamol and serum biliverdin concentrations were greatly increased in patients with fatal liver toxicity (Wardle and Williams, 1981). In addition, serum bile acid and ferritin concentrations were strikingly increased and these were proposed as sensitive indicators of the severity of liver damage (James *et al.*, 1975; Douglas *et al.*, 1976; Eastham *et al.*, 1976). The clearance of bromsulphthalein was reduced in patients who had taken an overdose of paracetamol and it competed with bromsulphthalein for uptake by the liver, conjugation with glutathione and biliary excretion (Davis *et al.*, 1975a).

Effects on Intermediary Metabolism

As shown by increased blood hydrogen ion concentrations, reduced blood pH and reduced plasma bicarbonate concentrations, metabolic acidosis was frequently observed in patients with severe paracetamol poisoning and in those who developed fulminant hepatic failure it was persistent and resistant to correction (Davidson and Eastham, 1966; Proudfoot and Wright, 1970; Prescott *et al.*, 1971; Clark *et al.*, 1973b, 1983; Benson and Boleyn, 1974; Emby and Fraser, 1977; Calvert and Linder, 1978; Cohen and Burk, 1978; Bickers and Roberts, 1979; Black *et al.*, 1982; Farah *et al.*, 1982; Zezulka and Wright, 1982; Prescott, 1984; Zabrodski and Schnurr, 1984; Flanagan and Mant, 1986; Gray *et al.*, 1987; Jakobsen *et al.*, 1987; Blake *et al.*, 1988; Kritharides *et al.*, 1988; van Vyve *et al.*, 1993). Early metabolic acidosis was also associated with impaired consciousness, hypotension and very high plasma paracetamol concentrations (Zezulka and Wright, 1982; Prescott, 1984; Flanagan and Mant, 1986). The acidosis was caused primarily by accumulation of lactate, which could not be cleared normally by the damaged liver (Record *et al.*, 1975b, 1981). Plasma lactate concentrations were increased in a substantial proportion of patients with paracetamol toxicity but the acidosis was often compensated and therefore not immediately obvious. Plasma lactate was correlated with plasma paracetamol concentrations (Figure 16.3) and the severity of the acidosis was an important prognostic factor (Gray *et al.*, 1987; O'Grady *et al.*, 1989). Because of intolerance to lactose in patients with hepatorenal failure, the use of lactose-based dialysate solutions could be harmful (Davenport *et al.*, 1990c). Very high plasma paracetamol concentrations inhibited mitochondrial respiration and this was proposed as a mechanism for the early metabolic acidosis (Esterline and Ji, 1989). Paradoxical alkalosis has been observed rarely in patients with paracetamol poisoning (Clark *et al.*, 1973b; Benson and Boleyn, 1974) and in one patient respiratory acidosis was probably due to respiratory depression caused by dextropropoxyphene taken with the paracetamol (Block *et al.*, 1992).

Hypoglycaemia was invariably associated with severe hepatic damage and liver failure and it indicated a very poor prognosis (Davidson and Eastham, 1966; Proudfoot and Wright, 1970; Prescott *et al.*, 1971; Clark *et al.*, 1973b; Record *et al.*, 1975a,b; Emby and Fraser, 1977; Cohen and Burk, 1978; Reikvam and Skjoto,

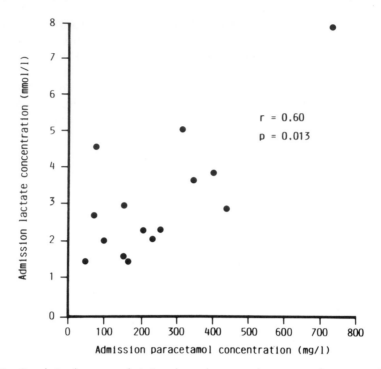

Figure 16.3 Correlation between admission plasma lactate and paracetamol concentrations in 16 patients with paracetamol poisoning (reproduced with permission of Oxford University Press, from Gray *et al.*, 1987).

1978; Wilson *et al.*, 1978; Bickers and Roberts, 1979; Weber and Cutz, 1980; Canalese *et al.*, 1981a; Black *et al.*, 1982; Greene *et al.*, 1983; Himmelstein *et al.*, 1984; Zabrodski and Schnurr, 1984; Kaysen *et al.*, 1985; Flanagan and Mant, 1986; Jakobsen *et al.*, 1987; Blake *et al.*, 1988; de Nardo *et al.*, 1988; Kritharides *et al.*, 1988; Block *et al.*, 1992; van Vyve *et al.*, 1993; Makin and Williams, 1994). Hyperglycaemia has also been observed in patients with liver damage following paracetamol overdosage (Thomson and Prescott, 1966; Pimstone and Uys, 1968; Toghill *et al.*, 1969; Peterson and Rumack, 1977; Scalley and Conner, 1978; Robertson *et al.*, 1986) and detailed studies revealed glucose intolerance, impaired gluconeogenesis and a paradoxical increase in plasma growth hormone concentrations in response to a glucose load (Record *et al.*, 1975a). Paracetamol could cause spurious and potentially dangerous changes in apparent blood glucose concentrations by interfering with its estimation by glucose oxidase methods (Burn, 1973; Farrance and Aldons, 1981; Fleetwood and Robinson, 1981; Farah *et al.*, 1982; Copland *et al.*, 1992). N-acetylcysteine given for the treatment of paracetamol poisoning could also cause interference resulting in spurious hyperglycaemia and ketonaemia (Williamson *et al.*, 1989). Blood ammonia concentrations were increased in patients with severe liver damage and hepatic encephalopathy (Nogen and Bremner, 1978; Bickers and Roberts, 1979; Weber and Cutz, 1980; Clark *et al.*, 1983; Blake *et al.*, 1988; de Nardo *et al.*, 1988). In such circumstances the hepatic production of urea was reduced resulting in low plasma urea concentrations that did not increase with the onset of renal failure (Emby and Fraser, 1977). Abnormal intermediary metabolism in patients with paracetamol-induced liver damage has been studied by high resolution proton nuclear magnetic resonance (Bales *et al.*, 1988) and ^{31}P magnetic resonance spectroscopy (Oberhaensli *et al.*, 1990; Dixon *et al.*, 1992).

Hypophosphataemia was another metabolic manifestation of paracetamol toxicity (Knell, 1975; Dawson *et al.*, 1987; Jones *et al.*, 1989; Makin and Williams, 1994). There was no correlation between the extent of hypophosphataemia and paracetamol dose or severity of liver damage, and as expected, hypophosphataemia did not occur in the presence of renal failure (Dawson *et al.*, 1987). However, in later reports, hypophosphataemia was correlated with liver and renal damage and the mechanism appeared to be increased renal loss of phosphate (Jones *et al.*, 1989; Florkowski *et al.*, 1994). Overdosage of paracetamol has also been associated with hyperphosphataemia but this was attributed to hypothermia caused by dextropropoxyphene taken with it (Block *et al.*, 1992).

Miscellaneous Abnormalities

Other biochemical abnormalities reported in patients with paracetamol-induced liver damage included decreased plasma prealbumin concentrations as a result of decreased hepatic synthesis (Hutchinson *et al.*, 1980) and impaired galactose elimination (Petersen and Vilstrup, 1979; Nagel *et al.*, 1991). Correlations were sought between the galactose elimination capacity and prothrombin index, and the lesions observed by electron microscopy in liver biopsies obtained from a patient on the first and fifth days after paracetamol overdosage. The chronological dissociation of abnormal liver function tests was reflected in the time sequence of the ultrastructural changes (Petersen and Vilstrup, 1979). Atypical pyroglutamic aciduria (5-oxoprolinuria) was probably caused by paracetamol toxicity (Creer *et al.*, 1989; Pitt, 1990; Pitt *et al.*, 1990) and this could have been due to relative deficiency of glycine caused by its diversion for cysteine synthesis (Persaud and Jackson, 1991). Serum hyaluronate concentrations rose rapidly with clinical deterioration in patients who developed encephalopathy following paracetamol poisoning and a reversible defect in hepatic endothelial cell hyaluronate receptors was proposed (Bramley *et al.*, 1991). Brown urine was described as though it was a new finding in patients with paracetamol poisoning and it was attributed to the presence of p-aminophenol (Clark *et al.*, 1986). p-Aminophenol has not been identified by others as a metabolite of paracetamol in man, and brown urine has been observed on many occasions following ingestion of paracetamol (Prescott *et al.*, 1968; MacLean *et al.*, 1968a; Boyer and Rouff, 1971; Sawyer *et al.*, 1977; Kleinman *et al.*, 1980; Jeffery and Lafferty, 1981).

Effects on Drug Metabolism

Acute liver damage caused by paracetamol resulted in impairment of hepatic drug metabolism. This was seen with paracetamol itself where reduced conjugation and prolongation of the plasma half-life was related to the severity of hepatic necrosis and prognosis (Prescott *et al.*, 1971; Prescott and Wright, 1973; Gazzard *et al.*, 1977; Prescott, 1979b, 1984; Saunders *et al.*, 1980). In patients with paracetamol-induced liver damage the capacity for glucuronide conjugation was reduced

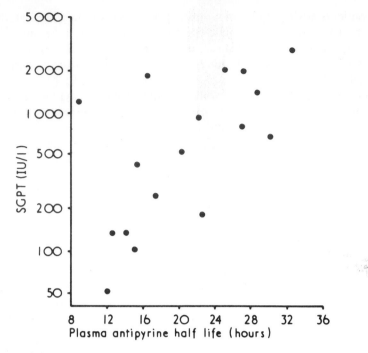

Figure 16.4 Correlation between the antipyrine half life and severity of liver damage as shown by the plasma alanine aminotransferase (SGPT) activity in patients with hepatic necrosis following paracetamol overdosage (reproduced with permission from Forrest *et al.*, 1974).

(Davidson *et al.*, 1976) and there was impaired metabolism of barbiturates (Stewart and Simpson, 1973; Pond *et al.*, 1982a) and caffeine (Nagel *et al.*, 1991). The antipyrine half life was also greatly prolonged and the increase was correlated with the prothrombin time, plasma bilirubin and plasma alanine aminotransferase activity (Figure 16.4). Antipyrine metabolism returned to normal after recovery (Forrest *et al.*, 1974). Reduced oxidation of [^{14}C]-aminopyrine as measured by breath test was proposed as a more reliable indicator of liver damage than the plasma paracetamol half life or conventional tests of liver function (Saunders *et al.*, 1980).

The appearance of 3-(cystein-S-yl) paracetamol protein adducts in the blood was considered a specific marker for paracetamol hepatotoxicity and there was a good correlation with plasma alanine aminotransferase activity indicating similar mechanisms of paracetamol hepatotoxicity in man and laboratory animals (Hinson *et al.*, 1990).

Fulminant Hepatic Failure

Paracetamol poisoning was the commonest cause of fulminant hepatic failure in the UK (Nagel *et al.*, 1991; Makin and Williams, 1994; Mutimer *et al.*, 1994; Williams, 1994). The clinical features differed in no way from those of hepatic failure from other causes (Clark *et al.*, 1973b) and survival was influenced by the presence of cerebral oedema, renal failure and uncompensated metabolic acidosis (O'Grady *et al.*, 1988). The prognosis was poor when the arterial blood pH was less than 7.30, the prothrombin time more than 100 s and the serum creatinine concentration exceeded 300 μmol l^{-1} (O'Grady *et al.*, 1989). Interpretation of the biochemical abnormalities in patients with hepatic failure caused by paracetamol was often made difficult because of co-existent renal failure.

The activity of acid protease (cathepsin D) in serum was increased about ten-fold in patients who died, and about four-fold in those who survived fulminant hepatic failure after paracetamol overdose and this was considered to be of prognostic value (Gove *et al.*, 1981). Hyponatraemia was partly due to haemodilution, but there was also a shift of sodium into the intracellular compartment as indicated by an increased concentration in leucocytes and this was inversely related to the plasma sodium concentration (Alam *et al.*, 1977a). Plasma human natriuretic factor was not increased except in patients with renal failure but there was an increase in plasma aldosterone concentrations (Panos *et al.*, 1991). Serum digoxin-like immunoreactive substances were increased in patients with paracetamol-induced hepatic failure, and the increase was correlated with renal failure as shown by the serum creatinine concentration (Yang *et al.*, 1988). Plasma concentrations of total and free carnitine, and long-chain acylcarnitine esters were also elevated, and again this seemed to be related to the presence of renal failure (Cooper *et al.*, 1991). There were significant deficiencies of complement in one patient with hepatic failure caused by paracetamol (Ellison *et al.*, 1990) and immune complexes were demonstrated in five of 22 such patients, while the clearance of [^{125}I]-microaggregated albumin was uniformly impaired (Canalese *et al.*, 1981b). Transiently raised serum concentrations of α-fetoprotein were observed in patients with hepatic damage due to paracetamol poisoning (Eleftheriou *et al.*, 1977), and in a more recent report, plasma hepatocyte growth factor and biliprotein concentrations were increased (Hughes *et al.*, 1994). The urinary excretion of epidermal growth factor was reduced, but this was to be expected in the presence of renal failure (Hughes *et al.*, 1990). The production of spontaneous and lipopolysaccharide-stimulated tumour necrosis factor was not increased (de la Mata *et al.*, 1990). Hepatocyte growth factor was produced by patients with fulminant hepatic failure but its action was suppressed by the presence of a low molecular weight inhibitor of hepatocyte DNA synthesis (Yamada *et al.*, 1994). Elevated brain concentrations of 1,4-benzodiazepines were detected in patients with fulminant hepatic failure caused by paracetamol who, apparently, had not taken these drugs (Basile *et al.*, 1991) and there was a weak but significant correlation between levels of diazepam and N-desmethyldiazepam receptor ligands and the severity of hepatic encephalopathy (Basile *et al.*, 1994).

Bleomycin-detectable iron was present in plasma from paracetamol overdose patients with hepatic failure and it was proposed that multi-organ failure was caused by circulating iron and copper ions that were catalytic for free radical reactions (Evans *et al.*, 1994). Gross impairment of drug metabolism would be expected in patients with hepatic failure but the clearance of atracurium was not reduced although there was accumulation of its major metabolite laudanosine (Bion *et al.*, 1993). The reduced clearance of caffeine and reduced galactose elimination capacity were not useful predictors of the outcome in patients with paracetamol-induced fulminant hepatic failure (Nagel *et al.*, 1991). Patients who died with fulminant hepatic failure had higher plasma bilirubin concentrations, lower total cholic acid and glycine cholic acid conjugation, and lower antipyrine clearance and galactose elimination capacity than survivors. A discriminant score based on these and other variables gave the best prediction of prognosis (Christensen *et al.*, 1984).

Haematological Abnormalities

Haemostasis was impaired in patients with acute paracetamol-induced liver damage as a result of reduced hepatic synthesis of clotting factors and in some it was compromised further by the development of disseminated intravascular coagulation. The degree of coagulopathy was directly related to the severity of liver damage, and it was an important guide to prognosis. The prothrombin time was widely used to assess the effect of paracetamol poisoning on haemostasis as it depended on the activity of the coagulation factors V, VII and X, as well as the capacity of thrombin to generate fibrin from fibrinogen. It was always prolonged in patients with moderate and severe liver damage (Prescott *et al.*, 1971; Clark *et al.*, 1973b; Benson and Boleyn, 1974; Gazzard *et al.*, 1974a; Goldfinger *et al.*, 1978; Black *et al.*, 1982; Haibach *et al.*, 1984; Bell *et al.*, 1987b; Mann *et al.*, 1989; Thornton and Losowsky, 1989, 1990; Eriksson *et al.*, 1992; Friedman *et al.*, 1993; Fischereder and Jaffe, 1994; and others) and the maximum increase usually occurred on the third or fourth day (Figure 16.2). The prothrombin time ratio was a useful guide to prognosis and there was a risk of hepatic failure if it exceeded 2.2 at 30 h (Clark *et al.*, 1973a,b; Davis and Williams, 1975; Gazzard *et al.*, 1975a, 1977; Hamlyn *et al.*, 1978). The prothrombin time ratio was also a useful guide to survival in patients with fulminant hepatic failure (O'Grady *et al.*, 1989; Harrison *et al.*, 1990b) and as a measure of the synthetic capacity of the liver, it was prolonged in parallel with impaired hepatic metabolism as shown by ^{31}P magnetic resonance spectroscopy (Dixon *et al.*, 1992). Following a hepatotoxic dose of paracetamol, the first manifestation of the decreased synthesis of clotting factors was a fall in the plasma concentration of factor VII followed in turn by decreases in the concentrations of factors V, X and II (prothrombin) (Clark *et al.*, 1973a). Other investigators have described reduced plasma concentrations of factors II, V, VII, VIII, IX and X in patients with paracetamol-induced hepatic necrosis (Gazzard *et al.*, 1974d, 1975a; Haibach *et al.*, 1984; Leist *et al.*, 1985; Denison *et al.*, 1987; Belin *et al.*, 1988; Pezzano *et al.*, 1988; Harrison *et al.*, 1990b; Viallon *et al.*, 1994). In addition to effects on the synthesis of clotting factors, it was also possible that paracetamol in overdosage could affect the vitamin K-dependent carboxylation of these factors (Malia *et al.*, 1985). The decrease in factor V concentrations and the ratio of the concentrations of factor VIII to factor V were proposed as guides to survival in patients with fulminant hepatic failure (Pereira *et al.*, 1992). Plasma concentrations of plasminogen and plasminogen activator were reduced (Hillenbrand *et al.*, 1974) and the partial thromboplastin time was prolonged in patients with severe liver damage (Clark *et al.*, 1973a; Benson and Boleyn, 1974; Haibach *et al.*, 1984; Leist *et al.*, 1985; Kartsonis *et al.*, 1986; Blake *et al.*, 1988; Minton *et al.*, 1988; Foust *et al.*, 1989; Mrvos *et al.*, 1992; Friedman *et al.*, 1993; Guccione *et al.*, 1993; Douidar *et al.*, 1994; Fischereder and Jaffe, 1994; Nadir *et al.*, 1994). There was a striking increase in plasma concentrations of specific plasminogen activator inhibitor (PAI-1) with smaller increases in tissue plasminogen activator (t-PA) and t-PA-PAI-1 complex (Leiper *et al.*, 1994). Antithrombin III concentrations were reduced (Sakai *et al.*, 1987; Eriksson *et al.*, 1992; Langley *et al.*, 1993) and an increased concentration of antithrombin III complex was taken to indicate disseminated intravascular coagulation (Langley *et al.*, 1990). Many investigators have demonstrated disseminated intravascular coagulation with increased plasma concentrations of fibrin degradation products and reduced platelets and fibrinogen in patients with moderate and severe paracetamol-induced hepatic necrosis (Clark *et al.*, 1973a; Gazzard *et al.*, 1974a, 1975a; Atwood, 1980; Licht *et al.*, 1980; Haibach *et al.*, 1984; Leist *et al.*, 1985; Sakai *et al.*, 1987; Shimazaki *et al.*, 1989; Thornton and Losowsky, 1990; Mrvos *et al.*, 1992; Friedman *et al.*, 1993; Guccione *et al.*, 1993; Langley *et al.*, 1993). The rate of fibrinogen synthesis was increased (Clark *et al.*, 1973a) and fibrinogen concentrations were only reduced in the presence of severe liver damage (Belin *et al.*, 1988; Thornton and Losowsky, 1990; Friedman *et al.*, 1993; Viallon *et al.*, 1994). Nevertheless, there were gross abnormalities of the fibrinolytic system in patients with paracetamol-induced fulminant hepatic failure (Pernambuco *et al.*, 1993).

In some patients with paracetamol-induced liver damage there was an initial leucocytosis (Prescott *et al.*, 1974; McJunkin *et al.*, 1976; Sawyer *et al.*, 1977; Wilson *et al.*, 1978; Jeffery and Lafferty, 1981; Prescott, 1981; Himmelstein *et al.*, 1984; Fleckenstein, 1985; Leist *et al.*, 1985; Sørensen *et al.*, 1986; Kher and Makker, 1987; Blake *et al.*, 1988; Shimazaki *et al.*, 1989) and reversible thrombocytopenia was a common finding after the second or third day (Clark *et al.*, 1973a; Benson and Boleyn, 1974; Gazzard *et al.*, 1974a; Goldfinger *et al.*, 1978; Atwood, 1980; Licht *et al.*, 1980; Haibach *et al.*, 1984; Yasunaga *et al.*, 1985; Kartsonis *et al.*, 1986; Sørensen *et al.*, 1986; Bell *et al.*, 1987a; Baeg *et al.*, 1988; Belin *et al.*, 1988; Blake *et al.*, 1988; Keaton, 1988; Foust *et al.*, 1989; Mann *et al.*, 1989; Eriksson *et al.*, 1992; Friedman *et al.*, 1993). Thrombocytopenia was related to the severity of liver damage but it was not always caused by disseminated intravascular coagulation (Fischereder and Jaffe, 1994). In some patients it was severe and associated with purpura and bleeding (Jensen, 1986; Kritharides *et al.*, 1988; Pezzano *et al.*, 1988; Thornton and Losowsky, 1990; Guccione *et al.*, 1993). In one young girl who was given excessive doses of paracetamol for a febrile illness, severe hepatotoxicity was complicated by leucopenia and thrombocytopenia and a bone marrow biopsy showed hypoplasia (Douidar *et al.*, 1994). In excessive doses, paracetamol did not cause clinically significant methaemoglobinaemia (Pimstone and Uys, 1968; Horwitz *et al.*, 1977; Mühlendahl and Krienke, 1980; Rabinovitz *et al.*, 1984).

Liver Pathology

Davidson and Eastham (1966) first described acute centrilobular hepatic necrosis at post-mortem in two patients who died following paracetamol overdosage. The necrosis extended throughout the lobule towards the peripheral areas with early degenerative changes even in peripheral hepatocytes surrounding the portal tracts and there was only a mild polymorphonuclear reaction. Similar abnormalities were observed in other early reports (MacLean *et al.*, 1968a; Pimstone and Uys, 1968; Rose, 1969; Toghill *et al.*, 1969; Proudfoot and Wright, 1970; Sanerkin, 1971; Clark *et al.*, 1973b). Davis and Williams (1975) described acute necrosis, collapse of the reticulin framework and a variable mononuclear cell infiltrate in a series of poisoned patients with liver damage. Follow-up biopsies 3–6 months later revealed remarkable recovery and restoration of the hepatic architecture although there was residual fibrosis in some of the most severely damaged patients. These changes were similar to those reported in animals treated with hepatotoxic doses of paracetamol (Boyd and Bereczky, 1966; Dixon *et al.*, 1971). In more detailed studies, Portmann *et al.* (1975) reviewed the histological abnormalities observed at post-mortem and in liver biopsies in 104 patients with paracetamol overdosage. The appearances depended on the severity of poisoning and the time after the overdose. In the mildest cases, seen between two and six days after the incident, there was cytoplasmic vacuolation, swelling of hepatocytes and occasional mitoses with binucleate cells and nuclear polymorphism. In more severely affected patients there was striking centrizonal confluent eosinophilic coagulative necrosis with variable cell loss. In biopsies performed later at 6–10 days after the overdose the necrotic cells had disappeared leaving areas of reticulin collapse with a lymphocytic or polymorphonuclear infiltrate and dense collections of pigment-laden macrophages. In the most severe and fatal cases the necrosis was very extensive and destroyed the limiting plates leaving only a rim of surviving hepatocytes round the portal tracts. In most of the biopsies with severe necrosis there was bile duct proliferation with cholestasis and at 8–10 days there was evidence of regeneration. In severely poisoned patients in whom liver biopsies had to be delayed for 15–42 days, there was interlobular bridging collapse with residual lipofuchsin-containing Kupffer cells and bile duct-like structures in the portal areas. In some patients there was extensive reticulin collapse, severe distortion of the architecture and apparent micronodule formation. Follow-up biopsies in three severely damaged patients revealed post-necrotic scarring in two and changes suggestive of incomplete septal cirrhosis in the third. In 27 less severely poisoned patients there was virtually complete recovery with only minor residual changes. The extent of damage was assessed quantitatively and the reduction in hepatocyte volume fraction was correlated with prognosis, mortality and the prothrombin time ratio and plasma bilirubin during the acute phase. There was no significant correlation with the plasma aspartate aminotransferase activity (Portmann *et al.*, 1975).

Similar findings were reported in another study of liver biopsies obtained from 100 patients with paracetamol poisoning. At follow-up after three months in 20 patients there was remarkable recovery with only minor residual changes in all but one severely damaged patient who showed persistent centrizonal condensation of reticulin with scarring (Lesna *et al.*, 1976b). In other reports on patients from the same centre, follow-up studies confirmed essentially complete recovery in all but those patients with very severe damage (Hamlyn *et al.*, 1977; Mathew *et al.*, 1994). Extensive centrilobular necrosis with loss of hepatocytes and limited regeneration in patients who took paracetamol in overdose are shown in Figures 16.5 and 16.6. Another patient was admitted with paracetamol overdoses on at least 31 occasions over a period of five years. On many occasions he presented late on purpose with severe poisoning and as a result suffered repeated episodes of severe liver damage (Prescott *et al.*, 1978a). Despite this, a liver biopsy obtained after the 31st overdose showed surprisingly little damage although there was some disturbance of the architecture with fibrous septa suggesting possible progression towards cirrhosis (Figure 16.7).

Many other investigators have reported centrilobular hepatic necrosis in patients with acute liver damage produced by paracetamol (Rose, 1969; Boyer and Rouff, 1971; Benson and Boleyn, 1974; van Heijst *et al.*, 1976; McJunkin *et al.*, 1976; Emby and Fraser, 1977; Sawyer *et al.*, 1977; Vilstrup *et al.*, 1977; Cohen and Burk, 1978; Reikvam and Skjoto, 1978; Silverman and Carithers, 1978; McClain *et al.*, 1980; Holzbecher *et al.*, 1981; Sutherland *et al.*, 1981; Agran *et al.*, 1983; Davis *et al.*, 1983; Zabrodski and Schnurr, 1984; O'Dell *et al.*, 1986; Sørensen *et al.*, 1986; Jakobsen *et al.*, 1987; Baeg *et al.*, 1988; Shimizu *et al.*, 1989; Mrvos *et al.*, 1992; Nadir *et al.*, 1994; and others). In some patients with severe damage, there was bridging necrosis (Ware *et al.*, 1978; Black *et al.*, 1982; Leist *et al.*, 1985; Yasunaga

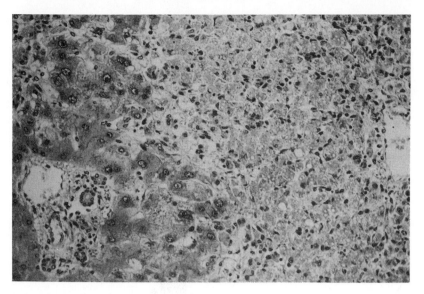

Figure 16.5   Massive hepatic necrosis in a patient who died with liver failure following paracetamol overdosage (reproduced with permission from Proudfoot and Prescott, 1977).

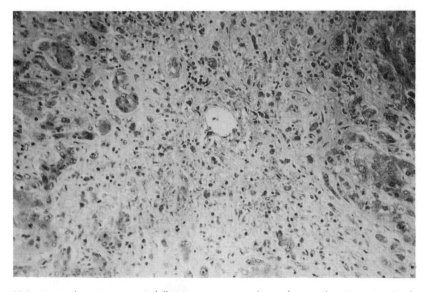

Figure 16.6   Acute hepatic necrosis following paracetamol overdosage showing extensive loss of hepatocytes with limited regeneration and sprouting of bile ducts.

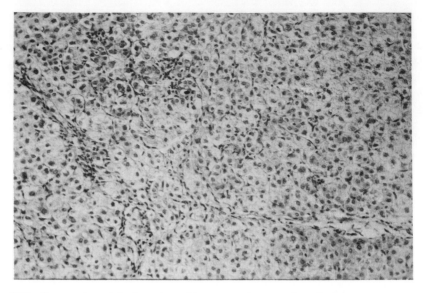

Figure 16.7 Preservation of the hepatic architecture with minimal residual damage in a liver biopsy from a young man who suffered multiple episodes of hepatic necrosis after taking paracetamol in overdosage on at least 31 occasions during the previous five years. The fibrous septa suggest progression towards cirrhosis but alcohol may have been a factor.

et al., 1985; Foust *et al.*, 1989; Price *et al.*, 1991; Patel, 1992) and collapse of the reticulin framework (Toghill *et al.*, 1969; Clark *et al.*, 1973b; Carloss *et al.*, 1978; Cohen and Burk, 1978; Kim and Dillman, 1978; Shimizu *et al.*, 1989; Price *et al.*, 1991). However, others have described preservation of the reticulin structure even in the presence of extensive necrosis (Benson and Boleyn, 1974; Leist *et al.*, 1985; Baeg *et al.*, 1988). As was observed in studies in animals, glycogen was depleted in the central necrotic areas (Petersen and Vilstrup, 1979). Many investigators noted a modest inflammatory reaction that was usually densest at the line of demarcation between the necrotic and viable hepatocytes (Pimstone and Uys, 1968; Sanerkin, 1971; Kim and Dillman, 1978; Ware *et al.*, 1978; Levinson, 1983; Kaysen *et al.*, 1985; Florén *et al.*, 1987; Foust *et al.*, 1989; Thornton and Losowsky, 1989). Macrophages and Kupffer cells, often laden with lipofuchsin, were also present in the areas of necrosis (Benson and Boleyn, 1974; Leist *et al.*, 1985; Baeg *et al.*, 1988). During the acute phase there was an increase in the population of Kupffer and parasinusoidal cells (Mathew *et al.*, 1994). Several days after the damage there was evidence of regeneration with mitotic figures, binucleate cells and enlarged hyperchromatic nuclei (MacLean *et al.*, 1968a; Pimstone and Uys, 1968; Benson and Boleyn, 1974; Kim and Dillman, 1978; Prescott *et al.*, 1978; Lesser *et al.*, 1986; Pezzano *et al.*, 1988). Regeneration and proliferation of residual cells was most marked 5–6 days after the overdose as shown by immunoreactivity with monoclonal antibody to proliferative cell nuclear antigen (NCL-PCNA) (Koukoulis *et al.*, 1992). In severely damaged livers there was proliferation of bile ducts (Sanerkin, 1971; Davis *et al.*, 1983; Lesser *et al.*, 1986; Shimizu *et al.*, 1989) and a cholestatic reaction (Pimstone and Uys, 1968; Toghill *et al.*, 1969; Benson and Boleyn, 1974; Cohen and Burk, 1978; Kim and Dillman, 1978; Olsson, 1978; Prescott *et al.*, 1978a; Wilson *et al.*,

1978; Gerber *et al.*, 1980; Symon *et al.*, 1982; Agran *et al.*, 1983; Kaysen *et al.*, 1985; Leist *et al.*, 1985). Minor degrees of fibrosis have been described in some patients but a causative role for paracetamol is doubtful as many were chronic alcoholics (Clark *et al.*, 1973b; Commandre *et al.*, 1976; Cohen and Burk, 1978; Olsson, 1978; Prescott *et al.*, 1978; Ware *et al.*, 1978; Wilson *et al.*, 1978; Gerber *et al.*, 1980; Black *et al.*, 1982; Davis *et al.*, 1983; Levinson, 1983; Leist *et al.*, 1985; Lesser *et al.*, 1986). A liver biopsy following an overdose of paracetamol in a 38-year-old alcoholic woman showed centrilobular necrosis but a further biopsy performed eight months later after she claimed to have been taking 6 g of paracetamol daily was said to show centrilobular necrosis and fibrosis. It was stated without evidence that the fibrosis was a consequence of the therapeutic use of paracetamol while consuming alcohol (O'Dell *et al.*, 1986). There have been occasional references to cirrhosis and micronodular cirrhosis but these lesions were usually seen only with very severe liver damage (Benson and Boleyn, 1974; Prescott *et al.*, 1978; Arthurs and Fielding, 1980; Lesser *et al.*, 1986; Luquel *et al.*, 1988). The extent of histological damage has been graded and correlated with biochemical abnormalities (James *et al.*, 1975; Portmann *et al.*, 1975; Lesna *et al.*, 1976b; Gazzard *et al.*, 1977; Hamlyn *et al.*, 1978, 1981).

Electron microscopy confirmed the presence of frank centrilobular necrosis with vacuolization of the endoplasmic reticulum, detachment of ribosomes, swelling and distortion of mitochondria, breakdown of plasma membranes, accumulation of amorphous cytoplasmic material and nuclear karyolysis (Ikejiri *et al.*, 1979; Petersen and Vilstrup, 1979; McCaul *et al.*, 1986). In other studies, ultrastructural abnormalities included abundant rough endoplasmic reticulum with smooth-surfaced vesicles on the smooth endoplasmic reticulum (Wilson *et al.*, 1978), dilatation of bile canaliculi with cholestasis, blunting of microvilli and myelin figures (Agran *et al.*, 1983) and disorganization of most of the hepatocyte organelles with variable amounts of electron-dense deposits in the matrix of the mitochondria (Weber and Cutz, 1980).

Renal Failure

Before the advent of effective treatment for paracetamol toxicity, acute renal failure requiring dialysis occurred in about 1 per cent of all unselected patients referred to hospital with paracetamol poisoning (Table 16.4) (Hamlyn *et al.*, 1978; Prescott, 1983). As shown in Table 16.3, the incidence in different series varied from 0 to about 10 per cent depending on the selection of patients and the efficacy of treatment. In a review of 2060 unselected patients seen over the period 1969–1980, the overall frequency of acute renal failure was 1.6 per cent. Patients who presented late (more than 10 h) after the overdose were more severely poisoned and 25 of 118 (21.2 per cent) such patients developed renal failure (Prescott *et al.*, 1982). The incidence was much higher (50–70 per cent) in patients who suffered fulminant hepatic failure (Wilkinson *et al.*, 1977; O'Grady *et al.*, 1988, 1991; Bray *et al.*, 1992a; Baudouin *et al.*, 1995; Makin and Williams, 1994). There were two distinct forms of nephrotoxicity following paracetamol overdosage. In the first, oliguric renal failure developed within 24–48 h and it was invariably accompanied by back pain, renal tenderness, proteinuria and microscopic haematuria. It usually occurred in association with hepatotoxicity, but was reported rarely in patients who only had mild liver damage with plasma aminotransferase activity less than 1000 units l^{-1} (Sawyer *et al.*, 1977; Kleinman *et al.*, 1980; Cobden *et al.*, 1982; Kleinknecht *et al.*, 1986b). Acute renal failure has also been reported in overdose patients who had no clinical or biochemical evidence of hepatotoxicity (Prescott *et al.*, 1982; Pillans and Hall, 1985; Kher and Makker, 1987; Duchene *et al.*, 1991; Campbell and Baylis, 1992). The renal failure was reversible and varied in severity from transient mild oliguria lasting only a few hours to the rapid onset of anuria necessitating treatment with haemodialysis. In some cases oliguria and impairment of renal function persisted for 7–14 days with a progressive increase in plasma creatinine concentrations before the onset of the diuretic phase and recovery (Figure 16.2) (Prescott, 1978, 1983; Stegeman-Castelen *et al.*, 1983; Dabbagh and Chesney, 1985; Davenport and Finn, 1988; McClain *et al.*, 1988). Urea production was greatly decreased in patients with severe liver damage and the plasma urea concentration could not be used as a guide to renal function. The degree of renal damage was related to hypophosphataemia, and phosphaturia and retinol binding proteinuria were proposed as sensitive markers of nephrotoxicity following paracetamol overdosage (Florkowski *et al.*, 1994). Case reports of patients with renal failure following paracetamol overdosage are summarized in Table 16.6, and the subject has recently been reviewed (Jones and Vale, 1993; Thomas, 1993). Renal failure has also been mentioned in many other reports of paracetamol poisoning (Proudfoot and Wright, 1970; Barnes and Prichard, 1972; Clark *et al.*, 1973b; Prescott and Wright, 1973; Stewart and Simpson, 1973; Douglas *et al.*, 1976; Prescott *et al.*, 1976c, 1979; Prescott, 1978, 1979, 1981; Vale *et al.*, 1979, 1981; Baumgarten *et al.*, 1983; Dawson *et al.*, 1987; Forbes *et al.*, 1989a; Hughes *et al.*, 1990; Weber *et al.*, 1990b; Panos *et al.*, 1991; Smilkstein *et al.*, 1991; Pereira *et al.*, 1992; Bion *et al.*, 1993).

The frequency of renal failure in patients with paracetamol-induced fulminant hepatic failure was no greater than in patients with hepatic failure from other causes. In a review of 160 such patients, the cause was paracetamol poisoning in 53, and other pathology including viral hepatitis in 107. Renal failure occurred in 28 of the paracetamol patients (53 per cent) and 41 (38 per cent) of the others, but this difference was not significant. In the paracetamol group, renal failure developed in 18 per cent of patients who survived compared with 62 per cent of those who died (Wilkinson *et al.*, 1977). Other investigators have shown that renal failure was an important adverse prognostic factor in patients with paracetamol-induced hepatic failure (Read *et al.*, 1986; O'Grady *et al.*, 1988, 1989, 1991; Pereira *et al.*, 1992; Boberg *et al.*, 1994). Renal failure often occurred in the setting of multi-organ failure, and endotoxaemia and disseminated intravascular coagulation were considered as possible aetiological factors. An increase in plasma renin activity was observed in most patients with paracetamol-induced hepatic failure irrespective of the development of renal failure (Wilkinson *et al.*, 1979). In another report, the increase in plasma renin activity was greatest in patients with more severe renal failure in whom there were also increased plasma concentrations of human atrial natriuretic factor and aldosterone (Panos *et al.*, 1991). The increase in plasma renin in patients with fulminant hepatic failure and renal failure was associated with marked renal vasoconstriction and reduced renal prostaglandin excretion (Guarner *et al.*, 1987). Not surprisingly, the fractional urinary excretion of β_2-microglobulin was decreased in patients with hepatic and renal failure following paracetamol poisoning (Hansen *et al.*, 1991). Histological examination of renal biopsies and autopsy specimens usually showed acute tubular necrosis (Rose, 1969; Toghill *et al.*, 1969; McJunkin *et*

Table 16.6 Case reports of acute renal failure following paracetamol overdosage.

Age and sex	Stated dose (g)	Plasma paracetamol (mg l⁻¹)	Time after ingestion (h)	Max. plasma creatinine (μmol l⁻¹)	Max. amino-transferase (u l⁻¹)	Renal histology[1]	Comments	Reference
40F	30	4.5	120	190[2]	7000	DTN	fatal hepatorenal failure	MacLean et al., 1968a
46M	37.5	–	–	137[2]	–	TN	fatal hepatorenal failure	Rose, 1969
33F	35	–	–	>300[2]	–	TN	fatal hepatorenal failure	Toghill et al., 1969
29F	19.5	–	–	792	4000	–	drug abuser	Boyer and Rouff, 1971
59M	90	152	36	–	>2000	TN	fatal hepatorenal failure	Benson and Boleyn, 1974
24F	13	–	–	392	8795	TN	?alcoholic, fatal hepatorenal failure	McJunkin et al., 1976
32F	25	220	?	–	2920	–	fatal hepatorenal failure, other drugs	van Heijst et al., 1976
31F	60	–	–	–	300	–	alcoholic, peritoneal dialysis, pancreatitis	Gilmore and Tourvas, 1977
54F	36	–	–	463	2520	–	recovered from hepatic failure	Merritt and Joyner, 1977
34M	50	–	–	450	438	–		Sawyer et al., 1977
20F	33	71	?	410	>5000	–	recovered from hepatic failure	Cohen and Burk, 1978
21F	30	–	–	997	9760	–		Cohen and Burk, 1978
18F	25	316[3]	14	–	8100	–	acute renal failure, late cysteamine treatment	Smith et al., 1978
21F	25	138[3]	15.5	–	7935	–	acute renal failure, late cysteamine treatment	Smith et al., 1978
??	50	208[3]	14	–	5145	–	hepatorenal failure, late cysteamine treatment	Smith et al., 1978
13F	?	98	36	160	>10000	–	fatal hepatorenal failure, on anticonvulsants	Wilson et al., 1978
50F	?	287	?	–	>8000	–	fatal hepatorenal failure	Hutchinson et al., 1980
26M	16	–	–	2136	146	TN	dextropropoxyphene, peritoneal dialysis	Kleinman et al., 1980
19F	50	3	70	979	9040	–	haemodialysis	Jeffery and Lafferty, 1981
19F	15	32	19	1006	11720	–	haemodialysis	Jeffery and Lafferty, 1981
45?	25	48	?	811	8280	–	oliguria	Cobden et al., 1982
18?	50	124	?	1240	732	TN	oliguria, peritoneal dialysis	Cobden et al., 1982
23F	17	34	?	1310	>1000	DTN	peritoneal dialysis	Cobden et al., 1982
20?	25	–	–	700	>2000	–	oliguria	Cobden et al., 1982
41?	29	–	–	1080	8440	–	peritoneal dialysis	Cobden et al., 1982
26?	10	–	–	1460	260	–	peritoneal dialysis	Cobden et al., 1982
38?	50	390	?	560	3980	–	oliguria	Cobden et al., 1982
17?	11	226	?	480	>5000	–	not oliguric	Cobden et al., 1982
19?	30	–	?	585	4200	–	oliguria	Cobden et al., 1982
25?	50	328	?	789	2150	–	oliguria	Cobden et al., 1982

(cont.)

Table 16.6 (cont.)

Age and sex	Stated dose (g)	Plasma paracetamol (mg l⁻¹)	Time after ingestion (h)	Max. plasma creatinine (μmol l⁻¹)	Max. amino-transferase (u l⁻¹)	Renal histology[1]	Comments	Reference
36F	30	60	48	1593	2284	–	oliguria, treated with cysteamine	Curry et al., 1982
21F	25	316	8	292	16 400	–	normal liver function tests	Harris, 1982
21M	15	–	–	256	normal	–	normal liver function tests, aspirin also taken	Prescott et al., 1982
22F	?	50	–	390	normal	–	normal liver function tests	Prescott et al., 1982
23M	?	86	11	450	normal	–	normal liver function tests	Prescott et al., 1982
28M	16	18	21	579	1296	–	also paraquat poisoning, fatal	Siefkin, 1982
38F	10	–	–	1000	–	TN	haemodialysis	Baumgarten et al., 1983
26M	25	–	–	1450	45[4]	AIN	overdose, haemodialysis	Pusey et al., 1983
26F	15	58	20	1150	>3000	–	poor nutrition	Stegeman-Castelen et al., 1983
42M	?	137	>48	917	894	TN	alcoholic, fatal hepatorenal failure	Himmelstein et al., 1984
29F	36	24	?	579	>1800	TN	alcoholic, fatal hepatorenal failure	Zabrodski and Schnurr, 1984
48F	?	45	?	472	4080	–	drug abuse, fatal hepatorenal failure	Zabrodski and Schnurr, 1984
19F	10	16	18	1317	16 336	–	epileptic, other drugs,[5] haemodialysis	Dabbagh and Chesney, 1985
16F	10	–	–	374	32	–	also took chlormezanone, oliguria	Pillans and Hall, 1985
51F	75	725	20	337	776	TN	other drugs, fatal	Clark et al., 1986
54M	50	302	15	486	7870	TN	other drugs, fatal	Clark et al., 1986
26F	40	50	36	908	>6000	–	haemodialysis	Clark et al., 1986
60F	25	–	–	600	8000	TN	fatal hepatorenal failure	Sorensen et al., 1986
39M	36	–	–	341	11 520	–	–	Bell et al., 1987b
44F	30	–	–	375	4695	–	–	Bell et al., 1987b
36M	24	–	–	519	23 660	–	–	Bell et al., 1987b
66F	?	–	–	723	24[6]	–	alcoholic	Denison et al., 1987, 1991
58F	?	408	17	239	16 000	–	fatal hepatorenal failure	Jakobsen et al., 1987
13½F	7.5	173	8	208	normal	–	normal liver function tests	Kher and Makker, 1987
30F	?	–	–	449	3360	–	drug abuse, cerebral atrophy	Sakai et al., 1987
37M	23	–	–	991	88[6]	–	also chlormezanone	Björck et al., 1988
35F	12.5	130	14	1000	15 456	TN	treated with N-acetylcysteine, haemodialysis	Davenport and Finn, 1988
33M	75	361	8	1353	16 000	TN	treated with N-acetylcysteine	Davenport and Finn, 1988
30F	?12	190	?	>600	4240	–	hypothermia, hypotension, haemofiltration	Kritharides et al., 1988
28F	30	235	7	1433	7920	–	also taking primidone and phenobarbitone	McClain et al., 1988

24F	50	–	–	481	11 300	–	alcoholic	McClain et al., 1988
20M	?	94	5.5	265	>5000	–	fatal hepatorenal failure, epileptic, also aspirin	Minton et al., 1988
31M	35	68	96	1095	18 726	–	fatal hepatorenal failure, cardiomyopathy	Mann et al., 1989
24F	4.8	47	8	–	119 200	–	haemodialysis, late cardiac failure	Ohtani et al., 1989
27M	6.4	–	–	632	5530	–	hepatic failure, plasma exchange, haemodialysis	Shimazaki et al., 1989
36F	3.2	–	–	454	6980	–	hepatic failure, plasma exchange, haemodialysis	Shimazaki et al., 1989
43M	37	–	–	710	13 600	–	fatal haemorrhage from acute varices	Thornton and Losowsky, 1989
14M	45	12	28	–	12 230	–	hepatic failure, haemodialysis, on phenytoin	McClements et al., 1990
19F	11.5	10	11.5	1610	209[6]	–	haemodialysis, N-acetylcysteine, on isoniazid	Murphy et al., 1990
23M	10	–	–	350	normal	–	normal liver function tests	Duchene et al., 1991
18F	10.5	5.5	72	709	5990	–	liver transplant, cardiomyopathy	Hoffmann et al., 1991
16F	15	154	11	872	9700	–	fatal hepatorenal failure	Price et al., 1991
15F	19.5	27	15	170	normal	–	treated with N-acetylcysteine	Campbell and Baylis, 1992
40F	17	12	?	–	5612	–	alcoholic, liver transplant	Mrvos et al., 1992
17M	31	134	12	1202	11 660	–	N-acetylcysteine, haemodialysis	Knoop et al., 1993
18F	8–20	–	–	1063	11 400	–	hepatic failure, haemodialysis	Boberg et al., 1994
18F	14	–	–	969	7740	–	failed liver transplant	Boberg et al., 1994
32F	29	106	12	1227	14 100	AIN	N-acetylcysteine, haemodialysis	Boberg et al., 1994
22M	16	–	–	1282	7840	–	haemodialysis	Brevet et al., 1994
21F	25	151	3	–	–	–	fatal hepatorenal failure	Cheung et al., 1994
46F	8	3	72	200	7780	–	hepatic failure, late N-acetylcysteine	Viallon et al., 1994

[1] Renal histology: TN = tubular necrosis, DTN = distal tubular necrosis, AIN = acute interstitial nephritis; [2] blood urea, mg 100 ml^{-1}; [3] inappropriate method of analysis giving false high results; [4] nine days after overdose; [5] also took valproate, carbamazepine and acetazolamide; [6] μkat l^{-1}

al., 1976; Baumgarten *et al.*, 1983; Himmelstein *et al.*, 1984; Zabrodski and Schnurr, 1984; Sørensen *et al.*, 1986; Davenport and Finn, 1988). The findings included coagulative necrosis of the proximal tubular cells, tubular dilatation, collections of cellular debris within damaged tubules, rupture of the tubular basement membranes, interstitial oedema and infiltration with lymphocytes and plasma cells (Wilkinson *et al.*, 1979; Kleinman *et al.*, 1980; Björck *et al.*, 1988; Price *et al.*, 1991). Electron microscopy showed additional loss of the tubular brush border with disorganization of the basolateral linear mitochondria (Kleinman *et al.*, 1980) as well as endothelial cell damage and evidence of regeneration (Björck *et al.*, 1988). In some reports there was mention of interstitial nephritis (Pusey *et al.*, 1983; Boberg *et al.*, 1994) and distal tubular damage (MacLean *et al.*, 1968a; Cobden *et al.*, 1982).

Other Complications

Cardiomyopathy

There have been several reports to the effect that paracetamol overdose caused myocardial damage. Pimstone and Uys (1968) described ST segment depression and sagging in the anterior chest leads of electrocardiographic recordings in a 26-year-old woman who died eight days after taking 30–40 g of paracetamol. At postmortem examination the myocardium showed diffuse damage with interstitial oedema and the fibres were described as thin, wispy and poorly stained. The most severe changes were subendocardial with band-like foci of necrosis and haemorrhage. The appearances were felt to represent severe cardiomyopathy although the patient had been hypotensive and had required ventilation for two days before death. The electrocardiogram of a 40-year-old woman who died of hepatic failure after taking an overdose of paracetamol showed striking ST segment depression, and in a 41-year-old man who took an overdose of paracetamol, phentermine and barbiturates, a pericardial friction rub was heard on the fifth day and the electrocardiogram showed generalized T wave flattening and inversion (MacLean *et al.*, 1968a). Unfortunately the myocardium for pathological examination in the first case was discarded, and as the abnormalities in the second were unchanged five months later it seems unlikely that paracetamol was the cause. In another report on a 15-year-old girl who died 40 h after taking paracetamol and chlormezanone, examination of the heart showed myocardial fatty degeneration, confluent early necrosis, irregular loss of staining and focal clumping of myofibrils (Sanerkin, 1971). A 19-year-old woman suffered mild liver damage (plasma aspartate aminotransferase 1350 units l^{-1}) after taking an overdose of paracetamol and electrocardiograms on the second and fourth days showed elevation of the ST segments in precordial leads, coronary sinus rhythm and T wave flattening in leads V5 and V6, which had reverted to normal by the seventh day (Will and Tomkins, 1971). These changes were probably due to a viral infection as she had a sore throat with atypical mononuclear cells in the blood. In other reports, electrocardiographic abnormalities and arrhythmias were seen as preterminal events in patients with fulminant hepatic failure (Clark *et al.*, 1973b; Benson and Boleyn, 1974; Jones and Thomas, 1977; Reikvam and Skjoto, 1978). A 15-year-old girl developed atrial and ventricular arrhythmias with hypotension, coma and ST segment depression and T wave inversion on the electrocardiogram before final cardiorespiratory arrest. At post-mortem examination there was almost complete hepatic necrosis and cerebral oedema with focal infiltration of neutrophils and occasional mast cells among necrotic myocardial muscle fibres (Wakeel *et al.*, 1987). As was pointed out later, the cardiovascular complications in this patient could have been due to cerebral oedema and fluid overload (Fagan *et al.*, 1988). In another patient aged 24 years, cardiac failure developed 16 days after paracetamol-induced liver damage and renal failure. Right heart catheterization revealed high pulmonary artery pressures and poor left ventricular function. Haemodialysis was performed to relieve pulmonary oedema and three months later a ventriculogram showed mild impairment of left ventricular function with an ejection fraction of 49 per cent (Ohtani *et al.*, 1989). It is difficult to see how paracetamol could cause myocardial damage as alleged in this patient more than two weeks after the overdose. Fatty change in the myocardium of a 31-year-old chronic alcoholic who died with hepatorenal failure was attributed to paracetamol (Mann *et al.*, 1989) and toxic myocarditis was suspected in an 18-year-old woman with hepatic failure who subsequently received a liver transplant (Hoffmann *et al.*, 1991). In some reports, the claims for paracetamol cardiotoxicity seem dubious to say the least. A 16-year-old girl died with hepatorenal failure nine days after taking an overdose of paracetamol. Her heart was transplanted into a young woman with congenital heart disease but she died two weeks later with sepsis. The transplanted heart showed extensive subendocardial necrosis that was stated to have been caused by the paracetamol rather than rejection, infection or multi-organ failure (Price *et al.*, 1991). In another report of 'paracetamol cardiotoxicity', a 29-year-old man who was receiving depot flupenthixol injections developed liver damage after taking an overdose of paracetamol. He recovered without further complications but an electrocardiogram on the second day showed ST segment and T wave changes with coronary sinus rhythm that had reverted to normal on the 10th day. The possible role of the flupenthixol was not considered and it was proposed without evidence that paracetamol caused functional coronary insufficiency resulting from inhibition of endothelium-derived relaxing factor secondary to depletion of sulphydryl groups (Armour and Slater, 1993).

Bradycardia (Manrique Larralde *et al.*, 1988), pericardial rub (Himmelstein *et al.*, 1984) and endocarditis (Yasunaga *et al.*, 1985) have been mentioned, and not surprisingly, frank cardiotoxicity has been observed with overdoses of combinations of dextropropoxyphene and paracetamol (Starkey and Lawson, 1978; Pond *et al.*, 1982b; Block *et al.*, 1992). Electrocardiographic abnormalities have occasionally been noted in patients with paracetamol poisoning who did not have fulminant hepatic failure but there was no clinical evidence of toxic myocarditis (Stewart and Simpson, 1973; Lesna *et al.*, 1976a; Hamlyn *et al.*, 1978, 1981; Prescott *et al.*, 1979). In 20 unselected cases of fatal paracetamol poisoning there was no evidence of myocardiopathy at post-mortem examination (Dixon, 1976). In a study of 106 patients with fulminant hepatic failure including 43 caused by paracetamol, cardiac arrhythmias and other abnormalities were observed in 92 per cent and were not related to the aetiology of the liver failure. Cardiovascular instability was probably related to increased intracranial pressure and arrhythmias were more likely to occur in the presence of acidosis, hypoxia and hypokalaemia, and in patients who required haemodialysis and ventilation. Significant cardiac abnormalities were not seen in patients who did not develop fulminant hepatic failure (Weston and Williams, 1976;

Weston *et al.*, 1976). The overall conclusion is that paracetamol is not cardiotoxic itself, but myocardial damage and cardiac arrhythmias occurred commonly with multi-organ failure in patients with paracetamol-induced fulminant hepatic failure.

Pancreatitis

Abnormal elevation of the plasma amylase activity was noted in 9 of 48 patients with paracetamol poisoning (Douglas *et al.*, 1976) and, soon after, acute pancreatitis was described following overdosage in a 31-year-old alcoholic barmaid who presented 54 h later with abdominal and back pain and absent bowel sounds. The serum amylase and aspartate aminotransferase were 1440 and 300 units l^{-1} respectively and she developed renal failure that was treated with peritoneal dialysis. Four weeks later a laparotomy was performed because of persistent abdominal pain, ileus and fever, and the pancreas was found to be oedematous and haemorrhagic with areas of fat necrosis (Gilmore and Tourvas, 1977). The delayed onset of what was referred to as acute pancreatitis has been described in several other patients with liver damage after paracetamol overdosage (Coward, 1977; Yasunaga *et al.*, 1985; Caldarola *et al.*, 1986; Hoffmann *et al.*, 1991). In another case, the diagnosis rested largely on the finding of decreased echogenicity on ultrasound examination, and associated abdominal distension with ileus could have been related to treatment (Mofenson *et al.*, 1991). Paracetamol hepatotoxicity has also been associated with alcoholic pancreatitis (Erickson and Runyon, 1984). There have been other reports of mild-to-moderate increases in plasma amylase activity without clinical or pathological evidence of pancreatitis (Cohen and Burk, 1978; Hamlyn *et al.*, 1978, 1981; Black *et al.*, 1982).

Muscle Damage

It was suggested that paracetamol poisoning might cause muscle or myocardial damage on the basis of increased plasma creatine phosphokinase activity (Hamlyn *et al.*, 1978; Pond *et al.*, 1982b; Kaysen *et al.*, 1985; Blake *et al.*, 1988; Mann *et al.*, 1989). Some of these patients were alcoholics or had taken other drugs, and in two others salicylate had also been taken with hyperpyrexia as a further significant complication (Reikvam and Skjoto, 1978; Bickers and Roberts, 1979). Raised plasma creatine kinase activity was found in 24 of 86 patients who had taken paracetamol in overdose. The greatest rise was generally seen 24 h after admission but the increases were minor (Hamlyn *et al.*, 1978). Subclinical rhabdomyolysis was reported following overdosage of paracetamol, caffeine and phenazone, but as shown by the plasma concentrations, the overdose was trivial (Michaelis *et al.*, 1991). Twenty-six patients with fulminant hepatic failure, including six in which the cause was paracetamol poisoning, were all found to have muscle necrosis at necropsy. The muscle damage had no specific histological features and was not associated with inflammation or vasculitis (Ojeda *et al.*, 1982).

Lung Damage

Acute lung damage was observed in 9 of 24 patients with fulminant hepatic failure following paracetamol overdosage. Lung injury would not be surprising in such circumstances and it was associated with circulatory failure and cerebral oedema but not with renal failure (Baudouin *et al.*, 1995).

Plasma Paracetamol Concentrations and Toxicity

In early reports, plasma concentrations of p-aminophenol produced by hydrolysis of paracetamol and its conjugates were measured in patients with paracetamol poisoning and not surprisingly there was no clear relationship with toxicity (Davidson and Eastham, 1966; Proudfoot and Wright, 1970; Brown, 1971). Measurement of urine p-aminophenol was also recommended as a screening test (Simpson and Stewart, 1973). A definitive relationship was established between plasma paracetamol concentrations, time after ingestion and biochemical liver damage in 30 overdose patients (Figure 7.4). Although a single measurement 4 h after ingestion was not always a reliable indicator of outcome, concentrations above 300 mg l^{-1} were always associated with severe liver damage (defined here as elevation of plasma aminotransferases above 1000 units l^{-1}) while there was none at concentrations below 120 mg l^{-1} at 4 h. A much clearer separation was observed at 12 h but the best correlation with liver function tests and prognosis was obtained with the plasma paracetamol half life. The mean half life was twice as long in the patients with hepatic necrosis than in those without, and liver damage was to be expected when the half life exceeded 4 h. In patients with fatal liver damage the half life exceeded 10–12 h and it increased progressively with time to 60 h or more (Prescott *et al.*, 1971; Prescott and Wright, 1973). Others have observed prolongation of the plasma paracetamol half life to more than 8–10 h in patients with severe and fatal liver damage (Gazzard *et al.*, 1974e; Davis and Williams, 1975; Saunders *et al.*, 1980; Zabrodski and Schnurr, 1984; Flanagan and Mant, 1986; Blake *et al.*, 1988). Unfortunately, it took time to determine the paracetamol half life and routine clinical measurement was not practicable.

These relationships were strengthened with observations from additional patients and a 'treatment line' joining plots on a semilogarithmic graph of 200 mg l^{-1} at 4 h and 30 mg l^{-1} at 15 h was proposed to identify patients at risk of liver damage who might benefit from treatment with cysteamine (Figure 16.8) (Prescott *et al.*, 1974). These data from Edinburgh were taken without the knowledge or permission of the originators and subsequently used to produce the much-quoted 'Rumack-Matthew nomogram' (Rumack and Matthew, 1975). Other investigators confirmed the relationship between plasma paracetamol concentrations, half life and hepatotoxicity, and the treatment line became established for determining prognosis and the need for specific antidotal therapy (Stewart and Simpson, 1973; James *et al.*, 1975; Douglas *et al.*, 1976; Prescott *et al.*, 1976c, 1979; Gazzard *et al.*, 1977; Prescott, 1978; National Poisons Information Service Monitoring Group, 1981). The treatment line shown in Figure 16.8 was based entirely on observations in these and earlier reports on patients who were admitted before effective treatment became available. It was stressed that as there was marked individual variation in susceptibility to the hepatotoxicity of paracetamol, the treatment line could only be used as a guide. One patient could develop liver damage with relatively low initial plasma paracetamol concentrations while another with concentrations several times higher could escape completely (Prescott and Critchley, 1983b). Plasma paracetamol concentrations could not be interpreted during the first 4 h because of uncertainty

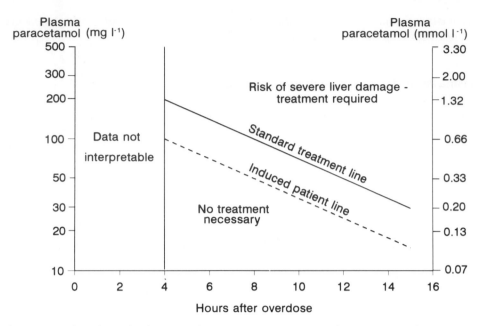

Plasma
paracetamol (mg l⁻¹)

Plasma
paracetamol (mmol l⁻¹)

Figure 16.8 The relationship between plasma concentrations, time after ingestion and the risk of liver damage following overdosage with paracetamol. Treatment with N-acetylcysteine would be indicated in patients with concentrations above the standard treatment line.

regarding absorption and there were also difficulties with interpretation when absorption was delayed by drugs such as central nervous system depressants and narcotic analgesics. Delayed absorption resulted in later higher concentrations and this no doubt explained in part the miraculous survival without disastrous toxicity reported in patients with high paracetamol concentrations admitted many hours after combined overdosage with dextropropoxyphene (Pond *et al.*, 1982b; Prescott, 1983; Ruane *et al.*, 1989; Block *et al.*, 1992). The paradox of paracetamol concentrations above and below the treatment line at different times in the same patient could also be explained by delayed absorption after combined overdosage with dextropropoxyphene (Tighe and Walter, 1994). In addition to dependence on absorption rate, the plasma paracetamol concentration-toxicity relationship also depended critically on accurate knowledge of the time of ingestion and this was subject to serious error. Indeed, some patients purposely gave the wrong times of ingestion to mislead medical staff (Prescott *et al.*, 1978a). It was assumed without good evidence that the same concentration-toxicity relationship applied in children, and many investigators extrapolated the treatment line into the no-man's-land beyond 15 h despite the fact that the limited data available clearly showed that the established relationships did not hold after this time (Helliwell and Essex, 1981; National Poisons Information Service Monitoring Group, 1981). The treatment line was also not appropriate for assessment of patients who had taken multiple doses of paracetamol over a period of time (Curry *et al.*, 1982; Smith *et al.*, 1986a; Blake *et al.*, 1988; Mathis *et al.*, 1988; Walson and Groth, 1993). In the light of all these problems, it was hardly surprising that the prognosis according to the treatment line did not always correspond to the subsequent outcome (Claass *et al.*, 1993; Cheung *et al.*, 1994).

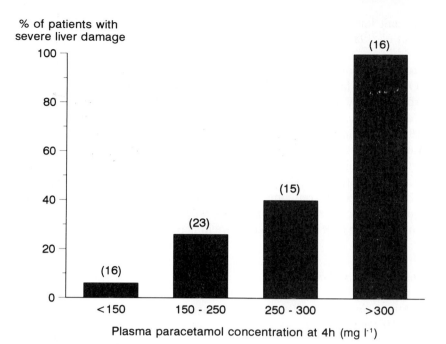

% of patients with
severe liver damage

Figure 16.9 The relationship between plasma concentrations at 4 h after overdosage and the risk of severe liver damage (plasma alanine aminotransferase activity exceeding 1000 u l^{-1}) following paracetamol overdosage. The numbers of patients in each group are given above each column. (Data from Prescott *et al.*, 1977a.)

The probability of severe liver damage with different plasma paracetamol concentrations 4 h after ingestion is shown in Figure 16.9 and there was a threshold effect with a disproportionate increase in the incidence as concentrations increased above 300 mg l^{-1}. It is widely believed that all patients with plasma paracetamol concentrations above the standard treatment line in Figure 16.8 would be doomed to suffer liver damage if not treated. Although this indicated absorption of at least 150 mg kg^{-1} of paracetamol, only about 60 per cent of patients would be at risk of severe liver damage with plasma aminotransferase activity exceeding 1000 units l^{-1}. Above a parallel line joining plots of 300 mg l^{-1} at 4 h and 45 mg l^{-1} at 15 h, patients had about a 90 per cent chance of severe liver damage while in the zone between these two lines the risk was only 25–30 per cent (Prescott *et al.*, 1979; Prescott, 1983). It was recommended that the treatment line should be lowered to 150 mg l^{-1} at 4 h and 5 mg l^{-1} at 24 h as an additional safety factor to allow for errors in timing of the overdose and analytical errors. This also allowed claims for superior results of treatment as more patients with lower concentrations at less risk of serious toxicity could be included in comparative trials against more severely poisoned patients with concentrations above the standard line (Rumack *et al.*, 1981; Rumack, 1983, 1985, 1986; Smilkstein *et al.*, 1988, 1991). Because of the belief that chronic alcoholics and patients taking inducing drugs were at greater risk of toxicity as a result of increased metabolic activation of paracetamol, it was also proposed that the treatment line should be lowered to 70 per cent (Smith *et al.*, 1986b), 60 per cent (Zwiers, 1993) or even 30 per cent (McClements *et al.*, 1990) of the original values. Although there was no evidence that the changes would be of any benefit, it was further suggested that the treatment line should be lowered to 100 mg l^{-1} at 4 h and 15 mg l^{-1} at 15 h (Minton *et al.*, 1988; Janes and Routledge, 1992; Ferner, 1993; Makin and Williams, 1994).

Patients who poisoned themselves with paracetamol often gave unreliable histories. On the one hand they may have purposely concealed the fact that they took an overdose (Emby and Fraser, 1977; Gazzard *et al.*, 1977; Gilmore and Tourvas, 1977; Canalese *et al.*, 1981a; Flanagan *et al.*, 1981b; Black *et al.*, 1982; Himmelstein *et al.*, 1984) while more often the amounts said to have been taken as a deliberate overdose were grossly overestimated (Ambre and Alexander, 1977; Shnaps *et al.*, 1980). In such circumstances the situation could only be clarified by measurement of the plasma concentration. The routine screening of self-poisoners for paracetamol was said not to affect the outcome (Mahoney *et al.*, 1990; Rygnestad *et al.*, 1990) but this would not necessarily apply in areas where paracetamol was the drug most commonly taken in overdose, or in unconscious patients.

Hepatotoxic Dose of Paracetamol

The minimum single hepatotoxic dose of paracetamol was accepted as 7.5 g in an adult, or 150 mg kg^{-1} but this was a very conservative estimate and in most individuals the dose would be much higher (Linden and Rumack, 1984; Ferner, 1993; Anker and Smilkstein, 1994; Chan *et al.*, 1994a). As calculated by the product of the plasma concentration at 3 h and an apparent volume of distribution of 0.8 l kg^{-1}, the amount of paracetamol absorbed showed a threshold effect with a disproportionate increase in liver damage as the dose increased above 250 mg kg^{-1} (Figure 16.10). This threshold dose of 250 mg kg^{-1} agreed well with a minimum toxic dose of about 15 g in an adult calculated on the basis of the hepatic glutathione content and the fraction of the dose that would be converted to the toxic metabolite (Mitchell *et al.*, 1974) . There have been many reports of liver damage in patients who were said to have taken much smaller doses of paracetamol in the therapeutic dose range (Tables 15.2, 15.3, 15.4, 16.5, 16.6 and 16.7). It can only be assumed that the drug histories were unreliable and in many cases the measured plasma paracetamol concentrations clearly indicated that substantial overdoses had been taken. Some reports, such as severe liver damage necessitating liver transplantation following the claimed ingestion of only 1.5 g of paracetamol (Rustgi *et al.*, 1993), and fatal liver failure in a 15-year-old girl who was said to have taken only 2.5 g (Patel, 1992) cannot be accepted. Even if the whole dose were converted to the toxic metabolite, it would be impossible to produce enough to cause critical depletion of hepatic glutathione and liver damage. In contrast to the alleged toxicity of such low doses in these and other reports, it was apparently considered safe and ethical to give healthy volunteers single doses of 5 g of paracetamol on four occasions in one study (Rose *et al.*, 1991), and single doses of 80 mg kg^{-1} on five occasions in another (Vance *et al.*, 1992).

Disposition and Kinetics of Paracetamol Following Overdosage

Paracetamol metabolism was impaired from the outset in patients who developed liver damage after taking an overdose, and the plasma half life was prolonged in

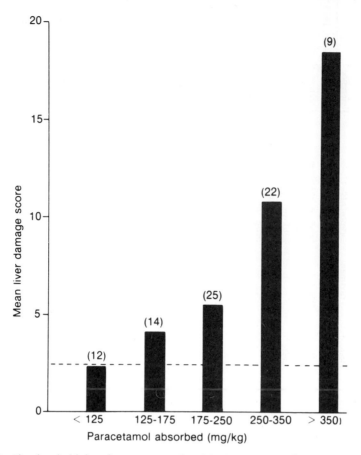

Figure 16.10 The threshold dose for paracetamol toxicity in man. Liver damage was assessed by an arbitrary score based on plasma aminotransferase activity, bilirubin and prothrombin time ratio and the upper normal limit is shown by the dotted line. The numbers of patients in each dose range are given above the columns (reproduced with permission from Prescott, 1983).

relation to the severity of hepatic injury (Prescott *et al.*, 1971; Prescott and Wright, 1973; Davis and Williams, 1975; Gazzard *et al.*, 1977; Saunders *et al.*, 1980; Melethil *et al.*, 1981; Zabrodski and Schnurr, 1984; Flanagan and Mant, 1986; Blake *et al.*, 1988). This impairment of paracetamol metabolism seemed to reflect almost immediate interference with hepatic function with the first passage of the overdose through the liver. Other studies have confirmed early depression of glucuronide conjugation with paracetamol-induced liver damage (Davidson *et al.*, 1976). In patients with very severe and fatal liver damage there was a progressive decrease in the rate of elimination of paracetamol and eventually its conjugation virtually ceased (Prescott and Wright, 1973). Rare patients who presented late with very high plasma concentrations of paracetamol and greatly prolonged half lives have escaped disastrous liver damage and this was presumably because toxic metabolic activation was also impaired (Zezulka and Wright, 1982; Prescott, 1984; Flanagan and Mant, 1986; Block *et al.*, 1992). In patients with liver damage, impaired glucuronide and sulphate conjugation resulted in an increased ratio of plasma concentrations of

Table 16.7 Reported cases of liver damage following acute paracetamol overdosage in chronic alcoholics.

Age and sex	Alleged dose (g)	Plasma paracetamol (mg l^{-1})	Time after ingestion (h)	Max. plasma amino-transferase (units l^{-1})	Max. plasma bilirubin (μmol l^{-1})	Max. prothrombin time ratio	Histology[1]	Treatment[2]	Comments	Reference
26M	25	690	2½	3600	68	–	–	CYS	late treatment	Scott and Stewart, 1975
30F	?	–	–	1250	612	–	AHN	PD	fatal, renal failure[3]	Alván et al., 1976
31F	10	–	–	3561	59	16%[4]	AHN	HF	acidosis, renal failure	Emby and Fraser, 1977
52M	14	–	–	13 160	36	–	AHN	–	acidosis, renal failure	Emby and Fraser, 1977
31F	30	–	–	300	102	5.2	–	–	pancreatitis, renal failure	Gilmore and Tourvas, 1977
24M	32.5	9.5	20	3900	27	1.3	–	–	drug abuse	Krenzelok et al., 1977
38F	6	<10	?	2350	51	1.3	–	HP	epileptic, phenobarbitone	Pond et al., 1982a
27M	32.5	63	?	5178	134	–	–	HD	renal failure	Himmelstein et al., 1984
29F	36	24	?	>1800	94	>5	AHN	HF	fatal, renal failure	Zabrodski and Schnurr, 1984
45M	8.4	–	–	10 100	163	2.3	–	NAC	renal failure	Fleckenstein, 1985
56F	20	24	24	10 670	55	40%[4]	–	–		Bell et al., 1987a
66F	?	–	–	24[5]	20	66%[4]	–	–	renal failure	Denison et al., 1987
30M	?	–	–	5[5]	9	92%[4]	–	–		Denison et al., 1987
31M	?	–	–	24[5]	24	41%[4]	–	–		Denison et al., 1987
38M	?	–	–	6[5]	5	130%[4]	–	–		Denison et al., 1987
55F	36	–	–	6160	37	3.1	–	–	fatal	McClain et al., 1988
24F	50	–	–	11 300	80	1.9	AHN; CF	NAC	renal failure	McClain et al., 1988
56M	14	–	–	8285	22	1.4	AHN	–		Foust et al., 1989
31M	35	68	?	18 726	236	6.5	AHN	–	fatal, renal failure[6]	Mann et al., 1989
40F	4.8	–	–	13 540	136	1.7	AHN	PE	fatal	Shimizu et al., 1989
22M	16	76	4	3460	340	5.2	–	–	fatal	McClements et al., 1990
45M	12	6	21	1928	–	15%[4]	–	NAC		Weber et al., 1990b
40F	17	12	?	5612	267	1.4	AHN	NAC	liver transplant	Mrvos et al., 1992
43F	40	80	10	9546	–	34%[4]	–	NAC		Coirault et al., 1993
21F	25	151	3		–	4.7	–	NAC	fatal, renal failure	Cheung et al., 1994

[1] Histology key: AHN = acute hepatic necrosis, CF = chronic fibrosis; [2] treatment key: CYS = cysteamine, NAC = N-acetylcysteine, HF = hepatic failure regime, PD = peritoneal dialysis, HP = haemoperfusion, HD = haemodialysis, PE = plasma exchange; [3] other drugs taken; [4] Quick, or International Ratio %; [5] μkat l^{-1}; [6] cardiomyopathy

unchanged to conjugated drug (Prescott and Wright, 1973) and the sulphate conjugation of paracetamol rapidly became saturated following an overdose irrespective of liver damage (Davis *et al.*, 1976b; Howie *et al.*, 1977; Prescott, 1979b, 1980; Forrest *et al.*, 1982). It was claimed that glucuronide conjugation was also saturated following overdosage and that liver damage occurred because an increased fraction of the dose was shunted through the toxic pathway of metabolism (Davis *et al.*, 1976b; Slattery and Levy, 1979a; Slattery *et al.*, 1987). No correlation could be demonstrated between paracetamol- or carbon tetrachloride-induced hepatotoxicity and prolongation of the paracetamol half life in mice and rats, and again it was concluded that the increased half life was due to saturation of conjugation (Siegers *et al.*, 1978). Glucuronide conjugation was a minor route of paracetamol metabolism in rats and might be readily saturable with toxic doses but it was not readily saturable in man. There was no evidence of transition from zero- to first-order kinetics as plasma paracetamol concentrations fell from high toxic to low therapeutic levels in poisoned patients (Figure 7.4) and essentially linear kinetics were observed in other reports (Peterson and Rumack, 1977; Melethil *et al.*, 1981; Pond *et al.*, 1982b; Haibach *et al.*, 1984; Lieh-Lai *et al.*, 1984; Roberts *et al.*, 1984; Edwards *et al.*, 1986; Blake *et al.*, 1988; Dawson *et al.*, 1989; Price *et al.*, 1991; Claass *et al.*, 1993). The pattern of urinary excretion of paracetamol metabolites after overdosage was said to show saturation of both sulphate and glucuronide conjugation (Davis *et al.*, 1976b) and these data were subsequently used to develop a model based on Michaelis-Menten kinetics (Slattery and Levy, 1979a). There was good agreement with this model between predicted and observed paracetamol concentrations in two overdose patients (Slattery and Levy, 1979b; Slattery *et al.*, 1981) but the data were also consistent with a linear model. In healthy volunteers given up to 3 g of paracetamol there was saturation of sulphate, but not glucuronide conjugation (Slattery *et al.*, 1987). Saturation of glucuronide conjugation has not been observed by other investigators although this could conceivably occur in patients with exceptionally high plasma paracetamol concentrations as shown in Figure 16.11. Even in this case the initial slow decline in concentrations could have been due to slow absorption or abnormally slow metabolism associated with hypotension, reduced liver blood flow or acidosis (Prescott, 1984).

In keeping with saturation kinetics, the proportional urinary recovery of the sulphate conjugate of paracetamol was greatly reduced following overdosage and this was associated with an increased excretion of glutathione-derived conjugates in patients who suffered hepatic necrosis (Davis *et al.*, 1976b; Howie *et al.*, 1977; Prescott, 1980). The reduced sulphate conjugation could be partially reversed by administration of precursors of inorganic sulphate such as cysteamine, methionine and N-acetylcysteine (Prescott, 1980; Slattery *et al.*, 1987). The fractional urinary excretion of paracetamol metabolites changed markedly over time with a fall in the proportion excreted as the glucuronide conjugate and an increase in the proportions recovered as the sulphate, cysteine and mercapturic acid conjugates (Prescott, 1979b, 1980). In metabolic studies in a newborn infant whose mother had taken an overdose of paracetamol before delivery, sulphate conjugation appeared to be the major route of metabolism and plasma concentrations of the cysteine and mercapturic acid conjugates were relatively low (Lederman *et al.*, 1983). In a similar case, the plasma paracetamol half life in the infant was prolonged to 10 h and the pattern of urinary metabolites resembled that in the mother with no evidence for dominant

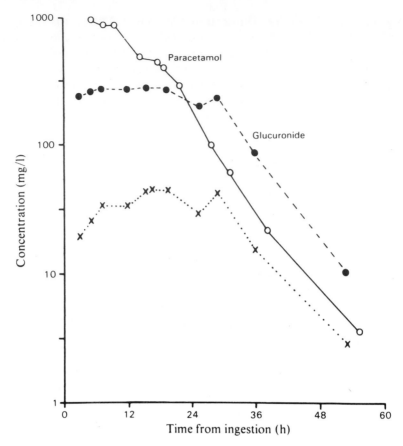

Figure 16.11 Plasma concentrations of paracetamol (○) and its glucuronide (●) and sulphate (×) conjugates in a 43-year-old woman following massive overdosage with paracetamol. Treatment with N-acetylcysteine was started 5 h after ingestion and she recovered without liver damage (reproduced with permission from Prescott, 1984).

sulphate conjugation (Roberts *et al.*, 1984). A 1-year-old boy ate 10 g of paracetamol and about half of this dose was recovered by dialysis and in the urine. The glucuronide conjugate was the major metabolite and about 12 per cent was recovered as cysteine and mercapturic acid conjugates (Lieh-Lai *et al.*, 1984).

Pharmacokinetic models and computer-assisted methods have been proposed for prediction of plasma paracetamol concentrations and prognosis but these approaches seemed to add little to direct measurement (Edwards *et al.*, 1986; Chung, 1989; Gentry *et al.*, 1994). By the use of simple exponential regression, it was possible to determine the prognosis and need for treatment without recourse to a graph (Jeyaranjan, 1991). Good agreement was reported between the observed and calculated urinary recovery of paracetamol in an overdose patient using a previously described pharmacokinetic model (Melethil *et al.*, 1981).

Post-mortem Drug Concentrations

Blood and tissue concentrations of paracetamol were determined in fatal poisonings involving paracetamol and in many cases other toxic agents had also been taken. As might be expected, paracetamol concentrations varied greatly and tended to be highest in the liver and kidney (Robinson *et al.*, 1977; Holzbecher *et al.*, 1981; Oliver *et al.*, 1981; Siefkin, 1982; Chaturvedi *et al.*, 1983; Haibach *et al.*, 1984; Steinmetz *et al.*, 1987; Cox and Pounder, 1992).

Factors Influencing the Hepatotoxicity of Paracetamol

Effects of Age

Accidental overdosage with paracetamol in young children under the age of 6 years is relatively common in some areas but serious toxicity is rare and children in this age group were thought to be less susceptible to toxicity than older children and adults (Rumack and Matthew, 1975; Crome *et al.*, 1976a; Meredith *et al.*, 1978b, 1979; Peterson and Rumack, 1981; Garnier *et al.*, 1982; Rumack, 1984, 1985, 1986; Riggs *et al.*, 1987; Kumar *et al.*, 1990; Flanagan and Meredith, 1991; Volans, 1991; Brotodihardjo *et al.*, 1992; Anker and Smilkstein, 1994). Accidental paracetamol poisoning occurred most commonly in the age range of 1–4 years (Meredith *et al.*, 1978b, 1979; Rumack, 1984; Jonville *et al.*, 1990; Kumar *et al.*, 1990). In this type of poisoning young children took smaller doses of paracetamol than with deliberate self-poisoning by older children and adults, and this was probably the most important factor in limiting toxicity (Meredith *et al.*, 1978b, 1979; Rumack and Peterson, 1978; Garnier *et al.*, 1982; Rumack, 1984, 1985, 1986; Jonville *et al.*, 1990). Of 52 young children with paracetamol poisoning, only three had plasma concentrations above the standard treatment line and they suffered minimal liver damage (Meredith *et al.*, 1978, 1979). There were similar consequences in two of 16 children in another report (Rumack and Peterson, 1978). In a study of 417 children under the age of 6 years, 55 had plasma paracetamol concentrations above the treatment line and 43 were treated with oral N-acetylcysteine. Only three children had liver damage, and treatment had been delayed in them all (Rumack, 1984, 1985, 1986; Riggs *et al.*, 1987). Many thousands of children at risk were said to have escaped liver damage (Rumack, 1984) and it was estimated that less than 5 per cent of children under the age of 6 years with paracetamol concentrations above the treatment line would develop transient hepatic abnormalities (Rumack, 1986). In a more recent study, there was no serious toxicity in 140 young children with paracetamol poisoning (Kumar *et al.*, 1990). The reasons for the apparent resistance of these young children to paracetamol toxicity was not known but they were more likely to vomit after ingestion than older children and adults (Peterson and Rumack, 1981; Rumack, 1984, 1985; Riggs *et al.*, 1987). There was no evidence for more rapid elimination or reduced formation of the toxic metabolite (Volans, 1991). Because serious toxicity was so rare in young children with accidental paracetamol overdose, no adequate data were available to establish the concentration-toxicity relationships and no specific recommendations could be made other than to use the standard treatment line as a guide to prognosis and the need for treatment. The plasma paracetamol half life in children without liver damage was probably the same as in adults (Peterson and Rumack, 1981; Taylor and Betts, 1983) but in a neonate it was prolonged to 10 h (Roberts *et al.*, 1984). In an 8-week-old infant with liver damage caused by iatrogenic paracetamol poisoning the half life was prolonged to 8 h

(Claass *et al.*, 1993). Above the age of about 6 years, the pattern and clinical features of paracetamol overdose were indistinguishable from those in adolescents and adults (Rumack, 1984, 1985, 1986).

In sharp contrast to the lack of serious toxicity after accidental overdose of paracetamol in young children, there have been many reports of major toxicity with its therapeutic use in this age group (Tables 15.3 and 15.4). In these cases excessive doses were administered by misguided parents and doctors, and toxicity often followed repeated overdosing for a minor febrile illness over a period of several days (Calvert and Linder, 1978; Bickers and Roberts, 1979; Agran *et al.*, 1983; Greene *et al.*, 1983; Swetnam and Florman, 1984; Smith *et al.*, 1986a; Fudin *et al.*, 1989; Henretig *et al.*, 1989; Chiossi *et al.*, 1991; Claass *et al.*, 1993; Douidar *et al.*, 1994). With oral administration, the dose absorbed could be limited by vomiting in the event of toxicity, but for many of these children there was no escape because the paracetamol was given by suppository (Montoya Cabrera *et al.*, 1982; Clark *et al.*, 1983; Smith *et al.*, 1986; de Nardo *et al.*, 1988; Henretig *et al.*, 1989; Chao, 1993; Claass *et al.*, 1993; Zwiener *et al.*, 1994). Many children were given grossly excessive doses and fatalities have been reported (Nogen and Bremner, 1978; Atwood, 1980; Mühlendahl and Krienke, 1980; Weber and Cutz, 1980; Montoya Cabrera *et al.*, 1982; Clark *et al.*, 1983; Blake *et al.*, 1988; de Nardo *et al.*, 1988; Chao, 1993; Nadir *et al.*, 1994). There were occasional reports of residual brain damage in children who survived (Augustin and Schmoldt, 1991b; Claass *et al.*, 1993). In one unusual case, a 3-year-old boy was said to have died from paracetamol poisoning after administration of large doses of benorylate (Symon *et al.*, 1982). Paracetamol has been used for deliberate non-accidental poisoning in children (Hickson *et al.*, 1983; Taylor and Betts, 1983). In the light of these reports of severe and fatal toxicity following the therapeutic use of paracetamol in young children, it was suggested that the margin of safety was much lower than previously appreciated (Penna and Buchanan, 1991). In adults, there was no evidence that age was an important factor in determining mortality or morbidity after paracetamol overdosage (Douglas *et al.*, 1976).

Pregnancy

Paracetamol passed readily into the fetal circulation (Levy *et al.*, 1975a; Lederman *et al.*, 1983; Roberts *et al.*, 1984; Wang *et al.*, 1986a) but the fetal liver did not appear to be particularly susceptible to toxicity. There have been several reports of maternal overdosage of paracetamol in late pregnancy just before delivery. In some, the mother suffered severe liver damage (Lederman *et al.*, 1983; Rosevear and Hope, 1989; Friedman *et al.*, 1993) while in others she did not (Roberts *et al.*, 1984; Ruthnum and Goel, 1984; Kumar *et al.*, 1990), but in all cases a normal infant was delivered with no evidence of hepatotoxicity. Fetal movements ceased when a 24-year-old woman took an overdose of paracetamol when 27–28 weeks pregnant. She subsequently suffered severe liver damage and was delivered of a stillborn infant five days later. There was autolysis of fetal tissues, including the liver and fetal death was attributed to the paracetamol although no plausible mechanism was put forward (Haibach *et al.*, 1984). In another report, a 31-year-old woman who was 35 weeks pregnant was admitted in coma with hypotension, seizures and haematemesis after taking aspirin, paracetamol, codeine and carisoprodol. Liver function tests were moderately abnormal but improved rapidly. A male infant was delivered five days later and he had seizures and an infratentorial haemorrhage that required treatment by craniotomy. For some reason these complications were attributed to the paracetamol (Kurzel, 1990). There have also been reports of maternal overdosage with paracetamol with and without severe liver damage in the first, second and early in the third trimesters of pregnancy. In all cases the infants were normal on delivery (Byer *et al.*, 1982; Stokes, 1984; Ludmir *et al.*, 1986; Robertson *et al.*, 1986). Despite the lack of evidence of major fetal toxicity of paracetamol, heroic emergency measures such as Caesarean section and exchange transfusion have been instituted following maternal overdosage (Lederman *et al.*, 1983; Roberts *et al.*, 1984; Friedman *et al.*, 1993).

During the period 1980–1983, enquiries were made concerning 111 women who took drug overdoses during pregnancy. Paracetamol was taken alone or in combination with other drugs by 18 and apparently there were no complications (Rayburn *et al.*, 1984). In a survey of 60 pregnant women with acute paracetamol overdosage, approximately one-third took it in each of the three trimesters. Twenty-four had plasma paracetamol concentrations above the standard treatment line and 10 were treated with oral N-acetylcysteine within 10 h. Of these, eight delivered normal infants and there were two elective abortions. Ten patients were treated 10–16 h after ingestion of the paracetamol and five had normal deliveries, two had elective abortions and three had spontaneous abortions. Of four women treated after 16 h, three suffered severe liver damage and one died as a result. In this group there was one elective and one spontaneous abortion, a stillbirth and a normal delivery. As with paracetamol poisoning generally, a good prognosis during pregnancy depended on early treatment with N-acetylcysteine (Riggs *et al.*, 1989). In another study, 48 of 115 pregnant women who took an overdose of paracetamol were followed up. There were no deaths and most pregnancies had a normal outcome. Four infants exposed during the third trimester had problems unrelated to paracetamol and two women had spontaneous abortions two weeks after the overdose (McElhatton *et al.*, 1990). Although there was no contraindication to the use of N-acetylcysteine for protection against paracetamol hepatotoxicity during pregnancy, it appeared not to cross the placenta in sheep and its ability to prevent liver toxicity in the human fetus was uncertain (Selden *et al.*, 1991).

Alcohol Consumption

It was widely believed that chronic alcoholics had an increased susceptibility to the hepatotoxicity of paracetamol and that they were at greater risk of liver damage after overdosage. This belief was based on animal studies which showed that chronic administration of ethanol increased the hepatotoxicity of paracetamol, together with numerous anecdotal reports of severe and fatal liver damage in chronic alcoholics following not only deliberate overdosage but also alleged therapeutic use of the drug. It was assumed that the mechanism of potentiation of toxicity was increased metabolic activation of paracetamol due to induction of hepatic drug metabolizing enzymes by ethanol. The severity of liver damage after paracetamol overdosage was compared in groups of eight potentially induced, and eight apparently not induced patients. The liver damage was greater, and the incidence of death and renal failure higher in the induced group, which included three chronic alcoholics (Wright and Prescott, 1973). Emby and Fraser (1977) then reported enhanced hepatotoxicity of paracetamol following overdosage with a fatal outcome in two chronic alcoholics. However convincing, this report was purely anecdotal, and the description did not differ materially from the original report of fatal paracetamol poisoning in two patients who presumably were not alcoholics (Davidson and Eastham, 1966). There followed further anecdotal accounts of liver damage with paracetamol poisoning in chronic alcoholics and an even greater number of reports of hepatotoxicity after its apparently innocent use with 'therapeutic intent' (Table 15.3). Cases of liver toxicity following overdosage in chronic alcoholics are summarized in Table 16.7. Although the incidence of renal failure might have been higher in these patients, the general pattern did not differ from that seen in poisoned patients who were not chronic alcoholics (Table 16.5).

Previous chronic treatment with ethanol invariably potentiated the hepatotoxicity of paracetamol in animals (Teschke *et al.*, 1979; Peterson *et al.*, 1980; Singletary *et al.*, 1980; Sato *et al.*, 1981a; Walker *et al.*, 1983b; Altomare *et al.*, 1984a; Tredger *et al.*, 1985; Carter, 1987; Lieber *et al.*, 1987; Lieber, 1990b; Prasad *et al.*, 1990) while an opposite effect was usually seen with acute administration (Wong *et al.*, 1980b; Sato *et al.*, 1981a; Altomare *et al.*, 1984a; Banda and Quart, 1984a,b; Tredger *et al.*, 1985; Serrar and Thevenin, 1987; Thummel *et al.*, 1988, 1989; Garrido *et al.*, 1989). It seemed that paracetamol metabolism was stimulated by chronic ethanol treatment and inhibited by its acute administration. The timing of acute administration of ethanol relative to dosing with paracetamol was critical. Protection was largely lost after a delay of 6 h (Serrar and Thevenin, 1987), and after 10–16 h the toxicity of paracetamol was actually potentiated (Strubelt *et al.*, 1978; Carter, 1987). In another report, acute ethanol reduced the antidotal efficacy of N-acetylcysteine in protecting against paracetamol-induced hepatotoxicity (Dalhoff *et al.*, 1991). The picture was further complicated as, depending on the timing, the effects of chronic and acute treatment with ethanol tended to cancel each other out (Altomare *et al.*, 1984a; Tredger *et al.*, 1985). It was also observed that the toxicity of paracetamol in hamsters was greatly reduced to well below control (untreated) levels when it was given 24 h after the chronic administration of ethanol had been discontinued (Singletary *et al.*, 1980). Chronic treatment of animals with ethanol increased the toxic metabolic activation of paracetamol as shown by increased urinary excretion of the cysteine and mercapturic acid conjugates (Sato *et al.*, 1981a; Lieber, 1983, 1990b; Tredger *et al.*, 1986b; Lieber *et al.*, 1987) and its glutathione conjugation was increased in isolated hepatocytes obtained from rats pretreated with ethanol for 6–8 weeks (Moldéus *et al.*, 1980a). However, in another study, chronic administration of ethanol had no effect on the production of glutathione-derived conjugates although the biliary excretion of conjugates was reduced (Vendemiale *et al.*, 1984). The protective effect of acute ethanol was probably due to decreased metabolic activation of paracetamol as shown by reduced formation of glutathione, cysteine and mercapturic acid conjugates in the intact animal (Sato and Lieber, 1981; Tredger *et al.*, 1986b; Lieber *et al.*, 1987; Thummel *et al.*, 1988, 1989; Sato *et al.*, 1991), liver microsomal preparations (Sato *et al.*, 1991) and the isolated perfused rat liver (Schlager *et al.*, 1987). Acute ethanol also inhibited the glucuronide conjugation of paracetamol, and this effect was dependent on fasting (Minnigh and Zemaitis, 1980; Minnigh and Zemaitis, 1982). In one study, acute ethanol protected against hepatotoxicity but it produced only a minor reduction in the formation of the cysteine conjugate of paracetamol (Prasad *et al.*, 1990). Similarly, ethanol had relatively little effect on the metabolic activation of paracetamol by human liver microsomes and any protective effect was probably indirect (Thummel *et al.*, 1989).

The evidence that chronic alcoholics have increased susceptibility to the hepatotoxicity of paracetamol is conflicting. In a retrospective study of selected patients with severe paracetamol-induced liver damage referred to a specialist liver unit, the prognosis was worse, and the incidence of renal failure was higher in 30 patients who took more than the maximum recommended amount of alcohol than in 49 patients who drank less (Bray *et al.*, 1991). These findings must be suspect because alcohol consumption was only assessed by retrospective inspection of case notes, and it was not known in an unstated number of patients. In a previous report from the same unit, previous intake of alcohol was not associated with a significantly worse prognosis (Read *et al.*, 1986). In other reports the severity of liver damage and prognosis in patients with paracetamol poisoning was not adversely affected by alcohol abuse (Rumack, 1983; Smilkstein *et al.*, 1989) and it was suggested that any potentiation of toxicity might be caused not so much by chronic consumption of alcohol as by dietary factors and fasting (Whitcomb and Block, 1994). It was proposed that all alcoholics who might have taken paracetamol should be treated with N-acetylcysteine regardless of the drug concentrations and the time since ingestion (Cheung *et al.*, 1994), but this was considered to be an unnecessary and retrograde step (Smilkstein *et al.*, 1994). The interacting effects of acute on chronic intake of ethanol would complicate matters even further. The form in which the alcohol was taken might also be important as ethanol given as beer produced much less induction of CYP2E1 in rats than the same doses given as a simple 10 per cent solution (Crankshaw and Hines, 1992).

If chronic alcoholism did potentiate the hepatotoxicity of paracetamol, the mechanism was unlikely to be induction of liver microsomal enzymes with increased formation of toxic metabolite. In chronic alcoholics with cirrhosis, the clearance of paracetamol and its glucuronide and sulphate conjugation were reduced (Porowski *et al.*, 1988) but in alcoholics with only mildly abnormal liver function tests the clearance of paracetamol was greater than in healthy non-alcoholic subjects (Dietz *et al.*, 1984). Similar enhanced clearance of paracetamol, consistent with induction of glucuronide conjugation, was observed in otherwise healthy chronic alcoholics on the third day of abstinence (Girre *et al.*, 1993). As judged by the urinary excretion of cysteine and mercapturic acid conjugates, the metabolic activation of paracetamol was increased in chronic alcoholics without obvious liver disease compared with control subjects but the fractional recoveries were still well within the normal range (Villeneuve *et al.*, 1983; Chern *et al.*, 1993). In another study, the excretion of these conjugates was not significantly increased in chronic alcoholics (Lauterburg and Velez, 1988). Contrary to expectations, there was no change in the fractional urinary recovery of the mercapturic acid conjugate of paracetamol in five chronic alcoholics after they had abstained from alcohol for at least 10 days. It was concluded that if chronic alcoholics were at increased risk of paracetamol hepatotoxicity, induction of microsomal enzyme activity was probably not an important mechanism (Skinner *et al.*, 1990). Drug metabolizing enzyme activity in liver biopsies from chronic alcoholics was not increased except in patients with active alcoholic liver disease, and otherwise, there was no evidence of induction in alcoholics (Hoensch, 1984). Other studies suggested that a more likely mechanism for increased susceptibility in alcoholics would be reduced capacity for glutathione synthesis (Guerri and Grisoli, 1978; Shaw *et al.*, 1983; Lauterburg *et al.*, 1984a,c; Lauterburg and Velez, 1988; Roseau, 1989). A single dose of ethanol decreased the overall rates of absorption and elimination of paracetamol in healthy men, although the metabolites were not measured (Wójcicki *et al.*, 1978), and it also markedly reduced the urinary excretion of the cysteine and mercapturic acid conjugates of paracetamol in healthy volunteers (Banda and Quart, 1982; Critchley *et al.*, 1983; Prescott and Critchley, 1983a; Altomare *et al.*, 1986). The acute ingestion of alcohol probably did protect against paracetamol-induced liver damage in man (Hartnell *et al.*, 1983; Rumack, 1983, 1984, 1986) and it seemed likely that many patients protected themselves unwittingly by taking alcohol before an overdose (Scott and Stewart, 1975; Critchley *et al.*, 1983; Prescott and Critchley, 1983a; Rumack, 1983). Some chronic alcoholics abused paracetamol regularly and a minority took excessive doses and might therefore be at risk of toxicity (Seifert *et al.*, 1993). Previously undiagnosed cirrhosis was observed in many chronic alcoholics who survived paracetamol-induced hepatic necrosis. It was implied that the paracetamol had caused cirrhosis, but no evidence was provided to substantiate this claim (Rothstein *et al.*, 1994).

It was commonly stated that increased metabolic activation and hepatotoxicity of paracetamol in chronic alcoholics was due to increased activity of ethanol-inducible isoforms of cytochrome P450 such as CYP2E1, which also had a high affinity for paracetamol (Black and Raucy, 1986; Zimmerman, 1986; Schenker and Maddrey, 1991). The liver content of CYP2E1 was increased in liver biopsies from heavy drinkers of alcohol (Perrot *et al.*, 1989), and the demonstration that human CYP2E1 also catalyzed the metabolic activation of paracetamol seemed to confirm this hypothesis (Black and Raucy, 1986; Zimmerman, 1986; Raucy *et al.*, 1989). Unfortunately, most of the relevant studies with paracetamol and ethanol were performed in rats and rabbits (Morgan *et al.*, 1983; Coon *et al.*, 1984; Coon and Koop, 1987; Lieber, 1988), and in man CYP2E1 was shown to have important activity against paracetamol at the very high concentration of 1500 mg l^{-1} (Raucy *et al.*, 1989). Subsequent studies at more clinically realistic concentrations indicated only a minor role for CYP2E1 in the metabolic activation of paracetamol in man and that other isoenzymes such as CYP3A4 made a more important contribution (Thummel *et al.*, 1993). Multiple isoforms of cytochrome P450 from human liver metabolized paracetamol, and CYP2E1, 1A2 and 3A4 showed the greatest activity (Patten *et al.*, 1993). A further complication was the demonstration of genetic polymorphism of CYP2E1 in patients with alcoholic liver disease (Tsutsumi *et al.*, 1994). As with hepatotoxicity following the alleged use of paracetamol with therapeutic intent, no positive challenge studies have been reported in chronic alcoholics who were supposed to have developed severe liver damage after small overdoses. Despite all the findings in animals treated chronically with ethanol and the specificity or otherwise of the isoforms of cytochrome P450, it has never been shown that the metabolic activation of paracetamol was significantly increased in chronic alcoholics to the point where hepatotoxicity would be potentiated. Indeed, in one patient who drank alcohol to excess, there was no evidence of liver damage despite the chronic consumption of 15–20 g of paracetamol daily for five years (Tredger *et al.*, 1995). At present, the mechanism of the presumed potentiation of the hepatotoxicity of paracetamol in chronic alcoholics must remain an open question.

Inducing Drugs

The pretreatment of animals with classical inducers of drug metabolizing enzymes such as phenobarbitone and 3-methylcholanthrene usually increased the hepatotoxicity of paracetamol by stimulating its metabolic activation, and it was easy to believe that similar potentiation would occur in man. Following the original report of increased liver damage following paracetamol overdosage in patients who had previously been taking drugs likely to cause induction of drug metabolizing enzymes (Wright and Prescott, 1973) there were anecdotal reports also claiming potentiation of hepatic and renal toxicity in patients who had been taking phenobarbitone and other anticonvulsants (Wilson *et al.*, 1978; Black *et al.*, 1982; Montoya Cabrera *et al.*, 1982; Pirotte, 1984; Dabbagh and Chesney, 1985; Marsepoil *et al.*, 1989; Smith *et al.*, 1986b; McClain *et al.*, 1988; Minton *et al.*, 1988; McClements *et al.*, 1990; Chiossi *et al.*, 1991). In a retrospective survey of selected patients with severe liver damage after paracetamol overdose referred to a specialist liver unit, it was claimed that the mortality was significantly greater in 18 patients taking anticonvulsants than in 394 control patients not taking these drugs (Bray *et al.*, 1992a). This report was criticized on the grounds that the unequal groups were not matched for plasma paracetamol concentrations, doses of paracetamol taken, use of alcohol or treatment with N-acetylcysteine (Buckley *et al.*, 1993). There was also no data to show that the metabolism of paracetamol was altered as implied in the patients taking anticonvulsants. As in the case of chronic alcoholics, it has never been shown that the metabolic activation of paracetamol was increased in such patients. Compared with healthy drug-free subjects, there was no significant increase in the clearance of paracetamol in six epileptic patients taking phenobarbitone, primidone, carbamazepine or diphenylhydantoin (Perucca and Richens, 1979), and in 15 induced patients taking anticonvulsants or rifampicin, the elimination of paracetamol was accelerated and its glucuronide conjugation was enhanced without increased formation of the cysteine and mercapturic acid conjugates (Prescott *et al.*, 1981).

Recently it was claimed that isoniazid caused induction of CYP2E1 in man, and that accordingly, it had potentiated hepatic and renal toxicity in a patient who had taken an overdose of paracetamol (Murphy *et al.*, 1990). Similar claims were made in the case of a 21-year-old woman taking isoniazid who developed severe liver damage after the alleged intake of only 3.25 g of paracetamol (Crippin, 1993). The possibility of a toxic interaction between paracetamol and isoniazid was suggested in two of 20 isoniazid-associated deaths, and a 3-year-old child who was receiving isoniazid died of liver failure after taking an unknown quantity of paracetamol (Moulding *et al.*, 1991). Again, isoniazid was metabolized in rats by the ethanol-inducible isoenzyme of cytochrome P450, CYP2E1 (Ryan *et al.*, 1986) and pretreatment with 1 g l^{-1} of isoniazid in the drinking water for 10 days potentiated the hepatotoxicity of paracetamol in rats also pretreated with phenobarbitone for four days (Burk *et al.*, 1990). However, the reports of enhanced paracetamol toxicity in patients taking isoniazid cannot be accepted because, in the doses used clinically, isoniazid has been recognized for years as a classical *inhibitor* of drug oxidation and as such it should have prevented rather than enhanced paracetamol toxicity. In keeping with this, isoniazid was shown to markedly inhibit the formation of the glutathione and catechol metabolites of paracetamol in man (Epstein *et al.*, 1991; Zand *et al.*, 1993). Rifampicin is a potent inducing drug and hepatotoxic reactions to paracetamol after overdosage and therapeutic use were reported in three women who were receiving rifampicin, isoniazid and other drugs for tuberculosis (Nolan *et al.*, 1994). No information was provided about the metabolism of paracetamol and in at least one case, the picture resembled isoniazid hepatotoxicity.

Fasting and Nutritional State

As discussed in Chapters 7 and 14, paracetamol metabolism and toxicity in animals were influenced by diet and nutritional state. In particular, fasting enhanced hepatotoxicity and an important mechanism appeared to be decreased hepatic glutathione synthesis. Fasting also reduced the glucuronide conjugation of paracetamol in rats, and toxicity was increased as a result of correspondingly enhanced metabolic activation (Price *et al.*, 1987; Price and Jollow, 1988, 1989a). The effects of fasting and enzyme induction on paracetamol-induced hepatotoxicity were additive (Pessayre *et al.*, 1980). It is not known to what extent these factors might apply in man. Barker *et al.* (1977) described liver toxicity in a 67-year-old cachectic woman with a bronchial carcinoma who was said to have been taking up to 6.5 g of paracetamol daily and this was attributed to reduced glutathione stores. On the other hand, a malnourished patient with anorexia nervosa weighing 43 kg was reported as escaping liver damage after an overdose of 15 g of paracetamol but this result might have been anticipated anyway as he was treated with N-acetylcysteine at 9 h (Newman and Bargman, 1979). Malnutrition, starvation and vomiting have been cited as predisposing factors for paracetamol toxicity in chronic alcoholics (Emby and Fraser, 1977; Erickson and Runyon, 1984; McClain *et al.*, 1988; Eriksson *et al.*, 1992) as well as individuals who apparently did not abuse alcohol (Ware *et al.*, 1978; Stegeman-Castelen *et al.*, 1983; Yasunaga *et al.*, 1985; Frisinette-Fich *et al.*, 1986; Chiossi *et al.*, 1991; Shriner and Goetz, 1992; Rustgi *et al.*, 1993). Of five patients with anorexia nervosa who took overdoses of paracetamol, two developed severe liver damage with aminotransferase activities of 1325 and 5220 units l^{-1} (Woolf and Gren, 1990) but this outcome could not be considered unusual. In a recent report it was proposed that fasting was more important than chronic alcohol consumption as a potentiating factor for liver damage following both overdosage and therapeutic use of paracetamol. Hepatotoxicity after claimed intake of 4–10 g daily was associated with fasting and, less commonly, with alcohol use, whereas patients who developed liver damage after apparently taking more than 10 g daily were alcohol users (Whitcomb and Block, 1994). In this study, 94 patients who had taken paracetamol were selected, but details were only presented for 49 who had liver damage. Information concerning the frequency of fasting and alcohol intake in another 42 patients who had taken paracetamol without hepatotoxicity would have been valuable control data but unfortunately no details were provided. It was presumed that paracetamol hepatotoxicity was enhanced by fasting as a result of impaired glucuronide conjugation with shunting of a larger fraction of the dose towards the pathway of toxic metabolic activation. No challenge studies were reported in patients who were supposed to have suffered liver damage after taking only small doses of paracetamol while fasting, and it is not known whether fasting has any effect on the metabolism of paracetamol or other drugs in man.

Other Factors

It was suggested that paracetamol hepatotoxicity might have been enhanced by psittacosis (Davis *et al.*, 1983), human immunodeficiency virus infection (Shriner and Goetz, 1992) and co-existing mercury intoxication (Zwiener *et al.*, 1994), but these reports were only anecdotal. Two weeks after halothane anaesthesia for a breast biopsy, a 40-year-old woman was admitted with mildly abnormal liver function tests and acute renal failure. She was said to have taken only 500 mg of paracetamol on the third and second days before admission and this toxicity was attributed, without evidence, to a synergistic reaction of halothane and paracetamol (Grinblat *et al.*, 1980). Any factor that decreased the rate of absorption or metabolic activation of paracetamol would reduce the rate of formation of the toxic metabolite and thus reduce the risk of liver damage. It was proposed that patients who took mixed overdoses of paracetamol and antimuscarinic drugs were less likely to suffer liver damage because gastric emptying and paracetamol absorption were delayed (Müller *et al.*, 1983). A similar effect could occur with combined overdosage with paracetamol and dextropropoxyphene or codeine and in some reports, associated hypothermia probably provided additional protection by slowing down the metabolic activation of paracetamol (Kritharides *et al.*, 1988; Block *et al.*, 1992). The fractional urinary recovery of the cysteine and mercapturic conjugates of paracetamol were significantly increased in subjects with Gilbert's disease (Esteban and Pérez-Mateo, 1993b) and patients with hepatocellular carcinoma (Leung and Critchley, 1991) suggesting that they would have increased susceptibility to hepatotoxicity.

General Management of Paracetamol Poisoning

The current management of paracetamol poisoning depended on prevention of further absorption, assessment of the risk of toxicity, institution of specific antidotal therapy if indicated, general measures and the treatment of major complications such as hepatic and renal failure.

Prevention of Further Absorption

Unless taken with other drugs that inhibit gastric emptying, such as dextropropoxyphene, paracetamol was usually absorbed rapidly and in the UK it was common practice to perform gastric lavage or induce emesis with syrup of ipecacuanha in patients who presented within 4 h. In other areas, the administration of activated charcoal was recommended routinely for the treatment of oral drug overdose (Hodgkinson *et al.*, 1991). The efficacy of these measures in practice was doubtful but in one uncontrolled study, severe liver damage was less likely in patients who had vomited or undergone gastric lavage within 6 h of taking an overdose than in those who had not (Gazzard *et al.*, 1977). The ratios of measured to predicted plasma concentrations of paracetamol were used to estimate the efficacy of emesis induced by ipecac in 50 children less than 5 years of age with accidental paracetamol poisoning and, not surprisingly, it was concluded that the prompt administration of syrup of ipecac resulted in greater reductions in plasma drug concentrations (Amitai *et al.*, 1987). In a simulated overdose in 10 volunteers, there was no difference between emesis induced by ipecac and administration of activated charcoal plus a cathartic in reducing the absorption of paracetamol (McNamara *et al.*, 1989). When emesis was produced in dogs 10 min after a dose of paracetamol, about 50 per cent was recovered in the vomit (Teshima *et al.*, 1990). In a comparative study of gastric lavage, ipecac-induced emesis and administration of activated charcoal in 60 adults who had taken more than 5 g of paracetamol, there was little to choose between lavage and emesis as judged by the subsequent percentage fall in plasma paracetamol concentrations. Activated charcoal was superior to both (Underhill *et al.*, 1990). A survey of plasma concentrations of paracetamol in children following overdosage in relation to the timing of induced emesis suggested that absorption could be reduced if vomiting occurred within 30 min of ingestion, but that it was useless when delayed for more than $1\frac{1}{2}$ h (Bond *et al.*, 1993). Endoscopy was used to assess the intragastric residue in 30 poisoned patients after emesis induced by ipecac or gastric lavage. Fourteen patients had taken paracetamol and overall, gastric lavage was less effective in emptying the stomach than emesis (Saetta and Quinton, 1991). Ultrasound examination was proposed as a means of detecting unabsorbed paracetamol tablets in the stomach following an overdose but this approach would hardly be feasible in practice (Amitai *et al.*, 1992). Twelve healthy volunteers were given a substantial overdose of 80 mg kg^{-1} of paracetamol on five occasions and absorption was determined in five different body positions. The mean maximum plasma paracetamol concentrations approached toxic levels but there was no mention of adverse effects or safety monitoring. Absorption was fastest in the right lateral, and slowest in the left lateral decubitus positions (Vance *et al.*, 1992). Disastrous gastrointestinal damage followed the overenthusiastic use of an excessively concentrated saline emetic in a patient who took an overdose of paracetamol and dextropropoxyphene (Calam *et al.*, 1982).

Activated charcoal was a powerful adsorbent of paracetamol (Bainbridge *et al.*, 1977; Boehm and Oppenheim, 1977; van de Graaff *et al.*, 1982; Rybolt *et al.*, 1986; Harou-Kouka *et al.*, 1989; Al-Shareef *et al.*, 1990; Eyer and Sprenger, 1991) and it effectively reduced paracetamol absorption in pigs when administered after a delay of one hour (Lipscomb and Widdop, 1975). The absorption of paracetamol was significantly reduced in healthy volunteers when activated charcoal was given up to 2 h afterwards (Dordoni *et al.*, 1973; Levy and Houston, 1976; Galinsky and Levy, 1984a; Remmert *et al.*, 1990; Eyer and Sprenger, 1991). In one study, healthy volunteers experienced nausea and flushing following administration of large single doses of 5 g of paracetamol and these adverse effects were not abolished when it was given with charcoal (Rose *et al.*, 1991). The optimum ratio of charcoal to paracetamol was at least 5 : 1 or 10 : 1 (Dordoni *et al.*, 1973; Levy and Houston, 1976; Galinsky and Levy, 1984a) and charcoal was more effective when given in suspension than as tablets or capsules (Remmert *et al.*, 1990). The addition of sorbitol as a cathartic did not enhance the inhibitory effect of charcoal on paracetamol absorption but it caused side effects and increased misery in the volunteers (McNamara *et al.*, 1988). Nevertheless, the use of charcoal with sorbitol to produce catharsis was still recommended as treatment for paracetamol poisoning (Eyer and Sprenger, 1991). Whole gut lavage with polyethylene glycol and electrolyte solution was also proposed for the treatment of paracetamol overdose on the basis of reduced absorption of doses of 4 g (but not 2 g) in volunteers when administered 30 min after the paracetamol was taken (Hassig *et al.*, 1993). When given 15 and 30 min after administration of

1 g of paracetamol in healthy volunteers, activated charcoal was more effective than emesis induced with syrup of ipecac in reducing absorption (Neuvonen *et al.*, 1983), but after a delay of one hour, there was no significant difference between emesis induced by ipecac and activated charcoal given with a cathartic (McNamara *et al.*, 1989). The practice of giving N-acetylcysteine orally in North America has caused a dilemma through fears that its absorption would be compromised by activated charcoal given at the same time. Although N-acetylcysteine and methionine were avidly bound by activated charcoal *in vitro* (Chinouth *et al.*, 1980; Klein-Schwartz and Oderda, 1981; Rybolt *et al.*, 1986), 50 g of charcoal did not significantly reduce the absorption of 140 mg kg^{-1} of N-acetylcysteine in volunteers when taken at the same time or 15 min later (North *et al.*, 1981; Renzi *et al.*, 1985). However, in a similar study with 100 g of charcoal in a larger number of subjects there was a 40 per cent reduction in the amount of N-acetylcysteine absorbed (Ekins *et al.*, 1987). An increased loading dose of oral N-acetylcysteine was recommended to reduce the loss incurred by the ingestion of charcoal (Chamberlain *et al.*, 1993) but this approach was criticized because the use of charcoal was probably unnecessary anyway, and larger doses of N-acetylcysteine would increase the risk of vomiting (Brent, 1993). In a study of 122 patients with paracetamol overdose, there was no evidence that the administration of activated charcoal reduced the hepatoprotective efficacy of oral N-acetylcysteine (Spiller *et al.*, 1994). Attention was drawn to the problems of assessment of the pharmacokinetics of N-acetylcysteine and the effects of charcoal on its absorption and efficacy (Watson and McKinncy, 1991), and there were considerable differences of opinion regarding the use of gastric lavage, induction of emesis and the use of activated charcoal together with oral N-acetylcysteine in patients with paracetamol poisoning (Fleisher *et al.*, 1991). It was recommended that activated charcoal should not be given with oral N-acetylcysteine (Antaki *et al.*, 1978; McBride and Rumack, 1992) and these problems could be avoided by the use of intravenous N-acetylcysteine. The use of activated charcoal for limiting paracetamol absorption following overdosage has been reviewed (Lewis and Paloucek, 1991). Cholestyramine protected rats against hepatic and renal toxicity and reduced the urinary recovery of paracetamol and its conjugates even when given as late as 4 and 24 h after the paracetamol (Siegers and Möller-Hartmann, 1989). Cholestyramine was more effective than activated charcoal in reducing the absorption of paracetamol given at the same time to healthy volunteers (Dordoni *et al.*, 1973).

Methods for Enhancing the Elimination of Paracetamol

Attempts to enhance the removal of paracetamol from the body after overdosage by techniques such as forced diuresis, dialysis, haemoperfusion and exchange transfusion have not provided significant benefit. Liver damage probably occurred very early as the overdose first passed through the liver during absorption (Prescott *et al.*, 1971; Prescott and Wright, 1973) and by the time that these measures could be instituted it would be far too late to influence the outcome. In addition, the early administration of N-acetylcysteine has been so successful in preventing liver damage that other treatment has become largely redundant.

Only a small fraction of a dose of paracetamol was normally excreted unchanged in the urine and its renal clearance was independent of urine pH. Although the clearance varied with urine flow rate, forced diuresis had no effect on the overall rate of elimination of paracetamol (Prescott and Wright, 1973; Prescott, 1980). The clearance of paracetamol by forced diuresis was reported as 1 ml min^{-1} compared with 40 and 90 ml min^{-1} with haemodialysis and haemoperfusion respectively (Lenz *et al.*, 1982). Despite the therapeutic futility and risks of forced diuresis, it has been employed with and without alkalinization in attempts to enhance paracetamol elimination in poisoned patients (Rose, 1969; Ambre and Alexander, 1977; Horwitz *et al.*, 1977; Baumgarten *et al.*, 1983; Weinberger *et al.*, 1994).

Haemodialysis was carried out in 15 patients with paracetamol overdose and the amounts said to be removed ranged from 0.75 to 5 g. Although liver damage was not prevented, haemodialysis was recommended for the treatment of paracetamol poisoning (Farid *et al.*, 1972). This report was criticized on the grounds that haemodialysis had been unnecessary in more than half of these patients as they had plasma paracetamol concentrations in the low therapeutic range and only trivial amounts could possibly have been removed by the procedure (Matthew, 1972; Prescott, 1972). In another report, the equivalent of less than one tablet of paracetamol was removed from a poisoned patient during 6 h of haemodialysis (van Heijst *et al.*, 1976). In studies of the removal of paracetamol by haemodialysis following a therapeutic dose of 650 mg in patients with renal failure, the extraction efficiency was 40–50 per cent and the mean dialysis clearance of the drug was 112 ml min^{-1} with blood flow rates of 170–280 ml min^{-1} (Lee *et al.*, 1981a). In another study in an overdose patient, the extraction ratio was 0.62 and removal of a total of 1.82 g of paracetamol by haemodialysis for 4 h did not prevent severe liver damage (Pond *et al.*, 1982b). Haemodialysis was performed in a seriously poisoned young child with recovery of 2.8 g of paracetamol. The extraction efficiency ranged from 20–72 per cent and the mean clearance was 18 ml min^{-1} (Lieh-Lai *et al.*, 1984). In one report, a patient was subjected to haemodialysis for 4 h even though the plasma paracetamol concentration at the start was only 22 mg l^{-1} (Ambre and Alexander, 1977). Despite lack of evidence of efficacy, haemodialysis was recommended for the treatment of paracetamol poisoning (Boukma, 1976; Lenz *et al.*, 1982) and it was still being used for this purpose (Weber *et al.*, 1990b). Paracetamol was removed effectively *in vivo* and *in vitro* in dogs with a sorbent suspension reciprocating dialyzer (Shihab-Eldeen *et al.*, 1988).

The same limitations as discussed above for haemodialysis apply to haemoperfusion. Paracetamol was effectively removed from pigs by charcoal haemoperfusion with an extraction efficiency of more than 90 per cent (Willson *et al.*, 1973) and biocompatibility was improved by the use of copolymer-coated charcoal granules (Gazzard *et al.*, 1974c). An average of only 612 mg of paracetamol was recovered by haemoperfusion for 1 or 2 h in dogs given an average dose of 7.2 g (Winchester *et al.*, 1975) and, in another report, the clearance of paracetamol by haemoperfusion in dogs ranged from 0 to 162 ml min^{-1} (Widdop *et al.*, 1975). The total body clearance of paracetamol in dogs could be doubled by haemoperfusion (Gelfand and Winchester, 1980) but the calculated amount removed could be greatly overestimated if the wrong kinetic model was used (Winchester *et al.*, 1974). There have been anecdotal reports of charcoal haemoperfusion in patients with paracetamol poisoning but again, liver damage was not prevented (Davis and Williams, 1975; Rigby *et al.*, 1978; Bismuth and Fournier, 1980; Bismuth *et al.*, 1981; Winchester *et al.*, 1981; Raper *et al.*, 1982; Bentur and Zonis, 1984). In one report the extraction ratio was only 50 per cent (Gelfand and Winchester, 1980). It was claimed that charcoal haemoperfusion had rapidly removed paracetamol and prevented liver damage following an overdose in a 53-year-old woman. The 'enormous, potentially fatal' concentrations of paracetamol in this patient were spurious because the method of assay was unsuitable as it included paracetamol conjugates, and in any event the patient had also received early treatment with cysteamine (Rigby *et al.*, 1978). In other reports, claims were made for the value of haemoperfusion in paracetamol poisoning, but it did not prevent severe and fatal liver damage, and in some cases insignificant amounts of drug were removed (Helliwell, 1980; Helliwell and Essex, 1981; Helliwell *et al.*, 1981a,b). In a controlled trial of haemoperfusion in eight poisoned patients, the plasma clearance of paracetamol was variable and disappointingly small. The amounts removed averaged less than the equivalent of three tablets and liver damage was more severe in the patients treated with charcoal haemoperfusion than in eight control patients (Gazzard *et al.*, 1974e). Haemoperfusion was still recommended for the treatment of paracetamol poisoning despite lack of evidence of efficacy (Hauss *et al.*, 1983; Rump and Keller, 1994). Charcoal haemoperfusion and daily high-flux dialysis were recommended for the removal of paracetamol on the basis of the results of treatment of 51 patients who had not received N-acetylcysteine within 15 h of an overdose. Comparisons were made with patients who presented after 42 h, but this was hardly valid and there were no proper control data. No information was provided about the amounts of paracetamol removed (Higgins *et al.*, 1993).

According to established pharmacokinetic principles, only a small fraction of the amount of paracetamol in the body could be removed readily by plasmapheresis and exchange transfusion. Plasmapheresis was carried out in a 39-year-old man who was thought to have taken 8 g of paracetamol, but no details were provided (Björck *et al.*, 1988), and exchange transfusion has been used in attempts to remove paracetamol in young children. In an 8-week-old infant exchange transfusion was performed when the plasma paracetamol concentration was in the therapeutic range (Claass *et al.*, 1993) and in other cases it had no obvious overall effect in reducing plasma paracetamol concentrations (Lederman *et al.*, 1983; Roberts *et al.*, 1984).

Other Measures

Because of the depletion of inorganic sulphate following toxic doses of paracetamol, the administration of sulphate was proposed to enhance elimination and reduce toxicity. Divided doses of sodium sulphate were better tolerated in volunteers than a single dose of 8 g that produced severe diarrhoea (Cocchetto and Levy, 1981). Activated charcoal did not alter the bioavailability of sodium sulphate given at the same time (Galinsky and Levy, 1984a), and magnesium sulphate was absorbed less completely than sodium sulphate and caused more adverse effects (Morris and Levy, 1983a). It is not known whether the administration of inorganic sulphate has any beneficial effect on the outcome of paracetamol poisoning in man.

Eleven patients referred for liver transplantation after paracetamol overdosage were treated with infusions of 30 μg h^{-1} of prostaglandin E$_1$ for an average of 5.8 days and all survived without transplantation (O'Brien *et al.*, 1992). It was implied that treatment with the prostaglandin was responsible but there was no evidence to support this claim. In another similar report, it was claimed that early treatment with intravenous prostaglandin E$_1$ increased survival from 37.5 to 54.5 per cent but proper assessment was impossible as no details were provided (Levy, 1993).

Cimetidine

Cimetidine is an inhibitor of microsomal drug oxidation and in most studies in animals it decreased the metabolic activation of paracetamol and protected against hepatotoxicity (Jackson, 1981, 1982; Mitchell *et al.*, 1981b, 1984b; Rudd *et al.*, 1981; Donn *et al.*, 1982; Drew *et al.*, 1982; Abernethy *et al.*, 1983; Peterson *et al.*, 1983; Lazarte *et al.*, 1984; Speeg *et al.*, 1985; Yurdakök *et al.*, 1985; Murase *et al.*, 1986; Okuno *et al.*, 1987; Speeg, 1987; Sachs and Kowalsky, 1988). In addition, cimetidine and N-acetylcysteine had additive protective effects (Speeg *et al.*, 1985; Speeg, 1987). On this basis, cimetidine was proposed as an antidote for the treatment of paracetamol poisoning in man (Ruffalo and Thompson, 1982; Mitchell *et al.*, 1984b; Black, 1987; Speeg, 1987; Sachs and Kowalsky, 1988; McClements *et al.*, 1990; Kiebler and Mowry, 1994). In healthy subjects, cimetidine significantly reduced the clearance of paracetamol by oxidation but it is doubtful whether this effect would protect against hepatotoxicity because cimetidine also significantly reduced the clearance by glucuronide conjugation (Mitchell *et al.*, 1984b). In other studies, cimetidine in clinical doses did not influence the kinetics or metabolic activation of paracetamol in man and it did not reduce the urinary recovery of the cysteine and mercapturic acid conjugates (Abernethy *et al.*, 1983a; Critchley *et al.*, 1983; Chen and Lee, 1985; Vendemiale *et al.*, 1987; Slattery *et al.*, 1989). Cimetidine has been used in patients with paracetamol poisoning in the hope that it might limit toxicity and there have been several anecdotal reports claiming benefit (Jackson, 1981, 1982; Kaysen *et al.*, 1985; Flanagan and Mant, 1986; Smith, 1986; Monteagudo and Folb, 1987; Kadri *et al.*, 1988; McClements *et al.*, 1990; Koga *et al.*, 1991; Rolband and Marcuard, 1991; Block *et al.*, 1992). At present there is no evidence that cimetidine has any useful effect in patients with paracetamol poisoning other than to reduce gastric acid secretion in patients with hepatic failure (Burkhart *et al.*, 1989; Lewis and Paloucek, 1991).

Fulminant Hepatic Failure

The management of fulminant hepatic failure following paracetamol overdose was a continuing challenge and major complications included hypoglycaemia, cerebral oedema, encephalopathy, renal failure, haemorrhage, hypotension, hypoxia and sepsis (Williams, 1988; Fingerote and Bain, 1993; Lee, 1993, 1994; Caraceni and van Thiel, 1995). However treatment continued to improve and the survival rate in patients with grade III to IV encephalopathy has risen to 64 per cent (Williams, 1994). Factors such as coagulopathy, acidosis, cerebral oedema and renal failure were primary indicators of prognosis (O'Grady *et al.*, 1988; Harrison *et al.*, 1990b; Langley *et al.*, 1990; Mulcahy and Hegarty, 1993; Boberg *et al.*, 1994) and transjugular liver biopsy also allowed an accurate prediction of the outcome (Donaldson *et al.*, 1993). Changes in flash visual evoked potentials correlated with the clinical grade and delta activity of the electroencephalogram in chronic liver disease, but not in patients with acute liver failure after paracetamol overdose (Levy *et al.*, 1990).

The administration of clotting factors did not completely reverse the defects in haemostasis (Gazzard *et al.*, 1974d) and controlled trials of heparin and fresh frozen plasma showed no benefit (Gazzard *et al.*, 1974a, 1975a). Nevertheless, treatment with fresh frozen plasma, clotting factor concentrates and platelets was recommended as necessary to control bleeding (Williams, 1988). A controlled trial of anti-thrombin III supplementation was also of no benefit and did not increase survival (Langley *et al.*, 1993). Prostacyclin was better than heparin as an extracorporeal anticoagulant in patients who required haemodialysis and haemofiltration. There was less haemorrhage and the life of the filters was prolonged (Davenport *et al.*, 1994). Renal failure was an important adverse factor. It was recommended that pumped haemodialysis should be avoided because of its undesirable effects on cerebral oedema and continuous veno-venous ultrafiltration was preferable (Davenport *et al.*, 1989b, 1990b; Wendon *et al.*, 1989; Makin and Williams, 1994). Membrane biocompatibility was also thought to play an important role in increasing the intracranial pressure during intermittent haemofiltration (Davenport *et al.*, 1989a). Ultrafiltration was used to control intracranial pressure but there could be a fatal rebound in pressure when it was discontinued (Davenport *et al.*, 1989c). In general, continuous modes of renal replacement were preferred to intermittent modes of therapy as they produced better cardiovascular control and better stability of intracranial pressure (Davenport *et al.*, 1993). Direct intravenous infusion of prostacyclin before the start of renal replacement treatment could be hazardous because it produced a fall in mean arterial pressure with a reduction in total cerebral oxygen delivery (Davenport *et al.*, 1991). Haemodialysis and haemoperfusion have been used in the treatment of fulminant hepatic failure for some time. It was reported that with early referral for charcoal haemoperfusion, 70 per cent of patients with paracetamol-induced fulminant hepatic failure survived (Gimson *et al.*, 1983). However, the patients who were referred early had less severe encephalopathy and there were no control data to allow assessment of the efficacy of haemoperfusion. In a controlled trial, haemoperfusion afforded little advantage and survival depended more on the absence of cerebral oedema, renal failure and acidosis (O'Grady *et al.*, 1988). It was also claimed that haemoperfusion, haemofiltration and plasmapheresis improved survival but again there were no control patients for comparison (Splendiani *et al.*, 1990). In another report, repeated high volume continuous plasma exchange was advocated on the basis of the survival of five patients with fulminant hepatic failure caused by paracetamol poisoning (Kondrup *et al.*, 1992). A system with partially purified glucuronyl transferase bonded to agarose beads was proposed as an extracorporeal assist device to enhance the glucuronide conjugation and removal of phenolic compounds such as paracetamol (Brunner *et al.*, 1979) and another extracorporeal liver assist device containing human hepatocytes cultured in a hollow fibre cartridge reversed paracetamol-induced fulminant hepatic failure in dogs (Sussman *et al.*, 1992). Regeneration of hepatocytes was an important element in the recovery from severe hepatic necrosis and Japanese investigators have used glucose-glucagon-insulin infusions in attempts to stimulate regeneration after paracetamol intoxication (Yasunaga *et al.*, 1985; Sakai *et al.*, 1987; Ohtani *et al.*, 1989; Yamakawa, 1992).

Cerebral oedema was the cause of death in about 80 per cent of patients who died from hepatic failure after taking an overdose of paracetamol (Makin and Williams, 1994). The prognosis was particularly poor in the presence of renal failure but it was claimed that survival was improved by the use of thiopentone to control intracranial pressure (Forbes *et al.*, 1989a). Mannitol infusion and controlled ventilation were normally used to reduce intracranial pressure (Vickers *et al.*, 1988) and atracurium was the preferred agent to induce paralysis for assisted ventilation as it did not accumulate in patients with hepatic failure (Bion *et al.*, 1993). In some circumstances, hyperventilation had adverse effects and it could reduce cerebral blood flow (Wendon *et al.*, 1994). Similarly, the head-up posture did not always reduce intracranial pressure, and this could be increased with a reduction in perfusion pressure (Davenport *et al.*, 1990a). Contrary to established belief, recovery was possible after a prolonged period of intracranial hypertension that was refractory to treatment and associated with reduced cerebral perfusion pressure. Four patients with fulminant hepatic failure induced by paracetamol in this condition survived, and such circumstances were normally regarded as a contraindication to liver transplantation because of the poor prognosis (Davies *et al.*, 1994a).

Orthotopic liver transplantation offered new hope of survival for patients with fulminant hepatic failure following an overdose of paracetamol but there were major problems with selection and about 50 per cent of such patients would be expected to recover without a transplant (De Knegt and Schalm, 1991; Lidofsky, 1993; Mutimer, 1993; Mutimer and Neuberger, 1993). The indications for transplantation were arterial pH less than 7.3 or a prothrombin time exceeding 100 s together with a plasma creatinine concentration above 300 μmol l^{-1} and grade III encephalopathy (Makin and Williams, 1994). Contraindications included sepsis, hypotension, impaired brainstem function and a history of repeated overdoses (Mulcahy and Hegarty, 1993). Of 73 patients with fulminant hepatic failure, 26 were considered for liver transplantation including four who had taken paracetamol. None of the latter received a transplant and two died while two recovered (Vickers *et al.*, 1988). Other patients have died because complications prevented successful transplantation (Rump and Keller, 1994) but, on the other hand, some recovered before suitable donors could be found (Viallon *et al.*, 1994). The benefits of liver transplantation in patients with paracetamol-induced fulminant hepatic failure have not been proven and the decision whether to transplant or not was particularly difficult (Florkowski *et al.*, 1991; Boberg *et al.*, 1994). There have been reports of successful liver transplantation in such patients (Bismuth *et al.*, 1987; Harry *et al.*, 1989; Hoffmann *et al.*, 1991; Mrvos *et al.*, 1992; Rustgi *et al.*, 1993). Thirty of 37 patients with fulminant hepatic failure after paracetamol overdose who were judged to have a reasonable prognosis without a liver transplant survived and 14 of 29 patients considered to have a poor prognosis were registered for transplantation. Four of six patients who received transplants survived, seven died and one survived without a transplant. Only three of the 15 patients with a poor prognosis who were not selected for a transplant died (O'Grady *et al.*, 1991). At another liver unit, 26 of 82 patients with paracetamol-induced fulminant hepatic failure who were not transplanted died, and a fatal outcome was associated with late presentation, prolongation of the prothrombin time, grade of coma, acidosis and renal failure. Most deaths were caused by cerebral oedema and sepsis. Liver transplantation was performed in 10 of 17 selected patients and seven of the 10 survived. Only one of those patients who were not transplanted survived (Mutimer *et al.*, 1994). In another report, an 18-year-old woman with fulminant hepatic failure after paracetamol overdosage was treated by total hepatectomy, hypothermia, plasma exchange and extracorporeal liver support consisting of plasma separation and perfusion through charcoal and a hollow fibre module containing matrix-attached pig hepatocytes. The patient was anhepatic for 14 h when she received an ABO incompatible liver transplant and this was replaced with a compatible organ eight days later (Rozga *et al.*, 1993).

Specific Antidotal Therapy

On the basis of studies in animals, specific treatment for paracetamol poisoning would logically be based on inhibition of the formation of N-acetyl-p-benzoquinoneimine or stimulation of the hepatic synthesis of glutathione. So far, only the latter approach has been successful clinically. Mitchell *et al.* (1973a,c, 1974) showed that paracetamol hepatotoxicity depended on depletion of hepatic gluta-thione, and that covalent binding could be reduced and hepatic necrosis prevented by supplying precursors such as L-cysteine and cysteamine. Glutathione itself could not be used as it did not enter cells readily and only partial protection against liver damage was afforded in animals even with unrealistically large doses (Gazzard *et al.*, 1974b; Benedetti *et al.*, 1975; Malnoë *et al.*, 1975). Furthermore, the oral bio-availability of glutathione in man was negligible (Witschi *et al.*, 1992). Glutathione synthesis depended on the availability of cysteine and in man, glutathione disap-peared rapidly from the circulation following intravenous administration and there was a transient increase in plasma cysteine concentrations (Trenti *et al.*, 1992). Japa-nese investigators have used intravenous glutathione for the treatment of paracetamol-induced liver damage but its efficacy is unknown and it was not able to prevent severe liver damage (Wakushima *et al.*, 1983; Ohtani *et al.*, 1989; Koga *et al.*, 1991; Yamakawa, 1992). Intravenous cysteine appeared to be as effective as cysteamine and methionine in preventing liver damage in patients with severe para-cetamol poisoning but it has been little used (Prescott *et al.*, 1978a; Prescott, 1979a,b). Amino-acid solutions containing cysteine have also been tried (Solomon *et al.*, 1977).

Cysteamine

Cysteamine (mercaptamine) was selected originally for trial in patients with parace-tamol poisoning and in dose-ranging studies in healthy volunteers it produced unpleasant and eventually incapacitating adverse effects (Prescott, 1979b). In a total dose of 3.2 g given intravenously over 20 h it completely prevented severe liver damage when administered within 10 h on seven occasions in five patients with severe paracetamol poisoning. In contrast, there was severe liver damage in all of 11 similarly poisoned patients who had been admitted previously and who did not receive cysteamine, and two died with hepatic failure (Prescott *et al.*, 1974). Cyste-amine was usually effective in preventing liver toxicity when given within 10 h of ingestion of the paracetamol but it was ineffective when treatment was delayed beyond 12 h (Scott and Stewart, 1975; van Heijst *et al.*, 1976; Eleftheriou *et al.*, 1977; Hamlyn *et al.*, 1977, 1978, 1980; Howie *et al.*, 1977; Jones and Thomas, 1977; Prescott *et al.*, 1978b; Rigby *et al.*, 1978; Starkey and Lawson, 1978; Saunders *et al.*, 1980; Harris, 1982). One patient with repetitive paracetamol overdosage received cysteamine on five separate occasions without suffering severe liver damage (Prescott *et al.*, 1978a). The crucial importance of the ingestion-treatment interval for the efficacy of cysteamine was not appreciated initially. In one report, cysteamine therapy was not thought to be of benefit, but this was because most patients had been treated too late for it to be effective (Douglas *et al.*, 1976). In another, mislead-ing and erroneous claims were made for the efficacy of cysteamine given late more than 12 h after the paracetamol. The confusion arose because a non-specific assay was used for the determination of plasma paracetamol and this gave spuriously high concentrations so that treatment was judged to be 'successful' in many patients who had never been at risk of toxicity in the first place (Smith *et al.*, 1978). Further studies established that cysteamine was very effective in preventing liver damage when given within 10 h of the overdose of paracetamol. It was partially effective after 10–12 h, but ineffective when treatment was delayed for more than 12 h (Prescott *et al.*, 1976a,c). Other comparative trials of cysteamine were reported in patients with paracetamol poisoning (Hughes *et al.*, 1976, 1977; James, 1976; Prescott *et al.*, 1976b; Solomon *et al.*, 1977; Hamlyn *et al.*, 1981). Cysteamine frequently caused nausea, vomiting and drowsiness and it was soon replaced. In animals, it increased gastric acid production and caused duodenal ulceration (Szabo, 1977). Cysteamine had complex kinetics (Kubalak *et al.*, 1986) and its protective action was probably related, at least in part, to inhibition of the toxic metabolic activation of paracetamol (Harvey and Goulding, 1974; Harvey and Levitt, 1976; Prescott, 1979a; Miller and Jollow, 1986a; Peterson *et al.*, 1989).

Dimercaprol and D-Penicillamine

Other thiols such as dimercaprol and D-penicillamine were investigated as potential protective agents but they did not seem to prevent liver and renal toxicity and were soon abandoned (Benson and Boleyn, 1974; Prescott and Wright, 1974; Wright and Benson, 1975; Hughes *et al.*, 1976, 1977; Prescott *et al.*, 1976b,c).

Methionine

L-methionine is a precursor of cysteine, and as such it stimulated glutathione synthesis and protected animals against paracetamol-induced liver toxicity (Maxwell *et al.*, 1975; McLean and Day, 1975; McLean *et al.*, 1976; Neuvonen *et al.*, 1985). The N-acetyl-DL-methionine ester of paracetamol also enhanced the hepatic synthesis of glutathione in mice and protected against paracetamol toxicity (Skoglund *et al.*, 1988). It was suggested that the problems of liver damage following paracetamol overdosage could be abolished simply by the addition of cysteine or methionine to the tablets (McLean, 1974; Neuvonen *et al.*, 1985, 1986). However, this would result in extensive unnecessary medication with many potential problems (Brandon, 1994). When given within 10 h, oral methionine in a dose of 2.5 g every 4 h to a total dose of 10 g was effective in preventing severe liver damage in 27 of 30 poisoned patients with plasma paracetamol concentrations above the standard treatment line (Crome *et al.*, 1976b). Similar results were reported previously (Crome *et al.*, 1976c) and early treatment with oral methionine was judged to be as effective as intravenous cysteamine (Hamlyn *et al.*, 1980, 1981). The efficacy of early treatment with oral methionine was confirmed in a larger study of 132 patients with severe paracetamol poisoning. Of 96 patients given methionine within 10 h, seven suffered severe liver damage but there were no deaths. Methionine was not effective when treatment was delayed for more than 12 h after the ingestion of paracetamol (Vale *et al.*, 1979, 1981). Similar results were obtained with intravenous methionine given in a total dose of 20 g over 20 h (Prescott *et al.*, 1976c). An alternative regimen for oral methionine of 3 g repeated three times was recommended by Swedish workers (Bæhrendtz *et al.*, 1976). Oral methionine was generally effective in reducing liver damage when given early within 10 h, but not when treatment was delayed (Fitzgerald and Drury, 1977; Lederman *et al.*, 1983; Flanagan and Mant, 1986; Jensen, 1986; Kondrup *et al.*, 1992). Amino-acid solutions containing methionine have been used (Andersson *et al.*, 1976; Solomon *et al.*, 1977; Vilstrup *et al.*, 1977) and there have been other reports of the use of intravenous methionine (Prescott *et al.*, 1978a; Petersen and Vilstrup, 1979). Oral methionine was considered to be as effective as intravenous N-acetylcysteine in preventing hepatic and renal toxicity in patients with paracetamol overdose and it was promoted as simple, safe and cheap treatment (Bæhrendtz and Werner, 1976; Crome *et al.*, 1976b; McLean, 1976; Meredith *et al.*, 1978a; Vale *et al.*, 1979, 1981; Hamlyn *et al.*, 1981). The major disadvantage was that absorption was likely to be compromised because nausea and vomiting occurred frequently in patients who had absorbed a toxic dose of paracetamol. For this reason, others preferred intravenous N-acetylcysteine (Prescott *et al.*, 1980; Canalese *et al.*, 1981a; Prescott, 1981; Monteagudo *et al.*, 1986; Read *et al.*, 1986). Late treatment with methionine increased the mortality of paracetamol in mice (Piperno *et al.*, 1978) and there were worries about its safety when given late in patients with impending hepatic failure. A further theoretical objection to the use of methionine rather than N-acetylcysteine was that several enzymic reactions were necessary for its conversion to the active form, cysteine. Two of these enzymes contained SH groups that could themselves be inactivated by paracetamol thus preventing the protective action of methionine. Unlike N-acetylcysteine and other thiols, methionine was unable to prevent direct covalent binding (Tredger *et al.*, 1980) or to reverse post-arylation damage to hepatocytes exposed for a short time to toxic concentrations of paracetamol (Tee *et al.*, 1986a; Tredger *et al.*, 1986a).

N-acetylcysteine

Prescott and Matthew (1974) first suggested that N-acetylcysteine might protect the liver against paracetamol-induced toxicity and it was subsequently shown to prevent liver damage and death from this cause in animals (Piperno and Berssenbruegge, 1976; Piperno *et al.*, 1978). Lyons *et al.* (1977) treated a 34-year-old man with large doses of oral N-acetylcysteine 15 h after he had taken an overdose of paracetamol but it failed to prevent severe liver damage. Peterson and Rumack (1977) described a 26-year-old woman who developed only minor elevation of the plasma aminotransferase activity after oral N-acetylcysteine was started 8 h after she had taken an overdose of paracetamol. The dose was 140 mg kg^{-1} followed by 70 mg kg^{-1} every 8 h for three days. In another study, N-acetylcysteine was given intravenously to 15 patients with severe paracetamol poisoning as shown by plasma paracetamol concentrations above the standard treatment line joining plots of 200 mg l^{-1} at 4 h and 30 mg l^{-1} at 15 h on a semilogarithmic graph. There was little or no hepatotoxicity in 11 who were treated early, but severe liver damage occurred in three in whom treatment was delayed for more than 10 h, and in one treated 7–9.5 h after ingestion of the paracetamol. The dose of intravenous N-acetylcysteine was 150 mg kg^{-1} given over 15 min followed by 50 mg kg^{-1} in 4 h and 100 mg kg^{-1} in 16 h (total 300 mg kg^{-1} over $20\frac{1}{4}$ h). It was well tolerated and there were no adverse effects of note (Prescott *et al.*, 1977b). In subsequent reports on 100 severely poisoned patients with plasma paracetamol concentrations above the standard treatment line, it was confirmed that intravenous N-acetylcysteine was remarkably effective in preventing liver damage. Only one of 62 patients treated within 10 h developed severe liver damage compared with 33 of 57 control patients studied retrospectively who had received supportive therapy alone. N-acetylcysteine also protected against renal failure and death but there was a critical ingestion-treatment interval of 8 h after which time efficacy diminished progressively. There was no evidence of protection after 15 h (Prescott *et al.*, 1979; Prescott, 1981). The importance of early treatment was illustrated by the outcome after treatment with intravenous N-acetylcysteine on six occasions in a 26-year-old man who repeatedly took paracetamol in overdosage. He escaped severe liver damage when treated within 10 h on four admissions but not on two occasions when he presented late and treatment was delayed for more than 12 h (Prescott *et al.*, 1978a). In a large American multicentre national study of oral N-acetylcysteine in 416 patients with paracetamol poisoning, only 112 had concentrations above the standard treatment line. Of these, 49 were treated within 10 h and eight (17 per cent) had severe liver damage while the corresponding incidences in 51 patients treated between 10 and 24 h and 12 treated after 24 h were 45 and 67 per cent respectively (Rumack and Peterson, 1978). The dose of oral N-acetylcysteine was 140 mg kg^{-1} followed by 70 mg kg^{-1} every 4 h for 17 doses (total 1330 mg kg^{-1}). In a subsequent report on this national study, the treatment line was lowered to 150 mg l^{-1} at 4 h and 18 mg l^{-1} at 16 h, and severe liver damage occurred in 7 per cent of 57 patients treated with oral N-acetylcysteine within 10 h compared with 43 per cent of 98 patients treated after this time (Rumack *et al.*, 1981, 1983). Oral N-acetylcysteine was given to 43 of 417 children less than 6 years of age who had taken paracetamol. Only three children developed severe liver damage and in all, treatment had been delayed for more than 16 h (Rumack, 1984). The latest report of the American national multicentre study involved 11 195 patients with suspected paracetamol poisoning but the vast majority were excluded from the analysis on the basis of the drug concentration measurements. Of the remainder, 2023 had paracetamol concentrations above the lower treatment line joining 150 mg l^{-1} at 4 h and 5 mg l^{-1} at 24 h. As before, early treatment with oral N-acetylcysteine was very effective in preventing liver damage and death, but these complications occurred increasingly frequently as treatment was delayed beyond 10 and 16 h. There was no difference in efficacy whether treatment was started up to 4 h or between 4 and 8 h after the paracetamol was taken, and there were no deaths when N-acetylcysteine was started within 16 h (Smilkstein *et al.*, 1988). In another study, N-acetylcysteine was given intravenously to 179 patients over a period of 48 h as a loading dose of 140 mg kg^{-1} followed by 12 doses of 70 mg kg^{-1} every 4 h. The same low treatment line starting at 150 mg kg^{-1} was used and despite the lack of appropriate control data, it was concluded that this high dose 48 h intravenous protocol for N-acetylcysteine was superior to the intravenous regimen used previously in more severely poisoned patients (Smilkstein *et al.*, 1991).

These different studies obviously cannot be compared directly, but the possibility was raised that treatment with N-acetylcysteine might be of some benefit up to 24 h after ingestion of the paracetamol. This was an important issue because late presentation and failure to provide late treatment with N-acetylcysteine were significant factors contributing to mortality in paracetamol poisoning (Canalese *et al.*, 1981a;

Meredith *et al.*, 1986; Read *et al.*, 1986; Tredger *et al.*, 1986). In 20 patients treated with standard intravenous N-acetylcysteine between 12 and 24 h after taking an overdose of paracetamol, severe liver damage occurred in three of 10 patients treated between 12 and 15 h, and in four of 10 treated between 15 and 24 h. The number of patients was small and there were no proper controls but these results were interpreted as showing that late treatment up to 24 h was of benefit (Parker *et al.*, 1990). There was also an anecdotal account of 'successful' treatment with N-acetylcysteine given as late as 72 h despite grossly abnormal liver function tests at the time (Viallon *et al.*, 1994). In an attempt to resolve the question of efficacy of late treatment, a retrospective study of intravenous N-acetylcysteine was carried out in 100 poisoned patients with fulminant hepatic failure referred to a specialist liver unit. The mortality rate was 37 per cent in 41 patients who received N-acetylcysteine during the period 10–36 h after ingestion compared to 58 per cent of 57 patients who did not receive N-acetylcysteine. Significantly fewer patients who were given N-acetylcysteine progressed to grade III/IV coma compared to those who did not receive the antidote (Harrison *et al.*, 1990a). This result was entirely to be expected because some patients who were treated with N-acetylcysteine between 10 and 15 and possibly 24 h would obviously have benefited. The median delay to treatment was 17 h but, unfortunately, no further information was given about these patients. In another study from the same unit, 50 patients with fulminant hepatic failure due to paracetamol overdosage were randomized to receive either continuous intravenous N-acetylcysteine at the standard rate until recovery from encephalopathy or death, or an equivalent volume of 5 per cent dextrose solution. The survival rate was higher in the N-acetylcysteine group (12 of 25 patients compared with 5 of 25 untreated patients) and there was a lower incidence of cerebral oedema and hypotension. No adverse effects were seen (Keays *et al.*, 1991). The beneficial effects of intravenous N-acetylcysteine in patients with fulminant hepatic failure were attributed to improved haemodynamics and oxygen delivery (Harrison *et al.*, 1991). An unusual potential application of the hepatoprotective action of N-acetylcysteine was targeted rescue of normal hepatocytes against lethal paracetamol cytotoxicity produced as chemotherapy for hepatocellular carcinoma (Wu *et al.*, 1985).

In healthy volunteers, an oral dose of 30 mg kg^{-1} of N-acetylcysteine produced a substantial increase in plasma concentrations of cysteine but there was no effect on concentrations of glutathione unless demand was increased as during the metabolism of paracetamol (Burgunder *et al.*, 1989). The administration of intravenous N-acetylcysteine in four healthy subjects and two patients with cirrhosis did not produce any change in the splanchnic efflux of glutathione and this was thought to indicate that circulating glutathione did not originate from the liver in man (Poulsen *et al.*, 1993). The standard infusion regimen for N-acetylcysteine used in the United Kingdom produced very high initial plasma concentrations (mean 554 mg l^{-1}) in 17 patients with paracetamol poisoning and concentrations were not different in patients with and without severe liver damage. It was possible that adverse effects of N-acetylcysteine could be related to these initial high concentrations and the risk might be reduced by simple modification of the dosage schedule (Prescott *et al.*, 1989a). Adverse reactions to intravenous N-acetylcysteine have been reported in up to 10 per cent of patients and seemed most likely to occur during the first hour when the plasma concentrations were highest (Mant *et al.*, 1984; Donovan *et al.*, 1987). Minor reactions were commonly referred to as 'anaphylactoid' and included nausea, vomiting, flushing, urticaria and pruritus. They usually subsided rapidly on slowing or discontinuing the infusion (Vale and Wheeler, 1982; Donovan *et al.*, 1987; Flanagan, 1987; Flanagan and Meredith, 1991; Monteagudo and Folb, 1987; Bonfiglio *et al.*, 1992; Chan and Critchley, 1994). These adverse effects may simply have reflected a dose-dependent pharmacological effect and were probably caused by release of histamine (Bateman *et al.*, 1984b). More severe reactions to N-acetylcysteine included bronchospasm, angioedema and hypotension and in some cases they were associated with the administration of excessive doses (Walton *et al.*, 1979; Ho and Beilin, 1983; Bateman *et al.*, 1984a; Mant *et al.*, 1984; Dawson *et al.*, 1989). In one patient, N-acetylcysteine caused severe asthma resulting in respiratory arrest that was fortunately reversible (Reynard *et al.*, 1992), and in a $3\frac{1}{2}$-year-old child, excessive fluid was given with the antidote and this produced water intoxication with convulsions (Mühlendahl, 1987). A serum sickness-like syndrome has also been reported (Mohammed *et al.*, 1994). Regrettably, in some reports of reactions to N-acetylcysteine the patients were not at risk of liver damage and there was no indication for its use in the first place (Vale and Buckley, 1983; Prescott and Critchley, 1984; Dawson *et al.*, 1989). Apart from nausea and vomiting, serious side effects have not been reported with oral N-acetylcysteine. At concentrations encountered clinically in patients with paracetamol poisoning, N-acetylcysteine caused vascular relaxation and this was proposed as a mechanism whereby it could cause hypotension (Sunman *et al.*, 1992). On the basis of findings with intradermal injection of very concentrated solutions, reactions to N-acetylcysteine were considered to be pseudoallergic in nature (Bateman *et al.*, 1984a).

There has been much discussion of the pros and cons of intravenous versus oral administration of N-acetylcysteine. The major problem with the oral route was the difficulty of administration in severely poisoned patients who were vomiting while with intravenous administration there was a greater risk of adverse effects. In one study where attempts were made to compare oral and intravenous N-acetylcysteine, the trial had to be abandoned because vomiting occurred in 77 per cent of 52 patients (Prescott, 1981). In another report based on telephone enquiries, vomiting was said to occur in only 16 per cent of patients with paracetamol poisoning (Adams *et al.*, 1980). N-acetylcysteine smelt of rotten eggs (Kiebler and Mowry, 1994) and because of vomiting, successful oral treatment in poisoned patients was considered to be a challenge (Smilkstein, 1994). Other investigators have experienced difficulty with the oral administration of N-acetylcysteine because of persistent vomiting (Maurer and Zeisler, 1978; Melethil *et al.*, 1981; Robertson *et al.*, 1986; Mann, 1988; Mrvos *et al.*, 1992) and in one case this probably resulted in a fatal outcome (Price *et al.*, 1991). Because of the problems of vomiting and the risk of unpredictable absorption, intravenous N-acetylcysteine was preferred to oral methionine (Nielsen and Pedersen, 1984; Davis, 1986; Jensen, 1986; Monteagudo *et al.*, 1986; Spearman *et al.*, 1993) and oral N-acetylcysteine (Kissun, 1981; Prescott, 1981; Poulsen and Ranek, 1984; Davis, 1986; Tenenbein, 1986; Brahm *et al.*, 1992; Janes and Routledge, 1992; Toledo and Borges, 1992; Birkland, 1993; Kiebler and Mowry, 1994; Makin and Williams, 1994). Odansetron has been used in attempts to stop protracted vomiting in patients with paracetamol poisoning to allow treatment with oral N-acetylcysteine (Tobias *et al.*, 1992; Reed and Marx, 1994). N-acetylcysteine was established as the treatment of choice for paracetamol poisoning in most countries (Oh and Shenfield, 1980; Pflüger, 1980; Breen *et al.*, 1982; Davis, 1986; Blanch *et al.*, 1987; Jaeger *et al.*, 1987; Jakobsen *et al.*, 1987; Rossini *et al.*,

1989; Weber *et al.*, 1990b; Harry and Varache, 1991; Bauer *et al.*, 1992; McBride and Rumack, 1992; Coirault *et al.*, 1993; Gaillard and Fréville, 1993; Mulcahy and Hegarty, 1993; Spearman *et al.*, 1993; van Vyve *et al.*, 1993; Jonville-Béra and Autret, 1994; van Berge Henegouwen and Savelkoul, 1994). Unfortunately, N-acetylcysteine was still used unnecessarily in patients who had taken only minor overdoses and who were not at risk of liver damage (Prescott and Critchley, 1984; Mühlendahl, 1987; Dawson *et al.*, 1989; Brotodihardjo *et al.*, 1992; Chan and Critchley, 1994).

References

Aanderud, L. and Bakke, O. M., 1983, Pharmacokinetics of antipyrine, paracetamol, and morphine in rat at 71 ATA, *Undersea Biomedical Research*, **10**, 193–201.

Aarbakke, J., 1994, Paracetamol, *Tidsskrift for den Norske Lægeforening*, **114**, 1168.

Aarbakke, J., Gadeholt, G. and Olsen, H., 1978, Lack of effect of fever on antipyrine oxidation in the rat, *European Journal of Pharmacology*, **49**, 31–37.

Abbadie, C. and Besson, J.–M., 1994, Chronic treatments with aspirin or acetaminophen reduce both the development of polyarthritis and Fos-like immunoreactivity in rat lumbar spinal cord, *Pain*, **57**, 45–54.

Abbott, C. J .A., Bouchier-Hayes, T. A. I. and Hunt, H. A., 1980, A comparison of the efficacy of naproxen sodium and a paracetamol/dextropropoxyphene combination in the treatment of soft-tissue disorders, *British Journal of Sports Medicine*, **14**, 213–218.

Abd Elbary, A., Ibrahim, S. A., Elsorady, H. and Abd Elmonem, H., 1983, Availability of paracetamol from different suppository bases. Part 2. Rectal absorption profile of paracetamol in humans, *Pharmazeutische Industrie*, **45**, 307–309.

Abdel-Halim, M. S., Sjöquist, B. and Änggård, E., 1978, Inhibition of prostaglandin synthesis in rat brain, *Acta Pharmacologica et Toxicologica*, **43**, 266–272.

Abeck, D., Gross, G. E., Kuwert, C., Steinkraus, V., Mensing, H. and Ring, J., 1992, Acetaminophen-induced progressive pigmentary purpura (Schamberg's disease), *Journal of the American Academy of Dermatology*, **27**, 123–124.

Abernethy, D. R., Divoll, M., Greenblatt, D. J. and Ameer, B., 1982a, Obesity, sex and acetaminophen disposition, *Clinical Pharmacology and Therapeutics*, **31**, 783–790.

Abernethy, D. R., Divoll, M., Ochs, H. R., Ameer, B. and Greenblatt, D. J., 1982b, Increased metabolic clearance of acetaminophen with oral contraceptive use, *Obstetrics and Gynecology*, **60**, 338–341.

Abernethy, D. R., Greenblatt, D. J., Ameer, B. and Shader, R. I., 1985, Probenecid impairment of acetaminophen and lorazepam clearance: direct inhibition of ether glucuronide formation, *Journal of Pharmacology and Experimental Therapeutics*, **234**, 345–349.

Abernethy, D. R., Greenblatt, D. J. and Divoll, M., 1982c, Differential effects of cimetidine on drug oxidation vs. conjugation: potential mode of therapy for acetaminophen hepatotoxicity, *Clinical Pharmacology and Therapeutics*, **31**, 198.

Abernethy, D. R., Greenblatt, D. J., Divoll, M., Ameer, B. and Shader, R. I., 1983a, Differential effect of cimetidine on drug oxidation (antipyrine and diazepam) vs. conjugation (acetaminophen and lorazepam): prevention of acetaminophen toxicity by cimetidine, *Journal of Pharmacology and Experimental Therapeutics*, **224**, 508–513.

Abernethy, D. R., Greenblatt, D. J., Divoll, M. and Shader, R. I., 1983b, Enhanced glucuronide conjugation of drugs in obesity: studies of lorazepam, oxazepam, and acetaminophen, *Journal of Laboratory and Clinical Medicine*, **101**, 873–880.

Abrams, S. M. L., Jackson, S. H. D., Johnston, A. and Turner, P., 1986, Does paracetamol modify frusemide diuresis? *British Journal of Clinical Pharmacology*, **89**, 718P.

Abramson, S. B., Cherksey, B., Gude, D., Leszczynska-Piziak, J., Philips, M. R., Blau, L. and Weissmann, G., 1990, Nonsteroidal antiinflammatory drugs exert differential effects on neutrophil function and plasma membrane viscosity: studies in human neutrophils and liposomes, *Inflammation*, **14**, 11–30.

Acharya, S. B., 1979, Cardiac effects of paracetamol, *Indian Journal of Physiology and Pharmacology*, **23**, 239–240.

Ackerman, Z., Flugelman, M. Y., Wax, Y., Shouval, D. and Levy, M., 1989, Hepatitis during measles in young adults: possible role of antipyretic drugs, *Hepatology*, **10**, 203–206.

Ackerman, Z. and Levy, M., 1988, Hepatotoxicity from therapeutic doses of paracetamol in different clinical situations, *Harefuah*, **115**, 334–336.

Ackermann, B. L., Watson, J. T., Newton, J. F., Hook, J. B. and Braselton, W. E., 1984, Application of fast atom bombardment mass spectrometry to biological samples: analysis of urinary metabolites of acetaminophen, *Biomedical Mass Spectrometry*, **11**, 502–511.

Acosta, D., Anuforo, D. C. and Smith, R. V., 1980, Cytotoxicity of acetaminophen and papaverine in primary cultures of rat hepatocytes, *Toxicology and Applied Pharmacology*, **53**, 306–314.

Adams, J. D., Lauterburg, B. H. and Mitchell, J. R., 1983, Plasma glutathione and glutathione disulfide in the rat: regulation and response to oxidative stress, *Journal of Pharmacology and Experimental Therapeutics*, **227**, 749–754.

Adams, R. H., Dallos, V., Daniels, R. G., Helps, P. J., Rogers, N. C., Guest, K. P., Rose, D., Wiseman, H. M. and Volans, G. N., 1980, Plasma concentrations of paracetamol, *British Medical Journal*, **280**, 560–561.

Adams, R. H. M., 1986, An accident and emergency department's view of self-poisoning: a retrospective study from the United Norwich Hospitals 1978–1982, *Human Toxicology*, **5**, 5–10.

Adams, S. S., 1960, Analgesic-antipyretics, *Journal of Pharmacy and Pharmacology*, **12**, 251–252.

Adamson, G. M. and Harman, A. W., 1988, Comparison of the susceptibility of hepatocytes from postnatal and adult mice to hepatotoxins, *Biochemical Pharmacology*, **37**, 4183–4190.

Adamson, G. M. and Harman, A. W., 1989, A role for the glutathione peroxidase/reductase enzyme system in the protection from paracetamol toxicity in isolated mouse hepatocytes, *Biochemical Pharmacology*, **38**, 3323–3330.

Adamson, G. M. and Harman, A. W., 1993, Oxidative stress in cultured hepatocytes exposed to acetaminophen, *Biochemical Pharmacology*, **45**, 2289–2294.

Adamson, G. M., Papadimitriou, J. M. and Harman, A. W., 1991, Postnatal mice have low susceptibility to paracetamol toxicity, *Pediatric Research*, **29**, 496–499.

Adelhøj, B., Petring, O. U., Brynnum, J., Ibsen, M. and Poulsen, H. E., 1985a, Effect of diazepam on drug absorption and gastric emptying in man, *British Journal of Anaesthesia*, **57**, 1107–1109.

Adelhøj, B., Petring, O. U., Erin-Madsen, J., Angelo, H. and Jelert, H., 1984, General anaesthesia with halothane and drug absorption. The effect of general anaesthesia with halothane and diazepam on postoperative gastric emptying in man, *Acta Anaesthesiologica Scandinavica*, **28**, 390–392.

Adelhøj, B., Petring, O. U., Frosig, F., Jensen, B. N., Ibsen, M. and Poulsen, H. E., 1987, The effect of spinal analgesia and surgery on preoperative drug absorption and gastric emptying in man, *Acta Anaesthesiologica Scandinavica*, **31**, 165–167.

Adelhøj, B., Petring, O. U., Ibsen, M., Brynnum, J. and Poulsen, H. E., 1985b, Buprenorphine delays drug absorption and gastric emptying in man, *Acta Anaesthesiologica Scandinavica*, **29**, 599–601.

Adithan, C., Danda, D., Swaminathan, R. P., Indhiresan, J., Shashindran, C. H., Bapna, J. S. and Chandrasekar, S., 1988, Effect of diabetes mellitus on salivary paracetamol elimination, *Clinical and Experimental Pharmacology and Physiology*, **15**, 465–471.

Adithan, C. and Thangam, J., 1982, A comparative study of saliva and serum paracetamol levels using a simple spectrophotometric method, *British Journal of Clinical Pharmacology*, **14**, 107–109.

Adjepon-Yamoah, K. K., Woolhouse, N. M. and Prescott, L. F., 1986, The effect of chloroquine on paracetamol disposition and kinetics, *British Journal of Clinical Pharmacology*, **21**, 322–324.

Adriaenssens, P. I. and Prescott, L. F., 1978, High performance liquid chromatographic estimation of paracetamol metabolites in man, *British Journal of Clinical Pharmacology*, **6**, 87–88.

Adriani, J., Minokadeh, S. and Naraghi, M., 1981, Effectiveness on mucous membranes of topically applied antipyretic analgesics, *Regional Anesthesia*, **6**, 47–50.

Aghababian, R. V., 1986, Comparison of diflunisal and acetaminophen with codeine in the management of grade 2 ankle sprain, *Clinical Therapeutics*, **8**, 520–526.

Agran, P. F., Zenk, K. E. and Romansky, S. G., 1983, Acute liver failure and encephalopathy in a 15-month-old infant, *American Journal of Diseases of Children*, **137**, 1107–1114.

Agudo, M. A., Ayuso, M. J. and Saenz, M. T., 1986, Actividad del paracetamol frente al dolor provocado por diferentes estimulos: influencia de mecanismos aminergicos, *Il Farmaco*, **41**, 274–278.

Aguilar, M. I., Hart, S. J. and Calder, I. C., 1988, Complete separation of urinary metabolites of paracetamol and substituted paracetamols by reversed-phase ion-pair high-performance liquid chromatography, *Journal of Chromatography: Biomedical Applications*, **426**, 315–333.

Ahlström, U., Fåhraeus, J., Quiding, H. and Ström, C., 1985, Multiple doses of paracetamol plus codeine taken immediately after oral surgery, *European Journal of Clinical Pharmacology*, **27**, 693–696.

Ahokas, J. T., Fehring, S. I., Davies, C., Ham, K. N., Emmerson, B. T. and Ravenscroft, P. J., 1984, The effect of tienilic acid on paracetamol toxicity, *IRCS Medical Science*, **12**, 971–972.

Ahonen, R., Enlund, H., Klaukka, T. and Martikainen, J., 1991, Consumption of analgesics and anti-inflammatory drugs in the nordic countries between 1978–1988, *European Journal of Clinical Pharmacology*, **41**, 37–42.

Ahonen, R., Enlund, H., Pakarinen, V. and Riihimäki, S., 1992, A 1-year follow-up of prescribing patterns of analgesics in primary health care, *Journal of Clinical Pharmacy and Therapeutics*, **17**, 43–47.

Aikawa, K., Satoh, T. and Kitagawa, H., 1977, Effect of acetaminophen on liver microsomal drug-metabolizing enzyme *in vitro* in mice, *Biochemical Pharmacology*, **26**, 893–895.

Aikawa, K., Satoh, T. and Kitagawa, H., 1978a, Comparison of effects of acetaminophen on liver microsomal drug metabolism and lipid peroxidation in rats and mice, *Japanese Journal of Pharmacology*, **28**, 485–491.

Aikawa, K., Satoh, T., Kobayashi, K. and Kitagawa, H., 1978b, Glutathione depletion by aniline analogs *in vitro* associated with liver microsomal cytochrome P-450, *Japanese Journal of Pharmacology*, **28**, 699–705.

Ajgaonkar, V. S., Marathe, S. N. and Virani, A. R., 1988, Dipyrone vs. paracetamol: a double-blind study in typhoid fever, *Journal of International Medical Research*, **16**, 225–230.

Akintonwa, A. and Essien, A. R., 1990, Protective effects of *Garcinia kola* seed extract against paracetamol-induced hepatotoxicity in rats, *Journal of Ethnopharmacology*, **29**, 207–211.

Alam, A. N., Wilkinson, S. P., Poston, L., Moodie, H. and Williams, R., 1977a, Intracellular electrolyte abnormalities in fulminant hepatic failure, *Gastroenterology*, **72**, 914–917.

Alam, S. N, Roberts, R. J. and Fischer, L. J., 1977b, Age-related differences in salicylamide and acetaminophen conjugation in man, *Journal of Pediatrics*, **90**, 130–135.

Albano, E., Poli, G., Chiarpotto, E., Biasi, R. and Dianzani, M. U., 1983, Paracetamol-stimulated lipid peroxidation in isolated rat and mouse hepatocytes, *Chemico-Biological Interactions*, **47**, 249–263.

Albano, E., Poli, G., Chiarpotto, E., D'Anelli, N. and Dianzani, M. U., 1981, Promethazine protection against paracetamol induced glutathione depletion in isolated hepatocytes, *IRCS Medical Science*, **9**, 961–962.

Albano, E., Rundgren, M., Harvison, P. J., Nelson, S. D. and Moldéus, P., 1985, Mechanisms of N-acetyl-p-benzoquinoneimine cytotoxicity, *Molecular Pharmacology*, **28**, 306–311.

Albert, K. S., Sedman, A. J. and Wagner, J. G., 1974a, Pharmacokinetics of orally administered acetaminophen in man, *Journal of Pharmacokinetics and Biopharmaceutics*, **2**, 381–393.

Albert, K. S., Sedman, A. J., Wilkinson, P., Stoll, R. G., Murray, W. J. and Wagner, J. G., 1974b, Bioavailability studies of acetaminophen and nitrofurantoin, *Journal of Clinical Pharmacology*, **14**, 264–270.

Albin, H., Demotes-Mainard, F., Vinçon, G., Bedjaoui, A. and Begaud, B., 1985, Effect of two antacids on the bioavailability of paracetamol, *European Journal of Clinical Pharmacology*, **29**, 251–253.

Alhava, E., Hassinen, K. and Nieminen, E., 1978, Toxicity of paracetamol in relation to age in mice, *Acta Pharmacologica et Toxicologica*, **42**, 317–319.

Ali, B. H., Bashir, A. A. and Wasfi, I. A., 1993, Effect of cysteamine and cimetidine on acetaminophen (paracetamol) pharmacokinetics in rabbits, *Medical Science Research*, **21**, 359–360.

Ali, B. H. and Sharif, S. I., 1993, Comparative study of salivary acetaminophen concentration in Libyans, Senegalese and Sudanese, *Pharmacology*, **47**, 24–27.

Ali, H. M., Homeida, M. M. A., Ford, J., Truman, C. A., Roberts, C. J. C. and Badwan, A. A., 1988, Paracetamol bioavailability from an elixir, a suspension and a new alcohol-free liquid dosage form in humans, *International Journal of Pharmaceutics*, **42**, 155–159.

Ali, M., Zamecnik, J., Cerskus, A. L., Stoessl, A. J., Barnett, W. H. and McDonald, J. W. D., 1977, Synthesis of thromboxane B$_2$ and prostaglandins by bovine gastric mucosal microsomes, *Prostaglandins*, **14**, 819–827.

Ali, N. A., Marshall, R. W., Allen, E. M., Graham, D. F. and Richens, A., 1985, Comparison of the effects of therapeutic doses of meptazinol and a dextropropoxyphene/paracetamol mixture alone and in combination with ethanol on ventilatory function and saccadic eye movements, *British Journal of Clinical Pharmacology*, **20**, 631–637.

Aliverti, V. and Zaninelli, P., 1980, Protective effect of oral acetylcysteine on hepatic acute toxicity of acetaminophen in the mouse, *Toxicology Letters*, **6**, 61.

Alkayer, M., Vallon, J. J., Pegon, Y. and Bichon, C., 1981, Dosage direct du paracetamol dans les milieux biologiques par polarographie sinusoidale, *Analytica Chimica Acta*, **124**, 113–119.

Alkhayat, A., 1986a, Modified enzymatic assay for acetaminophen, *Clinical Chemistry*, **32**, 699–700.

Alkhayat, A., 1986b, Interference of acetaminophen metabolites in the Glynn-Kendal method for acetaminophen, *Clinical Chemistry*, **32**, 2208.

Allain, P., Chaleil, D. and Larra, F., 1975, Activité radioprotectrice du N-acétyl p. aminophénol chez la souris, *Comptes Rendus des Séances de la Société de Biologie et de Ses Filiales*, **169**, 511–514.

Allen, R. C., Petty, R. E., Lirenman, D. S., Malleson, P. N. and Laxer, R. M., 1986, Renal papillary necrosis in children with chronic arthritis, *American Journal of Diseases of Children*, **140**, 20–22.

Almeida e Silva, T. C. and Pela, I. R., 1978, Changes in rectal temperature of the rabbit by intracerebroventricular injection of bradykinin and related kinins, *Agents and Actions*, **8**, 102–107.

Alonso, E. M., Sokol, R. J., Hart, J., Tyson, W., Allswang, M., Narkewicz, M. R. and Whitington, P. F., 1994, Unusual outbreak of fulminant hepatitis in young children: possible association with acetaminophen, *Hepatology*, **20**, 190A.

Alsén, M., Ekedahl, A., Löwenhielm, P., Niméus, A., Regnéll, G. and Träskman-Bendz, L., 1994, Medicine self-poisoning and the sources of the drugs in Lund, Sweden, *Acta Psychiatrica et Neurologica Scandinavica*, **89**, 255–261.

Al-Shareef, A. H., Buss, D. C. and Routledge, P. A., 1990, Drug adsorption to charcoals and anionic binding resins, *Human and Experimental Toxicology*, **9**, 95–97.

Altomare, E., Leo, M. A. and Lieber, C. S., 1984a, Interaction of acute ethanol administration with acetaminophen metabolism and toxicity in rats fed alcohol chronically, *Alcoholism*, **8**, 405–408.

Altomare, E., Leo, M. A., Sato, C., Vendemiale, G. and Lieber, C. S., 1984b, Interaction of ethanol with acetaminophen metabolism in the baboon, *Biochemical Pharmacology*, **33**, 2207–2212.

Altomare, E., Vendemiale, G., Trizio, T. and Albano, O., 1986, Does acute ethanol really protect against acetaminophen hepatotoxicity? *American Journal of Gastroenterology*, **81**, 91–93.

Altorjay, I., Sári, B., Imre, S., Balla, G. and és Dalmi, L., 1993, Paracetamol hatása a vörösvérsejtek savi haemolysisére különös tekintettel az intracellularis glutathion szintre, *Orvosi Hetilap*, **134**, 2259–2262.

Al-Turk, W. A. and Stohs, S. J., 1981, Hepatic glutathione content and aryl hydrocarbon hydroxylase activity of acetaminophen-treated mice as a function of age, *Drug and Chemical Toxicology*, **4**, 37–48.

Alubo, S. O., 1994, Death for sale: a study of drug poisoning and deaths in Nigeria, *Social Science and Medicine*, **38**, 97–103.

Alván, G., Evaldsson-Carlén, U. and Mellström, B., 1976, Paracetamolförgiftning – klinisk bild och behandlingsmöjligheter, *Läkartidningen*, **73**, 1723–1726.

Amadio, P., 1984, Peripherally acting analgesics, *American Journal of Medicine*, **77**, 17–26.

Amadio, P. and Cummings, D. M., 1983, Evaluation of acetaminophen in the management of osteoarthritis of the knee, *Current Therapeutic Research*, **34**, 59–66.

Ambre, J. and Alexander, M., 1977, Liver toxicity after acetaminophen ingestion. Inadequacy of the dose estimate as an index of risk, *Journal of the American Medical Association*, **238**, 500–501.

Amdekar, Y. K. and Desai, R. Z., 1985, Antipyretic activity of ibuprofen and paracetamol in children with pyrexia, *British Journal of Clinical Practice*, **39**, 140–143.

Ameer, B., 1993, Acetaminophen hepatotoxicity augmented by zidovudine, *American Journal of Medicine*, **95**, 342.

Ameer, B., Abernethy, D. R. and Greenblatt, D. J., 1984, Direct quantitation of glucuronide and sulfate metabolites of acetaminophen in urine, *Journal of Clinical Pharmacology*, **24**, 393–394.

Ameer, B., Divoll, M., Abernethy, D. R., Greenblatt, D. J. and Shargel, L., 1983, Absolute and relative bioavailability of oral acetaminophen preparations, *Journal of Pharmaceutical Sciences*, **72**, 955–958.

Ameer, B. and Greenblatt, D. J., 1977, Acetaminophen, *Annals of Internal Medicine*, **87**, 202–209.

Ameer, B., Greenblatt, D. J., Divoll, M., Abernethy, D. R. and Shargel, L., 1981, High-performance liquid determination of acetaminophen in plasma: single dose pharmacokinetic studies, *Journal of Chromatography: Biomedical Applications*, **226**, 224–230.

Ameer, B., James, M. O. and Saleh, J., 1992, Kinetic and inhibitor studies of acetaminophen and zidovudine glucuronidation in rat liver microsomes, *Drug and Chemical Toxicology*, **15**, 161–175.

Amitai, Y., Mitchell, A. A., McGuigan, M. A. and Lovejoy, F. H., 1987, Ipecac-induced emesis and reduction of plasma concentrations of drugs following accidental overdose in children, *Pediatrics*, **80**, 364–367.

Amitai, Y., Silver, B., Leikin, J. B. and Frischer, H., 1992, Visualization of ingested medications in the stomach by ultrasound, *American Journal of Emergency Medicine*, **10**, 18–23.

Amo, H. and Matsuyama, M., 1985, Subchronic and chronic effects of feeding large amounts of acetaminophen in B6C3F1 mice, *Japanese Journal of Hygiene*, **40**, 567–574.

Amor, B. and Benarrosh, C., 1988, A method for comparing analgesics: glafenine and paracetamol. Multicenter cross-over approach, *Clinical Rheumatology*, **7**, 492–497.

Amouyal, G., Larrey, D., Letteron, P., Genève, J., Labbe, G., Belghiti, J. and Pessayre, D., 1987, Effects of methoxsalen on the metabolism of acetaminophen in humans, *Biochemical Pharmacology*, **36**, 2349–2352.

Amsel, L. P. and Davison, C., 1972, Simultaneous metabolism of aspirin and acetaminophen in man, *Journal of Pharmaceutical Sciences*, **61**, 1474–1475.

Anania, V., Borroni, G. and Catanese, B., 1976, Ricerche comparative sull'assorbimento del paracetamolo e dell'aminofenazone nell'uomo dopo somministrazione per via orale o rettale, *Bollettino Chimico Farmaceutico*, **115**, 726–731.

Anantha Reddy, G., 1984, Effect of paracetamol on chromosomes of mouse bone marrow, *Caryologia*, **37**, 127–132.

Anantha Reddy, G. and Subramanyam, S., 1985, Cytogenetic response of meiocytes of Swiss albino mice to paracetamol, *Caryologia*, **38**, 355–374.

Anderson, A. B., Haynes, P. J., Fraser, I. S. and Turnbull, A. C., 1978, Trial of prostaglandin-synthetase inhibitors in primary dysmenorrhoea, *Lancet*, **1**, 345–348.

Anderson, K. E., Schneider, J., Pantuck, E. J., Pantuck, C. B., Mudge, G. H., Welch, R. M., Conney, A. H. and Kappas, A., 1983, Acetaminophen metabolism in subjects fed charcoal-broiled beef, *Clinical Pharmacology and Therapeutics*, **34**, 369–374.

Anderson, R. J., Weinshilboum, R. M., Phillips, S. F. and Broughton, D. D., 1981, Human platelet phenol sulphotransferase: assay procedure, substrate and tissue correlations, *Clinica Chimica Acta*, **110**, 157–167.

Andersson, B., Nordenskjöld, M., Rahimtula, A. and Moldéus, P., 1982, Prostaglandin synthetase-catalyzed activation of phenacetin metabolites to genotoxic products, *Molecular Pharmacology*, **22**, 479–485.

Andersson, B. S., Rundgren, M., Nelson, S. D. and Harder, S., 1990, N-acetyl-p-benzoquinoneimine-induced changes in the energy metabolism in hepatocytes, *Chemico-Biological Interactions*, **75**, 201–211.

Andersson, B. S., Rundgren, M., Porubek, D. J., Nicotera, P., Nelson, S. D. and Moldéus, P., 1989, Arylation and oxidation in paracetamol-induced hepatotoxicity, *Advances in the Biosciences*, **76**, 5–11.

Andersson, C., Leonhardt, T., Stubelius, L. and Svedberg, S., 1976, Ett fall av paracetamolintoxikation med reversibel leverskada -några reflexioner, *Läkartidningen*, **73**, 1726–1728.

Andreasen, P. B. and Hutters, L., 1979, Paracetamol (acetaminophen) clearance in patients with cirrhosis of the liver, *Acta Medica Scandinavica*, **624 (Suppl.)**, 99–105.

Andrews, D. J., Scott, P. H. and Lewin, D. J., 1982, Interference by levodopa and related compounds with paracetamol estimation, *Lancet*, **1**, 1193.

Andrews, R. S., Bond, C. C., Burnett, J., Saunders, A. and Watson, K., 1976, Isolation and identification of paracetamol metabolites, *Journal of International Medical Research*, **4 (Suppl. 4)**, 34–39.

Andrews, W. H. H. and Orbach, J., 1973, A study of compounds which initiate and block nerve impulses in the perfused rabbit liver, *British Journal of Pharmacology*, **49**, 192–204.

Angervall, L., Lehmann, L. and Bengtsson, U., 1964, The renal concentrating capacity in albino rats after long-term consumption of phenacetin, NAPA (N-acetyl-p-aminophenol) and acetylsalicylic acid, *Acta Medica Scandinavica*, **175**, 155–160.

Angervall, L., Lehmann, L. and Lincoln, K., 1962a, Induction of interstitial nephritis in rats fed phenacetin and NAPA (N-acetyl-p-aminophenol), *Acta Pathologica et Microbiologica Scandinavica*, **54**, 274–282.

Angervall, L., Lehmann, L. and Lincoln, K., 1962b, On the effect of phenacetin and NAPA (N-acetyl-p-aminophenol) on the development of bacterial interstitial nephritis in the rat, *Acta Pathologica et Microbiologica Scandinavica*, **Suppl. 154**, 61–64.

Angervall, L., Lehmann, L. and Lincoln, K., 1962c, On the action of NAPA (N-acetyl-p-aminophenol) on the induction of interstitial nephritis in rats, *Acta Pathologica et Microbiologica Scandinavica*, **54**, 283–286.

Anker, A. L. and Smilkstein, M. J., 1994, Acetaminophen: concepts and controversies, *Emergency Medicine Clinics of North America*, **12**, 335–349.

Ansari, R. A., Tripathi, S. C., Patnaik, G. K. and Dhawan, B. N., 1991, Antihepatotoxic properties of picroliv: an active fraction from rhizomes of *Picrorhiza kurrooa*, *Journal of Ethnopharmacology*, **34**, 61–68.

Ansher, S. S., Dolan, P. and Bueding, E., 1983, Chemoprotective effects of two dithiolthiones and of butylhydroxyanisole against carbon tetrachloride and acetaminophen toxicity, *Hepatology*, **3**, 932–935.

Antaki, A., Rollin, P., Weber, M. and Chicoine, L., 1978, L'intoxication à l'acétaminophène, *Union Médicale du Canada*, **107**, 670–673.

Antlitz, A. M. and Awalt, L. F., 1969, A double blind study of acetaminophen used in conjunction with oral anticoagulant therapy, *Current Therapeutic Research*, **11**, 360–361.

Antlitz, A. M., Mead, J. A. and Tolentino, M. A., 1968, Potentiation of oral anticoagulant therapy by acetaminophen, *Current Therapeutic Research*, **10**, 501–507.

Anundi, I., Högberg, J. and Stead, A. H., 1979, Glutathione depletion in isolated hepatocytes: its relation to lipid peroxidation and cell damage, *Acta Pharmacologica et Toxicologica*, **45**, 45–51.

Anundi, I., Lähteenmäki, T., Rundgren, M.., Moldéus, P. and Lindros, K. O., 1993, Zonation of acetaminophen metabolism and cytochrome P450 2E1-mediated toxicity studied in isolated periportal and perivenous hepatocytes, *Biochemical Pharmacology*, **45**, 1251–1259.

Anvik, J. O., 1984, Acetaminophen toxicosis in a cat, *Canadian Veterinary Journal*, **25**, 445–447.

Aoki, F. Y. and Sitar, D. S., 1992, Effects of chronic amantadine hydrochloride ingestion on its and acetaminophen pharmacokinetics in young adults, *Journal of Clinical Pharmacology*, **32**, 24–27.

Aoki, F. Y., Yassi, A., Cheang, M., Math, M., Murdzak, C., Hammond, G. W., Sekla, L. H. and Wright, B., 1993, Effects of acetaminophen on adverse effects of influenza vaccination in health care workers, *Canadian Medical Association Journal*, **149**, 1425–1430.

Apostolakis, J. C., Georgiou, C. A. and Koupparis, M.A., 1991, Use of ion-selective electrodes in kinetic flow injection: determination of phenolic and hydrazino drugs with 1-fluoro-2, 4-dinitrobenzene using a fluoride-selective electrode, *Analyst*, **116**, 233–237.

Ara, K. and Ahmad, K., 1980, Uptake of paracetamol into brain and liver of rats, *Bangladesh Medical Research Council Bulletin*, **6**, 39–44.

Arama, E., Michaud, P., Rouffiac, R. and Rodriguez, F., 1989, Biodisponsibilité de comprimés à libération prolongée de théophylline et de paracétamol formulés avec la pulpe de fruit du baobab (*Adansonia digitata* L.), *Pharmaceutica Acta Helvetiae*, **64**, 116–120.

Araya, H., Horie, T., Hayashi, M. and Awazu, S., 1987a, An alteration in the liver microsomal membrane of the rat following paracetamol overdose, *Journal of Pharmacy and Pharmacology*, **39**, 1047–1049.

Araya, H., Horie, T., Hayashi, M. and Awazu, S., 1987b, Alteration in rat liver microsomal membranes induced by acetaminophen, *Journal of Pharmacobiodynamics*, **10**, 296–301.

Araya, H., Mizuma, T., Horie, T., Hayashi, M. and Awazu, S., 1986, Heterogeneous distribution of the conjugation activity of acetaminophen and p-nitrophenol in isolated rat liver cells, *Journal of Pharmacobiodynamics*, **9**, 218–222.

Archer, C. T. and Richardson, R. A., 1980, An improved colorimetric method for the determination of plasma paracetamol, *Annals of Clinical Biochemistry*, **17**, 45–46.

Arena, J. M., Rourk, M. H. and Sibrack, C. D., 1978, Acetaminophen: report of an unusual poisoning, *Pediatrics*, **61**, 68–72.

Arendt-Nielsen, L., Nielsen, J. C. and Bjerring, P., 1991, Double-blind, placebo controlled comparison of paracetamol and paracetamol plus codeine – a quantitative evaluation by laser induced pain, *European Journal of Clinical Pharmacology*, **40**, 241–247.

Armour, A. and Slater, S. D., 1993, Paracetamol cardiotoxicity, *Postgraduate Medical Journal*, **69**, 52–54.

Arndt, K., Haschek, W. M. and Jeffery, E. H., 1989, Mechanism of dimethylsulfoxide protection against acetaminophen hepatotoxicity, *Drug Metabolism Reviews*, **20**, 261–269.

Arnman, R. and Olsson, R., 1978, Elimination of paracetamol in chronic liver disease, *Acta Hepato-Gastroenterologica*, **25**, 283–286.

Arnold, L., Collins, C. and Starmer, G. A., 1973, The short-term effects of analgesics on the kidney with special reference to acetylsalicylic acid, *Bulletin of the Postgraduate Committee in Medicine, University of Sydney*, **29**, 214–219.

Arnold, L., Collins, C. and Starmer, G. A., 1976, Studies on the modification of renal lesions due to aspirin and oxyphenbutazone in the rat and the effects on the kidney of 2:4 dinitrophenol, *Pathology*, **8**, 179–184.

Arthurs, Y. and Fielding, J. F., 1980, Paracetamol and chronic liver disease, *Journal of the Irish Medical Association*, **73**, 273–274.

Aselton, P., Jick, H., Milunsky, A., Hunter, J. R. and Stergachis, A., 1985, First-trimester drug use and congenital disorders, *Obstetrics and Gynecology*, **65**, 451–455.

Ashbourne, J. F., Olson, K. R. and Khayam-Bashi, H., 1989, Value of rapid screening for acetaminophen in all patients with intentional drug overdose, *Annals of Emergency Medicine*, **18**, 1035–1038.

Assem, E. S. K., 1976, Immunological and non-immunological mechanisms of some of the desirable and undesirable effects of anti-inflammatory and analgesic drugs, *Agents and Actions*, **6**, 212–218.

Atkins, C. E. and Johnson, R. K., 1975, Clinical toxicities of cats, *Veterinary Clinics of North America: Small Animal Practice*, **5**, 623–652.

Atwood, S. J., 1980, The laboratory in the diagnosis and management of acetaminophen and salicylate intoxication, *Pediatric Clinics of North America*, **27**, 871–879.

Augustin, C. and Schmoldt, A., 1991a, Zunahme der Paracetamolintoxikationen, *Beiträge zur Gerichtlichen Medizin*, **49**, 127–131.

Augustin, C. and Schmoldt, A., 1991b, Zunahme der Paracetamol-intoxikationen, *Pharmazeutische Zeitung*, **136**, 32–36.

Augustine, S. C., Schmelter, R. F., Nelson, K. L., Petersen, R. J. and Qualfe, M. A., 1983, Effect of acetaminophen on the leukocyte-labeling efficiency of indium oxine In[111], *American Journal of Hospital Pharmacy*, **40**, 1965–1967.

Aune, H., Bessesen, A., Olsen, H. and Mørland, J., 1983, Acute effects of halothane and enflurane on drug metabolism and protein synthesis in isolated rat hepatocytes, *Acta Pharmacologica et Toxicologica*, **53**, 363–368.

Aune, H., Hals, P.-A., Hansen, B. I. and Aarbakke, J., 1984, Effect of diethylether on the formation of paracetamol sulphate and glucuronide in isolated rat hepatocytes, *Pharmacology*, **28**, 67–73.

Aune, H., Olsen, H. and Mørland, J., 1981, Diethyl ether influence on the metabolism of antipyrine, paracetamol and sulphanilamide in isolated rat hepatocytes, *British Journal of Anaesthesia*, **53**, 621–626.

Austin, T. W. and Truant, G., 1978, Hyperthermia, antipyretics and function of polymorphonuclear leukocytes, *Canadian Medical Association Journal*, **118**, 493–495.

Autret, E., Breart, G., Jonville, A. P., Lassale, C. and Goehrs, J. M., 1994, Comparative efficacy and tolerance of ibuprofen syrup and acetaminophen syrup in children with pyrexia associated with infectious diseases and treated with antibiotics, *European Journal of Clinical Pharmacology*, **46**, 197–201.

Autret, E., Dutertre, J.-P., Breteau, M., Jonville, A.-P., Furet, Y. and Laugier, J., 1993, Pharmacokinetics of paracetamol in the neonate and infant after administration of propacetamol chlorhydrate, *Developmental Pharmacology and Therapeutics*, **20**, 129–134.

Avila, M. H., Walker, A. M., Romieu, I., Spiegelman, D. L., Perera, D. R. and Jick, H., 1988, Choice of non-steroidal anti-inflammatory drug in persons treated for dyspepsia, *Lancet*, **ii**, 556–559.

Avramova, J., 1989, Simultaneous determination of propyphenazone, paracetamol and caffeine in blood by high-performance liquid chromatography, *Journal of Pharmaceutical and Biomedical Analysis*, **7**, 1221–1224.

Aw, T. Y. and Jones, D. P., 1982, Secondary bioenergetic hypoxia. Inhibition of sulfation and glucuronidation reactions in isolated hepatocytes at low O_2 concentration, *Journal of Biological Chemistry*, **257**, 8997–9004.

Aw, T. Y. and Jones, D. P., 1984, Control of glucuronidation during hypoxia. Limitation by UDP-glucose pyrophosphorylase, *Biochemical Journal*, **219**, 707–712.

Aw, T. Y., Shan, X., Sillau, A. H. and Jones, D. P., 1991, Effect of chronic hypoxia on acetaminophen metabolism in the rat, *Biochemical Pharmacology*, **42**, 1029–1038.

Awni, W. M., St. Peter, J. V., Kovarik, J. M. and Matzke, G. R., 1990, Disposition of antipyrine and acetaminophen given alone and in combination to human subjects, *Pharmaceutical Research*, **7**, 204–207.

Axelsen, R. A., 1975, The induction of renal papillary necrosis in Gunn rats by analgesics and analgesic mixtures, *British Journal of Experimental Pathology*, **56**, 92–97.

Axelsen, R. A., 1980, Nephrotoxicity of mild analgesics in the Gunn strain of rat, *British Journal of Clinical Pharmacology*, **10 (Suppl. 2)**, 309S–312S.

Axworthy, D. B., Hoffmann, K.-J., Streeter, A. J., Calleman, C. J., Pascoe, G. A. and Baillie, T. A., 1988, Covalent binding of acetaminophen to mouse hemoglobin. Identification of major and minor adducts formed *in vivo* and implications for the nature of the arylating metabolites, *Chemico-Biological Interactions*, **68**, 99–116.

Aylward, M., Maddock, J., Parker, R. J. and Thomas, S. R., 1976, Evaluation of tolmetin in the treatment of arthritis: open and controlled double-blind studies, *Current Medical Research and Opinion*, **4**, 158–169.

Babhair, S. A. and Tariq, M., 1990, A study on bioavailability and pharmacological effects of acetaminophen in ethanolic and ethanol-free oral liquid preparations, *Research Communications in Substances of Abuse*, **11**, 65–68.

Bach, P. H. and Bridges, J. W., 1984, The role of metabolic activation of analgesics and non-steroidal anti-inflammatory drugs in the development of renal papillary necrosis and upper urothelial carcinoma, *Prostaglandins Leukotrienes and Medicine*, **15**, 251–274.

Bach, P. H. and Gregg, N. J., 1988, Experimentally induced renal papillary necrosis and upper urothelial carcinoma, *International Review of Experimental Pathology*, **30**, 1–54.

Bach, P. H., Gregg, N. J., Whittingham, A., Feldman, M., Pillai, K., Ijomah, P., Courtauld, E. and Hardy, T., 1988, Renal papillary necrosis and upper urothelial carcinoma, *Archives of Toxicology*, **62 (Suppl. 12)**, 137–142.

Bach, P. H. and Hardy, T. L., 1985, Relevance of animal models to analgesic-associated renal papillary necrosis in humans, *Kidney International*, **28**, 605–613.

Bachmann, K. A., 1989, The use of single-sample clearance estimates to probe hepatic drug metabolism in rats. IV. A model for possible application to phenotyping xenobiotic influences on human drug metabolism, *Xenobiotica*, **19**, 1449–1459.

Back, D. J., Madden, S. and L'Orme, M. E., 1990, Gastrointestinal metabolism of contraceptive steroids, *American Journal of Obstetrics and Gynecology*, **163**, 2138–2145.

Back, D. J. and Tjia, J. F., 1987, Single dose primaquine has no effect on paracetamol clearance, *European Journal of Clinical Pharmacology*, **32**, 203–205.

Badcock, N. R., Penna, A. C., Everett, D. S. and Sansom, L. N., 1984, Aspirin metabolites causing misinterpretation of paracetamol results, *Annals of Clinical Biochemistry*, **21**, 527–530.

Badr, M. Z., 1994, Controversial role of intracellular iron in the mechanisms of chemically-induced hepatotoxicity, *Journal of Biochemical Toxicology*, **9**, 25–29.

Baeg, N.-J., Bodenheimer, H. C. and Burchard, K., 1988, Long-term sequellae of acetaminophen-associated fulminant hepatic failure: relevance of early histology, *American Journal of Gastroenterology*, **83**, 569–571.

Bæhrendtz, S., Törnqvist, K. and Werner, B., 1976, Akut paracetamolförgiftning – dagsläget, *Läkartidningen*, **73**, 1729–1730.

Bæhrendtz, S. and Werner, B., 1976, Metionin – en replik, *Läkartidningen*, **73**, 2334.

Baekelandt, M., Vansteenberge, R., van der Spek, P., D'Haenens, P., Rollier, A. and Stockx, L., 1990, Rectal stenosis following the use of suppositories containing paracetamol and acetylsalicylic acid, *Gastrointestinal Radiology*, **15**, 171–173.

Baer, G. A., Rorarius, M. G. F., Kolemainen, S. and Selin, S., 1992, The effect of paracetamol or diclofenac administered before operation on postoperative pain and behaviour after adenoidectomy in small children, *Anaesthesia*, **47**, 1078–1080.

Bagnall, W. E., Kelleher, J., Walker, B. E. and Losowsky, M. S., 1979, The gastrointestinal absorption of paracetamol in the rat, *Journal of Pharmacy and Pharmacology*, **31**, 157–160.

Bailey, D. N., 1982, Colorimetry of serum acetaminophen (paracetamol) in uremia, *Clinical Chemistry*, **28**, 187–190.

Bailie, M. B., Federowicz, D. A., Dolce, K., Kahn, C., Mico, B. A. and Landi, M. S., 1987, Pharmacokinetics of acetaminophen, vancomycin, and antipyrine in the Hanford miniature swine, *Drug Metabolism and Disposition: The Biological Fate of Chemicals*, **15**, 729–730.

Bainbridge, C. A., Kelly, E. L. and Walkling, W. D., 1977, *In vitro* adsorption of acetaminophen onto activated charcoal, *Journal of Pharmaceutical Sciences*, **66**, 480–483.

Bajorek, P., Widdop, B. and Volans, G., 1978, Lack of inhibition of paracetamol absorption by codeine, *British Journal of Clinical Pharmacology*, **5**, 346–347.

Baker, M. D., Fosarelli, P. D. and Carpenter, R. O., 1987, Childhood fever: correlation of diagnosis with temperature response to acetaminophen, *Pediatrics*, **80**, 315–318.

Baker, R. C., Tiller, T., Bausher, J. C., Bellet, P. S., Cotton, W. H., Finley, A. H., Lenane, A. M., McHenry, C., Perez, K. K., Shapiro, R. A., Stephan, M. and Wason, S., 1989, Severity of disease correlated with fever reduction in febrile infants, *Pediatrics*, **83**, 1016–1019.

Bal, T. S., Hewitt, R. W., Hiscutt, A. A. and Johnson, B., 1989, Analysis of bone marrow and decomposed body tissue for the presence of paracetamol and dextropropoxyphene, *Journal of the Forensic Science Society*, **29**, 219–223.

Bales, J. R., Bell, J. D., Nicholson, J. K., Sadler, P. J., Timbrell, J. A., Hughes, R. D., Bennett, P. N. and Williams, R., 1988, Metabolic profiling of body fluids by proton NMR: self-poisoning episodes with paracetamol (acetaminophen), *Magnetic Resonance in Medicine*, **6**, 300–306.

Bales, J. R., Higham, D. P., Howe, I., Nicholson, J. K. and Sadler, P. J., 1984a, Use of high-resolution proton nuclear magnetic resonance spectroscopy for rapid multi-component analysis of urine, *Clinical Chemistry*, **30**, 426–432.

Bales, J. R., Nicholson, J. K. and Sadler, P. J., 1985, Two-dimensional proton nuclear magnetic resonance 'Maps' of acetaminophen metabolites in human urine, *Clinical Chemistry*, **31**, 757–763.

Bales, J. R., Sadler, P. J., Nicholson, J. K. and Timbrell, J. A., 1984b, Urinary excretion of acetaminophen and its metabolites as studied by proton NMR spectroscopy, *Clinical Chemistry*, **30**, 1631–1636.

Ballé, C. and Schollmeyer, P., 1990, Mo[rbidity of patients with analgesic-associated nephropathy on regular dialysis treatment and after renal transplantation, *Klinische Wochenschrift*, **68**, 38–42.

Banda, P. W. and Quart, B. D., 1982, The effect of mild alcohol consumption on the metabolism of acetaminophen in man, *Research Communications in Chemical Pathology and Pharmacology*, **38**, 57–70.

Banda, P. W. and Quart, B. D., 1984a, The effect of alcohol on the toxicity of acetaminophen in mice, *Research Communications in Chemical Pathology and Pharmacology*, **43**, 127–138.

Banda, P. W. and Quart, B. D., 1984b, The effect of alcohol on the toxicity of acetaminophen in mice, *Clinical Pharmacology and Therapeutics*, **35**, 227.

Banda, P. W. and Quart, B. D., 1987, The use of N-acetylcysteine long after an acetaminophen overdose in mice, *Toxicology Letters*, **36**, 89–94.

Bannwarth, B., Demotes-Mainard, F., Schæverbeke, T. and Dehais, J., 1993, Where are peripheral analgesics acting? *Annals of the Rheumatic Diseases*, **52**, 1–4.

Bannwarth, B. and Netter, P., 1994, Pharmacocinétique du paracétamol dans la liquide céphalorachidien, *Thérapie*, **49**, 157.

Bannwarth, B., Netter, P., Lapicque, F., Gillet, P., Péré, P., Boccard, E., Royer, R. J. and Gaucher, A., 1992, Plasma and cerebrospinal fluid concentrations of paracetamol after a single intravenous dose of propacetamol, *British Journal of Clinical Pharmacology*, **34**, 79–81.

Baños Gallardo, M., Claros González, I., Forascepi Roza, R. and Argüelles-Toraño, M., 1987, Nefritis intersticial aguda con fracaso renal secundario a drogas, *Revista Clínica Española*, **181**, 372–374.

Baños, J. E., Bosch, F., Ortega, F., Bassols, A. and Cañellas, M., 1989, Análisis del tratmeniento del dolor postoperatorio en tres hospitales, *Revista Clínica Española*, **184**, 177–181.

Baños, J. E., Bosch, F. and Toranzo, I., 1991, La automedicación con analgésicos. Estudio en el dolor odontológico, *Medicina Clinica*, **96**, 248–251.

Baraka, O. Z., Truman, C. A., Ford, J. M. and Roberts, C. J. C., 1990, The effect of propranolol on paracetamol metabolism in man, *British Journal of Clinical Pharmacology*, **29**, 261–264.

Barber, D. J., Fairhurst, S. and Horton, A. A., 1983, Effect of old age on paracetamol-induced lipid peroxidation in rat liver, *Toxicology Letters*, **15**, 283–287.

Barker, D. E. and Jacobs, A. G., 1982, Paracetamol estimation: a new approach to reducing salicylate interference, *Annals of Clinical Biochemistry*, **19**, 120–124.

Barker, J. D., de Carle, D. J. and Anuras, S., 1977, Chronic excessive acetaminophen use and liver damage, *Annals of Internal Medicine*, **87**, 299–301.

Barles, P. G., Garcia, F. D., Olmo, J. R. P., Aznar, J. P. and Alarma, J. L. E., 1988, Adverse reaction of acetaminophen as an alternative analgesic in A. A. S. Triad, *Allergologia et Immunopathologia (Madrid)*, **16**, 321–325.

Barnard, S., Kelly, D. F., Storr, R. C. and Park, B. K., 1993a, The effect of fluorine substitution on the hepatotoxicity and metabolism of paracetamol in the mouse, *Biochemical Pharmacology*, **46**, 841–849.

Barnard, S., McGoldrick, T. A., Park, B. K. and Hawksworth, G. M., 1993b, The effect of fluorine substitution on the hepatotoxicity of paracetamol *in vitro*, *British Journal of Clinical Pharmacology*, **36**, 147P.

Barnard, S., Storr, R. C., O'Neill, P. M. and Park, B. K., 1993c, The effect of fluorine substitution on the physicochemical properties and the analgesic activity of paracetamol, *Journal of Pharmacy and Pharmacology*, **45**, 736–744.

Barnes, P. and Prichard, J. S., 1972, Self-poisoning with paracetamol, *British Medical Journal*, **4**, 429–430.

Barraclough, M. A., 1972, Effect of vasopressin on the reabsorption of phenacetin and its metabolites from the tubular fluid in man, *Clinical Science*, **43**, 709–713.

Barraclough, M. A. and Nilam, F., 1973, Renal tubular reabsorption of acetaminophen after vasopressin administration in man, *Experientia*, **29**, 448–449.

Bartle, W. R. and Blakely, J. A., 1991, Potentiation of warfarin anticoagulation by acetaminophen, *Journal of the American Medical Association*, **265**, 1260.

Bartle, W. R., Paradiso, F. L., Derry, J. E. and Livingstone, D. J., 1989, Delayed acetaminophen toxicity despite acetylcysteine use, *Annals of Pharmacotherapy*, **23**, 509.

Bartolone, J. B., Beierschmitt, W. P., Birge, R. B., Emeigh Hart, S. G., Wyand, S., Cohen, S. D. and Khairallah, E. A., 1989a, Selective acetaminophen metabolite binding to hepatic and extrahepatic proteins: an *in vivo* and *in vitro* analysis, *Toxicology and Applied Pharmacology*, **99**, 240–249.

Bartolone, J. B., Birge, R. B., Bulera, S. J., Bruno, M. K., Nishanian, E. V., Cohen, S. D. and Khairallah, E. A., 1992, Purification, antibody production, and partial amino acid sequence of the 58-kDa acetaminophen-binding liver proteins, *Toxicology and Applied Pharmacology*, **113**, 19–29.

Bartolone, J. B., Birge, R. B., Sparks, K., Cohen, S. D. and Khairallah, E. A., 1988, Immunochemical analysis of acetaminophen covalent binding to proteins: partial characterization of the major acetaminophen-binding liver proteins, *Biochemical Pharmacology*, **37**, 4763–4774.

Bartolone, J. B., Cohen, S. D. and Khairallah, E. A., 1989b, Immunohistochemical localisation of acetaminophen-bound liver proteins, *Fundamental and Applied Toxicology*, **13**, 859–862.

Bartolone, J. B., Sparks, K., Cohen, S. D. and Khairallah, E. A., 1987, Immunochemical detection of acetaminophen-bound liver proteins, *Biochemical Pharmacology*, **36**, 1193–1196.

Bartsocas, C. S., Schulman, J. D. and Corash, L., 1982, Can acetaminophen cause hemolysis in G6PD deficiency? *Acta Haematologica*, **67**, 228.

Basile, A. S., Harrison, P. M., Hughes, R. D., Gu, Z.-Q., Pannell, L., McKinney, A., Jones, E. A. and Williams, R., 1994, Relationship between plasma benzodiazepine receptor ligand concentrations and severity of hepatic encephalopathy, *Hepatology*, **19**, 112–121.

Basile, A. S., Hughes, R. D., Harrison, P. M., Murata, Y., Pannell, L., Jones, E. A., Williams, R. and Skolnick, P., 1991, Elevated brain concentrations of 1,4-benzodiazepines in fulminant hepatic failure, *New England Journal of Medicine*, **325**, 473–478.

Bateman, D. N., Woodhouse, K. W. and Rawlins, M. D., 1984a, Adverse reactions to N-acetylcysteine, *Human Toxicology*, **3**, 393–398.

Bateman, D. N., Woodhouse, K. W. and Rawlins, M. D., 1984b, Adverse reactions to N-acetylcysteine, *Lancet*, **ii**, 228.

Bates, T. E., Williams, S. R., Busza, A. L., Gadian, D. G. and Proctor, E., 1988, A ^{31}P nuclear magnetic resonance study *in vivo* of metabolic abnormalities in rats with acute liver failure, *NMR in Biomedicine*, **1**, 67–73.

Batterman, R. C. and Grossman, A. J., 1955, Analgesic effectiveness and safety of N-acetyl-para-aminophenol, *Federation Proceedings*, **14**, 316–317.

Baty, J. D., Lindsay, R. M., Fox, W. R. and Willis, R. G., 1988, Stable isotopes as probes for the metabolism of acetanilide in man and the rat, *Biomedical and Environmental Mass Spectrometry*, **16**, 183–189.

Baty, J. D., Robinson, P. R. and Wharton, J., 1976, A method for the estimation of acetanilide, paracetamol and phenacetin in plasma and urine using mass fragmentography, *Biomedical and Environmental Mass Spectrometry*, **3**, 60–63.

Baudouin, S. V., Howdle, P., O'Grady, J. G. and Webster, N. R., 1995, Acute lung injury in fulminant hepatic failure following paracetamol poisoning, *Thorax*, **50**, 399–402.

Bauer, P., Weber, M., Renaud, D., Muller, F. and Lambert, H., 1992, L'Intoxication par le paracétamol. L'évolution est favorable si l'antidote spécifique est prescrit avant la 8ᵉ heure, *Revue du Praticien – Médecine Générale*, **6**, 45–48.

Bauguess, C. T., Fincher, J. H., Sadik, F. and Hartman, C. W., 1975a, Blood concentration profiles of acetaminophen following oral administration of fatty acid esters of acetaminophen with pancreatic lipase to dogs, *Journal of Pharmaceutical Sciences*, **64**, 1489–1492.

Bauguess, C. T., Sadik, F., Fincher, J. H. and Hartman, C. W., 1975b, Hydrolysis of fatty acid esters of acetaminophen in buffered pancreatic lipase systems I, *Journal of Pharmaceutical Sciences*, **64**, 117–120.

Bauman, J. E., Dean, B. S. and Krenzelok, E. P., 1989, Motor vehicles as a site of accidental poisonings, *Veterinary and Human Toxicology*, **31**, 563–566.

Baumann, J., von Bruchhausen, F. and Wurm, G., 1983a, Inhibition of prostaglandin synthetases derived from neuronal and glial cells and rat renal medulla by ortho-, meta- and para-substituted aminophenolic compounds, *Prostaglandins Leukotrienes and Medicine*, **10**, 319–329.

Baumann, J., von Bruchhausen, F. and Wurm, G., 1983b, Decreasing inhibitory potency of prostaglandin synthetase inhibitors during their cooxidative metabolism. Studies on aminophenols, pyrazolon derivatives and 1,3-diphenylisobenzofuran, *Pharmacology*, **27**, 267–280.

Baumann, J., von Bruchhausen, F. and Wurm, G., 1984, *In vitro* deacetylation studies of acetamidophenolic compounds in rat brain, liver and kidney, *Arzneimittel-Forschung*, **34**, 1278–1282.

Baumeler, H. R., Ettlin, Ch., Dubach, U. C. and Ladewig, D., 1975, Trendentwicklung der Ausscheidung von Analgetika im Urin beim gleichen Kollektiv 1968–1975, *Sozial- und Präventivmedizin*, **20**, 242–243.

Baumelou, E., Guiguet, M., Mary, J. Y. and French Cooperative Group for Epidemiological Study of Aplastic Anemia, 1993, Epidemiology of aplastic anemia in France: a case-control study. I. Medical history and medication use, *Blood*, **81**, 1471–1478.

Baumgarten, R., Schneider, W., Roschlau, G., Fengler, J.-D., Markus, R. and Binus, R., 1983, Parazetamolintoxikation: Klinik und Pharmakokinetik, *Zeitschrift für die Gesamte Innere Medizin und Ihre Grenzgebiete*, **38**, 472–475.

Beales, D., Hue, D. P. and McLean, A. E.M., 1985, Lipid peroxidation, protein synthesis, and protection by calcium EDTA in paracetamol injury to isolated hepatocytes, *Biochemical Pharmacology*, **34**, 19–23.

Beard, K., Belic, L., Aselton, P., Perera, D. R. and Jick, H., 1986, Outpatient drug-induced parenchymal liver disease requiring hospitalization, *Journal of Clinical Pharmacology*, **26**, 633–637.

Beaulac-Baillargeon, L., Auclair, A., Matte, L., Gaudreault, R. C. and Firest, J.-C., 1994, A novel approach for the determination of human milk/plasma ratios: correlation of *in vivo* and *in vitro* paracetamol milk/plasma ratios, *Drug Investigation*, **7**, 57–62.

Beaulac-Baillargeon, L. and Rocheleau, S., 1993, Paracetamol pharmacokinetics in pregnancy, *Drug Investigation*, **6**, 176–179.

Beaulac-Baillargeon, L. and Rocheleau, S., 1994, Paracetamol pharmacokinetics during the first trimester of human pregnancy, *European Journal of Clinical Pharmacology*, **46**, 451–454.

Beaulieu, P., 1994, Intravenous administration of paracetamol (propacetamol) for postoperative analgesia, *Anaesthesia*, **49**, 739–740.

Beaver, W. T., 1965, Mild analgesics. A review of their clinical pharmacology, *American Journal of the Medical Sciences*, **250**, 577–604.

Beaver, W. T., 1966, Mild analgesics. A review of their clinical pharmacology (Part II), *American Journal of the Medical Sciences*, **251**, 576–599.

Becherucci, C., Runci, F. M. and Segre, G., 1981, Gas chromatographic determination of paracetamol in plasma, *Farmaco (Prat)*, **36**, 312–316.

Becker, A., Berner, G., Leuschner, F. and Vögtle-Junkert, U., 1992, Pharmakokinetische Aspekte zur Kombination von Metoclopramid und Paracetamol. Ergebnisse einer Studie zur Humankinetik sowie Konsequenzen für den Migräne-patienten, *Arzneimittel-Forschung*, **42**, 552–555.

Becker, J., Beckmann, J., Bertelt, C., Gundert-Remy, U., Röhmel, J. and Ohlendorf, D., 1990, Doppelblindstudie über postoperative Analgetikawirkungen, *Deutsche Zahnärztliche Zeitschrift*, **45**, 36–38.

Beckett, G. J., Chapman, B. J., Dyson, E. H. and Hayes, J. D., 1985a, Plasma glutathione S-transferase measurements after paracetamol overdose: evidence for early hepatocellular damage, *Gut*, **26**, 26–31.

Beckett, G. J., Dyson, E. H., Chapman, B. J., Templeton, A. J. and Hayes, J. D., 1985b, Plasma glutathione S-transferase measurements by radioimmunoassay: a sensitive index of hepatocellular damage in man, *Clinica Chimica Acta*, **146**, 11–19.

Beckett, G. J., Foster, G. R., Hussey, A. J., Oliveira, D. B. G., Donovan, J. W., Prescott, L. F. and Proudfoot, A. T., 1989, Plasma glutathione S-transferase and F protein are more sensitive than alanine aminotransferase as markers of paracetamol (acetaminophen)-induced liver damage, *Clinical Chemistry*, **35**, 2186–2189.

Bedjaoui, A., Demotes-Mainard, F., Raynal, F., Vinçon, G., Galley, P. and Albin, H., 1984, Influence de l'âge et du sexe sur la pharmacocinétique du paracétamol, *Thérapie*, **39**, 353–359.

Begaud, B., Chaslerie, A., Carne, X., Bannwarth, B., Laporte, J. R., Sorbette, F. and Montastruc, P., 1993, Upper gastrointestinal bleeding associated with analgesics and NSAID use: a case-control study, *Journal of Rheumatology*, **20**, 1443–1444.

Behrendt, W. A. and Cserepes, J., 1985, Acute toxicity and analgesic action of a combination of buclizine, codeine and paracetamol ('Migraleve') in tablet and suppository form in rats, *Pharmatherapeutica*, **4**, 322–331.

Beierschmitt, W., Brady, J., Montelius, D., Meyers, L., Khairallah, E., Wyanci, S. and Cohen, S., 1986a, The effect of age on acetaminophen hepatotoxicity in mice, *Pharmacologist*, **28**, 125.

Beierschmitt, W. P., Brady, J. T., Bartolone, J. B., Wyand, D. S., Khairallah, E. A. and Cohen, S. D., 1989, Selective protein arylation and the age dependency of acetaminophen hepatotoxicity in mice, *Toxicology and Applied Pharmacology*, **98**, 517–529.

Beierschmitt, W. P., Keenan, K. P. and Weiner, M., 1986b, The development of acetaminophen-induced nephrotoxicity in male Fischer 344 rats of different ages, *Archives of Toxicology*, **59**, 206–210.

Beierschmitt, W. P., Keenan, K. P. and Weiner, M., 1986c, Age-related increased susceptibility of male Fischer 344 rats to acetaminophen nephrotoxicity, *Life Sciences*, **39**, 2335–2342.

Beierschmitt, W. P. and Weiner, M., 1986, Age-related changes in renal metabolism of acetaminophen in male Fischer 344 rats, *Age*, **9**, 7–13.

Bélanger, P. M., Lalande, M., Doré, F. and Labrecque, G., 1987, Time-dependent variations in the organ extraction ratios of acetaminophen in the rat, *Journal of Pharmacokinetics and Biopharmaceutics*, **15**, 133–143.

Belin, T., Kerouredan, V., Lanotte, R. and Perrotin, D., 1988, L'intoxication aiguë au paracetamol. Une urgence trompeuse, *Revue de Médecine de Tours*, **22**, 19–20.

Bell, H., Schjonsby, H. and Raknerud, N., 1987a, Alvorlig leverskade – etter terapeutisk dose av paracetamol, *Tidsskrift for den Norske Lægeforening*, **107**, 1037–1040.

Bell, H., Schjonsby, H. and Raknerud, N., 1987b, Alvorlig leverskade – etter inntak av paracetamol i suicidal hensikt, *Tidsskrift for den Norske Lægeforening*, **107**, 1041–1042.

Benedetti, M. S., Louis, A., Malnoë, A., Schneider, M., Lam, R., Kreber, L. and Smith, R. L., 1975, Prevention of paracetamol-induced liver damage in mice with glutathione, *Journal of Pharmacy and Pharmacology*, **27**, 629–632.

Benford, D. J., Dixit, M. and Foster, B., 1990, Variations in the response of cell lines to metabolism-mediated toxicity, *Toxicology in Vitro*, **4**, 506–508.

Bengtsson, U., Angervall, L., Ekman, H. and Lehmann, L., 1968, Transitional cell tumors of the renal pelvis in analgesic abusers, *Scandinavian Journal of Urology and Nephrology*, **2**, 145–150.

Bengtsson, U. and Lindholm, T., 1977, Paracetamol – ett harmlöst analgetikum? *Läkartidningen*, **74**, 1909–1910.

Benkirane-Agoumi, N., Belkhadir, J., Cherkaoui, O., Dadi-el Fassi Fihri, O. and Bensouda, J.

D., 1986, A propos d'un case d'agranulocytose au paracétamol, *Maroc Médical*, **9**, 470–474.

Bennett, A., 1989a, Gastric mucosal damage by nonsteroidal anti-inflammatory drugs, *International Journal of Tissue Reactions*, **11**, 53–57.

Bennett, A., 1989b, Some new aspects of gastric mucosal protection and damage, *Acta Physiologica Hungarica*, **73**, 179–183.

Bennett, A. and Curwain, B. P., 1977, Effects of aspirin-like drugs on canine gastric mucosal blood flow and acid secretion, *British Journal of Pharmacology*, **60**, 499–504.

Benoit, J. P., Boukari, A., Cavaillon, J. P., Girard, P., Haag, R., Lecointre, Cl. and Roussenque, P., 1986, Etude de l'activité et de la tolérance de l'association paracétamol-codéine comparée à la glafenine dans les douleurs post-opératoires en chirurgie buccale, *Information Dentaire*, **68**, 1707–1713.

Bensaude, I. and Modaï, J., 1982, Efficacité sur l'hyperthermie et tolérance du soluté buvable de paracétamol chez des enfants présentant une rougeole, *Semaine des Hôpitaux de Paris*, **58**, 693–694.

Benson, G. D., 1983, Acetaminophen in chronic liver disease, *Clinical Pharmacology and Therapeutics*, **33**, 95–101.

Benson, R. E. and Boleyn, T., 1974, Paracetamol overdose: a plan of management, *Anaesthesia and Intensive Care*, **2**, 334–339.

Benson, R. W., Pumford, N. R., McRae, T. A., Hinson, J. A. and Roberts, D. W., 1989, Development of a particle concentration fluorescence immunoassay for 3-(cystein-S-yl) acetaminophen adducts, *Toxicologist*, **9**, 47.

Bentley, K. C. and Head, T. W., 1987, The additive analgesic efficacy of acetaminophen, 1000 mg, and codeine, 60 mg, in dental pain, *Clinical Pharmacology and Therapeutics*, **42**, 634–640.

Bentur, Y. and Zonis, Z., 1984, Charcoal hemoperfusion in paracetamol poisoning, *Harefuah*, **107**, 333–334.

Benzick, A. E., Reddy, S. L., Gupta, S., Rogers, L. K. and Smith, C. V., 1994, Diquat- and acetaminophen-induced alterations of biliary efflux of iron in rats, *Biochemical Pharmacology*, **47**, 2079–2085.

Ben-Zvi, Z., Weissman-Teitellman, B., Katz, S. and Danon, A., 1990, Acetaminophen hepatotoxicity: is there a role for prostaglandin synthesis? *Archives of Toxicology*, **64**, 299–304.

Berg, K. J., 1994, Paracetamol – nyre og urinveier. Årsak til analgetikanefropati eller cancer? *Tidsskrift for den Norske Lægeforening*, **114**, 1169–1174.

Berg, K. J., Djøseland, O., Gjellan, A., Hundal, O., Knudsen, E. R., Rugstad, H. E. and Rønneberg, E., 1990, Acute effects of paracetamol on prostaglandin synthesis and renal function in normal man and in patients with renal failure, *Clinical Nephrology*, **34**, 255–262.

Berleur, M. P. and Cordier, S., 1992, Etude de l'association entre le cancer de la vessie et la consommation de phénacétine. Problèmes posés par une étude de pharmacoépidémiologie, *Thérapie*, **47**, 231–238.

Berlin, C. M., Yaffe, S. J. and Ragni, M., 1980, Disposition of acetaminophen in milk, saliva and plasma of lactating women, *Pediatric Pharmacology*, **1**, 135–141.

Bermejo, A. M., López-Rivadulla, M., Fernández, P. and Cruz, A., 1991, Application of second-derivative spectroscopy to the simultaneous identification and determination of plasma salicylate and paracetamol, *Analytical Letters*, **24**, 1147–1157.

Bernadou, J., Bonnafous, M., Labat, G., Loiseau, P. and Meunier, B., 1991, Model systems for metabolism studies: biomimetic oxidation of acetaminophen and ellipticine derivatives with water-soluble metalloporphyrins associated to potassium monopersulfate, *Drug Metabolism and Disposition: The Biological Fate of Chemicals*, **19**, 360–365.

Bernal, M. L., Sinues, B., Lanuza, J., Gracia, M., Mayayo, E. and Bartolome, M., 1993, Glutation reducido eritrocitario y tioeteres urinarios en niños tratados con paracetamol, *Anales Espanoles de Pediatria*, **39**, 501–505.

Bernard, A. M., de Russis, R., Amor, A. O. and Lauwerys, R. R., 1988, Potentiation of cadmium nephrotoxicity by acetaminophen, *Archives of Toxicology*, **62**, 291–294.

Berner, G. S, Staab, R. and Wagener, H. H., 1985, HPTLC-Bestimmung von Paracetamol im Serum, *Fresenius Zeitschrift für Analytische Chemie*, **321**, 601–602.

Berntzen, D., Fors, E. and Götestam, K. G., 1985, Effect of an analgesic drug (paralgin forte) upon laboratory pain under different cognitive manipulations: an experimental study, *Acta Neurologica Scandinavica*, **72**, 30–35.

Berry, F. N., Miller, J. M., Levin, H. M., Bare, W. W., Hopkinson, J. H. and Feldman, A. J., 1975, Relief of severe pain with acetaminophen in a new dose formulation vs. propoxyphene hydrochloride 65 mg and placebo: a comparative double-blind study, *Current Therapeutic Research*, **17**, 361–368.

Bertelli, A., Bertelli, A. A. E., Giovannini, L., Mian, M. and Spaggiari, P., 1990, Protective action of coenzyme A on paracetamol-induced tissue depletion of glutathione, *International Journal of Tissue Reactions*, **12**, 353–358.

Bertin, L., Pons, G., d'Athis, P., Lasfargues, G., Maudelonde, C., Duhamel, J. F. and Olive, G., 1991, Randomized, double-blind, multicenter, controlled trial of ibuprofen vs. acetaminophen (paracetamol) and placebo for treatment of symptoms of tonsillitis and pharyngitis in children, *Journal of Pediatrics*, **119**, 811–814.

Bethke, B. A. and Schubert, G. E., 1985, Kapillarosklerose der ableitenden Harnwege als Indiz eines Analgetika-Abusus. Häufigkeit bei unausgewählten Obduktionen in einer westdeutschen Großstadt, *Deutsche Medizinische Wochenschrift*, **110**, 343–346.

Betowski, L. D., Korfmacher, W. A., Lay, J. O., Potter, D. W. and Hinson, J. A., 1987, Direct analysis of rat bile for acetaminophen and two of its conjugated metabolites via thermospray liquid chromatography/mass spectrometry, *Biomedical and Environmental Mass Spectrometry*, **14**, 705–709.

Beutler, E., 1984, Acetaminophen and G-6-PD deficiency, *Acta Haematologica*, **72**, 211–212.

Bhargava, V. O., Emodi, S. and Hirate, J., 1988, Quantitation of acetaminophen and its metabolites in rat plasma after a toxic dose, *Journal of Chromatography: Biomedical Applications*, **426**, 212–215.

Bhargava, V. O. and Hirate, J., 1989, Gastrointestinal, liver and lung extraction ratio of acetaminophen in the rat after high dose administration, *Biopharmaceutics and Drug Disposition*, **10**, 389–396.

Bharija, S. C. and Kanwar, A. J., 1987, Fixed drug eruption due to paracetamol, *Australasian Journal of Dermatology*, **28**, 85.

Bhatia, V. and Bhatia, A., 1990, Morphological changes in the liver on chronic administration of small doses of paracetamol in albino rats, *Indian Journal of Pathology and Microbiology*, **33**, 221–223.

Bhatia, V., Bhatia, A. and Sood, S. K., 1988, Development of paracetamol induced hepatocellular tolerance in albino rats, *Indian Journal of Medical Research*, **88**, 181–186.

Bhatt, P. P., Rytting, J. H. and Topp, E. M., 1991, Influence of Azone and lauryl alcohol on the transport of acetaminophen and ibuprofen through shed snake skin, *International Journal of Pharmaceutics*, **72**, 219–226.

Bhattacharya, S. K. and Bhattacharya, D., 1983, Prostaglandin synthesis inhibitors reduce *Cannabis* and restraint stress induced increase in rat brain serotonin concentrations, *Zeitschrift für Naturforschung – Section C – Biosciences*, **38**, 337–338.

Bhattacharya, S. K., Goel, R. K., Bhattacharya, S. K. and Tandon, R., 1991, Potentiation of gastric toxicity of ibuprofen by paracetamol in the rat, *Journal of Pharmacy and Pharmacology*, **43**, 520–521.

Bhattacharya, S. K., Mohan Rao, P. J. R., Brumleve, S. J. and Parmar, S. S., 1986, Effects of intracerebroventricular administration of bradykinin on rat brain serotonin and prostaglandins, *Research Communications in Chemical Pathology and Pharmacology*, **54**, 355–366.

Bhattacharya, S. K., Mohan Rao, P. J. R., Das, N. and Das Gupta, G., 1988, Intracerebroventricularly administered bradykinin augments carrageenan-induced paw oedema in rats, *Journal of Pharmacy and Pharmacology*, **40**, 367–369.

Bhattacharya, S. K., Mohan Rao, P. J. R. and Das Gupta, G., 1989, Effect of centrally administered prostaglandin D_2 and some prostaglandin synthesis inhibitors on carageenan-induced paw oedema in rats, *Journal of Pharmacy and Pharmacology*, **41**, 569–571.

Bhounsule, S. A., Nevreker, P. R., Agshikar, N. V., Pal, M. N. and Dhume, V. G., 1990, A comparison of four analgesics in post-episiotomy pain, *Indian Journal of Physiology and Pharmacology*, **34**, 34–38.

Bickers, R. G. and Roberts, R. J., 1979, Combined aspirin/acetaminophen intoxication, *Journal of Pediatrics*, **94**, 1001–1003.

Bidault, I., Lagier, G., Garnier, R., Pallot, J. L. and Larrey, D., 1987, Les hépatites par toxicité subaiguë du paracétamol existent-elles? *Thérapie*, **42**, 387–388.

Bien, E., Vick, K. and Skorka, G., 1992, Effects of exogenous factors on the cerebral glutathione in rodents, *Archives of Toxicology*, **66**, 279–285.

Bijlani, R. L., Shukla, K., Narain, J. P. and Puri, P., 1992, Effect of coingestion of paracetamol on glycaemic response, *Indian Journal of Physiology and Pharmacology*, **36**, 215–218.

Bindra, D. S., Zhang, Y., Wilson, G. S., Sternberg, R., Thévenot, D. R., Moatti, D. and Reach, G., 1991, Design and *in vitro* studies of a needle-type glucose sensor for subcutaneous monitoring, *Analytical Chemistry*, **63**, 1692–1696.

Binková, B., Topinka, J. and Srám, R. J., 1990, The effect of paracetamol on oxidative damage in human peripheral lymphocytes, *Mutation Research*, **244**, 227–231.

Bion, J. F., Bowden, M. I., Chow, B., Honisberger, L. and Weatherley, B. C., 1993, Atracurium infusions in patients with fulminant hepatic failure awaiting liver transplantation, *Intensive Care Medicine*, **19 (Suppl. 2)**, S94–S98.

Bippi, H. and Frölich, J. C., 1990, Effects of acetylsalicylic acid and paracetamol alone and in combination on prostanoid synthesis in man, *British Journal of Clinical Pharmacology*, **29**, 305–310.

Birge, R. B., Bartolone, J. B., Cohen, S. D., Khairallah, E. A. and Smolin, L. A., 1991a, A comparison of proteins S-thiolated by glutathione to those arylated by acetaminophen, *Biochemical Pharmacology*, **42 Suppl.**, S197–S207.

Birge, R. B., Bartolone, J. B., Emeigh Hart, S. G., Nishanian, E. V., Tyson, C. A., Khairallah, E. A. and Cohen, S. D., 1990, Acetaminophen hepatotoxicity: correspondence of selective protein arylation in human and mouse liver *in vitro*, in culture, and *in vivo*, *Toxicology and Applied Pharmacology*, **105**, 472–482.

Birge, R. B., Bartolone, J. B., McCann, D. J., Mangold, J. B., Cohen, S. D. and Khairallah, E. A., 1989, Selective protein arylation by acetaminophen and 2,6-dimethylacetaminophen in cultured hepatocytes from phenobarbital-induced and uninduced mice: relationship to cytotoxicity, *Biochemical Pharmacology*, **38**, 4429–4438.

Birge, R. B., Bartolone, J. B., Nishanian, E. V., Bruno, M. K., Mangold, J. B., Cohen, S. D. and Khairallah, E. A., 1988, Dissociation of covalent binding from the oxidative effects of acetaminophen: studies using dimethylated acetaminophen derivatives, *Biochemical Pharmacology*, **37**, 3383–3393.

Birge, R. B., Bartolone, J. B., Tyson, C. A., Emeigh Hart, S. G., Cohen, S. D. and Khairallah, E. A., 1991b, Selective binding of acetaminophen (APAP) to liver proteins in mice and men, *Advances in Experimental Medicine and Biology*, **283**, 685–688.

Birge, R. B., Bulera, S. J., Bartolone, J. B., Ginsberg, G. L., Cohen, S. D. and Khairallah, E. A., 1991c, The arylation of microsomal membrane proteins by acetaminophen is associated with the release of a 44 kDa acetaminophen-binding mouse liver protein complex into the cytosol, *Toxicology and Applied Pharmacology*, **109**, 443–454.

Birkland, P., 1993, International update: alternative treatment for common but dangerous acetaminophen overdoses, *Journal of Emergency Nursing*, **19**, 32A–33A.

Birzle, H., Beck, K. and Dieterich, E., 1967, Die Wirkung gezielter Röntgentiefenbestrahlung der Leber auf die Bildung gepaarter Schwefelsäuren nach Belastung mit N-azetyl-p-aminophenol beim Kaninchen, *Strahlentherapie*, **133**, 602–609.

Bisby, R. H., Cundall, R. B. and Tabassum, N., 1985, Formation and reactivity of free radicals of acetaminophen formed by one electron oxidation, *Life Chemistry Reports*, **3**, 29–34.

Bisby, R. H. and Tabassum, N., 1988, Properties of the radicals formed by one-electron oxidation of acetaminophen – a pulse radiolysis study, *Biochemical Pharmacology*, **37**, 2731–2738.

Bismuth, C. and Fournier, P. E., 1980, Biological evaluation of hemoperfusion in acute poisoning, *Developments in Toxicology and Environmental Science*, **8**, 377–385.

Bismuth, C., Fournier, P. E. and Galliot, M., 1981, Biological evaluation of hemoperfusion in acute poisoning, *Clinical Toxicology*, **18**, 1213–1223.

Bismuth, C., Garnier, R., Fournier, P. E. and Baud, F., 1983, Sécurité des conditionnements nationaux de paracétamol: pas de mortalité française par intoxication aiguë, *Presse Médicale*, **12**, 1632–1634.

Bismuth, H., Samuel, D., Gugenheim, J., Castaing, D., Bernuau, J., Rueff, B. and Benhamou, J.-P., 1987, Emergency liver transplant for fulminant hepatitis, *Annals of Internal Medicine*, **107**, 337–341.

Bisordi, J. E., Schlondorff, D. and Hays, R. M., 1980, Interaction of vasopressin and prostaglandins in the toad urinary bladder, *Journal of Clinical Investigation*, **66**, 1200–1210.

Bito, L. Z. and Salvador, E. V., 1976, Effects of anti-inflammatory agents and some other drugs on prostaglandin biotransport, *Journal of Pharmacology and Experimental Therapeutics*, **198**, 481–488.

Bitzén, P.-O., Gustafsson, B., Jostell, K. G., Melander, A. and Wåhlin-Boll, E., 1981, Excretion of paracetamol in human breast milk, *European Journal of Clinical Pharmacology*, **20**, 123–125.

Bjerregaard, H. F., 1993, Electrophysiological measurements of a toad renal epithelial cell line (A6) as an assay to evaluate cellular toxicity *in vitro*, *Toxicology in Vitro*, **7**, 411–415.

Björck, S., Svalander, C. T. and Aurell, M., 1988, Acute renal failure after analgesic drugs including paracetamol (acetaminophen), *Nephron*, **49**, 45–53.

Björkman, R., Hallman, K. M., Hedner, J., Hedner, T. and Henning, M., 1994, Acetaminophen blocks spinal hyperalgesia induced by NMDA and substance P, *Pain*, **57**, 259–264.

Black, M., 1984, Acetaminophen hepatotoxicity, *Annual Review of Medicine*, **35**, 577–593.

Black, M., 1987, Hepatotoxic and hepatoprotective potential of histamine (H$_2$)-receptor antagonists, *American Journal of Medicine*, **83 (Suppl. 6A)**, 68–75.

Black, M., Cornell, J. F., Rabin, L. and Shachter, N., 1982, Late presentation of acetaminophen hepatotoxicity, *Digestive Diseases and Sciences*, **27**, 370–374.

Black, M. and Raucy, J., 1986, Acetaminophen, alcohol, and cytochrome P-450, *Annals of Internal Medicine*, **104**, 427–429.

Black, M. and Sprague, K., 1978, Rapid micromethod for acetaminophen determination in serum, *Clinical Chemistry*, **24**, 1288–1289.

Blackledge, H. M., O'Farrell, J., Minton, N. A. and McLean, A. E. M., 1991, The effect of therapeutic doses of paracetamol on sulphur metabolism in man, *Human and Experimental Toxicology*, **10**, 159–165.

Blackwell, G. J., Flower, R. J. and Vane, J. R., 1975, Some characteristics of the prostaglandin synthesizing system in rabbit kidney microsomes, *Biochimica Biophysica Acta*, **398**, 178–190.

Blair, D. and Rumack, B. H., 1977, Acetaminophen in serum and plasma estimated by high pressure liquid chromatography: a micro-scale method, *Clinical Chemistry*, **23**, 743–745.

Blair, I. A., Boobis, A. R., Davies, D. S. and Cresp, T. M., 1980, Paracetamol oxidation: synthesis and reactivity of N-acetyl-p-benzoquinoneimine, *Tetrahedron Letters*, **21**, 4947–4950.

Blair, J. B., Hinton, D. E. and Miller, M. R., 1989, Morphological changes in trout hepatocytes exposed to acetaminophen, *Marine Environmental Research*, **28**, 357–361.

Blaison, G., Bloch, J. G., Calvel, L., Kuntz, J. L. and Asch, L., 1991, Hypoglycémies induites par l'association chlorohydrate de dextropropoxyphène-paracétamol, *Semaine des Hôpitaux de Paris*, **67**, 1964–1966.

Blake, K. V., Bailey, D., Zientek, G. M. and Hendeles, L., 1988, Death of a child associated with multiple overdoses of acetaminophen, *Clinical Pharmacy*, **7**, 391–397.

Blakytny, R. and Harding, J. J., 1992, Prevention of cataract in diabetic rats by aspirin, paracetamol (acetaminophen) and ibuprofen, *Experimental Eye Research*, **54**, 509–518.

Blanch, R. R., Serra, B. and Muñiz, J. M., 1987, La N-acetilcisteïna en el tractament de la sobredosi per paracetamol, *Anales de Medicina*, **73**, 115–119.

Blanchi, A., Delchier, J.-C., Soulé, J.-C. and Bader, J.-P., 1984, Sténose anorectale liée à la prise de suppositoires associant dextropropoxyphène et paracétamol (Di-Antalvic), *Gastroentérologie Clinique et Biologique*, **8**, 579–580.

Block, R., Jankowski, J. A. Z., Lacoux, P. and Pennington, C. R., 1992, Does hypothermia protect against the development of hepatitis in paracetamol overdose? *Anaesthesia*, **47**, 789–791.

Blohmé, I. and Johansson, S., 1981, Renal pelvic neoplasms and atypical urothelium in patients with end-stage analgesic nephropathy, *Kidney International*, **20**, 671–675.

Bloomfield, S. S., Barden, T. P. and Mitchell, J., 1981, A comparison of pirprofen, aspirin, acetaminophen and placebo in postpartum uterine cramp pain, *Current Therapeutic Research*, **30 (Suppl.)**, S139–S145.

Blouin, R. A., Dickson, P., McNamara, P. J., Cibull, M. and McClain, C., 1987, Phenobarbital induction and acetaminophen hepatotoxicity: resistance in the obese Zucker rodent, *Journal of Pharmacology and Experimental Therapeutics*, **243**, 565–570.

Bluemle, L. W. and Goldberg, M., 1968, Renal accumulation of salicylate and phenacetin: possible mechanisms in the nephropathy of analgesic abuse, *Journal of Clinical Investigation*, **47**, 2507–2514.

Blume, H., Ali, S. L., Elze, M., Krämer, J., Wendt, G. and Scholz, M. E., 1994, Relative Bioverfügbarkeit von Paracetamol in Suppositorien-Zubereitungen im Vergleich zu Tabletten, *Arzneimittel-Forschung*, **44**, 1333–1338.

Blyden, G. T., Greenblatt, D. J., LeDuc, B. W. and Scavone, J. M., 1988, Effect of antipyrine coadministration on the kinetics of acetaminophen and lidocaine, *European Journal of Clinical Pharmacology*, **35**, 413–417.

Boardman, P. L. and Hart, F. D., 1967, Clinical measurement of the anti-inflammatory effects of salicylates in rheumatoid arthritis, *British Medical Journal*, **4**, 264–268.

Boberg, K. M., Schrumpf, E., Rogstad, B., Ganes, T. and Bergan, A., 1994, Behandling av paracetamol forgiftning: Indikasjon for levertransplantasjon? *Tidsskrift for den Norske Lægeforening*, **114**, 1199–1203.

Bock, K. W. and Bock-Hennig, B. S., 1987, Differential induction of human liver UDP-glucuronosyltransferase activities by phenobarbital-type inducers, *Biochemical Pharmacology*, **36**, 4137–4143.

Bock, K. W., Forster, A., Gschaidmeier, H., Brück, M., Münzel, P., Schareck, W., Fournel-Gigleux, S. and Burchell, B., 1993, Paracetamol glucuronidation by recombinant rat and human phenol UDP-glucuronosyltransferases, *Biochemical Pharmacology*, **45**, 1809–1814.

Bock, K. W., Schrenk, D., Forster, A., Griese, E-U., Mörike, K., Brockmeier, D. and Eichelbaum, M., 1994, The influence of environmental and genetic factors on CYP2D6, CYP1A2 and UDP-glucuronsyltransferases in man using sparteine, caffeine and paracetamol as probes, *Pharmacogenetics*, **4**, 209–218.

Bock, K. W., Wiltfang, J., Blume, R., Ullrich, D. and Bircher, J., 1987, Paracetamol as a test drug to determine glucuronide formation in man. Effects of inducers and of smoking, *European Journal of Clinical Pharmacology*, **31**, 677–683.

Bodd, E., Stuveseth, K., Kveseth, N., Mørland, J., Nordal, T. L. and Wickstrom, E., 1985, Kartlegging av acetylsalicylsyre- og paracetamol-forgiftninger i Norge, *Tidsskrift for den Norske Lægeforening*, **105**, 1774–1778.

Boehm, J. J. and Oppenheim, R. C., 1977, An *in vitro* study of the adsorption of various drugs by activated charcoal, *Australian Journal of Pharmaceutical Sciences*, **4**, 107–111.

Boeijinga, J. K., Boerstra, E. E., Ris, P., Breimer, D. D. and Jeletich-Bastiaanse, A., 1982, Interaction between paracetamol and coumarin anticoagulants, *Lancet*, **i**, 506.

Boeijinga, J. K., Boerstra, E. E., Ris, P., Breimer, D. D. and Jeletich-Bastiaanse, A., 1983, De invloed van paracetamol op antistollingsbehandeling met coumarinederivaten, *Pharmaceutisch Weekblad*, **118**, 209–212.

Boelsterli, U. A., 1993, Specific targets of covalent drug-protein interactions in hepatocytes and their toxicological significance in drug-induced liver injury, *Drug Metabolism Reviews*, **25**, 395–451.

Boissier, Ch., Perpoint, B., Laporte-Simitsidis, S., Mismetti, P., Hocquart, J., Gayet, J. L., Rambaud, C., Queneau, P. and Decousus, H., 1992, Acceptability and efficacy of two associations of paracetamol with a central analgesic (dextropropoxyphene or codeine): comparison in osteoarthritis, *Journal of Clinical Pharmacology*, **32**, 990–995.

Bolanowska, W. and Gessner, T., 1978, Drug interactions: inhibition of acetaminophen glucuronidation by drugs, *Journal of Pharmacology and Experimental Therapeutics*, **206**, 233–238.

Bolanowska, W. and Gessner, T., 1980, Drug interactions with acetaminophen: effects of phenobarbital, prednisone and 5-fluorouracil in normal and tumor-bearing rats, *Biochemical Pharmacology*, **29**, 1167–1175.

Bolcsfoldi, G., Johansson, M., Andersson, B. and Moldéus, P., 1981, Biotransformation of xenobiotics in isolated dog hepatocytes, *Acta Pharmacologica et Toxicologica*, **48**, 227–232.

Bomalaski, J. S., Alvarez, J., Touchstone, J. and Zurier, R. B., 1987, Alteration of uptake and distribution of eicosanoid precursor fatty acids by aspirin, *Biochemical Pharmacology*, **36**, 3249–3253.

Bonadio, W. A., Bellomo, T., Brady, W. and Smith, D., 1993, Correlating changes in body temperature with infectious outcome in febrile children who receive acetaminophen, *Clinical Pediatrics*, **32**, 343–346.

Bonanomi, L., Borgogelli, E. and Losa, M., 1982, Influenza dell'acetilcisteina sulla riduzione del glutatione epatico indotta nel topo da paracetamolo, *Rivista di Farmacologia e Terapia*, **13**, 205–210.

Bonati, M., 1991, An international survey on drug utilization during pregnancy, *International Journal of Risk and Safety in Medicine*, **2**, 345–350.

Bond, G. R., Krenzelok, E. P., Normann, S. A., Tendler, J. D., Morris-Kukoski, C. L., McCoy, D. J., Thompson, M. W., McCarthy, T., Roblez, J., Taylor, C., Dolan, M. A., Requa, R. K. and Curry, S. C., 1994, Acetaminophen ingestion in childhood: cost and relative risk of alternative referral strategies, *Journal of Toxicology. Clinical Toxicology*, **32**, 513–525.

Bond, G. R., Requa, R. K., Krenzelok, E. P., Normann, S. A., Tendler, J. D., Morris, C. L., McCoy, D. J., Thompson, M. W., McCarthy, T., Roblez, J., Taylor, C., Dolan, M. A. and Curry, S. C., 1993, Influence of time until emesis on the efficacy of decontamination using acetaminophen as a marker in a pediatric population, *Annals of Emergency Medicine*, **22**, 1403–1407.

Bonfiglio, M. F., Traegar, S. M., Hulisz, D. T. and Martin, B. R., 1992, Anaphylactoid reaction to intravenous acetylcysteine associated with electrocardiographic abnormalities, *Annals of Pharmacotherapy*, **26**, 22–25.

Bonham Carter, S. M., Rein, G., Glover, V., Sandler, M. and Caldwell, J., 1983, Human platelet phenolsulphotransferase M and P: substrate specificities and correlation with *in vivo* sulphoconjugation of paracetamol and salicylamide, *British Journal of Clinical Pharmacology*, **15**, 323–330.

Bonkovsky, H. L., Kane, R. E., Jones, D. P., Galinsky, R. E. and Banner, B., 1994, Acute hepatic and renal toxicity from low doses of acetaminophen in the absence of alcohol abuse or malnutrition: evidence for increased susceptibility to drug toxicity due to cardiopulmonary and renal insufficiency, *Hepatology*, **19**, 1141–1148.

Bonkowsky, H. L., Mudge, G. H. and McMurtry, R. J., 1978, Chronic hepatic inflammation and fibrosis due to low doses of paracetamol, *Lancet*, **i**, 1016–1018.

Boobis, A. R., Seddon, C. E., Nasseri-Sina, P. and Davies, D. S., 1990, Evidence for a direct role of intracellular calcium in paracetamol toxicity, *Biochemical Pharmacology*, **39**, 1277–1281.

Boobis, A. R., Tee, L. B. G., Hampden, C. E. and Davies, D. S., 1986, Freshly isolated hepatocytes as a model for studying the toxicity of paracetamol, *Food and Chemical Toxicology*, **24**, 731–736.

Boogaard, P. J., Mulder, G. J. and Nagelkerke, J. F., 1989, Isolated proximal tubular cells from rat kidney as an *in vitro* model for studies on nephrotoxicity: II. α-Methylglucose uptake as a sensitive parameter for mechanistic studies of acute toxicity by xenobiotics, *Toxicology and Applied Pharmacology*, **101**, 144–157.

Booy, R. H., 1972, Pijnbestrijding met eenvoudige analgetica in de tandheelkunde, *Nederlands Tijdschrift voor Tandheelkunde*, **79**, 69–75.

Boréus, L.-O. and Sandberg, F., 1953, A comparison of some pharmacological effects of acetophenetidin and N-acetyl p-aminophenol, *Acta Physiologica Scandinavica*, **28**, 261–265.

Boréus, L.-O., Sandberg, F. and Ågren, E., 1956, Experimental and clinical studies on the synergism and antagonism of oral analgesics, *Acta Odontologica Scandinavica*, **13**, 219–234.

Borin, M. T. and Ayres, J. W., 1989, Single dose bioavailability of acetaminophen following oral administration, *International Journal of Pharmaceutics*, **54**, 199–209.

Borm, P. L. A., Frankhuijzen-Sierevogel, A. and Noordhoek, J., 1983, Kinetics of *in vitro* O-deethylation of phenacetin and 7-ethoxycoumarin by rat intestinal mucosal cells and microsomes, *Biochemical Pharmacology*, **32**, 1573–1580.

Bosch, F., Toranzo, I. and Baños, J. E., 1990, Dental pain as a model for studying self-medication with analgesics, *European Journal of Pharmacology*, **183**, 1036–1037.

Boughton-Smith, N. K. and Whittle, B. J. R., 1983, Stimulation and inhibition of prostacyclin formation in the gastric mucosa and ileum *in vitro* by anti-inflammatory agents, *British Journal of Pharmacology*, **78**, 173–180.

Boukma, D. W., 1976, Acetaminophen toxicity, *Hospital Pharmacy*, **11**, 122–124.

Boureau, F. and Boccard, E., 1991, Placebo-controlled study of the analgesic efficacy of a combination of paracetamol and codeine in rheumatoid arthritis, *Acta Therapeutica*, **17**, 123–136.

Boureau, F. and Boccard, E., 1994, Étude controlleé vs. placebo de l'efficacité antalgique d'une association paracétamol 500 mg codeine 30 mg dans la polyarthrite rhumatoïde, *Rhumatologie*, **46**, 157–163.

Boureau, F., Joubert, J. M., Lassere, V., Prum, B. and Delecoeuillerie, G., 1994, Double-blind comparison of an acetaminophen 400 mg-codeine 25 mg combination vs. aspirin 1000 mg and placebo in acute migraine attack, *Cephalalgia*, **14**, 156–161.

Boxill, G. C., Nash, C. B. and Wheeler, A. G., 1958, Comparative pharmacological and toxicological evaluation of N-acetyl-p-aminophenol, salicylamide, and acetylsalicylic acid, *Journal of the American Pharmaceutical Association*, **47**, 479–487.

Boyd, E. M., 1970, Testicular atrophy from analgesic drugs, *Journal of Clinical Pharmacology*, **10**, 222–227.

Boyd, E. M. and Bereczky, G. M., 1966, Liver necrosis from paracetamol, *British Journal of Pharmacology*, **26**, 606–614.

Boyd, E. M. and Hogan, S. E., 1968, The chronic oral toxicity of paracetamol at the range of the $LD_{50(100 days)}$ in albino rats, *Canadian Journal of Physiology and Pharmacology*, **46**, 239–245.

Boyd, E. M. and Sheppard, E. P., 1966, Dose-response changes in organ weights and water contents following administration of toxic doses of paracetamol, *British Journal of Pharmacology and Chemotherapy*, **27**, 497–505.

Boyd, J. A. and Eling, T. E., 1981, Prostaglandin endoperoxide synthetase-dependent cooxidation of acetaminophen to intermediates which covalently bind *in vitro* to rabbit renal medullary microsomes, *Journal of Pharmacology and Experimental Therapeutics*, **219**, 659–664.

Boyd, J. C., Savory, M. G., Margrey, M., Herold, D. A., Shipe, J. R. and Savory, J., 1985, Adaptation of EMIT drug assays to a random-access automated clinical analyzer, *Annals of Clinical and Laboratory Science*, **15**, 39–44.

Boyer, T. D. and Rouff, S. L., 1971, Acetaminophen-induced hepatic necrosis and renal failure, *Journal of the American Medical Association*, **218**, 440–441.

Bozdogan, A., Kunt, G. K. and Acar, A. M., 1992, Simultaneous determination of acetaminophen and phenobarbital in suppositories by partial least-squares spectrophotometric calibration, *Analytical Letters*, **25**, 2051–2058.

Bradley, C. A., Wright, E. P. and Parl, F. F., 1983, Measurement of acetaminophen in serum with a microcentrifugal analyser, *Clinical Chemistry*, **29**, 1237.

Bradley, C. M. and Nicholson, A. N., 1987, Studies on performance with aspirin and paracetamol and with the centrally acting analgesics meptazinol and pentazocine, *European Journal of Clinical Pharmacology*, **32**, 135–139.

Bradley, H., Waring, R. H., Emery, P. and Arthur, V., 1991a, Metabolism of low-dose paracetamol in patients with rheumatoid arthritis, *Xenobiotica*, **21**, 689–693.

Bradley, J. D., Brandt, K. D., Katz, B. P., Kalasinski, L. A. and Ryan, S. I., 1991b, Comparison of an antiinflammatory dose of ibuprofen, an analgesic dose of ibuprofen, and acetaminophen in the treatment of patients with osteoarthritis of the knee, *New England Journal of Medicine*, **325**, 87–91.

Bradley, J. D., Brandt, K. D., Katz, B. P., Kalasinski, L. A. and Ryan, S. I., 1992, Treatment of knee osteoarthritis: relationship of clinical features of joint inflammation to the response to a nonsteroidal antiinflammatory drug or pure analgesic, *Journal of Rheumatology*, **19**, 1950–1954.

Brady, J. T., Birge, R. B., Khairallah, E. A. and Cohen, S. D., 1991, Post-treatment protection with piperonyl butoxide against acetaminophen hepatotoxicity is associated with changes in selective but not total covalent binding, *Advances in Experimental Medicine and Biology*, **283**, 689–692.

Brahm, J., Silva, G. and Palma, R., 1992, Sobredosis de paracetamol: una nueva forma de suicidio en Chile y el valor de la administracion de N-acetilcisteina, *Revista Médica de Chile*, **120**, 427–429.

Braiotta, E. A. and Buttery, J. E., 1982, Experience with a kit and a manual colorimetric method for plasma paracetamol, *Australian Journal of Medical Laboratory Science*, **3**, 109–113.

Braiotta, E. A. and Buttery, J. E., 1985, Enzymatic paracetamol measurement by a modified kit method, *Australian Journal of Medical Laboratory Science*, **6**, 82–84.

Bramley, P. N., Rathbone, B. J., Forbes, M. A., Cooper, E. H. and Losowsky, M. S., 1991, Serum hyaluronate as a marker of hepatic derangement in acute liver damage, *Journal of Hepatology*, **13**, 8–13.

Bramwell, H., Cass, A. E. G., Gibbs, P. N. B. and Green, M. J., 1990, Method for determining paracetamol in whole blood by chronoamperometry following enzymatic hydrolysis, *Analyst*, **115**, 185–188.

Brandon, G., 1993, The fatal paracetamol dosage – how low can you go? *Medicine, Science and the Law*, **33**, 274.

Brandon, G., 1994, Paracetamol overdose: the way forward, *Pharmaceutical Journal*, **252**, 804.

Bravo, M. E., Horwitz, I., Contreras, C., Olea, I. and Arancibia, A., 1987, Influencia del paracetamol en la farmacocinética del chloramfenicol en pacients con fiebre tifoídea,

Revista Chilena de Pediatria, **58**, 117–120.

Bravo-Fernández, E. F., Reddy, K. R., Jeffers, L. and Schiff, E. R., 1988, Hepatotoxicity after prolonged use of acetaminophen: a case report, *Boletin – Asociacion Medica de Puerto Rico*, **80**, 417–419.

Bray, G. P., 1993, Liver failure induced by paracetamol, *British Medical Journal*, **306**, 157–158.

Bray, G. P., Harrison, P. M., O'Grady, J. G., Tredger, J. M. and Williams, R., 1992a, Long-term anticonvulsant therapy worsens outcome in paracetamol-induced fulminant hepatic failure, *Human and Experimental Toxicology*, **11**, 265–270.

Bray, G. P., Mowat, C., Muir, D. F., Tredger, J. M. and Williams, R., 1991, The effect of chronic alcohol intake on prognosis and outcome in paracetamol overdose, *Human and Experimental Toxicology*, **10**, 435–438.

Bray, G. P., Tredger, J. M. and Williams, R., 1992b, S-adenosylmethionine protects against acetaminophen hepatotoxicity in two mouse models, *Hepatology*, **15**, 297–301.

Brazer, S. R., Tyor, M. P., Pancotto, F. S., Nickl, N. J., Wildermann, N. M., Harrell, F. E. and Pryor, D. B., 1990, Studies of gastric ulcer disease by communuity-based gastroenterologists, *American Journal of Gastroenterology*, **85**, 824–828.

Brazier, J. L., Ritter, J., Latour, J. F., Enoch, F., Khenfer, D. and Faucon, G., 1982, Allongement de la demi-vie du paracétamol et de l'hexobarbital en cas de cirrhose compensée et decompensée, *Thérapie*, **37**, 275–280.

Bredfeldt, J. E. and von Huene, C., 1984, Ranitidine, acetaminophen, and hepatotoxicity, *Annals of Internal Medicine*, **101**, 719.

Breen, K., Wandscheer, J.-C., Peignoux, M. and Pessayre, D., 1982a, *In situ* formation of the acetaminophen metabolite covalently bound in kidney and lung: supportive evidence provided by total hepatectomy, *Biochemical Pharmacology*, **31**, 115–116.

Breen, K. J., Bury, R. W., Desmond, P. V., Forge, B. H. R., Mashford, M. L. and Whelan, G., 1982b, Paracetamol self-poisoning – diagnosis, management, and outcome, *Medical Journal of Australia*, **1**, 77–79.

Brennan, R. J., Mankes, R. F., Lefevre, R., Raccio-Robak, N., Baevsky, R. H., Del Vecchio, J. A. and Zink, B. J., 1994, 4-Methylpyrazole blocks acetaminophen hepatotoxicity in the rat, *Annals of Emergency Medicine*, **23**, 487–494.

Brenner, A., Hodak, E., Dascalu, D., Lurie, R. and Wolf, R., 1990, A possible case of drug-induced familial pemphigus, *Acta Dermato-Venerologica*, **70**, 357–358.

Brent, J., 1993, Are activated charcoal-N-acetylcysteine interactions of clinical significance? *Annals of Emergency Medicine*, **22**, 1860–1862.

Brent, J. A. and Rumack, B. H., 1993, Role of free radicals in toxic hepatic injury. II. Are free radicals the cause of toxin-induced liver injury? *Journal of Toxicology. Clinical Toxicology*, **31**, 173–196.

Brevet, E. A., Hazzan, M. M. R., Reade, R. P., Bridoux, F., Dequiedt, P. C. M. and Lelièvre, G., 1994, Insuffisance rénale aiguë (IRA) secondaire à la prise de paracétamol, *Revue de Médecine Interne*, **15 (Suppl. 1)**, 181S.

Brewer, E. J., 1968, A comparative evaluation of indomethacin, acetaminophen and placebo as antipyretic agents in children, *Arthritis and Rheumatism*, **11**, 645–651.

Briant, R. H., Dorrington, R. E., Cleal, J. and Williams, F. M., 1976, The rate of acetaminophen metabolism in the elderly and the young, *Journal of the American Geriatrics Society*, **24**, 359–361.

Bridges, R. R., Kinniburgh, D. W., Keehn, B. J. and Jennison, T. A., 1983, An evaluation of common methods for acetaminophen quantitation for small hospitals, *Clinical Toxicology*, **20**, 1–17.

Briggs, D., Calder, I., Woods, R. and Tange, J., 1982, The influence of metabolic variation on analgesic nephrotoxicity: experiments with the Gunn rat, *Pathology*, **14**, 349–353.

British Pharmacopoeia, 1988, pp. 414–415, London: Her Majesty's Stationery Office.

Brodie, B. B. and Axelrod, J., 1948a, The estimation of acetanilide and its metabolic products aniline, N-acetyl p-aminophenol and p-aminophenol (free and total conjugated) in biological fluids and tissues, *Journal of Pharmacology and Experimental Therapeutics*, **94**, 22–28.

Brodie, B. B. and Axelrod, J., 1948b, The fate of acetanilide in man, *Journal of Pharmacology and Experimental Therapeutics*, **94**, 29–38.

Brodie, B. B. and Axelrod, J., 1949, The fate of acetophenetidin (phenacetin) in man and methods for the estimation of acetophenetidin and its metabolites in biological material, *Journal of Pharmacology and Experimental Therapeutics*, **97**, 58–67.

Brodie, M. J., Boobis, A. R., Hampden, C., McPherson, G. A. D., Benjamin, I. S. and Blumgart, L. H., 1981, Antipyrine and paracetamol metabolism in obstructive jaundice, *British Journal of Clinical Pharmacology*, **12**, 277P–278P.

Brodie, M. J., Boobis, A. R., Toverud, E-L., Ellis, W., Murray, S., Dollery, C. T., Webster, S. and Harrison, R., 1980, Drug metabolism in white vegetarians, *British Journal of Clinical Pharmacology*, **9**, 523–525.

Brodin, P. and Skoglund, L. A., 1987, Effects of salicylates and paracetamol compared to lidocaine on nerve conduction *in vitro*, *Neuropharmacology*, **26**, 1441–1444.

Bromm, B., Forth, W., Richter, E. and Scharein, E., 1992, Effects of acetaminophen and antipyrine on non-inflammatory pain and EEG activity, *Pain*, **50**, 213–221.

Bromm, B., Herrmann, M. W. and Scharein, E., 1988, Zur analgetischen Wirksamkeit von Paracetamol und Acetylsalicylsäure im experimentellen Schmerzmodell, *Schmerz Pain Douleur*, **9**, 5–11.

Bromm, B. and Scharein, E., 1993, Alterations in the human EEG induced by acetylsalicylic acid and related drugs, *Progress in Pharmacology and Clinical Pharmacology*, **10**, 23–40.

Brotodihardjo, A. E., Batey, R. G., Farrell, G. C. and Byth, K., 1992, Hepatotoxicity from paracetamol self-poisoning in western Sydney: a continuing challenge, *Medical Journal of Australia*, **157**, 382–385.

Brouwer, K. L. R., 1993, Acute phenobarbital administration alters the disposition of acetaminophen metabolites in the rat, *Drug Metabolism and Disposition: The Biological Fate of Chemicals*, **21**, 1129–1133.

Brouwer, K. L. R. and Jones, J. A., 1990, Altered hepatobiliary disposition of acetaminophen metabolites after phenobarbital pretreatment and renal ligation: evidence for impaired biliary excretion and a diffusional barrier, *Journal of Pharmacology and Experimental Therapeutics*, **252**, 657–664.

Brown, F., 1985, Paracetamol poisoning in cats, *The Veterinary Record*, **116**, 275.

Brown, F. L., Bodison, S., Dixon, J., Davis, W. and Nowoslawski, J., 1986, Comparison of diflunisal and acetaminophen with codeine in the treatment of initial or recurrent acute low back strain, *Clinical Therapeutics*, **9 (Suppl. C)**, 52–58.

Brown, K. A. and Collins, A. J., 1977, Action of nonsteroidal, anti-inflammatory drugs on human and rat peripheral leucocyte migration *in vitro*, *Annals of the Rheumatic Diseases*, **36**, 239–243.

Brown, P., Mehlisch, D. R. and Minn, F., 1990, Tramadol hydrochloride: efficacy compared to codeine sulfate, acetaminophen with dextropropoxyphene and placebo in dental-extraction pain, *European Journal of Pharmacology*, **183**, 1441.

Brown, R. A. G., 1968, Hepatic and renal damage with paracetamol overdosage, *Journal of Clinical Pathology*, **21**, 793.

Brown, R. C., Kelleher, J., Walker, B. E. and Losowsky, M. S., 1979, The effect of wheat bran and pectin on paracetamol absorption in the rat, *British Journal of Nutrition*, **41**, 455–464.

Brown, R. D., Wilson, J. T., Kearns, G. L., Eichler, V. F., Johnson, V. A. and Bertrand, K. M., 1992, Single-dose pharmacokinetics of ibuprofen and acetaminophen in febrile children, *Journal of Clinical Pharmacology*, **32**, 231–241.

Brown, S. S., 1971, Poisoning: clinical chemistry or chemical toxicology? *Annals of Clinical Biochemistry*, **8**, 98–104.

Brown, S. S., Campbell, R. S., Price, C. P., Rambohul, E., Widdop, B., Barbour, H. M., Roberts, J. G., Burnett, D., Atkinson, T., Scawen, M. D. and Hammond, P. M., 1983, Collaborative trial of an enzyme-based assay for the determination of paracetamol in plasma, *Annals of Clinical Biochemistry*, **20**, 353–359.

Bruchhausen, F. and Baumann, J., 1982, Inhibitory actions of desacetylation products of phenacetin and paracetamol on prostaglandin synthetases in neuronal and glial cell lines and rat renal medulla, *Life Sciences*, **30**, 1783–1791.

Bruguerolle, B., Bouvenot, G., Bartolin, R. and Pouyet, A., 1990, Chronokinetics of acetaminophen in elderly patients, *Annual Review of Chronopharmacology*, **7**, 265–268.

Brumas, V., Hacht, B., Filella, M. and Berthon, G., 1992, Can *N*-acetyl-L-cysteine affect zinc metabolism when used as a paracetamol antidote, *Agents and Actions*, **36**, 278–288.

Brunborg, G., Hongslo, J. K., Wiger, R. and Holme, J. A., 1994, Synergistic effects of paracetamol and UV on DNA repair and cell death in mammalian cells, *Pharmacology and Toxicology*, **74 (Suppl. 2)**, 21.

Brune, K., 1983, Prostaglandins and the mode of action of antipyretic analgesic drugs, *American Journal of Medicine*, **75 (5A)**, 19–23.

Brune, K., Aehringhaus, U. and Peskar, B. A., 1984, Pharmacological control of leukotriene and prostaglandin production from mouse peritoneal macrophages, *Agents and Actions*, **14**, 729–734.

Brune, K., Bucher, K. and Walz, D., 1974, The avian microcrystal arthitis. II. Central vs. peripheral effects of sodium salicylate, acetaminophen and colchicine, *Agents and Actions*, **4**, 27–33.

Brune, K., Bucher, K. and Walz, D., 1994, The avian microcrystal arthritis II. Central vs. peripheral effects of sodium salicylate, acetaminophen and colchicine, *Agents and Actions*, **43**, 211–217.

Brune, K. and Glatt, M., 1974, The avian microcrystal arthritis. IV. The impact of sodium salicylate, acetaminophen and colchicine on leucocyte invasion and enzyme liberation *in vivo*, *Agents and Actions*, **4**, 101–107.

Brune, K. and Lanz, R., 1984, Mode of action of peripheral analgesics, *Arzneimittel-Forschung*, **34**, 1060–1065.

Brune, K., Menzel-Soglowek, S. and Zeilhofer, H. U., 1993, New evidence for an additional (central) site of action of antipyretic analgesics, *Progress in Pharmacology and Clinical Pharmacology*, **10**, 41–50.

Brune, K. and Peskar, B. A., 1980, Paracetamol does not potentiate the acetylsalicylate inhibition of prostaglandin release from macrophages, *European Journal of Pharmacology*, **68**, 365–367.

Brune, K., Rainsford, K. D., Wagner, K. and Peskar, B. A., 1981, Inhibition by anti-inflammatory drugs of prostaglandin production in cultured macrophages, *Naunyn-Schmiedeberg's Archives of Pharmacology*, **315**, 269–278.

Brunner, F. P., Richtmann, L., Thiel, G. and Dubach, U. C., 1978, Tumoren der ableitenden Harnwege und Analgetika-Abusus, *Schweizerische Medizinische Wochenschrift*, **108**, 1013–1019.

Brunner, G., Holloway, C. J. and Lösgen, H., 1979, Large agarose beads for extracorporeal detoxification systems: preparation and enzymatic properties of agarose-bound UDP-glucuronyltransferase, *International Journal of Artificial Organs*, **2**, 163–169.

Bruno, M., Bartolone, J., Cohen, S. and Khairallah, E. A., 1985, Cultured mouse hepatocytes as a valid model for acetaminophen hepatotoxicity, *Pharmacologist*, **27**, 482.

Bruno, M. K., Cohen, S. D. and Khairallah, E. A., 1986, Pertubations in protein metabolism induced by acetaminophen are not the result of GSH depletion, *Federation Proceedings*, **45**, 1932.

Bruno, M. K., Cohen, S. D. and Khairallah, E. A., 1988, Antidotal effectiveness of N-acetylcysteine in reversing acetaminophen-induced hepatotoxicity: enhancement of the proteolysis of arylated proteins, *Biochemical Pharmacology*, **37**, 4319–4325.

Bruno, M. K., Cohen, S. D. and Khairallah, E. A., 1991, Selective alterations in the profiles of newly synthesized proteins by acetaminophen (APAP) and its dimethylated analogues: relationship to oxidative stress, *Advances in Experimental Medicine and Biology*, **283**, 257–260.

Bruno, M. K., Cohen, S. D. and Khairallah, E. A., 1992, Selective alterations in the patterns of newly synthesized proteins by acetaminophen and its dimethylated analogues in primary cultures of mouse hepatocytes, *Toxicology and Applied Pharmacology*, **112**, 282–290.

Bruschi, S. A. and Priestly, B. G., 1990, Implication of alterations in intracellular calcium ion homeostasis in the advent of paracetamol-induced cytotoxicity in primary mouse hepatocyte monolayer cultures, *Toxicology in Vitro*, **4**, 734–749.

Brusquet, Y., Nezri, M. and Bussereau, M., 1982, Contrôle de l'hyperthermie du jeune enfant par le soluté buvable de paracétamol, *Annales de Pédiatrie*, **29**, 429–431.

Brzeznicka, E. A. and Piotrowski, J. K., 1989, Dynamics of glutathione levels in liver and indicatory enzymes in serum in acetaminophen intoxication in mice, *Polish Journal of Occupational Medicine*, **2**, 15–22.

Büch, H., Eschrich, Ch. and Pfleger, K., 1966a, Zur Frage der Induzierbarkeit der Sulfurylierung des N-Acetyl-p-aminophenols (NAPAP), *Archiv für experimentelle Pathologie und Pharmakologie*, **255**, 6–7.

Büch, H., Gerhards, W., Pfleger, K., Rüdiger, W. and Rummel, W., 1967a, Metabolische Umwandlung von Phenacetin und N-Acetyl-p-aminophenol nach Vorbehandlung mit Phenobarbital, *Biochemical Pharmacology*, **16**, 1585–1599.

Büch, H., Häuser, H., Pfleger, K. and Rüdiger, W., 1966b, Bestimmung von Phenacetin und N-acetyl-p-aminophenol über Stoffwechselprodukte im Harn, *Zeitschrift für Klinische Chemie*, **4**, 288–290.

Büch, H., Pfleger, K. and Rummel, W., 1967b, Untersuchungen über den oxydativen Stoffwechsel des Phenacetins bei der Ratte, *Biochemical Pharmacology*, **16**, 2247–2256.

Büch, H., Pfleger, K. and Rüdiger, W., 1967c, Nachweis und Bestimmung von Phenacetin, N-acetyl-p-aminophenol sowie ihren Hauptumwandlungsprodukten in Harn und Serum, *Zeitschrift für Klinische Chemie*, **5**, 110–114.

Büch, H., Rummel, W., Pfleger, K., Eschrich, Ch. and Texter, N., 1968, Ausscheidung Freien und Konjugierten Sulfates bei Ratte und Menschen nach Verabreichung von N-acetyl-p-aminophenol, *Naunyn Schmiedeberg's Archiv für experimentelle Pathologie und Pharmakologie*, **259**, 276–289.

Buchanan, N. and Moodley, G. P., 1979, Interaction between chloramphenicol and paracetamol, *British Medical Journal*, **2**, 307–308.

Buchanan, T., Adriaenssens, P. and Stewart, M. J., 1979, A micromethod for the emergency estimation of plasma paracetamol concentrations using high performance liquid chromatography, *Clinica Chimica Acta*, **99**, 161–165.

Buchanan, W. J., 1991, A year of intentional self poisoning in Christchurch, *New Zealand Medical Journal*, **104**, 470–472.

Buckley, N., Whyte, I. and Dawson, A., 1993, Anticonvulsant use and paracetamol overdose, *Human and Experimental Toxicology*, **12**, 412.

Buckpitt, A. R., Rollins, D. E. and Mitchell, J. R., 1979, Varying effects of sulfhydryl nucleophiles on acetaminophen oxidation and sulfhydryl adduct formation, *Biochemical Pharmacology*, **28**, 2941–2946.

Buckpitt, A. R., Rollins, D. E., Nelson, S. D., Franklin, R. B. and Mitchell, J. R., 1977, Quantitative determination of the glutathione, cysteine, and N-acetyl cysteine conjugates of acetaminophen by high-pressure liquid chromatography, *Analytical Biochemistry*, **83**, 168–177.

Buhl, A. E., Waldon, D. J., Baker, C. A. and Johnson, G. A., 1990, Minoxidil sulfate is the active metabolite that stimulates hair follicles, *Journal of Investigative Dermatology*, **95**, 553–557.

Buhring, S., Hennighausen, G. and Jonas, L., 1991, The effects of paracetamol on the hepatic uptake of microparticles *in vivo* and *in vitro*, *Archives of Toxicology*, **14 (Suppl.)**, 181–184.

Bullingham, R. E. S., McQuay, H. J., Moore, R. A. and Weir, L., 1981, An oral buprenorphine and paracetamol combination compared with paracetamol alone: a single dose double-blind postoperative study, *British Journal of Clinical Pharmacology*, **12**, 863–867.

Buniva, G., Sassela, D. and Beretta, E., 1977, Plasma levels and urinary elimination of diftalone, paracetamol, and their metabolites after single oral administration in man, *International Journal of Clinical Pharmacology*, **15**, 460–467.

Burcham, P. C. and Harman, A. W., 1988, Effect of acetaminophen hepatotoxicity on hepatic mitochondrial and microsomal calcium contents in mice, *Toxicology Letters*, **44**, 91–99.

Burcham, P. C. and Harman, A. W., 1989, Paracetamol-induced stimulation of glycogenolysis in isolated mouse hepatocytes is not directly associated with cell death, *Biochemical Pharmacology*, **38**, 2357–2362.

Burcham, P. C. and Harman, A. W., 1990, Mitochondrial dysfunction in paracetamol hepatotoxicity: *in vitro* studies in isolated mouse hepatocytes, *Toxicology Letters*, **50**, 37–48.

Burcham, P. C. and Harman, A. W., 1991, Acetaminophen toxicity results in site-specific mitochondrial damage in isolated mouse hepatocytes, *Journal of Biological Chemistry*, **266**, 5049–5054.

Burger, D. M., Meenhorst, P. L., Koks, C. H. W. and Beijnen, J. H., 1994a, Pharmacokinetics of zidovudine and acetaminophen in a patient on chronic acetaminophen therapy, *Annals of Pharmacotherapy*, **28**, 327–330.

Burger, D. M., Meenhorst, P. L., Underberg, W. J. M., van der Heijde, J. F., Koks, C. H. W. and Beijnen, J. H., 1994b, Short-term, combined use of paracetamol and zidovudine does not alter the pharmacokinetics of either drug, *Netherlands Journal of Medicine*, **44**, 161–165.

Burgess, H. A., Merrington, D. M., Oliver, W. J., Thomson, A. and Rogers, H. J., 1985, The relative bioavailability of paracetamol after rectal administration of suppositories containing a mixture of paracetamol, codeine phosphate and buclizine hydrochloride in healthy volunteers, *Current Medical Research and Opinion*, **9**, 634–641.

Burgunder, J. M., Varriale, A. and Lauterburg, B. H., 1989, Effect of N-acetylcysteine on plasma cysteine and glutathione following paracetamol administration, *European Journal of Clinical Pharmacology*, **36**, 127–131.

Burk, R. F., Hill, K. E., Hunt, R. W. and Martin, A. E., 1990, Isoniazid potentiation of acetaminophen hepatotoxicity in the rat and 4-methylpyrazole inhibition of it, *Research Communications in Chemical Pathology and Pharmacology*, **69**, 115–118.

Burk, R. F. and Lane, J. M., 1983, Modification of chemical toxicity by selenium deficiency, *Fundamental and Applied Toxicology*, **3**, 218–221.

Burke, D. A., Wedd, D. J., Herriott, D., Bayliss, M. K., Spalding, D. J. M. and Wilcox, P., 1994, Evaluation of pyrazole and ethanol induced S9 fraction in bacterial mutagenicity testing, *Mutagenesis*, **9**, 23–29.

Burkhart, K., Janco, N., Kulig, K. and Rumack, B., 1989, Cimetidine as adjunctive treatment for acetaminophen overdose, *Veterinary and Human Toxicology*, **31**, 337.

Burn, R., 1973, Blood-glucose in paracetamol poisoning, *Lancet*, **i**, 728.

Burns, J. J. and Conney, A. H., 1965, Biochemical studies with phenacetin and related compounds, *Excerpta Medica International Congress Series 97: Proceedings of the European Society for the Study of Drug Toxicity*, **6**, 76–81.

Burrell, J. H. and Yong, J. L. C., 1991, Analgesic nephropathy in Fischer 344 rats: comparative effects of chronic treatment with either aspirin or paracetamol, *Pathology*, **23**, 107–114.

Burrell, J. H., Yong, J. L. C. and Macdonald, G. J., 1990, Experimental analgesic nephropathy: changes in renal structure and urinary concentrating ability in Fischer 344 rats given continuous low doses of aspirin and paracetamol, *Pathology*, **22**, 33–44.

Burrell, J. H., Yong, J. L. C. and Macdonald, G. J., 1991, Irreversible damage to the medullary interstitium in experimental analgesic nephropathy in F344 rats, *Journal of Pathology*, **164**, 329–338.

Burtis, C. A., Butts, W. C. and Rainey, W. T., 1970, Separation of the metabolites of phenacetin in urine by high-resolution anion exchange chromatography, *American Journal of Clinical Pathology*, **53**, 769–777.

Bush, J. P., Holmbeck, G. N. and Cockrell, J. L., 1989, Patterns of PRN analgesic drug administration in children following elective surgery, *Journal of Pediatric Psychology*, **14**, 433–448.

Buskin, J. N., Upton, R. A. and Williams, R. L., 1982, Improved acetaminophen assay sensitivity by modification of a high-performance liquid chromatography technique, *Journal of Chromatography: Biomedical Applications*, **230**, 443–447.

Buttar, H. S., 1976, Impairment in the hepatic clearance of [^{35}S]-bromosulphophthalein in paracetamol-intoxicated rats, *British Journal of Pharmacology*, **56**, 145–153.

Buttar, H. S., Chow, A. Y. K. and Downie, R. H., 1977, Glutathione alterations in rat liver after acute and subacute oral administration of paracetamol, *Clinical and Experimental Pharmacology and Physiology.*, **4**, 1–6.

Buttar, H. S., Nera, E. A. and Downie, R. H., 1976, Serum enzyme activities and hepatic triglyceride levels in acute and subacute acetaminophen-treated rats, *Toxicology*, **6**, 9–20.

Butters, L. and Howie, C. A., 1990, Awareness among pregnant women of the effect on the fetus of commonly used drugs, *Midwifery*, **6**, 146–154.

Butterworth, M., Upshall, D. G., Smith, L. L. and Cohen, G. M., 1992, Cysteine *iso*propylester protects against paracetamol-induced toxicity, *Biochemical Pharmacology*, **43**, 483–488.

Buttery, J. E., Boord, S. and Ludvigsen, N., 1988, Ascorbate interference in the urinary screen for acetaminophen, *Clinical Chemistry*, **34**, 769.

Buttery, J. E., Braiotta, E. A. and Pannall, P. R., 1982a, Correction for salicylate interference in the colorimetric paracetamol assay, *Clinica Chimica Acta*, **122**, 301–304.

Buttery, J. E., Braiotta, E. A. and Pannall, P. R., 1982b, Plasma acetaminophen results are method dependent, *Journal of Toxicology. Clinical Toxicology*, **19**, 1117–1122.

Buylaert, W. A., Calle, P., De Paepe, P., Verstraete, A. and Decruyenaere, J., 1994, Acute intoxicaties met paracetamol bij volwassenen, *Tijdschrift voor Geneeskunde*, **50**, 873–880.

Byer, A. J., Traylor, T. R. and Semmer, J. R., 1982, Acetaminophen overdose in the third trimester of pregnancy, *Journal of the American Medical Association*, **247**, 3114–3115.

Cabezas Cerrato, J., Jiménez de Diego, L. and Fernández-Cruz, A., 1970, Estudio sobre la antidiuresis farmacologica en la diabetes insipida. II. Acetaminophen and tegretol, *Revista Clínica Española*, **119**, 111–118.

Cade, L. and Ashley, J., 1993, Prophylactic paracetamol for analgesia after vaginal termination of pregnancy, *Anaesthesia and Intensive Care*, **21**, 93–96.

Cahn, A. and Hepp, P., 1886, Das Antifebrin, ein neues Fiebermittel, *Zentralblatt für Klinische Medizin*, **vii**, 561–564.

Cahn, A. and Hepp, P., 1887a, Ueber Antifebrin (Acetanilid) und verwandte Körper, *Berliner Klinische Wochenschrift*, **24**, 4–8.

Cahn, A. and Hepp, P., 1887b, Ueber Antifebrin (Acetanilid) und verwandte Körper, *Berliner Klinische Wochenschrift*, **24**, 26–30.

Cairns, F. J., Koelmeyer, T. D. and Smeeton, W. M. I., 1983, Deaths from drugs and poisons, *New Zealand Medical Journal*, **96**, 1045–1048.

Calam, J., Krasner, N. and Haqqani, M., 1982, Extensive gastrointestinal damage following a saline emetic, *Digestive Diseases and Sciences*, **27**, 936–940.

Calatayud, J. M. and Benito, C. G., 1990, Flow-injection spectrofluorimetric determination of paracetamol, *Analytica Chimica Acta*, **231**, 259–264.

Caldarola, V., Hasset, J. M., Hall, A. H., Bronstein, A. B., Kulig, K. W. and Rumack, B. H., 1986, Hemorrhagic pancreatitis associated with acetaminophen overdose, *American Journal of Gastroenterology*, **81**, 579–582.

Calder, I. C., Creek, M. J. and Williams, P. J., 1974, N-Hydroxyphenacetin as a precursor of 3-substituted 4-hydroxyacetanilide metabolites of phenacetin, *Chemico-Biological Interactions*, **8**, 87–90.

Calder, I. C., Funder, C. C., Green, C. R., Ham, K. N. and Tange, J. D., 1971, Comparative nephrotoxicity of aspirin and phenacetin derivatives, *British Medical Journal*, **4**, 518–521.

Calder, I. C., Hart, S. J., Healey, K. and Ham, K. N., 1981a, N-hydroxyacetaminophen: a postulated toxic metabolite of acetaminophen, *Journal of Medicinal Chemistry*, **24**, 988–993.

Calder, I. C., Hart, S. J., Smail, M. C. and Tange, J. D., 1981b, Hepatotoxicity of phenacetin and paracetamol in the Gunn rat, *Pathology*, **13**, 757–762.

Calder, I. C., Williams, P. J., Woods, R. A., Funder, C. C., Green, C. R., Ham, K. N. and Tange, J. D., 1975, Nephrotoxicity and molecular structure, *Xenobiotica*, **5**, 303–307.

Calder, I. C., Yong, A. C., Woods, R. A., Crowe, C. A., Ham, K. N. and Tange, J. D., 1979, The nephrotoxicity of p-aminophenol. II. The effect of metabolic inhibitors and inducers, *Chemico-Biological Interactions*, **21**, 245–254.

Caldwell, J., Davies, S. and Smith, R. L., 1980, Inter-individual differences in the conjugation of paracetamol with glucuronic acid and sulphate, *British Journal of Pharmacology*, **70**, 112P–113P.

Caldwell, J., Smith, R. L. and Davies, S. A., 1978, Drug metabolism in a case of progeria, *Gerontology*, **24**, 373–380.

Calvert, L. J. and Linder, C. W., 1978, Acetaminophen poisoning, *Journal of Family Practice*, **7**, 953–956.

Cameron, J. S., Specht, P. G. and Wendt, G. R., 1967, Effects of placebo and an acetaminophen-salicylamide combination on moods, emotions, and motivations, *Journal of Psychology*, **67**, 257–262.

Campbell, D. and Oates, R. K., 1992, Childhood poisoning: a changing profile with scope for prevention, *Medical Journal of Australia*, **156**, 238–240.

Campbell, N. R. C. and Baylis, B., 1992, Renal impairment associated with an acute paracetamol overdose in the absence of hepatotoxicity, *Postgraduate Medical Journal*, **68**, 116–118.

Campbell, R. S., Hammond, P. M., Scawen, M. D. and Price, C. P., 1983, The measurement of serum paracetamol using a discrete analyser, *Journal of Automatic Chemistry*, **5**, 146–149.

Campbell, R. S. and Price, C. P., 1986, Experience with a homogeneous immunoassay for paracetamol (acetaminophen), *Journal of Clinical Chemistry and Clinical Biochemistry*, **24**, 155–159.

Campbell, W. I., 1990, Analgesic side effects and minor surgery: which analgesic for minor and day-case surgery? *British Journal of Anaesthesia*, **64**, 617–620.

Campos, R., Garrido, A., Guerra, R. and Valenzuela, A., 1988, Acetaminophen hepatotoxicity in rats is attenuated by silybin dihemisuccinate, *Progress in Clinical and Biological Research*, **280**, 375–378.

Campos, R., Garrido, A., Guerra, R. and Valenzuela, A., 1989, Silybin dihemisuccinate protects against glutathione depletion and lipid peroxidation induced by acetaminophen on rat liver, *Planta Medica*, **55**, 417–419.

Campos, S. O., 1984, Estudo duplo-cego comparativo, em dose única de acetaminofen e dipirona no tratamento de doenças febris em crianças, *Folha Medica*, **88**, 133–138.

Canalese, J., Gimson, A. E. S., Davis, M. and Williams, R., 1981a, Factors contributing to mortality in paracetamol-induced hepatic failure, *British Medical Journal*, **282**, 199–201.

Canalese, J., Wyke, R. J., Vergani, D., Eddleston, A. L. W. F. and Williams, R., 1981b, Circulating immune complexes in patients with fulminant hepatic failure, *Gut*, **22**, 845–848.

Cantwell-Simmons, E., Druckro, P. N. and Richardson, W. D., 1993, A review of studies on the relationship of chronic analgesic use and chronic headaches, *Headache Quarterly, Current Treatment and Research*, **4**, 28–35.

Capetola, R. J., Shriver, D. A. and Rosenthale, M. E., 1980, Suprofen, a new peripheral analgesic, *Journal of Pharmacology and Experimental Therapeutics*, **214**, 16–23.

Caraceni, P. and van Thiel, D. H., 1995, Acute liver failure, *Lancet*, **345**, 163–168.

Caradoc-Davies, T. H., 1984, Nonsteroidal anti-inflammatory drugs, arthritis, and gastro-intestinal bleeding in elderly in-patients, *Age and Ageing*, **13**, 295–298.

Cardot, J.-M., Aiache, J.-M., Renoux, R., Aiache, S. and Sibaud, Y., 1985a, Etude de l'influence de l'alimentation sur la biodisponibilité du paracétamol, *Journal de Pharmacie Clinique*, **4**, 145–153.

Cardot, J.-M., Aiache, J.-M., Renoux, R. and Kantelip, J.-P., 1985b, Corrélation entre les taux salivaires et les taux plasmatiques de paracétamol intérêt pour les études de bio-disponibilité, *Sciences Techniques et Pratiques Pharmaceutiques*, **1**, 114–120.

Cardot, J. M., Beyssac, E., Renoux, R., Aiache, J. M., Kantelip, J. P. and Ducroux, P., 1986, Etude de la biodisponibilité du paracétamol au moyen de prélèvements salivaires, *Journal de Pharmacie Clinique*, **5**, 241–256.

Caretti, J. P., 1986, Single-blind study of an anti-inflammatory agent v. paracetamol in acute infections of the oral cavity and upper respiratory tract, *Clinical Trials Journal*, **23**, 372–381.

Carlin, G., Djursäter, R., Smedegård, G. and Gerdin, B., 1985, Effect of anti-inflammatory drugs on xanthine oxidase and xanthine oxidase induced depolymerization of hyaluronic acid, *Agents and Actions*, **16**, 377–384.

Carlo, P. E., Cambosos, N. M., Feeney, G. C. and Smith, P. K., 1955, Plasma levels after the oral administration of acetylsalicylic acid and N-acetyl-p-aminophenol in different forms to human subjects, *Journal of the American Pharmaceutical Association*, **44**, 396–399.

Carloss, H., Forrester, J., Austin, F. and Fuson, T., 1978, Acute acetaminophen intoxication, *Southern Medical Journal*, **71**, 906–908.

Carlson, R. W., Borrison, R. A., Sher, H. B., Eisenberg, P. D., Mowry, P. A. and Wolin, E. M., 1990, A multiinstitutional evaluation of the analgesic efficacy and safety of ketorolac tromethamine, acetaminophen plus codeine, and placebo in cancer pain, *Pharmacotherapy*, **10**, 211–216.

Carlsson, K.-H., Monzel, W. and Jurna, I., 1988, Depression by morphine and the non-opioid analgesic agents, metamizol (dipyrone), lysine acetylsalicylate, and paracetamol, of activity in rat thalamus neurones evoked by electrical stimulation of nociceptive afferents, *Pain*, **32**, 313–326.

Carlsson, K. H. and Jurna, I., 1987, Central analgesic effect of paracetamol manifested by depression of nociceptive activity in thalamic neurones of the rat, *Neuroscience Letters*, **77**, 339–343.

Carlton, W. W. and Engelhardt, J. A., 1989, Experimental renal papillary necrosis in the Syrian hamster, *Food and Chemical Toxicology*, **27**, 331–340.

Carpenter, H. M. and Mudge, G. H., 1981, Acetaminophen nephrotoxicity: studies on renal acetylation and deacetylation, *Journal of Pharmacology and Experimental Therapeutics*, **218**, 161–167.

Carson, D. J. L. and Carson, E. D., 1976, Dextropropoxyphene poisoning, *British Medical Journal*, **2**, 105–106.

Carter, E. A., 1987, Enhanced acetaminophen toxicity associated with prior alcohol consumption in mice: prevention by N-acetylcysteine, *Alcohol*, **4**, 69–71.

Casadevall, G., Morena, J. J., Franch, M. A. and Queralt, J., 1993, N-Acetyl-β-D-glucosaminidase (NAG) and alanine aminopeptidase (AAP) excretion after acute administration of acetaminophen, salsalate and aspirin in rats, *Research Communications in Chemical Pathology and Pharmacology*, **81**, 77–89.

Caslavska, J., Lienhard, S. and Thormann, W., 1993, Comparative use of three electrokinetic capillary methods for the determination of drugs in body fluids: prospects for rapid determination of intoxications, *Journal of Chromatography*, **638**, 335–342.

Cassidy, W. M. and Reynolds, T. B., 1994, Serum lactic dehydrogenase in the differential diagnosis of acute hepatocellular injury, *Journal of Clinical Gastroenterology*, **19**, 118–

121.

Castañeda-Hernández, G., Granados-Soto, V., Flores-Murrieta, F. J. and López-Muñoz, F. J., 1992, Pharmacokinetic/pharmacodynamic analysis of the interaction between acetaminophen and caffeine, *Proceedings of the Western Pharmacology Society*, **35**, 5–9.

Casterlin, M. E. and Reynolds, W. W., 1980, Fever and antipyresis in the crayfish *Cambarus bartoni*, *Journal of Physiology*, **303**, 417–421.

Cavallo-Perin, P., Aimo, G., Mazzillo, A., Riccardini, F. and Pagano, G., 1991, Gastric emptying of liquids and solids evaluated by acetaminophen test in diabetic patients with and without autonomic neuropathy, *Rivista Europea Per Le Scienze Mediche e Farmacologiche*, **13**, 205–209.

Cayanis, E., Gomperts, E. D., Balinsky, D., Disler, P. and Myers, A., 1975, G6PD Hillbrow: a new variant of glucose-6-phosphate dehydrogenase associated with drug-induced haemolytic anaemia, *British Journal of Haematology*, **30**, 343–349.

Cedrato, A. E., Passarelli, I., Cimollini, L. and Maccarone, H., 1989, Comparación del efecto antipiretico de una dosis de dipiroma, paracetamol y diclofenac resinato. ensayo clinico multicéntrico, *Medicina (Argentina)*, **49**, 635–636.

Cerretani, D., Micheli, L., Fiaschi, A. I., Romeo, M. R., Taddei, I. and Giorgi, G., 1994, MK-801 potentiates the glutathione depletion induced by acetaminophen in rat brain, *Current Therapeutic Research*, **55**, 707–717.

Chafee, F. H. and Settipane, G. A., 1967, Asthma caused by FD & C approved dyes, *Journal of Allergy*, **40**, 65–72.

Chafetz, L., Daly, R. E., Schriftman, H. and Lomner, J. J., 1971, Selective colorimetric determination of acetaminophen, *Journal of Pharmaceutical Sciences*, **60**, 463–466.

Chakrabarti, A. K. and Lloyd, G. H. T., 1973, Gross paracetamol overdosage with recovery, *Practitioner*, **210**, 408–411.

Chakrabarty, A. K., 1979, Interference by antibiotics in plasma paracetamol determination, *Annals of Clinical Biochemistry*, **16**, 217.

Chaleby, K., el-Yazigi, A. and Atiyeh, M., 1987, Decreased drug absorption in a patient with Behçet's syndrome, *Clinical Chemistry*, **33**, 1679–1681.

Chalmers, J. P., West, M. J., Wing, L. M. H., Bune, A. J. C. and Graham, J. R., 1984, Effects of indomethacin, sulindac, naproxen, aspirin, and paracetamol in treated hypertensive patients, *Clinical and Experimental Hypertension – Part A, Theory and Practice*, **6**, 1077–1093.

Chamberlain, J. M., Gorman, R. L., Oderda, G. M., Klein-Schwartz, W. and Klein, B. L., 1993, Use of activated charcoal in a simulated poisoning with acetaminophen: a new loading dose for N-acetylcysteine? *Annals of Emergency Medicine*, **22**, 1398–1402.

Chambers, R. E. and Jones, K., 1976, Comparison of a gas chromatographic and colorimetric method for the determination of plasma paracetamol, *Annals of Clinical Biochemistry*, **13**, 433–434.

Chan, J. C., Lai, F. M. and Critchley, J. A. J. H., 1991, A case of Stevens-Johnson syndrome, cholestatic hepatitis and haemolytic anaemia associated with use of mefenamic acid, *Drug Safety*, **6**, 230–234.

Chan, K. and McCann, J. F., 1979, Improved gas-liquid chromatography-electron capture detection technique for the determination of paracetamol in human plasma and urine, *Journal of Chromatography: Biomedical Applications*, **164**, 394–398.

Chan, T. Y. K., Chan, A. Y. W. and Critchley, J. A. J. H., 1993, Paracetamol poisoning and hepatotoxicity in Chinese – the Prince of Wales Hospital (Hong Kong) experience, *Singapore Medical Journal*, **34**, 299–302.

Chan, T. Y. K. and Critchley, J. A. J. H., 1994, Adverse reactions to intravenous N-acetylcysteine in Chinese patients with paracetamol (acetaminophen) poisoning, *Human and Experimental Toxicology*, **13**, 542–544.

Chan, T. Y. K., Critchley, J. A. J. H., Chan, J. C. N. and Tomlinson, B., 1994a, Metabolic activation and paracetamol hepatotoxicity: an update on the management of paracetamol (acetaminophen) poisoning, *Journal of the Hong Kong Medical Association*, **46**, 87–92.

Chan, T. Y. K., Critchley, J. A. J. H., Chan, J. C. N., Tomlinson, B., Lau, M. S. W., Anderson, P. J., Lau, G. S. N. and So, K. W. H., 1994b, Childhood poisoning in Hong Kong: experience of the Drug and Poisons Information Bureau from 1988 to 1992, *Journal of Paediatrics and Child Health*, **30**, 453–454.

Chan, T. Y. K., Critchley, J. A. J. H., Chan, M. T. V. and Yu, C. M., 1994c, Drug overdosage and other poisoning in Hong Kong: the Prince of Wales Hospital (Shatin) experience, *Human and Experimental Toxicology*, **13**, 512–515.

Chanda, S., Mangipudy, R. S., Warbritton, A., Bucci, T. J. and Mehendale, H. M., 1995, Stimulated hepatic tissue repair underlies heteroprotection by thioacetamide against acetaminophen-induced lethality, *Hepatology*, **21**, 477–486.

Chang, D. M., Baptiste, P. and Schur, P. H., 1990, The effect of antirheumatic drugs on interleukin 1 (IL-1) activity and IL-1 and IL-1 inhibitor production by human monocytes, *Journal of Rheumatology*, **17**, 1148–1157.

Chang, M. J. W., Kao, G. I. and Tsai, C. T., 1993, Biological monitoring of exposure to low dose aniline, *P*-aminophenol, and acetaminophen, *Bulletin of Environmental Contamination and Toxicology*, **51**, 494–500.

Channer, K. S. and Roberts, C. J. C., 1985, Effect of delayed esophageal transit on acetaminophen absorption, *Clinical Pharmacology and Therapeutics*, **37**, 72–76.

Chao, E. S., Dunbar, D. and Kaminsky, L. S., 1988, Intracellular lactate dehydrogenase concentration as an index of cytotoxicity in rat hepatocyte primary culture, *Cell Biology and Toxicology*, **4**, 1–11.

Chao, T. C., 1993, Adverse drug reactions: tales of a forensic pathologist, *Annals of the Academy of Medicine, Singapore*, **22**, 86–89.

Char, V. C., Chandra, R., Fletcher, A. B. and Avery, G. B., 1975, Polyhydramnios and neonatal renal failure – a possible association with maternal acetaminophen ingestion, *Journal of Pediatrics*, **86**, 638–639.

Chattopadhyay, R. R., Sarkar, S. K., Ganguly, S., Banerjee, R. N., Basu, T. K. and Mukherjee, A., 1992, Hepatoprotective activity of *Azadirachta indica* leaves on paracetamol induced hepatic damage in rats, *Indian Journal of Experimental Biology*, **30**, 738–740.

Chaturvedi, A. K., Rao, N. G. S. and Hurly, M. P., 1983, Toxicological findings in a multidrug death involving propoxyphene, caffeine, phenacetin, acetaminophen and salicylate, *Forensic Science International*, **23**, 255–264.

Chaudhary, I. P., Tuntaterdtum, S., McNamara, P. J., Robertson, L. W. and Blouin, R. A., 1993, Effect of genetic obesity and phenobarbital treatment on the hepatic conjugation pathways, *Journal of Pharmacology and Experimental Therapeutics*, **265**, 1333–1338.

Chen, J.-T., Hirai, Y., Yagi, H., Katase, K., Shimizu, Y., Nakayama, K., Teshima, H., Hamada, T., Fujimoto, I., Yamauchi, K., Hasumi, K. and Masubuchi, K., 1988, Effect of medical vagotomy on the CDDP induced nausea and vomiting evaluated by the chemotherapy-vomiting time (CV time), *Acta Obstetrica et Gynaecologica Japonica*, **40**, 1359–1364.

Chen, M.-M., Lee, C., Imamura, Y. and Perrin, J. H., 1983, Acetaminophen-aluminum hydroxide interaction in rabbits, *Journal of Pharmaceutical Sciences*, **72**, 828–830.

Chen, M. M. and Lee, C. S., 1985, Cimetidine-acetaminophen interaction in humans, *Journal of Clinical Pharmacology*, **25**, 227–229.

Chen, R. and Gillette, J. R., 1988, Pharmacokinetic procedures for the estimation of organ clearances for the formation of short-lived metabolites, *Drug Metabolism and Disposition: The Biological Fate of Chemicals*, **16**, 373–385.

Chen, T. S., Richie, J. P. J. and Lang, C. A., 1990, Life span profiles of glutathione and acetaminophen detoxification, *Drug Metabolism and Disposition: The Biological Fate of Chemicals*, **18**, 882–887.

Cheney-Thamm, J., Alianello, E. A., Freed, C. R. and Reite, M., 1987, *In vivo* electrochemical recording of acetaminophen in non human primate brain, *Life Sciences*, **40**, 375–379.

Cheng, L., 1992a, Acetaminophen-induced hepatotoxicity in an alcoholic, *Pharmacology and Therapeutics*, **17**, 1635.

Cheng, T., Li, T., Duan, Z., Cao, Z., Ma, Z. and Zhang, P., 1990, Acute toxicity of flesh oil of *Hippophae rhamnoides L.* and its protection against experimental hepatic injury, *Chung-Kuo Chung Yao Tsa Chih*, **15**, 45–7, 64.

Cheng, T.-J., 1992b, Protective action of seed oil of *Hippophae rhamnoides L.* (HR) against experimental liver injury in mice, *Chung-Hua Yu Fang i Hsueh Tsa Chih*, **26**, 227–229.

Chengelis, C. P., Dodd, D. C., Means, J. R. and Kotsonis, F. N., 1986, Protection by zinc against acetaminophen induced hepatotoxicity in mice, *Fundamental and Applied Toxicology*, **6**, 278–284.

Chern, I., Brent, J., Slattery, J., Ritvo, J., Kalhorn, T., Gomez, H., Downing, J., Benson, R. and Roberts, D., 1993, Is it safe to give acetaminophen to alcoholics? A metabolic study, *Veterinary and Human Toxicology*, **35**, 365.

Chesham, J. and Davies, G. E., 1985, The role of metabolism in the immunogenicity of drugs: production of antibodies to a horseradish peroxidase generated conjugate paracetamol, *Clinical and Experimental Immunology*, **61**, 224–231.

Chételat, A., Albertini, S. and Gocke, E., 1992, Alleged *in vivo* genotoxicity of paracetamol and green S, *Mutation Research: Genetic Toxicology Testing*, **298**, 139–140.

Cheung, L., Potts, R. G. and Meyer, K. C., 1994, Acetaminophen treatment nomogram, *New England Journal of Medicine*, **330**, 1907–1908.

Chichmanian, R. M., Taillan, B., Fuzibet, J. G., Vinti, H. and Dujardin, P., 1989, Agranulocytose due au paracétamol: un cas, avec réadministration positive, *Annales de Medécine Interne*, **140**, 332–333.

Childs, C. and Little, R. A., 1988, Acetaminophen (paracetamol) in the management of burned children with fever, *Burns*, **14**, 343–348.

Chinouth, R. W., Czajka, P. A. and Peterson, R. G., 1980, N-acetylcysteine adsorption by activated charcoal, *Veterinary and Human Toxicology*, **22**, 392–394.

Chiossi, M., Ferrea, G., Lattere, M., Di Pietro, P., Capurro, M. and Tarateta, A., 1991, Tossicità da paracetamolo a dosi terapeutiche come possibile spiegazione di insufficienza epatica acuta. Descrizione di un caso, *Rivista Italiana di Pediatria*, **17**, 245–246.

Chiou, W. L., 1975, Estimation of hepatic first-pass effect of acetaminophen in humans after oral administration, *Journal of Pharmaceutical Sciences*, **64**, 1734–1735.

Chipkin, R. E., Latranyi, M. B., Iorio, L. C. and Barnett, A., 1983, Determination of analgesic drug efficacies by modification of the Randall and Selitto rat yeast paw test, *Journal of Pharmacological Methods*, **10**, 223–229.

Chiu, S. and Bhakthan, N. M. G., 1978, Experimental acetaminophen-induced hepatic necrosis: biochemical and electron microscopic study of cysteamine protection, *Laboratory Investigation*, **39**, 193–203.

Cho, C., Raheja, K. L. and Linscheer, W. G., 1980, Prevention of acetaminophen (AAP) hepatotoxicity by propylthiouracil (PTU) in rats, *Laboratory Investigation*, **42**, 106.

Cho, C. H. and Ogle, C. W., 1990, Paracetamol potentiates stress-induced gastric ulceration in rats, *Journal of Pharmacy and Pharmacology*, **42**, 505–507.

Choffray, D. U., Crielaard, J. M., Albert, A. and Franchimont, P., 1987, Comparative study of high bio-availability glaphenine and paracetamol in cervical and lumbar arthrosis, *Clinical Rheumatology*, **6**, 518–525.

Choonara, I. A., 1987, Interaction between chloramphenicol and acetaminophen, *Archives of Disease in Childhood*, **62**, 319.

Chow, P., Tierney, M. G. and Dickinson, G. E., 1992, Acute intoxications. Cases presenting to an adult emergency department, *Canadian Family Physician*, **38**, 1379–1382.

Chow, W.-H., McLaughlin, J. K., Linet, M. S., Niwa, S. and Mandel, J. S., 1994, Use of analgesics and risk of renal cell cancer, *International Journal of Cancer*, **59**, 467–470.

Chrischilles, E. A., Lemke, J. H., Wallace, R. B. and Drube, G. A., 1990, Prevalence and characteristics of multiple analgesic drug use in an elderly study group, *Journal of the American Geriatrics Society*, **38**, 979–984.

Christensen, E., Bremmelgaard, A., Bahnsen, M., Andreasen, P. B. and Tygstrup, N., 1984, Prediction of fatality in fulminant hepatic failure, *Scandinavian Journal of Gastroenterology*, **19**, 90–96.

Christie, I., Leeds, S., Baker, M., Keedy, F. and Vadgama, P., 1993, Direct electrochemical determination of paracetamol in plasma, *Analytica Chimica Acta*, **272**, 145–150.

Chung, S. J., 1989, Computer-assisted predictive mathematical relationship among plasma acetaminophen concentration and time and hepatotoxicity in man, *Computer Methods and Programs in Biomedicine*, **28**, 37–43.

Claass, A., Gaude, M. and Schröder, H., 1993, Paracetamolvergiftung im Säuglingsalter, *Deutsche Medizinische Wochenschrift*, **118**, 898–902.

Clark, J. H., Russell, G. J. and Fitzgerald, J. F., 1983, Fatal acetaminophen toxicity in a 2-year-old, *Journal of the Indiana State Medical Association*, **76**, 832–835.

Clark, J. M. and Seager, S. J., 1983, Gastric emptying following premedication with glycopyrrolate or atropine, *British Journal of Anaesthesia*, **55**, 1195–1199.

Clark, P. M. S., Clark, J. D. A. and Wheatley, T., 1986, Urine discoloration after acetaminophen overdose, *Clinical Chemistry*, **32**, 1777–1778.

Clark, R., Borirakchanyavat, V., Gazzard, B. G., Rake, M. O., Shilkin, K. B., Flute, P. T. and Williams, R., 1973a, Disordered hemostasis in liver damage from paracetamol overdose, *Gastroenterology*, **65**, 788–795.

Clark, R., Thompson, R. P. H., Borirakchanyavat, V., Widdop, B., Davidson, A. R., Goulding, R. and Williams, R., 1973b, Hepatic damage and death from overdose of paracetamol, *Lancet*, **i**, 66–70.

Clark, R. A., Holdsworth, C. D., Rees, M. R. and Howlett, P. J., 1980, The effect on paracetamol absorption of stimulation and blockade of β-adrenoceptors, *British Journal of Clinical Pharmacology*, **10**, 555–559.

Clark, R. F. and Harchelroad, F., 1991, Toxicology screening of the trauma patient: a changing profile, *Annals of Emergency Medicine*, **20**, 151–153.

Clark, W. G., 1970, The antipyretic effects of acetaminophen and sodium salicylate on endotoxin-induced fever in cats, *Journal of Pharmacology and Experimental Therapeutics*, **175**, 469–475.

Clark, W. G. and Alderdice, M. T., 1972, Inhibition of leukocytic pyrogen-induced fever by intracerebroventricular administration of salicylate and acetaminophen in the cat, *Proceedings of the Society for Experimental Biology and Medicine*, **140**, 399–403.

Clark, W. G. and Coldwell, B. A., 1972, Competitive antagonism of leukocytic pyrogen by sodium salicylate and acetaminophen, *Proceedings of the Society for Experimental Biology and Medicine*, **141**, 669–672.

Clark, W. G., Holdeman, M. and Lipton, J. M., 1985, Analysis of the antipyretic action of α-melanocyte-stimulating hormone in rabbits, *Journal of Physiology*, **359**, 459–465.

Clark, W. G. and Moyer, S. G., 1972, The effects of acetaminophen and sodium salicylate on the release and activity of leucocyte pyrogen in the cat, *Journal of Pharmacology and Experimental Therapeutics*, **181**, 183–191.

Clavelou, P., Pajot, J., Dallel, R. and Raboisson, P., 1989, Application of the formalin test to the study of orofacial pain in the rat, *Neuroscience Letters*, **103**, 349–353.

Clements, J. A., Critchley, J. A. J. H. and Prescott, L. F., 1984, The role of sulphate conjugation in the metabolism and disposition of oral and intravenous paracetamol in man, *British Journal of Clinical Pharmacology*, **18**, 481–485.

Clements, J. A., Nimmo, W. S., Heading, R. C. and Prescott, L. F., 1978, Kinetics of acetaminophen absorption and gastric emptying in man, *Clinical Pharmacology and Therapeutics*, **24**, 420–431.

Clements, J. A. and Prescott, L. F., 1976, Data point weighting in pharmacokinetic analysis: intravenous paracetamol in man, *Journal of Pharmacy and Pharmacology*, **28**, 707–709.

Clothier, R. H., Balls, M., Hosty, G. S., Robertson, N. J. and Horner, S. A., 1982, Amphibian organ culture in experimental toxicology: the effects of paracetamol and phenacetin on cultured tissues from urodele and anuran amphibians, *Toxicology*, **25**, 31–40.

Clothier, R. H., Dewar, J. R., Santos, M. A., North, A. D., Foster, S. and Balls, M., 1981, A comparative study of the deacetylation of paracetamol by urodele and anuran amphibian organ cultures, *Xenobiotica*, **11**, 149–157.

Clyburn, P. A. and Rosen, M., 1989, Oral controlled-release morphine and gut function: a study in volunteers, *European Journal of Anaesthesiology*, **6**, 347–353.

Coakley, F., Hayes, C., Fennell, J. and Johnson, Z., 1994, A study of deliberate self-poisoning in a Dublin hospital 1986–1990, *Irish Journal of Psychological Medicine*, **11**, 70–72.

Cobden, I., Record, C. O., Ward, M. K. and Kerr, D. N. S., 1982, Paracetamol-induced acute renal failure in the absence of fulminant liver damage, *British Medical Journal*, **284**, 21–22.

Cocchetto, D. M. and Levy, G., 1981, Absorption of orally administered sodium sulfate in humans, *Journal of Pharmaceutical Sciences*, **70**, 331–333.

Cociglio, M. and Alric, R., 1988, Statistical validation of a liquid chromatographic assay of theophylline, caffeine and acetaminophen in plasma, *Journal de Pharmacie Clinique*, **7**, 305–312.

Coggon, D., Langman, M. J. S. and Spiegelhalter, D., 1982, Aspirin, paracetamol, and haematemesis and melaena, *Gut*, **23**, 340–344.

Cohen, G. M., Bakke, O. M. and Davies, D. S., 1974, 'First-pass' metabolism of paracetamol in rat liver, *Journal of Pharmacy and Pharmacology*, **26**, 348–351.

Cohen, H. A., Nussinovitch, M. and Frydman, M., 1992, Fixed drug eruption caused by acetaminophen, *Annals of Pharmacotherapy*, **26**, 1596–1597.

Cohen, S. B. and Burk, R. F., 1978, Acetaminophen overdoses at a county hospital: a year's experience, *Southern Medical Journal*, **71**, 1359–1365.

Coirault, C., Berton, C., Tritsch, L. and Richard, C., 1993, Intoxication aiguë par le paracétamol: l'administration précoce de N-acétylcystéine réduit les risques d'hépatotoxicité, *Revue du Praticien – Médecine Générale*, **7**, 35–38.

Coldwell, B. B., Thomas, B. H., Whitehouse, L. W., Wong, L. T. and Hynie, I., 1976, Metabolism of ^{14}C-acetaminophen in humans and laboratory animals, *Excerpta Medica International Congress Series 376: Proceedings of the European Society of Toxicology*, **17**, 269–276.

Cole, F. O. A., 1985, Urticaria from paracetamol, *Clinical and Experimental Dermatology*, **10**, 404.

Coles, B., Wilson, I., Wardman, P., Hinson, J. A., Nelson, S. D. and Ketterer, B., 1988, The spontaneous and enzymic reaction of N-acetyl-p-benzoquinone imine with glutathione: a stopped-flow kinetic study, *Archives of Biochemistry and Biophysics*, **264**, 253–260.

Colgan, M. T. and Mintz, A. A., 1957, The comparative antipyretic effect N-acetyl-p-aminophenol and acetylsalicylic acid, *Journal of Pediatrics*, **50**, 552–555.

Colin, P., Sirois, G. and Chakrabarti, S., 1986a, Effects of route of administration on the dose-dependent metabolism of acetaminophen in rats: relationship with its toxicity, *Archives Internationales de Pharmacodynamie et de Thérapie*, **281**, 181–191.

Colin, P., Sirois, G. and Chakrabarti, S., 1986b, Simultaneous determination of the major metabolites of styrene and acetaminophen, and of unchanged acetaminophen in urine by ion-pairing high-performance liquid chromatography, *Journal of Chromatography*, **377**, 243–251.

Colin, P., Sirois, G. and Chakrabarti, S., 1987, Rapid high-performance liquid chromatographic assay of acetaminophen in serum and tissue homogenates, *Journal of Chromatography: Biomedical Applications*, **413**, 151–160.

Collet, J.-P., 1992, Paracetamol or acetylsalicylic acid in young children? *European Journal of Clinical Pharmacology*, **43**, 327.

Collet, J. P., Bossard, N., Floret, D., Gillet, J., Honegger, D., Boissel, J. P. and the Epicrèche research group, 1991, Drug prescription in young children: results of a survey in France, *European Journal of Clinical Pharmacology*, **41**, 489–491.

Collins, E., 1981, Maternal and fetal effects of acetaminophen and salicylate in pregnancy, *Obstetrics and Gynecology*, **58**, 57S–62S.

Collins, S., 1993, Health prevention messages may have paradoxical effect, *British Medical Journal*, **306**, 926.

Colomes, M., Rispail, Y., Berlan, M., Pous, J. and Montastruc, J. L., 1990, Consommation médicamenteuse d'une population de retraités, *Thérapie*, **45**, 321–324.

Columb, M. O., Shah, M. V., Sproat, L. J., Sherratt, M. J. and Inglis, T. J., 1992, Assessment of gastric dysfunction: current techniques for the measurement of gastric emptying, *British Journal of Intensive Care*, **2**, 75–80.

Commandre, F., Pierre, M. and Kermarec, J., 1976, Tentative d'autolyse médicamenteuse: épreuve spontanée de toxicité aiguë, *Lyon Méditerranée Médical*, **12**, 2341–2344.

Concheiro, A., Vila Jato, J. L. and Llabrés, M., 1984, Application du Manova des moments statistiques dans une étude de la biodisponibilité de trois formulations de paracétamol, *Pharmaceutica Acta Helvetiae*, **59**, 109–111.

Concheiro, A., Vila, J. L. and Llabrés, M., 1982, Método densitométrico para la determinación de paracetamol en la orina, *Ciencia e Industria Farmaceutica*, **1**, 38–41.

Conney, A. H., Sansur, M., Soroko, F., Koster, R. and Burns, J. J., 1966, Enzyme induction and inhibition in studies on the pharmacological actions of acetophenetidin, *Journal of Pharmacology and Experimental Therapeutics*, **151**, 133–137.

Conti, M., Malandrino, S. and Magistretti, M. J., 1992, Protective activity of silipide on liver damage in rodents, *Japanese Journal of Pharmacology*, **60**, 315–321.

Coon, M. J. and Koop, D. R., 1987, Alcohol-inducible cytochrome P-450 (P-450$_{ALC}$), *Archives of Toxicology*, **60**, 16–21.

Coon, M. J., Koop, D. R., Reeve, L. E. and Crump, B. L., 1984, Alcohol metabolism and toxicity: role of cytochrome P-450, *Fundamental and Applied Toxicology*, **4**, 134–143.

Cooper, M. B., Forte, C. A., Hughes, R. D. and Williams, R., 1991, Elevated plasma carnitine content in acute (paracetamol-induced) liver damage in humans, *Medical Science Research*, **19**, 287–288.

Cooper, S. A. and Beaver, W. T., 1976, A model to evaluate mild analgesics in oral surgery outpatients, *Clinical Pharmacology and Therapeutics*, **20**, 241–250.

Cooper, S. A., Erlichman, M. C. and Mardirossian, G., 1986, Double-blind comparison of an acetaminophen-codeine-caffeine combination in oral surgery pain, *Anesthesia Progress*, **33**, 139–142.

Cooper, S. A., Firestein, A. and Cohn, P., 1988, Double-blind comparison of meclofenamate sodium with acetaminophen, acetaminophen with codeine and placebo for relief of post-surgical dental pain, *Journal of Clinical Dentistry*, **1**, 31–34.

Cooper, S. A. and Kupperman, A., 1991, The analgesic efficacy of flurbiprofen compared to acetaminophen with codeine, *Journal of Clinical Dentistry*, **2**, 70–74.

Cooper, S. A., Precheur, H., Rauch, D., Rosenheck, A., Ladov, M. and Engel, J., 1980, Evaluation of oxycodone and acetaminophen in treatment of postoperative dental pain, *Oral Surgery, Oral Medicine, Oral Pathology*, **50**, 496–501.

Cooper, S. A., Schachtel, B. P., Goldman, E., Gelb, S. and Cohn, P., 1989, Ibuprofen and acetaminophen in the relief of acute pain: a randomised double-blind, placebo-controlled study, *Journal of Clinical Pharmacology*, **29**, 1026–1030.

Copland, A. M., Mather, J., Ness, A. and Fulton, J. D., 1992, Apparent hyperglycaemia in paracetamol overdose, *British Journal of General Practice*, **42**, 259–260.

Corbett, M. D., Corbett, B. R., Hannothiaux, M.-H. and Quintana, S. J., 1989, Metabolic activation and nucleic acid binding of acetaminophen and related arylamine substrates by the respiratory burst of human granulocytes, *Chemical Research in Toxicology*, **2**, 260–266.

Corbett, M. D., Corbett, B. R., Hannothiaux, M.-H. and Quintana, S. J., 1992, The covalent binding of acetaminophen to cellular nucleic acids as the result of the respiratory burst of neutrophils derived from the HL-60 cell line, *Toxicology and Applied Pharmacology*, **113**, 80–86.

Corcoran, G. B., Bauer, J. A. and Lau, T.-W. D., 1988, Immediate rise in intracellular calcium and glycogen phosphorylase *a* activities upon acetaminophen covalent binding leading to hepatotoxicity in mice, *Toxicology*, **50**, 157–167.

Corcoran, G. B., Chung, S.-J. and Salazar, D. E., 1987a, Early inhibition of the Na^+/K^+-ATPase ion pump during acetaminophen-induced hepatotoxicity in rat, *Biochemical and Biophysical Research Communications*, **149**, 203–207.

Corcoran, G. B. and Mitchell, J. R., 1981, Evidence for redox cycling of acetaminophen and its reactive metabolite by endogenous microsomal systems, *Advances in Experimental Medicine and Biology*, **136**, 1085–1098.

Corcoran, G. B., Mitchell, J. R., Vaishnav, Y. N. and Horning, E. C., 1980, Evidence that acetaminophen and N-hydroxyacetaminophen form a common arylating intermediate, N-acetyl-p-benzoquinoneimine, *Molecular Pharmacology*, **18**, 536–542.

Corcoran, G. B., Racz, W. J., Smith, C. V. and Mitchell, J. R., 1985a, Effects of N-acetylcysteine on acetaminophen covalent binding and hepatic necrosis in mice, *Journal of Pharmacology and Experimental Therapeutics*, **232**, 864–872.

Corcoran, G. B., Todd, E. L., Racz, W. J., Hughes, H., Smith, C. V. and Mitchell, J. R., 1985b, Effects of N-acetylcysteine on the disposition and metabolism of acetaminophen in mice, *Journal of Pharmacology and Experimental Therapeutics*, **232**, 857–863.

Corcoran, G. B. and Wong, B. K., 1986, Role of glutathione in prevention of acetaminophen-induced hepatotoxicity by N-acetyl-L-cysteine *in vivo*: studies with N-acetyl-D-cysteine in mice, *Journal of Pharmacology and Experimental Therapeutics*, **238**, 54–61.

Corcoran, G. B. and Wong, B. K., 1987, Obesity as a risk factor in drug-induced organ injury: increased liver and kidney damage by acetaminophen in the obese overfed rat, *Journal of Pharmacology and Experimental Therapeutics*, **241**, 921–927.

Corcoran, G. B., Wong, B. K. and Neese, B. L., 1987b, Early sustained rise in total liver calcium during acetaminophen hepatotoxicity in mice, *Research Communications in Chemical Pathology and Pharmacology*, **58**, 291–305.

Corcoran, G. B., Wong, B. K., Shum, L. and Galinsky, R. E., 1987c, Acetaminophen sulfation deficit in obese rats overfed an energy-dense cafeteria diet, *Endocrine Research*, **13**, 101–121.

Corinaldesi, R., Fabbri, R., Casadio, R., Venturoli, L., Foresti, A. and Barbara, L., 1978, Studio comparativo dell'effetto del paracetamolo e dell'acido acetilsalicilico sulla esfoliazione gastrica, *Il Farmaco*, **33**, 131–135.

Cornely, D. A. and Ritter, J. A., 1956, N-acetyl-p-aminophenol (Tylenol elixir) as a pediatric antipyretic-analgesic, *Journal of the American Medical Association*, **160**, 1219–1221.

Costa, L. G. and Murphy, S. D., 1984, Interaction between acetaminophen and organophosphates in mice, *Research Communications in Chemical Pathology and Pharmacology*, **44**, 389–400.

Cottafava, F., Nieri, S., Franzone, G., Sanguinetti, M., Bertolazzi, L. and Ravera, G., 1990, Confronto in doppio cieco controllato tra placebo e paracetamolo in soggetti carenti di G-6-PD, *Pediatria Medica e Chirurgica*, **12**, 631–637.

Cotty, V. F., Sterbenz, F. J., Mueller, F., Melman, K., Ederma, H., Skerpac, J., Hunter, D. and Lehr, M., 1977, Augmentation of human blood acetylsalicylate concentrations by the simultaneous administration of acetaminophen with aspirin, *Toxicology and Applied Pharmacology*, **41**, 7–13.

Coughtrie, M. W. H. and Sharp, S., 1990, Purification and immunochemical characterization of a rat liver sulphotransferase conjugating paracetamol, *Biochemical Pharmacology*, **40**, 2305–2313.

Coughtrie, M. W. H., Sharp, S., Tan, T. M. C., Bamforth, K. J. and Wong, K. P., 1990, Liver-specific expression of paracetamol sulphotransferase, *Biochemical Society Trans-*

actions, **18**, 1209.

Coursin, D. B. and Kurtz, C. H., 1957, Acetaminophen: a new antipyretic-analgesic for pediatric use, *American Practitioner and Digest of Treatment*, **8**, 1415–1417.

Cove-Smith, J. R. and Knapp, M. S., 1978, Analgesic nephropathy: an important cause of chronic renal failure, *Quarterly Journal of Medicine*, **47**, 46–49.

Coward, R. A., 1977, Paracetamol-induced acute pancreatitis, *British Medical Journal*, **1**, 1086.

Cowell, D. C. and Ford, P. A. E., 1987, Interference in an electrochemical detection system for peroxidase-linked reactions based on a fluoride ion-selective electrode, *Clinical Chemistry*, **33**, 1458–1460.

Cox, D. E. and Pounder, D. J., 1992, Evaluating suspected co-proxamol overdose, *Forensic Science International*, **57**, 147–156.

Coxon, R. E., Gallacher, G., Landon, J. and Rae, C., 1988, Development of a specific polarization fluoroimmunoassay for paracetamol in serum, *Annals of Clinical Biochemistry*, **25**, 49–52.

Craig, R. M., 1980, How safe is acetaminophen? *Journal of the American Medical Association*, **244**, 272.

Crankshaw, D. L. and Hines, N. D., 1992, Hepatic microsomes from beer fed rats contain a cytochrome P-450 metabolic intermediate complex, *Biochemical and Biophysical Research Communications*, **189**, 899–905.

Cranston, W. I., Hellon, R. F. and Mitchell, D., 1975, Is brain prostaglandin synthesis involved in responses to cold? *Journal of Physiology*, **249**, 425–434.

Crawford, I. L., Kennedy, J. I., Lipton, J. M. and Ojeda, S. R., 1979, Effects of central administration of probenecid on fevers produced by leukocytic pyrogen and PGE_2 in the rabbit, *Journal of Physiology*, **287**, 519–533.

Creer, M. H., Lau, B. W. C., Jones, J. D. and Chan, K.-M., 1989, Pyroglutamic acidemia in an adult patient, *Clinical Chemistry*, **35**, 684–686.

Cretton, E. M. and Sommadossi, J.-P., 1991, Modulation of 3′-azido-3′-deoxythymidine catabolism by probenecid and acetaminophen in freshly isolated rat hepatocytes, *Biochemical Pharmacology*, **42**, 1475–1480.

Crippin, J. S., 1993, Acetaminophen hepatotoxicity: potentiation by isoniazid, *American Journal of Gastroenterology*, **88**, 590–592.

Critchley, J. A. J. H., Cregeen, R. J., Balali-Mood, M., Pentland, B. and Prescott, L. F., 1982, Paracetamol metabolism in heavy drinkers, *British Journal of Clinical Pharmacology*, **13**, 276P–277P.

Critchley, J. A. J. H., Dyson, E. H., Scott, A. W., Jarvie, D. R. and Prescott, L. F., 1983, Is there a place for cimetidine or ethanol in the treatment of paracetamol poisoning? *Lancet*, **i**, 1375–1376.

Critchley, J. A. J. H., Nimmo, G. R., Gregson, C. A., Woolhouse, N. M. and Prescott, L. F., 1986, Inter-subject and ethnic differences in paracetamol metabolism, *British Journal of Clinical Pharmacology*, **22**, 649–657.

Critchley, J. A. J. H., Smith, M. F. and Prescott, L. F., 1985, Distalgesic abuse and retroperitoneal fibrosis, *British Journal of Urology*, **57**, 486–487.

Crombie, D. L., Pinsent, R. J. F. H., Slater, B. C., Fleming, D. and Cross, K. W., 1970, Teratogenic drugs – R. C. G. P. survey, *British Medical Journal*, **4**, 178–179.

Crome, P., 1993, The toxicity of drugs used for suicide, *Acta Psychiatrica et Neurologica Scandinavica*, **87 (Suppl. 371)**, 33–37.

Crome, P., Vale, J. A., Volans, G. N. and Widdop, B., 1976a, Toxicity of paracetamol in children, *British Medical Journal*, **2**, 475.

Crome, P., Vale, J. A., Volans, G. N., Widdop, B. and Goulding, R., 1976b, Oral methionine in the treatment of severe paracetamol (acetaminophen) overdose, *Lancet*, **ii**, 829–830.

Crome, P., Volans, G. N., Vale, J. A., Widdop, B. and Goulding, R., 1976c, The use of methionine for acute paracetamol poisoning, *Journal of International Medical Research*, **4**

(Suppl. 4), 105–111.

Cronberg, S., Wallmark, E. and Söderberg, I., 1984, Effect on platelet aggregation of oral administration of 10 non-steroidal analgesics to humans, *Scandinavian Journal of Haematology*, **33**, 155–159.

Crook, D., Collins, A. J., Bacon, P. A. and Chan, R., 1976, Prostaglandin synthetase activity from human rheumatoid synovial microsomes. Effect of 'aspirin-like' drug therapy, *Annals of the Rheumatic Diseases*, **35**, 327–332.

Crowe, C. A., Yong, A. C., Calder, I. C., Ham, K. N. and Tange, J. D., 1979, The nephrotoxicity of p-aminophenol. I. The effect on microsomal cytochromes, glutathione and covalent binding in kidney and liver, *Chemico-Biological Interactions*, **27**, 235–243.

Crowe, M. T. I., 1989, Trends in fatal poisonings in Leeds, 1977 to 1987, *Medicine, Science and the Law*, **29**, 124–129.

Cullen, S., Kenny, D., Ward, O. C. and Sabra, K., 1989, Paracetamol suppositories: a comparative study, *Archives of Disease in Childhood*, **64**, 1504–1505.

Cummings, A. J., King, M. L. and Martin, B. K., 1967, A kinetic study of drug elimination: the excretion of paracetamol and its metabolites in man, *British Journal of Pharmacology and Chemotherapy*, **29**, 150–157.

Cunietti, E., Monti, M., Viganó, A., D'Aprile, E., Saligari, A., Scafuro, E. and Scaricabarozzi, I., 1993, Nimesulide in the treatment of hyperpyrexia in the aged: double-blind comparison with paracetamol, *Arzneimittel-Forschung*, **43**, 160–162.

Cunningham, J. L. and Price Evans, D. A., 1981, Acetanilide and paracetamol pharmacokinetics defore and during phenytoin administration: genetic control of induction? *British Journal of Clinical Pharmacology*, **11**, 591–595.

Cupit, G. C., 1982, The use of non-prescription analgesics in an older population, *Journal of the American Geriatrics Society*, **30**, S76–S80.

Curry, R. W., Robinson, J. D. and Sughrue, M. J., 1982, Acute renal failure after acetaminophen ingestion, *Journal of the American Medical Association*, **247**, 1012–1014.

Curtis, M. A., Pullen, R. H. and Kenna, K. M. C., 1991, HPLC determination of analgesics in human plasma and serum by direct injection on 80 Angstrom pore methyl bonded phase silica columns, *Journal of Liquid Chromatography*, **14**, 165–178.

Curzio, M., Flaccavento, C., Tesio, A., Primon, A. and Torrielli, M. V., 1980, Influenza del pretrattamento con tetrachloruro di carbonio sull 'epatottossicita' del paracetamolo, *Bollettino della Società Italiana di Biologia Sperimentale*, **56**, 2546–2552.

Czajka, P. A. and Whitington, G. L., 1982, Acetaminophen hepatotoxicity in a young child, *Veterinary and Human Toxicology*, **24**, 283.

Czapek, E. E., 1976, Aspirin, acetaminophen, and bleeding, *Journal of the American Medical Association*, **235**, 636.

Daas, M., Gupta, M. B., Gupta, G. P. and Bhargava, K. P., 1978, Role of biogenic amines in the ulcerogenic action of analgin and paracetamol in albino rats, *Indian Journal of Medical Research Section A - Infectious Diseases*, **67**, 677–681.

Dabbagh, S. and Chesney, R. W., 1985, Acute renal failure related to acetaminophen (paracetamol) overdose without fulminant hepatic disease, *International Journal of Pediatric Nephrology*, **6**, 221–224.

Daftary, S. N, Mehta, A. C. and Nanavati, M., 1980, A controlled comparison of dipyrone and paracetamol in post-episiotomy pain, *Current Medical Research and Opinion*, **6**, 614–618.

Dahlin, D. C., Miwa, G. T., Lu, A. Y. H. and Nelson, S. D., 1984, N-acetyl-p-benzoquinone imine: a cytochrome P-450-mediated oxidation product of acetaminophen, *Proceedings of the National Academy of Sciences of the United States of America*, **81**, 1327–1331.

Dahlin, D. C. and Nelson, S. D., 1982, Synthesis, decomposition kinetics, and preliminary toxicological studies of pure N-acetyl-p-benzoquinone imine, a proposed toxic metabolite of acetaminophen, *Journal of Medicinal Chemistry*, **25**, 885–886.

Dalens, B., 1991, La douleur aiguë de l'enfant et son traitement, *Annales Françaises d'Anesthésie et de Réanimation*, **10**, 38–61.

Dalhoff, K., Hansen, P. B., Ott, P., Loft, S. and Poulsen, H. E., 1991, Acute ethanol adminis-tration reduces the antidote effect of n-acetylcysteine after acetaminophen overdose in mice, *Human and Experimental Toxicology*, **10**, 431–433.

Dalhoff, K. and Poulsen, H. E., 1992, Effects of cysteine and acetaminophen on the syntheses of glutathione and adenosine 3′-phosphate 5′-phosphosulfate in isolated rat hepatocytes, *Biochemical Pharmacology*, **44**, 447–454.

Dalhoff, K. and Poulsen, H. E., 1993a, Inhibition of acetaminophen oxidation by cimetidine and the effects on glutathione and activated sulphate synthesis rates, *Pharmacology and Toxicology*, **73**, 215–218.

Dalhoff, K. and Poulsen, H. E., 1993b, Simultaneous measurements of glutathione and acti-vated sulphate (PAPS) synthesis rates and the effects of selective inhibition of glutathione conjugation or sulphation of acetaminophen, *Biochemical Pharmacology*, **46**, 383–388.

Dalhoff, K. and Poulsen, H. E., 1993c, Synthesis rates of glutathione and activated sulphate (PAPS) and response to cysteine and acetaminophen administration in glutathione-depleted rat hepatocytes, *Biochemical Pharmacology*, **46**, 1295–1297.

Daly, R. E., Moran, C. and Chafetz, L., 1972, Acetaminophen colorimetry as 2-nitro-4-aceta-midophenol, *Journal of Pharmaceutical Sciences*, **61**, 927–929.

Dange, S. V., Shah, K. U., Deshpande, A. S. and Shrotri, D. S., 1987, Bioavailability of acetaminophen after rectal administration, *Indian Pediatrics*, **24**, 331–332.

Dange, S. V., Shah, K. U., Ghongane, B. B. and Ranade, R. S., 1985, Potentiation of anti-pyretic effect of acetaminophen by concomitant administration of ascorbic acid, *Indian Journal of Physiology and Pharmacology*, **29**, 129–131.

Danninger, R., Jakse, R. and Beubler, E., 1993, Randomisierter Crossover-Vergleich von 2g- und 4g- Tagesdosen Paracetamol bei leicht- bis mittelgradigen Schmerzen von Tumoren im Kopf-Hals-Bereich, *European Journal of Pain*, **14**, 14–18.

Danon, A., Leibson, V. and Assouline, G., 1983, Effects of aspirin, indomethacin, flufenamic acid and paracetamol on prostaglandin output from rat stomach and renal papilla *in vitro* and *ex vivo*, *Journal of Pharmacy and Pharmacology*, **35**, 576–579.

Dascombe, M. J., 1984, Evidence that cyclic nucleotides are not mediators of fever in rabbits, *British Journal of Pharmacology*, **81**, 583–588.

Dascombe, M. J. and Milton, A. S., 1975, The effects of cyclic adenosine 3′,5′-monophosphate and other adenine nucleotides on body temperature, *Journal of Physiology*, **250**, 143–160.

Dascombe, M. J. and Milton, A. S., 1976, Cyclic adenosine 3′,5′-monophosphate in cerebro-spinal fluid during thermoregulation and fever, *Journal of Physiology*, **263**, 441–463.

Dasgupta, A. and Kinnaman, G., 1993, Microwave-induced rapid hydrolysis of acetamino-phen and its conjugates in urine for emergency toxicological screen, *Clinical Chemistry*, **39**, 2349–2350.

Datta, S. B., 1973, Fatal pancytopenia after administration of Fortagesic, *British Medical Journal*, **3**, 173.

Davenport, A., Davison, A. M. and Will, E. J., 1989a, Are changes in intracranial pressure during intermittent machine haemofiltration dependent upon membrane bio-compatibility? *International Journal of Artificial Organs*, **12**, 703–707.

Davenport, A. and Finn, R., 1988, Paracetamol (acetaminophen) poisoning resulting in acute renal failure without hepatic coma, *Nephron*, **50**, 55–56.

Davenport, A., Will, E. J. and Davison, A. M., 1990a, Effect of posture on intracranial pres-sure and cerebral perfusion pressure in patients with fulminant hepatic and renal failure after acetaminophen self-poisoning, *Critical Care Medicine*, **18**, 286–289.

Davenport, A., Will, E. J. and Davison, A. M., 1990b, Early changes in intracranial pressure during haemofiltration treatment in patients with grade 4 hepatic encephalopathy and acute oliguric renal failure, *Nephrology, Dialysis, Transplantation*, **5**, 192–198.

Davenport, A., Will, E. J. and Davison, A. M., 1990c, Paradoxical increase in arterial hydro-gen ion concentration in patients with hepatorenal failure given lactate-based fluids,

Nephrology, Dialysis, Transplantation, **5**, 343–346.

Davenport, A., Will, E. J. and Davison, A. M., 1991, Adverse effects on cerebral perfusion of prostacyclin administered directly into patients with fulminant hepatic failure and acute renal failure, *Nephron*, **59**, 449–454.

Davenport, A., Will, E. J. and Davison, A. M., 1993, Effect of renal replacement therapy on patients with combined acute renal and fulminant hepatic failure, *Kidney International*, **43 (Suppl. 41)**, S245–S251.

Davenport, A., Will, E. J. and Davison, A. M., 1994, Comparison of the use of standard heparin and prostacyclin anti-coagulation in spontaneous and pump-driven extracorporeal circuits in patients with combined acute renal and hepatic failure, *Nephron*, **66**, 431–437.

Davenport, A., Will, E. J., Davison, A. M., Swindells, S., Cohen, A. T., Miloszewski, K. J. A. and Losowsky, M. S., 1989b, Changes in intracranial pressure during haemofiltration in oliguric patients with Grade IV hepatic encephalopathy, *Nephron*, **53**, 142–146.

Davenport, A., Will, E. J. and Losowsky, M. S., 1989c, Rebound surges of intracranial pressure as a consequence of forced ultrafiltration used to control intracranial pressure in patients with severe hepatorenal failure, *American Journal of Kidney Diseases*, **14**, 516–519.

Davey, L. and Naidoo, D., 1993, Urinary screen for acetaminophen (paracetamol) in the presence of N-acetylcysteine, *Clinical Chemistry*, **39**, 2348–2349.

Davidson, A. R., Rojas-Bueno, A., Thompson, R. P. H. and Williams, R., 1976, Early unconjugated hyperbilirubinaemia after paracetamol overdosage, *Scandinavian Journal of Gastroenterology*, **11**, 623–628.

Davidson, D. G. D. and Eastham, W. N., 1966, Acute liver necrosis following overdose of paracetamol, *British Medical Journal*, **2**, 497–499.

Davidson, W., Bassist, L. and Shippey, W., 1973a, *In vitro* effects of aspirin and phenacetin metabolites on the metabolism of the dog renal medulla, *Clinical Research*, **21**, 227.

Davidson, W., Shippey, W. and Bassist, L., 1973b, Effect of aspirin and phenacetin metabolites on protein synthesis in dog renal medulla, *Clinical Research*, **21**, 683.

Davie, I. T. and Gordon, N. H., 1978, Comparative assessment of fenoprofen and paracetamol given in combination for pain after surgery, *British Journal of Anaesthesia*, **50**, 931–935.

Davies, D. J., Kennedy, A. and Roberts, C., 1970, The aetiology of renal medullary necrosis: a survey of adult cases in Liverpool, *Journal of Pathology*, **100**, 257–268.

Davies, D. S., Fawthrop, D. J., Nasseri-Sina, P., Wilson, J. W., Hardwick, S. J. and Boobis, A. R., 1992, Paracetamol toxicity and its prevention by cytoprotection with iloprost, *Toxicology Letters*, **64–65**, 575–580.

Davies, D. S., Tee, L. B. G., Hampden, C. and Boobis, A. R., 1986, Acetaminophen toxicity in isolated hepatocytes, *Advances in Experimental Medicine and Biology*, **197**, 993–1003.

Davies, M. H., Mutimer, D., Lowes, J., Elias, E. and Neuberger, J., 1994a, Recovery despite impaired cerebral perfusion in fulminant hepatic failure, *Lancet*, **343**, 1329–1330.

Davies, M. H., Ngong, J. M., Yucesoy, M., Acharya, S. K., Mills, C. O., Weaver, J. B., Waring, R. H. and Elias, E., 1994b, The adverse effect of pregnancy upon sulphation: a clue to the pathogenesis of intrahepatic cholestasis of pregnancy? *Journal of Hepatology*, **21**, 1127–1134.

Davies, M. H., Schamber, G. J. and Schnell, R. C., 1991, Oltipraz-induced amelioration of acetaminophen hepatotoxicity in hamsters. I. Lack of dependence on glutathione, *Toxicology and Applied Pharmacology*, **109**, 17–28.

Davies, M. H. and Schnell, R. C., 1991, Oltipraz-induced amelioration of acetaminophen hepatotoxicity in hamsters: II. Competitive shunt in metabolism via glucuronidation, *Toxicology and Applied Pharmacology*, **109**, 29–40.

Davis, A. and Perkins, M. N., 1993, The effects of capsaicin and conventional analgesics in two models of monoarthritis in the rat, *Agents and Actions*, **38**, C10–C12.

Davis, A. M., Helms, C. M., Mitros, F. A., Wong, Y. W. and LaBrecque, D. R., 1983, Severe hepatic damage after acetaminophen use in psittacosis, *Journal of the American Medical Association*, **74**, 349–352.

Davis, D. C., Potter, W. Z., Jollow, D. J. and Mitchell, J. R., 1974a, Species differences in hepatic glutathione depletion, covalent binding and hepatic necrosis after acetaminophen, *Life Sciences*, **14**, 2099–2109.

Davis, D. R., Fogg, A. G., Burns, D. T. and Wragg, J. S., 1974b, A colorimetric method for the determination of phenacetin and paracetamol, *Analyst*, **99**, 12–18.

Davis, M., 1986, Protective agents for acetaminophen overdose, *Seminars in Liver Disease*, **6**, 138–147.

Davis, M., Harrison, N. G., Ideo, G., Portmann, B., Labadarios, D. M. and Williams, R., 1976a, Paracetamol metabolism in the rat: relationship to covalent binding and hepatic damage, *Xenobiotica*, **6**, 249–255.

Davis, M., Ideo, G., Harrison, N. G. and Williams, R., 1975a, Hepatic glutathione depletion and impaired bromosulphthalein clearance early after paracetamol overdosage in man and the rat, *Clinical Science*, **49**, 495–502.

Davis, M., Ideo, G., Harrison, N. G. and Williams, R., 1975b, Early inhibition of hepatic bilirubin conjugation after paracetamol (acetaminophen) administration in the rat, *Digestion*, **13**, 42–48.

Davis, M., Simmons, C. J., Harrison, N. G. and Williams, R., 1976b, Paracetamol overdose in man: relationship between pattern of urinary metabolites and severity of liver damage, *Quarterly Journal of Medicine*, **45**, 181–191.

Davis, M. and Williams, R., 1975, Paracetamol and liver damage. In: Modern Trends in Gastroenterology. Read, A. E. Ed. Butterworths, London, pp. 318–344.

Davison, C., Dorrbecker, B. R. and Edelson, J., 1977, Comparative metabolism of benorylate and an equivalent mixture of aspirin and paracetamol in neonate and adult rabbits, *Xenobiotica*, **7**, 561–571.

Davison, C., Guy, J. L., Levitt, M. and Smith, P. K., 1961, The distribution of certain non-narcotic analgetic agents in the CNS of several species, *Journal of Pharmacology and Experimental Therapeutics*, **134**, 176–183.

Dawson, A. H., Henry, D. A. and McEwan, J., 1989, Adverse reactions to N-acetylcysteine during treatment for paracetamol poisoning, *Medical Journal of Australia*, **150**, 329–331.

Dawson, A. H. and Whyte, I. M., 1990, Compound analgesics, *Medical Journal of Australia*, **152**, 334.

Dawson, C. M., Rainbow, S. J. and Tickner, T. R., 1988a, Problems encountered with the use of the enzymic paracetamol assay on post-mortem blood samples, *Annals of Clinical Biochemistry*, **25 (Suppl.)**, 209S–210S.

Dawson, C. M., Wang, T. W. M., Rainbow, S. J. and Tickner, T. R., 1988b, A non-extraction HPLC method for the simultaneous determination of serum paracetamol and salicylate, *Annals of Clinical Biochemistry*, **25**, 661–667.

Dawson, D. J., Babbs, C., Warnes, T. W. and Neary, R. H., 1987, Hypophosphataemia in acute liver failure, *British Medical Journal*, **295**, 1312–1313.

Dawson, J., Knowles, R. G. and Pogson, C. I., 1990, Determination of glucuronidation in isolated rat liver cells by incorporation of ^{14}C from fructose, *Biochemical Society Transactions*, **18**, 1205.

Dawson, J., Knowles, R. G. and Pogson, C. I., 1991, Quantitative studies of sulphate conjugation by isolated rat liver cells using [^{35}S]sulphate, *Biochemical Pharmacology*, **42**, 45–49.

Dawson, J., Knowles, R. G. and Pogson, C. I., 1992, Measurement of glucuronidation by isolated rat liver cells using [^{14}C]fructose, *Biochemical Pharmacology*, **43**, 971–978.

Dawson, J. R., Norbeck, K., Anundi, I. and Moldéus, P., 1984, The effectiveness of N-acetylcysteine in isolated hepatocytes, against the toxicity of paracetamol, acrolein, and paraquat, *Archives of Toxicology*, **55**, 11–15.

Day, A. and Abbott, G. D., 1994, Chronic paracetamol poisoning in children: a warning to health professionals, *New Zealand Medical Journal*, **107**, 201.

De Beer, J. O., Jacobs, G. A., Janssens, G. and Martens, M. A., 1985, Impact of dilution on the pharmacokinetic behavior of acetaminophen in rabbits after oral administration, *Journal of Pharmaceutical Sciences*, **74**, 325–327.

de Gara, C., Taylor, M. and Hedges, A., 1982, Assessment of analgesic drugs in soft tissue injuries presenting to an accident and emergency department – a comparison of antrafenine, paracetamol and placebo, *Postgraduate Medical Journal*, **58**, 489–492.

de Gislain, C., Dumas, M., d'Athis, P., Chapuis, T., Mayer, F., Fargeot, P., Guerrin, J. and Escousse, A., 1990, Evolution de la créatininémie lors d'injections répétées de cisplatine: influence des associations médicamenteuses, *Thérapie*, **45**, 423–427.

De Knegt, R. J. and Schalm, S. W., 1991, Fulminant hepatic failure: to transplant or not to transplant, *Netherlands Journal of Medicine*, **38**, 131–141.

de la Mata, M., Meager, A., Rolando, N., Daniels, H. M., Nouri-Aria, K. T., Goka, A. K. J., Eddleston, A. L. W. F., Alexander, G. J. M. and Williams, R., 1990, Tumour necrosis factor production in fulminant hepatic failure: relation to aetiology and superimposed microbial infection, *Clinical and Experimental Immunology*, **82**, 479–484.

De Lange, E. C. M., Danhof, M., de Boer, A. G. and Breimer, D. D., 1993, The use of intracerebral microdialysis to study blood-brain barrier transport in health, after modification and in disease, *Advances in Experimental Medicine and Biology*, **331**, 257–262.

De Lange, E. C. M., Danhof, M., de Boer, A. G. and Breimer, D. D., 1994, Critical factors of intracerebral microdialysis as a technique to determine the pharmacokinetics of drugs in rat brain, *Brain Research*, **666**, 1–8.

de Morais, S. M. F., Chow, S. Y. M. and Wells, P. G., 1992a, Biotransformation and toxicity of acetaminophen in congenic RHA rats with or without a hereditary deficiency in bilirubin UDP-glucuronosyltransferase, *Toxicology and Applied Pharmacology*, **117**, 81–87.

de Morais, S. M. F., Uetrecht, J. P. and Wells, P. G., 1992b, Decreased glucuronidation and increased bioactivation of acetaminophen in Gilbert's syndrome, *Gastroenterology*, **102**, 577–586.

de Morais, S. M. F. and Wells, P. G., 1988, Deficiency in bilirubin UDP-glucuronyl transferase as a genetic determinant of acetaminophen toxicity, *Journal of Pharmacology and Experimental Therapeutics*, **247**, 323–331.

de Morais, S. M. F. and Wells, P. G., 1989, Enhanced acetaminophen toxicity in rats with bilirubin glucuronyl transferase deficiency, *Hepatology*, **10**, 163–167.

de Nardo, V., Lapadula, G. and Sioligno, O., 1988, Danno epatico e morte di una bambina di tre anni per intossicazione da paracetamolo, *Minerva Pediatrica*, **40**, 571.

de Paillerets, F. and Furioli, J., 1984, Action antipyrétique du soluté buvable de paracétamol chez l'enfant, *Annales de Pédiatrie*, **31**, 339–341.

de Toledo, C. F. and Borges, D. R., 1993, Plasma-kallikrein clearance by the liver of acetaminophen-intoxicated rats, *Life Sciences*, **52**, 1451–1459.

de Vos, M. and Barbier, F., 1985, La mesure de la différence de potentiel gastrique trans-épithéliale induite par l'acide acétylsalicylique tamponné. Effet due paracétamol et du sucralfate, *Gastroentérologie Clinique et Biologique*, **9**, 116–118.

de Vries, B. J., van der Kraan, P. M. and van den Berg, W. B., 1990, Decrease in inorganic blood sulfate following treatment with selected antirheumatic drugs: potential consequences for articular cartilage, *Agents and Actions*, **29**, 224–231.

de Vries, J., 1981, Hepatotoxic metabolic activation of paracetamol and its derivatives phenacetin and benorilate: oxygenation or electron transfer? *Biochemical Pharmacology*, **30**, 399–402.

de Vries, J., de Jong, J., Lock, F. M., van Bree, L., Mullink, H. and Veldhuizen, R. W., 1984, Protection against paracetamol-induced hepatotoxicity by acetylsalicylic acid in rats, *Toxicology*, **30**, 297–304.

de Vries, J., Jansen, J.-D., Kroese, E. D., van Bree, L. and van Ginneken, C. A. M., 1981, Protection against paracetamol-induced glutathione depletion following a paracetamol-acetylsalicylic acid mixture or benorilate in phenobarbital-treated rats, *Toxicology Letters*, **9**, 345–347.

Deakin, C. D., Gove, C. D., Fagan, E. A., Tredger, J. M. and Williams, R., 1991, Delayed calcium channel blockade with diltiazem reduces paracetamol hepatotoxicity in mice, *Human and Experimental Toxicology*, **10**, 119–123.

Dearden, J. C., O'Hara, J. H. and Townend, M. S., 1980, A double-peaked quantitative structure-activity relationship (QSAR) in a series of paracetamol derivatives, *Journal of Pharmacy and Pharmacology*, **32**, 102P.

Debets, A. J. J., van de Straat, R., Voogt, W. H., Vos, H., Vermeulen, N. P. E. and Frei, R. W., 1988, Simultaneous determination of glutathione, glutathione disulphide, paracetamol and its sulphur containing metabolites using HPLC and electrochemical detection with on-line generated bromine, *Journal of Pharmaceutical and Biomedical Analysis*, **6**, 329–336.

Dechtiaruk, W. A., Johnson, G. F. and Solomon, H. M., 1976, Gas-chromatographic method for acetaminophen (*N*-acetyl-*p*-aminophenol) based on sequential alkylation, *Clinical Chemistry*, **22**, 879–883.

Decousus, H., Laporte, S., Perpoint, B., Mismetti, P., Gaillet, J. L., Hocquart, J., Thomas, C. and Queneau, P., 1990, Comparison in 141 outpatients with osteoarthritis of two combinations of paracetamol with a narcotic analgesic: a controlled clinical trial, *European Journal of Pharmacology*, **183**, 1044.

Deeter, L. B., Martin, L. W. and Lipton, J. M., 1989, Antipyretic effect of central α-MSH summates with that of acetaminophen or ibuprofen, *Brain Research Bulletin*, **23**, 573–575.

Degen, J. and Maier-Lenz, H., 1984, Vergleichende Pharmakokinetik und Biolverfügbarkeit von Paracetamol aus Suppositorien, *Arzneimittel-Forschung*, **34**, 900–902.

Degen, J., Maier-Lenz, H. and Windorfer, A., 1982, Zur Pharmakokinetik und Bioverfügbarkeit von Paracetamol in Suppositorien für die Pädiatrie, *Arzneimittel-Forschung*, **32**, 420–422.

Delacroix, P., Kenesi, C. and Stoppa, R., 1985, Évaluation de l'efficacité antalgique du propacétamol vs. placebo chez des patients présentant une douleur post-opératoire, *Semaine des Hôpitaux de Paris*, **61**, 2739–2742.

Delaney, J. C., 1976, The diagnosis of aspirin idiosyncrasy by analgesic challenge, *Clinical Allergy*, **6**, 177–181.

Delaney, J. C., 1983, The effect of ketotifen on aspirin-induced asthmatic reactions, *Clinical Allergy*, **13**, 247–251.

DeLaurentis, M., Snyder, E., Chegwidden, K., Khanna, P. and Jaklitsch, A., 1982, Homogenous enzyme immunoassay for acetaminophen in human serum, *Clinical Chemistry*, **28**, 1664.

Demotes-Mainard, F., Vinçon, G., Jarry, C. and Albin, H., 1984, Dosage plasmatique du paracétamol par chromatographie liquide haute performance: application à une étude pharmacocinétique, *Annales de Biologie Clinique*, **42**, 9–13.

Deng, J. F., Spyker, D. A., Rall, T. W. and Steward, O., 1982, Reduction in caffeine toxicity by acetaminophen, *Journal of Toxicology. Clinical Toxicology*, **19**, 1031–1043.

Denison, H., Kaczynski, J. and Wallerstedt, S., 1987, Paracetamol medication and alcohol abuse: a dangerous combination for the liver and kidney, *Scandinavian Journal of Gastroenterology*, **22**, 701–704.

Denison, H., Kaczynski, J. and Wallerstedt, S., 1991, Paracetamol i terapeutiska doser kan ge svara lever-och njurskador hos alkoholister, *Läkartidningen*, **88**, 2664–2665.

Depot, M., Powell, J. R., Messenheimer, J. A., Cloutier, G. and Dalton, M. J., 1990, Kinetic effects of multiple oral doses of acetaminophen on a single oral dose of lamotrigine, *Clinical Pharmacology and Therapeutics*, **48**, 346–355.

Depré, M., van Hecken, A., Verbesselt, R., Tjandra-Maga, T. B., Gerin, M. and de Schepper, P. J., 1990, Tolerance and pharmacokinetics of propacetamol HCl, a paracetamol formulation for I.V. use, *European Journal of Pharmacology*, **183**, 388–389.

Depré, M., van Hecken, A., Verbesselt, R., Tjandra-Maga, T. B., Gerin, M. and de Schepper, P. J., 1992, Tolerance and pharmacokinetics of propacetamol, a paracetamol formulation for intravenous use, *Fundamental and Clinical Pharmacology*, **6**, 259–262.

Derby, L. E. and Jick, H., 1991, Renal parenchymal disease related to over-the-counter analgesic use, *Pharmacotherapy*, **11**, 467–471.

Derbyshire, N. D. J., Asscher, A. W. and Matthews, P. N., 1989, Hypercalcaemia as a manifestation of malignant urothelial change in analgesic nephropathy, *Nephron*, **52**, 79–80.

Derendorf, H., Drehsen, G. and Rohdewald, P., 1982, Cortical-evoked potentials and saliva levels as basis for the comparison of pure analgesics to analgesic combinations, *Pharmacology*, **25**, 227–236.

Dershewitz, R. A. and Levin, G. S., 1984, The effect of the Tylenol scare on parent's use of over-the-counter drugs, *Clinical Pediatrics*, **23**, 445–448.

Deshayes, P. and Mathieu, M., 1979, Essai d'un paracétamol effervescent dans le cadre d'un service de rééducation fonctionnelle, *Rhumatologie*, **31**, 43–47.

Deshpande, A. V., 1980, Effect of amino acids on bioavailability of paracetamol in rabbits, *Indian Journal of Experimental Biology*, **18**, 1498–1499.

Devalia, J. L. and McLean, A. E. M., 1982, Rapid method for the purification of [3,5-^{14}C] paracetamol, *Journal of Chromatography: Biomedical Applications*, **232**, 197–202.

Devalia, J. L. and McLean, A. E. M., 1983, Covalent binding and the mechanism of paracetamol toxicity, *Biochemical Pharmacology*, **32**, 2602–2603.

Devalia, J. L., Ogilvie, R. C. and McLean, A. E. M., 1982, Dissociation of cell death from covalent binding of paracetamol by flavones in a hepatocyte system, *Biochemical Pharmacology*, **31**, 3745–3749.

Devictor, D., Decimo, D., Sebire, G., Tardieu, M. and Hadchouel, M., 1992, Enhanced tumor necrosis factor alpha in coronavirus but not in paracetamol-induced acute hepatic necrosis in mice, *Liver*, **12**, 205–208.

Dey, P. K., Feldberg, W., Gupta, K. P., Milton, A. S. and Wendlandt, S., 1974, Further studies on the role of prostaglandin in fever, *Journal of Physiology*, **241**, 629–646.

Dey, P. K., Feldberg, W., Gupta, K. P. and Wendlandt, S., 1975, Lipid A fever in cats, *Journal of Physiology*, **253**, 103–119.

Dey, P. K. and Sharma, H. S., 1984, Influence of ambient temperature and drug treatments on brain oedema induced by impact injury on skull in rats, *Indian Journal of Physiology and Pharmacology*, **28**, 177–186.

D'Haens, G., Breysem, Y., Rutgeerts, P., van Besien, B. and Vantrappen, G., 1993, Proctitis and rectal stenosis induced by nonsteroidal antiinflammatory suppositories, *Journal of Clinical Gastroenterology*, **17**, 207–212.

Di Simplicio, P., Dolara, P. and Lodovici, M., 1984, Blood glutathione as a measure of exposure to toxic compounds, *Journal of Applied Toxicology*, **4**, 227–229.

Diaz, D., Fabre, I., Daujat, M., Saint Aubert, B., Bories, P., Michel, H. and Maurel, P., 1990, Omeprazole is an aryl hydrocarbon-like inducer of human hepatic cytochrome P450, *Gastroenterology*, **99**, 737–747.

Diener, H.-C., Dichgans, J., Scholz, E., Geiselhart, S., Gerber, W.-D. and Bille, A., 1989, Analgesic-induced chronic headache: long-term results of withdrawal therapy, *Journal of Neurology*, **236**, 9–14.

Diener, M., Bridges, R. J. and Büch, H. P., 1986, The effect of aniline derivatives on absorption of fluid, glucose and sodium in isolated duodenal segments from rats, *Naunyn-Schmiedeberg's Archives of Pharmacology*, **334**, 531–535.

Dieppe, P. A., Frankel, S. J. and Toth, B., 1993, Is research into the treatment of osteoarthritis with non-steroidal anti-inflammatory drugs misdirected? *Lancet*, **341**, 353–354.

Dieter, M. P., Maronpot, R. R., Jameson, C. W. and Ward, S. M., 1992, The effects of iodinated glycerol, trichlorfon, and acetaminophen on tumor progression in a Fischer rat leukemia transplant model, *Cancer Detection and Prevention*, **16**, 173–183.

Dietz, A. J., Carlson, J. D., Wahba Khalil, S. K. and Nygard, G., 1984, Effects of alcoholism on acetaminophen pharmacokinetics in man, *Journal of Clinical Pharmacology*, **24**, 205–208.

Dietz, A. J., Wahbe Khalil, S. K. and Nygard, G., 1982, Acetaminophen kinetics in the alcoholic, *Clinical Pharmacology and Therapeutics*, **31**, 218.

Diez Gómez, M. L., Alvarez Cuesta, E., Hinojosa Macias, M., Garcia Cañadillas, F. and Alcover Sánchez, R., 1984, Urticaria-angioedema inducidos por analgésicos-antiinflammatorios no esteroideos, *Allergologia et Immunopathologia (Madrid)*, **12**, 179–188.

Dikstein, S., Grotto, M., Zor, U., Tamari, M. and Sulman, F. G., 1966a, The stimulatory effect of paracetamol and its derivatives on growth and the rat tibia test, *Journal of Endocrinology*, **36**, 257–262.

Dikstein, S., Zor, U., Ruah, D. and Sulman, F. G., 1966b, Stimulatory effect of paracetamol on chicken growth, *Poultry Science*, **45**, 744–746.

Dills, R. L. and Klaassen, C. D., 1986, Effect of reduced hepatic energy state on acetaminophen conjugation in rats, *Journal of Pharmacology and Experimental Therapeutics*, **238**, 463–472.

Dimova, S. and Stoytchev, T., 1990, Effect of potassium ethylxanthogenate on the acetaminophen hepatotoxicity in mice, *Acta Physiologica et Pharmacologica Bulgarica*, **16**, 23–30.

Dimova, S. and Stoytchev, Ts., 1989, Effect of potassium ethylxanthogenate on the toxicity and analgesic effect of acetaminophen, *Acta Physiologica et Pharmacologica Bulgarica*, **15**, 9–16.

Dimova, S. and Stoytchev, Ts., 1994, Influence of rifampicin on the toxicity and the analgesic effect of acetaminophen, *European Journal of Drug Metabolism and Pharmacokinetics*, **19**, 311–317.

Dingeon, B., Charvin, M. A., Quenard, M. T. and Thome, H., 1988, Multi-wavelength analyses of second-derivative spectra for rapid determination of acetaminophen in serum, *Clinical Chemistry*, **34**, 1119–1121.

Dinis, T. C. P., Madeira, V. M. C. and Almeida, L. M., 1994, Action of phenolic derivatives (acetaminophen, salicylate, and 5-aminosalicylate) as inhibitors of membrane lipid peroxidation and as peroxyl radical scavengers, *Archives of Biochemistry and Biophysics*, **315**, 161–169.

Dinwoodie, A. J., 1978, Interferences in an emergency acetaminophen method and its modification, *Clinical Biochemistry*, **11**, 131–132.

Dionne, R., Campbell, R. A., Cooper, S. A., Hall, D. L. and Buckingham, B., 1983, Suppression of postoperative pain by preoperative administration of ibuprofen in comparison to placebo, acetaminophen, and acetaminophen plus codeine, *Journal of Clinical Pharmacology*, **23**, 37–43.

DiPasquale, G. and Mellace, D., 1977, Inhibition of arachidonic acid induced mortality in rabbits with several non-steroidal anti-inflammatory agents, *Agents and Actions*, **7**, 481–485.

Dittert, L. W., Irwin, G. M., Chong, C. W. and Swintosky, J. V., 1968, Acetaminophen prodrugs. II. Effect of structure and enzyme source on enzymatic and nonenzymatic hydrolysis of carbonate esters, *Journal of Pharmaceutical Sciences*, **57**, 780–783.

Divoll, M., Abernethy, D. R., Ameer, B. and Greenblatt, D. J., 1982a, Acetaminophen kinetics in the elderly, *Clinical Pharmacology and Therapeutics*, **31**, 151–156.

Divoll, M., Ameer, B., Abernethy, D. R. and Greenblatt, D. J., 1982b, Age does not alter acetaminophen absorption, *Journal of the American Geriatrics Society*, **30**, 240–244.

Divoll, M., Greenblatt, D. J., Ameer, B. and Abernethy, D. R., 1982c, Effect of food on acetaminophen absorption in young and elderly subjects, *Journal of Clinical Pharmacology*, **22**, 571–576.

Dixon, M. F., 1976, Paracetamol hepatotoxicity, *Lancet*, **i**, 35.

Dixon, M. F., Dixon, B., Aparicio, S. R. and Lowey, D. P., 1975a, Experimental paracetamol-induced hepatic necrosis: a light- and electron- microscope and histochemical study, *Journal of Pathology*, **116**, 17–29.

Dixon, M. F., Fulker, M. J., Walker, B. E., Kelleher, J. and Losowsky, M. S., 1975b, Serum transaminase levels after experimental paracetamol-induced hepatic necrosis, *Gut*, **16**, 800–807.

Dixon, M. F., Nimmo, J. and Prescott, L. F., 1971, Experimental paracetamol-induced hepatic necrosis – a histopathological study, *Journal of Pathology*, **103**, 225–229.

Dixon, R. M., Angus, P. W., Rajagopalan, B. and Radda, G. K., 1992, ^{31}P magnetic resonance spectroscopy detects a functional abnormality in liver metabolism after acetaminophen poisoning, *Hepatology*, **16**, 943–948.

Djimbo, M. and Moës, A. J., 1986, Influence de l'interaction de paracétamol-surfactifs non ioniques sur l'absorption rectale à partir de suppositoires, *Journal de Pharmacie de Belgique*, **41**, 393–401.

Djordjevic, S. P., Hayward, N. K. and Lavin, M. F., 1986, Effect of N-Hydroxyparacetamol on cell cycle progression, *Biochemical Pharmacology*, **35**, 3511–3516.

Doan, T. and Greenberger, P. A., 1993, Nearly fatal episodes of hypotension, flushing, and dyspnea in a 47-year-old woman, *Annals of Allergy*, **70**, 439–444.

Doggett, N. S. and Jawaharlal, K., 1977, Anorectic activity of prostaglandin precursors, *British Journal of Pharmacology*, **60**, 417–423.

Doherty, N. S., Beaver, T. H., Chan, K. Y., Dinerstein, R. J. and Diekema, K. A., 1990, The antinociceptive activity of paracetamol in zymosan-induced peritonitis in mice: the role of prostacyclin and reactive oxygen species, *British Journal of Pharmacology*, **101**, 869–874.

Dolara, P., Lodovici, M., Salvadori, M., Saltutti, C., Delle Rose, A., Selli, C. and Kriebel, D., 1988, Variations of cortisol hydroxylation and paracetamol metabolism in patients with bladder carcinoma, *British Journal of Urology*, **62**, 419–426.

Dolara, P., Lodovici, M., Salvadori, M., Zaccara, G. and Muscas, G. C., 1987, Urinary 6-beta-OH-cortisol and paracetamol metabolites as a probe for assessing oxidation and conjugation of chemicals in humans, *Pharmacological Research Communications*, **19**, 261–273.

Dolci, G., Ripari, M., Pacifici, L. and Umile, A., 1993, Efficacia analgesica e tollerabilità di piroxicam-β-ciclodestrina in confronto con piroxicam, paracetamolo e placebo nel trattamento del dolore post-estrattivo dentale, *Minerva Stomatologica*, **42**, 235–241.

Dolegeal-Vendrely, M. and Guernet, M., 1976, Dosage du paracétamol dans le plasma par spectrofluorimétrie, *Analusis*, **4**, 223–226.

Dolphin, C. T., Caldwell, J. and Smith, R. L., 1987, Effect of poly rI : rC treatment upon the metabolism of [^{14}C]-paracetamol in the BALB/cJ mouse, *Biochemical Pharmacology*, **36**, 3835–3840.

Donaldson, B. W., Gopinath, R., Wanless, I. R., Phillips, M. J., Cameron, R., Roberts, E. A., Greig, P. D., Levy, G. and Blendis, L. M., 1993, The role of transjugular liver biopsy in fulminant liver failure: relation to other prognostic indicators, *Hepatology*, **18**, 1370–1376.

Donatus, I. A., Vermeulen, S. and Vermeulen, N. P. E., 1990, Cytotoxic and cytoprotective activities of curcumin: effects on paracetamol-induced cytotoxicity, lipid peroxidation and glutathione depletion in rat hepatocytes, *Biochemical Pharmacology*, **39**, 1869–1875.

Done, A. K., 1959, Uses and abuses of antipyretic therapy, *Pediatrics*, **23**, 774–780.

Donn, K. H., Rudd, G. D., Grisham, J. W. and Koch, G. G., 1982, Prevention of acetaminophen-induced hepatic injury by cimetidine, *Clinical Pharmacology and Therapeutics*, **31**, 218–219.

Donnelly, P. J., Walker, R. M. and Racz, W. J., 1994, Inhibition of mitochrondrial respiration *in vivo* is an early event in acetaminophen-induced hepatotoxicity, *Archives of Toxicology*, **68**, 110–118.

Donovan, J. W., Jarvie, D. R., Prescott, L. F. and Proudfoot, A. T., 1987, Adverse reactions of

N-acetylcysteine and their relation to plasma levels, *Veterinary and Human Toxicology*, **29**, 470.

Doran, T. F., de Angelis, C., Baumgardner, R. A. and Mellits, E. D., 1989, Acetaminophen: more harm than good for chicken pox? *Journal of Pediatrics*, **114**, 1045–1048.

Dordoni, B., Willson, R. A., Thompson, R. P. H. and Williams, R., 1973, Reduction of absorption of paracetamol by activated charcoal and cholestyramine: a possible therapeutic measure, *British Medical Journal*, **3**, 86–87.

Dougall, J. R., Cunningham, B. and Nimmo, W. S., 1983, Paracetamol absorption from Paramax, Panadol and Solpadeine, *British Journal of Clinical Pharmacology*, **15**, 487–489.

Douglas, A. P., Hamlyn, A. N. and James, O., 1976, Controlled trial of cysteamine in treatment of acute paracetamol (acetaminophen) poisoning, *Lancet*, **i**, 111–115.

Douglas, A. P., Savage, R. L. and Rawlins, M. D., 1978, Paracetamol (acetaminophen) kinetics in patients with Gilbert's syndrome, *European Journal of Clinical Pharmacology*, **13**, 209–212.

Douidar, S. M. and Ahmed, A. E., 1982, Studies on simultaneous determination of acetaminophen, salicylic acid and salicyluric acid in biological fluids by high performance liquid chromatography, *Journal of Clinical Chemistry and Clinical Biochemistry*, **20**, 791–798.

Douidar, S. M. and Ahmed, A. E., 1987, A novel mechanism for the enhancement of acetaminophen hepatotoxicity by phenobarbital, *Journal of Pharmacology and Experimental Therapeutics*, **240**, 578–583.

Douidar, S. M., Al-Khalil, I. and Habersang, R. W., 1994, Severe hepatotoxicity, acute renal failure, and pancytopenia in a young child after repeated acetaminophen overdosing, *Clinical Pediatrics*, **33**, 42–45.

Douidar, S. M., Boor, P. J. and Ahmed, A. E., 1985, Potentiation of the hepatotoxic effect of acetaminophen by prior administration of salicylate, *Journal of Pharmacology and Experimental Therapeutics*, **233**, 242–248.

Douidar, S. M., Wolf, B., Al-Khalil, I. and Habersang, R., 1992, Severe hepatotoxicity, acute renal failure and pancytopenia in a young child following repeated acetaminophen (APAP) overdosing, *Veterinary and Human Toxicology*, **34**, 327.

Dray, A., Patel, I. A., Perkins, M. N. and Rueff, A., 1992, Bradykinin-induced activation of nociceptors: receptor and mechanistic studies on the neonatal rat spinal cord-tail preparation *in vitro*, *British Journal of Pharmacology*, **107**, 1129–1134.

Drehsen, G. and Rohdewald, P., 1981, Rapid high-performance thin-layer chromatography of salicylic acid, salicylamide, ethoxybenzamide and paracetamol in saliva, *Journal of Chromatography: Biomedical Applications*, **223**, 479–483.

Drenth, J. P. H., Frenken, L. A. M., Wuis, E. W. and van der Meer, J. W. M., 1994, Acute renal failure associated with paracetamol ingestion in an alcoholic patient, *Nephron*, **67**, 483–485.

Drew, R. and Miners, J. O., 1984, The effects of buthionine sulphoximine (BSO) on glutathione depletion and xenobiotic biotransformation, *Biochemical Pharmacology*, **33**, 2989–2994.

Drew, R., Rowell, J. and Miners, J. O., 1982, Prevention of paracetamol hepatic toxicity by cimetidine, *Clinical and Experimental Pharmacology and Physiology*, **9**, 471.

Drez, D., Ritter, M. and Rosenberg, T. D., 1987, Pain relief after arthroscopy: naproxen sodium compared to propoxyphene napsylate with acetaminophen, *Southern Medical Journal*, **80**, 440–443.

Drower, E. J., Stapelfeld, A., Mueller, R. A. and Hammond, D. L., 1987, The antinociceptive effects of prostaglandin antagonists in the rat, *European Journal of Pharmacology*, **133**, 249–256.

Drukker, W., Schwarz, A. and Vanherweghem, J.-L., 1986, Analgesic nephropathy: an underestimated cause of end-stage renal disease, *International Journal of Artificial Organs*, **9**, 219–246.

Drvota, V., Vesterqvist, O. and Gréen, K., 1991, Effects of non-steroidal anti-inflammatory drugs on the *in vivo* synthesis of thromboxane and prostacyclin in humans, *Advances in Prostaglandin, Thromboxane, and Leukotriene Research*, **21**, 153–156.

D'Souza, M. J., Solomon, H. M. and Lowance, D. C., 1989, Effect of chronic treatment with cyclosporine and prednisone on acetaminophen metabolism in renal transplant patients, *Transplantation*, **48**, 697–700.

Dubach, U. C., 1967a, P-Aminophenol-Bestimmung im Urin als Routinemthode zur Erfassung der Phenacetineinnahme, *Deutsche Medizinische Wochenschrift*, **92**, 211–215.

Dubach, U. C., 1967b, Nachweis und Ausscheidung von N-acetyl-p-aminophenol in Abhängigkeit der Niereninfunktion nach Einnahme von phenacetin, *Helvetica Medica Acta*, **47 (Suppl.)**, 107.

Dubach, U. C., 1968, Absorption, Schicksal und Ausscheidung von phenacetin und N-acetyl-p-aminophenol bei Niereninsuffizienz, *Klinische Wochenschrift*, **46**, 261–264.

Dubach, U. C., 1981, Die Bedeutung des Analgetikaabusus für chronische Harntraktinfektionen, *Therapiewoche*, **31**, 7890–7898.

Dubach, U. C., 1984, Harnwegsinfektionen bei Analgetika-Abusus, *Deutsche Gesundheitswesen*, **39**, 1606–1608.

Dubach, U. C., Levy, P. S. and Minder, F., 1968, Epidemiological study of analgesic intake and its relationship to urinary tract disorders in Switzerland, *Helvetica Medica Acta*, **34**, 297–312.

Dubach, U. C., Levy, P. S. and Müller, A., 1971, Relationships between regular analgesic intake and urorenal disorders in a working female population of Switzerland I. Initial results (1968), *American Journal of Epidemiology*, **93**, 425–434.

Dubach, U. C., Levy, P. S., Rosner, B., Baumeler, H. R., Müller, A., Peier, A. and Ehrensperger, T., 1975, Relation between regular intake of phenacetin-containing analgesics and laboratory evidence for urorenal disorders in a working female population of Switzerland, *Lancet*, **i**, 539–543.

Dubach, U. C., Rosner, B. and Pfister, E., 1983, Epidemiologic study of the abuse of analgesics containing phenacetin: renal morbidity and mortality (1968–1979), *New England Journal of Medicine*, **308**, 357–362.

Dubach, U. C., Rosner, B. and Stürmer, T., 1991, An epidemiologic study of abuse of analgesic drugs: effects of phenacetin and salicylate on mortality and cardiovascular morbidity (1968 to 1987), *New England Journal of Medicine*, **324**, 155–160.

DuBois, R. N., Hill, K. E. and Burk, R. F., 1983, Antioxidant effect of acetaminophen in rat liver, *Biochemical Pharmacology*, **32**, 2621–2622.

Duchene, A., Chadenas, D. and Marneffe-Lebrequier, H., 1991, Insuffisance rénal aiguë isoleé après intoxication volontaire par le paracétamol, *Presse Médicale*, **20**, 1684–1685.

Duer, G. T., 1979, Acetaminophen intoxication in the cat: a case report, *Southwestern Veterinarian*, **32**, 215–218.

Duffy, J. P. and Byers, J., 1979, Acetaminophen assay: the clinical consequences of a colorimetric vs. a high-pressure liquid chromatography determination in the assessment of two potentially poisoned patients, *Clinical Toxicology*, **15**, 427–435.

Duggan, J. M., 1980, Gastrointestinal toxicity of minor analgesics, *British Journal of Clinical Pharmacology*, **10 (Suppl. 2)**, 407S–410S.

Duggan, J. M., Dobson, A. J., Johnson, H. and Fahey, P., 1986, Peptic ulcer and non-steroidal anti-inflammatory agents, *Gut*, **27**, 929–933.

Duggin, G. G., 1977, Analgesic induced kidney disease, *Australian Journal of Pharmaceutical Sciences*, **6**, 44–48.

Duggin, G. G., 1980, Mechanisms in the development of analgesic nephropathy, *Kidney International*, **18**, 553–561.

Duggin, G. G., Caterson, R. J., Mohandas, J., Horvath, J. and Tiller, D., 1980, Biochemical basis of synergistic analgesic toxicity, *Australian and New Zealand Journal of Medicine*, **10**, 129–130.

Duggin, G. G., Mohandas, J., Horvath, J. S. and Tiller, D. J., 1982, Metabolic activation of paracetamol during renal prostaglandin biosynthesis, *Australian and New Zealand Journal of Medicine*, **12**, 344–345.

Duggin, G. G. and Mudge, G. H., 1975, Renal tubular transport of paracetamol and its conjugates in the dog, *British Journal of Pharmacology*, **54**, 359–366.

Duggin, G. G. and Mudge, G. H., 1976, Analgesic nephropathy: renal distribution of acetaminophen and its conjugates, *Journal of Pharmacology and Experimental Therapeutics*, **199**, 1–9.

Duggin, G. G. and Mudge, G. H., 1978, Effect of acute diuresis on the renal excretion of phenacetin and its major metabolites, *Journal of Pharmacology and Experimental Therapeutics*, **207**, 584–593.

Duhamel, G., Najman, A., Gorin, N.-C. and Stachowiak, J., 1977, Aspets actuels de l'agranulocytose (A propos de 15 observations), *Annales de Medécine Interne*, **128**, 303–306.

Duhamel, J. F., Guillot, M., Brouard, J., Debosque, S., Consten, L., Dresco, I., Perret, M. and Rezvani, Y., 1993, Effet antipyrétique de l'acide tiaprofénique chez l'enfant: étude comparative au paracétamol, *Pédiatrie*, **48**, 655–659.

Duhra, P. and Porter, D. I., 1990, Paracetamol-induced fixed drug eruption with positive immunofluorescence findings, *Clinical and Experimental Dermatology*, **15**, 293–295.

Duniec, Z., Robak, J. and Gryglewski, R., 1983, Antioxidant properties of some chemicals vs. their influence on cyclooxygenase and lipoxidase activities, *Biochemical Pharmacology*, **32**, 2283–2286.

Dunn, T. L., Gardiner, R. A., Seymour, G. J. and Lavin, M. F., 1987, Genotoxicity of analgesic compounds assessed by an *in vitro* micronucleus assay, *Mutation Research*, **189**, 299–306.

Dupin, J.-P., Gravier, D., Casadebaig, F., Boisseau, M. R. and Bernard, H., 1988, *In vitro* antiaggregant activity of paracetamol and derivatives, *Thrombosis Research*, **50**, 437–447.

Durán-Suárez, J. R., 1984, Anemias hemolíticas inducidas por medicamentos, *Medicina Clinica*, **82**, 816–821.

Dussarat, G. V., Dalger, J., Mafart, B. and Chagnon, A., 1988, Purpura vasculaire au paracétamol: une observation, *Presse Médicale*, **17**, 1587.

Dwivedi, Y., Rastogi, R., Garg, N. K. and Dhawan, B. N., 1991, Prevention of paracetamol-induced hepatic damage in rats by picroliv, the standardised active fraction from *Picrorhiza kurroa*, *Phytotherapy Research*, **5**, 115–119.

Dwyer, P. S. and Jones, I. F., 1984, Fatal self-poisoning in the UK and the paracetamol/dextropropoxyphene combination, *Human Toxicology*, **3 (Suppl.)**, 145S–174S.

Dybing, E., 1976, Inhibition of acetaminophen glucuronidation by oxazepam, *Biochemical Pharmacology*, **25**, 1421–1425.

Dybing, E., 1977, Activation of α-methyldopa, paracetamol and furosemide by human liver microsomes, *Acta Pharmacologica et Toxicologica*, **41**, 89–93.

Dybing, E., 1985, Metabolsk aktivering og kjemiske nyreskader, *Tidsskrift for den Norske Lægeforening*, **105**, 1610–1613.

Dybing, E., Holme, J. A., Gordon, W. P., Søderlund, E. J., Dahlin, D. C. and Nelson, S. D., 1984, Genotoxicity studies with paracetamol, *Mutation Research*, **138**, 21–32.

Eade, N. R. and Lasagna, L., 1967, A comparison of acetophenetidin and acetaminophen. II. Subjective effects in healthy volunteers, *Journal of Pharmacology and Experimental Therapeutics*, **155**, 301–308.

Eandi, M., Viano, I. and Ricci Gamalero, S., 1984, Absolute bioavailability of paracetamol after oral or rectal administration in healthy volunteers, *Arzneimittel-Forschung*, **34**, 903–907.

Eastham, E. J., Bell, J. I. and Douglas, A. P., 1976, Serum ferritin levels in acute hepatocellular damage from paracetamol overdosage, *British Medical Journal*, **1**, 750–751.

Ebel, S., Liedtke, R. and Mißler, B., 1980, Quantitative Bestimmung von Paracetamol im blutserum durch HPLC mit Direktinjektion, *Archiv der Pharmazie und Berichte der Deutschen pharmazeutischen Gesellschaft*, **313**, 324–329.

Ecobichon, D. J., D'Ver, A. S. and Ehrhart, W., 1988, Drug disposition and biotransformation in the developing beagle dog, *Fundamental and Applied Toxicology*, **11**, 29–37.

Ecobichon, D. J., Hidvegi, S., Comeau, A. M. and Varma, D. R., 1989, Acetaminophen metabolism *in vivo* by pregnant, fetal and neonatal guinea pigs, *Journal of Biochemical Toxicology*, **4**, 235–240.

Eden, A. N. and Kaufman, A., 1967, Clinical comparison of three antipyretic agents, *American Journal of Diseases of Children*, **144**, 284–287.

Eder, H., 1964, Chronic toxicity studies on phenacetin,, N-acetyl-p-aminophenol (NAPA) and acetylsalicylic acid on cats, *Acta Pharmacologica et Toxicologica*, **21**, 197–204.

Edinboro, L. E., Jackson, G. F., Jortani, S. A. and Poklis, A., 1991, Determination of serum acetaminophen in emergency toxicology: evaluation of newer methods: Abbott TDx and second derivative ultraviolet spectrophotometry, *Journal of Toxicology. Clinical Toxicology*, **29**, 241–255.

Edmondson, H. D. and Bradshaw, A. J., 1983, Analgesia following oral surgery: a comparative study of Solpadeine and a soluble form of dextropropoxyphene napsylate and paracetamol, *Journal of International Medical Research*, **11**, 228–231.

Edwards, A. M. and Lucas, C. M., 1985, Induction of γ-glutamyl transpeptidase in primary cultures of normal rat hepatocytes by liver tumor promoters and structurally related compounds, *Carcinogenesis*, **6**, 733–739.

Edwards, D. A., Fish, S. F., Lamson, M. J. and Lovejoy, F. H., 1986, Prediction of acetaminophen level from clinical history of overdose using a pharmacokinetic model, *Annals of Emergency Medicine*, **15**, 1314–1319.

Edwards, O. M., Edwards, P., Huskisson, E. C. and Taylor, R. T., 1971, Paracetamol and renal damage, *British Medical Journal*, **2**, 87–89.

Edwards, R. and Oliphant, J., 1992, Paracetamol toxicity in chronic alcohol abusers – a plea for greater consumer awareness, *New Zealand Medical Journal*, **105**, 174–175.

Edwardson, P. A. D., Nichols, J. D. and Sugden, K., 1989, Application of a modified colorimetric enzyme assay to monitor plasma paracetamol levels following single oral doses to non-patient volunteers, *Journal of Pharmaceutical and Biomedical Analysis*, **7**, 287–293.

Eisalo, A. and Talanti, S., 1961, Observations on the effect of phenacetin and N-acetyl-p-aminophenol on rat kidneys, *Acta Medica Scandinavica*, **169**, 655–660.

Eisner, E. V. and Shahidi, N. T., 1972, Immune thrombocytopenia due to a drug metabolite, *New England Journal of Medicine*, **287**, 376–381.

Ekins, B. R., Ford, D. C., Thompson, M. I. B., Bridges, R. R., Rollins, D. E. and Jenkins, R. D., 1987, The effect of activated charcoal on N-acetylcysteine absorption in normal subjects, *American Journal of Emergency Medicine*, **5**, 483–487.

Ekwall, B. and Acosta, D., 1982, *In vitro* comparative toxicity of selected drugs and chemicals in HeLa cells, Chang liver cells, and rat hepatocytes, *Drug and Chemical Toxicology*, **5**, 219–231.

El-Din, M. K. S., Abuirjeie, M. A. and Abdel-Hay, M. H., 1991, Simultaneous determination of acetaminophen with orphenadrine citrate, ibuprofen or chlorzoxazone in combined dosage forms by zero-crossing derivative spectrophotometry, *Analytical Letters*, **24**, 2187–2206.

El-Hage, A. N., Herman, E. H. and Ferrans, V. J., 1983, Examination of the protective effect of ICRF-187 and dimethyl sulfoxide against acetaminophen-induced hepatotoxicity in Syrian golden hamsters, *Toxicology*, **28**, 295–303.

El Mouelhi, M. and Buszewski, B., 1990, Application of solid-phase extraction to the isolation and determination of paracetamol and its metabolites, *Journal of Pharmaceutical and Biomedical Analysis*, **8**, 651–653.

El-Obeid, H. A. and Al-Badr, A. A., 1985, *Analytical Profiles of Drug Substances*, Acetaminophen, **14**, 551–596, Orlando: Academic Press.

El Turabi, H., El Sirag, O., Homeida, M. M. A., Harron, D. W. G. and Leahey, W. J., 1989, Paracetamol pharmacokinetics in patients with hepatosplenic schistosomiasis, *International Journal of Pharmaceutics*, **53**, 249–251.

Eleftheriou, N., Heathcote, J., Thomas, H. C. and Sherlock, S., 1977, Serum alpha-fetoprotein levels in patients with acute and chronic liver disease. Relation to hepatocellular regeneration and development of primary liver cell carcinoma, *Journal of Clinical Pathology*, **30**, 704–708.

Elfarra, A. A. and Anders, M. W., 1984, Renal processing of glutathione conjugates: role in nephrotoxicity, *Biochemical Pharmacology*, **33**, 3729–3732.

Eling, T. E., Thompson, D. C., Foureman, G. L., Curtis, J. F. and Hughes, M. F., 1990, Prostaglandin H synthase and xenobiotic oxidation, *Annual Review of Pharmacology and Toxicology*, **30**, 1–45.

Elkind, A. H., 1991, Drug abuse and headache, *Medical Clinics of North America*, **75**, 717–732.

Ellcock, C. T. H. and Fogg, A. G., 1975, Selective colorimetric determination of paracetamol by means of an indophenol reaction, *Analyst*, **100**, 16–18.

Elliott, D. P., 1990, Preventing upper gastrointestinal bleeding in patients receiving non-steroidal antiinflammatory drugs, *Drug Intelligence and Clinical Pharmacy, the Annals of Pharmacotherapy*, **24**, 954–958.

Ellis, M., Haydik, I., Gillman, S., Cummins, L. and Cairo, M. S., 1989, Immediate adverse reactions to acetaminophen in children: evaluation of histamine release and spirometry, *Journal of Pediatrics*, **114**, 654–656.

Ellison, R. T., Horsburgh, C. R. and Curd, J., 1990, Complement levels in patients with hepatic dysfunction, *Digestive Diseases and Sciences*, **35**, 231–235.

Ellmers, S. E., Parker, L. R. C., Notarianni, L. J. and Jones, R. W., 1993, Excretion of paracetamol in fit and frail elderly people, *British Journal of Clinical Pharmacology*, **31**, 596P–597P.

Ellouk-Achard, S., Levresse, V., Martin, C., Pham-Huy, C., Duterte-Catella, H., Thevenin, M., Warnet, J.-M. and Claude, J. R., 1994, *Ex vivo* and *in vivo* acetaminophen hepatotoxicity, relationships between glutathione depletion, oxidative stress and disturbances in calcium homeostasis and energy metabolism, *Toxicology Letters*, **74 (Suppl. 1)**, 22.

Elseviers, M. M. and de Broe, M. E., 1988, Is analgesic nephropathy still a problem in Belgium? *Nephrology, Dialysis, Transplantation*, **2**, 143–149.

Elseviers, M. M. and de Broe, M. E., 1994a, Which analgesics are nephrotoxic? *Journal of the American Society of Nephrology*, **5**, 392.

Elseviers, M. M. and de Broe, M. E., 1994b, Analgesic nephropathy in Belgium is related to the sales of particular analgesic mixtures, *Nephrology, Dialysis, Transplantation*, **9**, 41–46.

Emby, D. J. and Fraser, B. N., 1977, Hepatotoxicity of paracetamol enhanced by ingestion of alcohol, *South African Medical Journal*, **51**, 208–209.

Emeigh Hart, S. G., Beierschmitt, W. P., Bartolone, J. B., Wyand, D. S., Khairallah, E. A. and Cohen, S. D., 1991a, Evidence against deacetylation and for cytochrome P450-mediated activation in acetaminophen-induced nephrotoxicity in the CD-1 mouse, *Toxicology and Applied Pharmacology*, **107**, 1–15.

Emeigh Hart, S. G., Beierschmitt, W. P., Wyand, D. S., Khairallah, E. A. and Cohen, S. D., 1994, Acetaminophen nephrotoxicity in CD-1 mice. I. Evidence of a role for *in situ* activation in selective covalent binding and toxicity, *Toxicology and Applied Pharmacology*, **126**, 267–275.

Emeigh Hart, S. G., Birge, R. B., Cartun, R. W., Tyson, C. A., Dabbs, J. E., Nishanian, E. V., Wyand, D. S., Khairallah, E. A. and Cohen, S. D., 1991b, *In vivo* and *in vitro* evidence for *in situ* activation and selective covalent binding of acetaminophen (APAP) in mouse kidney, *Advances in Experimental Medicine and Biology*, **283**, 711–716.

Emeigh Hart, S. G., Cartun, R. W., Wyand, D. S., Khairallah, E. A. and Cohen, S. D., 1990,

Selective protein arylation by acetaminophen (APAP): immunohistochemical localization in mouse liver, lung and kidney, *Toxicologist*, **10**, 229.

Emery, S., Oldham, H. G., Norman, S. J. and Chenery, R. J., 1985, The effect of cimetidine and ranitidine on paracetamol glucuronidation and sulphation in cultured rat hepatocytes, *Biochemical Pharmacology*, **34**, 1415–1421.

Emslie, K. R., Calder, I. C., Hart, S. J. and Tange, J. D., 1981a, Induction of paracetamol metabolism in the isolated perfused kidney, *Xenobiotica*, **11**, 579–587.

Emslie, K. R., Calder, I. C., Hart, S. J. and Tange, J. D., 1982, Metabolism of paracetamol by the isolated perfused kidney of the homozygous Gunn rat, *Xenobiotica*, **12**, 77–82.

Emslie, K. R., Smail, M. C., Calder, I. C., Hart, S. J. and Tange, J. D., 1981b, Paracetamol and the isolated perfused kidney: metabolism and functional effects, *Xenobiotica*, **11**, 43–50.

Endo, T., Kano, S. and Nishida, A., 1988a, Forensico-toxicological investigation on acetaminophen-induced toxicity. 1. Dose-related morphological changes of hepatotoxicity, *Journal of Tokyo Medical College*, **46**, 24–28.

Endo, T., Kano, S. and Nishida, A., 1988b, Forensico-toxicological investigation on acetaminophen-induced toxicity. 2. Biochemical studies on aminoacid fractions in liver and kidney and biogenic amine metabolism, *Journal of Tokyo Medical College*, **46**, 29–33.

Engelhardt, G., 1984, Tierexperimentelle Untersuchungen zur Frage des Zusammenwirkens von Paracetamol und Acetylsalicylsäure, *Arzneimittel-Forschung*, **34**, 992–1001.

Engelking, L. R., Blyden, G. T., Lofstedt, J. and Greenblatt, D. J., 1987a, Pharmacokinetics of antipyrine, acetaminophen and lidocaine in fed and fasted horses, *Journal of Veterinary Pharmacology and Therapeutics*, **10**, 73–82.

Engelking, L. R., Lofstedt, J., Blyden, G. T. and Greenblatt, D. J., 1987b, Antipyrine and lidocaine are cleared faster in horses than in humans: acetaminophen may be handled similarly, *Pharmacology*, **34**, 192–200.

Enrico, J.-F. and Buchser, E., 1983, Les intoxications médicamenteuses volontaires, *Therapeutische Umschau*, **40**, 522–529.

Entacher, U., Stoffel, C., Lerchner, A. and Gadner, H., 1993, Paracetamolintoxikation, *Tägliche Praxis*, **34**, 523–527.

Epstein, M. M., Nelson, S. D., Slattery, J. T., Kalhorn, T. F., Wall, R. A. and Wright, J. M., 1991, Inhibition of the metabolism of paracetamol by isoniazid, *British Journal of Clinical Pharmacology*, **31**, 139–142.

Epton, J., 1979, Paracetamol: a report of a regional quality control scheme, *Annals of Clinical Biochemistry*, **16**, 265–270.

Erickson, R. A. and Runyon, B. A., 1984, Acetaminophen hepatotoxicity associated with alcoholic pancreatitis, *Archives of Internal Medicine*, **144**, 1509–1510.

Eriksson, L. S., Broomé, U., Kalin, M. and Lindholm, M., 1992, Hepatotoxicity due to repeated intake of low doses of paracetamol, *Journal of Internal Medicine*, **231**, 567–570.

Eskenazi, J., Nikiforidis, T., Livio, J. J. and Schelling, J. L., 1976, Effect of paracetamol, mephenoxalone and their combination on pain following bone surgery, *European Journal of Clinical Pharmacology*, **9**, 411–415.

Espey, L. L., 1983, Comparison of the effect of nonsteroidal and steroidal antiinflammatory agents on prostaglandin production during ovulation in the rabbit, *Prostaglandins*, **26**, 71–78.

Espey, L. L., Stein, V. I. and Dumitrescu, J., 1982, Survey of antiinflammatory agents and related drugs as inhibitors of ovulation in the rabbit, *Fertility and Sterility*, **38**, 238–247.

Essien, E. E., Ette, E. I. and Brown-Awala, E. A., 1988, Evaluation of the effect of co-administered paracetamol on the gastro-intestinal absorption and disposition of chloroquine, *Journal of Pharmaceutical and Biomedical Analysis*, **6**, 521–526.

Esteban, A., Calvo, R. and Pérez-Mateo, M., 1994, Acetaminophen (A) metabolism in two different ethnic Spanish populations, *Methods and Findings in Experimental and Clinical Pharmacology*, **16 (Suppl. 1)**, 121.

Esteban, A., Graells, M., Satorre, J. and Pérez-Mateo, M., 1992, Determination of paraceta-mol and its four major metabolites in mouse plasma by reversed-phase ion-pair high-performance liquid chromatography, *Journal of Chromatography: Biomedical Applications*, **573**, 121–126.

Esteban, A. and Pérez-Mateo, M., 1993a, El metabolismo del paracetamol en voluntarios sanos: estudio de una muestra en poblacion española, *Gastroenterologia y Hepatologia*, **16**, 55–60.

Esteban, A. and Pérez-Mateo, M., 1993b, Gilbert's disease: a risk factor for paracetamol overdosage? *Journal of Hepatology*, **18**, 257–258.

Esteban, A., Satorres, J., Graells, M. L. and Pérez-Mateo, M., 1993a, Estudio de los niveles plasmáticos de paracetamol y sus metabolitos tras sobrecarga oral o intraperitoneal en el ratón, *Gastroenterología y Hepatología*, **16**, 17–20.

Esteban, A., Satorres, J., Mayole, M. J., Graells, M. L. and Pérez-Mateo, M., 1993b, Liver damage and plasma concentrations of paracetamol and its metabolites after paracetamol overdosage in mice, *Methods and Findings in Experimental and Clinical Pharmacology*, **15**, 125–130.

Esterline, R. L. and Ji, S., 1989, Metabolic alterations resulting from the inhibition of mito-chondrial respiration by acetaminophen *in vivo*, *Biochemical Pharmacology*, **38**, 2390–2392.

Esterline, R. L., Ray, S. D. and Ji, S., 1989, Reversible and irreversible inhibition of hepatic mitochondrial respiration by acetaminophen and its toxic metabolite N-acetyl-p-benzo-quinoneimine (NAPQI), *Biochemical Pharmacology*, **38**, 2387–2390.

Estrela, J. M., Sáez, G. T., such, L. and Viña, J., 1983, The effect of cysteine and N-acetylcysteine on rat liver glutathione (GSH), *Biochemical Pharmacology*, **32**, 3483–3485.

Eswarasankaran, S., Ramakrishnan, P. N., Palanichamy, S. and Murugesh, N., 1982, Influ-ence of drugs on the transfer of paracetamol across everted rat intestine, *Indian Journal of Hospital Pharmacy*, **19**, 103–105.

Evans, M. A. and Harbison, R. D., 1977, GLC microanalyses of phenacetin and acetamino-phen plasma levels, *Journal of Pharmaceutical Sciences*, **66**, 1628–1629.

Evans, P. J., Evans, R. W., Bomford, A., Williams, R. and Halliwell, B., 1994, Metal ions catalytic for free radical reactions in the plasma of patients with fulminant hepatic failure, *Free Radical Research Communications*, **20**, 139–144.

Evans, P. J. D., McQuay, H. J., Rolfe, M., O'Sullivan, G., Bullingham, R. E. S. and Moore, R. A., 1982, Zomepirac, placebo and paracetamol/dextropropoxyphene combination com-pared in orthopaedic postoperative pain, *British Journal of Anaesthesia*, **54**, 927–933.

Ewah, B., Yau, K., King, M., Reynolds, F., Carson, R. J. and Morgan, B., 1993, Effect of epidural opioids on gastric emptying in labour, *International Journal of Obstetric Anes-thesia*, **2**, 125–128.

Eyanagi, R., Hisanari, Y. and Shigematsu, H., 1991, Studies of paracetamol/phenacetin tox-icity: isolation and characterization of p-aminophenol-glutathione conjugate, *Xeno-biotica*, **21**, 793–803.

Eyer, P. and Sprenger, M., 1991, Orale Verabreichung einer Ativkohle-Sorbit-Suspension als Erstmassnahme zur Verminderung der Giftresorption? *Klinische Wochenschrift*, **69**, 887–894.

Faber, J., 1980, Lack of effect of acetaminophen on serum T_4, T_3, reverse T_3, 3,3′-diiodothy-ronine and 3′,5′-diiodothyronine in man, *Hormone and Metabolic Research*, **12**, 637–638.

Factor, S. A., Hefti, F. and Weiner, W. J., 1988, Acetaminophen metabolism by cytochrome P-450 in Parkinson's disease, *Archives of Neurology*, **45**, 808–809.

Factor, S. A., Weiner, W. J. and Hefti, F., 1989, Acetaminophen metabolism by cytochrome P450 monooxygenases in Parkinson's disease, *Annals of Neurology*, **26**, 286–288.

Fagan, E., Forbes, A. and Williams, R., 1988, Toxic myocarditis in paracetamol poisoning, *British Medical Journal*, **296**, 63–64.

Fairbrother, J. E., 1974, Acetaminophen. In: Analytical Profiles of Drug Substances,

Volume 3. Florey, K. Ed. Academic Press, London, pp. 1–111.

Fairhurst, S., Barber, D. J., Clark, B. and Horton, A. A., 1982, Studies on paracetamol-induced lipid peroxidation, *Toxicology*, **23**, 249–259.

Fairhurst, S. and Horton, A. A., 1984, Paracetamol toxicity in isolated rat hepatocytes, *Biochemical Society Transactions*, **12**, 675–676.

Falkowski, A. and Wei, R., 1981, A simple electrochemical method for the quantitative determination of acetaminophen in serum, *Analytical Letters*, **14**, 1003–1012.

Falliers, C. J., 1983, Acetaminophen and aspirin challenges in subgroups of asthmatics, *Journal of Asthma*, **20(S-1)**, 39–49.

Falloon, I., Watt, D. C., Lubbe, K., MacDonald, A. and Shepherd, M., 1978, N-acetyl-p-amino-phenol (paracetamol, acetaminophen) in the treatment of acute schizophrenia, *Psychological Medicine*, **8**, 495–499.

Farag, M. M. and Abdel-Meguid, E. M., 1994, Hepatic glutathione and lipid peroxidation in rats treated with theophylline: effect of dose and combination with caffeine and acetaminophen, *Biochemical Pharmacology*, **47**, 443–446.

Farah, D. A., Boag, D., Moran, F. and McIntosh, S., 1982, Paracetamol interference with blood glucose analysis: a potentially fatal phenomenon, *British Medical Journal*, **285**, 172.

Farber, B. F. and Wolff, A. G., 1992, The use of nonsteroidal antiinflammatory drugs to prevent adherence of *Staphylococcus epidermidis* to medical polymers, *Journal of Infectious Diseases*, **166**, 861–865.

Farber, J. L. and Gerson, R. J., 1984, Mechanisms of cell injury with hepatotoxic chemicals, *Pharmacological Reviews*, **36 (Suppl. 2)**, 71S–75S.

Farber, J. L., Leonard, T. B., Kyle, M. E., Nakae, D., Serroni, A. and Rogers, S. A., 1988, Peroxidation-dependent and peroxidation-independent mechanisms by which acetaminophen kills cultured rat hepatocytes, *Archives of Biochemistry and Biophysics*, **267**, 640–650.

Farghali, H., Rossaro, L., Gavaler, J. S., van Thiel, D. H., Dowd, S. R., Williams, D. S. and Ho, C., 1992, ^{31}P-NMR spectroscopy of perifused rat hepatocytes immobilized in agarose threads: application to chemical-induced hepatotoxicity, *Biochimica Biophysica Acta*, **1139**, 105–114.

Farid, N. R., Glynn, J. P. and Kerr, D. N. S., 1972, Haemodialysis in paracetamol self-poisoning, *Lancet*, **ii**, 396–398.

Farmer, R. D. T., 1994, Suicide and poisons, *Human Psychopharmacology*, **9 (Suppl. 1)**, S11–S19.

Farrance, I. and Aldons, J., 1981, Paracetamol interference with YSI glucose analyser, *Clinical Chemistry*, **27**, 782–783.

Fascetti Testi, P., Rosini, S. and Silvestri, S., 1975, Studio dell'assorbimento, nell'uomo di una preparazione effervescente di N-acetil-p-aminofenolo (paracetamolo), *Farmaco – Edizione Pratica*, **30**, 437–444.

Faulkner, G., Prichard, P., Somerville, K. and Langman, M. J. S., 1988, Aspirin and bleeding peptic ulcers in the elderly, *British Medical Journal*, **297**, 1311–1313.

Faunø, P., Petersen, K. D. and Husted, S. E., 1993, Increased blood loss after preoperative NSAID: retrospective study of 186 hip arthroplasties, *Acta Orthopaedica Scandinavica*, **64**, 522–524.

Fauvelle, F., Leon, A., Niakate, M. T., Petitjean, O. and Guillevin, L., 1988, Pharmacokinetics of paracetamol, diclofenac and vidaribine during plasma exchange, *International Journal of Artificial Organs*, **11**, 195–200.

Fauvelle, F., Nicolas, P., Leon, A., Tod, M., Perret, G., Petitjean, O. and Guillevin, L., 1991, Diclofenac, paracetamol, and vidarabine removal during plasma exchange in polyarteritis nodosa patients, *Biopharmaceutics and Drug Disposition*, **12**, 411–424.

Fawthrop, D. J., Wilson, J., Hardwick, S., Thorgeirsson, S. S., Battula, N., Boobis, A. R. and Davies, D. S., 1992, Cycloheximide abolishes the cytoprotective effect of iloprost on paracetamol-treated RLER52H-16 cells, *Human and Experimental Toxicology*, **11**, 432–433.

Fayz, S., Cherry, W. F., Dawson, J. R., Mulder, G. J. and Pang, K. S., 1984, Inhibition of acetaminophen sulfation by 2,6-dichloro-4-nitrophenol in the perfused rat liver preparation: lack of a compensatory increase of glucuronidation, *Drug Metabolism and Disposition: The Biological Fate of Chemicals*, **12**, 323–329.

Fazio, A., 1991, Oral contraceptive drug interactions: important considerations, *Southern Medical Journal*, **84**, 997–1002.

Feinberg, S. M. and Feinberg, A. R., 1955, Useful drugs in the treatment of allergy, *Illinois Medical Journal*, **108**, 5–9.

Feldberg, W. and Gupta, K. P., 1973, Pyrogen fever and prostaglandin-like activity in cerebrospinal fluid, *Journal of Physiology*, **228**, 41–53.

Feldberg, W., Gupta, K. P., Milton, A. S. and Wendlandt, S., 1972, Effect of bacterial pyrogen and antipyretics on prostaglandin activity in cerebrospinal fluid of unanaesthetised cats, *British Journal of Pharmacology*, **46**, 550P–551P.

Feldberg, W., Gupta, K. P., Milton, A. S. and Wendlandt, S., 1973, Effect of pyrogen and antipyretics on prostaglandin activity in cisternal C.S.F. of unanaesthetized cats, *Journal of Physiology*, **234**, 279–303.

Feldberg, W. and Saxena, P. N., 1975, Prostaglandins, endotoxin and lipid A on body temperature in rats, *Journal of Physiology*, **249**, 601–615.

Feldman, S., 1975, Bioavalability of acetaminophen suppositories, *American Journal of Hospital Pharmacy*, **32**, 1173–1175.

Feller, K. and le Petit, G., 1977, On the distribution of drugs in saliva and blood plasma, *International Journal of Clinical Pharmacology and Biopharmacy*, **15**, 468–469.

Fenzy, A. and Bogomoletz, W. V., 1987, Anorectal ulceration due to abuse of dextropropoxyphene and paracetamol suppositories, *Journal of the Royal Society of Medicine*, **80**, 62.

Ferenc, F., Katalin, T. and János, K., 1994, Csecsemókori paracetamol mérgezés – veszélytelen-e a paracetamol? *Orvosi Hetilap*, **135**, 2487–2489.

Ferguson, D. R., Snyder, S. K. and Cameron, A. J., 1977, Hepatotoxicity in acetaminophen poisoning, *Mayo Clinic Proceedings*, **52**, 246–248.

Ferguson, D. V., Roberts, D. W., Han-Shu, H., Andrews, A., Benson, R. W., Bucci, T. J. and Hinson, J. A., 1990, Acetaminophen-induced alterations in pancreatic β cells and serum insulin concentrations in B6C3F1 mice, *Toxicology and Applied Pharmacology*, **104**, 225–234.

Ferguson, J. A., Sellar, C. and Goldacre, M. J., 1992, Some epidemiological observations on medicinal and non-medicinal poisoning in preschool children, *Journal of Epidemiology and Community Health*, **46**, 207–210.

Fernandez, E. and Fernandez-Brito, A. C., 1977, Acetaminophen toxicity, *New England Journal of Medicine*, **296**, 577.

Fernando, C. R., Calder, I. C. and Ham, K. N., 1980, Studies on the mechanism of toxicity of acetaminophen. Synthesis and reactions of N-acetyl-2,6-dimethyl- and N-acetyl-3,5-dimethyl-p-benzoquinone imines, *Journal of Medicinal Chemistry*, **23**, 1153–1158.

Ferner, R., 1993, Paracetamol poisoning: an update, *Prescribers' Journal*, **33**, 45–50.

Ferrari, R. A., Ward, S. J., Zobre, C. M., van Liew, D. K., Perrone, M. H., Connell, M. J. and Haubrich, D. R., 1990, Estimation of the *in vivo* effect of cyclooxygenase inhibitors on prostaglandin E_2 levels in mouse brain, *European Journal of Pharmacology*, **179**, 25–34.

Ferreira, S. H., Lorenzetti, B. B. and Correa, F. M. A., 1978, Central and peripheral anti-algesic action of aspirin-like drugs, *European Journal of Pharmacology*, **53**, 39–48.

Ferrell, W. J. and Goyette, G. W., 1982, Analysis of acetaminophen and salicylate by reversed phase HPLC, *Journal of Liquid Chromatography*, **5**, 93–96.

Fevery, J. and de Groote, J., 1969, Conjugation of N-acetyl-p-aminophenol (N.A.P.A.) in adult liver patients, *Acta Hepato-Splenologica*, **16**, 11–18.

Fiaschi, A. I., Micheli, L., Giorgi, G. and Runci, F. M., 1990, Recovery of normal hepatic glutathione levels lowered by acetaminophen in rat, *European Journal of Pharmacology*, **183**, 1347–1348.

Filtzer, H. S., 1980, Double-blind randomised comparison of naproxen sodium, acetaminophen and pentazocine in postoperative pain, *Current Therapeutic Research*, **27**, 293–302.

Finco, D. R., Duncan, J. R., Schall, W. D. and Prasse, K. W., 1975, Acetaminophen toxicosis in the cat, *Journal of the American Veterinary Medical Association*, **166**, 469–472.

Findlay, J. W. A., DeAngelis, R. L., Kearney, M. F., Welch, R. M. and Findlay, J. M., 1981, Analgesic drugs in breast milk and plasma, *Clinical Pharmacology and Therapeutics*, **29**, 625–633.

Finet, L., Saleme, R., Delcenserie, R. and Dupas, J. L., 1990, Ulcère oesophagien lié à la prise orale de Di-Antalvic (association de dextropropoxyphène et de paracétamol), *Gastroentérologie Clinique et Biologique*, **14**, 1033–1034.

Fingerote, R. J. and Bain, V. G., 1993, Fulminant hepatic failure, *American Journal of Gastroenterology*, **88**, 1000–1010.

Finkelstein, M. B., Baggs, R. B. and Anders, M. W., 1992, Nephrotoxicity of the glutathione and cysteine conjugates of 2-bromo-2-chloro-1,1-difluoroethene, *Journal of Pharmacology and Experimental Therapeutics*, **261**, 1248–1252.

Fischer, L. J., Green, M. D. and Harman, A. W., 1981, Levels of acetaminophen and its metabolites in mouse tissues after a toxic dose, *Journal of Pharmacology and Experimental Therapeutics*, **219**, 281–286.

Fischer, L. J., Green, M. D. and Harman, A. W., 1985a, Studies on the fate of the glutathione and cysteine conjugates of acetaminophen in mice, *Drug Metabolism and Disposition: The Biological Fate of Chemicals*, **13**, 121–126.

Fischer, T. J., Guilfoile, T. D., Kesarwala, H. H., Winant, J. G., Kearns, G. L., Gartside, P. S. and Moomaw, C. J., 1983, Adverse pulmonary responses to aspirin and acetaminophen in chronic childhood asthma, *Pediatrics*, **71**, 313–318.

Fischer, V., Harman, L. S., West, P. R. and Mason, R. P., 1986, Direct electron spin resonance detection of free radical intermediates during the peroxidase catalyzed oxidation of phenacetin metabolites, *Chemico-Biological Interactions*, **60**, 115–127.

Fischer, V. and Mason, R. P., 1984, Stable free radical and benzoquinone imine metabolites of an acetaminophen analogue, *Journal of Biological Chemistry*, **259**, 10284–10288.

Fischer, V., West, P. R., Harman, L. S. and Mason, R. P., 1985b, Free-radical metabolites of acetaminophen and a dimethylated derivative, *Environmental Health Perspectives*, **64**, 127–137.

Fischer, V., West, P. R., Nelson, S. D., Harvison, P. J. and Mason, R. P., 1985c, Formation of 4-aminophenoxyl free radical from the acetaminophen metabolite N-acetyl-p-benzoquinone imine, *Journal of Biological Chemistry*, **260**, 11446–11450.

Fischereder, M. and Jaffe, J. P., 1994, Thrombocytopenia following acute acetaminophen overdose, *American Journal of Hematology*, **45**, 258–259.

Fisherman, E. W. and Cohen, G. N., 1973, Aspirin and other cross-reacting small chemicals in known aspirin intolerant patients, *Annals of Allergy*, **31**, 476–484.

Fisker, N. J., Garcia, R. S. and Andersen, P. K., 1991, Bevidst selvforgiftning. Et 10 ars materiale fra en intensivafdeling, *Ugeskrift for Læger*, **153**, 840–844.

Fitzgerald, G. A. and Drury, M. I., 1977, Paracetamol poisoning – a brief report, *Journal of the Irish Medical Association*, **70**, 448–449.

Fitzpatrick, F. A. and Wynalda, M. A., 1976, *In vivo* suppression of prostaglandin biosynthesis by non-steroidal anti-inflammatory agents, *Prostaglandins*, **12**, 1037–1051.

Flaccavento, C., Drago, A., Pagliuca, C. and Torrielli, M. V., 1980a, Osservazioni sperimentale sul danno epatico conseguente alla sominstrazione di paracetamolo e tetracloruro di carbonio, *Bollettino della Società Italiana di Biologia Sperimentale*, **56**, 912–918.

Flaccavento, C., Rossi, M. A. and Torrielli, M. V., 1980b, Relationship between GSH depletion and 'in vitro' lipoperoxidative processes in liver of rats intoxicated with paracetamol, *Bollettino della Società Italiana di Biologia Sperimentale*, **56**, 42–48.

Flaks, A. and Flaks, B., 1983, Induction of liver cell tumours in IF mice by paracetamol, *Carcinogenesis*, **4**, 363–368.

Flaks, B., Flaks, A. and Shaw, A. P. W., 1985, Induction by paracetamol of bladder and liver tumours in the rat: effects on hepatocyte fine structure, *Acta Pathologica Microbiologica et Immunologica Scandinavica*, **93 Section A**, 367–377.

Flanagan, R. J., 1987, The role of acetylcysteine in clinical toxicology, *Medical Toxicology and Adverse Drug Experience*, **2**, 93–104.

Flanagan, R. J., Huggett, A., Saynor, D. A., Raper, S. M. and Volans, G. N., 1981a, Value of toxicological investigation in the diagnosis of acute drug poisoning in children, *Lancet*, **ii**, 682–685.

Flanagan, R. J. and Mant, T. G. K., 1986, Coma and metabolic acidosis early in severe acute paracetamol poisoning, *Human Toxicology*, **5**, 256–259.

Flanagan, R. J. and Meredith, T. J., 1991, Use of N-acetylcysteine in clinical toxicology, *American Journal of Medicine*, **91 (Suppl. 3C)**, 131S–139S.

Flanagan, R. J., Widdop, B. and Volans, G. N., 1981b, Factors contributing to mortality in paracetamol-induced hepatic failure, *British Medical Journal*, **282**, 905–906.

Flavell Matts, S. G. and Boston, P. F., 1983, Paracetamol plus metoclopramide ('Paramax') as an adjunct analgesic in the treatment of arthritis, *Current Medical Research and Opinion*, **8**, 547–552.

Fleckenstein, J. L., 1985, Nyquil and acute hepatic necrosis, *New England Journal of Medicine*, **313**, 48.

Fleetwood, J. A. and Robinson, S. M. A., 1981, Paracetamol interference with glucose analyser, *Clinical Chemistry*, **27**, 1945.

Fleisher, G. R., Kearney, T. E., Henretig, F. and Tenenbein, M., 1991, Gastric decontamination in the poisoned patient, *Pediatric Emergency Care*, **7**, 378–381.

Fletterick, C. G., Grove, T. H. and Hohnadel, D. C., 1979, Liquid-chromatographic determination of acetaminophen in serum, *Clinical Chemistry*, **25**, 409–412.

Flinn, F. B. and Brodie, B. B., 1948, The effect on the pain threshold of N-acetyl p-aminophenol, a product derived in the body from acetanilide, *Journal of Pharmacology and Experimental Therapeutics*, **94**, 76–77.

Florén, C.-H., Thesleff, P. and Nilsson, Å., 1987, Severe liver damage caused by therapeutic doses of acetaminophen, *Acta Medica Scandinavica*, **222**, 285–288.

Florkowski, C. M., Ferner, R. E. and Jones, A. F., 1991, Liver transplantation after paracetamol overdose, *British Medical Journal*, **303**, 420.

Florkowski, C. M., Jones, A. F., Guy, J. M., Husband, D. J. and Stevens, J., 1994, Retinol binding proteinuria and phosphaturia: markers of paracetamol-induced nephrotoxicity, *Annals of Clinical Biochemistry*, **31**, 331–334.

Flower, R. J. and Vane, J. R., 1972, Inhibition of prostaglandin synthetase in brain explains the anti-pyretic activity of paracetamol (4-acetamidophenol), *Nature*, **240**, 410–411.

Focella, A., Heslin, P. and Teitel, S., 1972, The synthesis of two phenacetin metabolites, *Canadian Journal of Chemistry*, **50**, 2025–2030.

Font, J., Nomdedeu, B., Martinez Orozco, F., Ingelmo, M. and Balcells, A., 1981, Amegakaryocytic thrombocytopenia and an analgesic, *Annals of Internal Medicine*, **95**, 783.

Foote, R. W., Achini, R. and Römer, D., 1988, FS 205–397: a new antipyretic analgesic with a paracetamol-like profile of activity but lack of acute hepatotoxicity in mice, *Life Sciences*, **43**, 905–912.

Forbes, A., Alexander, G. J. M., O'Grady, J. G., Keays, R., Gullan, R., Dawling, S. and Williams, R., 1989a, Thiopental infusion in the treatment of intracranial hypertension complicating fulminant hepatic failure, *Hepatology*, **10**, 306–310.

Forbes, J. A., 1994, Evaluation of two opioid-acetaminophen combinations and placebo in post-operative oral surgery pain, *Pharmacotherapy*, **14**, 139–146.

Forbes, J. A., Barkaszi, B. A., Ragland, R. N. and Hankle, J. J., 1984a, Analgesic effect of acetaminophen, phenyltoloxamine and their combination in postoperative oral surgery pain, *Pharmacotherapy*, **4**, 221–226.

Forbes, J. A., Butterworth, G. A., Burchfield, W. H. and Beaver, W. T., 1990a, Evaluation of ketorolac, aspirin and an acetaminophen-codeine combination in postoperative oral surgery pain, *Pharmacotherapy*, **10**, 77S–93S.

Forbes, J. A., Butterworth, G. A., Burchfield, W. H., Yorio, C. C., Selinger, L. R., Rosenmertz, S. K. and Beaver, W. T., 1989b, Evaluation of flurbiprofen, acetaminophen, an acetaminophen-codeine combination, and placebo in postoperative oral surgery pain, *Pharmacotherapy*, **9**, 322–330.

Forbes, J. A., Kehm, C. J., Grodin, C. D. and Beaver, W. T., 1990b, Evaluation of ketorolac, ibuprofen, acetaminophen, and an acetaminophen-codeine combination in postoperative oral surgery pain, *Pharmacotherapy*, **10**, 94S–105S.

Forbes, J. A., Kolodny, A. L., Beaver, W. T., Shackleford, R. W. and Scarlett, V. R., 1983, A 12-hour evaluation of the analgesic efficacy of diflunisal, acetaminophen, and an acetaminophen-codeine combination, and placebo in postoperative pain, *Pharmacotherapy*, **3**, 47S–54S.

Forbes, J. A., Kolodny, A. L., Chachich, B. M. and Beaver, W. T., 1984b, Nalbuphine, acetaminophen, and their combination in postoperative pain, *Clinical Pharmacology and Therapeutics*, **35**, 843–851.

Forfar, J. C., Pottage, A., Toft, A. D., Irvine, W. J., Clements, J. A. and Prescott, L. F., 1980, Paracetamol pharmacokinetics in thyroid disease, *European Journal of Clinical Pharmacology*, **18**, 269–273.

Forrest, J. A. H., Adriaenssens, P. I., Finlayson, N. D. C. and Prescott, L. F., 1979, Paracetamol metabolism in chronic liver disease, *European Journal of Clinical Pharmacology*, **15**, 427–431.

Forrest, J. A. H., Clements, J. A. and Prescott, L. F., 1982, Clinical pharmacokinetics of paracetamol, *Clinical Pharmacokinetics*, **7**, 93–107.

Forrest, J. A. H., Finlayson, N. D. C., Adjepon-Yamoah, K. K. and Prescott, L. F., 1977, Antipyrine, paracetamol and lignocaine elimination in chronic liver disease, *British Medical Journal*, **1**, 1384–1387.

Forrest, J. A. H., Roscoe, P., Prescott, L. F. and Stevenson, I. H., 1974, Abnormal drug metabolism following barbiturate and paracetamol overdose, *British Medical Journal*, **4**, 499–502.

Forster, C., Magerl, W., Beck, A., Geisslinger, G., Gall, T., Brune, K. and Handwerker, H. O., 1992, Differential effects of dipyrone, ibuprofen, and paracetamol on experimentally induced pain in man, *Agents and Actions*, **35**, 112–121.

Forsyth, B. W., Horwitz, R. I., Acampora, D., Shapiro, E. D., Viscoli, C. M., Feinstein, A. R., Henner, R., Holabird, N. B., Jones, B. A., Karabelas, A. D. E., Kramer, M. S., Miclette, M. and Wells, J. A., 1989, New epidemiological evidence confirming that bias does not explain the aspirin/Reye's syndrome association, *Journal of the American Medical Association*, **261**, 2517–2524.

Fort, D. J., Rayburn, J. R. and Bantle, J. A., 1992, Evaluation of acetaminophen-induced developmental toxicity using FETAX, *Drug and Chemical Toxicology*, **15**, 329–350.

Forte, A. J. and Nelson, S. D., 1980, Comparison of the distribution and covalent binding of acetaminophen and N-methylacetaminophen, *Pharmacologist*, **22**, 229.

Forte, A. J., Wilson, J. M., Slattery, J. T. and Nelson, S. D., 1984, The formation and toxicity of catechol metabolites of acetaminophen in mice, *Drug Metabolism and Disposition: The Biological Fate of Chemicals*, **12**, 484–491.

Forth, W., 1993, Zum Tod durch Paracetamol: eine besondere britische Variante? *Münchener Medizinische Wochenschrift*, **135**, 25.

Fortunati, E., Debetto, P., Borella, S. and Bianchi, V., 1993, Inhibition of cell growth and alteration of cytosolic calcium levels in the cytotoxicity evaluation of nine MEIC chemicals, *Toxicology in Vitro*, **7**, 511–516.

Fossa, A. A., Hadley, W. M. and Born, J. L., 1979, Decrease in acetaminophen toxicity in mice treated with metyrapone, *Toxicology Letters*, **4**, 379–384.

Fouse, B. L. and Hodgson, E., 1987, Effect of chlordecone and mirex on the acute hepato-toxicity of acetaminophen in mice, *General Pharmacology*, **18**, 623–630.

Foust, R. T., Reddy, K. R., Jeffers, L. J. and Schiff, E. R., 1989, Nyquil-associated liver injury, *American Journal of Gastroenterology*, **84**, 422–425.

Fowler, L. M., Moore, R. B., Foster, J. R. and Lock, E. A., 1991, Nephrotoxicity of 4-aminophenol glutathione conjugate, *Human and Experimental Toxicology*, **10**, 451–459.

Fowler, M. W. and Altmiller, D. H., 1978, A rapid, micromethod for the determination of acetaminophen in serum by high performance liquid chromatography, *Clinical Chemistry*, **24**, 1007.

Frachet, B., Genes, N. and Rezvani, Y., 1991, Efficacité et tolérance de l'acide tiaprofénique (Surgam) dans les sinusites aiguës de l'adulte. Résultats d'une étude randomisée contre paracétamol et contre placebo, *Annales d'Oto-Laryngologie et de Chirurgie Cervico-Faciale*, **108**, 364–369.

Frame, W. T., Allison, R. H., Moir, D. D. and Nimmo, W. S., 1984, Effect of naloxone on gastric emptying during labour, *British Journal of Anaesthesia*, **56**, 263–266.

Frame, J. W. and Rout, P. G. J., 1986, A comparison of the analgesic efficacy of flurbiprofen, diclofenac, dihydrocodeine/paracetamol and placebo following oral surgery, *British Journal of Clinical Practice*, **40**, 463–467.

Francavilla, A., Azzarone, A., Carrieri, G., Cillo, U., van Thiel, D., Subbottin, V. and Starzl, T. E., 1993, Administration of hepatic stimulatory substance alone or with other liver growth factors does not ameliorate acetaminophen-induced liver failure, *Hepatology*, **17**, 429–433.

Francavilla, A., Makowka, L., Polimeno, L., Barone, M., Demetris, J., Guglielmi, F. W., Ambrosino, G., van Thiel, D. H. and Starzl, T. E., 1988, A new model of acute hepatic failure in dogs with implications for transplantation research, *Transplantation Proceedings*, **20 (Suppl. 1)**, 713–715.

Francavilla, A., Makowka, L., Polimeno, L., Barone, M., Demetris, J., Prelich, J., van Thiel, D. H. and Starzl, T. E., 1989, A dog model for acetaminophen-induced fulminant hepatic failure, *Gastroenterology*, **96**, 470–478.

Frank, G. J. and Kefford, R. H., 1983, Report of a double-blind crossover study to compare flurbiprofen with paracetamol in the treatment of primary dysmenorrhoea, *Journal of International Medical Research*, **11 (Suppl. 2)**, 6–10.

Fraser, N. C., 1980, Accidental poisoning deaths in British children 1958–77, *British Medical Journal*, **280**, 1595–1598.

Frati, M. E., Marruecos, L., Porta, M., Martin, M. L. and Laporte, J.-R., 1983, Acute severe poisoning in Spain: clinical outcome related to the implicated drugs, *Human Toxicology*, **2**, 625–632.

Freeman, D. A. and Manoguerra, A. S., 1982, Outcome of salicylate and acetaminophen ingestions initially managed by a regional poison control center, *Veterinary and Human Toxicology*, **21 (Suppl.)**, 73–75.

Fregnan, G. B., Chieli, T. and Prada, M., 1982, The protective effect of dihydroxy-dibutyl-ether against acute drug-induced intoxication in rodents, *Acta Therapeutica*, **8**, 189–198.

Frerich, D. and Krumme, U., 1981, Comparison of the analgesic efficacy of fluproquazone, propoxyphene and paracetamol in post-hysterectomy pain, *Arzneimittel-Forschung*, **31**, 925–927.

Frey, H.-H. and Dengjel, C., 1976, Antagonism of arachidonic acid-induced broncho-constriction in cats by aspirin-like analgesics, *European Journal of Pharmacology*, **40**, 345–348.

Friederiszick, F. K. and Toussaint, W., 1966, Wirkungen von Phenazetin und NAPAP auf das Blutbild des Säuglings, *Medizinische Klinik*, **61**, 304–307.

Friedman, A. D. and Barton, L. L., 1990, Efficacy of sponging vs. acetaminophen for reduction of fever, *Pediatric Emergency Care*, **6**, 6–7.

Friedman, G. D. and Ury, H. K., 1980, Initial screening for carcinogenicity of commonly used drugs, *Journal of the National Cancer Institute*, **65**, 723–733.

Friedman, J. M., Little, B. B., Brent, R. L., Cordero, J. F., Hanson, J. W. and Shepard, T. H., 1990, Potential human teratogenicity of frequently prescribed drugs, *Obstetrics and Gynecology*, **75**, 594–599.

Friedman, S., Gatti, M. and Baker, T., 1993, Cesarean section after maternal acetaminophen overdose, *Anesthesia and Analgesia*, **77**, 632–634.

Friis, H. and Andreasen, P. B., 1992, Drug-induced hepatic injury: an analysis of 1100 cases reported to the Danish committee on adverse drug reactions between 1978 and 1987, *Journal of Internal Medicine*, **232**, 133–138.

Frings, C. S. and Saloom, J. M., 1979, Colorimetric method for the quantitative determination of acetaminophen in serum, *Clinical Toxicology*, **15**, 67–73.

Frisinette-Fich, C., Lundberg, M. and Sörensen, J., 1986, Avslutade fasta med vin och paracetamol. Patient fick lever- och njurskada, *Läkartidningen*, **83**, 2757–2758.

Fritz, A. K., Benziger, D. P., Peterson, J. E., Park, G. B. and Edelson, J., 1984, Relative bioavailability and pharmacokinetics: a combination of pentazocine and acetaminophen, *Journal of Pharmaceutical Sciences*, **73**, 326–331.

Frommel, Ed., Gold, Ph., Melkonian, D., Radouco, C., Delmonte, J., Valette, F. and de Quay, M.-B., 1953, Le N-acétyl p-aminophénol: comparaison de l'effet antithermique et analgésique de ce corps à celui de l'antipyrine, de la phénacétin, du pyramidon et de la quinine, *Praxis*, **42**, 968–972.

Fudin, R., Prego, J., Schwartz, M., Shostak, A., Jaichenko, J. and Gotloib, L., 1989, Sequential hemofiltration in MOF associated with paracetamol intoxication and gram-negative sepsis, *Intensive Care Medicine*, **15**, 328.

Fulkerson, J. P. and Folcik, M. A., 1986, Analgesia following arthroscopic surgery: comparison of diflunisal and acetaminophen with codeine, *Arthroscopy*, **2**, 108–110.

Fulton, B., James, O. and Rawlins, M. D., 1979, The influence of age on the pharmacokinetics of paracetamol, *British Journal of Clinical Pharmacology*, **7**, 418P.

Fulton, J. D. and McGonigal, G., 1989, Steroid responsive haemolytic anaemia due to dextropropoxyphene paracetamol combination, *Journal of the Royal Society of Medicine*, **82**, 228.

Funatsu, K., Ishii, M., Mizuno, Y., Oda, M. and Tsuchiya, M., 1987, Ultrastructural and biochemical study on acute liver injury induced by continuous intravenous infusion of acetaminophen in rats, *Journal of Clinical Electron Microscopy*, **20**, 569–570.

Furman, K. I., 1982, Paracetamol as a cause of analgesic nephropathy, *South African Medical Journal*, **62**, 885.

Furman, K. I., Galasko, G. T. F., Meyers, A. M. and Rabkin, R., 1976, Post-transplantation analgesic dependence in patients who formerly suffered from analgesic nephropathy, *Clinical Nephrology*, **5**, 54–56.

Furman, K. I., Kündig, H. and Lewin, J. R., 1981, Experimental paracetamol nephropathy and pyelonephritis in rats, *Clinical Nephrology*, **16**, 271–275.

Furuhama, K., Benson, R. W., Pumford, N. R., Rowland, K. L. and Hinson, J. A., 1989a, Immunochemical quantitation of 3-(cystein-S-yl)acetaminophen protein adducts in kidney of rats treated with nephrotoxic doses of acetaminophen and p-aminophenol, *Toxicologist*, **9**, 47.

Furuhama, K., Roberts, D. W., McRae, T. A. and Hinson, J. A., 1989b, Evidence that the nephrotoxicities of acetaminophen and p-aminophenol are not mediated by metabolism of the glutathione conjugates, *FASEB Journal*, **3**, A740.

Furukawa, N., Sato, M. and Suzuki, Y., 1986, Effects of O,O,O-tri-n-alkyl phosphorothioates on acetaminophene-induced hepatotoxicity in rats, *Toxicology Letters*, **34**, 95–98.

Fyfe, A. I. and Wright, J. M., 1990, Chronic acetaminophen ingestion associated with (1; 7) (p11; p11) translocation and immune deficiency syndrome, *American Journal of Medi-*

cine, **88**, 443–444.

Gabriel, J., Gawronska-Szklarz, B. and Wójcicki, J., 1985, Farmakokinetyka paracetamolo podanego doustnie chorym ze ze zwezeniem odzwiernika, *Polski Tygodnik Lekarski*, **40**, 1465–1468.

Gabriel, R., Caldwell, J. and Hartley, R. B., 1982, Acute tubular necrosis caused by therapeutic doses of paracetamol? *Clinical Nephrology*, **18**, 269–271.

Gadomski, A., 1994, Rational use of over-the-counter medications in young children, *Journal of the American Medical Association*, **272**, 1063–1064.

Gadomski, A. M., Permutt, T. and Stanton, B., 1994, Correcting respiratory rate for the presence of fever, *Journal of Clinical Epidemiology*, **47**, 1043–1049.

Gaillard, Y. and Fréville, J. C., 1993, Schéma d'un arbre décisionnel à propos d'une intoxication aiguë par le paracétamol, *Lyon Pharmaceutique*, **44**, 121–123.

Gainant, A., Sautereau, D., Rigault, M., Denax, A., Nouaille, Y., Pillegand, B. and Cubertafond, P., 1989, Sténose rectale iatrogène par suppositoires de Véganine, *Gastroentérologie Clinique et Biologique*, **13**, 951.

Gainsborough, N., Maskrey, V. L., Nelson, M. L., Keating, J., Sherwood, R. A., Jackson, S. H. D. and Swift, C. G., 1993a, The association of age with gastric emptying, *Age and Ageing*, **22**, 37–40.

Gainsborough, N., Maskrey, V. L., Nelson, M. L., Keating, J., Sherwood, R. A., Jackson, S. H. D. and Swift, C. G., 1993b, The association of age with gastric emptying, *Journal of Age Related Disorders*, **5**, 6–7.

Gale, G. R., Atkins, L. M., Smith, A. B., Lamar, C. and Walker, E. M., 1987, Acetaminophen-induced hepatotoxicity: antagonistic action of caffeine in mice, *Research Communications in Chemical Pathology and Pharmacology*, **55**, 203–225.

Gale, G. R., Atkins, L. M., Smith, A. B. and Walker, E. M., 1986a, Effects of caffeine on acetaminophen-induced hepatotoxicity and cadmium redistribution in mice, *Research Communications in Chemical Pathology and Pharmacology*, **51**, 337–350.

Gale, G. R., Atkins, L. M., Smith, A. B., Walker, E. M. and Fody, E. P., 1986b, Effect of acetaminophen on cadmium metabolism in mice, *Toxicology and Applied Pharmacology*, **82**, 368–377.

Gale, G. R. and Smith, A. B., 1988, Interaction of caffeine with acetaminophen in mice: schedule dependency of the antagonism by caffeine of acetaminophen hepatotoxicity and the effects of caffeine metabolites, allopurinol, and diethyl ether, *Research Communications in Chemical Pathology and Pharmacology*, **59**, 305–320.

Galinsky, R. E., 1986, Role of glutathione turnover in drug sulfation: differential effects of diethylmaleate and buthionine sulfoximine on the pharmacokinetics of acetaminophen in the rat, *Journal of Pharmacology and Experimental Therapeutics*, **236**, 133–139.

Galinsky, R. E., Alexander, D. P. and Franklin, M. R., 1987a, Effect of cyclosporine on hepatic oxidative and conjugative metabolism in rats, *Drug Metabolism and Disposition: The Biological Fate of Chemicals*, **15**, 731–733.

Galinsky, R. E. and Chalasinka, B., 1988, Effect of taurolithocholate on *in vivo* sulfation and glucuronidation of acetaminophen in rats, *Pharmaceutical Research*, **5**, 61–64.

Galinsky, R. E. and Corcoran, G. B., 1986, Influence of advanced age on the formation and elimination of acetaminophen metabolites by male rats, *Pharmacology*, **32**, 313–320.

Galinsky, R. E. and Corcoran, G. B., 1988, Suppression of acetaminophen conjugation and of conjugate elimination in the rat by metyrapone, a classical P-450 inhibitor, *Drug Metabolism and Disposition: The Biological Fate of Chemicals*, **16**, 348–354.

Galinsky, R. E., Johnson, D. H., Kane, R. E. and Franklin, M. R., 1990, Effect of aging on hepatic biotransformation in female Fischer 344 rats: changes in sulfotransferase activities are consistent with known gender-related changes in pituitary growth hormone secretion in aging animals, *Journal of Pharmacology and Experimental Therapeutics*, **255**, 577–583.

Galinsky, R. E., Kane, R. E. and Franklin, M. R., 1986, Effect of aging on drug-metabolizing enzymes important in acetaminophen elimination, *Journal of Pharmacology and Experimental Therapeutics*, **237**, 107–113.

Galinsky, R. E. and Levy, G., 1979, Effect of N-acetylcysteine on the pharmacokinetics of acetaminophen in rats, *Life Sciences*, **25**, 693–700.

Galinsky, R. E. and Levy, G., 1981, Dose and time-dependent elimination of acetaminophen in rats: pharmacokinetic implications of cosubstrate depletion, *Journal of Pharmacology and Experimental Therapeutics*, **219**, 14–20.

Galinsky, R. E. and Levy, G., 1982, Effect of cimetidine on acetaminophen pharmacokinetics in rats, *International Journal of Pharmaceutics*, **10**, 301–306.

Galinsky, R. E. and Levy, G., 1984a, Evaluation of activated charcoal-sodium sulfate combination for inhibition of acetaminophen absorption and repletion of inorganic sulfate, *Journal of Toxicology. Clinical Toxicology*, **22**, 21–30.

Galinsky, R. E. and Levy, G., 1984b, Absorption and metabolism of acetaminophen shortly after parturition, *Drug Intelligence and Clinical Pharmacy*, **18**, 977–979.

Galinsky, R. E., Manning, B. W., Kimura, R. E. and Franklin, M. R., 1992, Changes in conjugative enzyme activity and acetaminophen metabolism in young and senescent male F-344 rats following prolonged exposure to buthionine sulfoximine, *Experimental Gerontology*, **27**, 221–232.

Galinsky, R. E., Nelson, E. B. and Rollins, D. E., 1987b, Pharmacokinetic consequences and toxicological implications of metyrapone-induced alterations of acetaminophen elimination in man, *European Journal of Clinical Pharmacology*, **33**, 391–396.

Galinsky, R. E., Slattery, J. T. and Levy, G., 1979, Effect of sodium sulfate on acetaminophen elimination by rats, *Journal of Pharmaceutical Sciences*, **68**, 803–805.

Gallacher, G., Coxon, R., Landon, J., Rae, C. J. and Abukinesha, R., 1988, Design of the immunogen and label for use in a fluoroimmunoassay for paracetamol, *Annals of Clinical Biochemistry*, **25**, 42–48.

Gallardo, F. and Rossi, E., 1990, Analgesic efficacy of flurbiprofen as compared to acetaminophen and placebo after periodontal surgery, *Journal of Periodontology*, **61**, 224–227.

Gallego, N., Teruel, J. L., Mampaso, F., Gonzalo, A. and Ortuno, J., 1991, Acute interstitial nephritis superimposed on glomerulonephritis: report of a case, *Pediatric Nephrology*, **5**, 229–231.

Gandy, J., Millner, G. C., Bates, H. K., Casciano, D. A. and Harbison, R. D., 1990, Effects of selected chemicals on the glutathione status in the male reproductive system of rats, *Journal of Toxicology and Environmental Health*, **29**, 45–57.

Garcia Domínguez, M. D., Lucena González, M. I., Ramírez Torres, J. M., Andrade Bellido, R. J. and Sánchez de la Cuesta, F., 1992, Patrón de utilización de medicamentos en una población geriátrica ambulatoria, *Revista Clínica Española*, **191**, 412–415.

Garland, W. A., Hsaio, K. C., Pantuck, E. J. and Conney, A. H., 1977, Quantitative determination of phenacetin and its metabolite acetaminophen by GLC-chemical ionization mass spectrometry, *Journal of Pharmaceutical Sciences*, **66**, 340–344.

Garle, M. J., Khan, J. and Fry, J. R., 1988, Depletion of glutathione by the hepatotoxins paracetamol and bromobenzene, and their non-hepatotoxic analogues, in a fortified liver microsomal system, *Toxicology in Vitro*, **2**, 247–252.

Garnier, R. and Bismuth, C., 1993, Liver failure induced by paracetamol, *British Medical Journal*, **306**, 718.

Garnier, R., Riboulet-Delmas, G. and Efthymiou, M. L., 1982, Intoxications aiguës par le paracétamol soluble: étude rétrospective des donneés du Centre Anti-poisons de Paris 1974–1981, *Semaine des Hôpitaux de Paris*, **58**, 435–439.

Garrido, A., Arancibia, C., Campos, R. and Valenzuela, A., 1991, Acetaminophen does not induce oxidative stress in isolated rat hepatocytes: its probable antioxidant effect is potentiated by the flavonoid silybin, *Pharmacology and Toxicology*, **69**, 9–12.

Garrido, A., Fairlie, J., Guerra, R., Campos, R. and Valenzuela, A., 1989, The flavonoid silybin ameliorates the protective effect of ethanol on acetaminophen hepatotoxicity,

537

Research Communications in Substances of Abuse, **10**, 193–196.

Gates, T. N. and Temple, A. R., 1989, Analgesic use and chronic renal disease, *New England Journal of Medicine*, **321**, 1125.

Gaudreault, P., Guay, J., Nicol, O. and Dupuis, C., 1988, Pharmacokinetics and clinical efficacy of intrarectal solution of acetaminophen, *Canadian Journal of Anaesthesia*, **35**, 149–152.

Gault, M. H., Rudwal, T. C. and Redmond, N. I., 1968, Analgesic habits of 500 veterans: incidence and complications of abuse, *Canadian Medical Association Journal*, **98**, 619–626.

Gaunt, S. D., Baker, D. C. and Green, R. A., 1981, Clinicopathologic evaluation of N-acetylcysteine therapy in acetaminophen toxicosis in the cat, *American Journal of Veterinary Research*, **42**, 1982–1984.

Gautry, Ph. and Bussereau, M., 1984, L'hyperthermie de l'enfant, efficacité du soluté buvable de paracétamol, *Semaine des Hôpitaux de Paris*, **60**, 63–65.

Gawel, M. J., Szalai, J. F., Stiglick, A., Aimola, N. and Weiner, M., 1990, Evaluation of analgesic agents in recurring headache compared with other clinical pain models, *Clinical Pharmacology and Therapeutics*, **47**, 504–508.

Gawronska-Szklarz, B., Gabriel, J. and Wójcicki, J., 1988, Pharmacokinetics of paracetamol in patients with stomach cancer, *Polish Journal of Pharmacology and Pharmacy*, **40**, 41–45.

Gawronska-Szklarz, B., Stankowska-Chomicz, A., Wójcicki, J. and Bay, B., 1985, Farmakokinetyka paracetamolu u osób pozostajacych w pozycji lezacej, *Polski Tygodnik Lekarski*, **40**, 309–311.

Gazzard, B. G., Clark, R., Borirakchanyavat, V. and Williams, R., 1974a, A controlled trial of heparin therapy in the coagulation defect of paracetamol-induced hepatic necrosis, *Gut*, **15**, 89–93.

Gazzard, B. G., Davis, M., Spooner, J. B. and Williams, R., 1976a, Why do people use paracetamol for suicide? *British Medical Journal*, **1**, 212–213.

Gazzard, B. G., Ford-Hutchinson, A. W., Smith, M. J. H. and Williams, R., 1973, The binding of paracetamol to plasma proteins of man and pig, *Journal of Pharmacy and Pharmacology*, **25**, 964–967.

Gazzard, B. G., Henderson, J. M. and Williams, R., 1975a, Early changes in coagulation following a paracetamol overdose and a controlled trial of fresh frozen plasma therapy, *Gut*, **16**, 617–620.

Gazzard, B. G., Hughes, R. D., Mellon, P. J., Portmann, B. and Williams, R., 1975b, A dog model of fulminant hepatic failure produced by paracetamol administration, *British Journal of Experimental Pathology*, **56**, 408–411.

Gazzard, B. G., Hughes, R. D., Portmann, B., Dordoni, B. and Williams, R., 1974b, Protection of rats against the hepatotoxic effect of paracetamol, *British Journal of Experimental Pathology*, **55**, 601–605.

Gazzard, B. G., Hughes, R. D., Widdop, B., Goulding, R., Davis, M. and Williams, R., 1977, Early prediction of the outcome of a paracetamol overdose based on an analysis of 163 patients, *Postgraduate Medical Journal*, **53**, 243–247.

Gazzard, B. G., Langley, P. G., Weston, M. J., Dunlop, E. H. and Williams, R., 1974c, Polymer coating of activated charcoal and its effects on biocompatibility and paracetamol binding, *Clinical Science*, **479**, 97–104.

Gazzard, B. G., Lewis, M. L., Ash, G., Rizza, C. R., Bidwell, E. and Williams, R., 1974d, Coagulation factor concentrate in the treatment of the haemorrhagic diathesis of fulminant hepatic failure, *Gut*, **15**, 993–998.

Gazzard, B. G., Spooner, J. B. and Williams, R. S., 1976b, Why paracetamol? *Journal of International Medical Research*, **4 (Suppl. 4)**, 25–28.

Gazzard, B. G., Willson, R. A., Weston, M. J., Thompson, R. P. H. and Williams, R., 1974e, Charcoal haemoperfusion for paracetamol overdose, *British Journal of Clinical Pharma-*

cology, **1**, 271–275.

Geddes, S. M., Thorburn, J. and Logan, R. W., 1991, Gastric emptying following Caesarean section and the effect of epidural fentanyl, *Anaesthesia*, **46**, 1016–1018.

Gelfand, M. C. and Winchester, J. F., 1980, Hemoperfusion in drug overdosage: a technique when conservative management is not sufficient, *Clinical Toxicology*, **17**, 583–602.

Gelgor, L., Butkow, N. and Mitchell, D., 1992a, Effects of systemic non-steroidal anti-inflammatory drugs on nociception during tail ischaemia and on reperfusion hyper-algesia in rats, *British Journal of Pharmacology*, **105**, 412–416.

Gelgor, L., Cartmell, S. and Mitchell, D., 1992b, Intracerebroventricular micro-injections of non-steroidal anti-inflammatory drugs abolish reperfusion hyperalgesia in the rat's tail, *Pain*, **50**, 323–329.

Gemborys, M. W., Gribble, G. W. and Mudge, G. H., 1978, Synthesis of N-hydroxyacetaminophen, a postulated toxic metabolite of acetaminophen, and its phenol-ic sulfate conjugate, *Journal of Medicinal Chemistry*, **21**, 649–652.

Gemborys, M. W. and Mudge, G. H., 1981, Formation and disposition of the minor metabo-lites of acetaminophen in the hamster, *Drug Metabolism and Disposition: The Biological Fate of Chemicals*, **9**, 340–351.

Gemborys, M. W., Mudge, G. H. and Gribble, G. W., 1980, Mechanism of decomposition of N-hydroxyacetaminophen, a postulated toxic metabolite of acetaminophen, *Journal of Medicinal Chemistry*, **23**, 304–308.

Gentry, C. A., Paloucek, F. P. and Rodvold, K. A., 1994, Prediction of acetaminophen con-centrations in overdose patients using a Bayesian pharmacokinetic model, *Journal of Toxicology. Clinical Toxicology*, **32**, 17–30.

Georgiou, C. A. and Koupparis, M. A., 1990, Automated flow injection spectrophotometric determination of *para*- and *meta*-substituted phenols of pharmaceutical interest based on their oxidative condensation with 1-nitroso-2-naphthol, *Analyst*, **115**, 309–313.

Gérard, A., Roche, G., Presles, O., Canton, Ph. and Dureux, J.-B., 1982, Syndromes de Lyell médicamenteux: à propos de neuf observations, *Thérapie*, **37**, 475–480.

Gerber, J. G., MacDonald, J. S., Harbison, R. D., Villeneuve, J.-P., Wood, A. J. J. and Nies, A. S., 1977, Effect of N-acetylcysteine on hepatic covalent binding of paracetamol (acetaminophen), *Lancet*, **i**, 657–658.

Gerber, M. A., Kaufmann, H., Klion, F. and Alpert, L. I., 1980, Acetaminophen associated hepatic injury, *Human Pathology*, **11**, 37–42.

Gerhardt, C., 1853, Recherches sur les acides organiques anhydres, *Annales de Chimie*, **37**, 285–342.

Gerson, R. J., Casini, A., Gilfor, D., Serroni, A. and Farber, J. L., 1985, Oxygen-mediated cell injury in the killing of cultured hepatocytes by acetaminophen, *Biochemical and Bio-physical Research Communications*, **126**, 1129–1137.

Gertzbein, S. D., Tile, M., McMurty, R. Y., Kellam, J. F., Hunter, G. A., Keith, R. G., Har-sanyi, Z. and Luffman, J., 1986, Analysis of the analgesic efficacy of acetaminophen 1000 mg, codeine phosphate 60 mg, and the combination of acetaminophen 1000 mg and codeine phosphate in the relief of postoperative pain, *Pharmacotherapy*, **6**, 104–107.

Getek, T. A., Korfmacher, W. A., McRae, T. A. and Hinson, J. A., 1989, Utility of solution electrochemistry mass spectrometry for investigating the formation and detection of bio-logically important conjugates of acetaminophen, *Journal of Chromatography*, **474**, 245–256.

Ghauri, F. Y. K., McLean, A. E. M., Beales, D., Wilson, I. D. and Nicholson, J. K., 1993, Induction of 5-oxoprolinuria in the rat following chronic feeding with N-acetyl-4-amino-phenol (paracetamol), *Biochemical Pharmacology*, **46**, 953–957.

Ghosh, A. B. and De, M. K., 1983, Experimental studies in paracetamol induced hepatic necrosis, *Calcutta Medical Journal*, **80**, 122–126.

Gichner, T., Veleminský, J., Wagner, E. D. and Plewa, M. J., 1993, Inhibitory effects of aceta-minophen, 7,8-benzoflavone and methimazole towards N-nitrosodimethylamine mutagenesis in *Arabidopsis thaliana*, *Mutation Research*, **300**, 57–61.

Giellen, M. L. and Bussereau, M., 1985, The antipyretic efficacy of an oral solution of paracetamol in the young child, *Acta Therapeutica*, **11**, 199–208.

Gilani, A. H. and Janbaz, K. H., 1992, Prevention of acetaminophen-induced liver damage by Berberis aristata leaves, *Biochemical Society Transactions*, **20**, 347S.

Gilani, A. H. and Janbaz, K. H., 1993, Protective effect of *Artemisia scoparia* extract against acetaminophen-induced hepatotoxicity, *General Pharmacology*, **24**, 1455–1458.

Gilani, A. H., Janbaz, K. H. and Javed, M. H., 1993, Hepatoprotective activity of *Cichorium intybus*, an indigenous medicinal plant, *Medical Science Research*, **21**, 151–152.

Gilbert, M. M., De Sola Pool, N. and Schecter, C., 1976, Analgesic/calmative effects of acetaminophen and phenyltoloxamine in treatment of simple nervous tension accompanied by headache, *Current Therapeutic Research*, **20**, 53–58.

Gillette, J. R., 1974a, A perspective on the role of chemically reactive metabolites of foreign compounds in toxicity – I. Correlation of changes in covalent binding of reactive metabolites with changes in the incidence and severity of toxicity, *Biochemical Pharmacology*, **23**, 2785–2794.

Gillette, J. R., 1974b, A perspective on the role of chemically reactive metabolites of foreign compounds in toxicity – II. Alterations in the kinetics of covalent binding, *Biochemical Pharmacology*, **23**, 2927–2938.

Gillette, J. R., Nelson, S. D., Mulder, G. J., Jollow, D. J., Mitchell, J. R., Pohl, L. R. and Hinson, J. A., 1981, Formation of chemically reactive metabolites of phenacetin and acetaminophen, *Advances in Experimental Medicine and Biology*, **136 Pt B**, 931–950.

Gilman, A., 1964, Analgesic nephropathy. A pharmacological analysis, *American Journal of Medicine*, **36**, 167–173.

Gilmore, J. T. and Tourvas, E., 1977, Paracetamol-induced acute pancreatitis, *British Medical Journal*, **1**, 753–754.

Gimson, A. E. S., Braude, S., Mellon, P. J., Canalese, J. and Williams, R., 1983, Earlier charcoal haemoperfusion in fulminant hepatic failure, *Lancet*, **ii**, 681–683.

Gin, T., Cho, A. M. W., Lew, J. K. L., Lau, G. S. N., Yuen, P. M., Critchley, J. A. J. H. and Oh, T. E., 1991, Gastric emptying in the postpartum period, *Anaesthesia and Intensive Care*, **19**, 521–524.

Ginsberg, G. L. and Cohen, S. D., 1985, Plasma membrane alterations and covalent binding to organelles after an hepatotoxic dose of acetaminophen (APAP), *Toxicologist*, **5**, 154.

Ginsberg, G. L., Placke, M. E., Wyand, D. S. and Cohen, S. D., 1982, Protection against acetaminophen-induced hepatotoxicity by prior treatment with fenitrothion, *Toxicology and Applied Pharmacology*, **66**, 383–399.

Giri, A. K., 1993, The genetic toxicology of paracetamol and aspirin: a review, *Mutation Research*, **296**, 199–210.

Giri, A. K., Sai Sivam, S. and Khan, K. A., 1992, Sister-chromatid exchange and chromosome aberrations induced by paracetamol *in vivo* in bone-marrow cells of mice, *Mutation Research*, **278**, 253–258.

Girre, C., Hispard, E., Palombo, S., N'Guyen, C. and Dally, S., 1993, Increased metabolism of acetaminophen in chronically alcoholic patients, *Alcoholism: Clinical and Experimental Research*, **17**, 170–173.

Gjellan, K., Graffner, C. and Quiding, H., 1994, Influence of amount of hard fat in suppositories on the *in vitro* release rate and bioavailability of paracetamol and codeine. I. A comparison of three suppository compositions *in vivo*, *International Journal of Pharmaceutics*, **102**, 71–80.

Glazenburg, E. J., Jekel-Halsema, I. M. C., Scholtens, E., Barrs, A. J. and Mulder, G. J., 1983, Effects of variation in the dietary supply of cysteine and methionine on liver concentration of glutathione and 'active sulfate' (PAPS) and serum levels of sulfate, cystine, methionine and taurine: relation to the metabolism of acetaminophen, *Journal of Nutrition*, **113**, 1363–1373.

Gleiberman, A. S., Kuprina-Khramkova, N. I., Rudinskaya-Beloshapkina, T. D. and Abelev, G. I., 1983, Alpha-fetoprotein synthesis in relation to structural peculiarities in postnatal and regenerating mouse liver, *International Journal of Cancer*, **32**, 85–92.

Glenn, E. M., Bowman, B. J. and Rohloff, N. A., 1977, Anti-inflammatory and PG inhibitory effects of phenacetin and acetaminophen, *Agents and Actions*, **7**, 513–516.

Glynn, J. P. and Bastian, W., 1973, Salivary excretion of paracetamol in man, *Journal of Pharmacy and Pharmacology*, **25**, 420–421.

Glynn, J. P. and Kendal, S. E., 1975, Paracetamol measurement, *Lancet*, **i**, 1147–1148.

Gmyrek, D., Kalz, M. and Pietsch, I., 1971, Zur medikamentösen Prophylaxe der Neugebore-nenhyperbilirubinämie II. Mitteil. Einfluss des Induktors Phenylbutazon mit Paraceta-mol bei Frühgeborenen, *Deutsche Gesundheitswesen*, **26**, 1618–1622.

Gmyrek, D. and Klimmt, G., 1971, Ergebnisse einer peroralen Belastung mit Paracetamol bei der Hepatitis infectiosa im Kindesalter, *Deutsche Gesundheitswesen*, **26**, 503–508.

Godellas, C. V., Fabri, P. J., Knierim, T. H., Rosemurgy, A. S. and Gower, W. R., 1992, Hepatic function after porto-systemic shunt, *Journal of Surgical Research*, **52**, 157–160.

Goenechea, S., 1969, Nachweis von Paracetamol im Urin nach Einnahme von thera-peutischen Mengen phenacetinhaltiger Analgetika, *Zeitschrift für Klinische Chemie und Klinische Biochemie*, **7**, 346–349.

Goldberger, L. E. and Talner, L. B., 1975, Analgesic abuse syndrome: a frequently overlooked cause of reversible renal failure, *Urology*, **5**, 728–732.

Golden, D. P., Mosby, E. L., Smith, D. J. and Mackercher, P., 1981, Acetaminophen toxicity. Report of two cases, *Oral Surgery, Oral Medicine, Oral Pathology*, **51**, 385–389.

Golden, N. L., King, K. C. and Sokol, R. J., 1982, Propoxyphene and acetaminophen. Pos-sible effects on the fetus, *Clinical Pediatrics*, **21**, 752–754.

Golden, S. M. and Perman, K. I., 1980, Bilateral clinical anophthalmia: drugs as potential factors, *Southern Medical Journal*, **73**, 1404–1407.

Goldenthal, A. E., 1982, Acetaminophen-complicated nitrite toxicosis in a cat, *Veterinary Medicine – Small Animal Clinician*, **77**, 939–940.

Goldfinger, R., Ahmed, K. S., Pitchumoni, C. S. and Weseley, S. A., 1978, Concomitant alcohol and drug abuse enhancing acetaminophen toxicity, *American Journal of Gastro-enterology*, **70**, 385–388.

Goldhill, D. R., Whelpton, R., Winyard, J. A. and Wilkinson, K. A., 1995, Gastric emptying in patients the day after surgery, *Anaesthesia*, **50**, 122–125.

Goldstein, M. and Nelson, E. B., 1979, Metyrapone as a treatment for acetaminophen (paracetamol) toxicity in mice, *Research Communications in Chemical Pathology and Pharmacology*, **23**, 203–206.

Goldstraw, P. and Bach, P., 1981, Gastric emptying after oesophagectomy as assessed by plasma paracetamol concentrations, *Thorax*, **36**, 493–496.

Golovkin, V. O., 1980, Optimization of the technology and studies of rectal drug forms. IV. The pharmacokinetics and relative biological availability of paracetamol and amidopy-rine in the form of gelatin rectal capsules, *Farmatsevtichnii Zhurnal*, 47–49.

Gomez, M. R., Benzick, A. E., Rogers, L. K., Heird, W. C. and Smith, C. V., 1994, Attenuation of acetaminophen hepatotoxicity in mice as evidence for the bioavailability of the cys-teine in D-glucose-L-cysteine *in vivo*, *Toxicology Letters*, **70**, 101–108.

Gómez-Lechón, M. J., Montoya, A., López, P., Donato, T., Larrauri, A. and Castell, J. V., 1988, The potential use of cultured hepatocytes in predicting the hepatotoxicity of xeno-biotics, *Xenobiotica*, **18**, 725–735.

Gommaa, A. A. and Osman, F. H., 1983, Influence of acetaminophen-induced hepatic nec-rosis on the pharmacokinetics of levonorgestrel, *Contraception*, **28**, 149–157.

Gonwa, T. A., Corbett, W. T., Schey, H. M. and Buckalew, V. M., 1980, Analgesic-associated nephropathy and transitional cell carcinoma of the urinary tract, *Annals of Internal Medicine*, **93**, 249–252.

González, R., Pascual, C., Ancheta, O., Carreras, B., Remírez, D. and Pellón, R., 1992, Hepatoprotective effects of lobenzarit disodium on acetaminophen-induced liver damage in mice, *Agents and Actions*, **37**, 114–120.

González, R., Remirez, D., Rodriguez, S., González, A., Ancheta, O., Merino, N. and Pascual, C., 1994, Hepatoprotective effects of Propolis extract on paracetamol-induced liver damage in mice, *Phytotherapy Research*, **8**, 229–232.

Goodman, M. J., Kent, P. W. and Truelove, S. C., 1977, Inhibition of glucosamine synthesis by salicylates, hydrocortisone and two non-ulcerogenic drugs, *Archives Internationales de Pharmacodynamie et de Thérapie*, **226**, 4–10.

Goon, D. and Klaassen, C. D., 1990, Dose-dependent intestinal glucuronidation and sulfation of acetaminophen in the rat *in situ*, *Journal of Pharmacology and Experimental Therapeutics*, **252**, 201–207.

Goon, D. and Klaassen, C. D., 1992, Effects of microsomal enzyme inducers upon UDP-glucuronic acid concentration and UDP-glucuronosyltransferase activity in the rat intestine and liver, *Toxicology and Applied Pharmacology*, **115**, 253–260.

Gordon, M. J., Skillman, J. J., Edwards, B. G. and Silen, W., 1974, Effect of ethanol, acetylsalicylic acid, acetaminophen, and ferrous sulfate on gastric mucosal permeability in man, *Surgery*, **76**, 405–412.

Goresky, C. A., Pang, K. S., Schwab, A. J., Barker, F., Cherry, W. F. and Bach, G. G., 1992, Uptake of a protein-bound polar compound, acetaminophen sulfate, by perfused rat liver, *Hepatology*, **16**, 173–190.

Gotelli, G. R., Kabra, P. M. and Marton, L. J., 1977, Determination of acetaminophen and phenacetin in plasma by high-pressure liquid chromatography, *Clinical Chemistry*, **23**, 957–959.

Götte, R. and Liedtke, R., 1978, Zum antipyretischen Effekt von Paracetamol: klinische Untersuchungen mit zwei unterschiedlichen Applikationsformen, *Medizinische Klinik*, **73**, 28–33.

Goulding, R., 1993, The fatal paracetamol dosage – how low can you go? *Medicine, Science and the Law*, **33**, 274.

Goulding, R., Volans, G. N., Crome, P., Widdop, B. and Williams, R., 1976, Paracetamol hepatotoxicity, *Lancet*, **i**, 358.

Goulston, K. and Skyring, A., 1964, Effect of paracetamol (N-acetyl-p-aminophenol) on gastrointestinal bleeding, *Gut*, **5**, 463–466.

Gove, C. D., Wardle, E. N. and Williams, R., 1981, Circulating lysosomal enzymes and acute hepatic necrosis, *Journal of Clinical Pathology*, **34**, 13–16.

Grafström, R., Moldéus, P., Andersson, B. and Orrenius, S., 1979a, Xenobiotic metabolism by isolated rat small intestinal cells, *Medical Biology*, **57**, 287–293.

Grafström, R., Ormstad, K., Moldéus, P. and Orrenius, S., 1979b, Paracetamol metabolism in the isolated perfused rat liver with further metabolism of biliary paracetamol conjugate by the small intestine, *Biochemical Journal*, **28**, 3573–3579.

Graham, D. Y. and Smith, J. L., 1985, Effects of aspirin and an aspirin-acetaminophen combination on the gastric mucosa in normal subjects: a double-blind endoscopic study, *Gastroenterology*, **88**, 1922–1925.

Graham, N. M. H., Burrell, C. J., Douglas, R. M., Debelle, P. and Davies, L., 1990, Adverse effects of aspirin, acetaminophen, and ibuprofen on immune function, viral shedding, and clinical status in rhinovirus-infected volunteers, *Journal of Infectious Diseases*, **162**, 1277–1282.

Gramatté, T. and Richter, K., 1993, Paracetamol absorption from different sites in the human small intestine, *British Journal of Clinical Pharmacology*, **37**, 608–611.

Gramolini, C. and Manini, G., 1990, Farmacosorveglianza degli antipiretici. Valutazione del rapporto rischio-beneficio della associazione paracetamolo-sobrerolo. Monitoraggio di 3501 pazienti ambulatoriali, *La Clinica Terapeutica*, **132**, 151–166.

Granados-Soto, V., Flores-Murrieta, F. J., López-Muñoz, F. J., Salazar, L. A., Villarreal, J. E. and Castañeda-Hernández, G., 1992, Relationship between paracetamol plasma levels and its analgesic effect in the rat, *Journal of Pharmacy and Pharmacology*, **44**, 741–744.

Granados-Soto, V., López-Muñoz, F. J., Castañeda-Hernández, G., Salazar, L. A., Villarreal, J. E. and Flores-Murrieta, F. J., 1993, Characterisation of the analgesic effects of paracetamol and caffeine combinations in the pain-induced functional impairment model in the rat, *Journal of Pharmacy and Pharmacology*, **45**, 627–631.

Grant, I. S., Nimmo, W. S. and Clements, J. A., 1981, Lack of effect of ketamine analgesia on gastric emptying in man, *British Journal of Anaesthesia*, **53**, 1321–1323.

Grantham, P. H., Matsushima, T., Mohan, L., Weisburger, E. K. and Weisburger, J. H., 1972, Changes in the metabolism of labelled acetanilide and binding of isotope to serum and liver macromolecules during chronic administration, *Xenobiotica*, **2**, 551–565.

Grantham, P. H., Mohan, L. C., Weisburger, E. K., Fales, H. M., Sokoloski, E. A. and Weisburger, J. H., 1974, Identification of new water-soluble metabolites of acetanilide, *Xenobiotica*, **4**, 69–76.

Gray, T. A., Buckley, B. M. and Vale, J. A., 1987, Hyperlactataemia and metabolic acidosis following paracetamol overdose, *Quarterly Journal of Medicine*, **65**, 811–821.

Greaves, M. W. and McDonald-Gibson, W. J., 1972, Anti-inflammatory agents and prostaglandin biosynthesis, *British Medical Journal*, **3**, 527.

Green, C. E., Dabbs, J. E. and Tyson, C. A., 1984a, Metabolism and cytotoxicity of acetaminophen in hepatocytes isolated from resistant and susceptible species, *Toxicology and Applied Pharmacology*, **76**, 139–149.

Gréen, K., Drvota, V. and Vesterqvist, O., 1989, Pronounced reduction of *in vivo* prostacyclin synthesis in humans by acetaminophen (paracetamol), *Prostaglandins*, **37**, 311–315.

Green, M. D. and Fischer, L. J., 1981, Age- and sex-related differences in acetaminophen metabolism in the rat, *Life Sciences*, **29**, 2421–2428.

Green, M. D. and Fischer, L. J., 1984, Hepatotoxicity of acetaminophen in neonatal and young rats. II. Metabolic aspects, *Toxicology and Applied Pharmacology*, **74**, 125–133.

Green, M. D., Shires, T. K. and Fischer, L. J., 1984b, Hepatotoxicity of acetaminophen in neonatal and young rats. I. Age-related changes in susceptibility, *Toxicology and Applied Pharmacology*, **74**, 116–124.

Greenberg, L. A. and Lester, D., 1946, The metabolic fate of acetanilid and other aniline derivatives. I. Major metabolites of acetanilid appearing in the urine, *Journal of Pharmacology and Experimental Therapeutics*, **88**, 87–98.

Greenberg, L. A. and Lester, D., 1947, The metabolic fate of acetanilid and other aniline derivatives. III. The role of p-aminophenol in the production of methemoglobinemia after acetanilid, *Journal of Pharmacology and Experimental Therapeutics*, **90**, 150–153.

Greenblatt, D. J. and Engelking, L. R., 1988, Enterohepatic circulation of lorazepam and acetaminophen conjugates in ponies, *Journal of Pharmacology and Experimental Therapeutics*, **244**, 674–679.

Greene, J. M. and Winickoff, R. N., 1992, Cost-conscious prescribing of nonsteroidal anti-inflammatory drugs for adults with arthritis. A review and suggestions, *Archives of Internal Medicine*, **152**, 1995–2002.

Greene, J. W., Craft, L. and Ghishan, F., 1983, Acetaminophen poisoning in infancy, *American Journal of Diseases of Children*, **137**, 386–387.

Gregg, N. J., Elseviers, M. M., de Broe, M. E. and Bach, P. H., 1989, Epidemiology and mechanistic basis of analgesic-associated nephropathy, *Toxicology Letters*, **46**, 141–151.

Gregg, N. J., Robbins, M. E. C., Hopewell, J. W. and Bach, P. H., 1990, The effect of acetaminophen on pig kidneys with a 2-bromoethanamine-induced papillary necrosis, *Renal Failure*, **12**, 157–163.

Gregus, Z., Kim, H. J., Madhu, C., Liu, Y., Rozman, P. and Klaassen, C. D., 1994a, Sulfation of acetaminophen and acetaminophen-induced alterations in sulfate and 3′-phosphoadenosine 5′-phosphosulfate homeostasis in rats with deficient dietary intake of sulfur, *Drug Metabolism and Disposition: The Biological Fate of Chemicals*, **22**, 725–730.

Gregus, Z., Madhu, C., Goon, D. and Klaassen, C. D., 1988a, Effect of galactosamine-induced hepatic UDP-glucuronic acid depletion on acetaminophen elimination in rats, *Drug Metabolism and Disposition: The Biological Fate of Chemicals*, **16**, 527–533.

Gregus, Z., Madhu, C. and Klaassen, C. D., 1987, Species variation in biliary and urinary excretion of acetaminophen (AA) metabolites, *Toxicologist*, **7**, 116.

Gregus, Z., Madhu, C. and Klaassen, C. D., 1988b, Species variation in toxication and detoxication of acetaminophen *in vivo*: a comparative study of biliary and urinary excretion of acetaminophen metabolites, *Journal of Pharmacology and Experimental Therapeutics*, **244**, 91–99.

Gregus, Z., Madhu, C. and Klaassen, C. D., 1990, Effect of microsomal enzyme inducers on biliary and urinary excretion of acetaminophen metabolites in rats: decreased hepatobiliary and increased hepatovascular transport of acetaminophen-glucuronide after microsomal enzyme induction, *Drug Metabolism and Disposition: The Biological Fate of Chemicals*, **18**, 10–19.

Gregus, Z., Oguro, T. and Klaassen, C. D., 1994b, Nutritionally and chemically induced impairment of sulfate activation and sulfation of xenobiotiics *in vivo*, *Chemico-Biological Interactions*, **92**, 169–177.

Grewal, K. K. and Racz, W. J., 1993, Intracellular calcium disruption as a secondary event in acetaminophen-induced hepatotoxicity, *Canadian Journal of Physiology and Pharmacology*, **71**, 26–33.

Gribetz, B. and Cronley, S. A., 1987, Underdosing of acetaminophen by parents, *Pediatrics*, **80**, 630–633.

Griener, J. C., Msall, M. E., Cooke, R. E. and Corcoran, G. B., 1990, Noninvasive determination of acetaminophen disposition in Down's syndrome, *Clinical Pharmacology and Therapeutics*, **48**, 520–528.

Griffeth, L. K., Rosen, G. M. and Rauckman, E. J., 1985, Effects of model traumatic injury on hepatic drug metabolism in the rat. V. Sulfation and acetylation, *Drug Metabolism and Disposition: The Biological Fate of Chemicals*, **13**, 398–405.

Grinblat, J., Lewitus, Z. and Rosenfeld, J., 1980, Renal tubular necrosis and liver damage. A possible consequence of low dose of acetaminophen and halothane anesthesia, *Drug Intelligence and Clinical Pharmacy*, **14**, 431–435.

Groarke, J. F., Averett, J. M. and Hirschowitz, B. I., 1977, Acetaminophen and hepatic necrosis, *New England Journal of Medicine*, **296**, 233.

Groom, C. A. and Luong, J. H. T., 1993, Improvement of the selectivity of amperometric biosensors by using a permselective electropolymerized film, *Analytical Letters*, **26**, 1383–1390.

Gross, M., 1946, *Acetanilid: A Critical Bibliographic Review*, New Haven: Hillhouse Press.

Gross, P. A., Levandowski, R. A., Russo, C., Weksler, M., Bonelli, J., Dran, S., Munk, G., Deichmiller, S., Hilsen, R. and Panush, R. F., 1994, Vaccine immune response and side effects with the use of acetaminophen with influenza vaccine, *Clinical and Diagnostic Laboratory Immunology*, **1**, 134–138.

Grove, J., 1971, Gas-liquid chromatography of N-acetyl-p-aminophenol (paracetamol) in plasma and urine, *Journal of Chromatography*, **59**, 289–295.

Gruber, C. M., Baptisti, A., Bauer, R. O., Jain, A., Lash, A. F. and McMahon, F. G., 1977, A multicenter analgesic study using single doses of placebo, propoxyphene and acetaminophen, *Journal of Medicine*, **8**, 35–51.

Grupo de Trabajo DUP España, 1991a, Estudio multicéntrico sobre el uso de medicamentos durante el embarazo en España (II). Los fármacos utilizados durante la gestación, *Medicina Clinica*, **96**, 11–15.

Grupo de Trabajo DUP España, 1991b, Estudio multicéntrico sobre el uso de medicamentos durante el embarazo en España (III). Los fármacos utilizados durante el primer trimestre de la gestación, *Medicina Clinica*, **96**, 52–57.

Gruppo Italiano Studi Epidemiologici in Dermatologia (GISED), 1993, Cutaneous reactions to analgesic-antipyretics and nonsteroidal anti-inflammatory drugs, *Dermatology*, **186**,

164–169.

Grymonpre, R. E., Sitar, D. S., Montgomery, P. R., Mitenko, P. A. and Aoki, F. Y., 1991, Prescribing patterns for older heavy drug users living in the community, *Drug Intelligence and Clinical Pharmacy, the Annals of Pharmacotherapy*, **25**, 186–190.

Grzelewska-Rzymowska, I., Szmidt, M. and Rozniecki, J., 1992, Urticaria/angioedema-type sensitivity to aspirin and other nonsteroidal anti-inflammatory drugs. Diagnostic value of anamnesis and challenge test with acetylsalicylic acid, *Journal of Investigative Allergology and Clinical Immunology*, **2**, 191–195.

Gsell, O., Rechenberg, H. K. and Meischer, P., 1957, Die primar chronische interstitielle Nephritis. II. Die Pathogenese der interstitiellen Nephritis, *Deutsche Medizinische Wochenschrift*, **82**, 1718–1726.

Guarner, F., Broughton-Smith, N. K., Blackwell, G. J. and Moncada, S., 1988, Reduction by prostacyclin of acetaminophen-induced liver toxicity in the mouse, *Hepatology*, **8**, 248–253.

Guarner, F., Hughes, R. D., Gimson, A. E. S. and Williams, R., 1987, Renal function in fulminant hepatic failure: haemodynamics and renal prostaglandins, *Gut*, **28**, 1643–1647.

Guasch, J., Grau, M., Montero, J. L. and Felipe, A., 1990, Pharmaco-toxicological effects of acetaminophen in rodents. Battery of tests to screen potential analgesic acetaminophen derivatives, *Methods and Findings in Experimental and Clinical Pharmacology*, **12**, 141–148.

Guberman, D., 1990, Use of acetaminophen in the community, *Harefuah*, **118**, 17–19.

Guccione, J. L., Zemtsov, A., Cobos, E. and Neldner, K. H., 1993, Acquired purpura fulminans induced by alcohol and acetaminophen: successful treatment with heparin and vitamin K, *Archives of Dermatology*, **129**, 1267–1269.

Guerri, C. and Grisoli, S., 1978, Decreased glutathione in rats due to chronic intake of ethanol, *Federation Proceedings*, **37**, 1541.

Guérin, C., Casez, J. P., Vital-Durand, D. and Levrat, R., 1984, Allergie au paracétamol: un cas d'atteinte hépatique et cutanée, *Thérapie*, **39**, 47–49.

Guin, J. D. and Baker, G. F., 1988, Chronic fixed drug eruption caused by acetaminophen, *Cutis*, **41**, 106–108.

Guin, J. D., Haynie, L. S., Jackson, D. and Baker, G. F., 1987, Wandering fixed drug eruption: a mucocutaneous reaction to acetaminophen, *Journal of the American Academy of Dermatology*, **17**, 399–402.

Gülden, M., Seibert, H. and Voss, J.-U., 1994, The use of cultured skeletal muscle cells in testing for acute systemic toxicity, *Toxicology in Vitro*, **8**, 779–782.

Gumbrecht, J. R. and Franklin, M. R., 1983, The alteration of hepatic cytochrome P-450 subpopulations of phenobarbital-induced and uninduced rat by regioselective hepatotoxins, *Drug Metabolism and Disposition: The Biological Fate of Chemicals*, **11**, 312–318.

Gupta, R. N., 1982, Simpler colorimetry of serum acetaminophen, *Clinical Chemistry*, **28**, 1392–1393.

Gupta, R. N., Eng, F. and Keane, P. M., 1977, Thin-layer chromatographic method for the quantitative analysis of paracetamol (N-acetyl-p-aminophenol) in blood plasma, *Journal of Chromatography*, **143**, 112–114.

Gupta, R. N., Pickersgill, R. and Stefanec, M., 1983, Colorimetric determination of acetaminophen, *Clinical Biochemistry*, **16**, 220–221.

Gupta, S., 1994, Biliary excretion of lysosomal enzymes, iron, and oxidized protein in Fischer-344 and Sprague-Dawley rats and the effects of diquat and acetaminophen, *Toxicology and Applied Pharmacology*, **125**, 42–50.

Gustafsson, B., Hagström, G. and Schmidt, D., 1979, Jämförande toleransstudie med suppositorier av paracetamol och placebo, *Läkartidningen*, **76**, 1631–1632.

Gustafsson, I., Nyström, E. and Quiding, H., 1983, Effect of preoperative paracetamol on pain after oral surgery, *European Journal of Clinical Pharmacology*, **24**, 63–65.

Gustafsson, L. L. and Boëthius, G., 1982, Utilization of analgesics from 1970 to 1978. Prescription patterns in the county of Jämtland and in Sweden as a whole, *Acta Medica Scandinavica*, **211**, 419–425.

Gutknecht, J., 1992, Aspirin, acetaminophen and proton transport through phospholipid bilayers and mitochondrial membranes, *Molecular and Cellular Biochemistry*, **114**, 3–8.

Gutteridge, J. M. C. and Wardle, N., 1981, Peroxidation of liver and brain tissue of paracetamol poisoned rats, *Medical Laboratory Sciences*, **38**, 167–169.

Guzman, F., Braun, C., Lim, R. K. S., Potter, G. D. and Rodgers, D. W., 1964, Narcotic and non-narcotic analgesics which block visceral pain evoked by intra-arterial injection of bradykinin and other algesic agents, *Archives Internationales de Pharmacodynamie et de Thérapie*, **149**, 571–588.

Gwilt, J. R., Robertson, A., Goldman, L. and Blanchard, A. W., 1963a, The absorption characteristics of paracetamol tablets in man, *Journal of Pharmacy and Pharmacology*, **15**, 445–453.

Gwilt, J. R., Robertson, A. and McChesney, E. W., 1963b, Determination of blood and other tissue concentrations of paracetamol in dog and man, *Journal of Pharmacy and Pharmacology*, **15**, 440–444.

Gwilt, P. R., Lear, C. L., Tempero, M. A., Birt, D. D., Grandjean, A. C., Ruddon, R. W. and Nagel, D. L., 1994, The effect of garlic extract on human metabolism of acetaminophen, *Cancer Epidemiology,Biomarkers and Prevention*, **3**, 155–160.

Gwynn, J., Fry, J. R. and Bridges, J. W., 1979, The effect of paracetamol and other foreign compounds on protein synthesis in isolated adult rat hepatocytes, *Biochemical Society Transactions*, **7**, 117–118.

Haanaes, H. R., Benterud, U. J. and Skoglund, L. A., 1986, RF 46-790 vs. paracetamol: effect on post-operative pain, *International Journal of Clinical Pharmacology, Therapy and Toxicology*, **24**, 598–601.

Haapanen, E. J., 1982, Hemoperfusion in acute intoxication. Clinical experience with 48 cases, *Acta Medica Scandinavica*, **668 (Suppl.)**, 76–81.

Habib, S., Matthews, R. W., Scully, C., Levers, B. G. H. and Shepherd, J. P., 1990, A study of the comparative efficay of four common analgesics in the control of postsurgical dental pain, *Oral Surgery, Oral Medicine, Oral Pathology*, **70**, 559–563.

Habior, A., 1992, Effect of captopril on liver glutathione and hepatotoxicity of paracetamol in rats, *Polskie Archiwum Medycyny Wewnetrznej*, **87**, 332–340.

Hackett, L. P. and Dusci, L. J., 1977, Determination of paracetamol in human serum, *Clinica Chimica Acta*, **74**, 187–190.

Hagen, I. J., Haram, E. M. and Laake, K., 1991, Absorption of paracetamol from suppositories in geriatric patients with fecal accumulation in the rectum, *Aging*, **3**, 25–29.

Hagenlocher, M., Soliva, M., Wittwer, F., Ziegler, W. H. and Speiser, P., 1987, Absorption rate and bioavailability of acetaminophen from hard gelatin capsules, *Pharmazeutische Industrie*, **49**, 1290–1294.

Hagiwara, A. and Ward, J. M., 1986, The chronic hepatoxic, tumor-promoting and carcinogenic effects of acetaminophen in male B6C3F$_1$ mice, *Fundamental and Applied Toxicology*, **7**, 376–386.

Hahn, L. and Petruson, B., 1979, The influence of acetylsalicylic acid and paracetamol on menstrual blood loss in women with and without an intrauterine contraceptive device, *American Journal of Obstetrics and Gynecology*, **135**, 393–396.

Haibach, H., Akhter, J. E., Muscato, M. S., Cary, P. L. and Hoffmann, M. F., 1984, Acetaminophen overdose with fetal demise, *American Journal of Clinical Pathology*, **82**, 240–242.

Hajnal, J., Sharp, J. and Popert, A. J., 1959, A method for testing analgesics in rheumatoid arthritis using a sequential procedure, *Annals of the Rheumatic Diseases*, **18**, 189–206.

Hale, P. W. and Poklis, A., 1983, Evaluation of a modified colorimetric assay for the determination of acetaminophen in serum, *Journal of Analytical Toxicology*, **7**, 249–251.

Hale, W. E., May, F. E., Marks, R. G., Moore, M. T. and Stewart, R. B., 1989, Renal effects of nonsteroidal anti-inflammatory drugs in the elderly, *Current Therapeutic Research*, **46**,

173–179.

Hall, A. H., Kulig, K. W. and Rumack, B. H., 1986a, Acetaminophen hepatotoxicity, *Journal of the American Medical Association*, **256**, 1893–1894.

Hall, A. H., Kulig, K. W. and Rumack, B. H., 1986b, Acetaminophen hepatotoxicity in alcoholics, *Annals of Internal Medicine*, **105**, 624.

Hall, A. H., Kulig, K. W. and Rumack, B. H., 1987, Acetaminophen and alcoholics, *Digestive Diseases and Sciences*, **32**, 558.

Hall, A. K. and Curry, C., 1994, Changing epidemiology and management of deliberate self poisoning in Christchurch, *New Zealand Medical Journal*, **107**, 396–399.

Hall, R. C., Brown, D., Carter, R. and Kendall, M. J., 1976a, The effect of desmethylimipramine on the absorption of alcohol and paracetamol, *Postgraduate Medical Journal*, **52**, 139–142.

Hall, S. M., Plaster, P. A., Glasgow, J. F. T. and Hancock, P., 1988, Preadmission antipyretics in Reye's syndrome, *Archives of Disease in Childhood*, **63**, 857–866.

Hall, T. J., James, P. R. and Cambridge, G., 1993, Development of an *in vitro* hepatotoxicity assay for assessing the effects of chronic drug exposure, *Research Communications in Chemical Pathology and Pharmacology*, **79**, 249–256.

Hall, W. J., O'Donoghue, J. P., O'Regan, M. G. and Penny, W. J., 1976b, Endogenous prostaglandins, adenosine 3' : 5'-monophosphate and sodium transport across isolated frog skin, *Journal of Physiology*, **258**, 731–753.

Hallbach, J. and Guder, W. G., 1991, Mechanized toxicological serum tests in screening hospitalized patients, *European Journal of Clinical Chemistry and Clinical Biochemistry*, **29**, 537–547.

Hallworth, M. J., 1983, Enzymatic method for acetaminophen adapted to a centrifugal analyser, *Clinical Chemistry*, **29**, 2123–2124.

Halpern, J., Baerwald, H., Johnson, R., Takita, H. and Ambrus, J. L., 1985, Propoxyphene and acetaminophen mixture (Darvocet)-related radiation-induced pneumonitis, *Archives of Internal Medicine*, **145**, 1509–1510.

Halpin, T. J., Holtzhauer, F. J., Campbell, R. J., Hall, L. J., Correa-Villaseñor, A., Lanese, R., Rice, J. and Hurwitz, E. S., 1982, Reye's syndrome and medication use, *Journal of the American Medical Association*, **248**, 687–691.

Halstead, L. S., Feldman, S., Claus-Walker, J. and Patel, V. C., 1985, Drug absorption in spinal cord injury, *Archives of Physical Medicine and Rehabilitation*, **66**, 298–301.

Ham, K. N., Robinson, I. S., Calder, I. C., Mohandas, J., Duggin, G. G., Horvath, J. S. and Tiller, D. J., 1981, Chronic active hepatitis after prolonged paracetamol (acetaminophen) ingestion, *Medical Journal of Australia*, **1**, 538.

Hamilton, M. and Kissinger, P. T., 1982, Determination of acetaminophen metabolites in urine by liquid chromatography/electrochemistry, *Analytical Biochemistry*, **125**, 143–148.

Hamilton, M. and Kissinger, P. T., 1986, The metabolism of 2- and 3-hydroxyacetanilide: determination of metabolic products by liquid chromatography/electrochemistry, *Drug Metabolism and Disposition: The Biological Fate of Chemicals*, **14**, 5–12.

Hamlyn, A. N., Douglas, A. P. and James, O., 1978, The spectrum of paracetamol (acetaminophen) overdose: clinical and epidemiological studies, *Postgraduate Medical Journal*, **54**, 400–404.

Hamlyn, A. N., Douglas, A. P., James, O. F., Lesna, M. and Watson, A. J., 1977, Liver function and structure in survivors of acetaminophen poisoning. A follow-up study of serum bile acids and liver histology, *American Journal of Digestive Diseases*, **22**, 605–610.

Hamlyn, A. N., Lesna, M., Record, C. O., Smith, P. A., Watson, A. J., Meredith, T., Widdop, B., Volans, G. N. and Crome, P., 1980, Prevention of hepatic necrosis in severe paracetamol (acetaminophen) poisoning: prospective controlled trial of early treatment with cysteamine or methionine, *Gut*, **21**, A448.

Hamlyn, A. N., Lesna, M., Record, C. O., Smith, P. A., Watson, A. J., Meredith, T. J., Volans, G. N. and Crome, P., 1981, Methionine and cysteamine in paracetamol (acetaminophen) overdose, prospective controlled trial of early therapy, *Journal of International Medical Research*, **9**, 226–231.

Hammond, P. M., Scawen, M. D., Atkinson, T., Campbell, R. S. and Price, C. P., 1984, Development of an enzyme-based assay for acetaminophen, *Analytical Biochemistry*, **143**, 152–157.

Hammond, P. M., Scawen, M. D. and Price, C. P., 1981, Enzyme based paracetamol estimation, *Lancet*, **i**, 391–392.

Handa, S. S. and Sharma, A., 1990, Hepatoprotective activity of andrographolide against galactosamine and paracetamol intoxication in rats, *Indian Journal of Medical Research*, **92**, 284–292.

Hanel, A. M. and Lands, W. E. M., 1982, Modification of anti-inflammatory drug effectiveness by ambient lipid peroxides, *Biochemical Pharmacology*, **31**, 3307–3311.

Haney, A. F., Hughes, S. F. and Hughes, C. L., 1988, Effects of acetaminophen and non-steroidal anti-inflammatory drugs on progesterone production by porcine granulosa cells *in vitro*, *Reproductive Toxicology*, **1**, 285–291.

Hangartner, P. J., Bühler, H., Münch, R., Zaruba, K., Stamm, B. and Ammann, R., 1987, Chronische Pankreatitis als wahrschneinliche folge eines Analgetikaabusus: prospektive Untersuchung bei 95 Fällen mit chronischer Niereninsuffizienz mit bzw. ohne Analgetikaabusus, *Schweizerische Medizinische Wochenschrift*, **117**, 638–642.

Hanna, A. N., McDonald, J. S., Miller, C. H. and Couri, D., 1989, Pretreatment with paracetamol inhibits metabolism of enflurane in rats, *British Journal of Anaesthesia*, **62**, 429–433.

Hannothiaux, M. H., Houdret, N., Lhermitte, M., Izydorczak, J. and Roussel, P., 1986, High performance liquid chromatographic determination of paracetamol in human serum, *Annales de Biologie Clinique*, **44**, 139–141.

Hans, P., Brichant, J. F., Bonhomme, V. and Triffaux, M., 1993, Analgesic efficiency of propacetamol hydrochloride after lumbar disc surgery, *Acta Anaesthesiologica Belgica*, **44**, 129–133.

Hansen, P. B., Dalhoff, K., Joffe, P. and Olesen, B., 1991, Fractional excretion of beta-2-microglobulin in the urine of patients with normal or reduced renal function and hepatic coma, *Scandinavian Journal of Gastroenterology*, **26**, 36–42.

Hanson, L., 1993, Acute hepatic decompensation in an alcoholic, *Journal of the Tennessee Medical Association*, **86**, 448.

Hara, Y. and Murayama, S., 1992, Effects of analgesic-antipyretics on the spinal reflex potentials in cats: an analysis of the excitatory action of aminopyrine, *Folia Pharmacologica Japonica*, **100**, 383–390.

Harada, T., Maronpot, R. R., Morris, R. W. and Boorman, G. A., 1989, Observations on altered hepatocellular foci in National Toxicology Program two-year carcinogenicity studies in rats, *Toxicologic Pathology*, **17**, 690–706.

Harasawa, S., Kikuchi, K., Senoue, I., Nomiyama, T. and Miwa, T., 1982, Gastric emptying in patients with gastric ulcers: effects of oral and intramuscular administration of anticholinergic drug, *Tokai Journal of Experimental and Clinical Medicine*, **7**, 551–559.

Harasawa, S., Tani, N., Suzuki, S., Miwa, M., Sakita, R., Nomiyama, T. and Miwa, T., 1979, Gastric emptying in normal subjects and patients with peptic ulcer. A study using the acetaminophen method, *Gastroenterologia Japonica*, **14**, 1–10.

Harbison, R. D., James, R. C. and Roberts, S. M., 1991, Hepatic glutathione suppression by the α-adrenoreceptor stimulating agents phenylephrine and clonidine, *Toxicology*, **69**, 279–290.

Hardin, J. G. and Kirk, K. A., 1979, Comparative effectiveness of five analgesics for the pain of rheumatoid synovitis, *Journal of Rheumatology*, **6**, 405–412.

Harding, J. J., Egerton, M. and Harding, R., 1989, Protection against cataract by aspirin, paracetamol and ibuprofen, *Acta Ophthalmologica*, **67**, 518–524.

Harding, J. J. and van Heyningen, R., 1988, Drugs, including alcohol, that act as risk factors for cataract, and possible protection against cataract by aspirin-like analgesics and cyclopenthiazide, *British Journal of Ophthalmology*, **72**, 809–814.

Hardwick, S. J., Wilson, J. W., Fawthrop, D. J., Boobis, A. R. and Davies, D. S., 1992a, The role of [Ca^{2+}] in paracetamol toxicity: studies in isolated hamster hepatocytes, *Human and Experimental Toxicology*, **11**, 412.

Hardwick, S. J., Wilson, J. W., Fawthrop, D. J., Boobis, A. R. and Davies, D. S., 1992b, Paracetamol toxicity in hamster isolated hepatocytes: the increase in cytosolic calcium accompanies, rather than precedes, loss of viability, *Archives of Toxicology*, **66**, 408–412.

Hardwicke, C., Holt, L., James, R. and Smith, A. J., 1986, Trends in self-poisoning with drugs in Newcastle, New South Wales, 1980–1982, *Medical Journal of Australia*, **144**, 453–454.

Hargreaves, R. J., Evans, J. G., Pelling, D. and Butterworth, K. R., 1982, Studies on the effects of L-ascorbic acid on acetaminophen-induced hepatotoxicity. II. An *in vivo* assessment in mice of the protection afforded by various dosage forms of ascorbate, *Toxicology and Applied Pharmacology*, **64**, 380–392.

Harman, A. W., 1985, The effectiveness of antioxidants in reducing paracetamol-induced damage subsquent to paracetamol activation, *Research Communications in Chemical Pathology and Pharmacology*, **49**, 215–228.

Harman, A. W., Adamson, G. M. and Shaw, S. G., 1992a, Protection from oxidative damage in mouse liver cells, *Toxicology Letters*, **64–65**, 581–587.

Harman, A. W. and Fischer, L. J., 1983, Hamster hepatocytes in culture as a model for acetaminophen toxicity: studies with inhibitors of drug metabolism, *Toxicology and Applied Pharmacology*, **71**, 330–341.

Harman, A. W., Kyle, M. E., Serroni, A. and Farber, J. L., 1991, The killing of cultured hepatocytes by N-acetyl-p-benzoquinone imine (NAPQI) as a model of the cytotoxicity of acetaminophen, *Biochemical Pharmacology*, **41**, 1111–1117.

Harman, A. W., Mahar, S. O., Burcham, P. C. and Madsen, B. W., 1992b, Level of cytosolic free calcium during acetaminophen toxicity in mouse hepatocytes, *Molecular Pharmacology*, **41**, 665–670.

Harman, A. W. and McCamish, L. E., 1986, Age-related toxicity of paracetamol in mouse hepatocytes, *Biochemical Pharmacology*, **35**, 1731–1735.

Harman, A. W. and Self, G., 1986, Comparison of the protective effects of N-acetylcysteine, 2-mercaptopropionylglycine and dithiothreitol against acetaminophen toxicity in mouse hepatocytes, *Toxicology*, **41**, 83–93.

Haroldsen, P. E., Reilly, M. H., Hughes, H., Gaskell, S. J. and Porter, C. J., 1988, Characterization of glutathione conjugates by fast atom bombardment/tandem mass spectrometry, *Biomedical and Environmental Mass Spectrometry*, **15**, 615–621.

Harou-Kouka, M., Haguenoer, J. M., Erb, F., M'Bisi, R., Gayot, A., Traisnel, M., Mathieu, M. and Mathieu, D., 1989, Efficacité des charbons activés dans le traitement des intoxications médicamenteuses, *Journal de Toxicologie Clinique et Expérimentale*, **9**, 255–260.

Harris, A. L., 1982, Paracetamol-induced acute renal failure, *British Medical Journal*, **284**, 825.

Harris, C., Stark, K. L. and Juchau, M. R., 1988, On the prediction of chemical toxicity *in vitro*: biotransformation of acetaminophen (APAP) and 7-OH-acetylaminofluorene (7-OH-AAF), *Toxicologist*, **851**, 32.

Harris, C., Stark, K. L., Luchtel, D. L. and Juchau, M. R., 1989, Abnormal neurulation induced by 7-hydroxy-2-acetylaminofluorene and acetaminophen: evidence for catechol metabolites as proximate dysmorphogens, *Toxicology and Applied Pharmacology*, **101**, 432–446.

Harris, S. R. and Hamrick, M. E., 1993, Antagonism of acetaminophen hepatotoxicity by phospholipase A$_2$ inhibitors, *Research Communications in Chemical Pathology and Pharmacology*, **79**, 23–44.

Harrison, P. M., Keays, R., Bray, G. P., Alexander, G. J. M. and Williams, R., 1990a, Improved outcome of paracetamol-induced fulminant hepatic failure by late administration of acetylcysteine, *Lancet*, **335**, 1572–1573.

Harrison, P. M., O'Grady, J. G., Keays, R. T., Alexander, G. J. M. and Williams, R., 1990b, Serial prothrombin time as prognostic indicator in paracetamol induced fulminant hepatic failure, *British Medical Journal*, **301**, 964–966.

Harrison, P. M., Wendon, J. A., Gimson, A. E. S., Alexander, G. J. M. and Williams, R., 1991, Improvement by acetylcysteine of hemodynamics and oxygen transport in fulminant hepatic failure, *New England Journal of Medicine*, **324**, 1852–1857.

Harry, P., Bourrier, Ph., Bouachour, G., Varache, N. and Alquier, Ph., 1989, La prévention des hépatites fulminantes dues au paracétamol est-elle correctement assurée? (3 observations), *Journal de Toxicologie Clinique et Expérimentale*, **9**, 327–329.

Harry, P. and Varache, N., 1991, Intoxication aiguë par le paracétamol, *Revue du Praticien – Médecine Générale*, **5**, 1035–1036.

Hart, J. G. and Timbrell, J. A., 1979, The effect of age on paracetamol hepatotoxicity in mice, *Biochemical Pharmacology*, **28**, 3015–3017.

Hart, J. L., 1978, Effects of hyperbaric helium-oxygen on the antipyretic actions of aspirin and acetaminophen in rats, *Undersea Biomedical Research*, **5**, 53–62.

Hart, S., Calder, I., Ross, B. and Tange, J., 1980, Renal metabolism of paracetamol: studies in the isolated perfused rat kidney, *Clinical Science*, **58**, 379–384.

Hart, S. J., Calder, I. C. and Tange, J. D., 1982a, The metabolism and toxicity of paracetamol in Sprague-Dawley and Wistar rats, *European Journal of Drug Metabolism and Pharmacokinetics*, **7**, 203–222.

Hart, S. J., Healey, K., Smail, M. C. and Calder, I. C., 1982b, 3-Thiomethylparacetamol sulphate and glucuronide: metabolites of paracetamol and N-hydroxyparacetamol, *Xenobiotica*, **12**, 381–386.

Hart, S. J., Tontodonati, R. and Calder, I. C., 1981, Reversed-phase chromatography of urinary metabolites of paracetamol using ion suppression and ion pairing, *Journal of Chromatography: Biomedical Applications*, **225**, 387–405.

Hartleb, M., 1994, Do thyroid hormones promote hepatotoxicity to acetaminophen? *American Journal of Gastroenterology*, **89**, 1269–1270.

Hartnell, G. G., Cowan, R. A. and Baird, I. M., 1983, Ethanol in paracetamol poisoning, *Lancet*, **i**, 617–618.

Harvey, F. and Goulding, R., 1974, Action of cysteamine in paracetamol poisoning, *Lancet*, **ii**, 1082.

Harvey, F. D. and Levitt, T. E., 1976, Experimental evaluation of paracetamol antidotes, *Journal of International Medical Research*, **4 (Suppl. 4)**, 130–137.

Harvey, J. G. and Spooner, J. B., 1978, Paracetamol poisoning, *British Medical Journal*, **2**, 832–833.

Harvey, J. W., French, T. W. and Senior, D. F., 1986, Hematologic abnormalities associated with chronic acetaminophen administration in a dog, *Journal of the American Veterinary Medical Association*, **189**, 1334–1335.

Harvey, P. W., Routh, M. R., Rees, S. J., Healing, G., Rush, K. C., Purdy, K., Everett, D. J. and Cockburn, A., 1993, Steroid pre-treatments and subsequent hepatic response to paracetamol in rats: do glucocorticoids modulate liver toxicity? *Medical Science Research*, **21**, 165–167.

Harvison, P. J., Egan, R. W., Gale, P. H., Christian, G. D., Hill, B. S. and Nelson, S. D., 1988a, Acetaminophen and analogs as cosubstrates and inhibitors of prostaglandin H synthase, *Chemico-Biological Interactions*, **64**, 251–266.

Harvison, P. J., Egan, R. W., Gale, P. H. and Nelson, S. D., 1986a, Acetaminophen as a cosubstrate and inhibitor of prostaglandin H synthase, *Advances in Experimental Medicine and Biology*, **197**, 739–747.

Harvison, P. J., Forte, A. J. and Nelson, S. D., 1986b, Comparative toxicities and analgesic activities of three monomethylated analogues of acetaminophen, *Journal of Medicinal Chemistry*, **29**, 1737–1743.

Harvison, P. J., Guengerich, F. P., Rashed, M. S. and Nelson, S. D., 1988b, Cytochrome P-450 isozyme selectivity in the oxidation of acetaminophen, *Chemical Research in Toxicology*, **1**, 47–52.

Hasegawa, R., Furukawa, F., Toyoda, K., Jang, J. J., Yamashita, K., Sato, S., Takahashi, M. and Hayashi, Y., 1988, Study for tumor-initiating effect of acetaminophen in two-stage liver carcinogenesis of male F344 rats, *Carcinogenesis*, **9**, 755–759.

Hasegawa, R., Takahashi, S., Imaida, K., Yamaguchi, S., Shirai, T. and Ito, N., 1991, Age-dependent induction of preneoplastic liver cell foci by 2-acetylaminofluorene, phenobarbital and acetaminophen in F344 rats initially treated with diethylnitrosamine, *Japanese Journal of Cancer Research*, **82**, 293–297.

Hassig, S. R., Linscheer, W. G., Murthy, U. K., Miller, C. and Banerjee, A., 1993, Effects of PGE-Electrolyte (Colyte) lavage on serum acetaminophen concentrations: a model for treatment of acetaminophen overdose, *Digestive Diseases and Sciences*, **38**, 1395–1401.

Hassing, J. M., Rosenberg, H. and Stohs, S. J., 1979, Acetaminophen-induced glutathione depletion in diabetic rats, *Research Communications in Chemical Pathology and Pharmacology*, **25**, 3–11.

Hatamori, N., Nakaoka, T., Yoshida, H., Mimoto, H., Hirohata, T., Yun, S., Morita, S., Kasuga, M., Hayashi, Y. and Mizoguchi, Y., 1993, A case of prolonged liver injury caused by low dose of acetaminophen, *Japanese Journal of Gastroenterology*, **90**, 2945–2950.

Hatanaka, S., Kondoh, M., Kawarabayashi, K. and Furuhama, K., 1994, The measurement of gastric emptying in conscious rats by monitoring serial changes in serum acetaminophen level, *Journal of Pharmacological and Toxicological Methods*, **31**, 161–165.

Hathcock, J. N., 1990, Nutritional toxicology: basic principles and actual problems, *Food Additives and Contaminants*, **7 (Suppl. 1)**, S12–S18.

Hauser, A. C., Derfler, K. and Balcke, P., 1991, Progression of renal insufficiency in analgesic nephropathy: impact of continuous drug abuse, *Journal of Clinical Epidemiology*, **44**, 53–56.

Hauser, A. C., Derfler, K., Stockenhuber, F. and Balcke, P., 1990, Post-transplantation malignant disease in patients with analgesic nephropathy, *Lancet*, **335**, 58.

Häuser, H. and Pfleger, K., 1965, Untersuchung über orale und rectale Resorption von Phenacetin und N-Acetyl-p-Aminophenol, *Archiv für experimentelle Pathologie und Pharmakologie*, **251**, 108–109.

Hauss, S., Gabinski, Cl. and Favarel-Garrigues, J.–C., 1983, Conduite à tenir devant une intoxication aiguë par le paracétamol (PCM), *Bordeaux Médical*, **16**, 273–274.

Hawton, K. and Fagg, J., 1992a, Deliberate self-poisoning and self-injury in adolescents: a study of characteristics and trends in Oxford, 1976–89, *British Journal of Psychiatry*, **161**, 816–823.

Hawton, K. and Fagg, J., 1992b, Trends in deliberate self poisoning and self injury in Oxford, 1976–90, *British Medical Journal*, **304**, 1409–1411.

Hawton, K., Ware, C., Mistry, H., Hewitt, J., Kingsbury, S., Roberts, D. and Weitzel, H., 1995, Why patients choose paracetamol for self poisoning and their knowledge of its dangers, *British Medical Journal*, **310**, 164.

Hayashi, Y., 1992, Overview of genotoxic carcinogens and non-genotoxic carcinogens, *Experimental and Toxicologic Pathology*, **44**, 465–472.

Hayes, A. H., 1981, Therapeutic implications of drug interactions with acetaminophen and aspirin, *Archives of Internal Medicine*, **141**, 301–304.

Hayes, J. D., Gilligan, D., Chapman, B. J. and Beckett, G. J., 1983, Purification of human hepatic glutathione S-transferases and the development of a radioimmunoassay for their measurement in plasma, *Clinica Chimica Acta*, **134**, 107–121.

Hayes, M. A., Murray, C. A. and Rushmore, T. H., 1986, Influences of glutathione status on different cytocidal responses of monolayer rat hepatocytes exposed to aflatoxin B_1 or acetaminophen, *Toxicology and Applied Pharmacology*, **85**, 1–10.

Hayes, M. A. and Pickering, D. B., 1985, Comparative cytopathology of primary rat hepatocyte cultures exposed to aflatoxin B_1, acetaminophen, and other hepatotoxins, *Toxicology and Applied Pharmacology*, **80**, 345–356.

Hayes, M. A., Roberts, E., Roomi, M. W., Safe, S. H., Farber, E. and Cameron, R. G., 1984, Comparative influences of different PB-type and 3-MC-type polychlorinated biphenyl-induced phenotypes on cytocidal hepatotoxicity of bromobenzene and acetaminophen, *Toxicology and Applied Pharmacology*, **76**, 118–127.

Hayes, P. C. and Bouchier, I. A. D., 1989, Effect of acute and chronic propranolol administration on antipyrine and paracetamol clearance in patients with chronic liver disease, *American Journal of Gastroenterology*, **84**, 723–726.

Haylor, J., 1980, Prostaglandin synthesis and renal function in man, *Journal of Physiology*, **298**, 383–396.

Hazelton, G. A., Hjelle, J. J. and Klaassen, C. D., 1985, Effects of butylated hydroxyanisole on hepatic glucuronidation capacity in mice, *Toxicology and Applied Pharmacology*, **78**, 280–290.

Hazelton, G. A., Hjelle, J. J. and Klaassen, C. D., 1986a, Effects of cysteine pro-drugs on acetaminophen-induced hepatotoxicity, *Journal of Pharmacology and Experimental Therapeutics*, **237**, 341–349.

Hazelton, G. A., Hjelle, J. J. and Klaassen, C. D., 1986b, Effects of butylated hydroxyanisole on acetaminophen hepatotoxicity and glucuronidation *in vivo*, *Toxicology and Applied Pharmacology*, **83**, 474–485.

Heading, R. C., 1968, Purpura and paracetamol, *British Medical Journal*, **3**, 743–744.

Heading, R. C., Nimmo, J., Prescott, L. F. and Tothill, P., 1973, The dependence of paracetamol absorption on the rate of gastric emptying, *British Journal of Pharmacology*, **47**, 415–421.

Healey, K. and Calder, I. C., 1979, The synthesis and reactions of N-hydroxyparacetamol (N, 4′-dihydroxyacetanilide), *Australian Journal of Chemistry*, **32**, 1307–1316.

Healey, K., Calder, I. C., Hart, S. J., Smail, M. C., Emslie, K. R. and Tange, J. D., 1980, Formation and handling of the glutathione conjugate of paracetamol, *Clinical and Experimental Pharmacology and Physiology*, **7**, 439.

Healey, K., Calder, I. C., Yong, A. C., Crowe, C. A., Funder, C. C., Ham, K. N. and Tange, J. D., 1978, Liver and kidney damage induced by N-hydroxyparacetamol, *Xenobiotica*, **8**, 403–411.

Heath, M. F., Evans, R. J., Poole, A. W., Hayes, L. J., McEvoy, R. J. and Littler, R. M., 1994, The effects of aspirin and paracetamol on the aggregation of equine blood platelets, *Journal of Veterinary Pharmacology and Therapeutics*, **17**, 374–378.

Hedges, A. and Kaye, C. M., 1973, A comparison of the absorption of two formulations of paracetamol, *Journal of International Medical Research*, **1**, 548–550.

Hedges, A., Kaye, C. M., Maclay, W. P. and Turner, P., 1974, A comparison of the absorption of effervescent preparations of paracetamol and penicillin V (phenoxymethylpenicillin) with solid dose forms of these drugs, *Journal of Clinical Pharmacology*, **14**, 363–368.

Hedwall, P. and Heeg, E., 1961, Die Beeinflussung einer Staphylokokken-infektion der Rattenniere durch Analgetica, *Arzneimittel-Forschung*, **11**, 909–911.

Hegedus, Z. L. and Nayak, U., 1991, Para-aminophenol and structurally related compounds as intermediates in lipofuscin formation and in renal and other tissue toxicities, *Archives Internationales de Physiologie de Biochimie et de Biophysique*, **99**, 99–105.

Heidbreder, E., Schäfer, R. M., Götz, R., Heidland, A. and Romen, W., 1986, Akutes Nierenversagen nach Einnahme von antipyretischen Analgetika, *Medizinische Welt*, **37**, 297–302.

Heidrich, G., Slavic-Svircev, V. and Kaiko, R. F., 1985, Efficacy and quality of ibuprofen and acetaminophen plus codeine analgesia, *Pain*, **22**, 385–397.

Heilmann, E., Lenger, H. and Werner, W., 1976, Untersuchungen zum Nachweis von N-Acetyl-p-Aminophenol im Urin, *Verhandlungen der Deutschen Gesellschaft für Innere*

Medizin, **82**, 1686–1689.

Heintz, B., Bock, T. A., Kierdorf, H. and Maurin, N., 1989, Haemolytic crisis after acetaminophen in glucose-6-phosphate dehydrogenase deficiency, *Klinische Wochenschrift*, **67**, 1068.

Heirwegh, K. P. M. and Fevery, J., 1967, Determination of unconjugated and total N-acetyl-p-aminophenol (NAPA) in urine and serum, *Clinical Chemistry*, **13**, 215–219.

Heit, W. and Heimpel, H., 1982, Arzneimittel-induzierte Agranulozytose, *Fortschritte der Medizin*, **100**, 1844–1850.

Hekimoglu, S., Ayanoglu-Dulger, G. and Hincal, A. A., 1987, Comparative bioavailability of three commercial acetaminophen tablets, *International Journal of Clinical Pharmacology, Therapy and Toxicology*, **25**, 93.

Hekimoglu, S., Sahin, S., Sumnu, M. and Hincal, A. A., 1991, Comparative bioavailability of three batches of four commercial acetaminophen tablets, *European Journal of Drug Metabolism and Pharmacokinetics*, **Spec. 3**, 228–232.

Hekman, P., Russel, F. G. M. and van Ginneken, C. A. M., 1986, Renal transport of glucuronides of paracetamol and p-nitrophenol in the dog, *Drug Metabolism and Disposition: The Biological Fate of Chemicals*, **14**, 370–371.

Hellerstein, M. K. and Munro, H. N., 1988, Glycoconjugates as noninvasive probes of intrahepatic metabolism: III. Application to galactose assimilation by the intact rat, *Metabolism*, **37**, 312–317.

Helliwell, M., 1980, Severe barbiturate and paracetamol overdose: the simultaneous removal of both poisons by haemoperfusion, *Postgraduate Medical Journal*, **56**, 363–365.

Helliwell, M. and Essex, E., 1981, Hemoperfusion in 'late' paracetamol poisoning, *Clinical Toxicology*, **18**, 1225–1233.

Helliwell, M., Prior, J. and Volans, G. N., 1981a, Paracetamol-induced hepatic failure, *British Medical Journal*, **282**, 473.

Helliwell, M., Vale, A. and Goulding, R., 1981b, Haemoperfusion in 'late' paracetamol poisoning, *Human Toxicology*, **1**, 25–30.

Helliwell, T. R., Yeung, J. H. K. and Park, B. K., 1985, Hepatic necrosis and glutathione depletion in captopril-treated mice, *British Journal of Experimental Pathology*, **66**, 67–78.

Hemet, J., Leroy, A., Duprey, F., Rocher, W., Metayer, J. and Ducastelle, T., 1986, Sténose anorectale par suppositoires of dextropropoxyphène et de paracétamol (Di-Antalvic), *Gastroentérologie Clinique et Biologique*, **10**, 517–520.

Henderson, A., Wright, M. and Pond, S. M., 1993, Experience with 732 acute overdose patients admitted to an intensive care unit over six years, *Medical Journal of Australia*, **158**, 28–30.

Hendrix-Treacy, S., Wallace, S. M., Hindmarsh, K. W., Wyant, G. M. and Danilkewich, A., 1986, The effect of acetaminophen administration on its disposition and body stores of sulphate, *European Journal of Clinical Pharmacology*, **30**, 273–278.

Henne-Bruns, D., Artwohl, J., Broelsch, C. and Kremer, B., 1988a, Acetaminophen-induced acute hepatic failure in pigs: controversial results to other animal models, *Research in Experimental Medicine*, **188**, 463–472.

Henne-Bruns, D., Artwohl, J., Dziwisch, L. and Kremer, B., 1988b, Paracetamol-intoxikation im Schweinemodell, *Zeitschrift für Experimentelle Chirurgie, Transplantation, und Kunstliche Organe*, **21**, 255–263.

Hennighausen, G. and Engel, M., 1989, Depletion of hepatic glutathione in rats impairs phagocytosis *in vivo*, *Archives of Toxicology*, **Suppl. 13**, 326–329.

Henochowicz, S., 1986, Acetaminophen-induced asthma in a patient with aspirin idiosyncrasy, *Immunology and Allergy Practice*, **8**, 43–45.

Henretig, F. M., Selbst, S. M., Forrest, C., Kearney, T. K., Orel, H., Werner, S. and Williams, T. A., 1989, Repeated acetaminophen overdosing causing hepatotoxicity in children, *Clinical Pediatrics*, **28**, 525–528.

Henriques, C. C., 1970, Acetaminophen sensitivity and fixed dermatitis, *Journal of the Amer-*

ican Medical Association, **214**, 2336.

Henry, M. A., Sweet, R. S. and Tange, J. D., 1983, A new reproducible experimental model of analgesic nephropathy, *Journal of Pathology*, **139**, 23–32.

Henry, M. A. and Tange, J. D., 1984, Chronic renal lesions in the uninephrectomized Gunn rat after analgesic mixtures, *Pathology*, **16**, 278–284.

Henry, M. A. and Tange, J. D., 1987, Lesions of the renal papilla induced by paracetamol, *Journal of Pathology*, **151**, 11–19.

Hepler, B., Weber, J., Sutheimer, C. and Sunshine, I., 1984, Homogenous enzyme immunoassay of acetaminophen in serum, *American Journal of Clinical Pathology*, **81**, 602–610.

Herd, B., Wynne, H., Wright, P., James, O. and Woodhouse, K., 1991, The effect of age on glucuronidation and sulphation of paracetamol by human liver fractions, *British Journal of Clinical Pharmacology*, **32**, 768–770.

Hering, R. and Steiner, T. J., 1991, Abrupt outpatient withdrawal of medication in analgesic-abusing migraineurs, *Lancet*, **337**, 1442–1443.

Herrera, A. M., Scott, D. O. and Lunte, C. E., 1990, Microdialysis sampling for determination of plasma protein binding of drugs, *Pharmaceutical Research*, **7**, 1077–1081.

Hertz, F. and Cloarec, A., 1984, Pharmacology of free radicals: recent views on their relation to inflammatory mechanisms, *Life Sciences*, **34**, 713–720.

Hertz, F. and Deghenghi, R., 1983, Analgesic activity of a thiomethyl metabolite of paracetamol, *Journal of Pharmacy and Pharmacology*, **35**, 521–522.

Heubner, W., 1913, Studien über Methämoglobinbildung, *Archiv für experimentelle Pathologie und Pharmakologie*, **72**, 239–281.

Heymann, M. A., 1986, Non-narcotic analgesics. Use in pregnancy and fetal and perinatal effects, *Drugs*, **32 (Suppl. 4)**, 164–176.

Hickey, R. F. J., 1982, Chronic low back pain: a comparison of diflunisal with paracetamol, *New Zealand Medical Journal*, **95**, 312–314.

Hickson, G. B., Greene, J. W., Ghishan, F. K. and Craft, L. T., 1983, Apparent intentional poisoning of an infant with acetaminophen, *American Journal of Diseases of Children*, **137**, 917.

Hidvegi, S. and Ecobichon, D. J., 1986, Acetaminophen in the guinea pig: metabolite identification in blood urine and bile, *Canadian Journal of Physiology and Pharmacology*, **64**, 72–76.

Hierton, C., 1981, Effects of indometacin, naproxen and paracetamol on regional blood flow in rabbits: a microsphere study, *Acta Pharmacologica et Toxicologica*, **49**, 327–333.

Higgins, R., Goldsmith, D. J. A., Venning, M. C. and Ackrill, P., 1993, Charcoal haemoperfusion in acetaminophen poisoning, *Nephrology, Dialysis, Transplantation*, **8**, 992.

Higgins, T., 1987, Enzymic method for acetaminophen adapted to an Abbott ABA–200 analyzer, *Clinical Chemistry*, **33**, 612.

Hikal, A. H., Morad, A. R. M. and El-Houfy, S., 1983, Assay of acetaminophen in dosage forms and in blood by high performance liquid chromatography, *Pharmazeutische Industrie*, **45**, 426–428.

Hill, K. E. and Burk, R. F., 1984, Toxicity studies in isolated hepatocytes from selenium-deficient rats and vitamin E-deficient rats, *Toxicology and Applied Pharmacology*, **72**, 32–39.

Hill, R., 1983, Salicylate interference with measurement of acetaminophen, *Clinical Chemistry*, **29**, 575–576.

Hillenbrand, P., Parbhoo, S. P., Jedrychowski, A. and Sherlock, S., 1974, Significance of intravascular coagulation and fibrinolysis in acute hepatic failure, *Gut*, **15**, 83–88.

Himmelstein, D. U., Woolhandler, S. J. and Adler, R. D., 1984, Elevated SGOT/SGPT ratio in alcoholic patients with acetaminophen hepatotoxicity, *American Journal of Gastroenterology*, **79**, 718–720.

Hindmarsh, K. W., Mayers, D. J., Wallace, S. M., Danilkewich, A. and Ernst, A., 1991, Increased serum sulfate concentrations in man due to environmental factors: effects on acetaminophen metabolism, *Veterinary and Human Toxicology*, **33**, 441–445.

Hingorani, K., 1971, Orphenadrine/paracetamol in backache – a double-blind controlled trial, *British Journal of Clinical Practice*, **25**, 227–231.

Hinsberg, O. and Kast, A., 1887, Ueber die Wirkung des Acetphenetidins, *Zentralblatt für die Medizinischen Wissenschaften*, **25**, 145–148.

Hinsberg, O. and Treupel, G., 1894, Ueber die physiologische Wirkung des p-Amidophenols und einiger Derivate desselben, *Archiv für experimentelle Pathologie und Pharmakologie*, **33**, 216–250.

Hinson, J. A., 1980, Biochemical toxicology of acetaminophen. In: Reviews of Biochemical Toxicology, Vol. 2. Hodgson, E., Bend, J. R. and Philpot, R. M. Eds. Elsevier, Amsterdam, pp. 103–129.

Hinson, J. A., 1983, Reactive metabolites of phenacetin and acetaminophen: a review, *Environmental Health Perspectives*, **49**, 71–79.

Hinson, J. A. and Gillette, J. R., 1980, Evidence for more than one chemically reactive metabolite of acetaminophen formed by hamster liver microsomes, *Federation Proceedings*, **39**, 748.

Hinson, J. A., Han-Hsu, H., Mays, J. B., Holt, S. J., McLean, P. and Ketterer, B., 1984, Acetaminophen-induced alterations in blood glucose and blood insulin levels in mice, *Research Communications in Chemical Pathology and Pharmacology*, **43**, 381–391.

Hinson, J. A., Mays, J. B. and Cameron, A. M., 1983, Acetaminophen-induced hepatic glycogen depletion and hyperglycemia in mice, *Biochemical Pharmacology*, **32**, 1979–1988.

Hinson, J. A., Monks, T. J., Hong, M., Highet, R. J. and Pohl, L. R., 1982, 3-(Glutathion-S-yl) acetaminophen: a biliary metabolite of acetaminophen, *Drug Metabolism and Disposition: The Biological Fate of Chemicals*, **10**, 47–50.

Hinson, J. A., Nelson, S. D. and Gillette, J. R., 1979a, Metabolism of [p-^{18}O]–phenacetin: the mechanism of activation of phenacetin to reactive metabolites in hamsters, *Molecular Pharmacology*, **15**, 419–427.

Hinson, J. A., Nelson, S. D. and Mitchell, J. R., 1977, Studies on the microsomal formation of arylating metabolites of acetaminophen and phenacetin, *Molecular Pharmacology*, **13**, 625–633.

Hinson, J. A., Pohl, L. R. and Gillette, J. R., 1979b, N-hydroxyacetaminophen: a microsomal metabolite of N-hydroxyphenacetin but apparently not of acetaminophen, *Life Sciences*, **24**, 2133–2138.

Hinson, J. A., Pohl, L. R. and Gillette, J. R., 1980a, A simple high-pressure liquid chromatographic assay for the N-hydroxy derivatives of phenacetin, acetaminophen, 2-acetylaminofluorene, and other hydroxamic acids, *Analytical Biochemistry*, **101**, 462–467.

Hinson, J. A., Pohl, L. R., Monks, T. J. and Gillette, J. R., 1981, Acetaminophen-induced hepatotoxicity, *Life Sciences*, **29**, 107–116.

Hinson, J. A., Pohl, L. R., Monks, T. J., Gillette, J. R. and Guengerich, F. P., 1980b, 3-Hydroxyacetaminophen: a microsomal metabolite of acetaminophen. Evidence against an epoxide as the reactive metabolite of acetaminophen, *Drug Metabolism and Disposition: The Biological Fate of Chemicals*, **8**, 289–294.

Hinson, J. A., Roberts, D. W., Benson, R. W., Dalhoff, K., Loft, S. and Poulsen, H. E., 1990, Mechanism of paracetamol toxicity, *Lancet*, **335**, 732.

Hiraga, K. and Fujii, T., 1985, Carcinogenicity testing of acetaminophen in F344 rats, *Gann*, **76**, 79–85.

Hirate, J., Zhu, C., Horikoshi, I. and Bhargava, V. O., 1991, Age-dependent changes in first-pass metabolism of acetaminophen in rats, *Biopharmaceutics and Drug Disposition*, **12**, 119–126.

Hirate, J., Zhu, C.-Y., Horikoshi, I. and Bhargava, V. O., 1990, First-pass metabolism of acetaminophen in rats after low and high doses, *Biopharmaceutics and Drug Disposition*, **11**, 245–252.

Hirayama, C., Murawaki, Y., Yamada, S., Aoto, Y. and Ikeda, F., 1983, The target portion of acetaminophen induced hepatotoxicity in rats: modification by thiol compounds, *Research Communications in Chemical Pathology and Pharmacology*, **42**, 431–448.

Hirsch, J. F., Pichard, S., Flottes, P. and Negellen, J.-L., 1982, Agranulocytose et hyper-bilirubinémie au décours d'un traitement prolongée par le paracétamol, *Thérapie*, **37**, 593–594.

Hjelle, J. J., 1986, Hepatic UDP-glucuronic acid regulation during acetaminophen biotrans-formation in rats, *Journal of Pharmacology and Experimental Therapeutics*, **237**, 750–756.

Hjelle, J. J., Brzeznicka, E. A. and Klaassen, C. D., 1986, Comparison of the effects of sodium sulfate and N-acetylcysteine on the hepatotoxicity of acetaminophen in mice, *Journal of Pharmacology and Experimental Therapeutics*, **236**, 526–534.

Hjelle, J. J. and Grauer, G. F., 1986, Acetaminophen-induced toxicosis in dogs and cats, *Journal of the American Veterinary Medical Association*, **188**, 742–746.

Hjelle, J. J., Hazelton, G. A. and Klaassen, C. D., 1985a, Acetaminophen decreases adenosine 3′-phosphate 5′-phosphosulfate and uridine diphosphoglucuronic acid in rat liver, *Drug Metabolism and Disposition: The Biological Fate of Chemicals*, **13**, 35–41.

Hjelle, J. J., Hazelton, G. A. and Klaassen, C. D., 1985b, Increased UDP-glucuronosyltransferase activity and UDP-glucuronic acid concentration in the small intestine of butylated hydroxyanisole-treated mice, *Drug Metabolism and Disposition: The Biological Fate of Chemicals*, **13**, 68–70.

Hjelle, J. J. and Klaassen, C. D., 1984, Glucuronidation and biliary excretion of acetamino-phen in rats, *Journal of Pharmacology and Experimental Therapeutics*, **228**, 407–413.

Ho, S. W.-C. and Beilin, L. J., 1983, Asthma associated with N-acetylcysteine infusion and paracetamol poisoning; report of two cases, *British Medical Journal*, **287**, 876–877.

Hobi, V., Ladewig, D., Dubach, U. C., Miest, P.-Ch. and Ehrensberger, T., 1976, Analgesic abuse and personality characteristics, *International Journal of Clinical Pharmacology*, **13**, 36–41.

Höbel, M. and Talebian, M., 1960, Die Resorption von N-acetyl-p-aminophenol aus Gelatine-Suppositorien Kapseln, *Arzneimittel-Forschung*, **10**, 653–656.

Hodgkinson, D. W., Jellett, L. B. and Ashby, R. H., 1991, A review of the management of oral drug overdose in the accident and emergency department of the Royal Brisbane Hospi-tal, *Archives of Emergency Medicine*, **8**, 8–16.

Hoensch, H. P., 1984, Enzyminduktion der Leber durch chronischen Alkoholismus als Risi-kofaktor der Hepatotoxizität, *Zeitschrift für Gastroenterologie*, **22**, 1–8.

Hoernecke, R. and Doenicke, A., 1993, Behandlung des Migräneanfalls: die Kombination Dihydroergotamintartrat und Paracetamol im Vergleich zu den Einzelsubstanzen und Placebo, *Medizinische Klinik*, **88**, 642–648.

Hoffman, D. A., Wallace, S. M. and Verbeeck, R. K., 1990, Circadian rhythm of serum sulfate levels in man and acetaminophen pharmacokinetics, *European Journal of Clinical Phar-macology*, **39**, 143–148.

Hoffman, D. A., Wallace, S. M. and Verbeeck, R. K., 1991, Simple method for the determi-nation of inorganic sulfate in human serum and urine using single-column ion chroma-tography, *Journal of Chromatography*, **565**, 447–452.

Hoffmann, K.-J., Axworthy, D. B. and Baillie, T. A., 1990, Mechanistic studies on the meta-bolic activation of acetaminophen *in vivo*, *Chemical Research in Toxicology*, **3**, 204–211.

Hoffmann, K.-J. and Baillie, T. A., 1988, The use of alkoxycarbonyl derivatives for the mass spectral analysis of drug-thioether metabolites. Studies with the cysteine, mercapturic acid and glutathione conjugates of acetaminophen, *Biomedical and Environmental Mass Spectrometry*, **15**, 637–647.

Hoffmann, K.-J., Streeter, A. J., Axworthy, D. B. and Baillie, T. A., 1985a, Identification of the major covalent adduct formed *in vitro* and *in vivo* between acetaminophen and mouse liver proteins, *Molecular Pharmacology*, **27**, 566–573.

Hoffmann, K.-J., Streeter, A. J., Axworthy, D. B. and Baillie, T. A., 1985b, Structural charac-terization of the major covalent adduct formed *in vitro* between acetaminophen and bovine serum albumin, *Chemico-Biological Interactions*, **53**, 155–172.

Hoffmann, R. M., Forst, H., Schelling, G., Denecke, H. and Pape, G. R., 1991, Unklares Leberkoma bei einer 18 jährigen Patientin, *Internist*, **32**, 735–737.

Hoffmeister, F., Dycka, J. and Rämsch, K., 1980, Intragastric self-administration in the Rhesus monkey: a comparison of the reinforcing effects of codeine, phenacetin and paracetamol, *Journal of Pharmacology and Experimental Therapeutics*, **214**, 213–218.

Hofstra, A. H. and Uetrecht, J. P., 1993, Myeloperoxidase-mediated activation of xenobiotics by human leukocytes, *Toxicology*, **82**, 221–242.

Hoftiezer, J. W., O'Laughlin, J. C. and Ivey, K. J., 1982, The effects of 24 hours of aspirin, Bufferin, paracetamol and placebo on normal human gastroduodenal mucosa, *Gut*, **23**, 692–697.

Hogan, D. L., 1988, Damage and protection of the human gastric mucosa, *American Journal of Medicine*, **84 (Suppl. 2A)**, 35–40.

Högberg, J. and Kristoferson, A., 1977, A correlation between glutathione levels and cellular damage in isolated hepatocytes, *European Journal of Biochemistry*, **74**, 77–82.

Hoigné, R., D'Andrea Jaeger, M., Wymann, R., Egli, A., Müller, U., Hess, T., Galeazzi, R., Maibach, R. and Künzi, U. P., 1990, Time pattern of allergic reactions to drugs, *Agents and Actions*, **S29**, 39–58.

Hoivik, D. J., Manautou, J. E., Tveit, A., Emeigh Hart, S. G., Khairallah, E. A. and Cohen, S. D., 1995, Gender-related differences in susceptibility to acetaminophen-induced protein arylation and nephrotoxicity on the CD-1 mouse, *Toxicology and Applied Pharmacology*, **130**, 257–271.

Hoivik, H. O., Gundersen, R. and Osmundsen, K., 1986, Kombinasjonsanalgetica ved nakkemyalgi. En dobbletblind sammenligning av paracetamol + orfenadrincitrat (Norgesic) og paracetamol + kodein (Paralgin forte) i almenpraksis, *Tidsskrift for den Norske Lægeforening*, **106**, 126–128.

Holme, J. A., Dahlin, D. C., Nelson, S. D. and Dybing, E., 1984, Cytotoxic effects of N-acetyl-p-benzoquinone imine, a common arylating intermediate of paracetamol and N-hydroxyparacetamol, *Biochemical Pharmacology*, **33**, 401–406.

Holme, J. A., Hongslo, J. K., Bjørge, C. and Nelson, S. D., 1991, Comparative cytotoxic effects of acetaminophen (N-acetyl-p-aminophenol), a non-hepatotoxic regioisomer acetyl-m-aminophenol and their postulated reactive hydroquinone and quinone metabolites in monolayer cultures of mouse hepatocytes, *Biochemical Pharmacology*, **42**, 1137–1142.

Holme, J. A., Hongslo, J. K., Bjornstad, C., Harvison, P. J. and Nelson, S. D., 1988, Toxic effects of paracetamol and related structure in V79 chinese hamster cells, *Mutagenesis*, **3**, 51–56.

Holme, J. A. and Jacobsen, D., 1986, Mechanism of paracetamol toxicity, *Lancet*, **i**, 804–805.

Holme, J. A. and Søderlund, E., 1986, Species differences in cytotoxic and genotoxic effects of phenacetin and paracetamol in primary monolayer cultures of hepatocytes, *Mutation Research*, **164**, 167–175.

Holme, J. A., Wirth, P. J., Dybing, E. and Thorgeirsson, S. S., 1982a, Cytotoxic effects of N-hydroxyparacetamol in suspensions of isolated rat hepatocytes, *Acta Pharmacologica et Toxicologica*, **51**, 87–95.

Holme, J. A., Wirth, P. J., Dybing, E. and Thorgeirsson, S. S., 1982b, Modulation of N-hydroxyparacetamol cytotoxicity in suspensions of isolated rat hepatocytes, *Acta Pharmacologica et Toxicologica*, **51**, 96–102.

Holt, S., Heading, R. C., Carter, D. C., Prescott, L. F. and Tothill, P., 1979, Effect of gel fibre on gastric emptying and absorption of glucose and paracetamol, *Lancet*, **i**, 636–639.

Holt, S., Heading, R. C., Clements, J. A., Tothill, P. and Prescott, L. F., 1981, Acetaminophen absorption and metabolism in celiac disease and Crohn's disease, *Clinical Pharmacology and Therapeutics*, **30**, 232–238.

Holt, S., Robson, H. R., Heading, R. C. and Sidhu, M., 1992, A lack of an effect of bran and anti-diarrheal drugs on acetaminophen absorption in humans, *Journal of Pharmaceutical Medicine*, **2**, 217–222.

Holvoet, J., Terriere, L., Van Hee, W., Verbist, L., Fierens, E. and Hautekeete, M. L., 1991, Relation of upper gastrointestinal bleeding to non-steroidal anti-inflammatory drugs and aspirin: a case-control study, *Gut*, **32**, 730–734.

Holzbecher, M., Perry, R. A. and Ellenberger, H. S., 1981, Acetaminophen fatality – a case report, *Journal of the Canadian Society of Forensic Science*, **14**, 32–33.

Homann, J., Thilo-Körner, D. G. S., Oehler, G., Schroyens, W., Temmesfeld, B., Kroker, R., Matthias, R. and Matthes, K.-J., 1990, Akute Paracetamol-intoxikation: Pathophysiologie, Verlauf und Therapie, *Medizinische Welt*, **41**, 946–950.

Hong, R. W., Rounds, J. D., Helton, W.S., Robinson, M. K. and Wilmore, D. W., 1992, Glutamine preserves liver glutathione after lethal hepatic injury, *Annals of Surgery*, **215**, 114–119.

Hongslo, J. K., Bjørge, C., Schwarze, P., Mann, G., Thelander, L. and Holme, J. A., 1990a, Paracetamol inhibits replicative DNA synthesis and induces sister-chromatid exchanges by destruction of a tyrosyl radical or ribonucleotide reductase, *Mutation Research*, **234**, 412–413.

Hongslo, J. K., Bjørge, C., Schwarze, P. E., Brøgger, A., Mann, G., Thelander, L. and Holme, J. A., 1990b, Paracetamol inhibits replicative DNA synthesis and induces sister chromatid exchange and chromosomal aberrations by inhibition of ribonucleotide reductase, *Mutagenesis*, **5**, 475–480.

Hongslo, J. K., Bjørnstad, C., Schwarze, P. E. and Holme, J. A., 1989, Inhibition of replicative DNA synthesis by paracetamol in V79 Chinese hamster cells, *Toxicology in Vitro*, **3**, 13–20.

Hongslo, J. K., Brøgger, A., Bjørge, C. and Holme, J. A., 1991, Increased frequency of sister-chromatid exchange and chromatid breaks in lymphocytes after treatment of human volunteers with therapeutic doses of paracetamol, *Mutation Research*, **261**, 1–8.

Hongslo, J. K., Brunborg, G., Steffensen, I.-L. and Holme, J. A., 1993, Paracetamol inhibits UV-induced DNA repair in resting human mononuclear blood cells *in vitro*, *Mutagenesis*, **8**, 423–429.

Hongslo, J. K., Christenson, T., Brunborg, G., Bjørnstad, C. and Holme, J. A., 1988, Genotoxic effects of paracetamol in V79 chinese hamster cells, *Mutation Research*, **204**, 333–341.

Hongslo, J. K. and Holme, J. A., 1994, DNA-skader av paracetamol, *Tidsskrift for den Norske Lægeforening*, **114**, 1204–1206.

Hongslo, J. K., Smith, C. V., Brunborg, G., Søderlund, E. J. and Holme, J. A., 1994, Genotoxicity of paracetamol in mice and rats, *Mutagenesis*, **9**, 93–100.

Hopkins, C. S., Underhill, S. and Booker, P. D., 1990, Pharmacokinetics of paracetamol after cardiac surgery, *Archives of Disease in Childhood*, **65**, 971–976.

Hopkinson, J. H., Bartlett, F. H., Steffens, A. O., McGlumphy, T. H., Macht, E. L. and Smith, M., 1973, Acetaminophen vs. propoxyphene hydrochloride for relief of pain in episiotomy patients, *Journal of Clinical Pharmacology*, **13**, 251–263.

Hopkinson, J. H., Blatt, G., Cooper, M., Levin, H. M., Berry, F. N. and Cohn, H., 1976, Effective pain relief: comparative results with acetaminophen in a new dose formulation, propoxyphene napsylate-acetaminophen combination, and placebo, *Current Therapeutic Research*, **19**, 622–630.

Hopkinson, J. H., Smith, M. T., Bare, W. W., Levin, H. M. and Posatko, R. J., 1974, Acetaminophen (500 mg) vs. acetaminophen (325 mg) for the relief of pain in episiotomy patients, *Current Therapeutic Research*, **16**, 194–200.

Horner, S. A., Zucco, F., Fry, J. R., Clothier, R. H. and Balls, M., 1987, Investigation of the cytotoxicity produced by generation of short-lived reactive metabolites *in vitro*: a study with paracetamol, *Toxicology in Vitro*, **1**, 133–138.

Hornfeldt, C. S., 1992, Distinction made between toxicoses caused by acetaminophen and nonsteroidal anti-inflammatory drugs, *Journal of the American Veterinary Medical Association*, **201**, 1318–1319.

Horton, A. A. and Wood, J. M., 1989, Effects of inhibitors of phospholipase A_2, cyclo-oxygenase and thromboxane synthetase on paracetamol hepatotoxicity in the rat, *Eicosanoids*, **2**, 123–129.

Horton, A. A. and Wood, J. M., 1991, Prevention of paracetamol-induced hepatotoxicity in the rat by the thromboxane receptor antagonist, Sulotroban (BM 13177), *Journal of Lipid Mediators*, **4**, 245–248.

Horvitz, R. A. and Jatlow, P. I., 1977, Determination of acetaminophen concentrations in serum by high-pressure liquid chromatography, *Clinical Chemistry*, **23**, 1596–1598.

Horwitz, A., Tenhonsel, G., Thomas, P. and Kosenow, W., 1977, Arzneimittelschäden: Paracetamolintoxikation, *Gynäkologische Praxis*, **1**, 555–557.

Hossain, M. and Ayres, J. W., 1992, Pharmacokinetics and pharmacodynamics in the design of controlled-release beads with acetaminophen as model drug, *Journal of Pharmaceutical Sciences*, **81**, 444–448.

Houssein, I., Wilcox, H. and Barron, J., 1985, Effect of heat treatment on results for biochemical analysis of plasma and serum, *Clinical Chemistry*, **31**, 2028–2030.

Houston, J. B. and Levy, G., 1976, Drug biotransformation interactions in man VI: acetaminophen and ascorbic acid, *Journal of Pharmaceutical Sciences*, **65**, 1218–1221.

Howard, C. R., Howard, F. M. and Weitzman, M. L., 1994, Acetaminophen analgesia in neonatal circumcision: the effect on pain, *Pediatrics*, **93**, 641–646.

Howell, S. R. and Klaassen, C., 1991, Circadian variation of hepatic UDP-glucuronic acid and the glucuronidation of xenobiotics in mice, *Toxicology Letters*, **57**, 73–79.

Howie, D., Adriaenssens, P. I. and Prescott, L. F., 1977, Paracetamol metabolism following overdosage: application of high performance liquid chromatography, *Journal of Pharmacy and Pharmacology*, **29**, 235–237.

Hsiao, J. K., Ball, B. A., Morrison, P. F., Mefford, I. N. and Bungay, P. M., 1990, Effects of different semipermeable membranes on *in vitro* and *in vivo* performance of microdialysis probes, *Journal of Neurochemistry*, **54**, 1449–1452.

Hu, J. J., Lee, M.-J., Vapiwala, M., Reuhl, K., Thomas, P. E. and Yang, C. S., 1993a, Sex-related differences in mouse renal metabolism and toxicity of acetaminophen, *Toxicology and Applied Pharmacology*, **122**, 16–26.

Hu, O.Y.-P., Ho, S.-T., Wang, J.-J., Ho, W., Wang, H.-J. and Lin, C.-Y., 1993b, Evaluation of gastric emptying in severe, burn-injured patients, *Critical Care Medicine*, **21**, 527–531.

Huang, K. C., Wolfe, W. M., Tsueda, K., Simpson, P. M. and Caissie, K. F., 1986, Effects of meclofenamate and acetaminophen on abdominal pain following tubal occlusion, *American Journal of Obstetrics and Gynecology*, **155**, 624–629.

Huang, T. L., Villalobos, S. A. and Hammock, B. D., 1993, Effect of hepatotoxic doses of paracetamol and carbon tetrachloride on the serum and hepatic carboxylesterase activity in mice, *Journal of Pharmacy and Pharmacology*, **45**, 458–465.

Huang, W.-Y. and Liu, G.-T., 1989, Protective action of kopsinine against experimental liver injuries in mice, *Acta Pharmacologica Sinica*, **10**, 65–68.

Hucker, R. S., Smith, G. T. and Minty, P. S. B., 1984, Evaluation of enzymic assay for paracetamol: clinical and forensic experiences, *Journal of Pharmaceutical and Biomedical Analysis*, **2**, 549–554.

Hue, D. P., Griffith, K. L. and McLean, A. E. M., 1985, Hepatocytes in primary culture become susceptible to paracetamol injury after depletion of glutathione using DL-buthionine-SR-sulphoximine (BSO), *Biochemical Pharmacology*, **34**, 4341–4344.

Huggett, A., Andrews, P. and Flanagan, R. J., 1981, Rapid micro-method for the measurement of paracetamol in blood plasma or serum using gas-liquid chromatography with flame-ionisation detection, *Journal of Chromatography: Biomedical Applications*, **209**, 67–76.

Huggett, A. and Blair, I. A., 1983a, The mechanism of paracetamol-induced hepatotoxicity: implications for therapy, *Human Toxicology*, **2**, 399–405.

Huggett, A. and Blair, I. A., 1983b, Chromatographic analysis of synthetic N-acetyl-p-benzoquinoneimine: the putative reactive metabolite of paracetamol, *Journal of Chromatographic Science*, **21**, 254–258.

Huggett, A. C. and Blair, I. A., 1982, Detoxification of the putative reactive metabolite of paracetamol with glutathione, *Biochemical Society Transactions*, **10**, 519–520.

Hughes, H., Smith, C., Horning, E. and Mitchell, J., 1981, Direct identification *in vivo* of lipid hydroperoxides and hydroxy acids from mouse liver following CCl4 but not acetaminophen administration, *Pharmacologist*, **23**, 221.

Hughes, R. D., Gazzard, B. G., Hanid, M. A., Trewby, P. N., Murray-Lyon, I. M., Davis, M., Williams, R. and Bennett, J. R., 1977, Controlled trial of cysteamine and dimercaprol after paracetamol overdose, *British Medical Journal*, **2**, 1395.

Hughes, R. D., Gazzard, B. G., Murray-Lyon, I. and Williams, R. S., 1976, The use of cysteamine and dimercaprol, *Journal of International Medical Research*, **4 (Suppl. 4)**, 123–129.

Hughes, R. D., Gove, C. D. and Williams, R., 1991, Protective effects of propylene glycol, a solvent used pharmaceutically, against paracetamol-induced liver injury in mice, *Biochemical Pharmacology*, **42**, 710–713.

Hughes, R. D., Gregory, H., Willshire, I. R., Moore, K. P. and Williams, R., 1990, Urinary excretion of epidermal growth factor in acute liver failure: preliminary results, *Medical Science Research*, **18**, 515–516.

Hughes, R. D., Zhang, L., Tsubouchi, H., Daikuhara, Y. and Williams, R., 1994, Plasma hepatocyte growth factor and biliprotein levels and outcome in fulminant hepatic failure, *Journal of Hepatology*, **20**, 106–111.

Hultengren, N., Lagergren, C. and Ljungqvist, A., 1965, Carcinoma of the renal pelvis in renal papillary necrosis, *Acta Chirurgica Scandinavica*, **130**, 314–320.

Hunskaar, S., Berge, O.-G. and Hole, K., 1986a, Orphenadrine citrate increases and prolongs the antinociceptive effects of paracetamol in mice, *Acta Pharmacologica et Toxicologica*, **59**, 53–59.

Hunskaar, S., Berge, O.-G. and Hole, K., 1986b, A modified hot-plate test sensitive to mild analgesics, *Behavioural Brain Research*, **21**, 101–108.

Hunskaar, S., Fasmer, O. B. and Hole, K., 1985a, Acetylsalicylic acid, paracetamol and morphine inhibit behavioral responses to intrathecally administered substance P or capsaicin, *Life Sciences*, **37**, 1835–1841.

Hunskaar, S., Fasmer, O. B. and Hole, K., 1985b, Formalin test in mice, a useful technique for evaluating mild analgesics, *Journal of Neuroscience Methods*, **14**, 69–76.

Hunskaar, S. and Hole, K., 1987, The formalin test in mice: dissociation between inflammatory and non-inflammatory pain, *Pain*, **30**, 103–114.

Hunter, J., 1973, Study of antipyretic therapy in current use, *Archives of Disease in Childhood*, **48**, 313–315.

Hurden, E. L., Harvey, D. R. and Lewis, P. J., 1980, Excretion of paracetamol in human breast milk, *Archives of Disease in Childhood*, **55**, 969–970.

Hurvitz, H., Branski, D., Gross-Kieselstein, E., Klar, A. and Abrahamov, A., 1984, Acetaminophen hypersensitivity resembling Kawasaki disease, *Israel Journal of Medical Sciences*, **20**, 145–147.

Hurwitz, E. S., Barrett, M. J., Bregman, D., Gunn, W. J., Pinsky, P., Schonberger, L. B., Drage, J. S., Kaslow, R. A., Burlington, B., Quinnan, G. V., LaMontagne, J. R., Fairweather, W. R., Dayton, D. and Dowdle, W. R., 1987, Public Health Service study of Reye's syndrome and medications: report of the main study, *Journal of the American Medical Association*, **257**, 1905–1911.

Huseby, N. E., 1981, Increased amount of hydrophilic γ-glutamyltransferase in serum after liver necrosis due to paracetamol intoxication, *Journal of Clinical Chemistry and Clinical Biochemistry*, **19**, 705–706.

Hussain, A., Kulkarni, P. and Perrier, D., 1978, Prodrug approaches to enhancement of physicochemical properties of drugs IX: acetaminophen prodrug, *Journal of Pharmaceutical Sciences*, **67**, 545–546.

Hutabarat, R. M., Unadkat, J. D., Kushmerick, P., Aitken, M. L., Slattery, J.T . and Smith, A. L., 1991, Disposition of drugs in cystic fibrosis. III. Acetaminophen, *Clinical Pharmacology and Therapeutics*, **50**, 695–701.

Hutchinson, D. R., Schilds, A. F. and Parke, D. V., 1986, Liver function in patients on long-term paracetamol (co-proxamol) analgesia, *Journal of Pharmacy and Pharmacology*, **38**, 242–243.

Hutchinson, D. R., Smith, M. G. and Parke, D. V., 1980, Prealbumin as an index of liver function after acute paracetamol poisoning, *Lancet*, **ii**, 121–123.

Hutchison, G. L., Crofts, S. L. and Gray, I. G., 1990, Preoperative piroxicam for postoperative analgesia in dental surgery, *British Journal of Anaesthesia*, **65**, 500–503.

IARC Monograph, 1990, Paracetamol (acetaminophen), *IARC Monographs on the Evaluation of the Carcinogenic Risk of Chemicals to Humans*, **50**, 307–332.

Idoko, J. A., Akpam, J. E., Aguye, I. and Adesanya, C. O., 1986, Angioneurotic oedema following ingestion of paracetamol, *Transactions of the Royal Society of Tropical Medicine and Hygiene*, **80**, 175–176.

Iida, S., Mizuma, T., Sakuma, N., Hayashi, M. and Awazu, S., 1989, Transport of acetaminophen conjugates in isolated rat hepatocytes, *Drug Metabolism and Disposition: The Biological Fate of Chemicals*, **17**, 341–344.

Ikejiri, N., Matsumoto, H., Eguchi, T., Kawaguchi, M., Abe, H. and Tanikawa, K., 1979, Acetaminophen-induced liver injury, *Journal of Clinical Electron Microscopy*, **12**, 814–815.

Ilkiw, J. E. and Ratcliffe, R. C., 1987, Paracetamol toxicity in a cat, *Australian Veterinary Journal*, **64**, 245–247.

Imamura, Y., Nozaki, Y., Higucho, T. and Otagiri, M., 1991, Reactivity for prostaglandins and inhibition by nonsteroidal anti-inflammatory drugs of rabbit liver befunolol reductase, *Research Communications in Chemical Pathology and Pharmacology*, **71**, 49–57.

Imamura, Y., Wang, L. H., Lee, C. S. and Perrin, J. H., 1980, Effects of chlorpromazine and atropine on acetaminophen absorption in rabbits, *International Journal of Pharmaceutics*, **5**, 25–32.

Imamura, Y., Wang, L. H., Lee, C. S., Perrin, J. H., Shiozu, K. and Ichibagase, H., 1981, Acetaminophen-diphenhydramine interaction in rabbits, *International Journal of Pharmaceutics*, **8**, 277–284.

Imashuku, S. and LaBrosse, E. H., 1971, Differentiation of urinary N-acetyl-p-aminophenol from endogenous phenolic compounds, *Clinical Chemistry*, **17**, 122–124.

Imbimbo, B. P., Gardino, L., Palmas, F., Frascio, M., Canepa, G. and Scarpignato, C., 1990, Different effects of atropine and cimetropium bromide on gastric emptying of liquids and antroduodenal motor activity in man, *Hepato-Gastroenterology*, **37**, 242–246.

Indelicato, P. A., 1986, Comparison of diflunisal and acetaminophen with codeine in the treatment of mild to moderate pain due to strains and sprains, *Clinical Therapeutics*, **8**, 269–274.

Inoue, K., Kobatake, K., Haruma, K., Yamanaka, H., Fujimura, J., Yoshihara, M., Sumii, K. and Kajiyama, G., 1993, Gastric emptying in elderly patients with cerebral vascular diseases and the effect of trimebutine, *Japanese Journal of Geriatrics*, **30**, 41–45.

International Agranulocytosis and Aplastic Anemia Study, 1986, Risks of agranulocytosis and aplastic anemia: a first report of their relation to drug use with special reference to analgesics, *Journal of the American Medical Association*, **256**, 1749–1757.

Ioannides, C., Hall, D. E., Mulder, D. E., Steele, C. M., Spickett, J., Delaforge, M. and Parke, D. V., 1983a, A comparison of the protective effects of N-acetylcysteine and S-carboxymethylcysteine against paracetamol-induced hepatotoxicity, *Toxicology*, **28**, 313–321.

Ioannides, C., Lum, P. Y. and Parke, D. V., 1984, Cytochrome P-448 and the activation of toxic chemicals and carcinogens, *Xenobiotica*, **14**, 119–137.

Ioannides, C., Steele, C. M. and Parke, D. V., 1983b, Species variation in the metabolic activation of paracetamol to toxic intermediates: role of cytochromes P-450 and P-448, *Toxicology Letters*, **16**, 55–61.

Ipp, M. M., Gold, R., Greenberg, R. U. L., Goldbach, M., Kupfert, B. B., Lloyd, D. D., Maresky, D. C., Saunders, N. and Wise, S.A., 1987, Acetaminophen prophylaxis of adverse reactions following vaccination of infants with diphtheria-pertussis-tetanus toxoids-polio vaccine, *Pediatric Infectious Disease Journal*, **6**, 721–725.

Irshaid, Y. M., Gharaybeh, K. I., Ammari, F. F. and Rawashdeh, N. M., 1990, Glucuronidation of 7-hydroxy-4-methylcoumarin by human liver microsomes: inhibition by certain drugs, *European Journal of Drug Metabolism and Pharmacokinetics*, **15**, 295–301.

Irvine, G. H., Lutterloch, M. J. and Bowerman, J. E., 1982, Comparison of diflunisal and paracetamol in the management of pain following wisdom teeth removal, *British Dental Journal*, **152**, 18–20.

Isaacs, S. N., Axelrod, P. I. and Lorber, B., 1990, Antipyretic orders in a university hospital, *American Journal of Medicine*, **88**, 31–35.

Ishidate, M., Hayashi, M., Sawada, M., Matsuoka, A., Yoshikawa, K., Ono, M. and Nakadate, M., 1978, Cytotoxicity test on medical drugs: chromosome aberration tests with Chinese hamster cells *in vitro*, *Bulletin of the National Institute of Hygienic Sciences*, **96**, 55–61.

Ishidate, M. and Yoshikawa, K., 1980, Chromosome aberration tests with Chinese hamster cells *in vitro* with and without metabolic activation: a comparative study on mutagens and carcinogens, *Archives of Toxicology*, **4**, 41–44.

Ishikawa, M., Tanno, K., Sasaki, M., Takayanagi, Y. and Sasaki, K., 1990a, Antidotal effect of lipopolysaccharide against acetaminophen-induced mortality in mice, *Pharmacology and Toxicology*, **68**, 387–391.

Ishikawa, M., Tanno, K., Takayanagi, Y. and Sasaki, K., 1990b, Prevention of acetaminophen-induced hepatotoxicity by endotoxin in mice, *Research Communications in Chemical Pathology and Pharmacology*, **69**, 111–114.

Ismail, S., Back, D. J. and Edwards, G., 1992, The effect of malaria infection on 3'-azido-3'-deoxythymidine and paracetamol glucuronidation in rat liver microsomes, *Biochemical Pharmacology*, **44**, 1879–1882.

Ismail, S., Kokwaro, G. O., Back, D. J. and Edwards, G., 1994, Effect of malaria infection on the pharmacokinetics of paracetamol in rat, *Xenobiotica*, **24**, 527–533.

Ismail, S., Na Bangchang, K., Karbwang, J., Back, D. J. and Edwards, G., 1995, Paracetamol disposition in Thai patients during and after treatment of falciparum malaria, *European Journal of Clinical Pharmacology*, **48**, 65–69.

Ispano, M., Fontana, A., Scibilia, J. and Ortolani, C., 1993, Oral challenge with alternative nonsteroidal anti-inflammatory drugs (NSAIDs) and paracetamol in patients intolerant to these agents, *Drugs*, **46 (Suppl. 1)**, 253–256.

Issopoulos, P. B., 1990, Spectrophotometric determination of acetaminophen by reduction of molybdenum (VI), *Analytical Letters*, **23**, 1057–1068.

Itinose, A. M., Doi-Sakuno, M. L. and Bracht, A., 1994, N-acetylcysteine stimulates hepatic glycogen deposition in the rat, *Research Communications in Chemical Pathology and Pharmacology*, **83**, 87–92.

Itinose, A. M., Sakuno, M. L. D. and Bracht, A., 1989, Metabolic effects of acetaminophen. Studies in the isolated perfused rat liver, *Cell Biochemistry and Function*, **7**, 263–273.

Ito, Y., Suzuki, Y., Ogonuki, H., Hiraishi, H., Razandi, M., Terano, A., Harada, T. and Ivey, K. J., 1994, Role of iron and glutathione redox cycle in acetaminophen-induced cytotoxicity to cultured rat hepatocytes, *Digestive Diseases and Sciences*, **39**, 1257–1264.

Itoh, S., Matsuo, S., Shiomi, M. and Ichinoe, A., 1983, Cirrhosis following 12 years of treatment with acetaminophen, *Hepato-Gastroenterology*, **30**, 58.

Iversen, P. L. and Franklin, M. R., 1985, Microsomal cytochrome P-450 'handprints': five fractions from anion-exchange high-pressure liquid chromatography provide a rapid preliminary screen for selectivity in the induction and destruction of rat hepatic cytochrome

P-450 subpopulations, *Toxicology and Applied Pharmacology*, **78**, 1–9.

Ivey, K. J., 1983, Gastrointestinal effects of antipyretic analgesics, *American Journal of Medicine*, **75 (5A)**, 53–64.

Ivey, K. J., 1986, Gastrointestinal intolerance and bleeding with non-narcotic analgesics, *Drugs*, **32 (Suppl. 4)**, 71–89.

Ivey, K. J. and Settree, P., 1976, Effect of paracetamol (acetaminophen) on gastric ion fluxes and potential difference in man, *Gut*, **17**, 916–919.

Ivey, K. J., Silvoso, G. R. and Krause, W. J., 1978, Effect of paracetamol on gastric mucosa, *British Medical Journal*, **1**, 1586–1588.

Iwuagwu, M. A. and Aloko, K. S., 1992, Adsorption of paracetamol and chloroquine phosphate by some antacids, *Journal of Pharmacy and Pharmacology*, **44**, 655–658.

Jack, D., Thomas, M. and Skidmore, I. F., 1985, Ranitidine and paracetamol metabolism, *Lancet*, **ii**, 1067.

Jackson, J. E., 1981, Cimetidine protects against acetaminophen hepatoxicity, *Veterinary and Human Toxicology*, **23 (Suppl. 1)**, 7–9.

Jackson, J. E., 1982, Cimetidine protects against acetaminophen toxicity, *Life Sciences*, **31**, 31–35.

Jacobsen, D., Frederichsen, P. S., Knutsen, K. M., Sørum, Y., Talseth, T. and Ødegaard, O. R., 1984, Clinical course in acute self-poisonings: a prospective study of 1125 consecutively hospitalised adults, *Human Toxicology*, **3**, 107–116.

Jacobson, J. and Bertilson, S. O., 1987, Analgesic efficacy of paracetamol/codeine and paracetamol/dextropropoxyphene in pain after episiotomy and ruptures in connection with childbirth, *Journal of International Medical Research*, **15**, 89–95.

Jacqueson, A., Semont, H., Thevenin, M., Warnet, J.-M., Prost, R. and Claude, J. R., 1984, Effects of daily high doses of paracetamol given orally during spermatogenesis in the rat testes, *Archives of Toxicology*, **55 (Suppl. 7)**, 164–166.

Jaeger, A., Flesch, F., Kopferschmitt, J. and Sauder, Ph., 1987, Intoxication aiguë par le paracétamol, *Revue du Praticien*, **37**, 2881–2866.

Jaeschke, H., 1990, Glutathione disulfide formation and oxidant stress during acetaminophen-induced hepatotoxicity in mice *in vivo*: the protective effect of allopurinol, *Journal of Pharmacology and Experimental Therapeutics*, **255**, 935–941.

Jaeschke, H., Smith, C. W. and Farhood, A., 1991, Role of neutrophils in acetaminophen-induced liver injury, *Toxicologist*, **11**, 32.

Jaeschke, H., Werner, C. and Wendel, A., 1987, Disposition and hepatoprotection by phosphatidyl choline liposomes in mouse liver, *Chemico-Biological Interactions*, **64**, 127–137.

Jaffari, S. A. and Pickup, J. C., 1994, Nafion/polyurethane coating of glucose sensors to reduce interference by ascorbate and paracetamol, *Diabetic Medicine*, **11 (Suppl. 2)**, S34.

Jaffe, J. M., Colaizzi, J. L. and Barry, H., 1971, Effects of dietary components on GI absorption of acetaminophen tablets in man, *Journal of Pharmaceutical Sciences*, **60**, 1646–1650.

Jaffe, M. and Hilbert, P., 1888, Ueber Acetanilid und Acetoluid und ihr Verhalten im thierischen Stoffwechsel, *Hoppe Seyles Zeitschrift für Physiologische Chemie*, **12**, 295–321.

Jagenburg, O. R. and Toczko, K., 1964, The metabolism of acetophenetidine: isolation and characterisation of S-(1-acetamido-4-hydroxyphenyl)-cysteine, a metabolite of acetophenetidine, *Biochemical Journal*, **92**, 639–643.

Jagenburg, R., Nagy, A. and Rödjer, S., 1968, Separation of p-acetamidophenol metabolites by gel filtration on Sephadex G 10, *Scandinavian Journal of Clinical and Laboratory Investigation*, **22**, 11–16.

Jain, A. K., Ryan, J. R., McMahon, F. G. and Smith, G., 1986, Comparison of oral nalbuphine, acetaminophen, and their combination in postoperative pain, *Clinical Pharmacology and Therapeutics*, **39**, 295–299.

Jakobsen, D., Holme, J. A. and Wiik-Larsen, E., 1987, Paracetamolforgiftning: Mekanismer og klinisk behandling, *Tidsskrift for den Norske Lægeforening*, **107**, 1033–1036.

Jakobsen, J., Christensen, K. S. and Fallingborg, J., 1984, Accidentel paracetamolforgiftning,

Ugeskrift for Læger, **146**, 4033–4034.

James, A. J., Silbert, P. L. and Dunne, J. W., 1992, Paracetamol syrup induced diarrhoea, *Medical Journal of Australia*, **156**, 72.

James, O., 1976, A controlled trial of cysteamine in the treatment of acute paracetamol poisoning, *Journal of International Medical Research*, **4 (Suppl. 4)**, 118–122.

James, O., Lesna, M., Roberts, S. H., Pulman, L., Douglas, A. P., Smith, P. A. and Watson, A. J., 1975, Liver damage after paracetamol overdose. Comparison of liver-function tests, fasting serum bile acids, and liver histology, *Lancet*, **ii**, 579–581.

James, R. C., Harbison, R. D. and Roberts, S. M., 1993, Phenylpropanolamine potentiation of acetaminophen-induced hepatotoxicity: evidence for a glutathione-dependent mechanism, *Toxicology and Applied Pharmacology*, **118**, 159–168.

Janbu, T., Løkken, P. and Nesheim, B.-L., 1978, Effect of acetylsalicylic acid, paracetamol, and placebo on pain and blood loss in dysmenorrhoeic women, *European Journal of Clinical Pharmacology*, **14**, 413–416.

Janbu, T., Løkken, P. and Nesheim, B.-L., 1979, Effect of acetylsalicylic acid, paracetamol and placebo on pain and blood loss in dysmenorrheic women, *Acta Obstetricia et Gynecologica Scandinavica*, **87 (Suppl.)**, 81–85.

Janes, J. and Routledge, P. A., 1992, Recent developments in the management of paracetamol (acetaminophen) poisoning, *Drug Safety*, **7**, 170–177.

Jang, S. H., Lee, M. H. and Lee, M. G., 1994, Pharmacokinetics of acetaminophen after intravenous and oral administration to spontaneously hypertensive rats and normotensive Wistar rats, *Journal of Pharmaceutical Sciences*, **83**, 810–814.

Janicki, P. K., Erskine, W. A. R. and James, M. F. M., 1991, The route of morphine administration affects the development of tolerance in relation to gastric emptying in rats: is morphine-6-glucuronide involved? *Clinical and Experimental Pharmacology and Physiology*, **18**, 193–194.

Janjua, M. Z. and Draz, U., 1991, The effect of paracetamol on naprosyn induced damage to gastric mucosa in albino rat, *Journal of the Pakistan Medical Association*, **41**, 107–112.

Jarvis, M. R., Wasserman, A. L. and Todd, R. D., 1990, Acute psychosis in a patient with Epstein-Barr virus infection, *Journal of the American Academy of Child and Adolescent Psychiatry*, **29**, 468–469.

Jasiewicz, M. L. and Richardson, J. C., 1987, Absence of mutagenic activity of benorylate, paracetamol and aspirin in the Salmonella/mammalian microsome test, *Mutation Research*, **190**, 95–100.

Jaszewski, R. and Sheridan, V. L., 1987, Acetaminophen treatment protects against acetaminophen hepatotoxicity in mice, *Biochemical Archives*, **3**, 211–216.

Jaw, S. and Jeffery, E. H., 1993, Interaction of caffeine with acetaminophen. I. Correlation of the effect of caffeine on acetaminophen hepatotoxicity and acetaminophen bioactivation following treatment of mice with various cytochrome P-450 inducing agents, *Biochemical Pharmacology*, **46**, 493–501.

Jayasinghe, K. S. A., Roberts, C. J. C. and Read, A. E., 1986, Is biliary excretion of paracetamol significant in man? *British Journal of Clinical Pharmacology*, **22**, 363–366.

Jean, R., Lesbros, D. and Ariole, P., 1983, Activité antipyrétique du soluté buvable de paracétamol chez l'enfant, *Annales de Pédiatrie*, **30**, 807–809.

Jeevanandam, M., Novic, B., Savich, R. and Wagman, E., 1980, Serum acetaminophen assay using activated charcoal adsorption and gas chromatography without derivatization, *Journal of Analytical Toxicology*, **4**, 124–126.

Jefferson, S. G., 1986, Adaptation of an enzymatic kit for acetaminophen (paracetamol) to the Technicon RA-1000, *Clinical Chemistry*, **32**, 2101–2102.

Jeffery, E. H., Arndt, K. and Haschek, W. M., 1988, Mechanism of inhibition of hepatic bioactivation of paracetamol by dimethyl sulfoxide, *Drug Metabolism and Drug Interactions*, **6**, 413–424.

Jeffery, E. H., Arndt, K. and Haschek, W. M., 1991, The role of cytochrome P-450IIE1 in bioactivation of acetaminophen in diabetic and acetone-treated mice, *Advances in Experimental Medicine and Biology*, **283**, 249–251.

Jeffery, E. H. and Haschek, W. M., 1988, Protection by dimethylsulfoxide against acetaminophen-induced hepatic, but not respiratory toxicity in the mouse, *Toxicology and Applied Pharmacology*, **93**, 452–461.

Jeffery, W. H. and Lafferty, W. E., 1981, Acute renal failure after acetaminophen overdose: report of two cases, *American Journal of Hospital Pharmacy*, **38**, 1355–1358.

Jenny, R. W., 1985, Interlaboratory evaluations of salicylate interference in colorimetric acetaminophen methods and its clinical significance, *Clinical Chemistry*, **31**, 1158–1162.

Jensen, B. T., Theilade, P. and Kaa, E., 1987, Paracetamolforgiftninger med letalt forlob, *Ugeskrift for Læger*, **149**, 1360–1362.

Jensen, C. B., Price, V. F. and Jollow, D. J., 1986, Acetaminophen hepatotoxicity: species differences in the excretion of acetaminophen-cysteine conjugate as a metabolite of acetaminophen, *Pharmacologist*, **28**, 125.

Jensen, E., Falch, E. and Bundgaard, H., 1991, Water-soluble aminoalkylbenzoate esters of phenol as prodrugs. Synthesis, enzymatic hydrolysis and chemical stability of paracetamol esters, *Acta Pharmaceutica Nordica*, **3**, 31–40.

Jensen, F. M., Dahl, J. B. and Frigast, C., 1992, Direct spinal effect of intrathecal acetaminophen on visceral noxious stimulation in rabbits, *Acta Anaesthesiologica Scandinavica*, **36**, 837–841.

Jensen, K., 1986, Paracetamolforgiftning, *Ugeskrift for Læger*, **148**, 641–643.

Jepson, M. A., Davis, M. J. H., Horton, A. A. and Walker, D. G., 1987, Histochemical and biochemical observations on the cytotoxicity of paracetamol and its effects on glycogen metabolism in rat liver, *Toxicology*, **47**, 325–337.

Jespersen, T. W., Christensen, K. S., Kjaersgaard-Andersen, P., Sommer, S. and Juhl, B., 1989, Postoperativ smertebehandling med morfin vs. morfin og paracetamol: En dobbeltblind klinisk kontrolleret undersøgelse med placebo, *Ugeskrift for Læger*, **151**, 1615–1618.

Jeyaranjan, R., 1991, When does acetaminophen poisoning require treatment? *Postgraduate Medicine*, **90**, 272.

Jick, H., 1981, Effects of aspirin and acetaminophen in gastrointestinal hemorrhage, *Archives of Internal Medicine*, **141**, 316–321.

Jick, H., Holmes, L. B., Hunter, J. R., Madsen, S. and Stergachis, A., 1981, First-trimester drug use and congenital disorders, *Journal of the American Medical Association*, **246**, 343–346.

Johannessen, W., Gadeholt, G. and Aarbakke, J., 1981, Effects of diethyl ether anaesthesia on the pharmacokinetics of antipyrine and paracetamol in the rat, *Journal of Pharmacy and Pharmacology*, **33**, 365–368.

Johannessen, W. M., Tyssebotn, I. M. and Aarbakke, J., 1982, Antipyrine and acetaminophen kinetics in the rat: comparison of data based on blood samples from the cut tail and a cannulated femoral artery, *Journal of Pharmaceutical Sciences*, **71**, 1352–1356.

Johansson, S., Angervall, L., Bengtsson, U. and Wahlqvist, L., 1974, Uroepithelial tumors of the renal pelvis associated with the abuse of phenacetin-containing analgesics, *Cancer*, **33**, 743–753.

Johansson, S. L., 1981, Carcinogenicity of analgesics: long-term treatment of Sprague-Dawley rats with phenacetin, phenazone, caffeine and paracetamol (acetamidophen), *International Journal of Cancer*, **27**, 521–529.

Johansson, S. L., Radio, S. J., Saidi, J. and Sakata, T., 1989, The effects of acetaminophen, antipyrine and phenacetin on rat uroepithelial cell proliferation, *Carcinogenesis*, **10**, 105–111.

Johnson, G. K. and Tolman, K. G., 1977, Chronic liver disease and acetaminophen, *Annals of Internal Medicine*, **87**, 302–304.

Johnson, M. W., Friedman, P. A. and Mitch, W. E., 1981, Alcoholism, nonprescription drugs and hepatotoxicity: the risk from unknown acetaminophen ingestion, *American Journal of Gastroenterology*, **76**, 530–533.

Johnson, P. C. and Driscoll, T., 1981, Comparison of plain and buffered aspirin with acetaminophen in regard to gastrointestinal bleeding, *Current Therapeutic Research*, **30**, 79–84.

Jokl, P. and Warman, M., 1989, A comparison of the efficacy and tolerability of diflunisal and dextropropoxyphene napsylate with acetaminophen in the management of mild to moderate pain after arthroscopy of the knee, *Clinical Therapeutics*, **11**, 841–845.

Jollow, D. J., 1980, Glutathione thresholds in reactive metabolite toxicity, *Archives of Toxicology*, **Suppl. 3**, 95–110.

Jollow, D. J., Mitchell, J. R., Potter, W. Z., Davis, D. C., Gillette, J. R. and Brodie, B. B., 1973, Acetaminophen-induced hepatic necrosis. II. Role of covalent binding *in vivo*, *Journal of Pharmacology and Experimental Therapeutics*, **187**, 195–202.

Jollow, D. J., Roberts, S., Price, V. and Smith, C., 1981, Biochemical basis for dose response relationships in reactive metabolite toxicity, *Advances in Experimental Medicine and Biology*, **136**, 99–113.

Jollow, D. J., Thorgeirsson, S. S., Potter, W. Z., Hashimoto, M. and Mitchell, J. R., 1974, Acetaminophen-induced hepatic necrosis. VI. Metabolic disposition of toxic and non-toxic doses of acetaminophen, *Pharmacology*, **12**, 251–271.

Jones, A. C. and Doherty, M., 1992, The treatment of osteoarthritis, *British Journal of Clinical Pharmacology*, **33**, 357–363.

Jones, A. F., Harvey, J. M. and Vale, J. A., 1989, Hypophosphataemia and phosphaturia in paracetamol poisoning, *Lancet*, **ii**, 608–609.

Jones, A. F., McAleer, J. F., Braithwaite, R. A., Scott, L. D., Brown, S. S. and Vale, J. A., 1990, Rapid sideroom test for paracetamol, *Lancet*, **335**, 793–794.

Jones, A. F. and Vale, J. A., 1993, Paracetamol poisoning and the kidney, *Journal of Clinical Pharmacy and Therapeutics*, **18**, 5–8.

Jones, A. L., Hume, R., Bamforth, K. J. and Coughtrie, M. W. H., 1992a, Estrogen and phenol sulfotransferase activities in human fetal lung, *Early Human Development*, **28**, 65–77.

Jones, D. I. R., 1977, Self-poisoning with drugs: the past 20 years in Sheffield, *British Medical Journal*, **1**, 28–29.

Jones, D. P., Sundby, G.-B., Ormstad, K. and Orrenius, S., 1979, Use of isolated kidney cells for study of drug metabolism, *Biochemical Pharmacology*, **28**, 929–935.

Jones, G. and Thomas, P., 1977, Treatment of acute paracetamol poisoning, *British Medical Journal*, **2**, 1224.

Jones, G. R. and Pounder, D. J., 1987, Site dependence of drug concentrations in postmortem blood – a case study, *Journal of Analytical Toxicology*, **11**, 186–190.

Jones, R. D., Baynes, R. E. and Nimitz, C. T., 1992b, Nonsteroidal anti-inflammatory drug toxicosis in dogs and cats: 240 cases (1989–1990), *Journal of the American Veterinary Medical Association*, **201**, 475–477.

Jonker, D., Lee, V. S., Hargreaves, R. J. and Lake, B. G., 1988, Comparison of the effects of ascorbyl palmitate and l-ascorbic acid on paracetamol-induced hepatotoxicity in the mouse, *Toxicology*, **52**, 287–295.

Jonville, A. P., Autret, E., Majzoub, S., Furet, Y., Ernouf, D. and Breteau, M., 1988, Epidémiologie des intoxications au paracétamol en pédiatrie (analyse rétrospective des appels reçus au Centre Anti-Poisons de Tours), *Revue de Médecine de Tours*, **22**, 211–214.

Jonville, A. P., Autret, E., Majzoub, S., Furet, Y., Ernouf, D. and Breteau, M., 1990, Epidémiologie des intoxications au paracétamol en pédiatrie (analyse rétrospective des appels reçus au Centre Anti-Poisons de Tours), *Journal de Toxicologie Clinique et Expérimentale*, **10**, 21–25.

Jonville-Béra, A.-P. and Autret, E., 1994, Severe intoxication by paracetamol and salicylates, *Revue du Praticien*, **44**, 1797–1801.

Jørgensen, L., Thomsen, P. and Poulsen, H. E., 1988, Disulfiram prevents acetaminophen hepatotoxicity in rats, *Pharmacology and Toxicology*, **62**, 267–271.

Jørgensen, L. N., 1985, Overlevels efter selvforgiftning med 80 g paracetamol, *Ugeskrift for Læger*, **147**, 3610–3611.

Jorup-Rönström, C., Beerman, B., Wåhlin-Boll, E., Melander, A. and Britton, S., 1986, Reduction of paracetamol and aspirin metabolism during viral hepatitis, *Clinical Pharmacokinetics*, **11**, 250–256.

Joshi, S., Zenser, T. V., Mattammal, M. B., Herman, C. A. and Davis, B. B., 1978, Kidney metabolism of acetaminophen and phenacetin, *Journal of Laboratory and Clinical Medicine*, **92**, 924–931.

Joshi, Y. M., Sovani, V. B., Joshi, V. V., Navrange, J. R., Benakappa, D. G., Shivananda, P. and Sankaranarayanan, V. S., 1990, Comparative evaluation of the antipyretic efficacy of ibuprofen and paracetamol, *Indian Pediatrics*, **27**, 803–806.

Josting, D., Winne, D. and Bock, K. W., 1976, Glucuronidation of paracetamol, morphine and 1-naphthol in the rat intestinal loop, *Biochemical Pharmacology*, **25**, 613–616.

Joubert, P. H., Clark, E. C., Otto, A. C. and Pannall, P. R., 1977, Unreliable drug histories, analgesics, and changes in renal function, *South African Medical Journal*, **52**, 107–109.

Jouet, J. P., Huart, J. J., Bauters, F. and Goudenand, M., 1980, Le paracétamol cause méconnue d'agranulocytose aiguë médicamenteuse, *La Nouvelle Presse Médicale*, **9**, 1386–1387.

Jover, R., Ponsoda, X., Castell, J. V. and Gómez-Lechón, M. J., 1992, Evaluation of the cytotoxicity of ten chemicals on human cultured hepatocytes: predictability of human toxicity and comparison with rodent cell culture systems, *Toxicology in Vitro*, **6**, 47–52.

Joyave, J. L., Steinhauer, L. S., Dillehay, D. L., Born, C. K. and Hamrick, M. E., 1985, Alteration of chemically induced hepatotoxicity by copper (II) (3,5-diisopropylsalicylate)$_2$, *Biochemical Pharmacology*, **34**, 3915–3919.

Joyce, C. R. P., Zutshi, D. W., Hrubes, V. and Mason, R. M., 1975, Comparison of fixed interval and visual analogue scales for rating chronic pain, *European Journal of Clinical Pharmacology*, **8**, 415–420.

Judson, D. G., 1985, Paracetamol poisoning in cats, *The Veterinary Record*, **116**, 355.

Jung, D., 1985, Disposition of acetaminophen in protein-calorie malnutrition, *Journal of Pharmacology and Experimental Therapeutics*, **232**, 178–182.

Jung, D. and Zafar, N. U., 1985, Micro high-performance liquid chromatographic assay of acetaminophen and its major metabolites in plasma and urine, *Journal of Chromatography: Biomedical Applications*, **339**, 198–202.

Jurna, I., 1991, Zentrale analgetische Wirkungen nichtsteroidaler Antirheumatika (NSAR), *Zeitschrift für Rheumatolgie*, **50 (Suppl. 1)**, 7–13.

Jurna, I., Carlsson, K.-H., Kömen, W. and Bonke, D., 1990, Acute effects of vitamin B_6 and fixed combinations of vitamin B_1, B_6 and B_{12} on nociceptive activity evoked in the rat thalamus: dose-response relationship and combinations with morphine and paracetamol, *Klinische Wochenschrift*, **68**, 129–135.

Justice, J. L. and Kline, S. S., 1988, Analgesics and warfarin: a case that brings up questions and cautions, *Postgraduate Medicine*, **83**, 217–220.

Juzwiak, S., 1993, Doswiadczalna ocena wplywu wyciagu z pylkow kwiatowych na przebieg zatrucia paracetamolem, *Annales Academiae Medicae Stetinensis*, **39**, 57–69.

Juzwiak, S., Rainska, T., Dutkiewicz, T., Cioch, U., Olenderek, B., Krasowska, B., Rózewicka, L., Juzyszyn, Z., Wójcicki, J. and Samochowiec, L., 1992, Pollen extracts reduce the hepatotoxicity of paracetamol in mice, *Phytotherapy Research*, **6**, 141–145.

Kaa, E., 1980, Rapid gas chromatographic method for emergency determination of paracetamol in human serum, *Journal of Chromatography: Biomedical Applications*, **221**, 414–418.

Kadri, A. Z., Fisher, R. and Winterton, M. C., 1988, Cimetidine and paracetamol hepatotoxicity, *Human Toxicology*, **7**, 205.

Kahela, P., Laine, E. and Anttila, M., 1987, A comparison of the bioavailability of paracetamol from a fatty and a hydrous suppository base and the effect of storage on the absorption in man, *Drug Development and Industrial Pharmacy*, **13**, 213–224.

Kaito, T. and Sagara, K., 1974, Studies on fluorometric analysis of phenol derivatives. III. Fluorometric determination of acetaminophen. (2) Fluorometric analysis of p-aminophenol and its application to determination of acetaminophen, *Journal of the Pharmaceutical Society of Japan*, **94**, 639–644.

Kaito, T., Sagara, K., Yoshida, T. and Ito, Y., 1974, Studies on fluorometric analysis of phenol derivatives. II. Fluorometric determination of acetaminophen. (1), *Journal of the Pharmaceutical Society of Japan*, **94**, 633–638.

Kaka, J. S. and Al-Khamis, K. I., 1986, Effect of domperidone on acetyl salicylic acid and acetaminophen absorption in rabbits, *International Journal of Pharmaceutics*, **28**, 133–137.

Kakemi, M., Masuda, K., Ueda, M. and Koizuma, T., 1975, Pharmacokinetic analysis of pharmacological effects and drug disposition: acetaminophen and 4-aminoantipyrine, *Chemical and Pharmaceutical Bulletin*, **23**, 736–745.

Kalabis, G. M. and Wells, P. G., 1990, Biphasic modulation of acetaminophen bioactivation and hepatotoxicity by pretreatment with the interferon inducer polyinosinic-polycytidylic acid, *Journal of Pharmacology and Experimental Therapeutics*, **255**, 1408–1419.

Kalhorn, T. F., Lee, C. A., Slattery, J. T. and Nelson, S. D., 1990, Effect of methylxanthines on acetaminophen hepatotoxicity in various induction states, *Journal of Pharmacology and Experimental Therapeutics*, **252**, 112–116.

Kaloyanides, G. J., 1991, Metabolic interactions between drugs and renal tubulo-interstitial cells: role in nephrotoxicity, *Kidney International*, **39**, 531–540.

Kalra, J., Mamer, O. A., Gregory, B. and Gault, M. H., 1977, Interference by endogenous p-hydroxyphenylacetic acid with estimation of N-acetyl-p-aminophenol in urine by gas chromatography, *Journal of Pharmacy and Pharmacology*, **29**, 127–128.

Kalyoncu, A. F., 1994, Acetaminophen hypersensitivity and other analgesics, *Annals of Allergy*, **72**, 285.

Kamali, F., 1993, The effect of probenecid on paracetamol metabolism and pharmacokinetics, *European Journal of Clinical Pharmacology*, **45**, 551–553.

Kamali, F., Edwards, C. and Rawlins, M. D., 1992, The effect of pirenzepine on gastric emptying and salivary flow rate: constraints on the use of saliva paracetamol concentrations for the determination of paracetamol pharmacokinetics, *British Journal of Clinical Pharmacology*, **33**, 309–312.

Kamali, F., Fry, J. R. and Bell, G. D., 1987a, Salivary excretion of paracetamol in man, *Journal of Pharmacy and Pharmacology*, **39**, 150–152.

Kamali, F., Fry, J. R. and Bell, G. D., 1987b, Temporal variation in paracetamol absorption and metabolism in man, *Xenobiotica*, **17**, 635–642.

Kamali, F., Fry, J. R., Bell, G. D., Kitchingman, G. K., Standen, G. and Sokal, M., 1988, Hepatic drug metabolising ability and gastrointestinal absorption of drugs in patients undergoing high-dose methotrexate chemotherapy, *Journal of Drug Development*, **1**, 137–143.

Kamali, F., Fry, J. R., Smart, H. L. and Bell, G. D., 1985, A double-blind placebo controlled study to examine effects of sucralfate on paracetamol absorption, *British Journal of Clinical Pharmacology*, **19**, 113–114.

Kamali, F. and Herd, B., 1990, Liquid-liquid extraction and analysis of paracetamol (acetaminophen) and its major metabolites in biological fluids by reversed-phase ion-pair chromatography, *Journal of Chromatography: Biomedical Applications*, **530**, 222–225.

Kamali, F. and Rawlins, M. D., 1992, Influence of probenecid and paracetamol (acetaminophen) on zidovudine glucuronidation in human liver *in vitro*, *Biopharmaceutics and Drug Disposition*, **13**, 403–409.

Kamali, F., Thomas, S. H. L. and Ferner, R. E., 1993, Paracetamol elimination in patients with non-insulin dependent diabetes mellitus, *British Journal of Clinical Pharmacology*, **35**, 58–61.

Kamanabroo, D. and Schmitz-Landgraf, W., 1988, Plasma exchange in the successful treatment of severe drug-induced toxic epidermal necrolysis (Lyell's disease), *Plasma Therapy and Transfusion Technology*, **9**, 99–101.

Kamiyama, T., Sato, C., Liu, J., Tajiri, K., Miyakawa, H. and Marumo, F., 1993, Role of lipid peroxidation in acetaminophen-induced hepatotoxicity: comparison with carbon tetrachloride, *Toxicology Letters*, **66**, 7–12.

Kampffmeyer, H. G., 1971, Elimination of phenacetin and phenazone by man before and after treatment with phenobarbital, *European Journal of Clinical Pharmacology*, **3**, 113–118.

Kampffmeyer, H. G., 1974, Metabolic rate of phenacetin and of paracetamol in dogs before and after treatment with phenobarbital or SKF 525 A, *Biochemical Pharmacology*, **23**, 713–724.

Kane, R., Li, A., Brems, J. and Kaminsky, D., 1990a, Sulfation and glucuronidation of acetaminophen (APAP) by human hepatocytes cultured on Matrigel and type I collagen replicating *in vivo* metabolism, *Hepatology*, **12**, 1010.

Kane, R. E. and Chen, L. J., 1987, Influence of gonadal hormones upon rat hepatic acetaminophen sulfotransferases, *Drug Metabolism and Disposition: The Biological Fate of Chemicals*, **15**, 725–728.

Kane, R. E., Lamott, J., Franklin, M. R. and Galinsky, R. E., 1989, Perinatal cimetidine exposure has no apparent effect on hepatic drug oxidative or conjugative activity in adult male rat offspring, *Developmental Pharmacology and Therapeutics*, **12**, 96–105.

Kane, R. E., Tector, J., Brems, J. J., Li, A. and Kaminski, D., 1991, Sulfation and glucuronidation of acetaminophen by cultured hepatocytes reproducing *in vivo* sex-differences in conjugation on Matrigel and type 1 collagen, *In Vitro Cellular and Developmental Biology*, **27A**, 953–960.

Kane, R. E., Tector, J., Brems, J. J., Li, A. P. and Kaminski, D. L., 1990b, Sulfation and glucuronidation of acetaminophen by cultured hepatocytes replicating *in vivo* metabolism, *ASAIO Transactions*, **36**, M607–M610.

Kaneo, Y., Fujihara, Y., Tanaka, T., Kozawa, Y., Mori, H. and Iguchi, S., 1989a, Effects of glutathione, as the dextran conjugate, on acetaminophen-induced hepatotoxicity, *Chemical and Pharmaceutical Bulletin*, **37**, 218–220.

Kaneo, Y., Fujihara, Y., Tanaka, T., Kozawa, Y., Mori, H. and Iguchi, S., 1989b, Intrahepatic delivery of glutathione by conjugation to dextran, *Pharmaceutical Research*, **6**, 1025–1031.

Kaneo, Y., Ogawa, K., Tanaka, T., Fujihara, Y. and Iguchi, S., 1994, A protective effect of glutathione-dextran macromolecular conjugates on acetaminophen-induced hepatotoxicity dependent on molecular size, *Biological and Pharmaceutical Bulletin*, **17**, 1379–1384.

Kaniwa, N., Aoyagi, N., Ogata, H. and Ejima, A., 1988, Gastric emptying rates of drug preparations. I. Effects of size of dosage forms, food and species on gastric emptying rates, *Journal of Pharmacobiodynamics*, **11**, 563–570.

Kanui, T. I., Karim, F. and Towett, P. K., 1993, The formalin test in the naked mole-rat (*Heterocephalus glaber*): analgesic effects of morphine, nefopam and paracetamol, *Brain Research*, **600**, 123–126.

Kapetanovic, I. M., Kupferberg, H. J., Theodore, W. and Porter, R. J., 1981, Lack of effect of valproate on paracetamol (acetaminophen) disposition in epileptic patients, *British Journal of Clinical Pharmacology*, **11**, 391–393.

Kapetanovic, I. M. and Mieyal, J. J., 1979, Inhibition of acetaminophen-induced hepatotoxicity by phenacetin and its alkoxy analogs, *Journal of Pharmacology and Experimental Therapeutics*, **209**, 25–30.

Kaplowitz, N., Eberle, D. E., Petrini, J., Touloukian, J., Corvasce, M. C. and Kuhlenkamp, J., 1983, Factors influencing the efflux of hepatic glutathione into bile in rats, *Journal of Pharmacology and Experimental Therapeutics*, **224**, 141–147.

Kapur, V., Pillai, K. K., Hussian, S. Z. and Balani, D. K., 1994, Hepatoprotective activity of

'Jigrine' on liver damage caused by alcohol-carbon tetrachloride and paracetamol in rats, *Indian Journal of Pharmacology*, **26**, 35–40.

Kartsonis, A., Reddy, K. R. and Schiff, E. R., 1986, Alcohol, acetaminophen and hepatic necrosis, *Annals of Internal Medicine*, **105**, 138–139.

Karttunen, T., Autio-Harmainen, H. and Sutinen, S., 1982, Capillarosclerosis of the urinary tract associated with the use of paracetamol and cyclophosphamide, *Acta Pathologica Microbiologica et Immunologica Scandinavica – Section A, Pathology*, **90**, 391–392.

Kasai, S., Tanaka, K., Machimura, H., Takeda, H., Kaneshige, H., Sakai, H. and Harasawa, S., 1991, Effect of cisapride on gastric emptying in diabetic patients without gastrointestinal symptoms, *Tokai Journal of Experimental and Clinical Medicine*, **16**, 97–102.

Kasper, C. K. and Rapaport, S. I., 1972, Bleeding times and platelet aggregation after analgesics in hemophilia, *Annals of Internal Medicine*, **77**, 189–193.

Katyare, S. S. and Satav, J. G., 1989, Impaired mitochondrial oxidative energy metabolism following paracetamol-induced hepatotoxicity in the rat, *British Journal of Pharmacology*, **96**, 51–58.

Katyare, S. S. and Satav, J. G., 1991, Altered kinetic properties of liver mitochondrial membrane-bound enzyme activities following paracetamol hepatotoxicity in the rat, *Journal of Bioscience*, **16**, 71–79.

Katz, S., Pitt, W. W. and Mrochek, J. E., 1975, Comparative serum and urine analyses by dual-detector anion-exchange chromatography, *Journal of Chromatography*, **104**, 303–310.

Kauffman, R. E., Sawyer, L. A. and Scheinbaum, M. L., 1992, Antipyretic efficacy of ibuprofen vs. acetaminophen, *American Journal of Diseases of Children*, **146**, 622–625.

Kaufman, D. W., Kelly, J. P., Johannes, C. B., Sandler, A., Harmon, D., Stolley, P. D. and Shapiro, S., 1993, Acute thrombocytopenic purpura in relation to the use of drugs, *Blood*, **82**, 2714–2718.

Kaufmann-Raab, I., Jonen, H. G., Jähnchen, E., Kahl, G. F. and Groth, U., 1976, Interference by acetaminophen in the glucose oxidase-peroxidase method for blood glucose determination, *Clinical Chemistry*, **22**, 1729–1731.

Kawachi, T., Komatsu, T., Kada, T., Ishidate, M., Sasaki, M., Sugiyama, T. and Tazima, Y., 1980, Results of recent studies on the relevance of various short-term screening tests in Japan, *Applied Methods in Oncology*, **3**, 253–267.

Kawamoto, H., Yamamura, H., Tatsuta, M. and Okuda, S., 1985, Effect of glucagon on gastric motility examined by the acetaminophen absorption method and the endoscopic procedure, *Arzneimittel-Forschung*, **35**, 1475–1477.

Kayama, H. and Koh, K., 1991, Clinical and experimental studies on gastrointestinal motility following total colectomy: direct measurement (strain gauge force transducer method, barium method) and indirect measurement (hydrogen breath test, acetaminophen method), *Journal of Smooth Muscle Research*, **27**, 97–114.

Kaye, L., 1991, Warfarin and paracetamol, *Pharmaceutical Journal*, **246**, 692.

Kaysen, G. A., Pond, S. M., Roper, M. H., Menke, D. J. and Marrama, M. A., 1985, Combined hepatic and renal injury in alcoholics during therapeutic use of acetaminophen, *Archives of Internal Medicine*, **145**, 2019–2023.

Kazmierczyk, J., 1979, Pharmacokinetics of interaction of N-acetyl-p-aminophenol with the drugs affecting the secretory and motorial activity of the alimentary tract, *Annales Academiae Medicae Stetinensis*, **25**, 247–265.

Kearns, G. L., Bocchini, J. A., Brown, R. D., Cotter, D. L. and Wilson, J. T., 1985, Absence of a pharmacokinetic interaction between chloramphenicol and acetaminophen in children, *Journal of Pediatrics*, **107**, 134–139.

Keaton, M. R., 1988, Acute renal failure in an alcoholic during therapeutic acetaminophen ingestion, *Southern Medical Journal*, **81**, 1163–1166.

Keays, R., Harrison, P. M., Wendon, J. A., Forbes, A., Gove, C., Alexander, G. J. M. and Williams, R., 1991, Intravenous acetylcysteine in paracetamol induced fulminant hepatic failure: a prospective controlled trial, *British Medical Journal*, **303**, 1026–1029.

Keegan, C., Smith, C., Ungemach, F. and Simpson, J., 1984, A fluorescence polarization immunoassay for the quantitation of acetaminophen, *Clinical Chemistry*, **30**, 1025.

Keinänen, S., Hietula, M., Similä, S. and Kouvalainen, K., 1977, Antipyretic therapy: comparison of rectal and oral paracetamol, *European Journal of Clinical Pharmacology*, **12**, 77–80.

Keinänen-Kiukaanniemi, S., Similä, S., Luoma, P., Kangas, L. and Saukkonen, A.-L., 1979, Antipyretic effect and plasma concentrations of rectal acetaminophen and diazepam in children, *Epilepsia*, **20**, 607–612.

Kelemen, K. and Marko, R., 1988, Paracetamol-induced prostaglandin release in the heart, *Pharmacological Research Communications*, **20**, 97–98.

Kelemen, K. and Marko, R., 1992, Minor analgetics: blockers or stimulators of prostaglandin production? *Pharmacological Research*, **25 (Suppl. 2)**, 247–248.

Kelleher, J., McLachlan, M. S. F., Walker, B. E., Dixon, M. F. and Losowsky, M. S., 1977, Portal venous infusion of paracetamol and antipyrine in the rat, *Pharmacological Research Communications*, **9**, 701–710.

Kelleher, J., Walker, B. E., Keaney, N. P., Losowsky, M. S. and Dixon, M. F., 1976a, Modification of paracetamol toxicity by antioxidants, *Biochemical Society Transactions*, **4**, 292–294.

Kelleher, J., Walker, B. E., Losowsky, M. S. and Dixon, M. F., 1976b, Paracetamol hepatotoxicity and vitamin E, *International Journal for Vitamin and Nutrition Research*, **46**, 251–253.

Keller, R. J. and Hinson, J. A., 1991, Mechanism of acetaminophen-stimulated NADPH oxidation catalyzed by the peroxidase-H_2O_2 system, *Drug Metabolism and Disposition: The Biological Fate of Chemicals*, **19**, 184–187.

Kelley, M. T., Walson, P. D., Edge, J. H., Cox, S. and Mortensen, M. E., 1992, Pharmacokinetics and pharmacodynamics of ibuprofen isomers and acetaminophen in febrile children, *Clinical Pharmacology and Therapeutics*, **52**, 181–189.

Kelley, M. T., Walson, P. D., Hayes, J. R. and Edge, J. H., 1993, Safety of paracetamol and ibuprofen in febrile children, *Drug Investigation*, **6**, 48–56.

Kellmeyer, K., Yates, C., Parker, S. and Hilligoss, D., 1982, Bilirubin interference with kit determination of acetaminophen, *Clinical Chemistry*, **28**, 554–555.

Kellokumpu-lehtinen, P., Iisalo, E. and Nordman, E., 1989, Hepatotoxicty of paracetamol in combination with interferon and vinblastine, *Lancet*, **i**, 1143.

Kelly, C. and Galloway, R., 1992, Deliberate self-poisoning presenting at Craigavon Area Hospital: 1976 and 1986, *Ulster Medical Journal*, **61**, 12–18.

Kelly, J. H., Koussayer, T., He, D., Chong, M. G., Shang, T. A., Whisennand, H. H. and Sussman, N. L., 1992, An improved model of acetaminophen-induced fulminant hepatic failure in dogs, *Hepatology*, **15**, 329–335.

Kelly, R. C., Doshier, L. A. and Rubin, H. R., 1984, A convenient thin-layer chromatographic screening method for acetaminophen in serum, *Journal of Analytical Toxicology*, **8**, 54–58.

Kemp, R. B., Cross, D. M. and Meredith, R. W. J., 1988, Comparison of cell death and adenosine triphosphate content as indicators of acute toxicity *in vitro*, *Xenobiotica*, **18**, 633–639.

Kennedy, K. S., 1989, Quincke's disease after acetaminophen use, *Ear, Nose, and Throat Journal*, **68**, 721–722.

Kenny, D. and Ward, J., 1987, Determination of therapeutic concentrations of paracetamol in serum with the Cobas Fara analyser, *Annals of Clinical Biochemistry*, **24 (Suppl.)**, S1-72–S1-73.

Kerr, D., 1970, Phenacetin nephropathy, *British Medical Journal*, **4**, 363–364.

Kerr, D., 1973, Paracetamol overdosage, *Lancet*, **i**, 158.

Kerr, H. D., 1989, Self-poisoning with drugs, *Wisconsin Medical Journal*, **88**, 15–18.

Khairy, L., Isom, G. E. and Kildsig, D. O., 1983, Reversal of acetaminophen intoxication with an N-acetylcysteine-liposome preparation, *Research Communications in Chemical Pathology and Pharmacology*, **42**, 153–156.

Khalil, N., Bamil, I., Ahmed, O. and Shalaby, E., 1978, Paracetamol in hepatosplenic bilharziasis, *Journal of the Egyptian Medical Association*, **61**, 449–456.

Khani, S. C., Zaphiropoulos, P. G., Fujita, V. S., Porter, T. D., Koop, D. R. and Coon, M. J., 1987, cDNA and derived amino acid sequence of ethanol-inducible rabbit liver cytochrome P-450 isozyme 3a (P-450$_{ALC}$), *Proceedings of the National Academy of Sciences of the United States of America*, **84**, 638–642.

Khedun, S. M, Maharaj, B., Leary, W. P. and Naicker, T., 1993, The effect of therapeutic doses of paracetamol on liver function in the rat perfused liver, *Journal of Pharmacy and Pharmacology*, **45**, 566–569.

Kher, K. and Makker, S., 1987, Acute renal failure due to acetaminophen ingestion without concurrent hepatotoxicity, *American Journal of Medicine*, **82**, 1280–1281.

Kiebler, B. and Mowry, J. B., 1994, Acetaminophen's potential for morbidity and mortality, *Pediatric Nursing*, **20**, 491–494.

Kiersch, T. A., Halladay, S. C. and Hormel, P. C., 1994, A single-dose, double-blind comparison of naproxen sodium, acetaminophen, and placebo in postoperative dental pain, *Clinical Therapeutics*, **16**, 394–404.

Kiese, M. and Menzel, H., 1962, Hämiglobinbildung im Blute des Menschen nach einnahme von Phenacetin und von N-Acetyl-p-aminophenol, *Naunyn Schmiedeberg's Archiv für experimentelle Pathologie und Pharmakologie*, **242**, 551–554.

Kietzmann, D., Bock, K. W., Krähmer, B., Kettler, D. and Bircher, J., 1990, Paracetamol test: modification by renal function, urine flow and pH, *European Journal of Clinical Pharmacology*, **39**, 245–251.

Kim, D.-H. and Kobashi, K., 1986, The role of intestinal flora in metabolism of phenolic sulfate esters, *Biochemical Pharmacology*, **35**, 3507–3510.

Kim, H.-S. and Dillman, R. O., 1978, Acetaminophen overdose and hepatic necrosis, *Texas Medicine*, **74**, 56–59.

Kim, H. J., Rozman, P., Madhu, C. and Klaassen, C. D., 1992, Homeostasis of sulfate and 3'-phosphoadenosine 5'-phosphosulfate in rats after acetaminophen administration, *Journal of Pharmacology and Experimental Therapeutics*, **261**, 1015–1021.

Kimura, T., Kim, S. K. and Sezaki, H., 1981, Effect of taurine on drug absorption from the rat gastrointestinal tract, *Journal of Pharmacobio-Dynamics*, **4**, 35–41.

Kinberger, B. and Holmén, A., 1982, Simultaneous determination of acetaminophen, theophylline and salicylate in serum by high-performance liquid chromatography, *Journal of Chromatography: Biomedical Applications*, **229**, 492–497.

Kincaid-Smith, P., 1967, Pathogenesis of the renal lesion associated with the abuse of analgesics, *Lancet*, **i**, 859–862.

Kincaid-Smith, P., Saker, B. M., McKenzie, I. F. C. and Muriden, K. D., 1968, Lesions in the blood supply of the papilla in experimental analgesic nephropathy, *Medical Journal of Australia*, **1**, 203–206.

King, M.-T., Beikirch, H., Eckhardt, K., Gocke, E. and Wild, D., 1979, Mutagenicity studies with X-ray contrast media, analgesics, antipyretics, antirheumatics and some other pharmaceutical drugs in bacterial, Drosophila and mammalian test systems, *Mutation Research*, **66**, 33–43.

Kinney, C. D. and Kelly, J. G., 1987, Liquid chromatographic determination of paracetamol and dextropropoxyphene in plasma, *Journal of Chromatography: Biomedical Applications*, **419**, 433–437.

Kinsella, H. C., Smith, S., Rogers, H. J. and Toseland, P.A., 1979, Effect of paracetamol on amylobarbitone hydroxylation in man: a gas chromatographic method for simultaneous estimation of underivatised paracetamol and barbiturates, *Journal of Pharmacy and Pharmacology*, **31**, 153–156.

Kirby, M. G., Dukes, G. E., Heizer, W. D., Bryson, J. C. and Powell, J. R., 1989, Effect of metoclopramide, bethanecol and loperamide on gastric residence time, gastric emptying and mouth-to-cecum transit time, *Pharmacotherapy*, **9**, 226–231.

Kirkland, D. J., Dresp, J. H., Marshall, R. R., Baumeister, M., Gerloff, C. and Gocke, E., 1992, Normal chromosomal aberration frequencies in peripheral lymphocytes of healthy human volunteers exposed to a maximum daily dose of paracetamol in a double blind trial, *Mutation Research*, **279**, 181–194.

Kirshon, B., Moise, K. J. and Wasserstrum, N., 1989, Effect of acetaminophen on fetal acid-base balance in chorioamnionitis, *Journal of Reproductive Medicine*, **34**, 955–959.

Kissun, A. A., 1981, Paracetamol poisoning: the treatment of choice, *Australian Journal of Hospital Pharmacy*, **11**, 98–102.

Kitaguchi, S., Miyazawa, T., Minesita, M., Doi, M., Takahashi, K. and Yamakido, M., 1992, A case of acetaminophen-induced pneumonitis, *Japanese Journal of Thoracic Diseases*, **30**, 1322–1326.

Kitamura, Y., Kamisaki, Y. and Itoh, T., 1989, Hepatoprotective effects of cystathionine against acetaminophen-induced necrosis, *Journal of Pharmacology and Experimental Therapeutics*, **250**, 667–671.

Kitteringham, N. R., Lambert, C., Maggs, J. L., Colbert, J. and Park, B. K., 1988, A comparative study of the formation of chemically reactive drug metabolites by human liver microsomes, *British Journal of Clinical Pharmacology*, **26**, 13–21.

Kjaersgaard-Andersen, P., Nafei, A., Skov, O., Madsen, F., Andersen, H. M., Krøner, K., Hvass, I., Gjøderum, O., Pedersen, L. and Branebjerg, P. E., 1990, Codeine plus paracetamol vs. paracetamol in longer-term treatment of chronic pain due to osteoarthritis of the hip. A randomised, double-blind, multi-centre study, *Pain*, **43**, 309–318.

Klaassen, C. D., Bracken, W. M., Dudley, R. E., Goering, P. L., Hazelton, G. A. and Hjelle, J. J., 1985, Role of sulfhydryls in the hepatotoxicity of organic and metallic compounds, *Fundamental and Applied Toxicology*, **5**, 806–815.

Klein, B., Tiomny, A., Globerson, A., Elian, I., Notti, I. and Djaldetti, M., 1982, Effect of antiinflammatory drugs on the phagocytic activity of peripheral blood monocytes, *Prostaglandins Leukotrienes and Medicine*, **9**, 321–330.

Klein, G., Barkworth, M. F., Birkenfeld, A., Dyde, C. J., Rehm, K. D., Töberich, H. and Cierpka, H., 1986, Relative Bioverfügbarkeit von Paracetamol aus Tabletten und Zäpfchen sowie von Paracetamol und Codein aus einer Kombinationstablette, *Arzneimittel-Forschung*, **36**, 496–499.

Klein-Schwartz, W. and Oderda, G. M., 1981, Adsorption of oral antidotes for acetaminophen poisoning (methionine and N-acetylcysteine) by activated charcoal, *Clinical Toxicology*, **18**, 283–290.

Kleinknecht, D., Landais, P. and Goldfarb, B., 1986a, Les insuffisances rénales aiguës associées à des médicaments ou à des produits de contraste iodés: résultats d'une enquête coopérative multicentrique de la société de néphrologie, *Néphrologie*, **7**, 41–46.

Kleinknecht, D., Landais, P. and Goldfarb, B., 1986b, Analgesic and non-steroidal anti-inflammatory drug-associated acute renal failure: a prospective collaborative study, *Clinical Nephrology*, **25**, 275–281.

Kleinman, J. G., Breitenfield, R. V. and Roth, D. A., 1980, Acute renal failure associated with acetaminophen ingestion: report of a case and review of the literature, *Clinical Nephrology*, **14**, 201–205.

Klos, C., Koob, M., Kramer, C. and Dekant, W., 1992, p-Aminophenol nephrotoxicity: biosynthesis of toxic glutathione conjugates, *Toxicology and Applied Pharmacology*, **115**, 98–106.

Kluger, M. T., Plummer, J. L. and Owen, H., 1991, The influence of rectal cisapride on morphine-induced gastric stasis, *Anaesthesia and Intensive Care*, **19**, 346–350.

Klugmann, F. B., Decorti, G., Mallardi, F. and Baldini, L., 1984, Enhancement of paracetamol induced hepatotoxicity by prior treatment with carboxymethylcellulose, *Pharmaco-*

logical Research Communications, **16**, 313–318.

Klutch, A. and Bordun, M., 1968, Chromatographic methods for analysis of the metabolites of acetophenetidin (phenacetin), *Journal of Pharmaceutical Sciences*, **57**, 524–526.

Klutch, A., Levin, W., Chang, R. L., Vane, F. and Conney, A. H., 1978, Formation of a thiomethyl metabolite of phenacetin and acetaminophen in dogs and man, *Clinical Pharmacology and Therapeutics*, **24**, 287–293.

Klys, M. and Brandys, J., 1988, Wide-bore capillary column gas chromatography in toxicological analysis of biological samples from multidrug overdoses fatalities, *Forensic Science International*, **38**, 185–192.

Knapp, M. and Avioli, L. V., 1982, Analgesic nephropathy, *Archives of Internal Medicine*, **142**, 1197–1199.

Knell, A. J., 1975, Risk of hepatic coma in paracetamol poisoning, *Lancet*, **ii**, 1039.

Knepil, J., 1974, A sensitive, specific method for measuring N-acetyl-p-aminophenol (paracetamol) in blood, *Clinica Chimica Acta*, **52**, 369–372.

Knight, B. I. and Skellern, G. G., 1980, Measurement of the formation of paracetamol and p-nitrophenol glucuronides *in vitro*, by ion-pair high-performance liquid chromatography, *Journal of Chromatography*, **192**, 247–249.

Knights, K. M., Gourlay, G. K., Hall, P. and Cousins, M. J., 1983, The predictive value of changes in antipyrine pharmacokinetics in halothane and paracetamol induced hepatic necrosis in rats, *Research Communications in Chemical Pathology and Pharmacology*, **40**, 199–215.

Knoop, K. J., Snook, C. P., Stephan, M. and Wason, S., 1993, Failure of N-acetylcysteine (NAC) to prevent acetaminophen-induced renal failure, *Veterinary and Human Toxicology*, **35**, 336.

Knorr, L., 1884, Einwirkung von Acetessigester auf Hydrazinchinizinderivate, *Berichte der deutschen chemischen Gesellschaft*, **17**, 546–552.

Knox, J. H. and Jurand, J., 1977, Determination of paracetamol and its metabolites in urine by high-performance liquid chromatography using reversed-phased bonded supports, *Journal of Chromatography*, **142**, 651–670.

Knox, J. H. and Jurand, J., 1978, Determination of paracetamol and its metabolites in urine by high-performance liquid chromatography using ion-pair systems, *Journal of Chromatography*, **149**, 297–312.

Kobbe, K. and Goenechea, S., 1982, Toxikologisch-chemische Harnbefunde nach Einnahme phenacetin-(paracetamol)- und aspirinhalltiger Analgetica, *Beiträge zur Gerichtlichen Medizin*, **40**, 341–345.

Kobusch, A. B. and du Souich, P., 1990, Effect of diltiazem on acetaminophen and phalloidine hepatotoxicity, *Research Communications in Chemical Pathology and Pharmacology*, **68**, 143–157.

Koch, H. J., 1992, Analgesic drug prescription during the spondylodesis by the Harrington rod method, *European Journal of Clinical Pharmacology*, **43**, 325.

Koch, H. K., Gropp, A. and Oehlert, W., 1985, Drug-induced liver injury in liver biopsies of the years 1981 and 1983, their prevalence and type of presentation, *Pathology Research and Practice*, **179**, 469–477.

Kocisová, J., Rossner, P., Binková, B., Bavorová, H. and Srám, R. J., 1988, Mutagenicity studies on paracetamol in human volunteers. I. Cytogenetic analysis of peripheral lymphocytes and lipid peroxidation in plasma, *Mutation Research*, **209**, 161–165.

Kocisová, J. and Srám, R. J., 1990a, Mutagenicity studies on paracetamol in human volunteers. III. Cytokinesis block micronucleus method, *Mutation Research*, **244**, 27–30.

Kocisová, J. and Srám, R. J., 1990b, Mikronukleus test v lidskych perifernich lymfocytech, *Ceskoslovenská Farmacie*, **39**, 131–133.

Koebe, H. G., Pahernik, S., Eyer, P. and Schildberg, F.-W., 1994, Collagen gel immobilization: a useful cell culture technique for long-term metabolic studies on human hepatocytes, *Xenobiotica*, **24**, 95–107.

Koga, Y., Nakashima, Y., Kumashiro, R., Ueno, T., Sakisaka, S., Yasumoto, K., Sata, M., Abe, H., Tanikawa, K. and Kaku, N., 1991, A case of liver failure due to long-term ingestion of acetaminophen, *Acta Hepatologica Japonica*, **32**, 512–515.

Kogan, M. D., Pappas, G., Yu, S. M. and Kotelchuck, M., 1994, Over-the-counter medication use among US preschool-age children, *Journal of the American Medical Association*, **272**, 1025–1030.

Kohli, U., Sharma, S. K., Agarwal, S. S. and Sahib, M. K., 1982, Influence of nutritional status on acetaminophen metabolism in man, *Indian Journal of Medical Research Section A - Infectious Diseases*, **75**, 265–273.

Kohút, A., Mirossay, L., Siksová, K. and Lapsanská, L., 1992, Vplyv paracetamolu na zalúdocné lézie vyvolané indometacínom, ethanolom a imobilizacnym stresom u potkanov, *Ceskoslovenská Gastroenterologie a Vyziva*, **46**, 117–122.

Koizumi, F., Ebina, H., Kawamura, T., Ishimori, A. and Satoh, M., 1988a, Relationship between plasma acetaminophen concentrations measured by fluorescence polarization immunoassay and gastric emptying time in men, *Japanese Journal of Gastroenterology*, **85**, 2559–2562.

Koizumi, F., Kawamura, T. and Ishimori, A., 1989, Correlation between gastric emptying time and both plasma gastrin and pancreatic polypeptide in streptozotocin diabetic dogs, *Japanese Journal of Gastroenterology*, **86**, 1037–1043.

Koizumi, F., Kawamura, T., Ishimori, A., Ebina, H. and Satoh, M., 1988b, Plasma paracetamol concentrations measured by fluorescence polarization immunoassay and gastric emptying time, *Tohoku Journal of Experimental Medicine*, **155**, 159–164.

Kondo, K., Inoue, Y., Hamada, H., Yokoyama, A., Kohno, N. and Hiwada, K., 1993, Acetaminophen-induced eosinophilic pneumonia, *Chest*, **104**, 291–292.

Kondrup, J., Almdal, T., Vilstrup, H. and Tygstrup, N., 1992, High volume plasma exchange in fulminant hepatic failure, *International Journal of Artificial Organs*, **15**, 669–676.

Konturek, S. J., Brzozowski, T., Piastucki, I. and Radecki, T., 1982, Prevention of ethanol and aspirin-induced gastric mucosal lesions by paracetamol and salicylate in rats: role of endogenous prostaglandins, *Gut*, **23**, 536–540.

Konturek, S. J., Obtulowicz, W., Kwiecien, N. and Oleksy, J., 1984, Generation of prostaglandins in gastric mucosa of patients with peptic ulcer disease: effect of nonsteroidal anti-inflammatory compounds, *Scandinavian Journal of Gastroenterology*, **19 (Suppl. 101)**, 75–77.

Konturek, S. J., Obtulowicz, W., Sito, E., Olesky, J., Wilkon, S. and Kiec-Dembinska, A., 1981, Distribution of prostaglandins in gastric and duodenal mucosa of healthy subjects and duodenal ulcer patients: effects of aspirin and paracetamol, *Gut*, **22**, 283–289.

Koo, E. W. Y., Hayes, A., Wong, M. K. K. and Gotlieb, A. I., 1987, Aflatoxin B_1 and acetaminophen induce different cytoskeletal responses during prelethal hepatocyte injury, *Experimental and Molecular Pathology*, **47**, 37–47.

Korberly, B. H., Schreiber, G. F., Kilkuts, A., Orkand, R. K. and Segal, H., 1980, Evaluation of acetaminophen and aspirin in the relief of preoperative dental pain, *Journal of the American Dental Association*, **100**, 39–42.

Korduba, C. A. and Petruzzi, R. F., 1984, High-performance liquid chromatographic method for determination of trace amounts of acetaminophen in plasma, *Journal of Pharmaceutical Sciences*, **73**, 117–119.

Kornberg, A. and Polliack, A., 1978, Paracetamol-induced thrombocytopenia and hæmolytic anaemia, *Lancet*, **ii**, 1159.

Kosmeas, N. and Clerc, J. T., 1989, Schnelle DC-Methode zur simultanen quantitativen Bestimmung von Paracetamol, Caffeine, Phenobarbital und Propyphenazone in Plasma, *Pharmaceutica Acta Helvetiae*, **64**, 2–7.

Kotal, P., Perlík, F., Vlachová, E. and Kordac, V., 1989, Determination of paracetamol in the blood using high-performance liquid chromatography, *Ceskoslovenská Farmacie*, **38**, 195–197.

Koukoulis, G., Rayner, A., Tan, K.-C., Williams, R. and Portmann, B., 1992, Immunolocalization of regenerating cells after submassive liver necrosis using PCNA staining, *Journal of Pathology*, **166**, 359–368.

Koutsaimanis, K. G. and De Wardener, H. E., 1970, Phenacetin nephropathy, with particular reference to the effect of surgery, *British Medical Journal*, **4**, 131–134.

Kovach, I. M., Pitman, I. H. and Higuchi, T., 1981, Amino acid esters of phenols as prodrugs: synthesis and stability of glycine, β-aspartic acid, and α-aspartic acid esters of p-acetamidophenol, *Journal of Pharmaceutical Sciences*, **70**, 881–885.

Koymans, L., Donné-Op den Kelder, G. M., Te Koppele, J. M. and Vermeulen, N. P. E., 1993, Generalised cytochrome P-450-mediated oxidation and oxygenation reactions in aromatic substrates with activated N-H, O-H, C-H or S-H substituents, *Xenobiotica*, **23**, 633–648.

Koymans, L., van Lenthe, J. H., van de Straat, R., Donné-Op den Kelder, G. M. and Vermeulen, N. P. E., 1989, A theoretical study on the metabolic activation of paracetamol by cytochrome P-450: indications for a uniform oxidation mechanism, *Chemical Research in Toxicology*, **2**, 60–66.

Krack, G., Goethals, F., Deboyser, D. and Roberfroid, M., 1980, Interference of chemicals with glycogen metabolism in isolated hepatocytes, *Toxicology*, **18**, 213–223.

Kramer, M. S., Naimark, L. E., Roberts-Bräuer, R., McDougall, A. and Leduc, D. G., 1991, Risks and benefits of paracetamol antipyresis in young children with fever of presumed viral origin, *Lancet*, **337**, 591–594.

Kreiger, N., Marrett, L. D., Dodds, L., Hilditch, S. and Darlington, G. A., 1993, Risk factors for renal cell carcinoma: results of a population-based case-control study, *Cancer Causes and Control*, **4**, 101–110.

Krempien, W., Radetzky, B., Elsäßer, R., Seeling, P. and Seeling, W. D., 1994, Perioperative Analgesie in der Oralchirurgie: ein Vergleich von Ibuprofen, Lysinat und Paracetamol, *Zeitschrift für Allgemeinmedizin*, **70**, 78–83.

Krenzelok, E. P., Best, L. and Manoguerra, A. S., 1977, Acetaminophen toxicity, *American Journal of Hospital Pharmacy*, **34**, 391–394.

Krijgsheld, K. R., Scholtens, E. and Mulder, G. J., 1981, An evaluation of methods to decrease the availability of inorganic sulphate for sulphate conjugation in the rat *in vivo*, *Biochemical Pharmacology*, **30**, 1973–1979.

Krikler, D. M., 1967, Paracetamol and the kidney, *British Medical Journal*, **2**, 615–616.

Kritharides, L., Fassett, R. and Singh, B., 1988, Paracetamol-associated coma, metabolic acidosis, renal and hepatic failure, *Intensive Care Medicine*, **14**, 439–440.

Kruze, D., Fehr, K. and Böni, A., 1976, Effect of antirheumatic drugs on cathepsin B_1 from bovine spleen, *Zeitschrift für Rheumatolgie*, **35**, 95–102.

Kubalak, S., Jensen, C. and Jollow, D., 1986, Acetaminophen hepatotoxicity: studies on the mechanism of cysteamine protection, *Pharmacologist*, **28**, 125.

Kudeken, N., Kawakami, K., Kakazu, T., Takushi, Y., Kakazu, T., Fukuhara, H., Nakamura, H., Kaneshima, H., Saito, A. and Toda, T., 1993, A case of acetaminophen-induced pneumonitis, *Japanese Journal of Thoracic Diseases*, **31**, 1585–1590.

Kuhlman, J. J., Levine, B., Smith, M. L. and Hordinsky, J. R., 1991, Toxicological findings in Federal Aviation Administration general aviation accidents, *Journal of Forensic Sciences*, **36**, 1121–1128.

Kulmacz, R. J., Palmer, G. and Tsai, A.-L., 1991, Prostaglandin-H synthase: perturbation of the tyrosyl radical as a probe of anticyclooxygenase agents, *Molecular Pharmacology*, **40**, 833–837.

Kumar, A., Goel, K. M. and Rae, M. D., 1990, Paracetamol overdose in children, *Scottish Medical Journal*, **35**, 106–107.

Kumar, S. and Rex, D. K., 1991, Failure of physicians to recognize acetaminophen hepatotoxicity in chronic alcoholics, *Archives of Internal Medicine*, **151**, 1189–1191.

Kummer, M. and Mehlhaus, N., 1984, Zur Bioverfügbarkeit von Codein und Paracetamol aus einem Kombinationspräparat nach oraler und rektaler Applikation, *Fortschritte der Medizin*, **102**, 173–178.

Kuo, P. C. and Slivka, A., 1994, Nitric oxide decreases oxidant-mediated hepatocyte injury, *Journal of Surgical Research*, **56**, 594–600.

Kurata, Y., Tsuda, H., Tamano, S. and Ito, N., 1985, Inhibitory potential of acetaminophen and o-, m-, p-aminophenols for development of γ-glutamyltranspeptidase-positive liver cell foci in rats pretreated with diethylnitrosamine, *Cancer Letters*, **28**, 19–25.

Kuroda, T., Yoshihara, Y., Nakamura, H., Azumi, T., Inatome, T., Fukuzaki, H., Takanashi, H., Yogo, K. and Akima, M., 1992, Effects of cisapride on gastrointestinal motor activity and gastric emptying of disopyramide, *Journal of Pharmacobiodynamics*, **15**, 395–402.

Kurt, T. L., Zwiener, R. J., Day, L. C. and Timmons, C. F., 1993, Potentiation of hepatotoxicity in mercury poisoning by acetaminophen, *Clinical Pharmacology and Therapeutics*, **53**, 156.

Kurzel, R. B., 1990, Can acetaminophen excess result in maternal and fetal toxicity? *Southern Medical Journal*, **83**, 953–955.

Kwiatkowski, A., 1991, Wplyw estrogenow na farmakokinetyke fenazonu i N-acetylo-p-aminofenolu, *Annales Academiae Medicae Stetinensis*, **37**, 35–47.

Kyle, M. E., Miccadei, S., Nakae, D. and Farber, J. L., 1987, Superoxide dismutase and catalase protect cultured hepatocytes from the cytotoxicity of acetaminophen, *Biochemical and Biophysical Research Communications*, **149**, 889–896.

Kyle, M. E., Nakae, D., Serroni, A. and Farber, J. L., 1988, 1,3-(2-chloroethyl)-1-nitrosourea potentiates the toxicity of acetaminophen both in phenobarbital-induced rat and in hepatocytes cultured from such animals, *Molecular Pharmacology*, **34**, 584–589.

Kyle, M. E., Sakaida, I., Serroni, A. and Farber, J. L., 1990, Metabolism of acetaminophen by cultured rat hepatocytes: depletion of protein thiol groups without any loss of viability, *Biochemical Pharmacology*, **40**, 1211–1218.

Laake, K., Borchgrevink, Chr. F. and Kjeldaas, L., 1983, Aksidentelle overdoseringer ved kombinasjonen reseptfrie/reseptbelagte legemidler, *Tidsskrift for den Norske Lægeo rening*, **103**, 2061–2062.

Labadarios, D. M., Davis, M., Portmann, B. and Williams, R., 1977, Paracetamol-induced hepatic necrosis in the mouse – relationship between covalent binding, hepatic glutathione depletion and the protective effect of α-mercaptopropionylglycine, *Biochemical Pharmacology*, **26**, 31–35.

LaBrecque, D. R. and Mitros, F. A., 1980, Increased hepatotoxicity of acetaminophen in the alcoholic, *Gastroenterology*, **78**, 1310.

Lacotte, J., Perrin, C., Mosquet, B., Moulin, M. and Bazin, C., 1990, Agranulocytose au paracétamol. A propos d'un cas, *Thérapie*, **45**, 438–439.

Lacroix, J., Gaudreault, P. and Gauthier, M., 1989, Admission to a pediatric intensive care unit for poisoning: a review of 105 cases, *Critical Care Medicine*, **17**, 748–750.

Lacroix, R., Lacroix, J. and Proust, N., 1985, Des interactions médicamenteuses du paracétamol, *Journal de Pharmacie Clinique*, **4**, 467–481.

Ladds, G., Wilson, K. and Burnett, D., 1987, Automated liquid chromatographic method for the determination of paracetamol and six metabolites in human urine, *Journal of Chromatography: Biomedical Applications*, **414**, 355–364.

Ladwa, R. A. R., 1981, Comparison of Syndol and paracetamol in the relief of dental pain, *British Dental Journal*, **150**, 187–188.

Lages, B. and Weiss, H. J., 1989, Inhibition of human platelet function *in vitro* and *ex vivo* by acetaminophen, *Thrombosis Research*, **53**, 603–613.

Lake, B. G., Harris, R. A., Phillips, J. C. and Gangolli, S. D., 1981, Studies on the effects of L-ascorbic acid on acetaminophen-induced hepatotoxicity. 1. Inhibition of covalent binding of acetaminophen metabolites to hepatic microsomes *in vitro*, *Toxicology and Applied Pharmacology*, **60**, 229–240.

Lambert, G. H. and Thorgeirsson, S. S., 1976, Glutathione in the developing mouse liver – I.

Developmental curve and depletion after acetaminophen treatment, *Biochemical Pharmacology*, **25**, 1777–1781.

Landa Garcia, J. I., Torres, A., Ortega Medina, L., Cuberes, R., Morena Azcoita, M., Suarez, A., Silecchia, G., Balibrea Cantero, J. L. and Moreno Gonzalez, E., 1984, Allotrapianto epatico bisegmentario eterotopico: modello sperimentale di 'supporto temporaneo' in corso di epatite fulminante indotta nel cane con acetaminofene, *Chirurgia Gastroenterologica*, **18**, 187–195.

Landis, C. A., Robinson, C. R., Helms, C. and Levine, J. D., 1989, Differential effects of acetylsalicylic acid and acetaminophen on sleep abnormalities in a rat chronic pain model, *Brain Research*, **488**, 195–201.

Landon, E. J., Naukam, R. J. and Sastry, B. V. R., 1986, Effects of calcium channel blocking agents on calcium and centrilobular necrosis in the liver of rats treated with hepatotoxic agents, *Biochemical Pharmacology*, **35**, 697–705.

Lands, W. E. M. and Hanel, A. M., 1982, Phenolic anticyclooxygenase agents in anti-inflammatory and analgesic therapy, *Prostaglandins*, **24**, 271–277.

Lanfear, J., Fleming, J., Walker, M. and Harrison, P., 1993, Different patterns of regulation of the genes encoding the closely related 56 kDa selenium- and acetaminophen-binding proteins in normal tissues and during carcinogenesis, *Carcinogenesis*, **14**, 335–340.

Langley, P. G., Forbes, A., Hughes, R. D. and Williams, R., 1990, Thrombin-antithrombin III complex in fulminant hepatic failure: evidence for disseminated intravascular coagulation and relationship to outcome, *European Journal of Clinical Investigation*, **20**, 627–631.

Langley, P. G., Hughes, R. D., Forbes, A., Keays, R. and Williams, R., 1993, Controlled trial of antithrombin III supplementation in fulminant hepatic failure, *Journal of Hepatology*, **17**, 326–331.

Langman, M. J. S., Coggon, D. and Spiegelhalter, D., 1983, Analgesic intake and the risk of acute upper gastrointestinal bleeding, *American Journal of Medicine*, **74**, 79–82.

Langman, M. J. S., Weil, J., Wainwright, P., Lawson, D. H., Rawlins, M. D., Logan, R. F. A., Murphy, M., Vessey, M. P. and Colin-Jones, D. G., 1994, Risks of bleeding peptic ulcer associated with individual non-steroidal anti-inflammatory drugs, *Lancet*, **343**, 1075–1078.

Langrick, A. F. and Gunn, A. D. G., 1982, A comparison of naproxen sodium and a dextropropoxyphene/paracetamol combination in the treatment of primary dysmenorrhoea in University Health Centres, *British Journal of Clinical Practice*, **36**, 181–184.

Lanthier, P., Detry, R., Debongnie, J. C., Mahieu, P. and Vanheuverzwyn, R., 1987, Lésions solitaires du rectum dues à des suppositoires associant acide acétylsalicylique et paracétamol, *Gastroentérologie Clinique et Biologique*, **11**, 250–253.

Lanz, R., Polster, P. and Brune, K., 1986, Antipyretic analgesics inhibit prostaglandin release from astrocytes and macrophages similarly, *European Journal of Pharmacology*, **130**, 105–109.

Lanza, F. L., Royer, G. L., Nelson, R. S., Rack, M. F., Seckman, C. E. and Schwartz, J. H., 1986, Effect of acetaminophen on human gastric mucosal injury caused by ibuprofen, *Gut*, **27**, 440–443.

Laplanche, G., Grosshans, E., Heid, E., Jaeck, D. and Welsch, M., 1984, Ulcérations ano-recto-vaginales par suppositoires contenant du dextropropoxyphène, *Annales de Dermatologie et de Venereologie*, **111**, 347–355.

Laporte, J.-R., Carné, X., Vidal, X., Moreno, V. and Juan, J., 1991, Upper gastrointestinal bleeding in relation to previous use of analgesics and non-steroidal anti-inflammatory drugs, *Lancet*, **337**, 85–89.

Larrauri, A., Fabra, R., Gómez-Lechón, M. J., Trullenque, R. and Castell, J. V., 1989, Toxicity of paracetamol in human hepatocytes. Comparison of the protective effects of sulfhydryl compounds acting as glutathione precursors, *Molecular Toxicology*, **1**, 301–311.

Larrey, D., Amouyal, G., Tinel, M., Descatoire, V., Genève, J., Lettéron, P., Labbe, G. and

Pessayre, D., 1987, Effects of methoxsalen on hepatic cytochrome P-450 and on the metabolism of acetaminophen (paracetamol) in man, *Fundamental and Clinical Pharmacology*, **1**, 371.

Larrey, D., Lettéron, P., Foliot, A., Descatoire, V., Degott, C., Genève, J., Tinel, M. and Pessayre, D., 1986, Effects of pregnancy on the toxicity and metabolism of acetaminophen in mice, *Journal of Pharmacology and Experimental Therapeutics*, **237**, 283–291.

Larsen, B. H., Christiansen, L. V., Andersen, B. and Olesen, J., 1990, Randomized double-blind comparison of tolfenamic acid and paracetamol in migraine, *Acta Neurologica Scandinavica*, **81**, 464–467.

Larsson, R., Ross, D., Berlin, T., Olsson, L. I. and Moldéus, P., 1985, Prostaglandin synthetase catalysed metabolic activation of p-phenetidine and acetaminophen by microsomes isolated from rabbit and human kidney, *Journal of Pharmacology and Experimental Therapeutics*, **235**, 475–480.

Lasagna, L., Davis, M. and Pearson, J. W., 1967, A comparison of acetophenetidin and acetaminophen I. Analgesic effects in postpartum patients, *Journal of Pharmacology and Experimental Therapeutics*, **155**, 296–300.

Lasfargues, P. and Brehon, M., 1979, Surveillance de 13 femmes enceintes traitées par paracétamol effervescent, *Revue Française de Gynécologie et d'Obstetrique*, **74**, 619–620.

Laska, E. M., Sunshine, A., Mueller, F., Elvers, W. B., Siegel, C. and Rubin, A., 1984, Caffeine as an analgesic adjuvant, *Journal of the American Medical Association*, **251**, 1711–1718.

Laska, E. M., Sunshine, A., Zighelboim, I., Roure, C., Marrero, I., Wanderling, J. and Olson, N., 1983, Effect of caffeine on acetaminophen analgesia, *Clinical Pharmacology and Therapeutics*, **33**, 498–509.

Laskin, D. L., 1991, Parenchymal and non-parenchymal cell interactions in hepatotoxicity, *Advances in Experimental Medicine and Biology*, **283**, 499–505.

Laskin, D. L. and Pilaro, A. M., 1986, Potential role of activated macrophages in acetaminophen hepatotoxicity. I. Isolation and characterization of activated macrophages from rat liver, *Toxicology and Applied Pharmacology*, **86**, 204–215.

Laskin, D. L., Pilaro, A. M. and Ji, S., 1986, Potential role of activated macrophages in acetaminophen hepatotoxicity. II. Mechanism of macrophage accumulation and activation, *Toxicology and Applied Pharmacology*, **86**, 216–226.

Lau, G. S. N. and Critchley, J. A. J. H., 1994, The estimation of paracetamol and its major metabolites in both plasma and urine by a single high-performance liquid chromatography assay, *Journal of Pharmaceutical and Biomedical Analysis*, **12**, 1563–1572.

Lau, O.-W., Luk, S.-F. and Cheung, Y.-M., 1989, Simultaneous determination of ascorbic acid, caffeine and paracetamol in drug formulations by differential-pulse voltammetry using a glassy carbon electrode, *Analyst*, **114**, 1047–1051.

Lauriault, V. V. M. and O'Brien, P. J., 1991, Molecular mechanism for prevention of N-acetyl-p-benzoquinoneimine cytotoxicity by the permeable thiol drugs diethyldithiocarbamate and dithiothreitol, *Molecular Pharmacology*, **40**, 125–134.

Lauroba, J., Diez, I., Rius, M., Peraire, C. and Domenech, J., 1990, Study of the release process of drugs: suppositories of paracetamol, *International Journal of Clinical Pharmacology, Therapy and Toxicology*, **28**, 118–122.

Lauterburg, B. H., 1985, Arzneimittelschäden der Leber: Rolle von reaktiven Metaboliten und Pharmakokinetik, *Schweizerische Medizinische Wochenschrift*, **115**, 1306–1312.

Lauterburg, B. H., 1987, Early disturbance of calcium translocation across the plasma membrane in toxic liver injury, *Hepatology*, **7**, 1179–1183.

Lauterburg, B. H., Corcoran, G. B. and Mitchell, J. R., 1983, Mechanism of action of N-acetylcysteine in the protection against hepatotoxicity of acetaminophen in rats *in vivo*, *Journal of Clinical Investigation*, **71**, 980–991.

Lauterburg, B. H., Davies, S. and Mitchell, J. R., 1984a, Ethanol suppresses hepatic glutathione synthesis in rats *in vivo*, *Journal of Pharmacology and Experimental Therapeutics*, **230**, 7–11.

Lauterburg, B. H. and Mitchell, J. R., 1982, Toxic doses of acetaminophen suppress hepatic glutathione synthesis in rats, *Hepatology*, **2**, 8–12.

Lauterburg, B. H. and Mitchell, J. R., 1987, Therapeutic doses of paracetamol stimulate the turnover of cysteine and glutathione in man, *Journal of Hepatology*, **4**, 206–211.

Lauterburg, B. H. and Smith, C. V., 1986, Stimulation of hepatic efflux and turnover of glutathione by methionine in the rat, *European Journal of Clinical Investigation*, **16**, 494–499.

Lauterburg, B. H., Smith, C. V., Hughes, H. and Mitchell, J. R., 1984b, Biliary excretion of glutathione and glutathione disulfide in the rat, *Journal of Clinical Investigation*, **73**, 124–133.

Lauterburg, B. H., Vaishnav, Y., Stillwell, W. G. and Mitchell, J. R., 1980, The effect of age and glutathione depletion on hepatic glutathione turnover *in vivo* determined by acetaminophen probe analysis, *Journal of Pharmacology and Experimental Therapeutics*, **213**, 54–58.

Lauterburg, B. H. and Velez, M. E., 1988, Glutathione deficiency in alcoholics: risk factor for paracetamol hepatotoxicity, *Gut*, **29**, 1153–1157.

Lauterburg, B. H., Velez, M. E. and Mitchell, J. R., 1984c, Plasma glutathione (GSH) as an index of intrahepatic GSH in man: response to acetaminophen and chronic ethanol abuse, *Hepatology*, **4**, 1051.

Lavigne, J.-G., d'Auteuil, C. and Lavoie, J.-M., 1982, Influence of leukaemia on acetaminophen-induced hepatotoxicity in mice, *Revue Canadienne de Biologie Expérimentale*, **41**, 121–128.

Lawrence, A. H., 1987, Detection of drug residues on the hands of subjects by surface sampling and ion mobility spectrometry, *Forensic Science International*, **34**, 73–83.

Lawrence, J. N. and Benford, D. J., 1990, Toxicity of paracetamol and cyclophosphamide in monolayer cultures of rat and human hepatocytes, *Toxicology in Vitro*, **4**, 443–448.

Lawson, A. A. H. and McCallum, C. J., 1979, Trends in acute poisoning in a district medical unit, *Health Bulletin*, **37**, 121–127.

Lawson, G. R., Craft, A. W. and Jackson, R. H., 1983, Changing pattern of poisoning in children in Newcastle, 1974–81, *British Medical Journal*, **287**, 15–17.

Laxminarayana, D., Murthy, D. K. and Subramanyam, S., 1980, Cytogenetical action of paracetamol on meiotic cells of male mice, *Cytobios*, **27**, 27–34.

Lay, J. O., Potter, D. W. and Hinson, J. A., 1987, Fast atom bombardment mass spectrometry and fast atom bombardment mass spectrometry/mass spectrometry of three glutathione conjugates of acetaminophen, *Biomedical and Environmental Mass Spectrometry*, **14**, 517–521.

Lazarte, R. A., Bigelow, S. W., Nebert, D. W. and Levitt, R. C., 1984, Effects of cimetidine on theophylline, acetaminophen, and zoxazolamine toxicity in the intact mouse, *Developmental Pharmacology and Therapeutics*, **7**, 21–29.

Lecoeur, S., Bonierbale, E., Challine, D., Gautier, J.-C., Valadon, P., Dansette, P. M., Catinot, R., Ballet, F., Mansuy, D. and Beaune, P. H., 1994, Specificity of *in vitro* covalent binding of tienilic acid metabolites to human liver microsomes in relationship to the type of hepatotoxicity: comparison with two directly hepatotoxic drugs, *Chemical Research in Toxicology*, **7**, 434–442.

Lederman, S., Fysh, W. J., Tredger, M. and Gamsu, H. R., 1983, Neonatal paracetamol poisoning: treatment by exchange transfusion, *Archives of Disease in Childhood*, **58**, 631–633.

Lee, C. A., Thummel, K. E., Kalhorn, T. F., Nelson, S. D. and Slattery, J. T., 1991a, Inhibition and activation of acetaminophen reactive metabolite formation by caffeine: roles of cytochromes P-450IA1 and IIIA2, *Drug Metabolism and Disposition: The Biological Fate of Chemicals*, **19**, 348–353.

Lee, C. A., Thummel, K. E., Kalhorn, T. F., Nelson, S. D. and Slattery, J. T., 1991b, Activation of acetaminophen-reactive metabolite formation by methylxanthines and known cytochrome P-450 activators, *Drug Metabolism and Disposition: The Biological Fate of*

Chemicals, **19**, 966–971.

Lee, C. S., Wang, L. H., Marbury, T. C. and Cade, J. R., 1981a, Hemodialysis for acetaminophen detoxification, *Clinical Toxicology,* **18**, 431–439.

Lee, H. S., Ti, T. Y., Koh, Y. K. and Prescott, L. F., 1992, Paracetamol elimination in Chinese and Indians in Singapore, *European Journal of Clinical Pharmacology,* **43**, 81–84.

Lee, H. S., Ti, T. Y., Tan, C. C., Lai, W. C. and Tan, G. H., 1990, Paracetamol elimination in chronic renal failure patients, *European Journal of Pharmacology,* **183**, 1065–1066.

Lee, J.-S., Lee, C.K. and Choi, J.-W., 1993, Pharmacologic activities of saikosaponins(I) – effects on drug metabolising enzymes modification and liver toxicities due to acetaminophen, *Korean Journal of Pharmacognosy,* **24**, 69–77.

Lee, P., Anderson, J. A. and Buchanan, W. W., 1976, The status of current non-steroidal, antirheumatic drugs, *Australian and New Zealand Journal of Medicine,* **6**, 173.

Lee, P., Watson, M., Webb, J., Anderson, J. and Buchanan, W., 1975, Therapeutic effectiveness of paracetamol in rheumatoid arthritis, *International Journal of Clinical Pharmacology,* **11**, 68–75.

Lee, W. H., Kramer, W. G. and Granville, G. E., 1981b, The effect of obesity on acetaminophen pharmacokinetics in man, *Journal of Clinical Pharmacology,* **21**, 284–287.

Lee, W.M., 1993, Acute liver failure, *New England Journal of Medicine,* **329**, 1862–1872.

Lee, W. M., 1994, Acute liver failure, *American Journal of Medicine,* **96 (Suppl. 1A)**, 1A-3S–1A-9S.

Lee, W. M., Emerson, D. L., Young, W. O., Goldschmidt-Clermont, P. J., Jollow, D. J. and Galbraith, R. M., 1987, Diminished serum Gc (vitamin D-binding protein) levels and increased Gc : G-actin complexes in a hamster model of fulminant hepatic necrosis, *Hepatology,* **7**, 825–830.

Leeder, J. S., Cannon, M., Nakhooda, A. and Spielberg, S. P., 1988, Drug metabolite toxicity assessed in human lymphocytes with a purified, reconstituted cytochrome P-450 system, *Journal of Pharmacology and Experimental Therapeutics,* **245**, 956–962.

Leeling, J. L., Johnson, N. and Helms, R. J., 1981, Effect of paracetamol coadministration on aspirin-induced gastrointestinal bleeding in dogs, *Journal of Pharmacy and Pharmacology,* **33**, 61–62.

Leen, C. L. S. and Welsby, P. D., 1984, Paracetamol overdose as a cause of non-A, non-B hepatitis, *British Medical Journal,* **288**, 50–51.

Le Fur, J. M., Colin, A., Parent, P. and Castel, Y., 1983, Traitement de l'hyperthermie: efficacité du soluté buvable de paracétamol (1), *Ouest Médical,* **36**, 135–137.

Legallicier, B., Parent, B., Chamoun, S., Duparc, F., Lemoine, F., Lerebours, F. and Colin, R., 1991, Toxicité rectale des suppositoires de Véganine: un mode de révélation original, *Gastroentérologie Clinique et Biologique,* **15**, 92–93.

Leguen, M. A., 1985, Single-blind clinical trial comparing use of fentiazac and paracetamol in postendodontic periodontitis, *Clinical Therapeutics,* **7**, 145–150.

Lehmann, F.-M., Bretz, N., Bruchhausen, F. and Wurm, G., 1989, Substrates for arachidonic acid co-oxidation with peroxidase/hydrogen peroxide: further evidence for radical intermediates, *Biochemical Pharmacology,* **38**, 1209–1216.

Lehnert, S., Reuther, J., Wahl, G. and Barthel, K., 1990, Wirksamkeit von Paracetamol (Tylenol) und Acetylsalizylsäure (Aspirin) bei postoperativen Schmerzen, *Deutsche Zahnärztliche Zeitschrift,* **45**, 23–26.

Leibowitz, H. and Kuhn, J. A., 1980, Acetaminophen overdosage: a case presentation and review of current therapy, *Delaware Medical Journal,* **52**, 135–138.

Leiper, K., Croll, A., Booth, N. A., Moore, N. R., Sinclair, T. and Bennett, B., 1994, Tissue plasminogen activator, plaminogen activator inhibitors, and activator-inhibitor complex in liver disease, *Journal of Clinical Pathology,* **47**, 214–217.

Leist, M. H., Gluskin, L. E. and Payne, J. A., 1985, Enhanced toxicity of acetaminophen in alcoholics: report of three cases, *Journal of Clinical Gastroenterology,* **7**, 55–59.

Leng-Peschlow, E., 1988, Antagonisierung der Paracetamol-intoxikation durch Silibinin in der isoliert perfundierten Rattenleber, *Zeitschrift für Gastroenterologie*, **26**, 49.

Lenz, K., Resch, F., Druml, W., Gassner, A., Hruby, K., Kleinberger, G. and Pichler, M., 1982, Effektivität und Komplikationsrate von forcierter Diurese im Vergleich zu extrakorporalen Elininationsverfahren, *Intensivmedizin und Notfallmedizin*, **19**, 190–193.

Leonard, T. B. and Dent, J. G., 1984, Effects of H_2 receptor antagonists on the hepatotoxicity of various chemicals, *Research Communications in Chemical Pathology and Pharmacology*, **44**, 375–388.

Leonard, T. B., Morgan, D. G. and Dent, J. G., 1985a, Ranitidine-acetaminophen interaction: effects on acetaminophen-induced hepatotoxicity in Fischer 344 rats, *Hepatology*, **5**, 480–487.

Leonard, T. B., Morgan, D. G. and Dent, J. G., 1985b, Characterisation of ranitidine-acetaminophen (APAP) interactions in F344 rats: effects on hepatotoxicity, *Toxicologist*, **5**, 154.

Le Perdriel, F., Hanegraaff, C., Chastagner, N. and de Montety, E., 1968, Sur une nouvelle réaction colorée du paracétamol. Application à son dosage dans les formes médicamenteuses, *Annales Pharmaceutiques Françaises*, **26**, 227–237.

Lepine, R., 1886, Sur l'action de acétanilid (Antifébrine), *La Semaine Médicale (Paris)*, **6**, 473–474.

Lerner, W., Caruso, R., Faig, D. and Karpatkin, S., 1985, Drug-dependent and non-drug-dependent antiplatelet antibody in drug-induced immunologic thrombocytopenic purpura, *Blood*, **66**, 306–311.

Lesna, M., 1978, Paracetamol poisoning, *British Medical Journal*, **4**, 1785.

Lesna, M., Watson, A. J., Douglas, A. P., Hamlyn, A. N. and James, O., 1976a, Toxicity of paracetamol, *Lancet*, **i**, 191.

Lesna, M., Watson, A. J., Douglas, A. P., Hamlyn, A. N. and James, O. F. W., 1976b, Evaluation of paracetamol-induced damage in liver biopsies: acute changes and follow-up findings, *Virchows Archiv. A. Pathological Anatomy and Histopathology*, **370**, 333–344.

Lesser, P. B., Vietti, M. M. and Clark, W. D., 1986, Lethal enhancement of therapeutic doses of acetaminophen by alcohol, *Digestive Diseases and Sciences*, **31**, 103–105.

Lester, D. and Greenberg, L. A., 1947, The metabolic fate of acetanilid and other aniline derivatives. II. Major metabolites of acetanilid appearing in the blood, *Journal of Pharmacology and Experimental Therapeutics*, **90**, 68–75.

Letley, E., Fowle, A. S. A., Whiteman, P. and Land, G., 1980, Plasma paracetamol profile following oral administration of paracetamol tablets, *Farmaco – Edizione Pratica*, **35**, 571–574.

Letteron, P., Descatoire, V., Larrey, D., Degott, C., Tinel, M., Genève, J. and Pessayre, D., 1986, Pre- or post-treatment with methoxsalen prevents the hepatotoxicity of acetaminophen in mice, *Journal of Pharmacology and Experimental Therapeutics*, **239**, 559–567.

Leung, N. W. Y. and Critchley, J. A. J. H., 1991, Increased oxidative metabolism of paracetamol in patients with hepatocellular carcinoma, *Cancer Letters*, **57**, 45–48.

Leung, R., Plomley, R. and Czarny, D., 1992, Paracetamol anaphylaxis, *Clinical and Experimental Allergy*, **22**, 831–833.

Leuzinger, D., Lucas, E. and Seta, F., 1978, Hypoglycémie induite par l'association chlorhydrate de dextropropoxyphène – paracétamol, *La Nouvelle Presse Médicale*, **7**, 1122.

Le Van, D. and Grilliat, J. P., 1990, Anaphylactic shock induced by paracetamol, *European Journal of Clinical Pharmacology*, **38**, 389–390.

Le Van, D., Marciniak, R., Wach, P. and Grilliat, J. P., 1989, Choc anaphylactoïde au paracétamol, *Annales Médicales de Nancy et de l'Est*, **28**, 221–222.

Levin, H. M., Bare, W. W., Berry, F. N. and Miller, J. M., 1974, Acetaminophen with codeine for the relief of severe pain in postpartum patients, *Current Therapeutic Research*, **16**, 921–927.

Levine, R. A., Nandi, J. and King, R. L., 1991, Nonsalicylate nonsteroidal antiinflammatory drugs augment prestimulated acid secretion in rabbit parietal cells: investigation of the mechanisms of action, *Gastroenterology*, **101**, 756–765.

Levinson, M., 1983, Ulcer, back pain, and jaundice in an alcoholic, *Hospital Practice*, **18**, 48N–48S.

Levy, G., 1971, Comparative systemic availability of acetaminophen when administered orally as such and as acetophenetidin, *Journal of Pharmaceutical Sciences*, **60**, 499–500.

Levy, G., 1981, Comparative pharmacokinetics of aspirin and acetaminophen, *Archives of Internal Medicine*, **141**, 279–281.

Levy, G., 1986, Sulfate conjugation in drug metabolism: role of inorganic sulfate, *Federation Proceedings*, **45**, 2235–2240.

Levy, G., 1987, Pharmacokinetic analysis of the analgesic effect of a second dose of acetaminophen in humans, *Journal of Pharmaceutical Sciences*, **76**, 88–89.

Levy, G., Galinsky, R. E. and Lin, J. H., 1982, Pharmacokinetic consequences and toxicologic implications of endogenous cosubstrate depletion, *Drug Metabolism Reviews*, **13**, 1009–1020.

Levy, G., Garrettson, L. K. and Soda, D. M., 1975a, Evidence for placental transfer of acetaminophen, *Pediatrics*, **55**, 895.

Levy, G. and Houston, J. B., 1976, Effect of activated charcoal on acetaminophen absorption, *Pediatrics*, **58**, 432–435.

Levy, G., Khanna, N. N., Soda, D. M., Tsuzuki, O. and Stern, L., 1975b, Pharmacokinetics of acetaminophen in the human neonate: formation of acetaminophen glucuronide and sulfate in relation to plasma bilirubin concentration and D-glucaric acid excretion, *Pediatrics*, **55**, 818–825.

Levy, G. and Regårdh, C.-G., 1971, Drug biotransformation interactions in man: V. Acetaminophen and salicylic acid, *Journal of Pharmaceutical Sciences*, **60**, 608–611.

Levy, G. and Yamada, H., 1971, Drug biotransformation interactions in man III: acetaminophen and salicylamide, *Journal of Pharmaceutical Sciences*, **60**, 215–221.

Levy, G. A., 1993, Acute hepatic failure: University of Toronto experience, *Canadian Journal of Gastroenterology*, **7**, 542–544.

Levy, L. J., Bolton, R. P. and Losowsky, M. S., 1990, The visual evoked potential in clinical hepatic encephalopathy in acute and chronic liver disease, *Hepato-Gastroenterology*, **37 (Suppl. 2)**, 66–73.

Levy, M., Miller, D. R., Kaufman, D. W., Siskind, V., Schwingl, P., Rosenberg, L., Strom, B. and Shapiro, S., 1988, Major upper gastrointestinal tract bleeding. Relation to the use of aspirin and other nonnarcotic analgesics, *Archives of Internal Medicine*, **148**, 281–285.

Levy, M. and Oren, R., 1985, Paracetamol overdosage in Jerusalem, *Israel Journal of Medical Sciences*, **21**, 36–39.

Lew, H. and Quintanilha, A., 1991, Effects of endurance training and exercise on tissue antioxidative capacity and acetaminophen detoxification, *European Journal of Drug Metabolism and Pharmacokinetics*, **16**, 59–68.

Lewis, A. J., Nelson, D. J. and Sugrue, M. F., 1975, On the ability of prostaglandin E_1 and arachidonic acid to modulate experimentally induced oedema in the rat paw, *British Journal of Pharmacology*, **55**, 51–56.

Lewis, J. M., 1984, Pediatric dosing of acetaminophen, *Pediatric Pharmacology*, **4**, 253–254.

Lewis, K., Cherry, J. D., Sachs, M. H., Woo, D. B., Hamilton, R. C., Tarle, J. M. and Overturf, G. D., 1988, The effect of prophylactic acetaminophen administration on reactions to DTP vaccination, *American Journal of Diseases of Children*, **142**, 62–65.

Lewis, R. K. and Paloucek, F. P., 1991, Assessment and treatment of acetaminophen overdose, *Clinical Pharmacy*, **10**, 765–774.

Lewis, R. P., Dunphy, J. A. and Reilly, C. S., 1991, Paracetamol metabolism after general anaesthesia, *European Journal of Anaesthesiology*, **8**, 445–450.

Leyland, A. and O'Meara, A. F., 1974, Probable paracetamol toxicity in a cat, *The Veterinary Record*, **94**, 104–105.

Li, J.-Y., Wang, L. and Zhang, X.-J., 1994a, Cytoprotective effect of neurotensin on acetaminophen-induced liver injury in relation to glutathione system, *Acta Physiologica Sinica*, **46**, 168–175.

Li, Q.-J., Bessems, J. G. M., Commandeur, J. N. M., Adams, B. and Vermeulen, N. P. E., 1994b, Mechanism of protection of ebselen against paracetamol-induced toxicity in rat hepatocytes, *Biochemical Pharmacology*, **48**, 1631–1640.

Li, Y., Wang, E., Patten, C. J., Chen, L. and Yang, C. S., 1994c, Effects of flavonoids on cytochrome P-450-dependent acetaminophen metabolism in rats and human liver microsomes, *Drug Metabolism and Disposition: The Biological Fate of Chemicals*, **22**, 566–571.

Liashek, P., Desjardins, P. J. and Triplett, R. G., 1987, Effect of pretreatment with acetaminophen-propoxyphene for oral surgery pain, *Journal of Oral and Maxillofacial Surgery*, **45**, 99–103.

Licht, H., Seeff, L. B. and Zimmerman, H. J., 1980, Apparent potentiation of acetaminophen hepatotoxicity by alcohol, *Annals of Internal Medicine*, **92**, 511.

Lidofsky, S. D., 1993, Liver transplantation for fulminant hepatic failure, *Gastroenterology Clinics of North America*, **22**, 257–269.

Lieber, C. S., 1983, Microsomal ethanol oxidizing system (MEOS): interaction with ethanol, drugs and carcinogens, *Pharmacology, Biochemistry and Behavior*, **18 (Suppl. 1)**, 181–187.

Lieber, C. S., 1988, The microsomal ethanol oxidising system: its role in ethanol and xenobiotic metabolism, *Biochemical Society Transactions*, **16**, 232–239.

Lieber, C. S., 1990a, Mechanism of ethanol induced hepatic injury, *Pharmacology and Therapeutics*, **46**, 1–41.

Lieber, C. S., 1990b, Interaction of alcohol with other drugs and nutrients: implication for the therapy of alcoholic liver disease, *Drugs*, **40 (Suppl. 3)**, 23–44.

Lieber, C. S., Lasker, J. M., Alderman, J. and Leo, M. A., 1987, The microsomal ethanol oxidizing system and its interaction with other drugs, carcinogens, and vitamins, *Annals of the New York Academy of Sciences*, **492**, 11–24.

Liederman, P. C. and Boldus, R. A., 1967, Psychic side effects of a chlorzoxazone and acetaminophen mixture: a case report, *Journal of the American Medical Association*, **202**, 158–160.

Liedtke, R., Berne, G., Haase, W., Nicolai, W., Staab, R. and Wagener, H. H., 1979, Vergleichende Humanpharmakokinetik von Paracetamol nach oraler und rektaler Einmalapplikation, *Arzneimittel-Forschung*, **29**, 1607–1611.

Liedtke, R., Ebel, S., Missler, B., Haase, W. and Stein, L., 1980, Humanpharmakokinetik von Paracetamol und Salicylamide nach kombinierter rektaler Mehrfachverabreichung, *Arzneimittel-Forschung*, **30**, 1295–1298.

Lieh-Lai, M. W., Sarnaik, A. P., Newton, J. F., Miceli, J. N., Fleischmann, L. E., Hook, J. B. and Kauffman, R. E., 1984, Metabolism and pharmacokinetics of acetaminophen in a severely poisoned young child, *Journal of Pediatrics*, **105**, 125–128.

Ligumsky, M., Sestieri, M., Karmeli, F. and Rachmilewitz, D., 1986, Protection by mild irritants against indomethacin-induced gastric mucosal damage in the rat: role of prostaglandin synthesis, *Israel Journal of Medical Sciences*, **22**, 807–811.

Lillsunde, P. and Korte, T., 1991, Comprehensive drug screening in urine using solid-phase extraction and combined TLC and GC/MS identification, *Journal of Analytical Toxicology*, **15**, 71–81.

Lim, R. K. S., Guzman, F., Rodgers, D. W, Goto, K., Braun, G., Dickerson, G. D. and Engle, R. J., 1964, Site of action of narcotic and non-narcotic analgesics determined by blocking bradykinin-evoked visceral pain, *Archives Internationales de Pharmacodynamie et de Thérapie*, **152**, 25–58.

Lim, S. P., Andrews, F. J. and O'Brien, P. E., 1994, Misoprostol protection against acetaminophen-induced hepatotoxicity in the rat, *Digestive Diseases and Sciences*, **39**, 1249–1256.

Lin, J. H. and Levy, G., 1981, Sulfate depletion after acetaminophen administration and replenishment by infusion of sodium sulfate or N-acetylcysteine in rats, *Biochemical*

Pharmacology, **30**, 2723–2725.

Lin, J. H. and Levy, G., 1982, Effect of experimental renal failure on sulfate retention and acetaminophen pharmacokinetics in rats, *Journal of Pharmacology and Experimental Therapeutics*, **221**, 80–84.

Lin, J. H. and Levy, G., 1983a, Renal clearance of inorganic sulfate in rats: effect of acetaminophen-induced depletion of endogenous sulfate, *Journal of Pharmaceutical Sciences*, **72**, 213–217.

Lin, J. H. and Levy, G., 1983b, Effect of pregnancy on the pharmacokinetics of acetaminophen in rats, *Journal of Pharmacology and Experimental Therapeutics*, **225**, 653–659.

Lin, J. H. and Levy, G., 1986, Effect of prevention of inorganic sulfate depletion on the pharmacokinetics of acetaminophen in rats, *Journal of Pharmacology and Experimental Therapeutics*, **239**, 94–98.

Lin, S.-C., Lin, C.-C., Lin, Y.-H. and Chen, C.-H., 1994a, Protective and therapeutic effects of Ban-zhi-lian on hepatotoxin-induced liver injuries, *American Journal of Chinese Medicine*, **22**, 29–42.

Lin, S.-C., Lin, C.-C., Lin, Y.-H. and Shyuu, S.-J., 1994b, Hepatoprotective effects of Taiwan folk medicine: *Wedelia chinensis* on three hepatotoxin-induced hepatotoxicity, *American Journal of Chinese Medicine*, **22**, 155–168.

Lin, S.-Y. and Yang, J.-C., 1990, Effect of β-cyclodextrin on the *in vitro* permeation rate and *in vivo* rectal absorption of acetaminophen hydrogel preparations, *Pharmaceutica Acta Helvetiae*, **65**, 9–10.

Lin, S.-Y., Yang, J.-C., Lui, T.-Y. and Lin, C.-Y., 1989, Pharmacokinetic study of acetaminophen after conventional whole cell and acellular diphtheria-tetanus-pertussis vaccination in rats, *Current Therapeutic Research*, **46**, 1034–1044.

Linden, C. H. and Rumack, B. H., 1984, Acetaminophen overdose, *Emergency Medicine Clinics of North America*, **2**, 103–119.

Lindeneg, O., Fischer, S., Pederson, J. and Nissen, N. I., 1959, Necrosis of the renal papillae and prolonged abuse of phenacetin, *Acta Medica Scandinavica*, **165**, 321–328.

Lindenthal, J., Sinclair, J. F., Howell, S., Cargill, I., Sinclair, P. R. and Taylor, T., 1993, Toxicity of paracetamol in cultured chick hepatocytes treated with methotrexate, *European Journal of Pharmacology – Environmental Toxicology and Pharmacology Section*, **228**, 289–298.

Lindgren, L. and Saarnivaara, L., 1985, Comparison of paracetamol and aminophenazone plus diazepam suppositories for anxiety and pain relief after tonsillectomy in children, *Acta Anaesthesiologica Scandinavica*, **29**, 679–682.

Linhares, M. C. and Kissinger, P. T., 1992, *In vivo* sampling using loop microdialysis probes coupled to a liquid chromatograph, *Journal of Chromatography: Biomedical Applications*, **578**, 157–163.

Linhares, M. C. and Kissinger, P. T., 1993, Pharmacokinetic monitoring in subcutaneous tissue using *in vivo* capillary ultrafiltration probes, *Pharmaceutical Research*, **10**, 598–602.

Linhares, M. C. and Kissinger, P. T., 1994, Pharmacokinetic studies using microdialysis probes in subcutaneous tissue: effects of the co-administration of ethanol and acetaminophen, *Journal of Pharmaceutical and Biomedical Analysis*, **12**, 619–627.

Linscheer, W. G., Raheja, K. L., Cho, C. and Smith, N. J., 1980, Mechanisms of the protective effect of propylthiouracil against acetaminophen (Tylenol) toxicity in the rat, *Gastroenterology*, **78**, 100–107.

Lipscomb, D. J. and Widdop, B., 1975, Studies with activated charcoal in the treatment of drug overdosage using the pig as an animal model, *Archives of Toxicology*, **34**, 37–46.

Lipton, J. M., Rosenstein, J. and Sklar, F. H., 1981, Thermoregulatory disorders after removal of a craniopharyngioma from the third cerebral ventricle, *Brain Research Bulletin*, **7**, 369–373.

Litovitz, T., 1992, Implication of dispensing cups in dosing errors and pediatric poisonings: a report from the American Association of Poison Control Centers, *Annals of Phar-*

macotherapy, **26**, 917–918.

Litovitz, T. and Manoguerra, A., 1992, Comparison of pediatric poisoning hazards: an analysis of 3.8 million exposure incidents. A report from the American Association of Poison Control Centers, *Pediatrics*, **89**, 999–1006.

Litovitz, T. L., Bailey, K. M., Schmitz, B. F., Holm, K. C. and Klein-Schwartz, W., 1991, 1990 Annual report of the American Association of Poison Control Centers National Data Collection System, *American Journal of Emergency Medicine*, **9**, 461–509.

Litovitz, T. L., Holm, K. C., Bailey, K. M. and Schmitz, B. F., 1992, 1991 Annual report of the American Association of Poison Control Centres National Data Collection System, *American Journal of Emergency Medicine*, **10**, 452–505.

Litovitz, T. L., Martin, T. G. and Schmitz, B., 1987, 1986 Annual report of the American Association of Poison Control Centers National Data Collection System, *American Journal of Emergency Medicine*, **5**, 405–445.

Litovitz, T. L., Schmitz, B. F. and Bailey, K. M., 1990, 1989 Annual report of the American Association of Poison Control Centers National Data Collection System, *American Journal of Emergency Medicine*, **8**, 394–442.

Litovitz, T. L., Schmitz, B. F. and Holm, K. C., 1989, 1988 Annual report of the American Association of Poison Control Centers National Data Collection System, *American Journal of Emergency Medicine*, **7**, 495–545.

Little, J. A., 1976, Acetaminophen and Reye's syndrome? *Pediatrics*, **58**, 918.

Liu, G.-T. and Wei, H.-L., 1987, Protection by Fructus Schizandrae against acetaminophen hepatotoxicity in mice, *Acta Pharmaceutica Sinica*, **22**, 650–654.

Liu, J., Liu, Y. and Klaassen, C. D., 1994a, The effect of Chinese hepatoprotective medicines on experimental liver injury in mice, *Journal of Ethnopharmacology*, **42**, 183–191.

Liu, J., Liu, Y., Madhu, C. and Klaassen, C. D., 1993, Protective effects of oleanolic acid on acetaminophen-induced hepatotoxicity in mice, *Journal of Pharmacology and Experimental Therapeutics*, **266**, 1607–1613.

Liu, J., Liu, Y., Mao, Q. and Klaassen, C. D., 1994b, The effects of 10 triterpenoid compounds on experimental liver injury in mice, *Fundamental and Applied Toxicology*, **22**, 34–40.

Liu, J., Sato, C. and Marumo, F., 1991, Characterization of the acetaminophen-glutathione conjugation reaction by liver microsomes: species difference in the effects of acetone, *Toxicology Letters*, **56**, 269–274.

Liu, J., Sato, C., Miyakawa, H., Kamiyama, T., Tajiri, K., Goto, M. and Marumo, F., 1992a, Inhibition of acetaminophen hepatotoxicity by acetaldehyde in the rat, *Toxicology Letters*, **62**, 287–292.

Liu, J., Sato, C., Shigesawa, T., Kamiyama, T., Tajiri, K., Miyakawa, H. and Marumo, F., 1992b, Effects of caffeine on paracetamol activation in rat and mouse liver microsomes, *Xenobiotica*, **22**, 433–437.

Liu, P., Naughton, B. A., Naughton, G. K. and Gordon, A. S., 1981, The effect of acetaminophen and ethanol on hepatic erythropoietin production, *Anatomical Record*, **199**, 155A.

Liu, T.-Z. and Skale, J. S., 1985, Rapid spectrophotometric method for quantitation of acetaminophen in serum, *Journal of the Formosan Medical Association*, **84**, 693–699.

Liu, T. Z. and Bigler, W. N., 1983, A better method for eliminating salicylate interference with measurement of acetaminophen, *Clinical Chemistry*, **29**, 590.

Liu, T. Z. and Oka, K. H., 1980, Spectrophotometric screening method for acetaminophen in serum and plasma, *Clinical Chemistry*, **26**, 69–71.

Liu, Y.-P., Liu, J., Jia, X.-S., Mao, Q., Madhu, C. and Klaassen, C. D., 1992c, Protective effects of fulvotomentosides on acetaminophen-induced hepatotoxicity, *Acta Pharmacologica Sinica*, **13**, 209–212.

Lloyd, R. S., Costello, F., Eves, M. J., James, I. G. V. and Miller, A. J., 1992, The efficacy and tolerability of controlled-release dihydrocodeine tablets and combination dextropropoxphene/paracetamol tablets in patients with severe osteoarthritis of the hips, *Current Medical Research and Opinion*, **13**, 37–48.

Lloyd, T. W., 1961, Agranulocytosis associated with paracetamol, *Lancet*, **i**, 114–115.

Lo, L. Y. and Bye, A., 1979, Rapid determination of paracetamol in plasma by reversed-phase high-performance liquid chromatography, *Journal of Chromatography*, **173**, 198–201.

Lobo, I. B. and Hoult, J. R. S., 1994, Groups I, II and III extracellular phospholipases A$_2$: selective inhibition of group II enzymes by indomethacin but not other NSAIDs, *Agents and Actions*, **41**, 111–113.

Lock, A., Eckman, B. M. and Ayres, J., 1979, Antipyretic effect of acetaminophen suppositories in rats, *Journal of Pharmaceutical Sciences*, **68**, 1105–1107.

Lock, F. M., de Vries, J., Mullink, H. and van Bree, L., 1982, Protective effect of a simultaneous oral dose of acetylsalicylic acid against paracetamol-induced hepatotoxicity in rats, *Pharmaceutisch Weekblad. Scientific Edition*, **4**, 211.

Lockhart, S. P. and Baron, J. H., 1987, Changing ethnic and social characteristics of patients admitted for self-poisoning in West London during 1971/2 and 1983/4, *Journal of the Royal Society of Medicine*, **80**, 145–148.

Loebl, D. H., Craig, R. M., Culic, D. D., Ridolfo, A. S., Falk, J. and Schmid, F. R., 1977, Gastrointestinal blood loss. Effect of aspirin, fenoprofen, and acetaminophen in rheumatoid arthritis as determined by sequential gastroscopy and radioactive fecal markers, *Journal of the American Medical Association*, **237**, 976–981.

Loeser, W. and Siegers, C.-P., 1985, Effects of phenobarbital, phorone and carbon tetrachloride pretreatment on the biliary excretion of acetaminophen in rats, *Archives Internationales de Pharmacodynamie et de Thérapie*, **275**, 180–188.

Loew, G. H. and Goldblum, A., 1985, Metabolic activation and toxicity of acetaminophen and related analogs: a theoretical study, *Molecular Pharmacology*, **27**, 375–386.

Löf, A., Wallén, M. and Hjelm, E. W., 1990, Influence of paracetamol and acetylsalicylic acid on the toxicokinetics of toluene, *Pharmacology and Toxicology*, **66**, 138–141.

Logan, R. F. A., Little, J., Hawtin, P. G. and Hardcastle, J. D., 1993, Effect of aspirin and non-steroidal anti-inflammatory drugs on colorectal adenomas: case-control study of subjects participating in the Nottingham faecal occult blood screening programme, *British Medical Journal*, **307**, 285–289.

Lohmann, J., Lessing, U., Schriewer, H., Clemens, M. and Gerlach, U., 1984, The influence of paracetamol on the hepatic biosynthesis of lecithin, *Archives of Toxicology*, **55 (Suppl. 7)**, 236–239.

Lohse, E., 1985, Grenzwertbestimmung einiger Analgetica in Blut und Urin mit Hilfe der Dünnschichtchromatografie beim Einsatz von Adsorberharz Y$_{29}$, *Pharmazie*, **40**, 358–359.

Long, R. M. and Moore, L., 1988, Evaluation of the calcium mobilizing action of acetaminophen and bromobenzene in rat hepatocyte cultures, *Journal of Biochemical Toxicology*, **3**, 353–362.

Longlands, M. G. and Wiener, K., 1982, Minimisation of salicylate interference in the Glynn and Kendal paracetamol procedure, *Annals of Clinical Biochemistry*, **19**, 187–190.

López-Fiesco, A., Luján, M., Alvarez, J. M., Zamora Lopez, G. and Martínez, E. L., 1992, Evaluation of the analgesic efficacy of a combination of naproxen and paracetamol vs. dipyrone on the tourniquet test in healthy volunteers, *Proceedings of the Western Pharmacology Society*, **35**, 207–210.

López-Muñoz, F. J., Castañeda-Hernández, G., Villalón, C. M., Terrón, J. A. and Salazar, L. A., 1993, Analgesic effects of combinations containing opioid drugs with either aspirin or acetaminophen in the rat, *Drug Development Research*, **29**, 299–304.

Lornoy, W., 1994, Analgesic nephropathy: are analgesic mixtures without phenacetin or paracetamol also nephrotoxic? *Tijdschrift voor Geneeskunde*, **50**, 729–735.

Lou, Y.-J., Ying, Y., Wu, F.-W. and Bao, J.-H., 1993, Inductive effects of aspirin, paracetamol and ibuprofen on micronuclei of rat preimplanted blastocysts *in vivo*, *Chinese Journal of Pharmacology and Toxicology*, **7**, 297–300.

Loux, J. J., Smith, S. and Salem, H., 1977, Antiinflammatory activity: evaluation of a new screening procedure, *Inflammation*, **2**, 125–130.

Love, E. B., 1977, Measuring plasma-paracetamol, *Lancet*, **i**, 195.

Lovering, E. G., McGilveray, I. J., McMillan, I. and Tostowaryk, W., 1975, Comparative bioavailabilities from truncated blood level curves, *Journal of Pharmaceutical Sciences*, **64**, 1521–1524.

Lowenthal, D. T., Øie, S., van Stone, J. C., Briggs, W. A. and Levy, G., 1976, Pharmacokinetics of acetaminophen elimination by anephric patients, *Journal of Pharmacology and Experimental Therapeutics*, **196**, 570–578.

Lozano Gutierrez, F., Santa Maria De Saenz, F. J., Soria Monge, A., Jimena Medina, M. and Perez Miranda, M., 1984, Correlación bioquímico-etiopatogénica en 26 casos de hepatopatía por fármacos, *Revista Espanola de las Enfermedades del Aparato Digestivo*, **65**, 147–156.

Lu, H., Li, Y. and Liu, G.-T., 1994, Protection of acetylcorynoline against paracetamol hepatotoxicity in mice, *Chinese Journal of Pharmacology and Toxicology*, **8**, 171–174.

Lu, H.-H., Thomas, J. and Fleisher, D., 1992a, Influence of D-glucose-induced water absorption on rat jejunal uptake of two passively absorbed drugs, *Journal of Pharmaceutical Sciences*, **81**, 21–25.

Lu, H.-H., Thomas, J. D., Tukker, J. J. and Fleisher, D., 1992b, Intestinal water and solute absorption studies: comparison of *in situ* perfusion with chronic isolated loops in rats, *Pharmaceutical Research*, **9**, 894–900.

Lubawy, W. C. and Garrett, R. J. B., 1977, Effects of aspirin and acetaminophen on fetal and placental growth in rats, *Journal of Pharmaceutical Sciences*, **66**, 111–113.

Lubek, B. M., Avaria, M., Basu, P. K. and Wells, P. G., 1984, Ocular toxicity of acetaminophen and naphthalene, *Pharmacologist*, **26**, 200.

Lubek, B. M., Avaria, M., Basu, P. K. and Wells, P. G., 1988a, Pharmacological studies on the *in vivo* cataractogenicity of acetaminophen in mice and rabbits, *Fundamental and Applied Toxicology*, **10**, 596–606.

Lubek, B. M., Basu, P. K. and Wells, P. G., 1988b, Metabolic evidence for the involvement of enzymatic bioactivation in the cataractogenicity of acetaminophen in genetically susceptible (C57BL/6) and resistant (DBA/2) murine strains, *Toxicology and Applied Pharmacology*, **94**, 487–495.

Ludmir, J., Main, D. M., Landon, M. B. and Gabbe, S. G., 1986, Maternal acetaminophen overdose at 15 weeks of gestation, *Obstetrics and Gynecology*, **67**, 750–751.

Lum, J. T. and Wells, P. G., 1986, Pharmacological studies on the potentiation of phenytoin teratogenicity by acetaminophen, *Teratology*, **33**, 53–72.

Lunte, S. M., Radzik, D. M. and Kissinger, P. T., 1990, An introduction to the study of xenobiotic metabolism using electroanalytical techniques, *Journal of Pharmaceutical Sciences*, **79**, 557–567.

Lupo, S., Yodis, L. A., Mico, B. A. and Rush, G. F., 1987, *In vivo* and *in vitro* hepatotoxicity and metabolism of acetaminophen in Syrian hamsters, *Toxicology*, **44**, 229–239.

Luquel, L., Azzi, R., Desaint, B., Massart, J. D. and Offenstadt, G., 1988, Hépato-néphrite aiguë chez l'alcoolique après prise de paracétamol à dose thérapeutique, *Presse Médicale*, **17**, 1318.

Luttinger, D., 1985, Determination of antinociceptive efficacy of drugs in mice using different water temperatures in a tail-immersion test, *Journal of Pharmacological Methods*, **13**, 351–357.

Lykkesfeldt, J. and Poulsen, H. E., 1993, Nitrosamindannende håndkøbspræparater? *Ugeskrift for Læger*, **155**, 4106–4107.

Lyng, R. D., 1989, Test of six chemicals for embryotoxicity using fetal mouse salivary glands in culture, *Teratology*, **39**, 591–599.

Lyons, L., Studdiford, J. S. and Sommaripa, A.M., 1977, Treatment of acetaminophen overdosage with N-acetylcysteine, *New England Journal of Medicine*, **296**, 174–175.

Lysell, L. and Anzén, B., 1992, Pain control after third molar surgery – a comparative study of ibuprofen (Ibumetin) and a paracetamol/codeine combination (Citodon), *Swedish Dental Journal*, **16**, 151–160.

Maatz, H., 1990, Bioverfügbarkeits-Studien zu Paracetamol, *Krankenhauspharmazie*, **11**, 5–6.

MacDonald, M. G., McGrath, P. P., McMartin, D. N., Washington, G. C. and Hudak, G., 1984, Potentiation of the toxic effects of acetaminophen in mice by concurrent infection with influenza B virus: a possible mechanism for human Reye's syndrome? *Pediatric Research*, **18**, 181–187.

Mace, P. F. K. and Walker, G., 1976, Salicylate interference with plasma-paracetamol method, *Lancet*, **ii**, 1362.

Macfie, A. G., Magides, A. D., Richmond, M. N. and Reilly, C. S., 1991, Gastric emptying in pregnancy, *British Journal of Anaesthesia*, **67**, 54–57.

MacGregor, E. A., Wilkinson, M. and Bancroft, K., 1993, Domperidone plus paracetamol in the treatment of migraine, *Cephalalgia*, **13**, 124–127.

MacGregor, R. R., 1976, The effect of anti-inflammatory agents and inflammation on granulocyte adherence. Evidence for regulation by plasma factors, *American Journal of Medicine*, **61**, 597–607.

Macheras, P., Parissi-Poulos, M. and Poulos, L., 1989, Pharmacokinetics of acetaminophen after intramuscular administration, *Biopharmaceutics and Drug Disposition*, **10**, 101–105.

MacIntyre, A., Gray, J. D., Gorelick, M. and Renton, K., 1986, Salicylate and acetaminophen in donated blood, *Canadian Medical Association Journal*, **135**, 215–216.

MacKay, I. S. and Ananian, V., 1982, Analgesia following adult tonsillectomy: a comparative study of Solpadeine and a soluble form of dextropropoxyphene napsylate and paracetamol, *Journal of International Medical Research*, **10**, 109–112.

MacKinnon, H. and Menon, R.S., 1974, Reaction to acetaminophen, *Canadian Medical Association Journal*, **110**, 1237–1239.

MacLean, D., 1983, A comparison of flurbiprofen and paracetamol in the treatment of primary dysmenorrhoea, *Journal of International Medical Research*, **11 (Suppl. 2)**, 1–5.

MacLean, D., Peters, T. J., Brown, R. A. G., McCathie, M., Baines, G. F. and Robertson, P. G. C., 1968a, Treatment of acute paracetamol poisoning, *Lancet*, **ii**, 849–852.

MacLean, D., Robertson, P. G. C. and Bain, S., 1968b, Methaemoglobinaemia and paracetamol, *British Medical Journal*, **4**, 390.

MacLure, M. and MacMahon, B., 1985, Phenacetin and cancers of the urinary tract, *New England Journal of Medicine*, **313**, 1479.

Maddern, G., Miners, J., Collins, P. J. and Jamieson, G. G., 1985, Liquid gastric emptying assessed by direct and indirect techniques: radionuclide labelled liquid emptying compared with a simple paracetamol marker method, *Australian and New Zealand Journal of Surgery*, **55**, 203–206.

Maddrey, W. C., 1987, Hepatic effects of acetaminophen: enhanced toxicity in alcoholics, *Journal of Clinical Gastroenterology*, **9**, 180–185.

Madhu, C., Gregus, Z. and Klaassen, C. D., 1989, Biliary excretion of acetaminophen-glutathione as an index of toxic activation of acetaminophen: effect of chemicals that alter acetaminophen hepatotoxicity, *Journal of Pharmacology and Experimental Therapeutics*, **248**, 1069–1077.

Madhu, C. and Klaassen, C. D., 1991, Protective effect of pregnenolone-16α-carbonitrile on acetaminophen-induced hepatotoxicity in hamsters, *Toxicology and Applied Pharmacology*, **109**, 305–313.

Madhu, C., Liu, L., Kim, H., Parkinson, A. and Klaassen, C. D., 1992a, Mechanisms of zinc and selenium protection against acetaminophen-induced hepatotoxicity in hamsters, *Toxicologist*, **12**, 418.

Madhu, C., Maziasz, T. and Klaassen, C. D., 1992b, Effect of pregnenolone-16α-carbonitrile and dexamethasone on acetaminophen-induced hepatotoxicity in mice, *Toxicology and Applied Pharmacology*, **115**, 191–198.

Madhusudanarao, K., Bapna, J. S., Adithan, C., Ray, K., Venkatadri, N., Kamatchi, G. L.,

Seetharaman, M. L. and Bahadur, P., 1988a, Effect of short course chemotherapy on salivary paracetamol elimination, *Clinical and Experimental Pharmacology and Physiology*, **15**, 639–643.

Madhusudanarao, K., Bapna, J. S., Adithan, C., Ray, K., Venkatadri, N., Kamatchi, G. L., Seetharaman, M. L. and Bahadur, P., 1988b, Effect of pulmonary tuberculosis on salivary paracetamol elimination, *Medical Science Research*, **16**, 481.

Madusolumuo, M. A. and Okoye, Z. S. C., 1993, Effect of *Sacoglottis gabonensis* stem bark extract, a Nigerian palmwine additive, on serum levels of acetaminophen and acetylsalicylic acid, *Medical Science Research*, **21**, 603–604.

Mahadeva, S., Herxheimer, A. and Corne, S.J., 1986, Quantifying ease of swallowing: a comparison of a new lozenge formulation for paracetamol and placebo tablets, *British Journal of Clinical Pharmacology*, **21**, 79–80.

Mahar, A. F., Allen, S. J., Milligan, P., Suthumnirund, S., Chotpitayasunondh, T., Sabchareon, A. and Coulter, J. B. S., 1994, Tepid sponging to reduce temperature in febrile children in a tropical climate, *Clinical Pediatrics*, **33**, 227–231.

Mahoney, J. D., Gross, P. L., Stern, T. A., Browne, B. J., Pollack, M. H., Reder, V. and Mulley, A. G., 1990, Quantitative serum toxic screening in the management of suspected drug overdose, *American Journal of Emergency Medicine*, **8**, 16–22.

Main, J. and Ward, M. K., 1992, Potentiation of aluminium absorption by effervescent analgesic tablets in a haemodialysis patient, *British Medical Journal*, **304**, 1686.

Makin, A. and Williams, R., 1994, The current management of paracetamol overdosage, *British Journal of Clinical Practice*, **48**, 144–148.

Malan, J., Moncrieff, J. and Bosch, E., 1985, Chronopharmacokinetics of paracetamol in normal subjects, *British Journal of Clinical Pharmacology*, **19**, 843–845.

Malia, R. G., Kennedy, H. J., Park, B. K., Triger, D. R. and Preston, F. E., 1985, The effect of acetaminophen on the vitamin K dependent prothrombin complex, *Thrombosis and Haemostasis*, **54**, 205.

Malley, A. D., 1987, Paracetamol poisoning in a cat, *The Veterinary Record*, **121**, 528.

Malmberg, A. B. and Yaksh, T. L., 1992, Antinociceptive actions of spinal non-steroidal anti-inflammatory agents on the formalin test in the rat, *Journal of Pharmacology and Experimental Therapeutics*, **263**, 136–146.

Malmberg, A. B. and Yaksh, T. L., 1993, Spinal actions of non-steroidal anti-inflammatory drugs: evidence for a central role of prostanoids in nociceptive processing, *Progress in Pharmacology and Clinical Pharmacology*, **10**, 91–110.

Malmberg, A. B. and Yaksh, T. L., 1994, Capsaicin-evoked prostaglandin E_2 release in spinal cord slices: relative effect of cyclooxygenase inhibitors, *European Journal of Pharmacology*, **271**, 293–299.

Malnoë, A., Louis, A., Benedetti, M. S., Schneider, M., Smith, R. L., Kreber, L. and Lam, R., 1975, Effect of liposomal entrapment on the protective action of glutathione against paracetamol-induced liver necrosis, *Biochemical Society Transactions*, **3**, 730–732.

Malone, K., McCormack, G. and Malone, J. P., 1992, Non-fatal deliberate self-poisoning in Dublin's North inner city – an overview, *Irish Medical Journal*, **85**, 132–135.

Malvin, M. D., Vaughn, L. K. and Kluger, M. J., 1979, Blood pressure in unanesthetized bacterially infected rabbits: effects of antipyretic drug therapy, *Circulatory Shock*, **6**, 7–12.

Manara, A. R., Quinn, K. G. and Park, G. R., 1990, Oral metoclopramide does not speed the absorption of concurrently administered paracetamol, *European Journal of Anaesthesiology*, **7**, 1–7.

Manautou, J. E., Hoivik, D. J., Tveit, A., Emeigh Hart, S. G., Khairallah, E. A. and Cohen, S. D., 1994, Clofibrate pretreatment diminishes acetaminophen's selective covalent binding and hepatotoxicity, *Toxicology and Applied Pharmacology*, **129**, 252–263.

Mancilla, J., Valdes, E. and Gil, L., 1989, A novel isocratic HPLC method to separate and quantify acetanilide and its hydroxy aromatic derivatives: 2-, 3- and 4-

hydroxyacetanilide (paracetamol or acetaminophen), *European Journal of Drug Metabolism and Pharmacokinetics*, **14**, 241–244.

Mancini, R. E., Sonawane, B. R. and Yaffe, S. J., 1980, Developmental susceptibility to acetaminophen toxicity, *Research Communications in Chemical Pathology and Pharmacology*, **27**, 603–606.

Manekar, M. S. and Raul, A. R., 1983, Pharmacological study of ulcerogenic action of antipyretic analgesic agents and their interaction with sodium salicylate, *Indian Journal of Physiology and Pharmacology*, **27**, 151–156.

Mann, J. M., Pierre-Louis, M., Kragel, P. J., Kragel, A. N. and Roberts, W. C., 1989, Cardiac consequences of massive acetaminophen overdose, *American Journal of Cardiology*, **63**, 1018–1021.

Mann, K. V., 1988, Treatment of acetaminophen overdose when oral acetylcysteine therapy is not tolerated, *Clinical Pharmacy*, **7**, 563–564.

Mann, N. S. and Sachdev, A. J., 1977, Gastric effects of propoxyphene, acetaminophen, indomethacin, phenylbutazone, and naproxen, *Journal of the Kentucky Medical Association*, **75**, 21–2, 50.

Manna, S., Mandal, T. K., Chakraborty, A. K. and Gupta, R. D., 1994, Modification of the disposition kinetics of paracetamol by oxytetracycline and endotoxin-induced fever in goats, *Indian Journal of Animal Sciences*, **64**, 248–252.

Manning, B. W., Franklin, M. R. and Galinsky, R. E., 1991, Drug metabolizing enzyme changes after chronic buthionine sulfoximine exposure modify acetaminophen disposition in rats, *Drug Metabolism and Disposition: The Biological Fate of Chemicals*, **19**, 498–502.

Manno, B. R., Manno, J. E., Dempsey, C. A. and Wood, M. A. , 1981, A high-pressure liquid chromatographic method for the determination of N-acetyl-p-aminophenol (acetaminophen) in serum or plasma using a direct injection technique, *Journal of Analytical Toxicology*, **5**, 24–28.

Manor, E. , Marmor, A. , Kaufman, S. and Leiba, H. , 1976, Massive hemolysis caused by acetaminophen: positive determination by direct Coombs test, *Journal of the American Medical Association*, **236**, 2777–2778.

Manrique Larralde, A., Salvador Ballaz, B., Ramos Castro, J., Pueyo Labay, A., Madurga Pérez, P. and Maravi Poma, E., 1988, Necrosis aguda hepática por sobredosis de paracetamol, *Medicina Intensiva*, **12**, 47–48.

Mansini, E., Lodovici, M., Fantozzi, R., Brunelleschi, S., Conti, A. and Mannaioni, P. F., 1986, Histamine release by free radicals: paracetamol-induced histamine release from rat peritoneal mast cells after *in vitro* activation by monooxygenase, *Agents and Actions*, **18**, 85–88.

Mansor, S. M., Edwards, G., Roberts, P. J. and Ward, S. A., 1991, The effect of malaria infection on paracetamol disposition in the rat, *Biochemical Pharmacology*, **41**, 1707–1711.

Mansuy, D., Sassi, A., Dansette, P. M. and Plat, M., 1986, A new potent inhibitor of lipid peroxidation *in vitro* and *in vivo*, the hepatoprotective drug anisyldithiolthione, *Biochemical and Biophysical Research Communications*, **135**, 1015–1021.

Mant, T. G. K., Tempowski, J. H., Volans, G. N. and Talbot, J. C. C., 1984, Adverse reactions to acetylcysteine and effects of overdose, *British Medical Journal*, **289**, 217–219.

Maraninchi, D., Gastaut, J. A., Sebahoun, G. and Carcassonne, Y., 1981, Agranulocytose secondaire à la prise de paracétamol? Intérêt du test *in vitro* sur les progéniteurs granulocytaires, *La Nouvelle Presse Médicale*, **10**, 41.

Marbury, T. C., Wang, L.-H., Lee, C. S. and Ashouri, O., 1979, Hemodialysis of acetaminophen in uremic patients, *Clinical Research*, **27**, 738A.

Marbury, T. C., Wang, L.H. and Lee, C. S., 1980, Hemodialysis of acetaminophen in uremic patients, *International Journal of Artificial Organs*, **3**, 263–266.

Marcella, K. L., 1983, Acetaminophen poisoning in cats and man, *Journal of the American*

Veterinary Medical Association, **183**, 836.

March, L., Irwig, L., Schwarz, J., Simpson, J., Chock, C. and Brooks, P., 1994, N of 1 trials comparing a non-steroidal anti-inflammatory drug with paracetamol in osteoarthritis, *British Medical Journal*, **309**, 1041–1046.

Marchioni, C. F., Gramolini, C., Guerzoni, P., Corona, M. and Corradini, M., 1990, Efficacia e tollerabilità dell'associazione paracetamolo-sobrerolo nel paziente iperpiretico, *La Clinica Terapeutica*, **135**, 105–113.

Marhic, C., 1986, Etude de l'action antalgique d'une association de paracétamol (500 mg) – codéine (30 mg), *Comptes Rendus des Thérapie et Pharmacologie Clinique*, **4**, 10–21.

Markiewicz, A., 1975, The influence of anti-inflammatory drugs on the values of xylose test in man, *Polish Journal of Pharmacology and Pharmacy*, **27**, 265–272.

Marko, R. and Kelemen, K., 1992, Deprenyl and paracetamol: indirect stimulators of the calcium and sodium channels in the heart, *Pharmacological Research*, **25 (Suppl. 2)**, 142–143.

Maron, J. J. and Ickes, A. C., 1976, The antipyretic effectiveness of acetaminophen suppositories vs. tablets: a double blind study, *Current Therapeutic Research*, **20**, 45–52.

Maronpot, R. R., Pitot, H. C. and Peraino, C., 1989, Use of rat liver altered focus models for testing chemicals that have completed two-year carcinogenicity studies, *Toxicologic Pathology*, **17**, 651–662.

Marquez, L.A. and Dunford, H.B., 1993, Interaction of acetaminophen with myeloperoxidase intermediates: optimum stimulation of enzyme activity, *Archives of Biochemistry and Biophysics*, **305**, 414–420.

Marriott, J.F., Asquith, P.A. and Shorrock, C.J., 1993, The use of proprietary medicines by patients presenting with peptic ulcer haemorrhage, *British Journal of Clinical Pharmacology*, **35**, 451–454.

Marruecos, L., Nogué, S. and Reig, R., 1988, Intoxicación aguda por paracetamol: utilidad de los niveles plasmáticos, *Medicina Intensiva*, **12**, 396.

Marsepoil, T., Mahassani, B., Roudiak, N., Sebbah, J. L. and Caillard, G., 1989, Potentialisation de la toxicité hépatique et rénal du paracétamol par le phénobarbital, *Jeur*, **2**, 118–120.

Marsh, R. H. K., Spencer, R. and Nimmo, W. S., 1984, Gastric emptying and drug absorption before surgery, *British Journal of Anaesthesia*, **56**, 161–164.

Marteau, P., Flourié, B., Froguel, E., Contou, J. F., Galian, A. and Rambaud, J. C., 1990, Rectites secondaires à l'utilisation prolongée de suppositoires de dextropropoxyphène et de paracétamol: le risque persiste malgré le changement d'excipient, *Gastroentérologie Clinique et Biologique*, **14**, 102–103.

Martí, M. L., De Los Santos, A. R., Di Girolamo, G., Gil, M., Manero, E. O. and Fraga, C., 1993, Lysine clonixinate in minor dental surgery: double-blind randomized parallel study vs. paracetamol, *International Journal of Tissue Reactions*, **15**, 207–213.

Martin, U. and Prescott, L. F., 1994, The interaction of paracetamol with frusemide, *British Journal of Clinical Pharmacology*, **37**, 464–467.

Martin, U., Temple, R. M., Winney, R. J. and Prescott, L. F., 1991, The disposition of paracetamol and the accumulation of its glucuronide and sulphate conjugates during multiple dosing in patients with chronic renal failure, *European Journal of Clinical Pharmacology*, **41**, 43–46.

Martin, U., Temple, R. M., Winney, R. J. and Prescott, L. F., 1993, The disposition of paracetamol and its conjugates during multiple dosing in patients with end-stage renal failure maintained on haemodialysis, *European Journal of Clinical Pharmacology*, **45**, 141–145.

Martín, J. A., Lázaro, M., Cuevas, M. and Alvarez-Cuesta, E., 1993, Hipersensibilidad al paracetamol, *Medicina Clínica (Barc.)*, **100**, 158.

Martindale, 1993, *The Extra Pharmacopoeia*, 30th edn, London: The Pharmaceutical Press, pp. 27–28.

Martinelli, A. L. C., Meneghelli, U. G. and Zucoloto, S., 1993, Cytochrome P-450 and glutathione in the liver of rats under exclusive sucrose ingestion, *Brazilian Journal of Medical and Biological Research*, **26**, 989–998.

Martinelli, A. L. C., Meneghelli, U. G., Zucoloto, S. and Lima, S. O., 1989, Effect of the intake of an exclusive sucrose diet on acetaminophen hepatotoxicity in rats, *Brazilian Journal of Medical and Biological Research*, **22**, 1381–1387.

Maruyama, H., Takashima, Y., Murata, Y., Nakae, D., Eimoto, H., Tsutsumi, M., Denda, A. and Konishi, Y., 1990, Lack of hepatocarcinogenic potential of acetaminophen in rats with liver damage associated with a choline-devoid diet, *Carcinogenesis*, **11**, 895–901.

Maruyama, H. and Williams, G. M., 1988, Hepatotoxicity and chronic high dose administration of acetaminophen to mice: a critical review and implications for hazard assessment, *Archives of Toxicology*, **62**, 465–469.

Marzella, L., Muhvich, K. and Myers, R. A. M., 1986, Effect of hyperoxia on liver necrosis induced by hepatotoxins, *Virchows Archiv. B. Cell Pathology*, **51**, 497–507.

Marzo, A., Quadro, G., Treffner, E., Ripamonti, M., Meroni, G. and Lucarelli, C., 1990, High-pressure liquid chromatographic evaluation of cyclic paracetamol-acetylsalicylate and its active metabolites with results of a comparative pharmacokinetic investigation in the rat, *Arzneimittel-Forschung*, **40**, 813–817.

Mason, R. P. and Fischer, V., 1986, Free radicals of acetaminophen: their subsequent reactions and toxological significance, *Federation Proceedings*, **45**, 2493–2499.

Massarrat, S. and Strutwolf, H., 1979, Einfluss verscheidener Antirheumatika auf die elektrische Potentialdifferenz der Magenschleimhaut, *Therapiewoche*, **29**, 8890–8892.

Massey, T. E. and Racz, W. J., 1981, The effects of N-acetylcysteine on the metabolism, covalent binding and toxicity of acetaminophen in isolated mouse hepatocytes, *Toxicology and Applied Pharmacology*, **60**, 220–228.

Massey, T. E., Walker, R. M., McElligott, T. F. and Racz, W. J., 1982, Acetaminophen-induced hypothermia in mice: evidence for a central action of the parent compound, *Toxicology*, **25**, 187–200.

Master, D. R., 1973, Analgesic nephropathy associated with paracetamol, *Proceedings of the Royal Society of Medicine*, **66**, 36.

Masuda, Y. and Nakayama, N., 1982, Protective effect of diethyldithiocarbamate and carbon disulfide against liver injury induced by various hepatotoxic agents, *Biochemical Pharmacology*, **31**, 2713–2725.

Masui, T., Tsuda, H., Inoue, K., Ogiso, T. and Ito, N., 1986, Inhibitory effects of ethoxyquin, 4,4′-diaminodiphenylmethane and acetaminophen on rat hepatocarcinogenesis, *Japanese Journal of Cancer Research*, **77**, 231–237.

Masukawa, T., Sai, M. and Tochino, Y., 1989, Methods for depleting brain gluathione, *Life Sciences*, **44**, 417–424.

Matheson, I., Lunde, P. K .M. and Notarianni, L., 1985, Infant rash caused by paracetamol in breast milk? *Pediatrics*, **76**, 651–652.

Mathew, J., Hines, J. E., James, O. F. W. and Burt, A. D., 1994, Non-parenchymal cell responses in paracetamol (acetaminophen)-induced liver injury, *Journal of Hepatology*, **20**, 537–541.

Mathew, T. H., 1992, Drug-induced renal disease, *Medical Journal of Australia*, **156**, 724–729.

Mathieu, L., 1974, Essai clinique en odonto-stomatologie d'une association paracétamol-acide ascorbique sous forme effervescente, *Revue d'Odonto-Stomatologie*, **3**, 169–176.

Mathis, D. F. and Budd, R. D., 1988, Extraction of acetaminophen and theophylline from post-mortem tissues and urine for high-performance liquid chromatographic analysis, *Journal of Chromatography*, **439**, 466–469.

Mathis, R. D., Walker, J. S. and Kuhns, D. W., 1988, Subacute acetaminophen overdose after incremental dosing, *Journal of Emergency Medicine*, **6**, 37–40.

Matsis, P. P. and Easthope, R. N., 1994, Torsades de pointes ventricular tachycardia associated with terfenadine and paracetamol self medication, *New Zealand Medical Journal*, **107**, 402–403.

Mattammal, M. B., Zenser, T. V., Brown, W. W., Herman, C. A. and Davis, B. B., 1979, Mechanism of inhibition of renal prostaglandin production by acetaminophen, *Journal of Pharmacology and Experimental Therapeutics*, **210**, 405–409.

Matthew, H., 1972, Haemodialysis in paracetamol self-poisoning, *Lancet*, **ii**, 607.

Matthew, H., 1973, Acute acetaminophen poisoning, *Clinical Toxicology*, **6**, 9–11.

Matthews, R. W., Scully, C. M. and Levers, B. G. H., 1984, The efficacy of diclofenac sodium (Voltarol) with and without paracetamol in the control of post-surgical dental pain, *British Dental Journal*, **157**, 357–359.

Mattock, G. L. and McGilveray, I. J., 1973, The effect of food intake and sleep on the absorption of acetaminophen, *Revue Canadienne de Biologie*, **32 (Suppl.)**, 77–84.

Mattock, G. L., McGilveray, I. J. and Cook, D., 1971a, Acetaminophen I. A protocol for the comparison of physiological availabilities of ten different dosage forms, *Canadian Journal of Pharmaceutical Sciences*, **6**, 35–38.

Mattock, G. L., McGilveray, I. J. and Mainville, C. A., 1971b, Acetaminophen III: Dissolution studies of commercial tablets of acetaminophen and comparison with *in vivo* absorption parameters, *Journal of Pharmaceutical Sciences*, **60**, 561–564.

Matzner, Y., Drexler, R. and Levy, M., 1984, Effect of dipyrone, acetylsalicylic acid and acetaminophen on human neutrophil chemotaxis, *European Journal of Clinical Investigation*, **14**, 440–443.

Maurer, W. G. and Zeisler, J., 1978, Intravenous acetylcysteine as treatment for acetaminophen overdose, *American Journal of Hospital Pharmacy*, **35**, 1025–1030.

Maxwell, L. F., Cotty, V. F., Marcus, A. D. and Barnett, L., 1975, Prevention of acetaminophen (paracetamol) poisoning, *Lancet*, **ii**, 610–611.

Mazur, L. J., Jones, T. Mc. and Kozinetz, C. A., 1989, Temperature response to acetaminophen and risk of occult bacteremia: a case-control study, *Journal of Pediatrics*, **115**, 888–891.

Mazur, L. J. and Kozinetz, C. A., 1994, Diagnostic tests for occult bacteremia: temperature response to acetaminophen vs. WBC count, *American Journal of Emergency Medicine*, **12**, 403–406.

Mburu, D. N., 1991, Evaluation of the anti-inflammatory effects of a low dose of acetaminophen following surgery in dogs, *Journal of Veterinary Pharmacology and Therapeutics*, **14**, 109–111.

Mburu, D. N., Maitho, T. E. and Lökken, P., 1990, Acetylsalicylic acid or paracetamol? *East African Medical Journal*, **67**, 302–310.

Mburu, D. N., Mbugua, S. W., Skoglund, L. A. and Lökken, P., 1988, Effects of paracetamol and acetylsalicylic acid on the post-operative course after experimental orthopaedic surgery in dogs, *Journal of Veterinary Pharmacology and Therapeutics*, **11**, 163–171.

McBride, P. V. and Rumack, B. H., 1992, Acetaminophen intoxication, *Seminars in Dialysis*, **5**, 292–298.

McCaul, T. F., Fagan, E. A., Tovey, G., Portmann, B., Williams, R. and Zuckerman, A. J., 1986, Fulminant hepatitis: an ultrastructural study, *Journal of Hepatology*, **2**, 276–290.

McClain, C. J., Holtzman, J. L., Allen, J., Kromhout, J. P. and Shedlofsky, S., 1988, Clinical features of acetaminophen toxicity, *Journal of Clinical Gastroenterology*, **10**, 76–80.

McClain, C. J., Kromhout, J. P., Peterson, F. J. and Holtzman, J. L., 1980, Potentiation of acetaminophen hepatotoxicity by alcohol, *Journal of the American Medical Association*, **244**, 251–253.

McClements, B. M., Hyland, M., Callender, M. E. and Blair, T. L., 1990, Management of paracetamol poisoning complicated by enzyme induction due to alcohol or drugs, *Lancet*, **335**, 1526.

McCormick, C. P. and Shihabi, Z. K., 1990, HPLC of fluorescent products of acetaminophen reaction with peroxidase, *Journal of Liquid Chromatography*, **13**, 1159–1171.

McCoy, D. J. and Trestrail, J. H., 1988, Findings of ten years of clinical drug screening, *Veterinary and Human Toxicology*, **30**, 34–38.

McCrae, T. A., Furuhama, K., Roberts, D. W., Getek, T. A. and Hinson, J. A., 1989, Evaluation of 3-(cystein-S-yl) acetaminophen in the nephrotoxicity of acetaminophen in rats, *Toxicologist*, **9**, 47.

McCredie, M., Disney, A. P. S., Coates, M. S., Auld, J. J., Ford, J. M. and Stewart, J. H., 1990, Geographical distribution of cancers of the kidney and urinary tract and analgesic nephropathy in Australia and New Zealand, *Australian and New Zealand Journal of Medicine*, **20**, 684–688.

McCredie, M., Ford, J. M. and Stewart, J. H., 1988, Risk factors for cancer of the renal parenchyma, *International Journal of Cancer*, **42**, 13–16.

McCredie, M., Pommer, W., McLaughlin, J. K., Stewart, J. H., Lindblad, P., Mandel, J. S., Mellemgaard, A., Schlehofer, B. and Niwa, S., 1995, International renal-cell cancer study. II. Analgesics, *International Journal of Cancer*, **60**, 345–349.

McCredie, M. and Stewart, J. H., 1988, Does paracetamol cause urothelial cancer or renal papillary necrosis? *Nephron*, **49**, 296–300.

McCredie, M., Stewart, J. H., Carter, J. C., Turner, J. and Mahoney, J. F., 1986, Phenacetin and papillary necrosis: independent risk factors for renal pelvic cancer, *Kidney International*, **30**, 81–84.

McCredie, M., Stewart, J. H. and Day, N. E., 1993, Different roles for phenacetin and paracetamol in cancer of the kidney and renal pelvis, *International Journal of Cancer*, **53**, 245–249.

McCredie, M., Stewart, J. H. and Ford, J. M., 1983a, Analgesics and tobacco as risk factors for cancer of the ureter and renal pelvis, *Journal of Urology*, **130**, 28–30.

McCredie, M., Stewart, J. H., Ford, J. M. and MacLennan, R. A., 1983b, Phenacetin-containing analgesics and cancer of the bladder or renal pelvis in women, *British Journal of Urology*, **55**, 220–224.

McCredie, M., Stewart, J. H. and Mahoney, J. F., 1982, Is phenacetin responsible for analgesic nephropathy in New South Wales? *Clinical Nephrology*, **17**, 134–140.

McCredie, M., Stewart, J. H., Mathew, T. H., Disney, A. P. S. and Ford, J. M., 1989, The effect of withdrawal of phenacetin-containing analgesics on the incidence of kidney and urothelial cancer and renal failure, *Clinical Nephrology*, **31**, 35–39.

McDanell, R. E., Beales, D., Henderson, L. and Sethi, J.K., 1992, Effect of dietary fat on the *in vitro* hepatotoxicity of paracetamol, *Biochemical Pharmacology*, **44**, 1303–1306.

McDonald-Gibson, W. J. and Collier, H. O. J., 1979, Paracetamol potentiates acetylsalicylate in inhibiting prostaglandin synthesis, *European Journal of Pharmacology*, **58**, 497–500.

McElhatton, P. R., Sullivan, F. M., Volans, G. N. and Fitzpatrick, R., 1990, Paracetamol poisoning in pregnancy: an analysis of the outcomes of cases referred to the Teratology Information Service of the National Poisons Information Service, *Human and Experimental Toxicology*, **9**, 147–153.

McGaw, T., Raborn, W. and Grace, M., 1987, Analgesics in pediatric dental surgery: relative efficacy of aluminium ibuprofen suspension and acetaminophen elixir, *Journal of Dentistry for Children*, **54**, 106–109.

McGilveray, I. J. and Mattock, G. L., 1972, Some factors affecting the absorption of paracetamol, *Journal of Pharmacy and Pharmacology*, **24**, 615–619.

McGilveray, I. J., Mattock, G. L., Fooks, J. R., Jordan, N. and Cook, D., 1971, Acetaminophen II. A comparison of the physiological availabilities of different commercial dosage forms, *Canadian Journal of Pharmaceutical Sciences*, **6**, 38–42.

McGoldrick, M. D., Urizar, R. and Cerda, J., 1992, Drug poisoning patterns: the Albany experience, 1978 and 1988, *New York State Journal of Medicine*, **92**, 134–136.

McGrath, J., 1989, A survey of deliberate self-poisoning, *Medical Journal of Australia*, **150**, 317–324.

McGuinness, B.W., 1983, A double-blind comparison in general practice of a combination tablet containing orphenadrine citrate and paracetamol ('Norgesic') with paracetamol alone, *Journal of International Medical Research*, **11**, 42–45.

McGuinness, B. W., Lloyd-Jones, M. and Fowler, P. D., 1969, A double-blind comparative trial of 'parazolidin' and paracetamol, *British Journal of Clinical Practice*, **23**, 452–455.

McIntire, S. C., Rubenstein, R. C., Gartner, J. C., Gilboa, N. and Ellis, D., 1993, Acute flank pain and reversible renal dysfunction associated with non-steroidal anti-inflammatory drug use, *Pediatrics*, **92**, 459–460.

McIntosh, J. H., Byth, K., Nasiry, R. W. and Piper, D. W., 1991, Patterns of dyspepsia during the course of duodenal ulcer, *Journal of Clinical Gastroenterology*, **13**, 506–513.

McIntosh, J. H., Byth, K. and Piper, D. W., 1985, Environmental factors in aetiology of chronic gastric ulcer: a case control study of exposure variables before the first symptoms, *Gut*, **26**, 789–798.

McIntosh, J. H., Fung, C. S., Berry, G. and Piper, D. W., 1988, Smoking, nonsteroidal anti-inflammatory drugs, and acetaminophen in gastric ulcer: a study of associations and of the effects of previous diagnosis on exposure patterns, *American Journal of Epidemiology*, **128**, 761–770.

McIntyre, R. L. E., Irani, M. S. and Piris, J., 1981, Histological study of the effects of three anti-inflammatory preparations on the gastric mucosa, *Journal of Clinical Pathology*, **34**, 836–842.

McJunkin, B., Barwick, K. W., Little, W. C. and Winfield, J. B., 1976, Fatal massive hepatic necrosis following acetaminophen overdose, *Journal of the American Medical Association*, **236**, 1874–1875.

McLaughlin, J. K., Blot, W. J., Mandel, J. S., Schuman, L. M., Mehl, E. S. and Fraumeni, J. F., 1983, Etiology of cancer of the renal pelvis, *Journal of the National Cancer Institute*, **71**, 287–291.

McLaughlin, J. K., Blot, W. J., Mehl, E. S. and Fraumeni, J. F., 1985, Relation of analgesic use to renal cancer: population-based findings, *National Cancer Institute Monographs*, **69**, 217–222.

McLaughlin, J. K., Mandel, J. S., Blot, W. J., Schuman, L. M., Mehl, E. S. and Fraumeni, J. F., 1984, A population-based case-control study of renal cell carcinoma, *Journal of the National Cancer Institute*, **72**, 275–284.

McLaughlin, W. J. and Boroujerdi, M., 1987, BHA (2(3)-tert-butyl-4-hydroxyanisole)-mediated modulation of acetaminophen phase II metabolism *in vivo* in Fisher 344 rats, *Research Communications in Chemical Pathology and Pharmacology*, **56**, 321–333.

McLean, A. E. M., 1974, Prevention of paracetamol poisoning, *Lancet*, **i**, 729.

McLean, A. E. M., 1976, Treatment of paracetamol overdose, *Lancet*, **ii**, 362.

McLean, A. E. M., Armstrong, G. R. and Beales, D., 1989, Effect of d- or l-methionine and cysteine on the growth inhibitory effects of feeding 1% paracetamol to rats, *Biochemical Pharmacology*, **38**, 347–352.

McLean, A. E. M., Chenery, R., Fisher, C. and Nuttall, L., 1976, Dietary factors in renal and hepatic toxicity of paracetamol, *Journal of International Medical Research*, **4 (Suppl. 4)**, 79–82.

McLean, A. E. M. and Day, P., 1974, Increased hepatotoxicity of paracetamol in rats fed on low-protein diets or phenobarbital, and protection by selenate, *Biochemical Society Transactions*, **2**, 317.

McLean, A. E. M. and Day, P. A., 1975, The effect of diet on the toxicity of paracetamol and the safety of paracetamol-methionine mixtures, *Biochemical Pharmacology*, **24**, 37–42.

McLean, A. E. M. and Nuttall, L., 1976, Paracetamol injury to rat liver slices, and its subsequent prevention by some anti-oxidants, *Biochemical Society Transactions*, **4**, 655–656.

McLean, A. E. M. and Nuttall, L., 1978, An *in vitro* model of liver injury using paracetamol treatment of liver slices and prevention of injury by some antioxidants, *Biochemical Pharmacology*, **27**, 425–430.

McLean, A. E. M., Witts, D. J. and Tame, D., 1980, The influence of nutrition and inducers on mechanisms of toxicity in humans and animals. In: *Environmental Chemicals, Enzyme Function and Human Disease*, Ciba Foundation Symposium 76. Excerpta Medica,

Amsterdam, pp. 275–288.

McMurray, J. J., Northridge, D. B., Abernethy, V. A. and Lawson, A. A. H., 1987, Trends in analgesic self-poisoning in West-Fife, 1971–1985, *Quarterly Journal of Medicine*, **65**, 835–843.

McMurtry, R. J., Snodgrass, W. R. and Mitchell, J. R., 1978, Renal necrosis, glutathione depletion, and covalent binding after acetaminophen, *Toxicology and Applied Pharmacology*, **46**, 87–100.

McNamara, P. J., Burgio, D. and Yoo, S. D., 1991, Pharmacokinetics of acetaminophen, antipyrine, and salicylic acid in the lactating and nursing rabbit, with model predictions of milk to serum concentration ratios and neonatal dose, *Toxicology and Applied Pharmacology*, **109**, 149–160.

McNamara, R. M., Aaron, C. K. and Gemborys, M., 1988, Sorbitol catharsis does not enhance efficacy of charcoal in a simulated acetaminophen overdose, *Annals of Emergency Medicine*, **17**, 243–246.

McNamara, R. M., Aaron, C. K., Gemborys, M. and Davidheiser, S., 1989, Efficacy of charcoal cathartic vs. ipecac in reducing serum acetaminophen in a simulated overdose, *Annals of Emergency Medicine*, **18**, 934–938.

McNeill, M. J., Ho, E. T. and Kenny, G. N. C., 1990, Effect of i.v. metoclopramide on gastric emptying after opioid premedication, *British Journal of Anaesthesia*, **64**, 450–452.

McNicholl, B. P., 1992, Toxicity awareness and unintended suicide in drug overdoses, *Archives of Emergency Medicine*, **9**, 214–219.

McPhail, M. E., Dawson, J., Pogson, C. I. and Burchell, B., 1990, A comparison of N-acetyl-p-aminophenol metabolism in liver snips and isolated liver cells from male Wistar rats, *Biochemical Society Transactions*, **18**, 1216.

McPhail, M. E., Knowles, R. G., Salter, M., Dawson, J., Burchell, B. and Pogson, C. I., 1993, Uptake of acetaminophen (paracetamol) by isolated rat liver cells, *Biochemical Pharmacology*, **45**, 1599–1604.

McQuay, H. J., Carroll, D., Frankland, T., Harvey, M. and Moore, A., 1990, Bromfenac, acetaminophen, and placebo in orthopedic postoperative pain, *Clinical Pharmacology and Therapeutics*, **47**, 760–766.

McQuay, H. J., Carroll, D., Guest, P., Juniper, R. P. and Moore, R. A., 1992, A multiple dose comparison of combinations of ibuprofen and codeine and paracetamol, codeine and caffeine after third molar surgery, *Anaesthesia*, **47**, 672–677.

McQuay, H. J., Poppleton, P., Carroll, D., Summerfield, R. J., Bullingham, R. E. S. and Moore, R. A., 1986, Ketorolac and acetaminophen for orthopedic postoperative pain, *Clinical Pharmacology and Therapeutics*, **39**, 89–93.

McQueen, D. S., Iggo, A., Birrell, G. J. and Grubb, B. D., 1990, Effects of aspirin and paracetamol on high-threshold tarsal joint mechanoreceptors in anaesthetized rats with adjuvant-induced arthritis, *Journal of Physiology*, **425**, 35P.

McQueen, D. S., Iggo, A., Birrell, G. J. and Grubb, B. D., 1991, Effects of paracetamol and aspirin on neural activity of joint mechanonociceptors in adjuvant arthritis, *British Journal of Pharmacology*, **104**, 178–182.

McRae, T. A., Furuhama, K., Roberts, D. W., Getek, T. A. and Hinson, J. A., 1990, Evaluation of 3-(cystein-S-yl)-acetaminophen in the nephrotoxicity of acetaminophen in rats, *Toxicologist*, **9**, 47.

Meatherall, R. and Ford, D., 1988, Isocratic liquid chromatographic determination of theophylline, acetaminophen, chloramphenicol, caffeine, anticonvulsants, and barbiturates in serum, *Therapeutic Drug Monitoring*, **10**, 101–115.

Mehlisch, D. R. and Frakes, L. A., 1984, A controlled comparative evaluation of acetaminophen and aspirin in the treatment of postoperative pain, *Clinical Therapeutics*, **7**, 89–97.

Mehlisch, D. R., Sollecito, W. A., Helfrick, J. F., Leibold, D. G., Markowitz, R., Schow, C. E., Shultz, R. and Waite, D. E., 1990, Multicenter clinical trial of ibuprofen and acetaminophen in the treatment of postoperative dental pain, *Journal of the American Dental*

Association, **121**, 257–263.

Mehrotra, R., Nath, P., Chaturvedi, R. and Pandey, R. K., 1982, Experimental study on paracetamol induced hepatotoxicity, *Indian Journal of Medical Research Section A – Infectious Diseases*, **76**, 479–487.

Mehrotra, R., Nath, P., Pandey, R. and Chaturvedi, R., 1983, Histological & ultrastructural alterations in the livers of albino rats after prolonged administration of paracetamol, *Indian Journal of Medical Research*, **77**, 873–878.

Mehrotra, T. N. and Gupta, S. K., 1973, Paracetamol-induced haemolytic anaemia: report of a case, *Indian Journal of Medical Sciences*, **27**, 548–549.

Mehta, S., Nain, C. K., Sharma, B. and Mathur, V. S., 1982, Disposition of four drugs in malnourished children, *Drug-Nutrient Interactions*, **1**, 205–211.

Mehta, S., Nain, C. K., Yadav, D., Sharma, B. and Mathur, V. S., 1985, Disposition of acetaminophen in children with protein calorie malnutrition, *International Journal of Clinical Pharmacology, Therapy and Toxicology*, **23**, 311–315.

Meléndez, E., Reyes, J. L., Escalante, B. A. and Meléndez, M. A., 1990, Development of the receptors to prostaglandin E_2 in the rat kidney and neonatal renal functions, *Developmental Pharmacology and Therapeutics*, **14**, 125–134.

Melethil, S., Poklis, A. and Schwartz, H. S., 1981, Estimation of the amount of drug absorbed in acetaminophen poisoning: a case report, *Veterinary and Human Toxicology*, **23**, 421–423.

Melis, K. and Bochner, A., 1990, Acute poisoning in a children's hospital: an 8-year experience, *Acta Clinica Belgica*, **45 (Suppl. 13)**, 98–100.

Mellemgaard, A., Møller, H., Jensen, O. M., Halberg, P. and Olsen, J. H., 1992, Risk of kidney cancer in analgesics users, *Journal of Clinical Epidemiology*, **45**, 1021–1024.

Mellemgaard, A., Niwa, S., Mehl, E. S., Engholm, G., McLaughlin, J. K. and Olsen, J. H., 1994, Risk factors for renal cell carcinoma in Denmark: role of medication and medical history, *International Journal of Epidemiology*, **23**, 923–930.

Mellergård, P., 1992, Changes in human intracerebral temperature in response to different methods of brain cooling, *Neurosurgery*, **31**, 671–677.

Melzack, R., Bentley, K. C. and Jeans, M. E., 1985, Piroxicam vs. acetaminophen and placebo for the relief of postoperative dental pain, *Current Therapeutic Research*, **37**, 1134–1140.

Melzack, R., Jeans, M. E., Kinch, R. A. and Katz, J., 1983, Diflunisal (1000 mg single dose) vs. acetaminophen (650 mg) and placebo for the relief of post-episiotomy pain, *Current Therapeutic Research*, **34**, 929–939.

Menard, G., Allain, H., Le Roho, S., Morel, G. and Beneton, C., 1993, Enquête d'un jour en officine sur la consommation d'antalgiques et d'antipyrétiques, *Thérapie*, **48**, 263–267.

Mensing, H., 1993, Akute generalisierte exanthematische Pustulose (AGEP), *Zeitschrift für Hautkrankheiten*, **68**, 234–237.

Meola, J. M., 1978, Emergency determination of acetaminophen, *Clinical Chemistry*, **24**, 1642–1643.

Meredith, T. J., Crome, P., Volans, G. and Goulding, R., 1978a, Treatment of paracetamol poisoning, *British Medical Journal*, **1**, 1215–1216.

Meredith, T. J. and Goulding, R., 1980, Paracetamol, *Postgraduate Medical Journal*, **56**, 459–473.

Meredith, T. J., Newman, B. and Goulding, R., 1978b, Paracetamol poisoning in children, *British Medical Journal*, **2**, 478–479.

Meredith, T. J., Newman, B. and Goulding, R., 1979, Paracetamol (acetaminophen) poisoning in children, *Veterinary and Human Toxicology*, **21 (Suppl.)**, 101–102.

Meredith, T. J., Prescott, L. F. and Vale, J. A., 1986, Why do patients still die from paracetamol poisoning? *British Medical Journal*, **293**, 345–346.

Meredith, T. J. and Vale, J. A., 1984, Epidemiology of analgesic overdose in England and Wales, *Human Toxicology*, **3 (Suppl.)**, 61S–74S.

Meredith, T. J., Vale, J. A. and Goulding, R., 1981, The epidemiology of acute acetaminophen poisoning in England and Wales, *Archives of Internal Medicine*, **141**, 397–400.

Mereu, T., Appollonio, T., Sereni-Piceni, L. and Careddu, P., 1962, Excretion of N-acetil-p-aminophenol in the newborn, *Lancet*, **i**, 1300.

Mering, von J., 1893, Beiträge zur Kenntniss der Antipyretica, *Therapeutische Monatshefte*, **7**, 577–578.

Merritt, G. J. and Joyner, P. U., 1977, Acetaminophen toxicity: report of a case and review of the literature, *Drug Intelligence and Clinical Pharmacy*, **11**, 458–461.

Messick, R. T., 1979, Evaluation of acetaminophen, propoxyphene, and their combination in office practice, *Journal of Clinical Pharmacology*, **19**, 227–230.

Metz, U., Graben, N., Maruhn, D. and Bock, K. D., 1986, Urinary enzyme excretion after a single dose of phenacetin and paracetamol (acetaminophen) during antidiuresis and during water diuresis, *Clinica Chimica Acta*, **160**, 151–155.

Meyers, L. L., Beierschmitt, W. P., Khairallah, E. A. and Cohen, S. D., 1988, Acetaminophen-induced inhibition of hepatic mitochondrial respiration in mice, *Toxicology and Applied Pharmacology*, **93**, 378–387.

Meyrick Thomas, R. H. and Munro, D. D., 1986, Fixed drug eruption due to paracetamol, *British Journal of Dermatology*, **115**, 357–359.

Mezei, L. M., Berry, S. C. and Robb, W. P., 1983, Salicylate interference with measurement of acetaminophen – a reply, *Clinical Chemistry*, **29**, 987–988.

Miceli, J. N. and Aravind, M. K., 1980, A rapid, simple acetaminophen determination is available, *Clinical Chemistry*, **26**, 1627–1628.

Miceli, J. N., Aravind, M. K., Cohen, S. N. and Done, A. K., 1979a, Simultaneous measurement of acetaminophen and salicylate in plasma by liquid chromatography, *Clinical Chemistry*, **25**, 1002–1004.

Miceli, J. N., Aravind, M. K. and Done, A. K., 1979b, A rapid, simple acetaminophen spectrophotometric determination, *Pediatrics*, **63**, 609–611.

Michaelis, H. C., Sharifi, S. and Schoel, G., 1991, Rhabdomyolysis after suicidal ingestion of an overdose of caffeine, acetaminophen and phenazone as a fixed-dose combination (Spalt N), *Journal of Toxicology. Clinical Toxicology*, **29**, 521–526.

Micheli, L., Cerretani, D., Fiaschi, A. I., Giorgi, G., Romeo, M. R. and Runci, F. M., 1994, Effect of acetaminophen on glutathione levels in rat testis and lung, *Environmental Health Perspectives*, **102 (Suppl. 9)**, 63–64.

Micheli, L., Fiaschi, A. I., Cerretani, D. and Giorgi, G., 1993, Effect of acetaminophen on glutathione levels in several regions of the rat brain, *Current Therapeutic Research*, **53**, 730–736.

Micheli, L. and Giorgi, G., 1988, Variation of glutathione levels in liver of rats induced by acetaminophen, *Pharmacological Research Communications*, **20**, 427–428.

Michelson, P. A., 1975, Rash, weakness, and acetaminophen, *Annals of Internal Medicine*, **83**, 374.

Middleton, R. S. W., 1981, Double blind trial in general practice comparing the efficacy of 'Benylin Day and Night' and paracetamol in the treatment of the common cold, *British Journal of Clinical Practice*, **35**, 297–300.

Mielke, C. H., 1981, Comparative effects of aspirin and acetaminophen on hemostasis, *Archives of Internal Medicine*, **141**, 305–310.

Mielke, C. H. and Britten, A. F. H., 1970, Use of aspirin or acetaminophen in hemophilia, *New England Journal of Medicine*, **282**, 1270.

Mielke, C. H., Heiden, D., Britten, A. F., Hamos, J. and Flavell, P., 1976, Hemostasis, antipyretics, and mild analgesics: acetaminophen vs. aspirin, *Journal of the American Medical Association*, **235**, 613–616.

Miescher, P. and Studer, A., 1961, Weitere tierexperimentelle Untersuchungen zur Frage der Pathogenese der interstitiellen Nephritis, *Schweizerische Medizinische Wochenschrift*, **91**, 939–943.

Migliardi, J. R., Armellino, J. J., Friedman, M., Gillings, D. B. and Beaver, W. T., 1994,

Caffeine as an analgesic adjuvant in tension headache, *Clinical Pharmacology and Therapeutics*, **56**, 576–586.

Migliore-Samour, D., Delaforge, M., Jaouen, M., Mansuy, D. and Jollès, P., 1989, *In vivo* effects of immunostimulating lipopeptides on mouse liver microsomal cytochromes P-450 and on paracetamol-induced toxicity, *Experientia*, **45**, 882–886.

Mihatsch, M. J., Hofer, H. O., Gudat, F., Knüsli, C., Torhorst, J. and Zollinger, H. U., 1983, Capillary sclerosis of the urinary tract and analgesic nephropathy, *Clinical Nephrology*, **20**, 285–301.

Mihatsch, M. J., Hofer, H. O., Korteweg, E. and Zollinger, H. U., 1982, Phenacetinabusus V: Häufigkeit der Phenacetinabuser im Basler Autopsiegut 1978–1980. Ergebnisse einer prospektiven Studie, *Schweizerische Medizinische Wochenschrift*, **112**, 1245–1248.

Mihatsch, M. J. and Knüsli, C., 1982, Phenacetin abuse and malignant tumors: an autopsy study covering 25 years (1953–1977), *Klinische Wochenschrift*, **60**, 1339–1349.

Mihatsch, M. J., Manz, T., Knüsli, C., Hofer, H. O., Rist, M., Guetg, R., Rutishauser, G. and Zollinger, H. U., 1980a, Phenacetinabusus III. Maligne Harnwegtumoren bei phenacetinabusus in Basel 1963–1977, *Schweizerische Medizinische Wochenschrift*, **110**, 255–264.

Mihatsch, M. J., Schmidlin, P., Brunner, F. P., Hofer, H. O., Six, P. and Zollinger, H. U., 1980b, Phenacetinabusus II. Die chronische renale Niereinsuffizienz im Basler Autopsiegut, *Schweizerische Medizinische Wochenschrift*, **110**, 116–124.

Mikov, M., 1994, The metabolism of drugs by the gut flora, *European Journal of Drug Metabolism and Pharmacokinetics*, **19**, 201–207.

Mikov, M. and Caldwell, J., 1990, Metabolism of paracetamol 3-cysteine in conventional and germ-free mice: the crucial role of intestinal microflora, *European Journal of Pharmacology*, **183**, 1206–1207.

Mikov, M., Caldwell, J., Dolphin, C. T. and Smith, R. L., 1988, The role of intestinal microflora in the formation of the methylthio adduct metabolites of paracetamol: studies in neomycin-pretreated and germ-free mice, *Biochemical Pharmacology*, **37**, 1445–1449.

Milam, K. M. and Byard, J. L., 1985, Acetaminophen metabolism, cytotoxicity, and genotoxicity in rat primary hepatocyte cultures, *Toxicology and Applied Pharmacology*, **79**, 342–347.

Milch, G. and Szabó, E., 1991, Derivative spectrophotometric assay of acetaminophen and spectrofluorimetric determination of its main impurity, *Journal of Pharmaceutical and Biomedical Analysis*, **9**, 1107–1113.

Miller, D. J., Hickman, R., Fratter, R., Terblanche, J. and Saunders, S. J., 1976a, An animal model of fulminant hepatic failure: a feasibility study, *Gastroenterology*, **71**, 109–113.

Miller, D. J., Pichanick, G. G., Fiskerstrand, C. and Saunders, S. J., 1977, Experimental liver necrosis: hepatic erythrocyte sequestration as a cause of acute anemia, *American Journal of Digestive Diseases*, **22**, 1055–1059.

Miller, D. S., Talbot, C. A., Simpson, W. and Korey, A., 1987, A comparison of naproxen sodium, acetaminophen and placebo in the treatment of muscle contraction headache, *Headache*, **27**, 392–396.

Miller, L. and Shaw, J. S., 1981, The inhibitory effect of paracetamol on the electrically stimulated ileum of the guinea-pig, *Journal of Pharmacy and Pharmacology*, **33**, 188–189.

Miller, M. G., Beyer, J., Hall, G. L., DeGraffenried, L. A. and Adams, P. E., 1993a, Predictive value of liver slices for metabolism and toxicity *in vivo*: use of acetaminophen as a model hepatotoxicant, *Toxicology and Applied Pharmacology*, **122**, 108–116.

Miller, M. G. and Jollow, D. J., 1984, Effect of l-ascorbic acid on acetaminophen-induced hepatotoxicity and covalent binding in hamsters: evidence that *in vitro* covalent binding differs from that *in vivo*, *Drug Metabolism and Disposition: The Biological Fate of Chemicals*, **12**, 271–279.

Miller, M. G. and Jollow, D. J., 1986a, Acetaminophen hepatotoxicity: studies on the mechanism of cysteamine protection, *Toxicology and Applied Pharmacology*, **83**, 115–125.

Miller, M. G. and Jollow, D. J., 1986b, Relationship between sulfotransferase activity and susceptibility to acetaminophen-induced liver necrosis in the hamster, *Drug Metabolism and Disposition: The Biological Fate of Chemicals*, **15**, 143–150.

Miller, M. G., Price, V. F. and Jollow, D. J., 1986, Anomolous susceptibility of the fasted hamster to acetaminophen hepatotoxicity, *Biochemical Pharmacology*, **35**, 817–825.

Miller, M. R., Saito, N., Blair, J. B. and Hinton, D. E., 1993b, Acetaminophen toxicity in cultured trout liver cells. II. Maintenance of cytochrome P-450 1A1, *Experimental and Molecular Pathology*, **58**, 127–138.

Miller, M. R., Wentz, E., Blair, J. B., Pack, D. and Hinton, D. E., 1993c, Acetaminophen toxicity in cultured trout liver cells. I. Morphological alterations and effects on cytochrome P-450 1A1, *Experimental and Molecular Pathology*, **58**, 114–126.

Miller, R. P. and Fischer, L. J., 1974, Urinary excretion of acetaminophen by the rat, *Journal of Pharmaceutical Sciences*, **63**, 969–970.

Miller, R. P., Roberts, R. J. and Fischer, L. J., 1976b, Acetaminophen elimination kinetics in neonates, children, and adults, *Clinical Pharmacology and Therapeutics*, **19**, 284–294.

Milligan, K. R., Howe, J. P., McClean, E. and Dundee, J. W., 1988, Postoperative gastric emptying in outpatient anesthesia: the effect of opioid supplementation, *Journal of Clinical Anesthesia*, **1**, 9–11.

Milligan, T. P., Morris, H. C., Hammond, P. M. and Price, C. P., 1994, Studies on paracetamol binding to serum proteins, *Annals of Clinical Biochemistry*, **31**, 492–496.

Mills, D. C., 1989, The *in vitro* buffering capacity of soluble paracetamol, *Anaesthesia*, **44**, 967–969.

Milsom, I. and Andersch, B., 1984, Effects of ibuprofen, naproxen sodium and paracetamol on intrauterine pressure and menstrual pain in dysmenorrhoea, *British Journal of Obstetrics and Gynaecology*, **91**, 1129–1135.

Milton, A. S. and Wendlandt, S., 1968, The effect of 4-acetamidophenol in reducing fever produced by the intracerebral injection of 5-hydroxytryptamine and pyrogen in the conscious cat, *British Journal of Pharmacology*, **34**, 215P–216P.

Milton, A. S. and Wendlandt, S., 1971, The effects of 4-acetamidophenol (paracetamol) on the temperature response of the conscious rat to the intracerebral injection of prostaglandin E_1, adrenaline and pyrogen, *Journal of Physiology*, **217**, 33P–34P.

Minamide, Y., Hori, T. and Awazu, S., 1992, High molecular weight protein aggregates formed in the liver of the rat following large doses of paracetamol, *Journal of Pharmacy and Pharmacology*, **44**, 932–934.

Miner, D. J. and Kissinger, P. T., 1979a, Trace determination of acetaminophen in serum, *Journal of Pharmaceutical Sciences*, **68**, 96–97.

Miner, D. J. and Kissinger, P. T., 1979b, Evidence for the involvement of N-acetyl-p-quinoneimine in acetaminophen metabolism, *Biochemical Pharmacology*, **28**, 3285–3290.

Miner, D. J., Rice, J. R., Riggin, R. M. and Kissinger, P. T., 1981, Voltammetry of acetaminophen and its metabolites, *Analytical Chemistry*, **53**, 2258–2263.

Miners, J., Adams, J. F. and Birkett, D. J., 1984a, A simple HPLC assay for urinary paracetamol metabolites and its use to characterize the C3H mouse as a model for paracetamol metabolism studies, *Clinical and Experimental Pharmacology and Physiology*, **11**, 209–217.

Miners, J., Drew, R. and Birkett, D. J., 1984b, Effect of cimetidine on paracetamol activation in mice, *Biochemical Pharmacology*, **33**, 1996–1998.

Miners, J. O., Attwood, J. and Birkett, D. J., 1983, Influence of sex and oral contraceptive steroids on paracetamol metabolism, *British Journal of Clinical Pharmacology*, **16**, 503–509.

Miners, J. O., Attwood, J. and Birkett, D. J., 1984c, Determinants of acetaminophen metabolism: effects of inducers and inhibitors of drug metabolism on acetaminophen's metabolic pathways, *Clinical Pharmacology and Therapeutics*, **35**, 480–486.

Miners, J. O. and Birkett, D. J., 1993, The misuse of urinary metabolite excretion data in drug metabolism studies, *Pharmacogenetics*, **3**, 58–59.

Miners, J. O., Drew, R. and Birkett, D. J., 1984d, Mechanism of action of paracetamol protective agents in mice *in vivo*, *Biochemical Pharmacology*, **33**, 2995–3000.

Miners, J. O. and Lillywhite, K. J., 1991, Assessment of the drug inhibitor specificity of the human liver 4-methylumbelliferone UDP-glucuronosyltransferase activity, *Biochemical Pharmacology*, **41**, 838–841.

Miners, J. O., Lillywhite, K. J., Yoovathaworn, K., Pongmarutai, M. and Birkett, D. J., 1990, Characterization of paracetamol UDP-glucuronosyltransferase activity in human liver microsomes, *Biochemical Pharmacology*, **40**, 595–600.

Miners, J. O. and Mackenzie, P. I., 1991, Drug glucuronidation in humans, *Pharmacology and Therapeutics*, **51**, 347–369.

Miners, J. O., Osborne, N. J., Tonkin, A. L. and Birkett, D. J., 1992, Perturbation of paracetamol urinary metabolic ratios by urine flow rate, *British Journal of Clinical Pharmacology*, **34**, 359–362.

Miners, J. O., Penhall, R., Robson, R. A. and Birkett, D. J., 1988, Comparison of paracetamol metabolism in young adult and elderly males, *European Journal of Clinical Pharmacology*, **35**, 157–160.

Miners, J. O., Robson, R. A. and Birkett, D. J., 1986, Paracetamol metabolism in pregnancy, *British Journal of Clinical Pharmacology*, **22**, 359–362.

Mineshita, S., Eggers, R., Kitteringham, N. R. and Ohnhaus, E. E., 1986, Determination of phenacetin and its major metabolites in human plasma and urine by high-performance liquid chromatography, *Journal of Chromatography: Biomedical Applications*, **380**, 407–413.

Mineshita, S., Toyoshima, A. and Yazaki, T., 1989, Influence of phenacetin and its metabolites on renal function, *Japanese Journal of Nephrology*, **31**, 629–633.

Minnigh, M. B. and Zemaitis, M. A., 1980, The effect of acute ethanol administration and food deprivation on the glucuronide conjugation of acetaminophen, *Pharmacologist*, **22**, 279.

Minnigh, M. B. and Zemaitis, M. A., 1982, Altered acetaminophen disposition in fed and food-deprived rats after acute alcohol administration, *Drug Metabolism and Disposition: The Biological Fate of Chemicals*, **10**, 183–188.

Minton, N. A., Henry, J. A. and Frankel, R. J., 1988, Fatal paracetamol poisoning in an epileptic, *Human Toxicology*, **7**, 33–34.

Miranda, C. L., Henderson, M. C. and Buhler, D. R., 1985, Dietary butylated hydroxyanisole reduces covalent binding of acetaminophen to mouse tissue proteins *in vivo*, *Toxicology Letters*, **25**, 89–93.

Miranda, C. L., Henderson, M. C., Schmitz, J. A. and Buhler, D. R., 1983, Protective role of dietary butylated hydroxyanisole against chemical-induced acute liver damage in mice, *Toxicology and Applied Pharmacology*, **69**, 73–80.

Misra, R., Pandey, H., Chandra, M., Chandra, M., Agarwal, P. K. and Pandeya, S. N., 1990, Effect of commonly used non steroidal anti-inflammatory drugs on gastric mucosa: a clinical, endoscopic and histopathological study, *Journal of the Association of Physicians of India*, **38**, 636–638.

Mitchell, A. A., Lovejoy, F. H., Slone, D. and Shapiro, S., 1982, Acetaminophen and aspirin: prescription, use, and accidental ingestion among children, *American Journal of Diseases of Children*, **136**, 976–979.

Mitchell, D. B., Acosta, D. and Bruckner, J.V., 1985, Role of glutathione depletion in the cytotoxicity of acetaminophen in a primary culture system of rat hepatocytes, *Toxicology*, **37**, 127–146.

Mitchell, H., Cunningham, T. J., Mathews, J. D. and Muirden, K. D., 1984a, Further look at dextropropoxyphene with or without paracetamol in the treatment of arthritis, *Medical Journal of Australia*, **140**, 224–225.

Mitchell, I. M., Jamieson, M. P. G., Pollock, J. C. S. and Logan, R. W., 1991, Paracetamol suppositories after cardiac surgery, *Archives of Disease in Childhood*, **66**, 1004.

Mitchell, J. A., Akarasereenont, P., Thiemermann, C. and Flower, R. J., 1993, Selectivity of nonsteroidal antiinflammatory drugs as inhibitors of constitutive and inducible cyclo-oxygenase, *Proceedings of the National Academy of Sciences of the United States of America*, **90**, 11693–11697.

Mitchell, J. R., 1975a, Drug metabolism in the production of liver injury, *Medical Clinics of North America*, **59**, 877–885.

Mitchell, J. R., 1975b, Metabolic activation of drugs to toxic substances, *Gastroenterology*, **68**, 392–410.

Mitchell, J. R., 1988, Acetaminophen toxicity, *New England Journal of Medicine*, **319**, 1601–1602.

Mitchell, J. R., Corcoran, G. B., Smith, C. V., Hughes, H. and Lauterburg, B. H., 1981a, Alkylation and peroxidation injury from chemically reactive metabolites, *Advances in Experimental Medicine and Biology*, **136**, 199–223.

Mitchell, J. R., Jollow, D. J., Gillette, J. R. and Brodie, B. B., 1973a, Drug metabolism as a cause of drug toxicity, *Drug Metabolism and Disposition: The Biological Fate of Chemicals*, **1**, 418–423.

Mitchell, J. R., Jollow, D. J., Potter, W. Z., Davis, D. C., Gillette, J. R. and Brodie, B. B., 1973b, Acetaminophen-induced hepatic necrosis. I. Role of drug metabolism, *Journal of Pharmacology and Experimental Therapeutics*, **187**, 185–194.

Mitchell, J. R., Jollow, D. J., Potter, W. Z., Gillette, J. R. and Brodie, B. B., 1973c, Acetaminophen-induced hepatic necrosis. IV. Protective role of glutathione, *Journal of Pharmacology and Experimental Therapeutics*, **187**, 211–217.

Mitchell, J. R., McMurtry, R. J., Statham, C. N. and Nelson, S. D., 1977, Molecular basis for several drug-induced nephropathies, *American Journal of Medicine*, **62**, 518–526.

Mitchell, J. R., Thorgeirsson, S. S., Potter, W. Z., Jollow, D. J. and Keiser, H., 1974, Acetaminophen-induced hepatic injury: protective role of glutathione in man and rationale for therapy, *Clinical Pharmacology and Therapeutics*, **16**, 676–684.

Mitchell, M. C., Hamilton, R., Wacker, L. and Branch, R. A., 1989, Zonal distribution of paracetamol glucuronidation in the isolated perfused rat liver, *Xenobiotica*, **19**, 389–400.

Mitchell, M. C., Hanew, T., Meredith, C. G. and Schenker, S., 1983, Effects of oral contraceptive steroids on acetaminophen metabolism and elimination, *Clinical Pharmacology and Therapeutics*, **34**, 48–53.

Mitchell, M. C., Schenker, S., Avant, G. R. and Speeg, K. V., 1981b, Cimetidine protects against acetaminophen hepatotoxicity in rats, *Gastroenterology*, **81**, 1052–1060.

Mitchell, M. C., Schenker, S. and Speeg, K. V., 1984b, Selective inhibition of acetaminophen oxidation and toxicity by cimetidine and other histamine H_2-receptor antagonists *in vivo* and *in vitro* in the rat and in man, *Journal of Clinical Investigation*, **73**, 383–391.

Mitra, A., Kulkarni, A. P., Ravikumar, V. C. and Bourcier, D. R., 1991, Effect of ascorbic acid esters on hepatic glutathione levels in mice treated with a hepatotoxic dose of acetaminophen, *Journal of Biochemical Toxicology*, **6**, 93–100.

Mitra, A., Ravikumar, V. C., Bourn, W. and Bourcier, D. R., 1988, Influence of ascorbic acid esters on acetaminophen-induced hepatotoxicity in mice, *Toxicology Letters*, **44**, 39–46.

Miyazaki, K., Takemoto, C., Satoh, T., Ueno, K., Igarashi, T. and Kitagawa, H., 1983, Toxicity and biotransformation of acetaminophen in rat hepatocytes (I). Uptake and release, *Research Communications in Chemical Pathology and Pharmacology*, **39**, 77–86.

Mizuma, T., Araya, H., Hayashi, M. and Awazu, S., 1984, Multiple forms of aryl sulfotransferase for acetaminophen sulfate conjugation in rat liver cytosol, *Journal of Pharmacobiodynamics*, **7**, 784–789.

Mizuma, T., Hayashi, M. and Awazu, S., 1985, Factors influencing drug sulfate and glucuronic acid conjugation rates in isolated rat hepatocytes: significance of preincubation time, *Biochemical Pharmacology*, **34**, 2573–2575.

Mizuta, H., Kawazoe, Y., Haga, K. and Ogawa, K., 1990a, Effects of meals on gastric emptying and small intestinal transit times of a suspension in the beagle dog assessed using acetaminophen and salicylazosulfapyridine as markers, *Chemical and Pharmaceutical Bulletin*, **38**, 2224–2227.

Mizuta, H., Kawazoe, Y., Ikeda, Y. and Ogawa, K., 1991, Gastrointestinal absorption of nitrofurantoin: evaluation of a newly developed method for determination of the gastro-intestinal transit time in dogs, *Journal of the Pharmaceutical Society of Japan*, **111**, 794–799.

Mizuta, H., Kawazoe, Y. and Ogawa, K., 1990b, Gastrointestinal absorption of chlorothia-zide: evaluation of a method using salicylazosulfapyridine and acetaminophen as the marker compounds for determination of the gastrointestinal transit time in the dog, *Chemical and Pharmaceutical Bulletin*, **38**, 2810–2813.

Mizuta, H., Kawazoe, Y. and Ogawa, K., 1990c, Effect of small intestinal transit time on gastrointestinal absorption of 2-[3-(3,5-di-*tert*-butyl-4-hydroxyphenyl)-1*H*-pyrazolo[3,4-*b*]pyridin-1-yl]ethyl acetate, a new non-steroidal anti-inflammatory agent, *Chemical and Pharmaceutical Bulletin*, **38**, 2825–2828.

Moatti-Sirat, D., Poitout, V., Thomé, V., Gangnerau, M. N., Zhang, Y., Hu, Y., Wilson, G. S., Lemonnier, F., Klein, J. C. and Reach, G., 1994, Reduction of acetaminophen inter-ference in glucose sensors by a composite Nafion membrane: demonstration in rats and man, *Diabetologia*, **37**, 610–616.

Moatti-Sirat, D., Velho, G. and Reach, G., 1992, Evaluating *in vitro* and *in vivo* the inter-ference of ascorbate and acetaminophen on glucose detection by a needle-type glucose sensor, *Biosensors and Bioelectronics*, **7**, 345–352.

Mochizuki, H., Morikawa, A., Tokuyama, K., Kuroume, T. and Chao, A. C., 1994, The effect of non-steroidal anti-inflammatory drugs on the electrical properties of cultured dog tracheal epithelial cells, *European Journal of Pharmacology*, **252**, 183–188.

Moertel, C. G., Ahmann, D. L., Taylor, W. F. and Schwartau, N., 1972, A comparative evalu-ation of marketed analgesic drugs, *New England Journal of Medicine*, **286**, 813–815.

Moës, A., 1974a, Méthode d'évaluation de l'excrétion urinaire du N-acétyl-p-aminophénol total chez l'homme, *Journal de Pharmacie de Belgique*, **29**, 105–112.

Moës, A., 1974b, Étude de l'influence de l'excipient sur la 'biodisponibilité' du N-acétyl-p-aminophénol administré par voie rectale, *Journal de Pharmacie de Belgique*, **29**, 319–332.

Moës, A. and Jaminet, F., 1976, Influence of aging of suppositories on rectal absorption of paracetamol, *Pharmaceutica Acta Helvetiae*, **51**, 119–125.

Mofenson, H. C. and Caraccio, T. R., 1992, Is activated charcoal useful for acetaminophen overdose beyond two hours after ingestion? *Annals of Emergency Medicine*, **21**, 894.

Mofenson, H. C., Caraccio, T. R., Nawaz, H. and Steckler, G., 1991, Acetaminophen induced pancreatitis, *Journal of Toxicology. Clinical Toxicology*, **29**, 223–230.

Mohamed, A. E., Segal, I. and Riedel, L., 1990, Analgesics and gastric ulcers: a case-control study in an urbanized black population, *South African Medical Journal*, **77**, 135–137.

Mohammed, S., Jamal, A. Z. and Robison, L. R., 1994, Serum sickness-like illness associated with N-acetylcysteine therapy, *Annals of Pharmacotherapy*, **28**, 285.

Mohandas, J., Calder, I. C. and Duggin, G. G., 1977, Renal oxidative metabolism of drugs in C57BL6J mouse, *Proceedings of the Australian Society of Medical Research*, **10**, 49.

Mohandas, J., Chensee, Q. S., Mohamed, S. and Calder, I. C., 1979, NADPH independent metabolism of paracetamol and protein covalent binding in rabbit kidney, *Proceedings of the Australian Society of Medical Research*, **12**, 57.

Mohandas, J., Duggin, G. G., Horvath, J. S. and Tiller, D. J., 1981a, Metabolic oxidation of acetaminophen (paracetamol) mediated cytochrome P-450 mixed-function oxidase and prostaglandin endoperoxidase synthetase in rabbit kidney, *Toxicology and Applied Phar-macology*, **61**, 252–259.

Mohandas, J., Duggin, G. G., Horvath, J. S. and Tiller, D. J., 1981b, Regional differences in peroxidative activation of paracetamol (acetaminophen) mediated by cytochrome P-450 and prostaglandin endoperoxide synthetase in rabbit kidney, *Research Communications in Chemical Pathology and Pharmacology*, **34**, 69–80.

Mohandas, J., Marshall, J. J., Duggin, G. G., Horvath, J. S. and Tiller, D. J., 1984, Differential distribution of glutathione and glutathione-related enzymes in rabbit kidney, *Biochemical Pharmacology*, **33**, 1801–1807.

Mohapatra, D., Mishra, S. C., Parija, S. C. and Mishra, S. N., 1993, Paracetamol-induced hepatotoxicity in broiler birds, *Indian Veterinary Journal*, **70**, 914–916.

Mohr, T., Küster, G., de Vries, J. X., Waldherr, R., Walter-Sack, J., Rieser, P.-F. and Ritz, E., 1990, Epidemiologische Untersuchungen zur Häufigkeit des Analgetika-Abusus, *Deutsche Medizinische Wochenschrift*, **115**, 129–132.

Mohrland, J. S., Johnson, E. E. and VonVoigtlander, P. F., 1983, An ultrasound-induced tail-flick procedure: evaluation of nonsteroidal antiinflammatory analgesics, *Journal of Pharmacological Methods*, **9**, 279–282.

Moldéus, P., 1978, Paracetamol metabolism and toxicity in isolated hepatocytes from rat and mouse, *Biochemical Pharmacology*, **27**, 2859–2863.

Moldéus, P., Andersson, B. and Gergely, V., 1979, Regulation of glucuronidation and sulfate conjugation in isolated hepatocytes, *Drug Metabolism and Disposition: The Biological Fate of Chemicals*, **7**, 416–419.

Moldéus, P., Andersson, B., Norling, A. and Ormstad, K., 1980a, Effect of chronic ethanol administration on drug metabolism in isolated hepatocytes with emphasis on paracetamol activation, *Biochemical Pharmacology*, **29**, 1741–1745.

Moldéus, P., Andersson, B., Rahimtula, A. and Berggren, M., 1982a, Prostaglandin synthetase catalyzed activation of paracetamol, *Biochemical Pharmacology*, **31**, 1363–1368.

Moldéus, P., Dock, L., Cha, Y.-N., Berggren, M. and Jernström, B., 1982b, Elevation of conjugation capacity in isolated hepatocytes from BHA-treated mice, *Biochemical Pharmacology*, **31**, 1907–1910.

Moldéus, P. and Gergely, V., 1980b, Effect of acetone on the activation of acetaminophen, *Toxicology and Applied Pharmacology*, **53**, 8–13.

Moldéus, P., Jones, D. P., Ormstad, K. and Orrenius, S., 1978, Formation and metabolism of a glutathione-S-conjugate in isolated rat liver and kidney cells, *Biochemical and Biophysical Research Communications*, **83**, 195–200.

Moldéus, P. and Rahimtula, A., 1980, Metabolism of paracetamol to a glutathione conjugate catalyzed by prostaglandin synthetase, *Biochemical and Biophysical Research Communications*, **96**, 469–475.

Moldéus, P., von Bahr, C. and Rane, A., 1980c, Metabolism of a glutathione conjugate in human fetal and adult tissues, *Developmental Pharmacology and Therapeutics*, **1**, 83–89.

Molla, A. L. and Donald, J. F., 1974, A comparative study of ibuprofen and paracetamol in primary dysmenorrhoea, *Journal of International Medical Research*, **2**, 395–399.

Molland, E. A., 1978, Experimental renal papillary necrosis, *Kidney International*, **13**, 5–14.

Möller-Hartmann, W. and Siegers, C.-P., 1991, Nephrotoxicity of paracetamol in the rat – mechanistic and therapeutic aspects, *Journal of Applied Toxicology*, **11**, 141–146.

Momma, K. and Takao, A., 1990, Transplacental cardiovascular effects of four popular analgesics in rats, *American Journal of Obstetrics and Gynecology*, **162**, 1304–1310.

Momma, K. and Takeuchi, H., 1983, Constriction of fetal ductus arteriosus by non-steroidal anti-inflammatory drugs, *Prostaglandins*, **26**, 631–643.

Monks, T. J. and Lau, S. S., 1988, Reactive intermediates and their toxicological significance, *Toxicology*, **52**, 1–53.

Monshouwer, M., Witkamp, R. F., Pijpers, A., Verheijden, J. H. M. and van Mier, A. S. J. P. A. M., 1994, Dose-dependent pharmacokinetic interaction between antiyrine and paracetamol *in vivo* and *in vitro* when administered as a cocktail in pigs, *Xenobiotica*, **24**, 347–355.

Monteagudo, F. S. E. and Folb, P. I., 1987, Paracetamol poisoning at Groote Schuur Hospital. A 5-year experience, *South African Medical Journal*, **72**, 773–776.

Monteagudo, F. S. E., Straughan, J. L. and van der Merwe, L. P., 1986, The choice between intravenous N-acetylcysteine and oral methionine in paracetamol poisoning, *South African Medical Journal*, **69**, 279.

Montegue, A., Revol, A., Greefe, J. and Mathieu, P., 1994, Le p-acetylaminophénol (paracétamol) est-il une substance endogène produite chez l'homme? *Presse Médicale*, **23**, 1775.

Monto, G. L., Scheuer, P. J., Hansing, R. L. and Burroughs, A. K., 1994, Attenuation of acetaminophen hepatitis by prostaglandin E_2 : a histo-pathological study, *Digestive Diseases and Sciences*, **39**, 957–960.

Montoya Cabrera, M. A., Alemán Velázquez, P., Isunza Muñiz, M., Ravelo Méndez, E. H. and Dumois Nuñez, R., 1982, Intoxicación mortal por acetaminofén. (Informe del primer caso en México), *Revista Médica del Instituto Mexicano del Seguro Social*, **20**, 293–298.

Moolenaar, F., 1980, Biopharmaceutics of rectal administration of drugs in man, *Pharmaceutisch Weekblad*, **115**, 477–487.

Moolenaar, F. and Cox, H. L. M., 1980, Resorptiesnelheid en biologische beschikbaarheid van paracetamolzetpillen bereid met handelskwaliteiten paracetamol van verschillende deeltjesgrootte in een lipofiele basis, *Pharmaceutisch Weekblad*, **115**, 585–586.

Moolenaar, F., Olthof, L. and Huizinga, T., 1979a, Biopharmaceutics of rectal administration of drugs in man. 3. Absorption rate and bioavailability of paracetamol from rectal aqueous suspensions, *Pharmaceutisch Weekblad. Scientific Edition*, **1**, 25–30.

Moolenaar, F., Schoonen, A. J. M., Everts, A. and Huizinga, T., 1979b, Biopharmaceutics of rectal administration of drugs in man. 4. Absorption rate and bioavailability of paracetamol from fatty suppositories, *Pharmaceutisch Weekblad. Scientific Edition*, **1**, 89–94.

Moore, M., Thor, H., Moore, G., Nelson, S., Moldéus, P. and Orrenius, S., 1985a, The toxicity of acetaminophen and N-acetyl-p-benzoquinone imine in isolated hepatocytes is associated with thiol depletion and increased cytosolic Ca^{2+}, *Journal of Biological Chemistry*, **260**, 13035–13040.

Moore, P. A., Acs, G. and Hargreaves, J. A., 1985b, Postextraction pain relief in children: a clinical trial of liquid analgesics, *International Journal of Clinical Pharmacology, Therapy and Toxicology*, **23**, 573–577.

Moore, U., Seymour, R. A., Williams, F. M., Nicholson, E. and Rawlins, M. D., 1989, The efficacy of benorylate in postoperative dental pain, *European Journal of Clinical Pharmacology*, **36**, 35–38.

Moore, U. J., Seymour, R. A. and Rawlins, M. D., 1992, The efficacy of locally applied aspirin and acetaminophen in postoperative pain after third molar surgery, *Clinical Pharmacology and Therapeutics*, **52**, 292–296.

Moorjani, P. A., Miller, J. J. and Bock, G. R., 1985, The effects of paracetamol on frusemide ototoxicity, *Audiology*, **24**, 269–274.

Morato, G. S., Lemos, T. and Morato, E. F., 1992, Effects of indomethacin, aspirin, and acetaminophen on ethanol diuresis in rats, *Alcoholism: Clinical and Experimental Research*, **16**, 38–40.

Moreau, X., Cottineau, C., Cocaud, J., Rod, B. and Granry, J. C., 1990, Analgésie peropératoire en chirurgie veineuse périphérique, *Cahiers d'Anesthésiologie*, **38**, 403–407.

Moreau, X., Le Quay, L., Granry, J. C., Boishardy, N. and Delhumeau, A., 1993, Pharmacocinétique du paracétamol dans la liquide céphalorachidien de sujets âgés, *Thérapie*, **48**, 393–396.

Morgan, E. T., Koop, D. R. and Coon, M. J., 1982, Catalytic activity of cytochrome P-450 isozyme 3a isolated from liver microsomes of ethanol-treated rabbits, *Journal of Biological Chemistry*, **257**, 13951–13957.

Morgan, E. T., Koop, D. R. and Coon, M. J., 1983, Comparison of six rabbit liver cytochrome P-450 isozymes in formation of a reactive metabolite of acetaminophen, *Biochemical and Biophysical Research Communications*, **112**, 8–13.

Morgan, L. M., Tredger, J. A., Madden, A., Kwasowski, P. and Marks, V., 1985, The effect of guar gum on carbohydrate-, fat- and protein-stimulated gut hormone secretion: modification of postprandial gastric inhibitory polypeptide and gastrin responses, *British Journal of Nutrition*, **53**, 467–475.

Morgan, L. M., Tredger, J. A., Wright, J. and Marks, V., 1990, The effect of soluble- and insoluble-fibre supplementation on post-prandial glucose tolerance, insulin and gastric inhibitory polypeptide secretion in healthy subjects, *British Journal of Nutrition*, **64**, 103–110.

Morgan, L. M., Tredger, J. A. T., Hampton, S. M., French, A. P., Peake, J. C. F. and Marks, V., 1988, The effect of dietary modification and hyperglycaemia on gastric emptying and gastric inhibitory polypeptide (GIP) secretion, *British Journal of Nutrition*, **60**, 29–37.

Morgan, M. E. and Freed, C. R., 1981, Acetaminophen as an internal standard for calibrating *in vivo* electrochemical electrodes, *Journal of Pharmacology and Experimental Therapeutics*, **219**, 49–53.

Mörner, K. A. H., 1889, Stoffwechselprodukte des Acetanilids im menschlichen Körper, *Hoppe Seyles Zeitschrift für Physiologische Chemie*, **13**, 12–25.

Morris, H. C., Overton, P. D., Ramsay, J. R., Campbell, R. S., Hammond, P. M., Atkinson, T. and Price, C. P., 1990, Development and validation of an automated enzyme assay for paracetamol (acetaminophen), *Clinica Chimica Acta*, **187**, 95–104.

Morris, M. E., Galinsky, R. E. and Levy, G., 1984, Depletion of endogenous inorganic sulfate in the mammalian central nervous system by acetaminophen, *Journal of Pharmaceutical Sciences*, **73**, 853.

Morris, M. E., Gengo, F. M., Kinkel, W. R., Castellani, D. A. and Levy, G., 1986, Effect of acetaminophen on inorganic sulfate concentrations in human cerebrospinal fluid, *Journal of Pharmaceutical Sciences*, **75**, 722–723.

Morris, M. E. and Levy, G., 1983a, Absorption of sulfate from orally administered magnesium sulfate in man, *Journal of Toxicology. Clinical Toxicology*, **20**, 107–114.

Morris, M. E. and Levy, G., 1983b, Serum concentration and renal excretion by normal adults of inorganic sulfate after acetaminophen, ascorbic acid, or sodium sulfate, *Clinical Pharmacology and Therapeutics*, **33**, 529–536.

Morris, M. E. and Levy, G., 1984, Renal clearance and serum protein binding of acetaminophen and its major conjugates in humans, *Journal of Pharmaceutical Sciences*, **73**, 1038–1041.

Morrison, M. H. and Hawksworth, G. M., 1984, Glucuronic acid conjugation by hepatic microsomal fractions isolated from streptozotocin-induced diabetic rats, *Biochemical Pharmacology*, **33**, 3833–3838.

Morrison, N. A. and Repka, M. X., 1994, Ketorolac vs. acetaminophen or ibuprofen in controlling post-operative pain in patients with strabismus, *Opthalmology*, **101**, 915–918.

Morrison, P. F., Bungay, P. M., Hsiao, J. K., Ball, B. A., Mefford, I. N. and Dedrick, R. L., 1991, Quantitative microdialysis: analysis of transients and application to pharmacokinetics in brain, *Journal of Neurochemistry*, **57**, 103–119.

Morse, H. N., 1878, Ueber eine neue Darstellungsmethode der Acetylamidophenole, *Berichte der Deutschen Chemischen Gesellschaft*, **11**, 232–233.

Mostafa, M. H., Sheweita, S. A. and Abdel-Moneam, N. M., 1990, Influence of some anti-inflammatory drugs on the activity of aryl hydrocarbon hydroxylase and the cytochrome P-450 content, *Environmental Research*, **52**, 77–82.

Moulding, T. S., Redeker, A. G. and Kanel, G. C., 1991, Acetaminophen, isoniazid, and hepatic toxicity, *Annals of Internal Medicine*, **114**, 431.

Mourelle, M., Beales, D. and McLean, A. E. M., 1990, Electron transport and protection of liver slices in the late stage of paracetamol injury, *Biochemical Pharmacology*, **40**, 2023–2028.

Mourelle, M., Beales, D. and McLean, A. E. M., 1991, Prevention of paracetamol-induced liver injury by fructose, *Biochemical Pharmacology*, **41**, 1831–1837.

Mourelle, M. and McLean, A. E. M., 1989, Electron transport and protection of liver slices in the late stage of paracetamol injury of the liver, *British Journal of Pharmacology*, **98**

Suppl, 825P.

Mrochek, J. E., Katz, S., Christie, W. H. and Dinsmore, S. R., 1974, Acetaminophen metabolism in man, as determined by high-resolution liquid chromatography, *Clinical Chemistry*, **20**, 1086–1096.

Mrvos, R., Schneider, S. M., Dean, B. S. and Krenzelok, E. P., 1992, Orthotopic liver transplants necessitated by acetaminophen-induced hepatotoxicity, *Veterinary and Human Toxicology*, **34**, 425–427.

Mucklow, J. C., Fraser, H. S., Bulpitt, C. J., Kahn, C., Mould, G. and Dollery, C. T., 1980, Environmental factors affecting paracetamol metabolism in London factory and office workers, *British Journal of Clinical Pharmacology*, **10**, 67–74.

Mudge, G. H., 1982, Analgesic nephropathy: renal drug distribution and metabolism. In: *Nephrotoxic Mechanisms of Drugs and Environmental Toxins*, Porter, G. Ed. Plenum Publishing Corporation, New York pp. 209–225.

Mudge, G. H., Gemborys, M. W. and Duggin, G. G., 1978, Covalent binding of metabolites of acetaminophen to kidney protein and depletion of renal glutathione, *Journal of Pharmacology and Experimental Therapeutics*, **206**, 218–226.

Mugford, C. A. and Tarloff, J. B., 1995, Contribution of oxidation and deacetylation to the bioactivation of acetaminophen *in vitro* in liver and kidney from male and female Sprague-Dawley rats, *Drug Metabolism and Disposition: The Biological Fate of Chemicals*, **23**, 290–294.

Mugnier, A., 1978, Effervescent Paracetamol in odonto-stomatology for children, *Revue d'Odonto-Stomatologie*, **7**, 301–306.

Mugnier, A., Schneck, G., Champion, P. and Mignon, H., 1984, Douleurs postopératoires: étude comparative d'action antalgique du naproxène sodique et du paracétamol, *Presse Médicale*, **13**, 429–431.

Mühlendahl, K. E., 1987, Überbehandlung bei einer vermeintlichen Paracetamolvergiftung, *Tägliche Praxis*, **28**, 69–71.

Mühlendahl, K. E. and Krienke, E. G., 1980, Paracetamolvergiftung, *Intensivmedizinische Praxis*, **2**, 23–26.

Mulcahy, H. E. and Hegarty, J. E., 1993, Paracetamol hepatotoxicity, *Irish Journal of Medical Science*, **162**, 1–2.

Muller, H., 1983, Influence of paracetamol (acetaminophen) on cadmium-induced lipid peroxidation in hepatocytes from starved rats, *Toxicology Letters*, **15**, 159–165.

Müller, B. W., Franzky, H.-J., Kölln, C.-J. and Mengel, W., 1984, Vergleichende Untersuchungen zur Bioverfügbarkeit von Paracetamol aus Suppositorien, *Arzneimittel-Forschung*, **34**, 1319–1322.

Müller, F. O., van Achterbergh, S. M. and Hundt, H. K. L., 1983, Paracetamol overdose: protective effect of concomitantly ingested antimuscarinic drugs and codeine, *Human Toxicology*, **3**, 473–477.

Müller, G. J., Hoffman, B. A. and Lamprecht, J. H., 1993, Drug and poison information – the Tygerberg experience, *South African Medical Journal*, **83**, 395–399.

Müller, L., Kasper, P. and Madle, S., 1991, Further investigations on the clastogenicity of paracetamol and acetylsalicylic acid *in vitro*, *Mutation Research*, **263**, 83–92.

Müller, P., Dammann, H.-G. and Simon, B., 1988, Endoskopische Untersuchungen zur Magenverträglichkeit von Paracetamol und Acetylsalicylsäure: eine Plazebo-kontrollierte Doppelblindstudie an gesunden Probanden, *Arzneimittel-Forschung*, **38**, 831–832.

Müller, P., Simon, B., Weise, D. and Dammann, H. G., 1990, Endoskopische Untersuchungen zur Magenverträglichkeit einer mehrtägigen Gabe von Paracetamol und Acetylsalicylsäure: eine Plazebo-kontrollierte Doppelblindstudie an gesunden Probanden, *Arzneimittel-Forschung*, **40**, 316–318.

Mulley, B. A., Potter, B. I., Rye, R. M. and Takeshita, K., 1978, Interactions between diazepam and paracetamol, *Journal of Clinical Pharmacy*, **3**, 25–35.

Munck, L. K., Christensen, C. B., Pedersen, L., Larsen, U., Branebjerg, P. E. and Kampmann,

J. P., 1990, Codeine in analgesic doses does not depress respiration in patients with severe chronic obstructive lung disease, *Pharmacology and Toxicology*, **66**, 335–340.

Munoz, F. G. and Fearon, Z., 1984, Sex related differences in acetaminophen toxicity in the mouse, *Journal of Toxicology. Clinical Toxicology*, **22**, 149–155.

Munson, J. W. and Abdine, H., 1978, Direct determination of acetaminophen in plasma by differential pulse voltammetry, *Journal of Pharmaceutical Sciences*, **67**, 1775–1776.

Munson, J. W., Weierstall, R. and Kostenbauder, H. B., 1978, Determination of acetaminophen in plasma by high-performance liquid chromatography with electrochemical detection, *Journal of Chromatography: Biomedical Applications*, **145**, 328–331.

Murase, T., Hazama, H., Okuno, H., Shiozaki, Y. and Sameshima, Y., 1986, Effect of H_2-receptor antagonists on acetaminophen-induced hepatic injury, *Japanese Journal of Pharmacology*, **41**, 467–473.

Muriel, P., Garciapiña, T., Perez-Alvarez, V. and Mourelle, M., 1992, Silymarin protects against paracetamol-induced lipid peroxidation and liver damage, *Journal of Applied Toxicology*, **12**, 439–442.

Muriel, P., Quintanar, M. E. and Perez-Alvarez, V., 1993, Effect of colchicine on acetaminophen-induced liver damage, *Liver*, **13**, 217–221.

Murphy, D. F., Nally, B., Gardiner, J. and Unwin, A., 1984a, Effect of metoclopramide on gastric emptying before elective and emergency Caesarian section, *British Journal of Anaesthesia*, **56**, 1113–1116.

Murphy, G. J. J., McAleer, J. J. A. and O'Connor, F. A., 1984b, Drug overdoses – a three-year study at Altnagelvin Hospital, Londonderry, *Ulster Medical Journal*, **53**, 131–139.

Murphy, P. J., Badia, P., Myers, B. L., Boecker, M. R. and Wright, K. P., 1994, Nonsteroidal anti-inflammatory drugs affect normal sleep patterns in humans, *Physiology and Behavior*, **55**, 1063–1066.

Murphy, R., Swartz, R. and Watkins, P. B., 1990, Severe acetaminophen toxicity in a patient receiving isoniazid, *Annals of Internal Medicine*, **113**, 799–800.

Murray, M. D., Brater, D. C., Tierney, W. M., Hui, S. L. and McDonald, C. J., 1990, Ibuprofen-associated renal impairment in a large general internal medicine practice, *American Journal of the Medical Sciences*, **299**, 222–229.

Murray, S. and Boobis, A. R., 1986, An assay for paracetamol, produced by the O-deethylation of phenacetin *in vitro*, using gas chromatography/electron capture negative ion chemical ionization mass spectrometry, *Biomedical and Environmental Mass Spectrometry*, **13**, 91–93.

Murray, S. and Boobis, A. R., 1991, Combined assay for phenacetin and paracetamol in plasma using capillary column gas chromatography-negative-ion mass spectrometry, *Journal of Chromatography: Biomedical Applications*, **568**, 341–350.

Murray, T. G., Stolley, P. D., Anthony, J. C., Schinnar, R., Hepler-Smith, R. and Jeffreys, J. L., 1983, Epidemiological study of regular analgesic use and end-stage renal disease, *Archives of Internal Medicine*, **143**, 1687–1693.

Muscari, M. E., 1987, Adolescent suicide attempts by acetaminophen ingestion, *American Journal of Maternal Child Nursing*, **12**, 32–35.

Muscat, J. E., Stellman, S. D. and Wynder, E. L., 1994, Nonsteroidal antiinflammatory drugs and colorectal cancer, *Cancer*, **74**, 1847–1854.

Mushambi, M. C., Rowbotham, D. J. and Bailey, S. M., 1992, Gastric emptying after minor gynaecological surgery. The effect of anaesthetic technique, *Anaesthesia*, **47**, 297–299.

Mutimer, D., 1993, Paracetamol overdose – is there a role for liver transplantation? *Journal of Clinical Pharmacy and Therapeutics*, **18**, 303–307.

Mutimer, D. and Neuberger, J., 1993, Acute liver failure: improving the outcome despite a paucity of treatment options, *Quarterly Journal of Medicine*, **86**, 409–411.

Mutimer, D. J., Ayres, R. C. S., Neuberger, J. M., Davies, M. H., Holguin, J., Buckels, J. A. C., Mayer, A. D., McMaster, P. and Elias, E., 1994, Serious paracetamol poisoning and the results of liver transplantation, *Gut*, **35**, 809–814.

Mwangi, M. W. and Sixsmith, D. G., 1982, The bioavailability of some paracetamol tablets manufactured in Kenya, *East African Medical Journal*, **59**, 513–516.

Myers, J. B., Smith, A. J., Elliott, R. L. and MacAskill, P., 1981, Self-poisoning with drugs: a $3\frac{1}{2}$-year study in Newcastle, NSW, *Medical Journal of Australia*, **2**, 402–405.

Myers, T. G., 1994, Preferred orientations in the binding of 4'-hydroxyacetanilide (acetaminophen) to cytochrome P-450 1A1 and 2B1 isoforms as determined by ^{13}C- and ^{15}N-NMR relaxation studies, *Journal of Medicinal Chemistry*, **37**, 860–867.

Myers, W. C., Otto, T. A., Harris, E., Diaco, D. and Moreno, A., 1992, Acetaminophen overdose as a suicidal gesture: a survey of adolescents' knowledge of its potential for toxicity, *Journal of the American Academy of Child and Adolescent Psychiatry*, **31**, 686–690.

Nadir, A., McFadden, R., Griggs, J., Wright, H. I., Fagiuoli, S. and van Thiel, D. H., 1994, Parental and medical over-administration of acetaminophen causing lethal hepatotoxicity in a 10-year-old, *Journal of the Oklahoma Medical Association*, **87**, 216–263.

Naga Rani, M. A., Joseph, T. and Narayanan, R., 1989, Placental transfer of paracetamol, *Journal of the Indian Medical Association*, **87**, 182–183.

Nagasawa, H. T., Goon, D. J., Muldoon, W. P. and Zera, R. T., 1984, 2-Substituted thiazolidine-4(R)-carboxylic acids as prodrugs of L-cysteine. Protection of mice against acetaminophen hepatotoxicity, *Journal of Medicinal Chemistry*, **27**, 591–596.

Nagasawa, H. T., Goon, D. J. W., Zera, R. T. and Yuzon, D. L., 1982, Prodrugs of L-cysteine as liver-protective agents: 2(RS)-methylthiazolidine-4(R)-carboxylic acid, a latent cysteine, *Journal of Medicinal Chemistry*, **25**, 489–491.

Nagayama, S., Yokoi, T., Kawaguchi, Y. and Kamataki, T., 1994, Occurrence of autoantibody to protein disulphide isomerase in rats with xenobiotic-induced hepatitis, *Journal of Toxicological Sciences*, **19**, 155–161.

Nagel, R. A., Hayllar, K. M., Tredger, J. M. and Williams, R., 1991, Caffeine clearance and galactose elimination capacity as prognostic indicators in fulminant hepatic failure, *European Journal of Gastroenterology and Hepatology*, **3**, 907–913.

Nahata, M. C., Powell, D. A., Durrell, D. E. and Miller, M. A., 1984, Acetaminophen accumulation in pediatric patients after repeated therapeutic doses, *European Journal of Clinical Pharmacology*, **27**, 57–59.

Naidu, M. U. R., Kumar, T. R., Jagdishchandra, U. S., Babu, P. A., Rao, M. M., Babhulkar, S. S., Rao, P. T., Risbud, Y. and Shah, R., 1994, Evaluation of ketorolac, ibuprofen-paracetamol, and dextropropoxyphene-paracetamol in postoperative pain, *Pharmacotherapy*, **14**, 173–177.

Nakae, D., Oakes, J. W. and Farber, J. L., 1988, Potentiation in the intact rat of the hepatotoxicity of acetaminophen by 1,3-bis(2-chloroethyl)-1-nitrosourea, *Archives of Biochemistry and Biophysics*, **267**, 651–659.

Nakae, D., Yamamoto, K., Yoshiji, H., Kinugasa, T., Maruyama, H., Farber, J. L. and Konishi, Y., 1990a, Liposome-encapsulated superoxide dismutase prevents liver necrosis induced by acetaminophen, *American Journal of Pathology*, **136**, 787–795.

Nakae, D., Yoshiji, H., Yamamoto, K., Maruyama, H., Kinugasa, T., Takashima, Y., Denda, A. and Konishi, Y., 1990b, Influence of timing of administration of liposome-encapsulated superoxide dismutase on its prevention of acetaminophen-induced liver cell necrosis in rats, *Acta Pathologica Japonica*, **40**, 568–573.

Nakagawa, M. and Okabe, S., 1987, Lack of cytoprotection by acetaminophen against ethanol-, HCl-ethanol and HCl-aspirin-induced gastric mucosal lesions in rats, *Japanese Journal of Pharmacology*, **43**, 469–472.

Nakamura, J., Baba, S., Nakamura, T., Sasaki, H. and Shibasaki, J., 1987a, A method for the preparation of calibration curves for acetaminophen glucuronide and acetaminophen sulfate in rabbit urine without use of authentic compounds in high-performance liquid chromatography, *Journal of Pharmacobiodynamics*, **10**, 673–677.

Nakamura, J., Nakamura, T., Podder, S. K., Sasaki, H. and Shibasaki, J., 1987b, Intestinal first-pass metabolism of phenacetin, acetaminophen, ethenzamide and salicylamide in rabbits pretreated with 3,4-benzo[a]pyrene, *Biochemical Pharmacology*, **36**, 1171–1174.

Nakanishi, S. and Okuno, H., 1990, Comparison of inhibitory effects of new quinolones on drug metabolizing activity in the liver, *Japanese Journal of Pharmacology*, **53**, 81–96.

Nakano, M., Nakano, N. I., Funada, S. and Iwasaka, K., 1988, Correlation between salivary and plasma levels of acetaminophen, *Japanese Journal of Clinical Pharmacology and Therapeutics*, **19**, 549–553.

Nakra, B. R., Lee, F. E. and Gaind, R., 1973, Risk of paracetamol abuse, *Lancet*, **2**, 451–452.

Nanra, R. S., 1979, Paracetamol and analgesic nephropathy, *Current Therapeutics*, **20**, 163–164.

Nanra, R. S., 1980, Clinical and pathological aspects of analgesic nephropathy, *British Journal of Clinical Pharmacology*, **10 (Suppl. 2)**, 359S–368S.

Nanra, R. S., 1983, Renal effects of antipyretic analgesics, *American Journal of Medicine*, **75(5A)**, 70–81.

Nanra, R. S., 1993, Analgesic nephropathy in the 1990s – an Australian perspective, *Kidney International*, **44 (Suppl. 42)**, S-86–S-92.

Nanra, R. S., Chirawong, P., Jackson, B. and Kincaid-Smith, P., 1970a, Experimental papillary necrosis due to analgesic mixtures, *Australasian Annals of Medicine*, **19**, 88–89.

Nanra, R. S., Chirawong, P. and Kincaid-Smith, P., 1973a, Medullary ischaemia in experimental analgesic nephropathy – the pathogenesis of renal papillary necrosis. In: *Internationales Symposium über Probleme des Phenacetin Abusus*, Haschek, H. (Ed.) Vienna: Facta Publication, pp. 45–66.

Nanra, R. S., Chirawong, P. and Kincaid-Smith, P., 1973b, Medullary ischaemia in experimental analgesic nephropathy – the pathogenesis of renal papillary necrosis, *Australian and New Zealand Journal of Medicine*, **3**, 580–586.

Nanra, R. S., Daniel, V. and Howard, M., 1980, Analgesic nephropathy induced by common proprietary mixtures, *Medical Journal of Australia*, **1**, 486–487.

Nanra, R. S., Hicks, J. D., McNamara, J. H., Lie, J. T., Leslie, D. W., Jackson, B. and Kincaid-Smith, P., 1970b, Seasonal variation in the post-mortem incidence of renal papillary necrosis, *Medical Journal of Australia*, **1**, 293–296.

Nanra, R. S. and Kincaid-Smith, P., 1970, Papillary necrosis in rats caused by aspirin and aspirin-containing mixtures, *British Medical Journal*, **3**, 559–561.

Nanra, R. S. and Kincaid-Smith, P., 1973, Experimental renal papillary necrosis (RPN) with non-steroid anti-inflammatory analgesics. In: *Internationales Symposium über Probleme des Phenacetin Abusus*, Haschek, H. (Ed.) Vienna: Facta Publication, pp. 67–88.

Nanra, R. S. and Kincaid-Smith, P., 1975, Renal papillary necrosis in rheumatoid arthritis, *Medical Journal of Australia*, **1**, 194–197.

Nanra, R. S., Stuart-Taylor, J., de Leon, A. H. and White, K. H., 1978, Analgesic nephropathy: etiology, clinical syndrome, and clinicopathologic correlations in Australia, *Kidney International*, **13**, 79–92.

Nappi, C., Nolfe, G., La Pinta, M., Colace, G., Ruotolo, C. and Affinito, P., 1993, Trattamento del dolore postoperatorio nella chirurgia ostetrico-ginecologica. Studio comparativo tra ST-679 e paracetamolo, *Clinical Therapeutics*, **142**, 47–52.

Narisawa, S., Nagata, M., Danyoshi, C., Yoshino, H., Murata, K., Hirakawa, Y. and Noda, K., 1994, An organic acid-induced sigmoidal release system for oral controlled-release preparations, *Pharmaceutical Research*, **11**, 111–116.

Nash, R. M., Stein, L., Penno, M. B., Passananti, G. T. and Vesell, E. S., 1984a, Sources of interindividual variations in acetaminophen and antipyrine metabolism, *Clinical Pharmacology and Therapeutics*, **36**, 417–430.

Nash, S. L. and Oehme, F. W., 1984, A review of acetaminophen's effect on methemoglobin, glutathione, and some related enzymes, *Veterinary and Human Toxicology*, **26**, 123–132.

Nash, S. L., Savides, M. C., Oehme, F. W. and Johnson, D. E., 1984b, The effect of acetaminophen on methemoglobin and blood glutathione parameters in the cat, *Toxicology*, **31**, 329–334.

Nasseri-Sina, P., Boobis, A. R. and Davies, D. S., 1987, Cytoprotection against paracetamol-induced toxicity in isolated hepatocytes, with iloprost, a stable analogue of prostacyclin, *Human Toxicology*, **6**, 429–430.

Nasseri-Sina, P., Fawthrop, D. J., Wilson, J., Boobis, A. R. and Davies, D. S., 1992, Cytoprotection by iloprost against paracetamol-induced toxicity in hamster isolated hepatocytes, *British Journal of Pharmacology*, **105**, 417–423.

Nasseri-Sina, P., Seddon, C. E., Boobis, A. R. and Davies, D. S., 1988, Cytoprotective effects of 16,16-dimethyl prostaglandin E_2 on paracetamol toxicity in isolated hepatocytes, *Biochemical Society Transactions*, **16**, 641–642.

National Poisons Information Service Monitoring Group, 1981, Analgesic poisoning: a multi-centre, prospective survey, *Human Toxicology*, **1**, 7–23.

Navelet, Y., Girier, B., Clouzeau, J., Devictor, D. and Wood, Ch., 1990, Insuffisance hépatocellulaire aiguë grave de l'enfant: aspects EEG pronostiques, *Neurophysiologique Cliniques*, **20**, 237–245.

Nazareth, W. M. A., Sethi, J. K. and McLean, A. E. M., 1991, Effect of paracetamol on mitochondrial membrane function in rat liver slices, *Biochemical Pharmacology*, **42**, 931–936.

Nebert, D. W., Thorgeirsson, S. S. and Lambert, G. H., 1976, Genetic aspects of toxicity during development, *Environmental Health Perspectives*, **18**, 35–45.

Negro, F., Curzio, M., Flaccavento, C., Paradisi, L. and Torrielli, M. V., 1981, Suscettibilita' del fegato alla perossidazione lipidica dopo trattamento con paracetamolo, *Bollettino della Società Italiana di Biologia Sperimentale*, **57**, 283–289.

Nelson, E. and Morioka, T., 1963, Kinetics of the metabolism of acetaminophen by humans, *Journal of Pharmaceutical Sciences*, **52**, 864–868.

Nelson, E. B., 1980, The pharmacology and toxicology of meta-substituted acetanilide I: acute toxicity of 3-hydroxyacetanilide in mice, *Research Communications in Chemical Pathology and Pharmacology*, **28**, 447–456.

Nelson, E. B., Abernethy, D. R., Greenblatt, D. J. and Ameer, B., 1986, Paracetamol absorption from a feeding jejunostomy, *British Journal of Clinical Pharmacology*, **22**, 111–113.

Nelson, E. B., Montes, M. and Goldstein, M., 1980a, Effectiveness of metyrapone in the treatment of acetaminophen toxicity in mice, *Toxicology*, **17**, 73–81.

Nelson, M. M. and Forfar, J. O., 1971, Associations between drugs administered during pregnancy and congenital abnormalities of the fetus, *British Medical Journal*, **1**, 523–527.

Nelson, S. D., 1982, Metabolic activation and drug toxicity, *Journal of Medicinal Chemistry*, **25**, 753–765.

Nelson, S. D., 1990, Molecular mechanisms of the hepatotoxicity caused by acetaminophen, *Seminars in Liver Disease*, **10**, 267–278.

Nelson, S. D., Dahlin, D. C., Rauckman, E. J. and Rosen, G. M., 1981a, Peroxidase-mediated formation of reactive metabolites of acetaminophen, *Molecular Pharmacology*, **20**, 195–199.

Nelson, S. D., Forte, A. J. and Dahlin, D. C., 1980b, Lack of evidence for N-hydroxyacetaminophen as a reactive metabolite of acetaminophen *in vitro*, *Biochemical Pharmacology*, **29**, 1617–1620.

Nelson, S. D., Forte, A. J. and McMurtry, R. J., 1978, Decreased toxicity of the N-methyl analogs of acetaminophen and phenacetin, *Research Communications in Chemical Pathology and Pharmacology*, **22**, 61–71.

Nelson, S. D. and Pearson, P. G., 1990, Covalent and noncovalent interactions in acute lethal cell injury caused by chemicals, *Annual Review of Pharmacology and Toxicology*, **30**, 169–195.

Nelson, S. D., Tirmenstein, M. A., Rashed, M. S. and Myers, T. G., 1991, Acetaminophen and protein thiol modification, *Advances in Experimental Medicine and Biology*, **283**, 579–588.

Nelson, S. D., Vaishnav, Y., Kambara, H. and Baillie, T. A., 1981b, Comparative electron impact, chemical ionization and field desorption mass spectra of some thioether metabolites of acetaminophen, *Biomedical and Environmental Mass Spectrometry*, **8**, 244–251.

Nesbitt, J. A. A. and Minuk, G. Y., 1988, Adult Reye's syndrome, *Annals of Emergency Medicine*, **17**, 155–158.

Neuberger, J., Davis, M. and Williams, R., 1980, Long-term ingestion of paracetamol and liver disease, *Journal of the Royal Society of Medicine*, **73**, 701–707.

Neumann, C. M. and Zannoni, V. G., 1988, Acsorbic acid deficiency and hepatic UDP-glucuronyltransferase, *Drug Metabolism and Disposition: The Biological Fate of Chemicals*, **16**, 551–556.

Neuvonen, P. J., Lehtovaara, R., Bardy, A. and Elomaa, E., 1979, Antipyretic analgesics in patients on antiepileptic drug therapy, *European Journal of Clinical Pharmacology*, **15**, 263–268.

Neuvonen, P. J. and Olkkola, K. T., 1988, Oral activated charcoal in the treatment of intoxications: role of single and repeated doses, *Medical Toxicology*, **3**, 33–58.

Neuvonen, P. J., Simell, O. and Tokola, O., 1986, Why not add methionine to paracetamol tablets? *British Medical Journal*, **293**, 958.

Neuvonen, P. J., Tokola, O., Toivonen, M.-L. and Simell, O., 1985, Methionine in paracetamol tablets, a tool to reduce paracetamol toxicity, *International Journal of Clinical Pharmacology, Therapy and Toxicology*, **23**, 497–500.

Neuvonen, P. J., Vartiainen, M. and Tokola, O., 1983, Comparison of activated charcoal and ipecac syrup in prevention of drug absorption, *European Journal of Clinical Pharmacology*, **24**, 557–562.

New Zealand Rheumatism Association Study, 1974, Aspirin and the kidney, *British Medical Journal*, **1**, 593–596.

Newman, T. J. and Bargman, G. J., 1979, Acetaminophen hepatotoxicity and malnutrition, *American Journal of Gastroenterology*, **72**, 647–650.

Newton, D. R. L. and Tanner, J. M., 1956, N-Acetyl-para-aminophenol as an analgesic: a controlled trial using the method of sequential analysis, *British Medical Journal*, **2**, 1096–1099.

Newton, J. F., Bailie, M. B. and Hook, J. B., 1983a, Acetaminophen nephrotoxicity in the rat. Renal metabolic activation *in vitro*, *Toxicology and Applied Pharmacology*, **70**, 433–444.

Newton, J. F., Braselton, W. E., Kuo, C.-H., Kluwe, W. M., Gemborys, M. W., Mudge, G. H. and Hook, J. B., 1982a, Metabolism of acetaminophen by the isolated perfused kidney, *Journal of Pharmacology and Experimental Therapeutics*, **221**, 76–79.

Newton, J. F., Hoefle, D., Gemborys, M. W., Mudge, G. H. and Hook, J. B., 1986, Metabolism and excretion of a glutathione conjugate of acetaminophen in the isolated perfused rat kidney, *Journal of Pharmacology and Experimental Therapeutics*, **237**, 519–524.

Newton, J. F., Kuo, C.-H., DeShone, G. M., Hoefle, D., Bernstein, J. and Hook, J. B., 1985a, The role of p-aminophenol in acetaminophen-induced nephrotoxicity: effect of bis(p-nitrophenyl) phosphate on acetaminophen and p-aminophenol nephrotoxicity and metabolism in Fischer 344 rats, *Toxicology and Applied Pharmacology*, **81**, 416–430.

Newton, J. F., Kuo, C.-H., Gemborys, M. W., Mudge, G. H. and Hook, J. B., 1982b, Nephrotoxicity of p-aminophenol, a metabolite of acetaminophen, in the Fischer 344 rat, *Toxicology and Applied Pharmacology*, **65**, 336–344.

Newton, J. F., Pasino, D. A. and Hook, J. B., 1985b, Acetaminophen nephrotoxicity in the rat: quantitation of renal metabolic activation *in vivo*, *Toxicology and Applied Pharmacology*, **78**, 39–46.

Newton, J. F., Yoshimoto, M., Bernstein, J., Rush, G. F. and Hook, J. B., 1983b, Acetaminophen nephrotoxicity in the rat. I. Strain differences in nephrotoxicity and metabolism, *Toxicology and Applied Pharmacology*, **69**, 291–306.

Newton, J. F., Yoshimoto, M., Bernstein, J., Rush, G. F. and Hook, J. B., 1983c, Acetaminophen nephrotoxicity in the rat. II. Strain differences in nephrotoxicity and metabolism of p-aminophenol, a metabolite of acetaminophen, *Toxicology and Applied Pharmacology*, **69**, 307–318.

Nicholls-Grzemski, F. A., Calder, I. C. and Priestly, B. G., 1992, Peroxisome proliferators protect against paracetamol hepatotoxicity in mice, *Biochemical Pharmacology*, **43**, 1395–1396.

Nicholson, J. K., Timbrell, J. A., Bales, J. R. and Sadler, P. J., 1985, A high resolution proton nuclear magnetic resonance approach to the study of hepatocyte and drug metabolism. Application to acetaminophen, *Molecular Pharmacology*, **27**, 634–643.

Nickel, B. and Zerrahn, H., 1987, Pharmaco-electroencephalography in the rat as a method for characterization of different types of analgesics, *Postgraduate Medical Journal*, **63 (Suppl. 3)**, 45–47.

Nicotera, P., Hinds, T. R., Nelson, S. D. and Vincenzi, F. F., 1990, Differential effects of arylating and oxidizing analogs of N-acetyl-p-benzoquinoneimine on red blood cell membrane proteins, *Archives of Biochemistry and Biophysics*, **283**, 200–205.

Nicotera, P., Rundgren, M., Porubek, D. J., Cotgreave, I., Moldéus, P., Orrenius, S. and Nelson, S. D., 1989, On the role of Ca^{2+} in the toxicity of alkylating and oxidising quinone imines in isolated hepatocytes, *Chemical Research in Toxicology*, **2**, 46–50.

Nielsen, A. S. and Nielsen, B., 1992, Mønstret i præparatvalg ved intenderede selvforgiftninger: med særligt henblik på oendringer i ordinationsmonstret, *Ugeskrift for Læger*, **154**, 1972–1976.

Nielsen, I. and Pedersen, R. S., 1984, Paracetamolforgiftning. Specifik behandling med metionin eller N-acetylcystein? *Ugeskrift for Læger*, **146**, 1500–1502.

Nielsen, J. B. and Lings, S., 1993, Nitrosamindannende håndkøbspræparater? *Ugeskrift for Læger*, **155**, 2783–2785.

Nielsen, J. C., Bjerring, P. and Arendt-Nielsen, L., 1991, A comparison of the hypoalgesic effect of paracetamol in slow-release and plain tablets on laser-induced pain, *British Journal of Clinical Pharmacology*, **31**, 267–270.

Nielsen, J. C., Bjerring, P., Arendt-Nielsen, L. and Petterson, K.-J., 1992, Analgesic efficacy of immediate and sustained release paracetamol and plasma concentration of paracetamol. Double blind, placebo-controlled evaluation using painful laser stimulation, *European Journal of Clinical Pharmacology*, **42**, 261–264.

Nielsen-Kudsk, F., 1980, HPLC-determination of some antiinflammatory, weak analgesic and uricosuric drugs in human blood plasma and its application to pharmacokinetics, *Acta Pharmacologica et Toxicologica*, **47**, 267–273.

Nimmo, J., Dixon, M. F. and Prescott, L. F., 1973a, Effects of mepyramine, promethazine and hydrocortisone on paracetamol-induced hepatic necrosis in the rat, *Clinical Toxicology*, **6**, 75–81.

Nimmo, J., Heading, R. C., Tothill, P. and Prescott, L. F., 1973b, Pharmacological modification of gastric emptying: effects of propantheline and metoclopramide on paracetamol absorption, *British Medical Journal*, **1**, 587–589.

Nimmo, W. S., 1978, The measurement of gastric emptying during labour, *Journal of International Medical Research*, **6 (Suppl. 1)**, 52–53.

Nimmo, W. S., 1982, Gastrointestinal function following surgery, *Regional Anesthesia*, **7 (Suppl. 4)**, S105–S109.

Nimmo, W. S., 1984, Effect of anaesthesia on gastric motility and emptying, *British Journal of Anaesthesia*, **56**, 29–36.

Nimmo, W. S., Heading, R. C., Wilson, J. and Prescott, L. F., 1979a, Reversal of narcotic-induced delay in gastric emptying and paracetamol absorption by naloxone, *British Medical Journal*, **2**, 1189.

Nimmo, W. S., Heading, R. C., Wilson, J., Tothill, P. and Prescott, L. F., 1975a, Inhibition of gastric emptying and drug absorption by narcotic analgesics, *British Journal of Clinical Pharmacology*, **2**, 509–513.

Nimmo, W. S., King, I. S. and Prescott, L. F., 1979b, Paracetamol and aspirin absorption from Safapryn and Safapryn-Co, *British Journal of Clinical Pharmacology*, **7**, 219–220.

Nimmo, W. S., Littlewood, D. G., Scott, D. B. and Prescott, L. F., 1978, Gastric emptying following hysterectomy with extradural analgesia, *British Journal of Anaesthesia*, **50**,

559–561.

Nimmo, W. S. and Prescott, L. F., 1978, The influence of posture on paracetamol absorption, *British Journal of Clinical Pharmacology*, **5**, 348–349.

Nimmo, W. S., Todd, J. G. and Vogel, J., 1986, Effect of meptazinol on drug absorption and gastric emptying, *European Journal of Anaesthesiology*, **3**, 295–298.

Nimmo, W. S., Wilson, J. and Prescott, L. F., 1975b, Narcotic analgesics and delayed gastric emptying during labour, *Lancet*, **i**, 890–892.

Nivaud-Guernet, E., Guernet, M., Ivanovic, D. and Medenica, M., 1994, Effect of eluent pH on the ionic and molecular forms of the non-steroidal anti-inflammatory agents in reversed-phase high-performance liquid chromatography, *Journal of Liquid Chromatography*, **17**, 2343–2357.

Niwa, H. and Nakayama, T., 1968, Studies on the combination of drugs. IV. Effect of 4-hydroxyantipyrine and N-acetyl-p-aminophenol on the metabolism of phenylbutazone, oxyphenbutazone and ketophenylbutazone, *Journal of the Pharmaceutical Society of Japan*, **88**, 838–842.

Nogen, A. G. and Bremner, J. E., 1978, Fatal acetaminophen overdosage in a young child, *Journal of Pediatrics*, **92**, 832–833.

Nolan, C. M., Sandblom, R. E., Thummel, K. E., Slattery, J. T. and Nelson, S. D., 1994, Hepatotoxicity associated with acetaminophen usage in patients receiving multiple drug therapy for tuberculosis, *Chest*, **105**, 408–411.

Nordenfeldt, O. and Ringertz, N., 1961, Phenacetin takers dead with renal failure, *Acta Medica Scandinavica*, **170**, 385–402.

Nordenskjöld, M. and Moldéus, P., 1983, Induction of DNA-strand breaks in cultured human fibroblasts by reactive metabolites, *Annals of the New York Academy of Sciences*, **407**, 460–462.

Nordin, M., Wieslander, A., Martinson, E. and Kjellstrand, P., 1991, Effects of exposure period of acetylsalicylic acid, paracetamol and isopropanol on L929 cytotoxicity, *Toxicology in vitro*, **5**, 449–450.

Nørgaard, N. and Jensen, O. M., 1990, Fenacetin, paracetamol og blærecancer, *Ugeskrift for Læger*, **152**, 3687–3691.

Nørrelund, N., Christiansen, L. V. and Plantener, S., 1989, Tolfenamsyre vs. paracetamol ved migræneanfald. En dobbeltblind undersogelse i almen praksis ce, *Ugeskrift for Læger*, **151**, 2436–2438.

North, D. S., Peterson, R. G. and Krenzelok, E. P., 1981, Effects of activated charcoal administration on acetylcysteine serum levels in humans, *American Journal of Hospital Pharmacy*, **38**, 1022–1024.

Northover, B. J. and Subramanian, G., 1961, Some inhibitors of histamine-induced and formaldehyde-induced inflammation in mice, *British Journal of Pharmacology*, **16**, 163–169.

Notarianni, L. J., Oldham, H. G. and Bennett, P. N., 1987, Passage of paracetamol into breast milk and its subsequent metabolism by the neonate, *British Journal of Clinical Pharmacology*, **24**, 63–67.

Notarianni, L. J., Oldham, H. G., Bennett, P. N., Southgate, C. C. B. and Parfitt, R. T., 1981, Epoxides from paracetamol – a possible explanation for paracetamol toxicity, *Advances in Experimental Medicine and Biology*, **136**, 1077–1083.

Nouchi, T., Lasker, J. M. and Lieber, C. S., 1986, Activation of acetaminophen oxidation in rat liver microsomes by caffeine, *Toxicology Letters*, **32**, 1–8.

Novotony, R. E. and Elser, R. C., 1984, Indophenol method for acetaminophen in serum examined, *Clinical Chemistry*, **30**, 884–886.

Nozawa, I., Suzuki, Y. and Sato, S., 1991, Application of a thermo-responsive membrane to the transdermal delivery of non-steroidal anti-inflammatory drugs and antipyretic drugs, *Journal of Controlled Release*, **15**, 29–37.

Nusynowitz, M. L. and Forsham, P. H., 1966, The antidiuretic effect of acetaminophen, *Amer-*

ican Journal of the Medical Sciences, **252**, 429–435.

Nusynowitz, M. L., Wegienka, L. C., Bower, B. F. and Forsham, P. H., 1966, Effect on vasopressin action of analgesic drugs *in vitro*, *American Journal of the Medical Sciences*, **252**, 424–428.

Nyström, E., Gustafsson, I. and Quiding, H., 1988, The pain intensity at analgesic intake, and the efficacy of diflunisal in single doses and effervescent acetaminophen in single and repeated doses, *Pharmacotherapy*, **8**, 201–209.

Obafunwa, J. O. and Busuttil, A., 1994, Deaths from substance overdose in the Lothian and Borders region of Scotland (1983–1991), *Human and Experimental Toxicology*, **13(6)**, 401–406.

Oberhaensli, R., Rajagopalan, B., Galloway, G. J., Taylor, D. J. and Radda, G. K., 1990, Study of human liver disease with P-31 magnetic resonance spectroscopy, *Gut*, **31**, 463–467.

Oberholzer, B., Hoigné, R., Hartmann, K., Capaul, R., Egli, A., Wymann, R., Galeazzi, R. L., Kuhn, M., Künzi, U. P. and Maibach, R., 1993, Die Häufigkeit von unerwünschten Arzneimittelwirkung nach Symptomen und Syndromen. Aus den Erfahrungen des CHDM und der SANZ. Als Beispiel: die allergischen und pseudoallergischen Reactionen unter leichten analgetica und NSAIDs, *Therapeutische Umschau*, **50**, 13–19.

O'Brien, C. B., Henzel, B. S., Naji, A. and Brass, C. A., 1992, Prostaglandin E1 infusion is effective in the late treatment of patients with acetaminophen induced acute hepatic failure referred for liver transplantation, *Gastroenterology*, **102**, A862.

O'Brien, P. J., Khan, S. and Jatoe, S. D., 1991, Formation of biological reactive intermediates by peroxidases: Halide mediated acetaminophen oxidation and cytotoxicity, *Advances in Experimental Medicine and Biology*, **283**, 51–64.

O'Brien, W. F., Krammer, J., O'Leary, T. D. and Mastrogiannis, D. S., 1993, The effect of acetaminophen on prostacyclin production in pregnant women, *American Journal of Obstetrics and Gynecology*, **168**, 1164–1169.

Ochs, H. R., Greenblatt, D. J., Abernethy, D. R., Arendt, R. M., Gerloff, J., Eichelkraut, W. and Hahn, N., 1985, Cerebrospinal fluid uptake and peripheral distribution of centrally acting drugs: relation to lipid solubility, *Journal of Pharmacy and Pharmacology*, **37**, 428–431.

Ochs, H. R., Greenblatt, D. J., Verburg-Ochs, B., Abernethy, D. R. and Knüchel, M., 1984, Differential effects of isoniazid and oral contraceptive steroids on antipyrine oxidation and acetaminophen conjugation, *Pharmacology*, **28**, 188–195.

Ochs, H. R., Schuppan, U., Greenblatt, D. J. and Abernethy, D. R., 1983, Reduced distribution and clearance of acetaminophen in patients with congestive heart failure, *Journal of Cardiovascular Pharmacology*, **5**, 697–699.

O'Connell, S. E. and Zurzola, F. J., 1982, A rapid quantitative determination of acetaminophen in plasma, *Journal of Pharmaceutical Sciences*, **71**, 1291–1294.

O'Connell, T. and Feeley, J., 1993, Medical messages on television: grapevine effect, *British Medical Journal*, **306**, 1415–1416.

O'Dell, J. R., Zetterman, R. K. and Burnett, D. A., 1986, Centrilobular hepatic fibrosis following acetaminophen-induced hepatic necrosis in an alcoholic, *Journal of the American Medical Association*, **255**, 2636–2637.

Oder, W., Oder, B., Kollegger, H., Spatt, J., Zeiler, K., Aull, S., Mraz, M. and Wessely, P., 1994, Hemorheologic dysfunction in analgesic-induced chronic headache? Results of a pilot study, *Clinical Hemorheology*, **14**, 339–346.

Odièvre, M., Huguet, P. and Congard, B., 1990, Convulsions fébriles chez l'enfant: conduit à tenir, *Annales de Pédiatrie*, **37**, 570–573.

O'Grady, J. G., Alexander, G. J. M., Hayllar, K. M. and Williams, R., 1989, Early indicators of prognosis in fulminant hepatic failure, *Gastroenterology*, **97**, 439–445.

O'Grady, J. G., Gimson, A. E. S., O'Brien, C. J., Pucknell, A., Hughes, R. D. and Williams, R., 1988, Controlled trials of charcoal hemoperfusion and prognostic factors in fulminant hepatic failure, *Gastroenterology*, **94**, 1186–1192.

O'Grady, J. G., Wendon, J., Tan, K. C., Potter, D., Cottam, S., Cohen, A. T., Gimson, A. E. S. and Williams, R., 1991, Liver transplantation after paracetamol overdose, *British Medical Journal*, **303**, 221–223.

Ogunbode, O., 1987, A comparative trial of piroxicam and paracetamol after episiotomy wound repair, *Current Therapeutic Research*, **41**, 89–94.

Oguro, T., Gregus, Z., Madhu, C., Liu, L. and Klaassen, C. D., 1994, Molybdate depletes hepatic 3-phosphoadenosine 5-phosphosulfate and impairs the sulfation of acetaminophen in rats, *Journal of Pharmacology and Experimental Therapeutics*, **270**, 1145–1151.

Oh, T. H. and Shenfield, G. M., 1980, Intravenous N-acetylcysteine for paracetamol poisoning, *Medical Journal of Australia*, **1**, 664–665.

Ohta, T., Oribe, H., Ide, M. and Takitani, S., 1988a, Formation of N-acetyl-p-benzoquinoneimine, the well-known toxic metabolite of acetaminophen, by the reaction of acetaminophen with nitrite under model stomach conditions, *Chemical and Pharmaceutical Bulletin*, **36**, 4634–4637.

Ohta, T., Oribe, H., Kameyama, T., Goto, Y. and Takitani, S., 1988b, Formation of a diazoquinone-type mutagen from acetaminophen treated with nitrite under acidic conditions, *Mutation Research*, **209**, 95–98.

Ohtani, N., Matsuzaki, M., Anno, Y., Ogawa, H., Matsuda, Y. and Kusukawa, R., 1989, A case of myocardial damage following acute paracetamol poisoning, *Japanese Circulation Journal*, **53**, 278–282.

Øie, S., Lowenthal, D. T., Briggs, W. A. and Levy, G., 1975, Effect of hemodialysis on kinetics of acetaminophen elimination by anephric patients, *Clinical Pharmacology and Therapeutics*, **18**, 680–686.

Ojeda, V. J., Shilkin, K. B., Wright, E. A. and Williams, R., 1982, Massive hepatic necrosis and focal necrotising myopathy, *Lancet*, **i**, 172–173.

Okano, C. K., Hokama, Y. and Chou, S. C., 1984, The effects of aspirin and acetaminophen on tetrahymena pyriformis GL growth and macromolecular synthesis, *Research Communications in Chemical Pathology and Pharmacology*, **45**, 293–296.

Okuno, H., Murase, T., Hazama, H., Shiozaki, Y. and Sameshima, Y., 1987, The effects of cimetidine on acute liver injuries induced by acetaminophen, CCl4 and galactosamine, *Acta Hepatologica Japonica*, **28**, 154–163.

Okuyama, S. and Aihara, H., 1984a, Inhibition of electrically-induced vocalization in adjuvant arthritic rats as a novel method for evaluating analgesic drugs, *Japanese Journal of Pharmacology*, **34**, 67–77.

Okuyama, S. and Aihara, H., 1984b, The mode of action of analgesic drugs in adjuvant arthritic rats as an experimental model of chronic inflammatory pain: possible central analgesic action of acidic nonsteroidal antiinflammatory drugs, *Japanese Journal of Pharmacology*, **35**, 95–103.

Okuyama, S. and Aihara, H., 1985, Hyperalgesic action in rats of intracerebroventricularly administered arachidonic acid, PG E_2 and PG $F_{2\alpha}$: effects of analgesic drugs on hyperalgesia, *Archives Internationales de Pharmacodynamie et de Therapie*, **278**, 13–22.

Okuyama, S., Hashimoto, S., Amanuma, F. and Aihara, H., 1984c, Effect of various types of analgesic drugs on an experimental model of chronic inflammatory pain in mice, *Folia Pharmacologica Japonica*, **83**, 513–521.

Oldham, J. W., Preston, R. F. and Paulson, J. D., 1986, Mutagenicity testing of selected analgesics in Ames *salmonella* strains, *Journal of Applied Toxicology*, **6**, 237–243.

Oliver, J. S., Smith, H. and Yehia, B., 1981, Poisoning by dextropropoxyphene and paracetamol, *Journal of the Forensic Science Society*, **21**, 207–210.

Olling, M. and Rauws, A. G., 1986, Evaluation program BIOTEST applied to bioavailability tests of paracetamol preparations, *Methods and Findings in Experimental and Clinical Pharmacology*, **8**, 629–631.

Olson, K. R., Kearney, T. E., Dyer, J. O., Benowitz, N. L. and Blanc, P. D., 1994, Seizures associated with poisoning and drug overdose, *American Journal of Emergency Medicine*, **12**, 392–395.

Olsson, R., 1978, Increased hepatic sensitivity to paracetamol, *Lancet*, **ii**, 152–153.

Olstad, O. A. and Skjelbred, P., 1986a, The effects of indoprofen vs paracetamol on swelling, pain and other events after surgery, *International Journal of Clinical Pharmacology, Therapy and Toxicology*, **24**, 34–38.

Olstad, O. A. and Skjelbred, P., 1986b, Comparison of the analgesic effect of a corticsteroid and paracetamol in patients with pain after oral surgery, *British Journal of Clinical Pharmacology*, **22**, 437–442.

Olumide, Y., 1979, Fixed drug eruption. A lesson in drug usage, *International Journal of Dermatology*, **18**, 818–821.

Omura, H., Kamisaki, Y., Kawasaki, H. and Itoh, T., 1994, Effect of acetaminophen on stress-induced gastric mucosal lesions in rats, *Research Communications in Molecular Pathology and Pharmacology*, **86**, 297–310.

Ordog, G. J., 1987, Transcutaneous electrical nerve stimulation vs. oral analgesic: a randomized double-blind controlled study in acute traumatic pain, *American Journal of Emergency Medicine*, **5**, 6–10.

Oren, R. and Levy, M., 1992, Paracetamol overdose in Jerusalem, 1984–89, *Israel Journal of Medical Sciences*, **28**, 795–796.

Oren, R. and Levy, M., 1993, Paracetamol overdosage in Jerusalem 1984–89, *Israel Journal of Medical Sciences*, **29**, 118.

Orkin, L. R., Joseph, S. I. and Helrich, M., 1957, Effects of mild analgesics in postpartum pain: a method for evaluating analgesics, *New York State Journal of Medicine*, **57**, 71–73.

Orlowski, J. P., Campbell, P. and Goldstein, S., 1990, Reye's syndrome: a case control study of medication use and associated viruses in Australia, *Cleveland Clinic Journal of Medicine*, **57**, 323–329.

Orme, M. and Back, D. J., 1991, Oral contraceptive steroids: pharmacological issues of interest to the prescribing physician, *Advances in Contraception*, **7**, 325–331.

Ortega, L., Landa Garcia, J. I., Torres Garcia, A., Silecchia, G., Arenas, J., Suarez, A., Moreno Azcoitia, M., Sanz Esponera, J., Moreno Gonzalez, E. and Balibrea Cantero, J. L., 1985, Acetaminophen-induced fulminant hepatic failure in dogs, *Hepatology*, **5**, 673–676.

Osborne, N. J., Tonkin, A. L. and Miners, J. O., 1991, Interethnic differences in drug glucuronidation: a comparison of paracetamol metabolism in Caucasians and Chinese, *British Journal of Clinical Pharmacology*, **32**, 765–767.

Osselton, M. D., Blackmore, R. C., King, L. A. and Moffat, A. C., 1984, Poisoning-associated deaths for England and Wales between 1973 and 1980, *Human Toxicology*, **3**, 201–221.

Osterlind, P.-O. and Bucht, G., 1991, Drug consumption during the last decade among persons born in 1902 in Umeå, Sweden, *Drugs and Ageing*, **1**, 477–486.

Osterloh, J. and Yu, S., 1988, Simultaneous ion-pair and partition liquid chromatography of acetaminophen, theophylline and salicylate with application to 500 toxicologic specimens, *Clinica Chimica Acta*, **175**, 239–248.

Ota, S., Razandi, M., Sekhon, S., Terando, A., Hiraishi, H. and Ivey, K. J., 1988, Cytoprotective effect of acetaminophen against taurocholate-induced damage to rat gastric monolayer cultures, *Digestive Diseases and Sciences*, **33**, 938–944.

Ott, P., Dalhoff, K., Hansen, P. B., Loft, S. and Poulsen, H. E., 1990a, Consumption, overdose and death from analgesics during a period of over-the-counter availability of paracetamol in Denmark, *Journal of Internal Medicine*, **227**, 423–428.

Ott, P., Hansen, P. B., Dalhoff, K. P., Loft, S. H. and Poulsen, H. E., 1990b, Analgetikaforbrug, –overdosering og -dodsfald i Danmark 1979–1986, *Ugeskrift for Læger*, **152**, 250–252.

Ottinger, M. L., Kinney, K. W., Black, J. R. and Wittenberg, M., 1990, Comparison of flurbiprofen and acetaminophen with codeine in postoperative foot pain, *Journal of the American Podiatric Medical Association*, **80**, 266–270.

Ou, C.-N. and Frawley, V. L., 1982, Theophylline, dyphylline, caffeine, acetaminophen, salicylate, acetylsalicylate, procainamide and N-acetylprocainamide determined in serum with a single liquid-chromatographic assay, *Clinical Chemistry*, **28**, 2157–2160.

Ouvina, G. B., Lemberg, A. and Bengochea, L. A., 1994, Changes in liver drug glucuronidation during cholestasis are non predictable, *Archives Internationales de Physiologie de Biochimie et de Biophysique*, **102**, 121–123.

Ouviña, G., Pavese, A., Lemberg, A. and Bengochea, L., 1993, Aumento de la capacidad de conjugacion del acetaminofene en colestasis experimental, *Acta Gastroenterologica Latinoamericana*, **23**, 71–74.

Owen, S. G., Francis, H. W. and Roberts, M. S., 1994, Disappearance kinetics of solutes from synovial fluid after intra-articular injection, *British Journal of Clinical Pharmacology*, **38**, 349–355.

Ozaki, S., Nagaoka, H., Kisara, K. and Niwa, H., 1972, Effect of N-acetyl-p-aminophenol sulfate in augmenting the analgesic effect and acute toxicity of aminopyrine, *Folia Pharmacologica Japonica*, **68**, 521–528.

Özdemirler, G., Aykaç, G., Uysal, M. and Öz, H., 1994, Liver lipid peroxidation and glutathione-related defence enzyme systems in mice treated with paracetamol, *Journal of Applied Toxicology*, **14**, 297–299.

Ozoux, J. P., De Calan, L., Vannier, J., Rivallain, B., Gandet, O. and Brizon, J., 1987, Sténose rectale après utilisation prolongée de suppositoires de veganine, *Gastroentérologie Clinique et Biologique*, **11**, 349–350.

Pacifici, G. M., Back, D. J. and Orme, M. L'E., 1988, Sulphation and glucuronidation of paracetamol in human liver: assay conditions, *Biochemical Pharmacology*, **37**, 4405–4407.

Padmore, G. R. A. and Padmore, S. F., 1987, Factors affecting urinary screens for acetaminophen, *Clinical Chemistry*, **33**, 1695–1696.

Pagay, S. N., Poust, R. I. and Colaizzi, J. L., 1974, Influence of vehicle dielectric properties on acetaminophen bioavailability from polyethylene glycol suppositories, *Journal of Pharmaceutical Sciences*, **63**, 44–47.

Pagella, P. G., Faini, D. and Turba, C., 1980, Attivita'del tiazolidincarbossilato di arginine nei confronti dell'intossicazione acuta da paracetamolo nel topo, *Bollettino Chimico Farmaceutico*, **119**, 237–240.

Pakuts, A. P., Whitehouse, L. W. and Paul, C. J., 1988, Plasma sorbitol dehydrogenase determination in experimental hepatotoxicity using the Abbott bichromatic analyzer, *Journal of Clinical Chemistry and Clinical Biochemistry*, **26**, 693–695.

Paller, M. S., 1990, Drug-induced nephropathies, *Medical Clinics of North America*, **74**, 904–917.

Palmas, F., Brazioli, D., Guerra, P., Gardino, L., Aimo, G., Rocca, N. and Verme, G., 1985, Test di svuotamento gastrico con paracetamolo, *Recenti Progressi in Medicina*, **77**, 33–37.

Palmas, F., Brazioli, D., Guerra, P., Gardino, L., Aimo, G., Rocca, N. and Verme, G., 1986, Gastric emptying test by acetaminophen, *Italian Journal of Medicine*, **2**, 37–41.

Palmer, J. L., 1986, Novel method of sample preparation for the determination of paracetamol in plasma by high performance liquid chromatography with electrochemical detection, *Journal of Chromatography: Biomedical Applications*, **382**, 338–342.

Palmer, R. H., Frank, W. O., Nambi, P., Wetherington, J. D. and Fox, M. J., 1991, Effects of various concomitant medications on gastric alcohol dehydrogenase and the first-pass metabolism of ethanol, *American Journal of Gastroenterology*, **86**, 1749–1755.

Pan, T.-H., Wollack, A. R. and DeMarco, J. A., 1975, Malignant hyperthermia associated with enflurane anesthesia: a case report, *Anesthesia and Analgesia*, **54**, 47–49.

Panella, C., Makowka, L., Barone, M., Polimeno, L., Rizzi, S., Demetris, J., Bell, S., Guglielmi, F. W., Prelich, J. G., van Thiel, D. H., Starzl, T. E. and Francavilla, A., 1990, Effect of ranitidine on acetaminophen-induced hepatotoxicity in dogs, *Digestive Diseases and Sciences*, **35**, 385–391.

Pang, K. S., Cherry, W. F., Accaputo, J., Schwab, A. J. and Goresky, C. A., 1988a, Combined hepatic arterial-portal venous and hepatic arterial-hepatic venous perfusions to probe the abundance of drug metabolizing activities: perihepatic venous O-deethylation activity for phenacetin and periportal sulfation activity for acetaminophen in the once-through rat liver preparation, *Journal of Pharmacology and Experimental Therapeutics*, **247**, 690–700.

Pang, K. S. and Gillette, J. R., 1978a, Kinetics of metabolite formation and elimination in the perfused rat liver preparation: differences between the elimination of preformed acetaminophen and acetaminophen formed from phenacetin, *Journal of Pharmacology and Experimental Therapeutics*, **207**, 178–194.

Pang, K. S. and Gillette, J. R., 1978b, Complications in the estimation of hepatic blood flow *in vivo* by pharmacokinetic parameters: the area under the curve after concomitant intravenous and intraperitoneal (or intraportal) administration of acetaminophen in the rat, *Drug Metabolism and Disposition: The Biological Fate of Chemicals*, **6**, 567–576.

Pang, K. S. and Gillette, J. R., 1979, Sequential first-pass elimination of a metabolite derived from a precursor, *Journal of Pharmacokinetics and Biopharmaceutics*, **7**, 275–290.

Pang, K. S., Kong, P., Terrell, J. A. and Billings, R. E., 1985, Metabolism of acetaminophen and phenacetin by isolated rat hepatocytes. A system in which the spatial organization inherent in the liver is disrupted, *Drug Metabolism and Disposition: The Biological Fate of Chemicals*, **13**, 42–50.

Pang, K. S., Lee, W.-F., Cherry, W. F., Yuen, V., Accaputo, J., Fayz, S., Schwab, A. J. and Goresky, C. A., 1988b, Effects of perfusate flow rate on measured blood volume, Disse space, intracellular water space, and drug extraction in the perfused rat liver preparation: characterization by the multiple indicator dilution technique, *Journal of Pharmacokinetics and Biopharmaceutics*, **16**, 595–632.

Pang, K. S. and Mulder, G. J., 1990, The effect of hepatic blood flow on formation of metabolites, *Drug Metabolism and Disposition: The Biological Fate of Chemicals*, **18**, 270–275.

Pang, K. S., Sherman, I. A., Schwab, A. J., Geng, W., Barker, F., Dlugosz, J. A., Cuerrier, G. and Goresky, C. A., 1994, Role of the hepatic artery in the metabolism of phenacetin and acetaminophen: an intravital microscopic and multiple-indicator dilution study in perfused rat liver, *Hepatology*, **20**, 672–683.

Pang, K. S., Strobl, K. and Gillette, J. R., 1979a, A method for the estimation of the fraction of a precursor that is converted to a metabolite in rat *in vivo* with phenacetin and acetaminophen, *Drug Metabolism and Disposition: The Biological Fate of Chemicals*, **7**, 366–372.

Pang, K. S., Taburet, A. M., Hinson, J. A. and Gillette, J. R., 1979b, High-performance liquid chromatographic assay for acetaminophen and phenacetin in the presence of their metabolites in biological fluids, *Journal of Chromatography*, **174**, 165–175.

Pang, K. S. and Terrell, J. A., 1981a, Retrograde perfusion to probe the heterogeneous distribution of hepatic drug metabolizing enzymes in rats, *Journal of Pharmacology and Experimental Therapeutics*, **216**, 339–346.

Pang, K. S. and Terrell, J. A., 1981b, Conjugation kinetics of acetaminophen by the perfused rat liver preparation, *Biochemical Pharmacology*, **30**, 1959–1965.

Pang, K. S., Waller, L., Horning, M. G. and Chan, K. K., 1982, Metabolite kinetics: formation of acetaminophem from deuterated and non-deuterated phenacetin and acetanilide on acetaminophen sulfation kinetics in the perfused rat liver preparation, *Journal of Pharmacology and Experimental Therapeutics*, **222**, 14–19.

Pang, K. S., Xu, N., Chow, A. and Goresky, C. A., 1990, Effects of varying retrograde flows on drug extraction in the perfused rat liver, *European Journal of Pharmacology*, **183**, 1645.

Pang, K. S., Yuen, V., Fayz, S., Te Koppele, J. M. and Mulder, G. J., 1986, Absorption and metabolism of acetaminophen by the *in situ* perfused rat small intestine preparation, *Drug Metabolism and Disposition: The Biological Fate of Chemicals*, **14**, 102–111.

Panos, M. Z., Anderson, J. V., Forbes, A., Payne, N., Slater, J. D. H., Rees, L. and Williams, R., 1991, Human atrial natriuretic factor and renin-aldosterone in paracetamol induced fulminant hepatic failure, *Gut*, **32**, 85–89.

Pantuck, E. J., Pantuck, C. B., Anderson, K. E., Wattenberg, L. W., Conney, A. H. and Kappas, A., 1984, Effect of brussels sprouts and cabbage on drug conjugation, *Clinical Pharmacology and Therapeutics*, **35**, 161–169.

Pantuck, E. J., Pantuck, C. B., Kappas, A., Conney, A. H. and Anderson, K. E., 1991, Effects of protein and carbohydrate content of diet on drug conjugation, *Clinical Pharmacology and Therapeutics*, **50**, 254–258.

Pantuck, E. J., Weissman, C., Pantuck, C. B. and Lee, Y. J., 1989, Effects of parenteral amino acid nutritional regimens on oxidative and conjugative drug metabolism, *Anesthesia and Analgesia*, **69**, 727–731.

Panush, R. S., 1976, Effects of certain antirheumatic drugs on normal human peripheral blood lymphocytes. Inhibition of mitogen- and antigen-stimulated incorporation of tritiated thymidine, *Arthritis and Rheumatism*, **19**, 907–917.

Panush, R. S. and Ossakow, S. J., 1979, Effects of acetaminophen on normal human peripheral blood lymphocytes: enhancement of mitogen- and antigen-stimulated incorporation of tritiated thymidine, *Clinical and Experimental Immunology*, **38**, 539–548.

Parier, J. L., Picard, O., Bonhomme, L., Fredj, G., Ringard, J. and Gluck, C., 1988, Biodisponsibilité du paracétamol selon la forme pharmaceutique après administration orale unique, *Journal de Pharmacie de Belgique*, **43**, 287–291.

Park, G. R. and Weir, D., 1984, A comparison of the effect of oral controlled release morphine and intramuscular morphine on gastric emptying, *Anaesthesia*, **39**, 645–648.

Park, Y., Smith, R. d., Combs, A. B. and Kehrer, J. P., 1988, Prevention of acetaminophen-induced hepatotoxicity by dimethyl sulfoxide, *Toxicology*, **52**, 165–175.

Parker, D., White, J. P., Paton, D. and Routledge, P. A., 1990, Safety of late acetylcysteine treatment in paracetamol poisoning, *Human and Experimental Toxicology*, **9**, 25–27.

Parker, R. S., Morrissey, M. T., Moldéus, P. and Selivonchick, D. P., 1981, The use of isolated hepatocytes from rainbow trout (*Salmo gairdneri*) in the metabolism of acetaminophen, *Comparative Biochemistry and Physiology – B Comparative Biochemistry*, **70**, 631–633.

Parker, R. W. and Shaw, R. E., 1975, Analgesic abuse in urological practice, *British Journal of Surgery*, **62**, 298–302.

Parkhouse, J. and Hallinon, P., 1967, A comparison of aspirin and paracetamol, *British Journal of Anaesthesia*, **39**, 146–154.

Pascoe, G. A., Calleman, C. J. and Baillie, T. A., 1988, Identification of S-(2,5-dihydroxyphenyl)-cysteine and S-(2,5-dihydroxyphenyl)-N-acetyl-cysteine as urinary metabolites of acetaminophen in the mouse. Evidence for p-benzoquinone as a reactive metabolite in acetaminophen metabolism, *Chemico-Biological Interactions*, **68**, 85–98.

Pasquale, G., Scaricabarozzi, I., D'Agostino, R., Taborelli, G. and Vallarino, R., 1993, An assessment of the efficacy and tolerability of nimesulide vs paracetamol in children after adenotonsillectomy, *Drugs*, **46 (Suppl. 1)**, 234–237.

Pataki, A., Hodel, C., Rentsch, G. and Donatsch, P., 1974, Morphological and functional changes in the thyroid after chronic treatment of rats with aniline analgesics, *Excerpta Medica International Congress Series 289: Proceedings of the European Society for the Study of Drug Toxicity*, **15**, 307–312.

Patel, F., 1992, The fatal paracetamol dosage – how low can you go? *Medicine, Science and the Law*, **32**, 303–310.

Patel, H. V. and Morton, D. J., 1988, Specificity of a colorimetric paracetamol assay technique for use in cases of overdose, *Journal of Clinical Pharmacy and Therapeutics*, **13**, 233–238.

Patel, M., Tang, B. K. and Kalow, W., 1992, Variability of acetaminophen metabolism in Caucasians and Orientals, *Pharmacogenetics*, **2**, 38–45.

Patierno, S. R., Lehman, N. L., Henderson, B. E. and Landolph, J. R., 1989, Study of the ability of phenacetin, acetaminophen, and aspirin to induce cytotoxicity, mutation, and morphological transformation in C3H/10T$\frac{1}{2}$ clone 8 mouse embryo cells, *Cancer Research*, **49**, 1038–1044.

Patten, C. J., Thomas, P. E., Guy, R. L., Lee, M., Gonzalez, F. J., Guengerich, F. P. and Yang, C. S., 1993, Cytochrome P-450 enzymes involved in acetaminophen activation by rat and human liver microsomes and their kinetics, *Chemical Research in Toxicology*, **6**, 511–518.

Paulozzi, L. J., 1983, Seasonality of reported poison exposures, *Pediatrics*, **71**, 891–893.

Paulsen, H. and Kreilgård, B., 1984, Bioavailability of paracetamol after single oral and rectal administration, *Archives of Pharmaceutical Chemistry Sciences Edition*, **12**, 97–102.

Pavlovich, D., Uzunova, P., Galabova, T., Peneva, V., Sokolova, Z., Koracevic, D., Tsanev, R. and Ribarov, S., 1991, Paracetamol as a radical scavenger, *Journal of Clinical Biochemistry and Nutrition*, **11**, 171–182.

Pawlak, D. F., Itkin, A. B., Lapeyrolerie, F. M. and Zweig, B., 1978, Clinical effects of aspirin and acetaminophen on hemostasis after exodontics, *Journal of Oral Surgery*, **36**, 944–947.

Pearce, I., Frank, G. J. and Pearce, J. M. S., 1983, Ibuprofen compared with paracetamol in migraine, *Practitioner*, **277**, 465–467.

Pearson, H. A., 1978, Comparative effects of aspirin and acetaminophen on hemostasis, *Pediatrics*, **62 (Suppl.)**, 926–929.

Peatfield, R. C., Petty, R. G. and Rose, F. C., 1983, Double blind comparison of mefenamic acid and acetaminophen (paracetamol) in migraine, *Cephalalgia*, **3**, 129–134.

Pedersen, C. M., Rasmussen, H. B., Jensen, P. B. and Jørgensen, K. A., 1993, Akut nyresvigt foråsaget af paracetamolforgiftning, *Ugeskrift for Læger*, **155**, 1720–1721.

Pedraz, J. L., Alonso, E., Calvo, M. B., Lanao, J. M. and Dominguez-Gil, A., 1988a, Bioequivalence study of two oral formulations of paracetamol, *International Journal of Clinical Pharmacology, Therapy and Toxicology*, **26**, 232–236.

Pedraz, J. L., Calvo, M. B., Lanao, J. M. and Dominguez-Gil, A., 1988b, Choice of optimum pharmacokinetic model of orally administered paracetamol, *Biopharmaceutics and Drug Disposition*, **9**, 389–396.

Peggins, J. O., McMahon, T. F., Beierschmitt, W. P. and Weiner, M., 1987, Comparison of hepatic and renal metabolism of acetaminophen in male and female miniature swine, *Drug Metabolism and Disposition: The Biological Fate of Chemicals*, **15**, 270–273.

Pegon, Y. and Vallon, J. J., 1981, Extraction du paracétamol par relargage de solvant et application au dosage par chromatographie en phase gazeuse dans le plasma, *Analytica Chimica Acta*, **130**, 405–408.

Peleg, I. I., Maibach, H. T., Brown, S. H. and Wilcox, C. M., 1994, Aspirin and nonsteroidal anti-inflammatory drug use and the risk of subsequent colorectal cancer, *Archives of Internal Medicine*, **154**, 394–399.

Pélissier, T., Alloui, A., Caussade, F., Cloarec, A., Lavarenne, J. and Eschallier, A., 1994, Evidence for a spinal tropisetron-inhibited antinociceptive effect of paracetamol, *Fundamental and Clinical Pharmacology*, **8**, 263.

Pendergrass, P. B., Ream, L. J., Scott, J. N. and Agna, M. A., 1984, Do aspirin and acetaminophen affect total menstrual loss? *Gynecologic and Obstetric Investigation*, **18**, 129–133.

Pendergrass, P. B., Scott, J. N., Ream, L. J. and Agna, M. A., 1985, Effect of small doses of aspirin and acetaminophen on total menstrual loss and pain of cramps and headache, *Gynecologic and Obstetric Investigation*, **19**, 32–37.

Penna, A. and Buchanan, N., 1991, Paracetamol poisoning in children and hepatotoxicity, *British Journal of Clinical Pharmacology*, **32**, 143–149.

Penna, A. C., Dawson, K. P. and Penna, C. M., 1993, Is prescribing paracetamol 'pro re nata' acceptable? *Journal of Paediatrics and Child Health*, **29**, 104–106.

Pereira, L. M. M. B., Langley, P. G., Hayllar, K. M., Tredger, J. M. and Williams, R., 1992, Coagulation factor V and VIII/V ratio as predictors of outcome in paracetamol induced fulminant hepatic failure: relation to other prognostic indicators, *Gut*, **33**, 98–102.

Perkins, M. N. and Campbell, E. A., 1992, Capsazepine reversal of the antinociceptive action of capsaicin *in vivo*, *British Journal of Pharmacology*, **107**, 329–333.

Perlík, F., Janku, I. and Kordac, V., 1988, The effect of guaiphenesin on absorption and bioavailability of paracetamol from composite analgesic preparations, *International Journal of Clinical Pharmacology, Therapy and Toxicology*, **26**, 413–416.

Pernambuco, J. R. B., Langley, P. G., Hughes, R. D., Izumi, S. and Williams, R., 1993, Activation of the fibrinolytic system in patients with fulminant liver failure, *Hepatology*, **18**, 1350–1356.

Perneger, T. V., Whelton, P. K. and Klag, M. J., 1994, Risk of kidney failure associated with the use of acetaminophen, aspirin, and non-steroidal antiinflammatory drugs, *New England Journal of Medicine*, **331**, 1675–1679.

Perrot, N., Nalpas, B., Yang, C. S. and Beaune, P. H., 1989, Modulation of cytochrome P-450 isozymes in human liver, by ethanol and drug intake, *European Journal of Clinical Investigation*, **19**, 549–555.

Persaud, C. and Jackson, A. A., 1991, 5-L-oxoprolinuria and glycine sufficiency, *Clinical Chemistry*, **37**, 1660–1661.

Persaud, N., Johnson, E. S., Merrington, D. and Oliver, W., 1985, The relative bioavailability of paracetamol and codeine after oral administration of a combination of buclizine, paracetamol and codeine, with or without docusate, and of paracetamol alone in healthy volunteers, *Current Medical Research and Opinion*, **9**, 626–633.

Persson, H., 1991, Forgiftningsrisk vid subakut 'terapeutisk' overdosering av paracetamol, *Läkartidningen*, **88**, 3678–3681.

Perucca, E. and Richens, A., 1979, Paracetamol disposition in normal subjects and in patients treated with antiepileptic drugs, *British Journal of Clinical Pharmacology*, **7**, 201–206.

Peskar, B. M., 1977, On the synthesis of prostaglandins by human gastric mucosa and its modification by drugs, *Biochimica et Biophysica Acta*, **487**, 307–314.

Pessayre, D., Dolder, A., Artigou, J.-Y., Wandscheer, J.-C., Descatoire, V., Degott, C. and Benhamou, J.-P., 1979, Effect of fasting on metabolite-mediated hepatotoxicity in the rat, *Gastroenterology*, **77**, 264–271.

Pessayre, D., Wandscheer, J.-C., Cobert, B., Level, R., Degott, C., Batt, A. M., Martin, N. and Benhamou, J.-P., 1980, Additive effects of inducers and fasting on acetaminophen hepatotoxicity, *Biochemical Pharmacology*, **29**, 2219–2223.

Peters, B. H., Fraim, C. J. and Masel, B. E., 1983, Comparison of 650 mg aspirin and 1000 mg acetaminophen with each other, and with placebo in moderately severe headache, *American Journal of Medicine*, **74**, 36–42.

Peters, G., Baechtold-Fowler, N., Bonjour, J. P., Chométy-Diézi, F., Filloux, B., Guidoux, R., Guignard, J. P., Peters-Haefeli, L., Roch-Ramel, F., Schelling, J.-L., Hedinger, C. and Weber, E., 1972, General and renal toxicity of phenacetin, paracetamol and some antimitotic agents in the rat, *Archives of Toxicology*, **28**, 225–269.

Petersen, K.-U., 1993, Omeprazol und das cytochrom P-450-System der Leber, *Leber Magen Darm*, **23**, 186–192.

Petersen, P. and Vilstrup, H., 1979, Relation between liver function and hepatocyte ultrastructure in a case of paracetamol intoxication, *Digestion*, **19**, 415–419.

Peterson, F. J., Holloway, D. E., Erickson, R. R., Duquette, P. H., McClain, C. J. and Holtzman, J. L., 1980, Ethanol induction of acetaminophen toxicity and metabolism, *Life Sciences*, **27**, 1705–1711.

Peterson, F. J. and Knodell, R. G., 1984, Ascorbic acid protects against acetaminophen- and cocaine-induced hepatic damage in mice, *Drug-Nutrient Interactions*, **3**, 33–41.

Peterson, F. J., Knodell, R. G., Lindemann, N. J. and Steele, N. M., 1983, Prevention of acetaminophen and cocaine hepatotoxicity in mice by cimetidine treatment, *Gastroenterology*, **85**, 122–129.

Peterson, F. J., Lindemann, N. J., Duquette, P. H. and Holtzman, J. L., 1992, Potentiation of acute acetaminophen lethality by selenium and vitamin E deficiency in mice, *Journal of Nutrition*, **122**, 74–81.

Peterson, R. G., 1985, Antipyretics and analgesics in children, *Developmental Pharmacology and Therapeutics*, **8**, 68–84.

Peterson, R. G. and Rumack, B. H., 1977, Treating acute acetaminophen poisoning with acetylcysteine, *Journal of the American Medical Association*, **237**, 2406–2407.

Peterson, R. G. and Rumack, B. H., 1978, Pharmacokinetics of acetaminophen in children, *Pediatrics*, **62 (Suppl.)**, 877–879.

Peterson, R. G. and Rumack, B. H., 1981, Age as a variable in acetaminophen overdose, *Archives of Internal Medicine*, **141**, 390–393.

Peterson, T. C. and Brown, I. R., 1992, Cysteamine in combination with N-acetylcysteine prevents acetaminophen-induced hepatotoxicity, *Canadian Journal of Physiology and Pharmacology*, **70**, 20–28.

Peterson, T. C., Peterson, M. R. and Williams, C. N., 1989, The role of heme oxygenase and aryl hydrocarbon hydroxylase in the protection by cysteamine from acetaminophen hepatotoxicity, *Toxicology and Applied Pharmacology*, **97**, 430–439.

Petring, O. U., Adelhøj, B., Crawford, M., Angelo, H. and Jelert, H., 1988, The effect of droperidol on fentanyl-influenced gastric emptying in man, *Acta Anaesthesiologica Scandinavica*, **32**, 21–23.

Petring, O. U., Adelløj, B., Erin-Madsen, J., Angelo, H. and Jelert, H., 1984, Epidural anaesthesia does not delay early postoperative gastric emptying in man, *Acta Anaesthesiologica Scandinavica*, **28**, 393–395.

Petring, O. U., Adelhøj, B., Ibsen, M., Brynnum, J. and Poulsen, H. E., 1985, Abstaining from cigarette smoking has no major effect on gastric emptying in habitual smokers, *British Journal of Anaesthesia*, **57**, 1104–1106.

Petring, O. U., Adelhøj, B., Ibsen, M. and Poulsen, H. E., 1986, The relationship between gastric emptying of semisolids and paracetamol absorption, *British Journal of Clinical Pharmacology*, **22**, 659–662.

Petring, O. U., Adelhøj, B., Ibsen, M. and Poulsen, H. E., 1987, Effect of chlorpromazine on drug absorption and gastric emptying in man, *Canadian Journal of Anaesthesia*, **34**, 563–565.

Petring, O. U. and Flachs, H., 1990, Inter- and intrasubject variability of gastric emptying in healthy volunteers measured by scintigraphy and paracetamol absorption, *British Journal of Clinical Pharmacology*, **29**, 703–708.

Petrus, M., 1983, Essai du soluté buvable de paracétamol chez l'enfant fébrile, *Annales de Pédiatrie*, **30**, 131–133.

Petruson, B., Hahn, L., Korsan-Bengtsen, K. and Hallberg, L., 1977, Influence of acetylsalicylic acid and paracetamol on menstrual blood loss, *Haemostasis*, **6**, 266–268.

Petti, A., 1985, Postoperative pain relief with pentazocine and acetaminophen: comparison with other analgesic combinations and placebo, *Clinical Therapeutics*, **8**, 126–133.

Pezzano, M., Richard, Ch., Lampl, E., Pelletier, G., Fabre, M., Rimailho, A. and Auzépy, Ph., 1988, Toxicité hépatique et rénal du paracétamol chez l'alcoolique chronique, *Presse Médicale*, **17**, 21–24.

Pflüger, K.-H., 1980, Toxikologie und Therapie der Paracetamolvergiftung, *Internist*, **21**, 735–738.

Phadke, M. A., Paranjape, P. V. and Joshi, A. S., 1985, Ibuprofen in children with infective disorders – antipyretic efficacy, *British Journal of Clinical Practice*, **39**, 437–440.

Phillips, S., Hutchinson, S. and Ruggier, R., 1993, *Zingiber officinale* does not affect gastric emptying rate. A randomized, placebo-controlled, crossover trial, *Anaesthesia*, **48**, 393–395.

Piatkowski, T. S., Day, W. W. and Weiner, M., 1993, Increased renal drug metabolism in treadmill-exercised Fischer-344 male rats, *Drug Metabolism and Disposition: The Biological Fate of Chemicals*, **21**, 474–479.

Picciòla, G., Zavaglio, G., Ravenna, F., Gentili, P., Tempra-Gabbiati, G., Carenini, G. and Riva, M., 1986, Derivati della metionina ad attività epatoprotettrice, *Farmaco – Edizione*

Scientifica, **41**, 758–780.

Pickworth, W. B., Klein, S. A., George, F. R. and Henningfield, J. E., 1992, Acetaminophen fails to inhibit ethanol-induced subjective effects in human volunteers, *Pharmacology, Biochemistry and Behavior*, **41**, 189–194.

Picozzi, A. and Ross, N. M., 1989, A survey of dentists' drug prescribing practices, *American Journal of Dentistry*, **2**, 338–340.

Pietsch, I., Gmyrek, D., David, H., Behrisch, D. and Syllm-Rapoport, I., 1972, Paracetamol-belastung zur Beurteilung der reifenden Glukuronidierungsfunktion bei Frühgeborenen, *Pädiatrie und Grenzgebiete*, **11**, 171–178.

Piguet, V., Desmeules, J. A., Collart, L. and Dayer, P., 1994, Quelle posologie antalgique du paracétamol? *Schweizerische Medizinische Wochenschrift*, **124**, 2196–2198.

Piletta, P., Porchet, H. C. and Dayer, P., 1990, L'effet analgésique central du paracétamol, *Schweizerische Medizinische Wochenschrift*, **120**, 1950–1951.

Piletta, P., Porchet, H. C. and Dayer, P., 1991, Central analgesic effect of acetaminophen but not of aspirin, *Clinical Pharmacology and Therapeutics*, **49**, 350–354.

Pillans, P. and Hall, C., 1985, Paracetamol-induced acute renal failure in the absence of severe liver damage, *South African Medical Journal*, **67**, 791–792.

Pimstone, B. L. and Uys, C. J., 1968, Liver necrosis and myocardiopathy following paracetamol overdosage, *South African Medical Journal*, **42**, 259–262.

Piper, D. W., McIntosch, J. H., Greig, M. and Shy, C. M., 1982, Environmental factors and chronic gastric ulcer. A case control study of the association of smoking, alcohol, and heavy analgesic ingestion with the exacerbation of chronic gastric ulcer, *Scandinavian Journal of Gastroenterology*, **17**, 721–729.

Piper, D. W. and McIntosh, J. H., 1988, Paracetamol and peptic ulcer, *Lancet*, **ii**, 1192.

Piper, D. W., McIntosh, J. H., Ariotti, D. E., Fenton, B. H. and MacLennan, R., 1981, Analgesic ingestion and chronic peptic ulcer, *Gastroenterology*, **80**, 427–432.

Piper, J. M., Matanoski, G. M. and Tonascia, J., 1986, Bladder cancer in young women, *American Journal of Epidemiology*, **123**, 1033–1042.

Piper, J. M., Tonascia, J. and Matanoski, G. M., 1985, Heavy phenacetin use and bladder cancer in women aged 20 to 49 years, *New England Journal of Medicine*, **313**, 292–295.

Piperno, E. and Berssenbruegge, D. A., 1976, Reversal of experimental paracetamol toxicosis with N-acetylcysteine, *Lancet*, **ii**, 738–739.

Piperno, E., Mosher, A. H., Berssenbruegge, D. A., Winkler, J. D. and Smith, R. B., 1978, Pathophysiology of acetaminophen overdosage toxicity: implications for management, *Pediatrics*, **62 (Suppl.)**, 880–889.

Pircio, A. W., Buyniski, J. P. and Roebel, L. E., 1978, Pharmacological effects of a combination of butorphanol and acetaminophen, *Archives Internationales de Pharmacodynamie et de Thérapie*, **235**, 116–123.

Pirotte, J. H., 1984, Apparent potentiation by phenobarbital of hepatotoxicity from small doses of acetaminophen, *Annals of Internal Medicine*, **101**, 403.

Pitt, J. J., 1990, Association between paracetamol and pyroglutamic aciduria, *Clinical Chemistry*, **36**, 173–174.

Pitt, J. J., Brown, G. K., Clift, V. and Christodoulou, J., 1990, Atypical pyroglutamic aciduria: possible role of paracetamol, *Journal of Inherited Metabolic Disease*, **13**, 755–756.

Pitts, J., 1979, False-positive paracetamol assay, *Lancet*, **i**, 213–214.

Pizziketti, R. J., Pressman, N. S., Geller, E. B., Cowan, A. and Adler, M. W., 1985, Rat cold water tail-flick: a novel analgesic test that distinguishes opioid agonists from mixed agonist-antagonists, *European Journal of Pharmacology*, **119**, 23–29.

Placke, M. E., Ginsberg, G. L., Wyand, D. S. and Cohen, S. D., 1987a, Ultrastructural changes during acute acetaminophen-induced hepatotoxicity in the mouse: a time and dose study, *Toxicologic Pathology*, **15**, 431–438.

Placke, M. E., Wyand, D. S. and Cohen, S. D., 1987b, Extrahepatic lesions induced by acetaminophen in the mouse, *Toxicologic Pathology*, **15**, 381–387.

Plakogiannis, F. M. and Saad, A. M., 1978, Quantitative determination of acetaminophen in plasma, *Journal of Pharmaceutical Sciences*, **67**, 531.

Platt, S., Hawton, K., Kreitman, N., Fagg, J. and Foster, J., 1988, Recent clinical and epidemiological trends in parasuicide in Edinburgh and Oxford: a tale of two cities, *Psychological Medicine*, **18**, 405–418.

Pletscher, A., Studer, A. and Miescher, P., 1958, Experimentelle Untersuchungen über Erythrocyten- und Organveränderungen durch N-acetyl-p-aminophenol und Phenacetin, *Schweizerische Medizinische Wochenschrift*, **88**, 1214–1216.

Ploin, M., 1990, Le paracétamol en 1990: un centenaire en pleine santé, *Gazette Médicale de France*, **97**, 76.

Plotz, P. H. and Kimberly, R. P., 1981, Acute effects of aspirin and acetaminophen on renal function, *Archives of Internal Medicine*, **141**, 343–348.

Podder, S. K., Nakamura, T., Nakashima, M., Sazaki, H., Nakamura, J. and Shibasaki, J., 1988, Comparison of salicylamide and acetaminophen and their prodrug disposition in dogs, *Journal of Pharmacobiodynamics*, **11**, 324–329.

Poelma, F. G. J., Breäs, R. and Tukker, J. J., 1990, Intestinal absorption of drugs. III. The influence of taurocholate on the disappearance kinetics of hydrophilic and lipophilic drugs from the small intestine of the rat, *Pharmaceutical Research*, **7**, 392–397.

Poelma, F. G. J., Breäs, R., Tukker, J. J. and Crommelin, D. J. A., 1991, Intestinal absorption of drugs. The influence of mixed micelles on on the disappearance kinetics of drugs from the small intestine of the rat, *Journal of Pharmacy and Pharmacology*, **43**, 317–324.

Pohl, L. R., 1993, An immunochemical approach of identifying and characterizing protein targets of toxic reactive metabolites, *Chemical Research in Toxicology*, **6**, 786–793.

Polidori, G., Titti, G., Pieragostini, P., Comito, A. and Scaricabarozzi, I., 1993, A comparison of nimesulide and paracetamol in the treatment of fever due to inflammatory diseases of the upper respiratory tract in children, *Drugs*, **46 (Suppl. 1)**, 231–233.

Polity, M. P., Patzina, E. A. and Unger, C. P., 1993, Estudo da eficácia, início de açao e tolerabilidade de dose única de 750 mg de paracetamol no controle sintomático da cefaléia, em pacientes ambulatoriais, *Revista Brasileira de Medicina*, **50**, 229–231.

Pomiersky, Ch. and Blaich, E., 1985, Arzneimittelbedingte Hepatitis mit Cholestase nach Therapie mit Chlormezanon, *Zeitschrift für Gastroenterologie*, **23**, 684–686.

Pommer, W., Bronder, E., Greiser, E., Helmert, U., Jesdinsky, H. J., Klimpel, A., Borner, K. and Molzahn, M., 1989, Regular analgesic intake and the risk of end-stage renal failure, *American Journal of Nephrology*, **9**, 403–412.

Pommer, W., Glaeske, G. and Molzahn, M., 1986, The analgesic problem in the Federal Republic of Germany: analgesic consumption, frequency of analgesic nephropathy and regional differences, *Clinical Nephrology*, **26**, 273–278.

Pond, S., Jacob, P., Humphreys, M., Weiss, R. and Tong, T., 1982a, Impaired metabolism of methylphenobarbital after a combined drug overdose: treatment by resin hemoperfusion, *Journal of Toxicology. Clinical Toxicology*, **19**, 187–196.

Pond, S. M., Tong, T. G., Kaysen, G. A., Menke, D. J., Galinsky, R. E., Roberts, S. M. and Levy, G., 1982b, Massive intoxication with acetaminophen and propoxyphene: unexpected survival and unusual pharmacokinetics of acetaminophen, *Journal of Toxicology. Clinical Toxicology*, **19**, 1–16.

Pons, G., Badoual, J. and Olive, G., 1990, Posologie optimale du paracétamol chez l'enfant, *Archives Françaises Pédiatrie*, **47**, 539–542.

Ponsoda, X., Jover, R., Gómez-Lechón, M. J., Fabra, R., Trullenque, R. and Castell, J. V., 1991, Intracellular glutathione in human hepatocytes incubated with S-adenosyl-L-methionine and GSH-depleting drugs, *Toxicology*, **70**, 293–302.

Poon, Y. K., Cho, C. H. and Ogle, C. W., 1988a, Sub-diaphragmatic vagotomy attenuates the protective action of paracetamol against ethanol-induced gastric damage in rats, *Medical Science Research*, **16**, 1285.

Poon, Y. K., Cho, C. H. and Ogle, C. W., 1988b, Paracetamol confers resistance to ethanol-induced gastric mucosal damage in rats, *Journal of Pharmacy and Pharmacology*, **40**, 478–481.

Poon, Y. K., Cho, C. H. and Ogle, C. W., 1989, The protective mechanisms of paracetamol against ethanol-induced gastric mucosal damage in rats, *Journal of Pharmacy and Pharmacology*, **41**, 563–565.

Pootrakul, P. and Panich, V., 1983, Effect of acetaminophen on glucose-6-phosphate dehydrogenase, Mahidol variant, *Acta Haematologica*, **69**, 358–359.

Porowski, P., Joeres, R., Zilly, W. and Richter, E., 1988, Metabolitausscheidung von Paracetamol bei Patienten mit alkoholtoxischer Lebercirrhose, *Zeitschrift für Gastroenterologie*, **26**, 60.

Porpaczy, P. and Schramek, P., 1981, Analgesic nephropathy and phenacetin-induced transitional cell carcinoma – analysis of 300 patients with long-term consumption of phenacetin-containing drugs, *European Urology*, **7**, 349–354.

Porta, P., Aebi, S., Summer, K. and Lauterburg, B. H., 1991, L-2-Oxothiazolidine-4-carboxylic acid, a cysteine prodrug: pharmacokinetics and effects on thiols in plasma and lymphocytes in human, *Journal of Pharmacology and Experimental Therapeutics*, **257**, 331–334.

Portenoy, R. K. and Kanner, R. M., 1985, Patterns of analgesic prescription and consumption in a university-affiliated community hospital, *Archives of Internal Medicine*, **145**, 439–441.

Porter, J. D. H., Robinson, P. H., Glasgow, J. F. T., Banks, J. H. and Hall, S. M., 1990, Trends in the incidence of Reye's syndrome and the use of aspirin, *Archives of Disease in Childhood*, **65**, 826–829.

Porter, K. E. and Dawson, A. G., 1979, Inhibition of respiration and gluconeogenesis by paracetamol in rat kidney preparations, *Biochemical Pharmacology*, **28**, 3057–3062.

Portmann, B., Talbot, I. C., Day, D. W., Davidson, A. R., Murray-Lyon, I. M. and Williams, R., 1975, Histopathological changes in the liver following a paracetamol overdose: correlation with clinical and biochemical parameters, *Journal of Pathology*, **117**, 169–181.

Porubek, D. J., Rundgren, M., Harvison, P. J., Nelson, S. D. and Moldéus, P., 1987, Investigation of mechanisms of acetaminophen toxicity in isolated rat hepatocytes with acetaminophen analogues 3,5-dimethylacetaminophen and 2,6-dimethylacetaminophen, *Molecular Pharmacology*, **31**, 647–653.

Poss, W. B., Vernon, D. D. and Dean, J. M., 1994, A reemergence of Reye's syndrome, *Archives of Pediatrics and Adolescent Medicine*, **148**, 879–882.

Pottage, A., Nimmo, J. and Prescott, L. F., 1974, The absorption of aspirin and paracetamol in patients with achlorhydria, *Journal of Pharmacy and Pharmacology*, **26**, 144–145.

Potter, D. W. and Hinson, J. A., 1986a, Reactions of N-acetyl-p-benzoquinoneimine with reduced glutathione, acetaminophen, and NADPH, *Molecular Pharmacology*, **30**, 33–41.

Potter, D. W. and Hinson, J. A., 1986b, Reactions of glutathione with oxidative intermediates of acetaminophen, *Advances in Experimental Medicine and Biology*, **197**, 763–772.

Potter, D. W. and Hinson, J. A., 1987a, Mechanisms of acetaminophen oxidation to N-acetyl-p-benzoquinoneimine by horseradish peroxidase and cytochrome P-450, *Journal of Biological Chemistry*, **262**, 966–973.

Potter, D. W. and Hinson, J. A., 1987b, The 1- and 2-electron oxidation of acetaminophen catalyzed by prostaglandin H synthase, *Journal of Biological Chemistry*, **262**, 974–980.

Potter, D. W. and Hinson, J. A., 1989, Acetaminophen peroxidation reactions, *Drug Metabolism Reviews*, **20**, 341–358.

Potter, D. W., Miller, D. W. and Hinson, J. A., 1985, Identification of acetaminophen polymerization products catalyzed by horseradish peroxidase, *Journal of Biological Chemistry*, **260**, 12174–12180.

Potter, D. W., Miller, D. W. and Hinson, J. A., 1986, Horseradish peroxidase-catalyzed oxidation of acetaminophen to intermediates that form polymers or conjugate with glutathione, *Molecular Pharmacology*, **29**, 155–162.

Potter, D. W., Pumford, N. R., Hinson, J. A., Benson, R. W. and Roberts, D. W., 1989, Epitope characterization of acetaminophen bound to protein and nonprotein sulhydryl groups by an enzyme-linked immunosorbent assay, *Journal of Pharmacology and Experimental Therapeutics*, **248**, 182–189.

Potter, W. Z., Davis, D. C., Mitchell, J. R., Jollow, D. J., Gillette, J. R. and Brodie, B. B., 1973, Acetaminophen-induced hepatic necrosis. III. Cytochrome P-450-mediated covalent binding *in vitro*, *Journal of Pharmacology and Experimental Therapeutics*, **187**, 203–210.

Potter, W. Z., Thorgeirsson, S. S., Jollow, D. J. and Mitchell, J. R., 1974, Acetaminophen-induced hepatic necrosis. V. Correlation of hepatic necrosis, covalent binding and glutathione depletion in hamsters, *Pharmacology*, **12**, 129–143.

Poulsen, H. E. and Andreasen, P. B., 1980, Dissociation of subcellular functions in paracetamol induced liver damage in the rat, *Gastroenterology*, **79**, 1120.

Poulsen, H. E., Jørgensen, L. and Thomsen, P., 1987, Prevention of acetaminophen hepatotoxicity by disulfiram, *Pharmacology and Therapeutics*, **33**, 83.

Poulsen, H. E., Lerche, A. and Pedersen, N. T., 1985a, Potentiated hepatotoxicity from concurrent administration of acetaminophen and allyl alcohol to rats, *Biochemical Pharmacology*, **34**, 727–731.

Poulsen, H. E., Lerche, A. and Pedersen, N. T., 1985b, Phenobarbital induction does not potentiate hepatotoxicity but accelerates liver cell necrosis from acetaminophen overdose in the rat, *Pharmacology*, **30**, 100–108.

Poulsen, H. E., Lerche, A. and Skovgaard, L. T., 1985c, Acetaminophen metabolism by the perfused rat liver twelve hours after acetaminophen overdose, *Biochemical Pharmacology*, **34**, 3729–3733.

Poulsen, H. E., Petersen, P. and Vilstrup, H., 1981, Quantitative liver function and morphology after paracetamol administration to rats, *European Journal of Clinical Investigation*, **11**, 161–164.

Poulsen, H. E. and Ranek, L., 1984, Paracetamolforgiftning, *Ugeskrift for Læger*, **146**, 4030–4033.

Poulsen, H. E., Ranek, L. and Jørgensen, L., 1991, The influence of disulfiram on acetaminophen metabolism in man, *Xenobiotica*, **21**, 243–249.

Poulsen, H. E. and Thomsen, P., 1988, Long-term administration of toxic doses of paracetamol (acetaminophen) to rats, *Liver*, **8**, 151–156.

Poulsen, H. E., Vilstrup, H., Almdal, T. and Dalhoff, K., 1993, No net splanchnic release of glutathione in man during N-acetylcysteine infusion, *Scandinavian Journal of Gastroenterology*, **28**, 408–412.

Pounder, D. J. and Yonemitsu, K., 1991, Postmortem absorption of drugs and ethanol from aspirated vomitus: an experimental model, *Forensic Science International*, **51**, 189–195.

Pour, A. M., McMillan, D. A., Blacker, A. and Schnell, R. C., 1985, Amelioration of acetaminophen hepatotoxicity in male rats by zinc, *Toxicologist*, **5**, 154.

Power, I., Easton, J. C., Todd, J. G. and Nimmo, W. S., 1989, Gastric emptying after head injury, *Anaesthesia*, **44**, 563–566.

Powers, B. J., Cattau, E. L. and Zimmerman, H. J., 1986, Chlorzoxazone hepatotoxic reactions. An analysis of 21 identified or presumed cases, *Archives of Internal Medicine*, **146**, 1183–1186.

Powis, G., Svingen, B. A., Dahlin, D. C. and Nelson, S. D., 1984, Enzymatic and non-enzymatic reduction of N-acetyl-p-benzoquinone imine and some properties of the N-acetyl-p-benzoquinone imine radical, *Biochemical Pharmacology*, **33**, 2367–2370.

Pradeep Kumar, N., Sethuraman, K. R., Chandrasekar, S., Ray, K., Adithan, C. and Shashindran, C. H., 1987, Salivary paracetamol elimination in patients with congestive cardiac failure, *Clinical and Experimental Pharmacology and Physiology*, **14**, 731–734.

Pradeep Kumar, N., Sethuraman, K. R., Chandrasekar, S., Ray, K., Shashindran, C. H. and Adithan, C., 1989, Paracetamol elimination in patients with tricuspid regurgitation without cardiac failure, *Indian Journal of Physiology and Pharmacology*, **33**, 70–71.

628

Prakongpan, S., Puncoke, R. and Nagai, T., 1993, Comparative bioavailability study of aceta-minophen solutions used in hospital formulary, *Biological and Pharmaceutical Bulletin*, **16**, 613–615.

Prasad, J. S., Chen, N., Liu, Y., Goon, D. J. W. and Holtzman, J. L., 1990, Effects of ethanol and inhibitors on the binding and metabolism of acetaminophen and N-acetyl-p-benzo-quinoneimine by hepatic microsomes from control and ethanol-treated rats, *Biochemical Pharmacology*, **40**, 1989–1995.

Prasuhn, L. W., 1983, Tylenol poisoning in the cat, *Journal of the American Veterinary Medical Association*, **182**, 4.

Pratt, S. and Ioannides, C., 1985, Mechanisms of the protective action of n-acetylcysteine and methionine against paracetamol toxicity in the hamster, *Archives of Toxicology*, **57**, 173–177.

Prescott, L. F., 1965, Effects of acetylsalicylic acid, phenacetin, paracetamol, and caffeine on renal tubular epithelium, *Lancet*, **ii**, 91–96.

Prescott, L. F., 1966a, The nephrotoxicity of analgesics, *Journal of Pharmacy and Pharmacology*, **18**, 331–344.

Prescott, L. F., 1966b, Analgesic abuse and renal disease in Northeast Scotland, *Lancet*, **ii**, 1143–1145.

Prescott, L. F., 1969, The metabolism of phenacetin in patients with renal disease, *Clinical Pharmacology and Therapeutics*, **10**, 383–394.

Prescott, L. F., 1971a, Gas-liquid chromatographic estimation of phenacetin and paracetamol in plasma and urine, *Journal of Pharmacy and Pharmacology*, **23**, 111–115.

Prescott, L. F., 1971b, Gas-liquid chromatographic estimation of paracetamol, *Journal of Pharmacy and Pharmacology*, **23**, 807–808.

Prescott, L. F., 1972, Haemodialysis in paracetamol self-poisoning, *Lancet*, **ii**, 652.

Prescott, L. F., 1974, Gastrointestinal absorption of drugs, *Medical Clinics of North America*, **58**, 907–916.

Prescott, L. F., 1978, Prevention of hepatic necrosis following paracetamol overdosage, *Health Bulletin*, **36**, 204–212.

Prescott, L. F., 1979a, Paracetamol poisoning: prevention of liver damage, *Médecine et Chirurgie Digestives*, **8**, 391–393.

Prescott, L. F., 1979b, The nephrotoxicity and hepatotoxicity of analgesics, *British Journal of Clinical Pharmacology*, **7**, 453–462.

Prescott, L. F., 1980, Kinetics and metabolism of paracetamol and phenacetin, *British Journal of Clinical Pharmacology*, **10 (Suppl. 2)**, 291S–298S.

Prescott, L. F., 1981, Treatment of severe acetaminophen poisoning with intravenous acetyl-cysteine, *Archives of Internal Medicine*, **141**, 386–389.

Prescott, L. F., 1982a, Analgesic nephropathy: a reassessment of the role of phenacetin and other analgesics, *Drugs*, **23**, 75–149.

Prescott, L. F., 1982b, Analgesic overdosage – an overview of the problem, *Royal Society of Medicine International Congress and Symposium Series*, **52**, 19–26.

Prescott, L. F., 1983, Paracetamol overdosage: pharmacological considerations and clinical management, *Drugs*, **25**, 290–314.

Prescott, L. F., 1984, Drug conjugation in clinical toxicology, *Biochemical Society Transactions*, **12**, 96–99.

Prescott, L. F., 1986a, Liver damage with non-narcotic analgesics, *Medical Toxicology*, **1 (Suppl. 1)**, 44–56.

Prescott, L. F., 1986b, Effects of non-narcotic analgesics on the liver, *Drugs*, **32 (Suppl. 4)**, 129–147.

Prescott, L. F., 1995, unpublished observations.

Prescott, L. F. and Critchley, J. A. J. H., 1983a, Drug interactions affecting analgesic toxicity, *American Journal of Medicine*, **75 (5A)**, 113–116.

Prescott, L. F. and Critchley, J. A. J. H., 1983b, The treatment of acetaminophen poisoning,

Annual Review of Pharmacology and Toxicology, **23**, 87–101.

Prescott, L. F. and Critchley, J. A. J. H., 1984, Asthma associated with N-acetylcysteine infusion and paracetamol poisoning, *British Medical Journal*, **288**, 151.

Prescott, L. F., Critchley, J. A. J. H., Balali-Mood, M. and Pentland, B., 1981, Effects of microsomal enzyme induction on paracetamol metabolism in man, *British Journal of Clinical Pharmacology*, **12**, 149–153.

Prescott, L. F., Donovan, J. W., Jarvie, D. R. and Proudfoot, A. T., 1989a, The disposition and kinetics of intravenous N-acetylcysteine in patients with paracetamol overdosage, *European Journal of Clinical Pharmacology*, **37**, 501–506.

Prescott, L. F. and Highley, M. S., 1985, Drugs prescribed for self-poisoners, *British Medical Journal*, **290**, 1633–1636.

Prescott, L. F., Howie, D., Darrien, I. and Adriaenssens, P., 1977a, Paracetamol hepatotoxicity in man. In: *Alfred Benzon Symposium X*, Drug Design and Adverse Reactions. Bundgaard, H., Juul, P. and Kofod, H. Eds. Munksgaard, Copenhagen, pp. 99–108.

Prescott, L. F., Illingworth, R. N., Critchley, J. A. J. H. and Proudfoot, A. T., 1980, Intravenous N-acetylcysteine: still the treatment of choice for paracetamol poisoning, *British Medical Journal*, **280**, 46–47.

Prescott, L. F., Illingworth, R. N., Critchley, J. A. J. H., Stewart, M. J., Adam, R. D. and Proudfoot, A. T., 1979, Intravenous N-acetylcysteine: the treatment of choice for paracetamol poisoning, *British Medical Journal*, **2**, 1097–1100.

Prescott, L. F. and Matthew, H., 1974, Cysteamine for paracetamol overdosage, *Lancet*, **i**, 998.

Prescott, L. F., Mattison, P., Menzies, D. G. and Manson, L. M., 1990, The comparative effects of paracetamol and indomethacin on renal function in healthy female volunteers, *British Journal of Clinical Pharmacology*, **29**, 403–412.

Prescott, L. F., Newton, R. W., Swainson, C. P., Wright, N., Forrest, A. R. W. and Matthew, H., 1974, Successful treatment of severe paracetamol overdosage with cysteamine, *Lancet*, **i**, 588–592.

Prescott, L. F. and Nimmo, J., 1971, Drug therapy: physiological considerations, *Journal Mondial de Pharmacie*, **14**, 253–260.

Prescott, L. F., Oswald, I. and Proudfoot, A. T., 1978a, Repeated self-poisoning with paracetamol, *British Medical Journal*, **2**, 1399.

Prescott, L. F., Park, J., Ballantyne, A., Adriaenssens, P. and Proudfoot, A. T., 1977b, Treatment of paracetamol (acetaminophen) poisoning with N-acetylcysteine, *Lancet*, **ii**, 432–434.

Prescott, L. F., Park, J. and Proudfoot, A. T., 1976a, Cysteamine for paracetamol poisoning, *Lancet*, **i**, 357.

Prescott, L. F., Park, J. and Proudfoot, A. T., 1976b, Cysteamine, L-methionine and D-penicillamine in paracetamol poisoning, *Journal of International Medical Research*, **4 (Suppl. 4)**, 112–117.

Prescott, L. F., Park, J., Sutherland, G. R., Smith, I. J. and Proudfoot, A. T., 1976c, Cysteamine, methionine and penicillamine in the treatment of paracetamol poisoning, *Lancet*, **ii**, 109–114.

Prescott, L. F., Proudfoot, A. T. and Cregeen, R. J., 1982, Paracetamol-induced acute renal failure in the absence of fulminant liver damage, *British Medical Journal*, **284**, 421–422.

Prescott, L. F., Sansur, M., Levin, W. and Conney, A. H., 1968, The comparative metabolism of phenacetin and N-acetyl-p-aminophenol in man, with particular reference to effects on the kidney, *Clinical Pharmacology and Therapeutics*, **9**, 605–614.

Prescott, L. F., Speirs, G. C., Critchley, J. A. J. H., Temple, R. M. and Winney, R. J., 1989b, Paracetamol disposition and metabolite kinetics in patients with chronic renal failure, *European Journal of Clinical Pharmacology*, **36**, 291–297.

Prescott, L. F., Steel, R. F. and Ferrier, W. R., 1970, The effects of particle size on the absorption of phenacetin in man: a correlation between plasma concentration of phenacetin and effects on the nervous system, *Clinical Pharmacology and Therapeutics*, **11**, 496–504.

Prescott, L. F., Stewart, M. J. and Proudfoot, A. T., 1978b, Cysteamine or N-acetylcysteine for paracetamol poisoning? *British Medical Journal*, **2**, 856.

Prescott, L. F. and Wright, N., 1973, The effects of hepatic and renal damage on paracetamol metabolism and excretion following overdosage, *British Journal of Pharmacology*, **49**, 602–613.

Prescott, L. F. and Wright, N., 1974, B. A. L. in paracetamol poisoning, *Lancet*, **ii**, 833–834.

Prescott, L. F., Wright, N., Roscoe, P. and Brown, S. S., 1971, Plasma-paracetamol half-life and hepatic necrosis in patients with paracetamol overdosage, *Lancet*, **i**, 519–522.

Prescott, L. F., Yoovathaworn, K., Makarananda, K., Saivises, R. and Sriwatanakul, K., 1993, Impaired absorption of paracetamol in vegetarians, *British Journal of Clinical Pharmacology*, **36**, 237–240.

Price, C. P., Campbell, R. S., Hammond, P. M., Scawen, M. D. and Atkinson, T., 1986a, Specificity of enzymic paracetamol assay, *Annals of Clinical Biochemistry*, **23**, 358.

Price, C. P., Hammond, P. M. and Scawen, M. D., 1983, Evaluation of an enzymic procedure for the measurement of acetaminophen, *Clinical Chemistry*, **29**, 358–361.

Price, L. M., Poklis, A. and Johnson, D. E., 1991, Fatal acetaminophen poisoning with evidence of subendocardial necrosis of the heart, *Journal of Forensic Sciences*, **36**, 930–935.

Price, R. A., Cox, N. J., Spielman, R. S., Van Loon, J. A., Maidak, B. L. and Weinshilboum, R. M., 1988, Inheritance of human platelet thermolabile phenol sulfotransferase (TL PST) activity, *Genetic Epidemiology*, **5**, 1–15.

Price, V. F. and Gale, G. R., 1987, Effects of caffeine on biotransformation and elimination kinetics of acetaminophen in mice, *Research Communications in Chemical Pathology and Pharmacology*, **57**, 249–260.

Price, V. F. and Jollow, D. J., 1982, Increased resistance of diabetic rats to acetaminophen-induced hepatotoxicity, *Journal of Pharmacology and Experimental Therapeutics*, **220**, 504–513.

Price, V. F. and Jollow, D. J., 1983, Mechanism of ketone-induced protection from acetaminophen hepatotoxicity in the rat, *Drug Metabolism and Disposition: The Biological Fate of Chemicals*, **11**, 451–457.

Price, V. F. and Jollow, D. J., 1984, Role of UDPGA flux in acetaminophen clearance and hepatotoxicity, *Xenobiotica*, **14**, 553–559.

Price, V. F. and Jollow, D. J., 1986, Strain differences in susceptibility of normal and diabetic rats to acetaminophen hepatotoxicity, *Biochemical Pharmacology*, **35**, 687–695.

Price, V. F. and Jollow, D. J., 1988, Mechanism of decreased acetaminophen glucuronidation in the fasted rat, *Biochemical Pharmacology*, **37**, 1067–1075.

Price, V. F. and Jollow, D. J., 1989a, Effect of glucose and gluconeogenic subtrates on fasting-induced suppression of acetaminophen glucuronidation in the rat, *Biochemical Pharmacology*, **38**, 289–297.

Price, V. F. and Jollow, D. J., 1989b, Effects of sulfur-amino acid-deficient diets on acetaminophen metabolism and hepatotoxicity in rats, *Toxicology and Applied Pharmacology*, **101**, 356–369.

Price, V. F., Miller, M. G. and Jollow, D. J., 1987, Mechanisms of fasting-induced potentiation of acetaminophen hepatotoxicity in the rat, *Biochemical Pharmacology*, **36**, 427–433.

Price, V. F., Schulte, J. M., Spaethe, S. M. and Jollow, D. J., 1986b, Mechanism of fasting-induced suppression of acetaminophen glucuronidation in the rat, *Advances in Experimental Medicine and Biology*, **197**, 697–706.

Priego, J. G., Maroto, M. L., Ortega, M. P. and Armijo, M., 1983, Salicylic acid and paracetamol serum levels following the oral administration of eterilate, *Archivos de Farmacologia y Toxicologia*, **9**, 39–46.

Priestly, B. G., Nicholls-Grzemski, F. A. and Calder, I. C., 1993, Clofibrate dose- and time-dependence for paracetamol hepatoprotection in mice, *Clinical and Experimental Phar-*

macology and Physiology, **(Suppl. 1)**, 57.

Prieto, L., Pastor, A., Palop, A., Castro, J., Paricio, A. and Piquer, A., 1986, Rinitis con intolerancia a antiinflamatorios no esteroideos: Comunicación de tres casos, *Allergologia et Immunopathologia (Madrid)*, **14**, 147–153.

Primosch, R. E., Antony, S. J. and Courts, F. J., 1993, The efficacy of preoperative analgesic administration for postoperative pain management of pediatric dental patients, *Anesthesia and Pain Control in Dentistry*, **2**, 102–106.

Proctor, R. A. and Kunin, C. M., 1978, Salicylate-induced enzymuria: comparison with other anti-inflammatory agents, *American Journal of Medicine*, **65**, 987–993.

Prokopczyk, J., Piekarczyk, A., Mankowski, T., Wankowicz, B., Kaminska, E. and Zimak, J., 1993, Badania metabolizmu i farmakokinetyki paracetamolu u szczurów w róznym wieku, *Pediatria Polska*, **68**, 13–19.

Proudfoot, A. T. and Park, J., 1978, Changing pattern of drugs used for self-poisoning, *British Medical Journal*, **1**, 90–93.

Proudfoot, A. T. and Prescott, L. F., 1977, Poisoning with paraquat, salicylate and paracetamol. In: *Recent Advances in Intensive Therapy*, I. Ledingham, I. McA. Ed. Churchill Livingstone, Edinburgh, pp. 217–229.

Proudfoot, A. T. and Wright, N., 1970, Acute paracetamol poisoning, *British Medical Journal*, **3**, 557–558.

Prudencio, M. C. R., Calva de Moro, B. R-R. and Varela-Moreiras, G., 1994, Effects of short and long-term administration of acetylsalicylic acid, acetaminophen or phenacetin on diet utilization in rats, *Nutrition Research*, **14**, 399–410.

Pruss, T. P., Gardocki, J. F., Taylor, R. J. and Muschek, L. D., 1980, Evaluation of the analgesic properties of zomepirac, *Journal of Clinical Pharmacology*, **20**, 216–222.

Pumford, N. R., Hinson, J. A., Benson, R. W. and Roberts, D. W., 1990a, Immunoblot analysis of protein containing 3-(cystein-S-yl)acetaminophen adducts in serum and subcellular liver fractions from acetaminophen-treated mice, *Toxicology and Applied Pharmacology*, **104**, 521–532.

Pumford, N. R., Hinson, J. A., Potter, D. W., Rowland, K. L., Benson, R. W. and Roberts, D. W., 1989, Immunochemical quantitation of 3-(cystein-S-yl)acetaminophen adducts in serum and liver proteins of acetaminophen-treated mice, *Journal of Pharmacology and Experimental Therapeutics*, **248**, 190–196.

Pumford, N. R., Martin, B. M. and Hinson, J. A., 1992, A metabolite of acetaminophen covalently binds to the 56 kDa selenium binding protein, *Biochemical and Biophysical Research Communications*, **182**, 1348–1355.

Pumford, N. R., Roberts, D. W., Benson, R. W. and Hinson, J. A., 1990b, Immunochemical quantitation of 3-(cystein-S-yl)acetaminophen protein adducts in subcellular liver fractions following a hepatotoxic dose of acetaminophen, *Biochemical Pharmacology*, **40**, 573–579.

Pusey, C. D., Saltissi, D., Bloodworth, L., Rainford, D. J. and Christie, J. L., 1983, Drug associated acute interstitial nephritis: clinical and pathological features and the response to high dose steroid therapy, *Quarterly Journal of Medicine*, **52**, 194–211.

Putcha, L. and Cintrón, N. M., 1991, Pharmacokinetic consequences of spaceflight, *Annals of the New York Academy of Sciences*, **618**, 615–618.

Puy Montbrun, T., Delechenault, P., Ganansia, R. and Denis, J., 1990, Rectal stenosis due to veganine suppositories, *Gastrointestinal Radiology*, **15**, 169–170.

Qamar, M. A. and Alam, S. M., 1988, An experimental study of analgesic nephropathy in rabbit: a light microscopic study, *Journal of the Pakistan Medical Association*, **38**, 113–116.

Quattrone, A. J. and Putnam, R. S., 1981, A single liquid-chromatographic procedure for therapeutic monitoring of theophylline, acetaminophen, or ethosuximide, *Clinical Chemistry*, **27**, 129–132.

Quiding, H. and Häggquist, S.-O., 1983, Visual analogue scale and the analysis of analgesic action, *European Journal of Clinical Pharmacology*, **24**, 475–478.

Quiding, H., Oikarinen, V., Huitfeldt, B., Koskimo, M., Leikomaa, H. and Nyman, C., 1982a, An analgesic study with repeated doses of phenazone, phenazone plus dextropropoxyphene, and paracetamol, using a visual analogue scale, *International Journal of Oral Surgery*, **11**, 304–309.

Quiding, H., Oikarinen, V., Sane, J. and Sjöblad, A.-M., 1984, Analgesic efficacy after single and repeated doses of codeine and acetaminophen, *Journal of Clinical Pharmacology*, **24**, 27–34.

Quiding, H., Oksala, E., Happonen, R.-P., Lehtimäki, K. and Ojala, T., 1981, The visual analog scale in multiple-dose evaluations of analgesics, *Journal of Clinical Pharmacology*, **21**, 424–429.

Quiding, H., Persson, G., Ahlström, U., Bångens, S., Hellem, S., Johanssen, G., Jönsson, E. and Nordh, P. G., 1982b, Paracetamol plus supplementary doses of codeine. An analgesic study of repeated doses, *European Journal of Clinical Pharmacology*, **23**, 315–319.

Raabe, J. J., Perarnau, J. M. and Arbogast, J., 1987, Hépatotoxicité de l'association dextropropoxyphène-paracétamol (Di-Antalvic) en prise prolongeé, *Gastroentérologie Clinique et Biologique*, **11**, 820.

Rabinovitz, M., Garty, M. and Rosenfeld, J. B., 1984, Rare side effects following paracetamol poisoning, *Harefuah*, **105**, 127–128.

Rachtan, R. and Starek, A., 1990, Przeciwgoraczkowe dzialanie pochodnych aniliny u szczurow w roznych porach doby, *Folia Medica Cracoviensia*, **31**, 289–302.

Raclot, G. and Minazzi, H., 1993, Fistule recto-vaginale après prise prolongée de suppositoires de dextropropoxyphène et de paracétamol (Di-Antalvic), *Gastroentérologie Clinique et Biologique*, **17**, 872.

Radack, K. L., Deck, C. C. and Bloomfield, S. S., 1987, Ibuprofen interferes with the efficacy of antihypertensive drugs. A randomized, double-blind, placebo-controlled trial of ibuprofen compared with acetaminophen, *Annals of Internal Medicine*, **107**, 628–635.

Rademaker, M. and Salmon, P., 1994, Fixed drug eruption due to paracetamol, *New Zealand Medical Journal*, **107**, 295–296.

Rafeiro, E., Barr, S. G., Harrison, J. J. and Racz, W. J., 1994, Effects of N-acetylcysteine and dithiothreitol on glutathione and protein thiol replenishment during acetaminophen induced toxicity in isolated mouse hepatocytes, *Toxicology*, **93**, 209–224.

Ragot, J.-P., 1991, Comparaison de l'activité antalgique de l'acide méfénamique et du paracétamol dans le traitement de la douleur après extraction d'une 3eme molaire inférieure incluse, *Information Dentaire*, **73**, 1659–1664.

Raheja, K. L., Cho, C. and Hirose, N., 1987, Effect of nutritional status on propylthiouracil-induced protection against acetaminophen hepatotoxicity in the rat, *Drug-Nutrient Interactions*, **5**, 21–31.

Raheja, K. L., Landaw, S. A., Linscheer, W. G. and Cho, C., 1984, Effect of acetaminophen toxicity on erythrocyte osmotic fragility in the Fisher rat, *Comparative Biochemistry and Physiology*, **79**, 27–30.

Raheja, K. L., Linscheer, W. G. and Cho, C., 1983a, Prevention of acetaminophen hepatotoxicity by propylthiouracil in the glutathione depleted rat, *Comparative Biochemistry and Physiology*, **76**, 9–14.

Raheja, K. L., Linscheer, W. G. and Cho, C., 1983b, Hepatotoxicity and metabolism of acetaminophen in male and female rats, *Journal of Toxicology and Environmental Health*, **12**, 143–158.

Raheja, K. L., Linscheer, W. G., Cho, C. and Coulson, R., 1985, Failure of exogenous prostaglandin to afford complete protection against acetaminophen-induced hepatotoxicity in the rat, *Journal of Toxicology and Environmental Health*, **15**, 477–484.

Raheja, K. L., Linscheer, W. G., Cho, C. and Mahany, D., 1982, Protective effect of propylthiouracil independent of its hypothyroid effect on acetaminophen toxicity in the rat, *Journal of Pharmacology and Experimental Therapeutics*, **220**, 427–432.

Raheja, K. L., Turkki, P. R., Linscheer, W. G. and Cho, C., 1983c, Effect of riboflavin status on acetaminophen toxicity in the rat, *Drug-Nutrient Interactions*, **2**, 183–191.

Rahman, A., Segasothy, M. and Samad, S. A., 1993a, Analgesic abuse and analgesic nephropathy in patients with chronic headache, *Headache*, **33**, 283.

Rahman, A., Segasothy, M., Samad, S. A., Zulfiqar, A. and Rani, M., 1993b, Analgesic use and chronic renal disease in patients with headache, *Headache*, **33**, 442–445.

Raiford, D. S. and Thigpen, M. C., 1994, Kupffer cell stimulation with *Corynebacterium parvum* reduces some cytochrome P-450-dependent activities and diminishes acetaminophen and carbon tetrachloride-induced liver injury in the rat, *Toxicology and Applied Pharmacology*, **129**, 36–45.

Rainska, T., Juzwiak, S., Dutkiewicz, T., Krasowska, B., Olenderek, B., Rozéwicka, L., Samochowiec, L. and Juzyszyn, Z., 1992, Caffeine reduces the hepatotoxicity of paracetamol in mice, *Journal of International Medical Research*, **20**, 331–342.

Rajaonarison, J. F., Lacarelle, B., Catalin, J., Placidi, M. and Rahmani, R., 1992, 3'-azido-3'-deoxythymidine drug interactions. Screening for inhibitors in human liver microsomes, *Drug Metabolism and Disposition: The Biological Fate of Chemicals*, **20**, 578–584.

Rajaonarison, J. F., Lacarelle, B., De Sousa, G., Catalin, J. and Rahmani, R., 1991, *in vitro* glucuronidation of 3'-azido-3'-deoxythymidine by human liver. Role of UDP-glucuronosyltransferase 2 form, *Drug Metabolism and Disposition: The Biological Fate of Chemicals*, **19**, 809–815.

Raje, R. R. and Bhattacharya, S., 1990, Lovastatin-acetaminophen subchronic toxicity in mice, *Research Communications in Chemical Pathology and Pharmacology*, **69**, 373–376.

Rajpurohit, R. and Krishnaswamy, K., 1984, Lack of effect of paracetamol on the pharmacokinetics of chloramphenicol in adult human subjects, *Indian Journal of Pharmacology*, **16**, 124–128.

Ramachander, G., Williams, F. D. and Emele, J. F., 1973, Effect of concurrent administration of choline salicylate and acetaminophen on their mutual biotransformation in the rat, *Journal of Pharmaceutical Sciences*, **62**, 1498–1500.

Ramakrishna Rao, D. N., Fischer, V. and Mason, R. P., 1990, Glutathione and ascorbate reduction of the acetaminophen radical formed by peroxidase. Detection of the glutathione disulfide radical anion and the ascorbyl radical, *Journal of Biological Chemistry*, **265**, 844–847.

Ramakrishna, B. S., Gee, D., Weiss, A., Pannall, P., Roberts-Thomson, I. C. and Roediger, W. E. W., 1989, Estimation of phenolic conjugation by colonic mucosa, *Journal of Clinical Pathology*, **42**, 620–623.

Ramboer, C. and Verhamme, M., 1987, Rectale stenose door analgetische suppositoria, *Tijdschrift voor Geneeskunde*, **43**, 925–928.

Ramos Fernandez de Soria, R., Martín Núñez, G. and Sánchez Gil, F., 1994, Agranulocitosis inducida por drogas. Rapida recuperacion con el uso precoz de G-CSF, *Sangre*, **39**, 145–146.

Rampton, D. S., McNeil, N. I. and Sarner, M., 1983, Analgesic ingestion and other factors preceding relapse in ulcerative colitis, *Gut*, **24**, 187–189.

Ramsay, R. R., Rashed, M. S. and Nelson, S. D., 1989, *In vitro* effects of acetaminophen metabolites and analogs on the respiration of mouse liver mitochondria, *Archives of Biochemistry and Biophysics*, **273**, 449–457.

Rane, A. and Orrenius, S., 1985, Paracetamol och leverskador i ny belysning: Är fynd av tumörer hos mus och rattå relevanta för kliniska situationen? *Läkartidningen*, **82**, 1497.

Rao, C. S., Muralidhar, N., Naidu, M. U. R., Junnarkar, A. Y. and Singh, P. P., 1991, A rapid method for evaluation of analgesic and anti-inflammatory activity in rats, *Indian Journal of Experimental Biology*, **29**, 120–122.

Rao, G. H. R., Reddy, K. R. and White, J. G., 1982, Effect of acetaminophen and salicylate on aspirin-induced inhibition of human platelet cyclo-oxygenase, *Prostaglandins Leukotrienes and Medicine*, **9**, 109–115.

Rao, P. G. M., Gurumadhava, R., Ramnarayan, K. and Srinivasan, K. K., 1993, Effect of heptagard on paracetamol induced liver injury in male albino rats, *Indian Drugs*, **30**, 40–47.

Rao, S. S. and Saifi, A. Q., 1985, Influence of testosterone on indomethacin and paracetamol induced analgesia in albino rats, *Indian Journal of Pharmacology*, **17**, 136–139.

Raper, S., Crome, P., Vale, A., Helliwell, M. and Widdop, B., 1982, Experience with activated carbon-bead haemoperfusion columns in the treatment of severe drug intoxication. A preliminary report, *Archives of Toxicology*, **49**, 303–310.

Rashed, M. S., Myers, T. G. and Nelson, S. D., 1990, Hepatic protein arylation, glutathione depletion, and metabolite profiles of acetaminophen and a non-hepatotoxic regioisomer, 3′-hydroxyacetanilide, in the mouse, *Drug Metabolism and Disposition: The Biological Fate of Chemicals*, **18**, 765–770.

Rashed, M. S. and Nelson, S. D., 1989a, Characterization of glutathione conjugates of reactive metabolites of 3′-hydroxyacetanilide, a non-hepatotoxic positional isomer of acetaminophen, *Chemical Research in Toxicology*, **2**, 41–45.

Rashed, M. S. and Nelson, S. D., 1989b, Use of thermospray liquid chromatography-mass spectrometry for characterization of reactive metabolites of 3′-hydroxyacetanilide, a non-hepatotoxic regioisomer of acetaminophen, *Journal of Chromatography: Biomedical Applications*, **474**, 209–222.

Rashid, M. U. and Bateman, D. N., 1990, Effect of intravenous atropine on gastric emptying, paracetamol absorption, salivary flow and heart rate in young and fit elderly volunteers, *British Journal of Clinical Pharmacology*, **30**, 25–34.

Rasmussen, B. K., Jensen, R. and Olesen, J., 1992, Impact of headache on sickness absence and utilization of medical services: a Danish population study, *Journal of Epidemiology and Community Health*, **46**, 443–446.

Rattie, E. S., Shami, E. G., Dittert, L. W. and Swintosky, J. V., 1970, Acetaminophen prodrugs. 3. Hydrolysis of carbonate and carboxylic acid esters in aqueous buffers, *Journal of Pharmaceutical Sciences*, **59**, 1738–1741.

Rauck, R. L., Ruoff, G. E. and McMillen, J. I., 1994, Comparison of tramadol and acetaminophen with codeine for long-term pain management in elderly patients, *Current Therapeutic Research*, **55**, 1417–1431.

Raucy, J. L., Lasker, J. M., Kraner, J. C., Salazar, D. E., Lieber, C. S. and Corcoran, G. B., 1991, Induction of cytochrome P-450 IIE1 in the obese overfed rat, *Molecular Pharmacology*, **39**, 275–280.

Raucy, J. L., Sker, J. M. L., Lieber, C. S. and Black, M., 1989, Acetaminophen activation by human liver cytochromes P-450 IIE1 and P-450 IA2, *Archives of Biochemistry and Biophysics*, **271**, 270–283.

Rawlins, M. D., Henderson, D. B. and Hijab, A. R., 1977, Pharmacokinetics of paracetamol (acetaminophen) after intravenous and oral administration, *European Journal of Clinical Pharmacology*, **11**, 283–286.

Ray, J. E., Stove, J. and Williams, K. M., 1987, A rapid urinary screen for acetaminophen modified to avoid false-negative results, *Clinical Chemistry*, **33**, 718.

Ray, K., Adithan, C., Bapna, J. S., Kamatchi, G. L., Ray, K. and Mehta, R. B., 1986, Effect of halothane anaesthesia on salivary elimination of paracetamol, *European Journal of Clinical Pharmacology*, **30**, 371–373.

Ray, K., Adithan, C., Bapna, J. S., Kangle, P. R., Ray, K. and Ramakrishnan, S., 1985, Effect of short surgical procedures on salivary paracetamol elimination, *British Journal of Clinical Pharmacology*, **20**, 174–176.

Ray, K., Sahana, C. C., Chaudhuri, S. B., De, G. C. and Chatterjee, K., 1993a, Effects of trichloroethylene anaesthesia on salivary paracetamol elimination, *Indian Journal of Physiology and Pharmacology*, **37**, 79–81.

Ray, S. D., Kamendulis, L. M., Gurule, M. W., Yorkin, R. D. and Corcoran, G. B., 1993b, Ca^{2+} antagonists inhibit DNA fragmentation and toxic cell death induced by acetaminophen, *FASEB Journal*, **7**, 453–463.

Ray, S. D., Sorge, C. L., Raucy, J. L. and Corcoran, G. B., 1990, Early loss of large genomic DNA *in vivo* with accumulation of Ca^{2+} in the nucleus during acetaminophen-induced liver injury, *Toxicology and Applied Pharmacology*, **106**, 346–351.

Ray, S. D., Sorge, C. L., Tavacoli, A., Raucy, J. L. and Corcoran, G. B., 1991, Extensive alteration of genomic DNA and rise in nuclear Ca^{2+} *in vivo* early after hepatotoxic acetaminophen overdose in mice, *Advances in Experimental Medicine and Biology*, **283**, 699–705.

Rayburn, W., Aronow, R., DeLancey, B. and Hogan, M. J., 1984, Drug overdose during pregnancy: an overview from a metropolitan poison control center, *Obstetrics and Gynecology*, **64**, 611–614.

Rayburn, W., Shukla, U., Stetson, P. and Piehl, E., 1986, Acetaminophen pharmacokinetics: comparison between pregnant and nonpregnant women, *American Journal of Obstetrics and Gynecology*, **155**, 1353–1356.

Read, R. B., Tredger, J. M. and Williams, R., 1986, Analysis of factors responsible for continuing mortality after paracetamol overdose, *Human Toxicology*, **5**, 201–206.

Record, C. O., Chase, R. A., Alberti, K. G. M. M. and Williams, R., 1975a, Disturbances in glucose metabolism in patients with liver damage due to paracetamol overdose, *Clinical Science*, **49**, 473–479.

Record, C. O., Chase, R. A., Williams, R. and Appleton, D., 1981, Disturbances of lactate metabolism in patients with liver damage due to paracetamol overdose, *Metabolism*, **30**, 638–643.

Record, C. O., Iles, R. A., Cohen, R. D. and Williams, R., 1975b, Acid-base and metabolic disturbances in fulminant hepatic failure, *Gut*, **16**, 144–149.

Reed, M. D. and Marx, C. M., 1994, Ondansetron for treating nausea and vomiting in the poisoned patient, *Annals of Pharmacotherapy*, **28**, 331–333.

Reed, R. G., Guiney, W. R. and Collier, S. A., 1982, Salicylate interference with measurement of acetaminophen, *Clinical Chemistry*, **28**, 2178–2179.

Reel, J. R., Lawton, A. D. and Lamb, J. C., 1992, Reproductive toxicity evaluation of acetaminophen in Swiss CD-1 mice using a continuous breeding protocol, *Fundamental and Applied Toxicology*, **18**, 233–239.

Regal, R. E., 1986, Acetaminophen chronic toxicity, *Drug Intelligence and Clinical Pharmacy*, **20**, 507.

Regdon, G., Szikszay, M., Gebri, G. and Regdon, G. Jr., 1994, Paracetamol-tartalmu kupok es *in vivo* vizsgalata, *Acta Pharmaceutica Hungarica*, **64**, 45–49.

Reicks, M., Calvert, R. J. and Hathcock, J. N., 1988, Effects of prolonged acetaminophen ingestion and dietary methionine on mouse liver glutathione, *Drug-Nutrient Interactions*, **5**, 351–363.

Reicks, M. and Hathcock, J. N., 1989, Prolonged acetaminophen ingestion in mice: effects on the availability of methionine for metabolic functions, *Journal of Nutrition*, **119**, 1042–1049.

Reicks, M. M. and Crankshaw, D., 1993, Effects of D-limonene on hepatic microsomal monooxygenase activity and paracetamol-induced glutathione depletion in mouse, *Xenobiotica*, **23**, 809–819.

Reicks, M. M., Fullerton, F. R., Poirier, L. A., Whittaker, P. and Hathcock, J. N., 1992, Prolonged acetaminophen ingestion by mice fed a methionine-limited diet does not affect iron-induced liver lipid peroxidation or *S*-adenosylmethionine, *Journal of Nutrition*, **122**, 1738–1743.

Reicks, M. M. and Hathcock, J. N., 1984, Effects of dietary methionine and ethanol ingestion on acetaminophen hepatotoxicity in mice, *Drug-Nutrient Interactions*, **3**, 43–51.

Reicks, M. M. and Hathcock, J. N., 1987, Effects of methionine deficiency and ethanol ingestion on acetaminophen metabolism in mice, *Journal of Nutrition*, **117**, 572–579.

Reid, S., Shackleton, C., Wu, K., Kaempfer, S. and Hellerstein, M. K., 1990, Liquid chromatography/mass spectrometry of plasma glucose and secreted glucuronate for metabolic studies in humans, *Biomedical and Environmental Mass Spectrometry*, **19**, 535–540.

Reijntjes, R. J., Boering, G., Wesseling, H. and van Rijn, L. J., 1987, Suprofen versus paracetamol after oral surgery, *International Journal of Oral and Maxillofacial Surgery*, **16**, 45–49.

Reikvam, A. and Skjoto, J., 1978, Paracetamolintoksikasjon – leverskade, *Tidsskrift for den Norske Lægeforening*, **98**, 441–443.

Reilly, C. S. and Nimmo, W. S., 1984, Drug absorption after general anaesthesia for minor surgery, *Anaesthesia*, **39**, 859–861.

Reiter, C. and Weinshilboum, R., 1982a, Platelet phenol sulfotransferase activity: correlation with sulfate conjugation of acetaminophen, *Clinical Pharmacology and Therapeutics*, **32**, 612–621.

Reiter, C. and Weinshilboum, R. M., 1982b, Acetaminophen and phenol: substrates for both a thermostable and a thermolabile form of human platelet phenol sulfotransferase, *Journal of Pharmacology and Experimental Therapeutics*, **221**, 43–51.

Reiter, Ch. and Naudorf, M., 1987, The influence of oral N-acetylcysteine (NAC) on the sulfate turnover and the sulfate conjugation of acetaminophen (AC) in man, *Clinical Research*, **35**, 843A.

Reiter, R. and Wendel, A., 1983, Drug-induced lipid peroxidation in mice – IV. *In vitro* hydrocarbon evolution, reduction of oxygen and covalent binding of acetaminophen, *Biochemical Pharmacology*, **32**, 665–670.

Remmert, H. P., Olling, M., Slob, W., van der Giesen, W. F., van Dijk, A. and Rauws, A. G., 1990, Comparative antidotal efficacy of activated charcoal tablets, capsules and suspension in healthy volunteers, *European Journal of Clinical Pharmacology*, **39**, 501–505.

Ren, F.-L. and Cong, Z., 1994, Influences of dimethyl sulfoxide on acetaminophen-induced injury of rat hepatocytes in primary culture, *Chinese Journal of Pharmacology and Toxicology*, **8**, 56–59.

Renault, H., Rohrbach, Ph. and Dugniolle, J., 1956, Propriétés pharmacodynamiques du N-acétyl-p aminophénol, métabolite de la phénacétine et de l'acétanilide, *Thérapie*, **11**, 300–307.

Renic, M., Culo, F., Bilic, A., Bukovec, Z., Sabolovic, D. and Zupanovic, Z., 1993, The effect of interleukin 1α on acetaminophen-induced hepatotoxicity, *Cytokine*, **5**, 192–197.

Renic, M., Culo, F., Bilic, A., Culjak, K., Sabolovic, D. and Jagic, V., 1992, Protection of acetaminophen-induced heptotoxicity in mice, *Croatian Journal of Gastroenterology and Hepatology*, **1**, 59–64.

Renton, K. W. and Dickson, G., 1984, The prevention of acetaminophen-induced hepatotoxicity by the interferon inducer poly(rI. rC), *Toxicology and Applied Pharmacology*, **72**, 40–45.

Renzi, F. P., Donovan, J. W., Martin, T. G., Morgan, L. and Harrison, E. F., 1985, Concomitant use of activated charcoal and N-acetylcysteine, *Annals of Emergency Medicine*, **14**, 568–572.

Resta, O., Foschino-Barbaro, M. P., Carnimeo, N., Bavoso, P. and Picca, V., 1984, Asthma relieved by acetylsalicylic acid and non-steroid anti-inflammatory drugs, *Respiration*, **46**, 121–127.

Reuter, S. H. and Montgomery, W. W., 1964, Aspirin vs. acetaminophen after tonsillectomy, *Archives of Otolaryngology*, **80**, 214–217.

Rex, D. K. and Kumar, S., 1992, Recognizing acetaminophen hepatotoxicity in chronic alcoholics, *Postgraduate Medicine*, **91**, 241–245.

Reyes, J. L. and Meléndez, E., 1990, Effects of eicosanoids on the water and sodium balance of the neonate, *Pediatric Nephrology*, **4**, 630–634.

Reyes, J. L., Meléndez, E., Escalante, B. A. and Namorado, M. C., 1989, Effect of synthesis inhibitors of thromboxane A_2 and prostaglandin E_2 on the regulation of sodium and water, *Journal of Pharmacology and Experimental Therapeutics*, **251**, 694–699.

Reynard, K., Riley, A. and Walker, B. E., 1992, Respiratory arrest after N-acetylcysteine for paracetamol overdose, *Lancet*, **340**, 675.

Rhodes, K. F. and Waterfall, J. F., 1977, The effects of paracetamol on temperature and cardiovascular changes caused by pyrogenic contamination of chronically implanted arterial cannulae in the conscious, renal hypertensive cat, *Journal of Pharmacy and Pharmacology*, **29**, 304–305.

Richard, A. M., Hongslo, J. K., Boone, P. F. and Holme, J. A., 1991, Structure-activity study of paracetamol analogues: inhibition of replicative DNA synthesis in V79 Chinese hamster cells, *Chemical Research in Toxicology*, **4**, 151–156.

Richie, J. P. and Lang, C. A., 1985, Aging effects on acetaminophen toxicity and glutathione status in the mosquito, *Drug Metabolism and Disposition: The Biological Fate of Chemicals*, **13**, 14–17.

Richie, J. P., Lang, C. A. and Chen, T. S., 1992, Acetaminophen-induced depletion of glutathione and cysteine in the aging mouse kidney, *Biochemical Pharmacology*, **44**, 129–135.

Richman, D. D, Fischl, M. A., Grieco, M. H., Gottlieb, M. S., Volberding, P. A., Laskin, O. L., Leedom, J. M., Groopman, J. E., Mildvan, D., Hirsch, M. S., Jackson, G. G., Durack, D. T. and Nusinoff-Lehrman, S., 1987, The toxicity of azidothymidine (AZT) in the treatment of patients with AIDS and AIDS-related complex, *New England Journal of Medicine*, **317**, 192–197.

Richter, A. and Smith, S. E., 1974, Bioavailability of different preparations of paracetamol, *British Journal of Clinical Pharmacology*, **1**, 495–498.

Rigby, R. J., Thomson, N. M., Parkin, G. W. and Cheung, T. P. F., 1978, The treatment of paracetamol overdose with charcoal haemoperfusion and cysteamine, *Medical Journal of Australia*, **1**, 396–399.

Riggin, R. M., Schmidt, A. L. and Kissinger, P. T., 1975, Determination of acetaminophen in pharmaceutical preparations and body fluids by high-performance liquid chromatography with electrochemical detection, *Journal of Pharmaceutical Sciences*, **64**, 680–683.

Riggs, B. S., Bronstein, A. C., Kulig, K., Archer, P. G. and Rumack, B. H., 1989, Acute acetaminophen overdose during pregnancy, *Obstetrics and Gynecology*, **74**, 247–253.

Riggs, B. S., Kulig, K. and Rumack, B. H., 1987, Current status of aspirin and acetaminophen intoxication, *Pediatric Annals*, **16**, 886–898.

Rikans, L. E., 1989, Influence of aging on chemically induced hepatotoxicity: role of age-related changes in metabolism, *Drug Metabolism Reviews*, **20**, 87–110.

Rikans, L. E., 1991, Age-related differences in the susceptibility to drug-induced hepatotoxicity, *International Congress Series: Liver and Aging*, **940**, 59–74.

Rikans, L. E. and Moore, D. R., 1988, Acetaminophen hepatotoxicity in aging rats, *Drug and Chemical Toxicology*, **11**, 237.

Riley, M. L. and Harding, J. J., 1993, The reaction of malondialdehyde with lens proteins and the protective effect of aspirin, *Biochimica Biophysica Acta*, **1158**, 107–112.

Riley, R. J., Spielberg, S. P. and Leeder, J. S., 1993, A comparative study of the toxicity of chemically reactive xenobiotics towards adherent cell cultures: selective attenuation of menadione toxicity by buthionine sulphoximine pretreatment, *Journal of Pharmacy and Pharmacology*, **45**, 263–267.

Rinaldi, M. R., Colianni, R., D'Agata, A., Leggio, T. and Musumeci, S., 1989, La sindrome di Reye: osservazione di sette casi nel quinquennio 1982–1987, *Pediatria Medica e Chirurgica*, **11**, 205–208.

Ring, E. F. J., Collins, A. J., Bacon, P. A. and Cosh, J. A., 1974, Quantitation of thermography in arthritis using multi-isothermal analysis. II. Effect of nonsteroidal anti-inflammatory therapy on the thermographic index, *Annals of the Rheumatic Diseases*, **33**, 353–356.

Robak, J., Kostka-Trabka, E. and Duniec, Z., 1980, The influence of three prostaglandin biosynthesis stimulators on carrageenin-induced edema of rat paw, *Biochemical Pharmacology*, **29**, 1863–1865.

Robak, J., Wieckowski, A. and Gryglewski, R., 1978, The effect of 4-acetaminophenol on prostaglandin synthetase activity in bovine and ram seminal vesicle microsomes, *Biochemical Pharmacology*, **27**, 393–396.

Roberts, D. W., Benson, R. W., Hinson, J. A. and Kadlubar, F. F., 1991a, Critical considerations in the immunochemical detection and quantitation of antigenic biomarkers, *Biomedical and Environmental Sciences*, **4**, 113–129.

Roberts, D. W., Bucci, T. J., Benson, R. W., Warbritton, A. R., McRae, T. A., Pumford, N. R. and Hinson, J. A., 1991b, Immunohistochemical localization and quantification of the 3-(cystein-*S*-yl)acetaminophen protein adduct in acetaminophen hepatotoxicity, *American Journal of Pathology*, **138**, 359–371.

Roberts, D. W., Hinson, J. A., Benson, R. W., Pumford, N. R., Warbritton, A. R., Crowell, J. A. and Bucci, T. J., 1989, Immunohistochemical localization of 3-(cystein-S-yl)acetaminophen protein adducts in livers of mice treated with acetaminophen, *Toxicologist*, **9**, 47.

Roberts, D. W., Pumford, N. R., Potter, D. W., Benson, R. W. and Hinson, J. A., 1987a, A sensitive immunochemical assay for acetaminophen-protein adducts, *Journal of Pharmacology and Experimental Therapeutics*, **241**, 527–533.

Roberts, I., Byrne, T., Grennan, A. and McDowell, D., 1985, The effects of salicylate metabolites on the interpretation of paracetamol results, *Annals of Clinical Biochemistry*, **22**, 654.

Roberts, I., Robinson, M. J., Muchal, M. Z., Ratcliffe, J. G. and Prescott, L. F., 1984, Paracetamol metabolites in the neonate following maternal overdose, *British Journal of Clinical Pharmacology*, **18**, 201–206.

Roberts, J. C., Charyulu, R. L., Zera, R. T. and Nagasawa, H. T., 1992, Protection against acetaminophen hepatotoxicity by ribose-cysteine (RibCys), *Pharmacology and Toxicology*, **70**, 281–285.

Roberts, J. C., Nagasawa, H. T., Zera, R. T., Fricke, R. F. and Goon, D. J. W., 1987b, Prodrugs of l-cysteine as protective agents against acetaminophen-induced hepatotoxicity. 2-(Polyhydroxyalkyl)- and 2-(polyacetoxyalkyl)thiazolidine-4(R)-carboxylic acids, *Journal of Medicinal Chemistry*, **30**, 1891–1896.

Roberts, M. S. and Rowland, M., 1986, A dispersion model of hepatic elimination: 3. Application to metabolite formation and elimination kinetics, *Journal of Pharmacokinetics and Biopharmaceutics*, **14**, 289–308.

Roberts, S. A., Price, V. F. and Jollow, D. J., 1986, The mechanisms of cobalt chloride-induced protection against acetaminophen hepatotoxicity, *Drug Metabolism and Disposition: The Biological Fate of Chemicals*, **14**, 25–33.

Roberts, S. A., Price, V. F. and Jollow, D. J., 1990, Acetaminophen structure-toxicity studies: *in vivo* covalent binding of a nonhepatotoxic analog, 3-hydroxyacetanilide, *Toxicology and Applied Pharmacology*, **105**, 195–208.

Robertson, A., Glynn, J. P. and Watson, A. K., 1972, The absorption and metabolism in man of 4-acetamidophenyl-2-acetoxybenzoate (benorylate), *Xenobiotica*, **2**, 339–347.

Robertson, D. R. C., Higginson, I., Macklin, B. S., Renwick, A. G., Waller, D. G. and George, C. F., 1991, The influence of protein containing meals on the pharmacokinetics of levodopa in healthy volunteers, *British Journal of Clinical Pharmacology*, **31**, 413–417.

Robertson, D. R. C., Renwick, A. G., Macklin, B., Jones, S., Waller, D. G., George, C. F. and Fleming, J. S., 1992, The influence of levodopa on gastric emptying in healthy elderly volunteers, *European Journal of Clinical Pharmacology*, **42**, 409–412.

Robertson, D. R. C., Renwick, A. G., Wood, N. D., Cross, N., Macklin, B. S., Fleming, J. S., Waller, D. G. and George, C. F., 1990, The influence of levodopa on gastric emptying in man, *British Journal of Clinical Pharmacology*, **29**, 47–53.

Robertson, R. G., Van Cleave, B. L. and Collins, J. J., 1986, Acetaminophen overdose in the second trimester of pregnancy, *Journal of Family Practice*, **23**, 267–268.

Robinson, A. E., Sattar, H., McDowall, R. D., Holder, A. T. and Powell, R., 1977, Forensic toxicology of some deaths associated with the combined use of propoxyphene and acetaminophen (paracetamol), *Journal of Forensic Sciences*, **22**, 708–717.

Robinson, D. R., McGuire, M. B., Bastian, D., Kantrowitz, F. and Levine, L., 1978, The effects of anti-inflammatory drugs on prostaglandin production by rheumatoid synovial tissue, *Prostaglandins and Medicine*, **1**, 461–477.

Roblot, P., Gouet, D., Cazenave, F., Breuil, K. and Sudre, Y., 1987, Choc anaphylactique au paracétamol, *Revue Française d'Allergie et d'Immunologie Clinique*, **27**, 87.

Roddis, M. J., 1981, Paracetamol interference with glucose analysis, *Lancet*, **ii**, 634–635.

Rodière, M. and Astruc, J., 1990, La fièvre chez l'enfant une urgence? *Concours Médicale*, **112**, 3193–3195.

Rodrigo, C., Chau, M. and Rosenquist, J., 1989, A comparison of paracetamol and diflunisal for pain control following 3rd molar surgery, *International Journal of Oral and Maxillofacial Surgery*, **18**, 130–132.

Rodrigo, M. R. C., Rosenquist, J. B. and Cheung, L. K., 1987, Paracetamol and diflunisal for pain relief following third molar surgery in Hong Kong Chinese, *International Journal of Oral and Maxillofacial Surgery*, **16**, 566–571.

Rodriguez, F., Arama, E., Magbi, M., Paulin, T. and Rouffiac, R., 1990, Application de la fonction de Weibull à l'étude des corrélations *in vivo/in vitro*, *Journal de Pharmacie de Belgique*, **45**, 173–183.

Roe, A. L., Snawder, J. E., Benson, R. W., Roberts, D. W. and Casciano, D. A., 1993, HEPG2 Cells: an *in vitro* model for P-450-dependent metabolism of acetaminophen, *Biochemical and Biophysical Research Communications*, **190**, 15–19.

Rogers, S. A., Gale, K. C., Newton, J. F., Dent, J. G. and Leonard, T. B., 1988, Inhibition by ranitidine of acetaminophen conjugation and its possible role in ranitidine potentiation of acetaminophen-induced hepatotoxicity, *Journal of Pharmacology and Experimental Therapeutics*, **245**, 887–894.

Rogers, S. A., Newton, J. F., Dent, J. G. and Leonard, T. B., 1985, Ranitidine (RA) potentiation of acetaminophen (APAP)-induced hepatotoxicity in F344 rats: role of metabolism, *Toxicologist*, **5**, 154.

Rogers, S. M., Back, D. J. and Orme, M. L'E., 1987a, Intestinal metabolism of ethinyloestradiol and paracetamol *in vitro*: studies using Ussing chambers, *British Journal of Clinical Pharmacology*, **23**, 727–734.

Rogers, S. M., Back, D. J., Stevenson, P. J., Grimmer, S. F. M. and Orme, M. L'E., 1987b, Paracetamol interaction with oral contraceptive steroids: increased plasma concentrations of ethinyloestradiol, *British Journal of Clinical Pharmacology*, **23**, 721–725.

Rohdewald, P., Derendorf, H., Drehsen, G., Elger, C. E. and Knoll, O., 1982, Changes in cortical evoked potentials as correlates of the efficacy of weak analgesics, *Pain*, **12**, 329–341.

Rolband, G. C. and Marcuard, S. P., 1991, Cimetidine in the treatment of acetaminophen overdose, *Journal of Clinical Gastroenterology*, **13**, 79–82.

Rollins, D. E. and Buckpitt, A. R., 1979, Liver cytosol catalyzed conjugation of reduced glutathione with a reactive metabolite of acetaminophen, *Toxicology and Applied Pharmacology*, **47**, 331–339.

Rollins, D. E., von Bahr, C., Glaumann, H., Moldéus, P. and Rane, A., 1979, Acetaminophen: potentially toxic metabolite formed by human fetal and adult liver microsomes and isolated fetal liver cells, *Science*, **205**, 1414–1416.

Romanelli, L., Valeri, P., Morrone, L. A. and Pimpinella, G., 1991, Ocular disposition of acetaminophen and its metabolites following intravenous administration in rabbits, *Journal of Ocular Pharmacology*, **7**, 339–350.

Romano, M., Razandi, M. and Ivey, K. J., 1988a, Acetaminophen directly protects human gastric epithelial cell monolayers against damage induced by sodium taurocholate, *Digestion*, **40**, 181–190.

Romano, M., Razandi, M., Raza, A., Szabo, S. and Ivey, K. J., 1991, Sulphydryl mediation in the protection of gastric mucosal cells in tissue culture by acetaminophen, *Italian Journal of Gastroenterology*, **23**, 481–486.

Romano, M., Razandi, M., Sekhon, S., Krause, W. J. and Ivey, K. J., 1988b, Human cell line for study of damage to gastric epithelial cells *in vitro*, *Journal of Laboratory and Clinical Medicine*, **111**, 430–440.

Romero-Ferret, C., Mottot, G., Legros, J. and Margetts, G., 1983, Effect of vitamin C on acute paracetamol poisoning, *Toxicology Letters*, **18**, 153–156.

Rònai, K., Földes, K. and Gachályi, B., 1990, Paracetamol meghatarozasa vizeletbol folyadekkromatografiaval, *Acta Pharmaceutica Hungarica*, **60**, 156–161.

Roos, R. A. C., Steenvoorden, J. M. C., Mulder, G. J. and van Kemperen, G. M. J., 1993, Acetaminophen sulfation in patients with Parkinson's disease or Huntington's disease is not impaired, *Neurology*, **43**, 1373–1376.

Ros, S. P. and Conrad, H. A., 1994, Baseline liver function tests following acetaminophen ingestion: what is the utility? *Clinical Pediatrics*, **33**, 569–570.

Rosa, H., Prudente, M. S. and Cardoso, V. M., 1984, Paracetamol hepatic necrosis and its prevention by cholestyramine, *Arquivos de Gastroenterologia*, **21**, 164–166.

Roschlau, G., 1986, Virushepatitis gegen Arzneimittelhepatitis, *Zeitschrift fur Klinische Medizin*, **41**, 817–819.

Rose, P. G., 1969, Paracetamol overdose and liver damage, *British Medical Journal*, **1**, 381–382.

Rose, S. R., Gorman, R. L., Oderda, G. M., Klein-Schwartz, W. and Watson, W. A., 1991, Simulated acetaminophen overdose: pharmacokinetics and effectiveness of activated charcoal, *Annals of Emergency Medicine*, **20**, 1064–1068.

Roseau, G., 1989, Hépatotoxicité du paracétamol chez l'alcoolique par déficit en glutathion, *Presse Médicale*, **18**, 510.

Rosen, G. M., Rauckman, E. J., Ellington, S. P., Dahlin, D. C., Christie, J. L. and Nelson, S. D., 1984, Reduction and glutathione conjugation reactions of N-acetyl-p-benzoquinoneimine and two dimethylated analogues, *Molecular Pharmacology*, **25**, 151–157.

Rosen, G. M., Singletary, W. V., Rauckman, E. J. and Killenberg, P. G., 1983, Acetaminophen hepatotoxicity: an alternative mechanism, *Biochemical Pharmacology*, **32**, 2053–2059.

Rosen, M., Absi, E. G. and Webster, J. A., 1985, Suprofen compared to dextropropoxyphene hydrochloride and paracetamol (Cosalgesic) after extraction of wisdom teeth under general anaesthesia, *Anaesthesia*, **40**, 639–641.

Rosenbaum, J. M., Broer, H. H. and Shields, J., 1980, Misleading results in cases of coexisting acetaminophen and salicylate overdose, *Clinical Chemistry*, **26**, 673–674.

Rosenbaum, S. E., Carlo, J. R. and Boroujerdi, M., 1984, Protective action of 2(3)-tert-butyl-4-hydroxyanisole (BHA) on acetaminophen-induced liver necrosis in male A/J mice, *Research Communications in Chemical Pathology and Pharmacology*, **46**, 425–435.

Rosenberg, D. M., Meyer, A. A., Manning, I. H. and Neelon, F. A., 1977, Acetaminophen and hepatic dysfunction in infectious mononucleosis, *Southern Medical Journal*, **70**, 660–661.

Rosenberg, D. M. and Neelon, F. A., 1978, Acetaminophen and liver disease, *Annals of Internal Medicine*, **88**, 129.

Rosevear, S. K. and Hope, P. L., 1989, Favourable neonatal outcome following maternal paracetamol overdose and severe fetal distress. Case report, *British Journal of Obstetrics and Gynaecology*, **96**, 491–493.

Rosner, I., Romero-Ferret, C. and Mottot, G., 1973, Treatment of acute paracetamol poisoning, *Lancet*, **ii**, 1273–1274.

Rosner, J., 1974, Néphropathies expérimentales aux analgésiques, *Thérapie*, **29**, 483–505.

Ross, B., Tange, J., Emslie, K., Hart, S., Smail, M. and Calder, I., 1980, Paracetamol metabolism by the isolated perfused rat kidney, *Kidney International*, **18**, 562–570.

Ross, D., Albano, E., Nilsson, U. and Moldéus, P., 1984, Thiyl radicals – formation during peroxidase-catalyzed metabolism of acetaminophen in the presence of thiols, *Biochemical and Biophysical Research Communications*, **125**, 109–115.

Ross, D. and Moldéus, P., 1985, Generation of reactive species and fate of thiols during peroxidase-catalyzed metabolic activation of aromatic amines and phenols, *Environmental Health Perspectives*, **64**, 253–257.

Ross, R. K., Paganini-Hill, A., Landolph, J., Gerkins, V. and Henderson, B. E., 1989, Analgesics, cigarette smoking and other risk factors for cancer of the renal pelvis and ureter, *Cancer Research*, **49**, 1045–1048.

Rossi, L., MacGirr, L. G., Silva, J. and O'Brien, P. J., 1988, The metabolism of N-acetyl-3,5-dimethyl-p-benzoquinone imine in isolated hepatocytes involves N-deacetylation, *Molecular Pharmacology*, **34**, 674–681.

Rossini, D., Alessandri, M. G. and Scalori, V., 1989, Intossicazione da paracetamolo, *Acta Toxicologica et Therapeutica*, **10**, 153–166.

Rotenberg, A., Chauveinc, L., Rault, P., Rozenberg, H., Nemeth, J. and Potet, F., 1988, Lésions rectales secondaires à l'abus de suppositoires de dextropropoxyphène et paracétamol. Deux nouvelles observations, *Presse Médicale*, **17**, 1545.

Roth, J. L. A., Valdes-Dapena, A., Pieses, P. and Buchman, E., 1963, Topical action of salicylates in gastrointestinal erosion and hemorrhage, *Gastroenterology*, **44**, 146–158.

Rothstein, K. D., Black, M., Lim, J., Mital, D., Yang, S. L., Badosa, F. and Morris, H., 1994, Identification of previously undiagnosed cirrhosis in patients who survive fulminant hepatic failure due to acetaminophen and alcohol, *Hepatology*, **20**, 391A.

Roupe, G., Ahlmen, M., Fagerberg, B. and Suurküla, M., 1986, Toxic epidermal necrolysis with extensive mucosal erosions of the gastrointestinal and respiratory tracts, *International Archives of Allergy and Applied Immunology*, **80**, 145–151.

Routh, J. I., Shane, N. A., Arredondo, F. G. and Paul, W. D., 1968, Determination of N-acetyl-p-aminophenol in plasma, *Clinical Chemistry*, **14**, 882–889.

Rowbotham, D. J., Bamber, P. A. and Nimmo, W. S., 1988, Comparison of the effect of cisapride and metoclopramide on morphine-induced delay in gastric emptying, *British Journal of Clinical Pharmacology*, **26**, 741–746.

Rowbotham, D. J. and Nimmo, W. S., 1987, Effect of cisapride on morphine-induced delay in gastric emptying, *British Journal of Anaesthesia*, **59**, 536–539.

Rowbotham, D. J., Parnacott, S. and Nimmo, W. S., 1992, No effect of cisapride on paracetamol absorption after oral simultaneous administration, *European Journal of Clinical Pharmacology*, **42**, 235–236.

Roy, A. C., Yeang, M. and Karim, S. M. M., 1981, Inhibition of serum oxytocinase activity by prostaglandins, *Prostaglandins and Medicine*, **6**, 577–587.

Roy, A. C., Yeang, M. and Karim, S. M. M., 1982, pH Dependent inhibition of serum oxytocinase activity by prostaglandins and cyclic GMP, *Prostaglandins Leukotrienes and Medicine*, **8**, 173–179.

Rozga, J., Podesta, L., LePage, E., Hoffman, A., Morsiani, E., Sher, L., Woolf, G. M., Makowka, L. and Demetriou, A. A., 1993, Control of cerebral oedema by total hepatectomy and extracorporeal liver support in fulminant hepatic failure, *Lancet*, **342**, 898–899.

Ruane, B. J., Glover, G. and Varma, M. P. S., 1989, Survival after an overdose of Distalgesic (dextropropoxyphene and paracetamol), *Ulster Medical Journal*, **58**, 187–189.

Rubin, A. and Winter, L., 1984, A double-blind randomized study of an aspirin/caffeine combination vs. acetaminophen/aspirin conbination vs. acetaminophen vs. placebo in patients with moderate to severe post-partum pain, *Journal of International Medical Research*, **12**, 338–345.

Ruch, R. J. and Klaunig, J. E., 1986, Effects of tumor promoters, genotoxic carcinogens and hepatocytotoxins on mouse hepatocyte intercellular communication, *Cell Biology and Toxicology*, **2**, 469–483.

Ruchirawat, M., Aramphongphan, A., Tanphaichitr, V. and Bandittanukool, W., 1981, The effect of thiamine deficiency on the metabolism of acetaminophen (paracetamol), *Biochemical Pharmacology*, **30**, 1901–1906.

Rudd, G. D., Donn, K. H. and Grisham, J. W., 1981, Prevention of acetaminophen-induced hepatic necrosis by cimetidine in mice, *Research Communications in Chemical Pathology and Pharmacology*, **32**, 369–372.

Rudolph, A. M., 1981, Effects of aspirin and acetaminophen in pregnancy and in the newborn, *Archives of Internal Medicine*, **141**, 358–363.

Ruffalo, R. L. and Thompson, J. F., 1982, Cimetidine and acetylcysteine as antidotes for acetaminophen overdose, *Southern Medical Journal*, **75**, 954–958.

Rumack, B. H., 1983, Acetaminophen overdose, *American Journal of Medicine*, **75 (Suppl. 5A)**, 104–112.

Rumack, B. H., 1984, Acetaminophen overdose in young children: treatment and effects of alcohol and other additional ingestants in 417 cases, *American Journal of Diseases of Children*, **138**, 428–433.

Rumack, B. H., 1985, Acetaminophen: acute overdose toxicity in children, *Drug Intelligence and Clinical Pharmacy*, **19**, 911–912.

Rumack, B. H., 1986, Acetaminophen overdose in children and adolecents, *Pediatric Clinics of North America*, **33**, 691–701.

Rumack, B. H. and Matthew, H., 1975, Acetaminophen poisoning and toxicity, *Pediatrics*, **55**, 871–876.

Rumack, B. H. and Peterson, R. G., 1978, Acetaminophen overdose: incidence, diagnosis and management in 416 patients, *Pediatrics*, **62 (Suppl.)**, 898–903.

Rumack, B. H., Peterson, R. G., Koch, G. C. and Amara, I. A., 1981, Acetaminophen overdose. 662 cases with evaluation of oral acetylcysteine treatment, *Archives of Internal Medicine*, **141**, 380–385.

Rumble, R. H., Roberts, M. S. and Denton, M. J., 1991, Effects of posture and sleep on the pharmacokinetics of paracetamol (acetaminophen) and its metabolites, *Clinical Pharmacokinetics*, **20**, 167–173.

Rumore, M. M. and Blaiklock, R. G., 1992, Influence of age-dependent pharmacokinetics and metabolism on acetaminophen hepatotoxicity, *Journal of Pharmaceutical Sciences*, **81**, 203–207.

Rump, L. C. and Keller, E., 1994, Behandlung der Paracetamolvergiftung, *Intensivmedizin und Notfallmedizin*, **31**, 6–11.

Rundgren, M., Harder, S., Nelson, S. D. and Andersson, B. S., 1990, Oxidant-induced changes in the cellular energy homeostasis: a study with 3,5-dimethyl N-acetyl-p-benzoquinone imine and isolated hepatocytes, *Biochemical Pharmacology*, **40**, 239–243.

Rundgren, M., Porubek, D. J., Harvison, P. J., Cotgreave, I. A., Moldéus, P. and Nelson, S. D., 1988, Comparative cytotoxic effects of N-acetyl-p-benzoquinoneimine and two dimethylated analogues, *Molecular Pharmacology*, **34**, 566–572.

Rush, G. F., Smith, J. H., Newton, J. F. and Hook, J. B., 1984, Chemically induced nephrotoxicity: role of metabolic activation, *CRC Critical Reviews in Toxicology*, **13**, 99–160.

Rustgi, V. K., Manzarbeitia, C., Jonsson, J., Pinto, S., Oyloe, V. K., Cooper, J. N. and Scudera, P., 1993, Low dose acetaminophen resulting in fulminant hepatic failure, *Hepatology*, **18**, 321A.

Rustum, A. M., 1989, Determination of acetaminophen in human plasma by ion-pair reversed-phase high-performance liquid chromatography. Application to a single dose pharmacokinetic study, *Journal of Chromatographic Science*, **27**, 18–22.

Rusy, L. M., Houck, C. S., Sullivan, L. J., Ohlms, L. A., Jones, D. T., McGill, T. J. and Berde, C. B., 1995, A double-blind evaluation of ketorolac tromethamine vs. acetaminophen in pediatric tonsillectomy: analgesia and bleeding, *Anesthesia and Analgesia*, **80**, 226–229.

Ruthnum, P. and Goel, K. M., 1984, ABC of poisoning: paracetamol, *British Medical Journal*, **289**, 1538–1539.

Ruvalcaba, R. H. A., Limbeck, G. A. and Kelley, V. C., 1966, Acetaminophen and hypoglycemia, *American Journal of Diseases of Children*, **112**, 558–560.

Ryan, D. E., Koop, D. R., Thomas, P. E., Coon, M. J. and Levin, W., 1986, Evidence that isoniazid and ethanol induce the same microsomal cytochrome P-450 in rat liver, an isozyme homologous to rabbit liver cytochrome P-450 isoenzyme 3a, *Archives of Biochemistry and Biophysics*, **246**, 633–644.

Ryan, P. B., Rush, D. R., Nicholas, T. A. and Graham, D. G., 1987, A double-blind comparison of fenoprofen calcium, acetaminophen, and placebo in the palliative treatment of common nonbacterial upper respiratory infections, *Current Therapeutic Research*, **41**, 17–23.

Rybolt, T. R., Burrell, D. E., Shults, J. M. and Kelley, A. K., 1986, *In vitro* coadsorption of acetaminophen and N-acetylcysteine onto activated carbon powder, *Journal of Pharmaceutical Sciences*, **75**, 904–906.

Rygnestad, T., 1989, A comparative prospective study of self-poisoned patients in Trondheim, Norway between 1978 and 1987: epidemiology and clinical data, *Human Toxicology*, **8**, 475–482.

Rygnestad, T., Aastad, K., Gustafsson, K. and Jenssen, U., 1990, The clinical value of drug analyses in deliberate self-poisoning, *Human and Experimental Toxicology*, **9**, 221–230.

Saano, V., Elo, H. A. and Paronen, P., 1990, Effect of central muscle relaxants on single-dose pharmacokinetics of peroral paracetamol in man, *International Journal of Clinical Pharmacology, Therapy and Toxicology*, **28**, 39–45.

Saano, V., Koskiniemi, J., Tuomisto, J. and Airaksinen, M. M., 1983a, Absorption of paracetamol from two suppositories containing 100 mg of paracetamol, *Acta Pharmaceutica Fenniae*, **92**, 259–264.

Saano, V., Tuomisto, J. and Airaksinen, M. M., 1983b, Paracetamol absorption from an effervescent and two conventional tablets, *Acta Pharmaceutica Fenniae*, **92**, 77–83.

Saano, V., Tuomisto, J. and Airaksinen, M. M., 1983c, Absorption of paracetamol from five suppositories marketed in Finland, *Acta Pharmaceutica Fenniae*, **92**, 181–186.

Saarnivaara, L., 1984, Comparison of paracetamol and pentazocine suppositories for pain relief after tonsillectomy in adults, *Acta Anaesthesiologica Scandinavica*, **28**, 315–318.

Sabater, J., Domenéch, J. and Obach, R., 1993, Pharmacokinetic study of 4'-acetamidophenyl-2-(5'-p-toluyl-1'-methylpyrrole) acetate in the rat, *Arzneimittel-Forschung*, **43**, 154–159.

Sabater, J., Peraire, C., Obach, R., Moreno, J. and Domenech, J., 1991, Reduction of oral bioavailability of paracetamol by tolmetin in rat, *European Journal of Drug Metabolism and Pharmacokinetics*, **3**, 61–65.

Sabol, K. E. and Freed, C. R., 1988, Brain acetaminophen measurement by *in vivo* dialysis, *in vivo* electrochemistry and tissue assay: a study of the dialysis technique in the rat, *Journal of Neuroscience Methods*, **24**, 163–168.

Sacher, M. and Thaler, H., 1977, Toxic hepatitis after therapeutic doses of benorylate and D-penicillamine, *Lancet*, **i**, 481–482.

Sachs, G. and Kowalsky, S. F., 1988, Acetaminophen interaction with cimetidine and ranitidine: a critical analysis of the literature, *Advances in Therapy*, **5**, 257–272.

Saeed, S. A. and Cuthbert, J., 1977, On the mode of action and biochemical properties of anti-inflammatory drugs – II, *Prostaglandins*, **13**, 565–575.

Saeger, S., Preidel, W. and Ruprecht, L., 1992, Influence of paracetamol, sulfanilamide and ascorbic acid on the electrocatalytic glucose sensor, *Hormone and Metabolic Research*, **24**, 504–507.

Saenz de Santa Maria, J., Perez Miranda, M., Soria, A., Lozano, F., Martinena, E. and Gomez de Tejanda, R., 1983, Lesión hepática por acetaminofen: a propósito de un caso con infrecuente participación portal, *Revista Clínica Española*, **168**, 355–356.

Saetta, J. P. and Quinton, D. N., 1991, Residual gastric content after gastric lavage and ipecacuanha-induced emesis in self-poisoned patients: an endoscopic study, *Journal of the Royal Society of Medicine*, **84**, 35–38.

Sagne, S., Henrikson, P.-A., Kahnberg, K.-E., Thilander, H. and Bertilson, S. O., 1987, Analgesic efficacy and side-effect profile of paracetamol/codeine and paracetamol/dextropropoxyphene after surgical removal of a lower wisdom tooth, *Journal of International Medical Research*, **15**, 83–88.

Sahajwalla, C. G. and Ayres, J. W., 1991, Multiple-dose acetaminophen pharmacokinetics, *Journal of Pharmaceutical Sciences*, **80**, 855–860.

Saito, T., Asai, Y., Ikeda, K., Ohno, T., Kohno, A., Sakaizumi, K., Hasegawa, K., Higaki, M., Furuya, H., Matsumoto, A., Watanuki, K., Komori, N. and Ariizumi, M., 1990, A critical consideration for 'the standardization of evaluation of analgesics efficiency in toothache': clinical study of acetaminophen, *Oral Therapeutics and Pharmacology*, **9**, 28–38.

Sakai, K., Akima, M., Hinohara, Y., Sasaki, M. and Niki, R., 1980, Vascularly perfused rat small intestine: a research model for drug absorption, *Japanese Journal of Pharmacology*, **30**, 231–241.

Sakai, M., Iida, S., Morishita, T., Yoshida, K., Hashiguchi, O., Akahoshi, M., Fujiyama, S., Sagara, K. and Sato, T., 1987, A successfully treated case with brain atrophy and fulminant hepatitis induced by overdosage of taking analgesics on the market, *Acta Hepatologica Japonica*, **28**, 1238–1243.

Sakaida, I., Kayano, K., Kubota, M., Mori, K., Takenaka, K., Yasunaga, M. and Okita, K., 1992, Protective effect of deferoxamine for acetaminophen induced liver injury, *Gastroenterologia Japonica*, **27**, 426.

Sakaida, I., Kayano, K., Wasaki, S., Nagatomi, A., Matsumara, Y. and Okita, K., 1995, Protection against acetaminophen-induced liver injury *in vivo* by an iron chelator, deferoxamine, *Scandinavian Journal of Gastroenterology*, **30**, 61–67.

Sakellariou, G., Koukoudis, P., Karpouzas, J., Alexopoulos, E., Papadopoulou, D., Chrisomalis, F., Skenteris, N., Tsakaris, D. and Papadimitriou, M., 1991, Plasma exchange (PE) treatment in drug-induced toxic epidermal necrolysis (TEN), *International Journal of Artificial Organs*, **14**, 634–638.

Sakr, S. A., 1993, Effect of Thiola on acetaminophen induced hepatic necrosis in mice, *Bulletin of Environmental Contamination and Toxicology*, **51**, 808–813.

Sakurai, E., Hikichi, N. and Niwa, H., 1985, Alteration of histamine, serotonin and primary prostaglandin in case of diarrhea induced by endotoxin and gastrointestinal absorption of drug, *Journal of Pharmacobiodynamics*, **8**, 186–192.

Salvadó, A., Cemeli, J. and Del Pozo, A., 1988, Puesta a punto de un método analítico para la determinación del paracetamol en plasma humano, *Ciencia e Industria Farmaceutica*, **7**, 206–209.

Salvadó, A., Obach, R., Moreno, J. and Doménech, J., 1990, Biodisponibilité relative du paracétamol chez l'homme, *Sciences Techniques et Pratiques Pharmaceutiques*, **6**, 148–152.

Sánchez, J., Martínez, L., García-Barbal, J., Roser, R., Bartlett, A. and Sagarra, R., 1989, The influence of gastric emptying on droxicam pharmacokinetics, *Journal of Clinical Pharmacology*, **29**, 739–745.

Sánchez-Guisande, D., Arcocha, V., Novoa, D. and Romero, R., 1989, Fracaso renal agudo (FRA) con hepatopatia leve tras la administración de acetaminofeno a dosis terapéuticas, *Galicia Clínica*, **61**, 175–176.

Sandler, D. P., Smith, J. C., Weinberg, C. R., Buckalew, V. M., Dennis, V. W., Blythe, W. B. and Burgess, W. P., 1989, Analgesic use and chronic renal disease, *New England Journal of Medicine*, **320**, 1238–1243.

Sanerkin, N. G., 1971, Acute myocardial necrosis in paracetamol poisoning, *British Medical Journal*, **3**, 478.

Sangster, G., McCulloch, D. K. and Lawson, A. A. H., 1981, Medically serious self-poisoning in West Fife, 1970–1979, *Clinical Toxicology*, **18**, 1005–1014.

Saracino, M., Flowers, J. and Lovejoy, F. H., 1980, The epidemiology of poisoning from drug products, *American Journal of Diseases of Children*, **134**, 763–765.

Sarkar, A. K., Chakraborti, A., Saha, U. K., Bose, S. K. and Sengupta, D., 1989, Effects of aspirin and paracetamol on ATPases of human fetal brain: an *in vitro* study, *Indian Journal of Experimental Biology*, **27**, 802–804.

Sarre, S., van Belle, K., Smolders, I., Krieken, G. and Michotte, Y., 1992, The use of microdialysis for the determination of plasma protein binding of drugs, *Journal of Pharmaceutical and Biomedical Analysis*, **10**, 735–739.

Sasaki, M., 1986, Enhancing effect of acetaminophen on mutagenesis, *Progress in Clinical and*

Biological Research, **209A**, 365–372.

Sato, C. and Izumi, N., 1989, Mechanism of increased hepatotoxicity of acetaminophen by the simultaneous administration of caffeine in the rat, *Journal of Pharmacology and Experimental Therapeutics*, **248**, 1243–1247.

Sato, C., Izumi, N., Nouchi, T., Hasumara, Y. and Takeuchi, J., 1985, Increased hepatotoxicity of acetaminophen by concomitant administration of caffeine in the rat, *Toxicology*, **34**, 95–101.

Sato, C. and Lieber, C. S., 1981, Mechanism of the preventive effect of ethanol on acetaminophen-induced hepatotoxicity, *Journal of Pharmacology and Experimental Therapeutics*, **218**, 811–815.

Sato, C., Liu, J., Miyakawa, H., Nouchi, T., Tanaka, Y., Uchihara, M. and Marumo, F., 1991, Inhibition of acetaminophen activation by ethanol and acetaldehyde in liver microsomes, *Life Sciences*, **49**, 1787–1791.

Sato, C. and Marumo, F., 1991, Synergistic effect of NADH on NADH-dependent acetaminophen activation in liver microsomes and its inhibition by cyanide, *Life Sciences*, **48**, 2423–2427.

Sato, C., Matsuda, Y. and Lieber, C. S., 1981a, Increased hepatotoxicity of acetaminophen after chronic ethanol consumption in the rat, *Gastroenterology*, **80**, 140–148.

Sato, C., Nakano, M. and Lieber, C. S., 1981b, Prevention of acetaminophen-induced hepatotoxicity by acute ethanol administration in the rat: comparison with carbon tetrachloride-induced hepatotoxicity, *Journal of Pharmacology and Experimental Therapeutics*, **218**, 805–810.

Satoh, T., Aikawa, K. and Kitagawa, H., 1979, The metabolism and the mechanism for appearance of toxicity of acetaminophen in mice, *Journal of Toxicological Sciences*, **4**, 314–315.

Sattler, F. R., Ko, R., Antoniskis, D., Shields, M., Cohen, J., Nicoloff, J., Leedom, J. and Koda, R., 1991, Acetaminophen does not impair clearance of zidovudine, *Annals of Internal Medicine*, **114**, 937–940.

Saunders, J. B., Wright, N. and Lewis, K. O., 1980, Predicting outcome of paracetamol poisoning by using ^{14}C-aminopyrine breath test, *British Medical Journal*, **280**, 279–280.

Savage, R. L., Moller, P. W., Ballantyne, C. L. and Wells, J. E., 1993, Variation in the risk of peptic ulcer complications with nonsteroidal antiinflammatory drug therapy, *Arthritis and Rheumatism*, **36**, 84–90.

Savides, M. C. and Oehme, F. W., 1983, Acetaminophen and its toxicity, *Journal of Applied Toxicology*, **3**, 96–111.

Savides, M. C., Oehme, F. W. and Leipold, H. W., 1985, Effects of various antidotal treatments on acetaminophen toxicosis and biotransformation in cats, *American Journal of Veterinary Research*, **46**, 1485–1489.

Savides, M. C., Oehme, F. W., Nash, S. L. and Leipold, H. W., 1984, The toxicity and biotransformation of single doses of acetaminophen in dogs and cats, *Toxicology and Applied Pharmacology*, **74**, 26–34.

Saville, J. G., Davidson, C. P., D'Adrea, G. H., Born, C. K. and Hamrick, M. E., 1988, Inhibition of acetaminophen hepatotoxicity by chlorpromazine in fed and fasted mice, *Biochemical Pharmacology*, **37**, 2467–2471.

Savina, P. M. and Brouwer, K. L. R., 1992, Probenecid-impaired biliary excretion of acetaminophen glucuronide and sulfate in the rat, *Drug Metabolism and Disposition: The Biological Fate of Chemicals*, **20**, 496–501.

Sawas-Dimopoulou, C. and Soulpi, C., 1987, An approach to the early detection of liver dysfunction in acute paracetamol overdose by the use of ^{99m}Tc-mebrofenin, *Nuklearmedizin*, **26**, 132.

Sawyer, P. R., Cowart, T. D., Hurwitz, G. A., Halushka, P. V. and Jollow, D. J., 1977, Acetaminophen overdosage, *Journal of the South Carolina Medical Association*, **73**, 474–480.

Scalley, R. D. and Conner, C. S., 1978, Acetaminophen poisoning: a case report of the use of acetylcysteine, *American Journal of Hospital Pharmacy*, **35**, 964–967.

Scavone, J. M., Blyden, G. T. and Greenblatt, D. J. 1989, Lack of effect of influenza vaccine on the pharmacokinetics of antipyrine, alprazolam, paracetamol (acetaminophen) and lorazepam, *Clinical Pharmacokinetics*, **16**, 180–185.

Scavone, J. M., Greenblatt, D. J., Blyden, G. T., Luna, B. G. and Harmatz, J. S., 1990a, Validity of a two-point acetaminophen pharmacokinetic study, *Therapeutic Drug Monitoring*, **12**, 35–39.

Scavone, J. M., Greenblatt, D. J., Blyden, G. T., Luna, B. G. and Harmatz, J. S., 1990b, Acetaminophen pharmacokinetics in women receiving conjugated estrogen, *European Journal of Clinical Pharmacology*, **38**, 97–98.

Scavone, J. M., Greenblatt, D. J., LeDuc, B. W., Blyden, G. T., Luna, B. G. and Harmatz, J. S., 1990c, Differential effect of cigarette smoking on antipyrine oxidation versus acetaminophen conjugation, *Pharmacology*, **40**, 77–84.

Scavone, J. M., Greenblatt, D. J., Matlis, R. and Harmatz, J. S., 1986, Interaction of oxaprozin with acetaminophen, cimetidine and ranitidine, *European Journal of Clinical Pharmacology*, **31**, 371–374.

Scemama, M., 1972, Paracétamol: détermination des taux sanguins, *Annales Pharmaceutiques Françaises*, **30**, 861–864.

Schachtel, B. P., Fillingim, J. F., Thoden, W. R., Lane, A. C. and Baybutt, R. I., 1988, Sore throat pain in the evaluation of mild analgesics, *Clinical Pharmacology and Therapeutics*, **44**, 704–711.

Schachtel, B. P. and Thoden, W. R., 1993, A placebo-controlled model for assaying systemic analgesics in children, *Clinical Pharmacology and Therapeutics*, **53**, 593–601.

Schachtel, B. P., Thoden, W. R. and Baybutt, R. I., 1989, Ibuprofen and acetaminophen in the relief of postpartum episiotomy pain, *Journal of Clinical Pharmacology*, **29**, 550–553.

Schachtel, B. P., Thoden, W. R., Konerman, J. P., Brown, A. and Chaing, D. S., 1991, Headache pain model for assessing and comparing the efficacy of over-the-counter analgesic agents, *Clinical Pharmacology and Therapeutics*, **50**, 322–329.

Schechter, M. S., 1980, Dosage of aspirin and acetaminophen, *Journal of Pediatrics*, **96**, 1124.

Scheinberg, I. H., 1979, Thrombocytopenic reaction to aspirin and acetaminophen, *New England Journal of Medicine*, **300**, 678.

Schenker, S. and Maddrey, W. C., 1991, Subliminal drug-drug interactions: users and their physicians take notice, *Hepatology*, **13**, 995–998.

Schernitski, P., Bootman, J. L., Byers, J., Likes, K. and Hughes, J. H., 1980, Demographic characteristics of elderly drug overdose patients admitted to a hospital emergency department, *Journal of the American Geriatrics Society*, **28**, 544–546.

Schlager, J. J., LaCreta, F. P., Hurst, H. E. and Williams, W. M., 1987, Effect of ethanol on acetaminophen elimination by the isolated perfused rat liver, *Federation Proceedings*, **46**, 1138.

Schmid, J., Fedorcak, A. and Koss, F. W., 1980, Eine empfindliche, spezifische kolorimetrische Methode zur Bestimmung von Paracetamol im Humanplasma, *Arzneimittel-Forschung*, **30**, 996–998.

Schmid, W. H., 1977, Acetaminophen-induced bronchospasm, *Southern Medical Journal*, **70**, 590–612.

Schmitt, K. and Cilento, G., 1990, The peroxidase-promoted metabolic activation of acetaminophen produces electronically excited species, *Photochemistry and Photobiology*, **51**, 719–723.

Schnaiderman, D., Lahat, E., Sheefer, T. and Aladjem, M., 1993, Antipyretic effectiveness of acetaminophen in febrile seizures: ongoing prophylaxis versus sporadic usage, *European Journal of Pediatrics*, **152**, 747–749.

Schnell, R. C., Bozigian, H. P., Davies, M. H., Merrick, B. A. and Johnson, K. L., 1983, Circadian rhythm in acetaminophen toxicity: role of nonprotein sulfhydryls, *Toxicology and Applied Pharmacology*, **71**, 353–361.

Schnell, R. C., Bozigian, H. P., Davies, M. H., Merrick, B. A., Park, K. S. and McMillan, D. A., 1984, Factors influencing circadian rhythms in acetaminophen lethality, *Pharmacology*, **29**, 149–157.

Schnell, R. C., Park, K. S., Davis, M. H., Merrick, B. A. and Weir, S. W., 1988, Protective effects of selenium on acetaminophen-induced hepatotoxicity in the rat, *Toxicology and Applied Pharmacology*, **95**, 1–11.

Schnider, P., Aull, S., Feucht, M., Mraz, M., Travniczek, A., Zeiler, K. and Wessely, P., 1994, Use and abuse of analgesics in tension–type headache, *Cephalalgia*, **14**, 162–167.

Schnitzer, B. and Smith, E. B., 1966, Effects of the metabolites of phenacetin on the rat, *Archives of Pathology*, **81**, 264–267.

Schnitzer, T. J., 1993, Osteoarthritis treatment update. Minimising pain while limiting patient risk, *Postgraduate Medicine*, **93**, 89–92,95.

Schoots, A. C., Koomen, G. C. M., Struijk, D. G., Krediet, R. T. and Arisz, L., 1990, Isolation, identification, and analysis of 4-acetylaminophenol-glucuronide in body fluids of dialyzed renal patients: a molecular mass marker for peritoneal diffusive transport, *Clinica Chimica Acta*, **188**, 15–30.

Schor, N., Voos, A., Stella, R. C. R., Ribeiro, A. B. and Ramos, O. L., 1983, Effects of cyclooxygenase inhibitors on plasma and urinary kallikrein, *Hypertension*, **5 (Suppl. V)**, V-48–V-52.

Schubert, G. E. and Bethke, B. A., 1986, Capillarosclerosis of the renal pelvis: autopsy study for estimating the incidence of phenacetin and paracetamol abuse, *European Urology*, **12**, 327–330.

Schulz, W., 1990, Die Analgetika-niere, *Nieren- und Hochdruckkrankheiten*, **19**, 37–44.

Schurizek, B. A., 1991, The effects of general anaesthesia on antroduodenal motility, gastric pH and gastric emptying in man, *Danish Medical Bulletin*, **38**, 347–365.

Schurizek, B. A., Kraglund, K., Andreasen, F., Jensen, L. V. and Juhl, B., 1988, Gastrointestinal motility and gastric pH and emptying following ingestion of diazepam, *British Journal of Anaesthesia*, **61**, 712–719.

Schurizek, B. A., Kraglund, K., Andreasen, F., Vinter-Jensen, L. and Juhl, B., 1989a, Antroduodenal motility and gastric emptying. Gastroduodenal motility and pH following ingestion of paracetamol, *Alimentary Pharmacology and Therapeutics*, **3**, 93–101.

Schurizek, B. A., Willacy, L. H. O., Kraglund, K., Andreasen, F. and Juhl, B., 1989b, Effects of general anaesthesia with enflurane on antroduodenal motility, pH and gastric emptying rate in man, *European Journal of Anaesthesiology*, **6**, 265–279.

Schurizek, B. A., Willacy, L. H. O., Kraglund, K., Andreasen, F., Juhl, B., 1989c, Effects of general anaesthesia with halothane on antroduodenal motility, pH and gastric emptying rate in man, *British Journal of Anaesthesia*, **62**, 129–137.

Schurizek, B. A., Willacy, L. H. O., Kraglund, K., Andreasen, F. and Juhl, B., 1989d, Antroduodenal motility, pH and gastric emptying during balanced anaesthesia: comparison of pethidine and fentanyl, *British Journal of Anaesthesia*, **62**, 674–682.

Schwartz, J. G., Stuckey, J. H., Prihoda, T. J., Kazen, C. M. and Carnahan, J. J., 1990, Hospital-based toxicology: patterns of use and abuse, *Texas Medicine*, **86**, 44–51.

Schwarz, A., 1987, Analgesic-associated nephropathy, *Klinische Wochenschrift*, **65**, 1–16.

Schwarz, A., Faber, U., Borner, K., Keller, F., Offermann, G. and Molzahn, M., 1984, Reliability of drug history in analgesic users, *Lancet*, **ii**, 1163–1164.

Schwarz, A., Keller, F., Kunzendorf, U., Kühn-Freitag, G., Heinemeyer, G., Pommer, W. and Offermann, G., 1988, Characteristics and clinical course of hemodialysis patients with analgesic-associated nephropathy, *Clinical Nephrology*, **6**, 299–306.

Schwarz, A., Kunzendorf, U., Keller, F. and Offermann, G., 1989, Progression of renal failure in analgesic-associated nephropathy, *Nephron*, **53**, 244–249.

Schwarz, A., Offermann, G. and Keller, F., 1992, Analgesic nephropathy and renal transplantation, *Nephrology, Dialysis, Transplantation*, **7**, 427–432.

Schwarz, A., Pommer, W., Kühn-Freitag, G., Keller, F., Molzahn, M. and Offermann, G.,

1985, Merkmale der terminalen Analgetika-Nephropathie, *Schweizerische Medizinische Wochenschrift*, **115**, 790–795.

Schweizer, A. and Brom, R., 1985, Differentiation of peripheral and central effects of analgesic drugs, *International Journal of Tissue Reactions*, **7**, 79–83.

Scott, C. R. and Stewart, M. J., 1975, Cysteamine treatment in paracetamol overdose, *Lancet*, **i**, 452–453.

Scott, D. O., Sorensen, L. R. and Lunte, C. E., 1990, *In vivo* microdialysis sampling coupled to liquid chromatography for the study of acetaminophen metabolism, *Journal of Chromatography*, **506**, 461–469.

Scott, D. O., Sorenson, L. R., Steele, K. L., Puckett, D. L. and Lunte, C. E., 1991, *In vivo* microdialysis sampling for pharmacokinetic investigations, *Pharmaceutical Research*, **8**, 389–392.

Seddon, C. E., Boobis, A. R. and Davies, D. S., 1987, Comparative activation of paracetamol in the rat, mouse and man, *Archives of Toxicology*, **Suppl. 11**, 305–309.

Seddon, M. J., Spraul, M., Wilson, I. D., Nicholson, J. K. and Lindon, J. C., 1994, Improvement in the characterisation of minor drug metabolites from HPLC-NMR studies through the use of quantified maximum entropy processing of NMR spectra, *Journal of Pharmaceutical and Biomedical Analysis*, **12**, 419–424.

Seeff, L. B., Cuccherini, B. A., Zimmerman, H. J., Adler, E. and Benjamin, S. B., 1986, Acetaminophen hepatotoxicity in alcoholics. A therapeutic misadventure, *Annals of Internal Medicine*, **104**, 399–404.

Seegers, A. J. M., Jager, L. P. and van Noordwijk, J., 1978, Gastric erosions induced by analgesic drug mixtures in the rat, *Journal of Pharmacy and Pharmacology*, **30**, 84–87.

Seegers, A. J. M., Jager, L. P. and van Noordwijk, J., 1979, Effects of phenacetin, paracetamol and caffeine on the erosive activity of acetylsalicylic acid in the rat stomach: dose-response relationships, time course of erosion development and effects on acid secretion, *Journal of Pharmacy and Pharmacology*, **31**, 840–848.

Seegers, A. J. M., Jager, L. P. and van Noordwijk, J., 1980a, An hypothesis concerning the action of paracetamol against the erosive activity of acetylsalicylic acid in the rat stomach, *Advances in Prostaglandin and Thromboxane Research*, **8**, 1547–1551.

Seegers, A. J. M., Jager, L. P., Zandberg, P. and van Noordwijk, J., 1981, The anti-inflammatory, analgesic and antipyretic activities of non-narcotic analgesic drug mixtures in rats, *Archives Internationales de Pharmacodynamie et de Thérapie*, **251**, 237–254.

Seegers, A. J. M., Olling, M., Jager, L. P. and van Noordwijk, J., 1980b, Interactions of aspirin with acetaminophen and caffeine in rat stomach: pharmacokinetics of absorption and accumulation in gastric mucosa, *Journal of Pharmaceutical Sciences*, **69**, 900–906.

Seegers, A. J. M., Olling, M., Jager, L. P. and van Noordwijk, J., 1982, The influence of paracetamol on the erosive activity of indomethacin in the rat stomach, *Agents and Actions*, **12**, 247–253.

Segasothy, M., Cheong, I., Kong, B. C. T., Suleiman, A. B. and Morad, Z., 1986a, Further evidence of analgesic nephropathy in Malaysia, *Medical Journal of Malaysia*, **41**, 377–379.

Segasothy, M., Kong Chiew Tong, B., Kamal, A., Murad, Z. and Suleiman, A. B., 1984, Analgesic nephropathy associated with paracetamol, *Australian and New Zealand Journal of Medicine*, **14**, 23–26.

Segasothy, M., Muhaya, H. M., Musa, A., Rajagopalan, K., Lim, K. J., Fatimah, Y., Kamal, A. and Ahmad, K. S., 1986b, Analgesic use by leprosy patients, *International Journal of Leprosy and Other Mycobacterial Diseases*, **54**, 399–402.

Segasothy, M., Samad, S. A., Zulfigar, A. and Bennett, W. M., 1994a, Chronic renal disease and papillary necrosis associated with the long term use of nonsteroidal anti-inflammatory drugs as the sole or predominant analgesic, *American Journal of Kidney Diseases*, **24**, 17–24.

Segasothy, M., Samad, S. A., Zulfiqar, A., Shaariah, W., Morad, Z. and Menon, S. P., 1994b,

Computed tomography and ultrasonography: a comparative study in the diagnosis of analgesic nephropathy, *Nephron*, **66**, 62–66.

Segasothy, M., Suleiman, A. B., Puvaneswary, M. and Rohana, A., 1988, Paracetamol: a cause for analgesic nephropathy and end-stage renal disease, *Nephron*, **50**, 50–54.

Seideman, P., 1991, Lack of effect of paracetamol on the pharmacokinetics of indomethacin and paracetamol in humans, *Journal of Clinical Pharmacology*, **31**, 804–807.

Seideman, P., 1993a, Paracetamol in rheumatoid arthritis, *Agents and Actions*, **44**, 7–12.

Seideman, P., 1993b, Additive effect of combined naproxen and paracetamol in rheumatoid arthritis, *British Journal of Rheumatology*, **32**, 1077–1082.

Seideman, P., Alván, G., Andrews, R. S. and Labross, A., 1980, Relative bioavailability of a paracetamol suppository, *European Journal of Clinical Pharmacology*, **17**, 465–468.

Seideman, P. and Melander, A., 1988, Equianalgesic effects of paracetamol and indomethacin in rheumatoid arthritis, *British Journal of Rheumatology*, **27**, 117–122.

Seideman, P., Samuelson, P. and Neander, G., 1993, Naproxen and paracetamol compared with naproxen only in coxarthrosis: increased effect of the combination in 18 patients, *Acta Orthopaedica Scandinavica*, **64**, 285–288.

Seifert, C. F., Lucas, D. S., Vondracek, T. G., Kastens, D. J., McCarty, D. L. and Bui, B., 1993, Patterns of acetaminophen use in alcoholic patients, *Pharmacotherapy*, **13**, 391–395.

Sekikawa, H., Ito, K., Arita, T., Hori, R. and Nakano, M., 1979, Effects of macromolecular additives and urea on the intestinal absorption of acetaminophen in rats, *Chemical and Pharmaceutical Bulletin*, **27**, 1106–1111.

Selbst, S. M., 1992, Analgesia in children: why is it underused in emergency departments? *Drug Safety*, **7**, 8–13.

Selbst, S. M. and Henretig, F. M., 1989, The treatment of pain in the emergency department, *Pediatric Clinics of North America*, **36**, 965–978.

Selden, B. S., Curry, S. C., Clark, R. F., Johnson, B. C., Meinhart, R. and Pizziconi, V. B., 1991, Transplacental transport of N-acetylcysteine in an ovine model, *Annals of Emergency Medicine*, **20**, 1069–1072.

Sengupta, A. and Peat, M. A., 1977, Propoxyphene overdosage: a study of cases involving analgesic preparations containing dextropropoxyphene, *Archives of Toxicology*, **37**, 123–133.

Seppälä, E., Laitinen, O. and Vapaatalo, H., 1983, Comparative study on the effects of acetylsalicylic acid, indomethacin and paracetamol on metabolites of arachidonic acid in plasma, serum and urine in man, *International Journal of Clinical Pharmacology Research*, **3**, 265–269.

Seppälä, E., Nissilä, M., Isomäki, H., Wuorela, H. and Vapaatalo, H., 1990, Effects of non-steroidal anti-inflammatory drugs and prednisolone on synovial fluid white cells, prostaglandin E_2, leukotriene B_4 and cyclic AMP in patients with rheumatoid arthritis, *Scandinavian Journal of Rheumatology*, **19**, 71–75.

Serfontein, W. J., Coetzee, M., de Villiers, L. S. and Botha, D., 1976, GLC determination of paracetamol and d-propoxyphene, *South African Journal of Medical Sciences*, **41**, 297–304.

Serrar, D. and Thevenin, M., 1987, Toxicité du paracétamol chez la souris Swiss traitée par l'alcool éthylique en aigu ou à court terme, *Revue de l'Alcoolisme*, **32**, 105–111.

Settipane, R. A., Schrank, P. J., Simon, R. A., Mathison, D. A., Christiansen, S. C. and Stevenson, D. D., 1994, Prevalence of cross-sensitivity with acetaminophen in aspirin-sensitive subjects with asthma, *Journal of Allergy and Clinical Immunology*, **93**, 266.

Settipane, R. A. and Stevenson, D. D., 1989, Cross sensitivity with acetaminophen in aspirin-sensitive subjects with asthma, *Journal of Allergy and Clinical Immunology*, **84**, 26–33.

Sewell, R. D. E., Gonzalez, J. P. and Pugh, J., 1984, Comparison of the relative effects of aspirin, mefenamic acid, dihydrocodeine, dextropropoxyphene and paracetamol on visceral pain, respiratory rate and prostaglandin biosynthesis, *Archives Internationales de*

Pharmacodynamie et de Thérapie, **268**, 325–334.

Seymour, R. A., 1983, Efficacy of paracetamol in reducing post-operative pain after periodontal surgery, *Journal of Periodontology*, **10**, 311–316.

Seymour, R. A., Blair, G. S. and Wyatt, F. A. R., 1983, Postoperative dental pain and analgesic efficacy: part II. Analgesic usage and efficacy after dental surgery, *British Journal of Oral Surgery*, **21**, 298–303.

Seymour, R. A. and Rawlins, M. D., 1981, Pharmacokinetics of parenteral paracetamol and its analgesic effects in post-operative dental pain, *European Journal of Clinical Pharmacology*, **20**, 215–218.

Seymour, R. A., Williams, F. M., Oxley, A., Ward, A., Fearns, M., Brighan, K., Rawlins, M. D. and Jones, P. M., 1984, A comparative study of the effects of aspirin and paracetamol (acetaminophen) on platelet aggregation and bleeding time, *European Journal of Clinical Pharmacology*, **26**, 567–571.

Shaffer, J. E., Cagen, L. M. and Malik, K. U., 1981, Attenuation by acetaminophen of arachidonic acid-induced coronary vasodilation and output of prostaglandins in the isolated rat heart, *European Journal of Pharmacology*, **72**, 57–61.

Shah, M., Rosen, M. and Vickers, M. D., 1984, Effect of premedication with diazepam, morphine or nalbuphine on gastrointestinal motility after surgery, *British Journal of Anaesthesia*, **56**, 1235–1238.

Shalabi, E. A., 1992, Acetaminophen inhibits the human polymorphonuclear leukocyte function *in vitro*, *Immunopharmacology*, **24**, 37–46.

Shamszad, M., Soloman, H., Mobarhan, S. and Iber, F. L., 1975, Abnormal metabolism of acetaminophen in patients with alcoholic liver disease, *Gastroenterology*, **69**, 865.

Shangraw, R. F. and Walkling, W. D., 1971, Effect of vehicle dielectric properties on rectal absorption of acetaminophen, *Journal of Pharmaceutical Sciences*, **60**, 600–602.

Shanks, I., Sowray, J. H. and Mustill, T. A., 1987, Double-blind crossover comparison of suprofen and dextropropoxyphene plus paracetamol in post-operature dental pain, *Acta Therapeutica*, **13**, 325–331.

Shann, F., 1993, Paracetamol: when, why and how much, *Journal of Paediatrics and Child Health*, **29**, 84–85.

Shannon, M., Saladino, R., McCarty, D., Parker, K. M., Scott, L., Brown, G. and Vaughn, P., 1990, Clinical evaluation of an acetaminophen meter for the rapid diagnosis of acetaminophen intoxication, *Annals of Emergency Medicine*, **19**, 1133–1136.

Sharma, D. B., Lahori, U. C. and Gupta, R. C., 1979, Acute acetaminophen hypersensitivity in infancy, *Indian Pediatrics*, **16**, 1139–1141.

Sharma, S., Bhatia, A. and Das, P. K., 1983, Role of microsomal drug detoxifying enzyme systems in paracetamol induced liver injury in rats, *Indian Journal of Medical Research*, **78**, 134–141.

Sharman, J. R., 1981, OV-225 as a stationary phase for the determination of anticonvulsants, mexiletine, barbiturates, and acetaminophen, *Journal of Analytical Toxicology*, **5**, 153–156.

Sharon, R., Menczel, J. and Kidroni, G., 1982, Incidence of acetaminophen in donated blood, *Vox Sanguinis*, **43**, 138–141.

Sharp, G., 1915, A short history of the synthetic aniline alkaloidal derivatives – phenazone, phenacetine, and acetanilide, *Pharmaceutical Journal*, **95**, 197–198.

Shavila, J., Ioannides, C., King, L. J. and Parke, D. V., 1994, Effect of high fat diet on liver microsomal oxygenations in ferret, *Xenobiotica*, **24**, 1063–1076.

Shaw, S., Rubin, K. P. and Lieber, C. S., 1983, Depressed hepatic gluathione and increased diene conjugates in alcoholic liver disease, *Digestive Diseases and Sciences*, **28**, 585–589.

Shelley, J. H., 1978, Pharmacological mechanisms of analgesic nephropathy, *Kidney International*, **13**, 15–26.

Shelton, D. W. and Weber, L. J., 1981, Quantification of the joint effects of mixtures of hepatotoxic agents: evaluation of a theoretical model in mice, *Environmental Research*,

26, 33–41.

Shen, W., Kamendulis, L. M., Ray, S. D. and Corcoran, G. B., 1991, Acetaminophen-induced cytotoxicity in cultured mouse hepatocytes: correlation of nuclear Ca^{2+} accumulation and early DNA fragmentation with cell death, *Toxicology and Applied Pharmacology*, **111**, 242–254.

Shen, W., Kamendulis, L. M., Ray, S. D. and Corcoran, G. B., 1992, Acetaminophen-induced cytotoxicity in cultured mouse hepatocytes: effects of Ca^{2+}-endonuclease, DNA repair, and glutathione depletion inhibitors on DNA fragmentation and cell death, *Toxicology and Applied Pharmacology*, **112**, 32–40.

Shenoy, M. A. and Gopalakrishna, K., 1977, Some mechanisms involved in the radio-sensitization of *E. coli* B/r by paracetamol, *International Journal of Radiation Biology & Related Studies in Physics, Chemistry and Medicine*, **31**, 577–587.

Sheth, U. K., Gupta, K., Paul, T. and Pispati, P. K., 1980, Measurement of antipyretic activity of ibuprofen and paracetamol in children, *Journal of Clinical Pharmacology*, **20**, 672–675.

Shibasaki, J., Konishi, R., Kitasaki, T. and Koizumi, T., 1979, Relationship between blood levels and analgesic effects of acetaminophen in mice, *Chemical and Pharmaceutical Bulletin*, **27**, 129–138.

Shibasaki, J., Konishi, R., Takeda, Y. and Koizumi, T., 1971, Drug absorption, metabolism, and excretion. VII. Pharmacokinetics on formation and excretion of the conjugates of N-acetyl-p-aminophenol in rabbits, *Chemical and Pharmaceutical Bulletin*, **19**, 1800–1808.

Shibasaki, J., Konishi, R. and Yamada, K., 1980, Fluorometric determination of acetaminophen and its conjugates in whole blood, *Chemical and Pharmaceutical Bulletin*, **28**, 669–672.

Shibasaki, J., Konishi, R., Yamada, K. and Matsuda, S., 1982, Improved fluorometric determination of acetaminophen and its conjugates with 1-nitroso-2-naphthol in whole blood and urine, *Chemical and Pharmaceutical Bulletin*, **30**, 358–361.

Shichi, H., Gaasterland, D. E., Jensen, N. M. and Nebert, D. W., 1978, Ah Locus: genetic differences in susceptibility to cataracts induced by acetaminophen, *Science*, **200**, 539–541.

Shichi, H., Tanaka, M., Jensen, N. M. and Nebert, D. W., 1980, Genetic differences in cataract and other ocular abnormalities induced by paracetamol and naphthalene, *Pharmacology*, **20**, 229–241.

Shih, V. E., Nikiforov, V. and Carney, M. M., 1985, Acetaminophen metabolite interferes in analysis for amino acids, *Clinical Chemistry*, **31**, 148.

Shihab-Eldeen, A. A., Peck, G. E., Ash, S. R. and Kaufman, G., 1988, Evaluation of the sorbent suspension reciprocating dialyser in the treatment of overdose of paracetamol and phenobarbitone, *Journal of Pharmacy and Pharmacology*, **40**, 381–387.

Shihabi, Z. K. and David, R. M., 1984, Colorimetric assay for acetaminophen in serum, *Therapeutic Drug Monitoring*, **6**, 449–453.

Shim, C.-K. and Jung, B.-H., 1992a, Inter- and intrasubject variations of multiple saliva peaks of acetaminophen after oral administration of tablets, *International Journal of Pharmaceutics*, **82**, 233–237.

Shim, C.-K. and Jung, B.-H., 1992b, Noncontribution of enterohepatic recycling to multiple plasma peaks of acetaminophen in rats, *International Journal of Pharmaceutics*, **83**, 257–262.

Shim, C.-K., Kim, K.-M., Kim, Y.-I. and Kim, C.-K., 1990a, Development of controlled release oral drug delivery system by membrane-coating method – I: preparation and pharmaceutical evaluation of controlled release acetaminophen tablets, *Archives of Pharmaceutical Research*, **13**, 151–160.

Shim, C.-K., Kim, M.-A., Lee, M.-H. and Kim, S.-K., 1990b, Development of controlled release oral drug delivery system by membrane-coating method – II. Correlation between acetaminophen concentrations in plasma and saliva samples in man, *Journal of*

Korean Pharmaceutical Sciences, **20**, 29–33.

Shim, C.-K. and Suh, M.-K., 1992, Multiple plasma peaks of acetaminophen and ranitidine after simultaneous oral administration to rats, *Archives of Pharmaceutical Research*, **15**, 246–250.

Shimame, Y., 1985, Mutagenicity of acetaminophen on Chinese hamster V79 cells, *Shigaku*, **72**, 1175–1187.

Shimazaki, M., Sugihara, J.-I., Murakami, N., Kuboi, H., Imamine, T., Onishi, H., Saito, K., Moriwaki, H., Tomita, E., Muto, Y., Adachi, N., Shimizu, M., Takai, T. and Takahashi, Y., 1989, Three cases of severe acetaminophen overdose, *Acta Hepatologica Japonica*, **30**, 1520–1525.

Shimizu, M., Tokita, H., Koshino, Y., Hosiyama, N., Yamada, M., Takahashi, Y. and Nishikawa, Y., 1989, An autopsy case of acute hepatic failure caused by ingesting a small dose of acetaminophen in a drinker, *Acta Hepatologica Japonica*, **30**, 690–694.

Shiohama, N., Sugita, Y., Imamura, N., Sato, T. and Mizuno, Y., 1993, Type II citrullinemia triggered by acetaminophen, *Brain and Nerve*, **45**, 865–870.

Shiohara, T., Sagawa, Y. and Nagashima, M., 1992, Systemic release of interferon-γ in drug-induced cutaneous vasculitis, *Lancet*, **339**, 933.

Shirhatti, V. and Krishna, G., 1985, A simple and sensitive method for monitoring drug-induced cell injury in cultured cells, *Analytical Biochemistry*, **147**, 410–418.

Shively, C. A. and Vesell, E. S., 1975, Temporal variations in acetaminophen and phenacetin half-life in man, *Clinical Pharmacology and Therapeutics*, **18**, 413–424.

Shnaps, Y., Halkin, H., Dany, S. and Tirosh, M., 1980, Inadequacy of reported intake in assessing the potential hepatotoxicity of acetaminophen overdose, *Israel Journal of Medical Sciences*, **16**, 752–755.

Shnaps, Y., Kaplinsky, N., Frankel, O. and Tirosh, M., 1981, Acute hepatocellular damage due to paracetamol, *Harefuah*, **101**, 358–359.

Shoenfeld, Y., Shaklai, M., Livni, E. and Pinkhas, J., 1980, Thrombocytopenia from acetaminophen, *New England Journal of Medicine*, **303**, 47.

Shorr, R. I., Kao, K.-J., Pizzo, S. V., Rauckman, E. J. and Rosen, G. M., 1985, *In vitro* effects of acetaminophen and its analogues on human platelet aggregation and thromboxane B_2 synthesis, *Thrombosis Research*, **38**, 33–43.

Shrady, G. F., 1886, Another new antipyretic – Antifebrin, *Medical Record (New York)*, **30**, 294.

Shrewsbury, R. P. and White, L. G., 1990, The effect of moderate hemodilution with Fluosol-DA or normal saline on acetaminophen disposition in the rat, *Experientia*, **46**, 213–217.

Shriner, K. and Goetz, M. B., 1992, Severe hepatotoxicity in a patient receiving both acetaminophen and zidovudine, *American Journal of Medicine*, **93**, 94–96.

Shrivastava, R., Delomenie, C., Chevalier, A., John, G., Ekwall, B., Walum, E. and Massingham, R., 1992, Comparison of *in vivo* acute lethal potency and *in vitro* cytotoxicity of 48 chemicals, *Cell Biology and Toxicology*, **8**, 157–170.

Shrivastava, R., John, G., Chevalier, A., Beaughard, M., Rispat, G., Slaoui, M. and Massingham, R., 1994, Paracetamol potentiates isaxonine toxicity *in vitro*, *Toxicology Letters*, **73**, 167–173.

Shufman, N. and Machtey, I., 1979, Liver function tests following paracetamol administration, *Harefuah*, **97**, 110–111.

Shukla, B., Visen, P. K. S., Patnaik, G. K., Kapoor, N. K. and Dhawan, B. N., 1992a, Hepatoprotective effect of an active constituent isolated from the leaves of *Ricinus communis* Linn, *Drug Development Research*, **26**, 183–193.

Shukla, B., Visen, P. K. S., Patnaik, G. K., Tripathi, S. C., Srimal, R. C., Dayal, R. and Dobhal, P. C., 1992b, Hepatoprotective activity in the rat of ursolic acid isolated from Eucalyptus hybrid, *Phytotherapy Research*, **6**, 74–79.

Shukla, S. R., 1982, Fixed drug eruption to paracetamol, *Indian Medical Gazette*, **116**, 263–264.

Shulman, G. I., Cline, G., Schumann, W. C., Chandramouli, V., Kumaran, K. and Landau, B. R., 1990, Quantitative comparison of pathways of hepatic glycogen repletion in fed and fasted humans, *American Journal of Physiology*, **259**, E335–E341.

Shyadehi, A. Z. and Harding, J. J., 1991, Investigations of ibuprofen and paracetamol binding to lens proteins to explore their protective role against cataract, *Biochemical Pharmacology*, **42**, 2077–2084.

Sicardi, S. M., Martiarena, J. L. and Iglesias, M. T., 1991, Mutagenic and analgesic activities of aniline derivatives, *Journal of Pharmaceutical Sciences*, **80**, 761–764.

Sidhu, P. K., Srivastava, A. K., Kwatra, M. S. and Bal, M. S., 1993, Plasma levels, disposition kinetics and dosage regimen of paracetamol in buffalo calves, *Indian Journal of Animal Sciences*, **63**, 1160–1162.

Sidler, J., Frey, B. and Baerlocher, K., 1990, A double blind comparison of ibuprofen and paracetamol in juvenile pyrexia, *British Journal of Clinical Practice*, **44 (Suppl. 70)**, 22–25.

Siefkin, A. D., 1982, Combined paraquat and acetaminophen toxicity, *Journal of Toxicology. Clinical Toxicology*, **19**, 483–491.

Siegel, M. I., McConnell, R. T., Porter, N. A. and Cuatrecasas, P., 1980, Arachidonate metabolism via lipoxygenase and 12L-hydroperoxy-5,8, 10,14-icosatetraenoic acid peroxidase sensitive to anti-inflammatory drugs, *Proceedings of the National Academy of Sciences of the United States of America*, **77**, 308–312.

Siegers, C.-P., 1973, Effects of caffeine on the absorption and analgesic efficacy of paracetamol in rats, *Pharmacology*, **10**, 19–27.

Siegers, C.-P., 1978a, Antidotal effects of dimethyl sulphoxide against paracetamol-bromobenzene- and thioacetamide-induced hepatotoxicity, *Journal of Pharmacy and Pharmacology*, **30**, 375–377.

Siegers, C.-P., 1978b, Influence of dithiocarb on the biliary excretion of paracetamol and bilirubin in rats, *Experientia*, **34**, 1318–1319.

Siegers, C.-P., Bartels, L. and Riemann, D., 1989, Effects of fasting and glutathione depletors on the GSH-dependent enzyme system in the gastrointestinal mucosa of the rat, *Pharmacology*, **38**, 121–128.

Siegers, C.-P., Jeß, U. and Younes, M., 1983a, Effects of phenobarbital, GSH-depletors, CCl$_4$ and ethanol on the biliary efflux of glutathione in rats, *Archives Internationales de Pharmacodynamie et de Therapie*, **266**, 315–325.

Siegers, C.-P. and Klaassen, C. D., 1984, Biliary excretion of acetaminophen in ureter-ligated rats, *Pharmacology*, **28**, 177–180.

Siegers, C.-P., Loeser, W., Gieselmann, J. and Oltmanns, D., 1984, Biliary and renal excretion of paracetamol in man, *Pharmacology*, **29**, 301–303.

Siegers, C.-P., Loeser, W. and Younes, M., 1985, Biliary excretion of acetaminophen in diabetic and hyperthyroid rats, *Research Communications in Chemical Pathology and Pharmacology*, **47**, 345–355.

Siegers, C.-P. and Möller-Hartmann, W., 1989, Cholestyramine as an antidote against paracetamol-induced hepato- and nephrotoxicity in the rat, *Toxicology Letters*, **47**, 179–184.

Siegers, C.-P., Oltmanns, D. and Younes, M., 1981, Effect of alcohol and chronic liver disease on the metabolic disposal of acetaminophen in man, *Hepato-Gastroenterology*, **28**, 304.

Siegers, C.-P., Rozman, K. and Klaassen, C. D., 1983b, Biliary excretion and enterohepatic circulation of paracetamol in the rat, *Xenobiotica*, **13**, 591–596.

Siegers, C.-P. and Schütt, A., 1979, Dose-dependent biliary and renal excretion of paracetamol in the rat, *Pharmacology*, **18**, 175–179.

Siegers, C.-P., Steffen, B. and Younes, M., 1988, Antidotal effects of deferrioxamine in experimental liver injury – role of lipid peroxidation, *Pharmacological Research Communications*, **20**, 337–343.

Siegers, C.-P., Strubelt, O. and Schütt, A., 1978, Relations between hepatotoxicity and pharmacokinetics of paracetamol in rats and mice, *Pharmacology*, **16**, 273–278.

Siegers, C.-P. and Younes, M., 1979, Einfluss von 2-Dimethylaminoethanol auf die hepato-toxischen Wirkungen von paracetamol bei Ratten und Mäusen, *Arzneimittel-Forschung*, **29**, 520–523.

Siegers, C.-P., Younes, M. and Oltmanns, D., 1980, Hemmende und fördernde Einflüsse auf den Paracetamol-Metabolismus bei Ratten, *Arzneimittel-Forschung*, **30**, 804–807.

Silberbush, J., Lenstra, J. B., Leynse, B. and Gerbrandy, J., 1974, The influence of paracetamol loading on its excretion by the kidney, *Netherlands Journal of Medicine*, **17**, 108–114.

Silverman, J. J. and Carithers, R. L., 1978, Acetaminophen overdose, *American Journal of Psychiatry*, **135**, 114–115.

Sim, S. M., Back, D. J. and Breckenridge, A. M., 1991, The effect of various drugs on the glucuronidation of zidovudine (azidothymidine; AZT) by human liver microsomes, *British Journal of Clinical Pharmacology*, **32**, 17–21.

Similä, S., Kouvalainen, K. and Keinänen, S., 1976, Oral antipyretic therapy – evaluation of ibuprofen, *Scandinavian Journal of Rheumatology*, **5**, 81–83.

Similä, S., Kouvalainen, K. and Keinänen, S., 1977, Oral antipyretic therapy: evaluation of mefenamic acid, *Arzneimittel-Forschung*, **27**, 687–688.

Similä, S. and Kylmämaa, T., 1985, Antipyretic effect of tenoxicam and paracetamol in febrile children, *Drugs Under Experimental and Clinical Research*, **11**, 731–734.

Simmons, R. L. L., Owen, S., Abbott, C. J. A., Bouchier-Hayes, T. A. I. and Hunt, H. A., 1982, Naproxen sodium and paracetamol/dextropropoxyphene in sports injuries – a multi-centre comparative study, *British Journal of Sports Medicine*, **16**, 91–95.

Simon, H. B., 1976, Extreme pyrexia, *Journal of the American Medical Association*, **236**, 2419–2421.

Simon, P. and Meyrier, A., 1982, Drug-induced hepatic injury in maintenance hemodialysis patients, *Dialysis and Transplantation*, **11**, 774–779.

Simon, R. A., Meltsez, E. O. and Settipane, R. A., 1988, Systemic anaphylaxis following inges-tion of acetaminophen (Tylenol), *Journal of Allergy and Clinical Immunology*, **81**, 223.

Simpson, E. and Stewart, M. J., 1973, Screening for paracetamol poisoning, *Annals of Clinical Biochemistry*, **10**, 171–178.

Simpson, K. H. and Stakes, A. F., 1987, Effect of anxiety on gastric emptying in preoperative patients, *British Journal of Anaesthesia*, **59**, 540–544.

Simpson, K. H., Stakes, A. F. and Miller, M., 1988, Pregnancy delays paracetamol absorption and gastric emptying in patients undergoing surgery, *British Journal of Anaesthesia*, **60**, 24–27.

Sinclair, J., Lindenthal, J., Howell, S., Taylor, T., Cargill, I. and Sinclair, P., 1987, Increased toxicity of acetaminophen in the presence of methotrexate, *Toxicologist*, **7**, 116.

Singh, P. P., Junnarkar, A. Y., Rao, C. S., Varma, R. K. and Shridhar, D. R., 1983, Acetic acid and phenylquinone writhing test: a critical study in mice, *Methods and Findings in Experimental and Clinical Pharmacology*, **5**, 601–606.

Singh, V., Visen, P. K. S., Patnaik, G. K., Kapoor, N. K. and Dhawan, B. N., 1992, Effect of picroliv on low density lipoprotein receptor binding of rat hepatocytes in hepatic damage induced by paracetamol, *Indian Journal of Biochemistry and Biophysics*, **29**, 428–432.

Singletary, W. V., Rauckman, E. J., Rosen, G. M. and Killenberg, P. G., 1980, Protection from acetaminophen hepatotoxicity following discontinuation of ethanol intake, *Gastro-enterology*, **78**, 1322.

Sirén, A.-L. and Karppanen, H., 1980, Influence of analgesic antipyretics on the central car-diovascular effects of clonidine in rats, *Prostaglandins*, **20**, 285–296.

Sivaloganathan, K., Johnson, P. A., Bray, G. P. and Williams, R., 1993, Pericoronitis and accidental paracetamol overdose: a cautionary tale, *British Dental Journal*, **174**, 69–71.

Skakun, N. P. and Shmanko, V. V., 1984, Lipid peroxidation and bile formation in paracetamol-induced liver injury, *Farmakologiya i Toksikologiya*, **47**, 105–108.

Skingle, M. and Tyers, M. B., 1979, Evaluation of antinociceptive activity using electrical stimulation of the tooth pulp in the conscious dog, *Journal of Pharmacological Methods*, **2**, 71–80.

Skinner, M. H., Matano, R., Hazle, W. and Blaschke, T. F., 1990, Acetaminophen metabolism in recovering alcoholics, *Methods and Findings in Experimental and Clinical Pharmacology*, **12**, 513–515.

Skjelbred, P., Album, B. and Løkken, P., 1977, Acetylsalicylic acid vs. paracetamol: effects on post-operative course, *European Journal of Clinical Pharmacology*, **12**, 257–264.

Skjelbred, P. and Løkken, P., 1979, Paracetamol versus placebo: effects on post-operative course, *European Journal of Clinical Pharmacology*, **15**, 27–33.

Skjelbred, P. and Løkken, P., 1982, Codeine added to paracetamol induced adverse effects but did not increase analgesia, *British Journal of Clinical Pharmacology*, **14**, 539–543.

Skjelbred, P. and Løkken, P., 1993, Antiinflammatoriske midler ved akutte vevstraumer, *Tidsskrift for den Norske Lrening*, **113**, 439–443.

Skjoto, J. and Reikvam, A., 1979, Hyperthermia and rhabdomyolysis in self-poisoning with paracetamol and salicylates, *Acta Medica Scandinavica*, **205**, 473–476.

Skoglund, L. A., 1986, A new paracetamol/paracetamol-methionine ester combination effects on postoperative course, *European Journal of Clinical Pharmacology*, **31**, 45–48.

Skoglund, L. A., Eidsaunet, W. and Pettersen, N., 1989, The anti-oedematous efficacy of oxindanac equals that of paracetamol in acute postoperative inflammation: are weak cyclooxygenase inhibitors more effective than strong inhibitors? *International Journal of Clinical Pharmacology Research*, **9**, 371–375.

Skoglund, L. A., Ingebrigtsen, K., Lausund, P. and Nafstad, I., 1992, Plasma concentration of paracetamol and its major metabolites after p.o. dosing with paracetamol or concurrent administration of paracetamol and its N-acetyl-DL-methionine ester in mice, *General Pharmacology*, **23**, 155–158.

Skoglund, L. A., Ingebrigtsen, K. and Nafstad, I., 1987, Time development of distribution and toxicity following single toxic APAP doses in male BOM : NMRI mice, *Journal of Applied Toxicology*, **7**, 1–6.

Skoglund, L. A., Ingebrigtsen, K., Nafstad, I. and Aalen, O., 1986, Efficacy of paracetamol-esterified methionine vs. cysteine or methionine on paracetamol-induced hepatic GSH depletion and plasma ALAT level in mice, *Biochemical Pharmacology*, **35**, 3071–3075.

Skoglund, L. A., Ingebrigtsen, K., Nafstad, I. and Aalen, O., 1988, *In vivo* studies on toxic effects of concurrent administration of paracetamol and its N-acetyl-dl-methionine ester (SUR 2647 combination), *General Pharmacology*, **19**, 213–217.

Skoglund, L. A. and Pettersen, N., 1991, Effects of acetaminophen after bilateral oral surgery: double dose twice daily vs. standard dose four times daily, *Pharmacotherapy*, **11**, 370–375.

Skoglund, L. A. and Skjelbred, P., 1984, Comparison of a traditional paracetamol medication and a new paracetamol/paracetamol-methionine ester combination, *European Journal of Clinical Pharmacology*, **26**, 573–577.

Skoglund, L. A., Skjelbred, P. and Fyllingen, G., 1991, Analgesic efficacy of acetaminophen 1000 mg, acetaminophen 2000 mg, and the combination of acetaminophen 1000 mg and codeine phosphate 60 mg vs. placebo in acute postoperative pain, *Pharmacotherapy*, **11**, 364–369.

Skokan, J. D., Hewlett, J. S. and Hoffman, G. C., 1973, Thrombocytopenic purpura associated with ingestion of acetaminophen (Tylenol), *Cleveland Clinic Quarterly*, **40**, 89–91.

Sköld, A. and Rönnborg, P.-E., 1984, Paracetamol orsakar leverskador hos kroniska alkoholister? *Läkartidningen*, **81**, 1314.

Skoulis, N. P., James, R. C., Harbison, R. D. and Roberts, S. M., 1989, Depression of hepatic glutathione by opioid analgesic drugs in mice, *Toxicology and Applied Pharmacology*, **99**, 139–147.

Skovlund, E., Fyllingen, G., Landre, H. and Nesheim, B.-I., 1991a, Comparison of postpartum pain treatments using a sequential trial design. I. Paracetamol versus placebo, *European*

Journal of Clinical Pharmacology, **40**, 343–347.

Skovlund, E., Fyllingen, G., Landre, H. and Nesheim, B.-I., 1991b, Comparison of post-partum pain treatments using a sequential trial design: II. Naproxen versus paracetamol, *European Journal of Clinical Pharmacology*, **40**, 539–542.

Slater, S., 1987, Paracetamol analysis: evaluation of a new kit for enzymatic assay, *Pathology*, **19**, 77–79.

Slattery, J. T., Koup, J. R. and Levy, G., 1981, Acetaminophen pharmacokinetics after over-dose, *Clinical Toxicology*, **18**, 111–117.

Slattery, J. T. and Levy, G., 1977, Reduction of acetaminophen toxicity by sodium sulfate in mice, *Research Communications in Chemical Pathology and Pharmacology*, **18**, 167–170.

Slattery, J. T. and Levy, G., 1979a, Acetaminophen kinetics in acutely poisoned patients, *Clinical Pharmacology and Therapeutics*, **25**, 184–195.

Slattery, J. T. and Levy, G., 1979b, Pharmacokinetic model of acetaminophen elimination, *American Journal of Hospital Pharmacy*, **36**, 440.

Slattery, J. T., McRorie, T. I., Reynolds, R., Kalhorn, T.F., Kharasch, E. D. and Eddy, A. C., 1989, Lack of effect of cimetidine on acetaminophen disposition in humans, *Clinical Pharmacology and Therapeutics*, **46**, 591–597.

Slattery, J. T., Wilson, J. M., Kalhorn, T. F. and Nelson, S. D., 1987, Dose-dependent phar-macokinetics of acetaminophen: evidence for glutathione depletion in humans, *Clinical Pharmacology and Therapeutics*, **41**, 413–418.

Smail, M. C., Ham, K. N. and Calder, I. C., 1981, A histochemical study of paracetamol toxicity, *Clinical and Experimental Pharmacology and Physiology*, **8**, 413–414.

Smilgin, Z., Drozdzik, M., Gawronska-Szklarz, B., Wójcicki, J., Tustanowski, S. and Górnik, W., 1993, Farmakokinetyka N-acetylo-p-aminofenolu u osób narazonych zawodowo na dzialanie polichlorku winylu modyfikowanego plastyfikatorami, *Medycyna Pracy*, **44**, 423–429.

Smilkstein, M. J., 1994, A new loading dose for N-acetylcysteine? The answer is no, *Annals of Emergency Medicine*, **24**, 538.

Smilkstein, M. J., Bronstein, A. C., Linden, C., Augenstein, W. L., Kulig, K. W. and Rumack, B. H., 1991, Acetaminophen overdose: a 48-hour intravenous N-acetylcysteine treatment protocol, *Annals of Emergency Medicine*, **20**, 1058–1063.

Smilkstein, M. J., Douglas, D. R. and Daya, M. R., 1994, Acetaminophen poisoning and liver function, *New England Journal of Medicine*, **331**, 1310–1311.

Smilkstein, M. J., Knapp, G. L., Kulig, K. W. and Rumack, B. H., 1988, Efficacy of oral N-acetylcysteine in the treatment of acetaminophen overdose: analysis of the national multicenter study (1976–1985), *New England Journal of Medicine*, **319**, 1557–1562.

Smilkstein, M. J., Knapp, G. L., Kulig, K. W. and Rumack, B. H., 1989, N-Acetylcysteine in the treatment of acetaminophen overdose, *New England Journal of Medicine*, **320**, 1418.

Smith, A. P., 1971, Response of aspirin-allergic patients to challenge by some analgesics in common use, *British Medical Journal*, **2**, 494–496.

Smith, C. and Jollow, J., 1976, Potentiation of acetaminophen-induced liver necrosis in ham-sters by galactosamine, *Pharmacologist*, **18**, 156.

Smith, C. L. and Jollow, D. J., 1977, Enhancement of acetaminophen-induced liver necrosis in hamsters by borneol, *Pharmacologist*, **19**, 162.

Smith, C. V., Chang, A., Welty, S. E. and Rogers, L. K., 1992, Hepatotoxic doses of acetamin-ophen cause marked decreases in histone messenger RNA in mouse livers, *Pediatric Research*, **31**, 66A.

Smith, C. V., Hughes, H. and Mitchell, J. R., 1984, Free radicals *in vivo*: covalent binding to lipids, *Molecular Pharmacology*, **26**, 112–116.

Smith, C. V. and Jaeschke, H., 1989, Effect of acetaminophen on hepatic content and biliary efflux of glutathione disulfide in mice, *Chemico-Biological Interactions*, **70**, 241–248.

Smith, C. V. and Mitchell, J. R., 1985, Acetaminophen hepatotoxicity *in vivo* is not accompa-nied by oxidant stress, *Biochemical and Biophysical Research Communications*, **133**,

329–336.

Smith, C. V., Tsokos-Kuhn, J. O., Hughes, H., Lauterburg, B. H. and Mitchell, J. R., 1985, Oxidant stress and acute lethal injury *in vivo*: BCNU pretreatment potentiates the hepatotoxicity of diquat but not acetaminophen, *Pharmacologist*, **27**, 157.

Smith, D. W., Isakson, G., Frankel, L. R. and Kerner, J. A., 1986a, Hepatic failure following ingestion of multiple doses of acetaminophen in a young child, *Journal of Pediatric Gastroenterology and Nutrition*, **5**, 822–825.

Smith, F. A., 1981, Therapeutic drug monitoring of theophylline, salicylates and acetaminophen, *Clinics in Laboratory Medicine*, **1**, 559–579.

Smith, G. E. and Griffiths, L. A., 1976, Comparative metabolic studies of phenacetin and structurally-related compounds in the rat, *Xenobiotica*, **6**, 217–236.

Smith, G. M. and Smith, P. H., 1985, Effects of doxylamine and acetaminophen on postoperative sleep, *Clinical Pharmacology and Therapeutics*, **37**, 549–557.

Smith, J. A. E., Hine, I. D., Beck, P. and Routledge, P. A., 1986b, Paracetamol toxicity: is enzyme induction important? *Human Toxicology*, **5**, 383–385.

Smith, J. M., Roberts, W. O., Hall, S. M., White, T. A. and Gilbertson, A. A., 1978, Late treatment of paracetamol poisoning with mercaptamine, *British Medical Journal*, **1**, 331–333.

Smith, J. N. and Williams, R. T., 1948, Studies in detoxication. 16. The metabolism of acetanilide in the rabbit, *Biochemical Journal*, **42**, 538–544.

Smith, J. N. and Williams, R. T., 1949, Studies in detoxication. 22. The metabolism of phenacetin (p-ethoxyacetanilide) in the rabbit and a further observation on acetanilide metabolism, *Biochemical Journal*, **44**, 239–242.

Smith, J. P., 1986, Drug overdose: changing concepts for modern drugs, *Southern Medical Journal*, **79**, 1230–1233.

Smith, M. and Payne, R. B., 1979, Re-examination of effect of paracetamol on serum uric acid measured by phosphotungstic acid reduction, *Annals of Clinical Biochemistry*, **16**, 96–99.

Smith, M. A., Acosta, D. and Bruckner, J. V., 1986c, Development of a primary culture system of rat kidney cortical cells to evaluate the nephrotoxicity of xenobiotics, *Food and Chemical Toxicology*, **24**, 551–556.

Smith, M. T., Levin, H. M., Bare, W. W., Berry, F. N. and Miller, J. M., 1975, Acetaminophen extra strength capsules vs. propoxyphene compound-65 vs. placebo: a double-blind study of effectiveness and safety, *Current Therapeutic Research*, **17**, 452–459.

Smith, P. K., 1958, *Acetophenetidin: A Critical Bibliographic Review*, New York: Interscience Publishers.

Smith, R. L. and Timbrell, J. A., 1974, Factors affecting the metabolism of phenacetin. I. Influence of dose, chronic dosage, route of administration and species on the metabolism of [1-^{14}C-acetyl]phenacetin, *Xenobiotica*, **4**, 489–501.

Smith, R. M. and Nelsen, L. A., 1991, Hmong folk remedies: limited acetylation of opium by aspirin and acetaminophen, *Journal of Forensic Sciences*, **36**, 280–287.

Smolarek, T. A., Higgins, C. V. and Amacher, D. E., 1990, Metabolism and cytotoxicity of acetaminophen in hepatocyte cultures from rat, rabbit, dog and monkey, *Drug Metabolism and Disposition: The Biological Fate of Chemicals*, **18**, 659–663.

Snawder, J. E., Benson, R. W., Leakey, J. E. A. and Roberts, D. W., 1993, The effect of propylene glycol on the P-450-dependent metabolism of acetaminophen and other chemicals in subcellular fractions of mouse liver, *Life Sciences*, **52**, 183–189.

Snawder, J. E., Roe, A. L., Benson, R. W., Casciano, D. A. and Roberts, D. W., 1994a, Cytochrome P-450-dependent metabolism of acetaminophen in four human transgenic lymphoblastoid cell lines, *Pharmacogenetics*, **4**, 43–46.

Snawder, J. E., Roe, A. L., Benson, R. W. and Roberts, D. W., 1994b, Loss of CYP2E1 and CYP1A2 activity as a function of acetaminophen dose: relation to toxicity, *Biochemical and Biophysical Research Communications*, **203**, 532–539.

Solomon, A. E., Briggs, J. D., Knepil, J., Henry, D. A., Winchester, J. F. and Birrell, R., 1977,

Therapeutic comparison of thiol compounds in severe paracetamol poisoning, *Annals of Clinical Biochemistry*, **14**, 200–202.

Somaja, L. and Thangam, J., 1987, Salivary paracetamol elimination kinetics during the menstrual cycle, *British Journal of Clinical Pharmacology*, **23**, 348–350.

Sommers, De K., Moncrieff, J. and Avenant, J. C., 1987, Paracetamol conjugation: an inter-ethnic and dietary study, *Human Toxicology*, **6**, 407–409.

Sommers, De K., van Staden, D. A., Moncrieff, J. and Schoeman, H. S., 1985, Paracetamol metabolism in African villagers, *Human Toxicology*, **4**, 385–389.

Sommers, De K., van Wyk, M., Snyman, J. R. and Moncrieff, J., 1992, The effects of erythromycin base and terbinafine on gastric emptying and the oro-caecal transit time, *Medical Science Research*, **20**, 139.

Sommers, De K., van Wyk, M., Snyman, J. R. and Moncrieff, J., 1993, The influence of octreotide and metoclopramide on gastric emptying, the oro-caecal transit time and theophylline absorption from a sustained-release formulation, *Medical Science Research*, **21**, 725–727.

Sommers, De K., van Wyk, M., Snyman, J. R. and Moncrieff, J., 1994, Influence of granisetron, ondansetron and metoclopramide on gastric emptying, oro-caecal transit time and theophylline absorption from a sustained-release formulation, *Medical Science Research*, **22**, 329–331.

Somogyi, A., Bochner, F. and Chen, Z. R., 1991, Lack of effect of paracetamol on the pharmacokinetics and metabolism of codeine in man, *European Journal of Clinical Pharmacology*, **41**, 379–382.

Sonawane, B., Sills, M., Schrager, R. and Yaffe, S., 1981, Acute starvation and acetaminophen toxicity in young vs. adult mice, *Pediatric Research*, **15**, 502.

Sonawane, B. R., Mancini, R. E. and Yaffe, S. J., 1980, Toxicity of acetaminophen during postnatal development, *Federation Proceedings*, **39**, 862.

Sonne, J., 1993, Factors and conditions affecting the glucuronidation of oxazepam, *Pharmacology and Toxicology*, **73 (Suppl. 1)**, 1–23.

Sonne, J., Boesgaard, S., Poulsen, H. E., Loft, S., Hansen, J. M., Døssing, M. and Andreasen, F., 1990, Pharmacokinetics and pharmacodynamics of oxazepam and metabolism of paracetamol in severe hypothyroidism, *British Journal of Clinical Pharmacology*, **30**, 737–742.

Sonne, J., Poulsen, H. E. and Andreasen, P. B., 1986, Single dose oxazepam has no effect on acetaminophen clearance or metabolism, *European Journal of Clinical Pharmacology*, **30**, 127–129.

Sonne, J., Poulsen, H. E., Loft, S., Døssing, M., Vollmer-Larsen, A., Simonsen, K., Thyssen, H. and Lundstrøm, K., 1988, Therapeutic doses of codeine have no effect on acetaminophen clearance or metabolism, *European Journal of Clinical Pharmacology*, **35**, 109–111.

Sood, S. P. and Green, V. I., 1987, Routine methods in toxicology and therapeutic drug monitoring by high-performance liquid chromatography. I. Rapid method for determination of acetaminophen in plasma, including a STAT procedure, *Therapeutic Drug Monitoring*, **9**, 248–254.

Sørensen, F. B., Landbo, B. and Marcussen, N., 1986, Paracetamolforgiftning med letal levernekrose, *Ugeskrift for Læger*, **148**, 2689–2690.

Soslow, A. R., 1981, Acute drug overdose: one hospital's experience, *Annals of Emergency Medicine*, **10**, 18–21.

Sotiropoulos, J. B., Deutsch, T. and Plakogiannis, F. M., 1981, Comparative bioavailability of three commercial acetaminophen tablets, *Journal of Pharmaceutical Sciences*, **70**, 422–425.

Spano, R. and Stacchino, C., 1979, Some pharmacological activities of a new derivative of 4-acetamidophenol, *Bollettino Chimico Farmaceutico*, **118**, 567–570.

Spearman, C. W., Robson, S. C., Kirsch, R. E. and Pillans, P., 1993, Paracetamol poisoning, *South African Medical Journal*, **83**, 825–826.

Speck, R. F. and Lauterburg, B. H., 1991, Fish oil protects mice against acetaminophen hepatotoxicity *in vivo*, *Hepatology*, **13**, 557–561.

Speck, R. F., Schranz, C. and Lauterburg, B. H., 1993, Prednisolone stimulates hepatic gluta- thione synthesis in mice: protection by prednisolone against acetaminophen hepato- toxicity *in vivo*, *Journal of Hepatology*, **18**, 62–67.

Spector, S. L., Wangaard, C. H. and Farr, R. S., 1979, Aspirin and concomitant idiosyncrasies in adult asthmatic patients, *Journal of Allergy and Clinical Immunology*, **64**, 500–506.

Speeg, K. V., 1987, Potential use of cimetidine for treatment of acetaminophen overdose, *Pharmacotherapy*, **7**, 125S–133S.

Speeg, K. V., Christian, D. C. and Mitchell, M. C., 1984, Ranitidine and acetaminophen hepatotoxicity, *Annals of Internal Medicine*, **100**, 315–316.

Speeg, K. V., Mitchell, M. C. and Maldonado, A. L., 1985, Additive protection of cimetidine and N-acetylcysteine treatment against acetaminophen-induced hepatic necrosis in the rat, *Journal of Pharmacology and Experimental Therapeutics*, **234**, 550–554.

Speranza, R., Martino, R., Laveneziana, D. and Sala, B., 1992, Ossicodone vs. paracetamolo in premedicazione per os negli interventi di colecistectomia, *Minerva Anestesiologica*, **58**, 191–194.

Spielberg, S. P., 1980, Acetaminophen toxicity in human lymphocytes *in vitro*, *Journal of Pharmacology and Experimental Therapeutics*, **213**, 395–398.

Spielberg, S. P., 1983, *In vitro* human pharmacogenetics of reactive drug metabolite detoxifi- cation, *Progress in Clinical and Biological Research*, **135**, 107–118.

Spielberg, S. P., 1984, Acetaminophen toxicity in lymphocytes heterozygous for glutathione synthetase deficiency, *Canadian Journal of Physiology and Pharmacology*, **63**, 468–471.

Spielberg, S. P., 1985, Acetaminophen toxicity in lymphocytes heterozygous for glutathione synthetase deficiency, *Canadian Journal of Physiology and Pharmacology*, **63**, 468–471.

Spielberg, S. P. and Gordon, G. B., 1981, Glutathione synthetase-deficient lymphocytes and acetaminophen toxicity, *Clinical Pharmacology and Therapeutics*, **29**, 51–55.

Spika, J. S. and Aranda, J. V., 1987, Interaction between chloramphenicol and acetamino- phen, *Archives of Disease in Childhood*, **62**, 1087–1088.

Spika, J. S., Davies, D. J., Martin, S. R., Beharry, K., Rex, J. and Aranda, J. V., 1986, Inter- action between chloramphenicol and acetaminophen, *Archives of Disease in Childhood*, **61**, 1121–1124.

Spiller, H. A., Krenzelok, E. P., Grande, G. A., Safir, E. F. and Diamond, J. J., 1994, A prospective evaluation of the effect of activated charcoal before oral N-acetylcysteine in acetaminophen overdose, *Annals of Emergency Medicine*, **23**, 519–523.

Splendiani, G., Tancredi, M., Daniele, M. and Giammaria, U., 1990, Treatment of acute liver failure with hemodetoxification techniques, *International Journal of Artificial Organs*, **13**, 370–374.

Spooner, J. B. and Harvey, J. G., 1976, The history and usage of paracetamol, *Journal of International Medical Research*, **4 (Suppl. 4)**, 1–6.

Spooner, J. B. and Harvey, J. G., 1978, Paracetamol poisoning, *British Medical Journal*, **2**, 1369.

Spooner, J. B. and Harvey, J. G., 1993, Paracetamol overdosage – facts not misconceptions, *Pharmaceutical Journal*, **250**, 706–707.

Spooner, R. J., Reavey, P. C. and McIntosh, L., 1976, Rapid estimation of paracetamol in plasma, *Journal of Clinical Pathology*, **29**, 663.

Spühler, O. and Zollinger, H. U., 1953, Die chronische interstitielle Nephritis, *Zeitschrift fur Klinische Medizin*, **151**, 1–50.

Spurway, T. D., Gartland, K. P. R., Warrander, A., Pickford, R., Nicholson, J. K. and Wilson, I. D., 1990, Proton nuclear magnetic resonance of urine and bile from paracetamol dosed rats, *Journal of Pharmaceutical and Biomedical Analysis*, **8**, 969–973.

Srám, R. J., Kocisová, J., Rössner, P., Binková, B., Topinka, J. and Bavorová, H., 1989, Mutagenní aktivita paracetamolu. Studie na dobrovolnících, *Casopis Lekaru Ceskych*,

128, 1230–1234.

Srám, R. J., Kocisová, J., Rössner, P., Binková, B., Topinka, J. and Bavorová, H., 1990, Mutagenic activity of paracetamol. A study conducted on volunteers, *Czechoslovak Medicine*, **13**, 114–123.

Srinivasan, R. S., Bourne, D. W. A. and Putcha, L., 1994, Application of physiologically based pharmacokinetic models for assessing drug disposition in space, *Journal of Clinical Pharmacology*, **34**, 692–698.

Srivastava, D. N., Bhattacharya, S. K. and Sanyal, A. K., 1978, Effect of some prostaglandin synthesis inhibitors on the antinociceptive action of morphine in albino rats, *Clinical and Experimental Pharmacology and Physiology*, **5**, 503–509.

St. Omer, V. E. V. and Mohammad, F. K., 1984, Effect of antidotal N-acetylcysteine on the pharmacokinetics of acetaminophen in dogs, *Journal of Veterinary Pharmacology and Therapeutics*, **7**, 277–281.

St. Omer, V. V. and McKnight, E. D., 1980, Acetylcysteine for treatment of acetaminophen toxicosis in the cat, *Journal of the American Veterinary Medical Association*, **176**, 911–913.

Stableforth, P. G., 1977, Mefenamic acid and dextropropoxyphene with paracetamol as analgesics in the accident department, *Current Medical Research and Opinion*, **5**, 189–191.

Stacher, G., Bauer, P., Ehn, I. and Schreiber, E., 1979, Effects of tolmetin, paracetamol, and of two combinations of tolmetin and paracetamol as compared to placebo on experimentally induced pain. A double blind study, *International Journal of Clinical Pharmacology and Biopharmacy*, **17**, 250–255.

Stachura, J., Tarnawski, A., Ivey, K. J., Ruwart, M. J., Rush, B. D., Friedle, N. M., Szczudrawa, J. and Mach, T., 1981, 16,16 Dimethyl prostaglandin E_2 protection of rat liver against acute injury by galactosamine, acetaminophen, ethanol and ANIT, *Gastroenterology*, **80**, 1349.

Stage, J., Jensen, J. H. and Bonding, P., 1988, Post-tonsillectomy haemorrhage and analgesics. A comparative study of acetylsalicylic acid and paracetamol, *Clinical Otolaryngology*, **13**, 201–204.

Stamm, D., 1994, Paracétamol et autres antalgiques antipyrétiques: doses optimales en pédiatrie, *Archives de Pédiatrie*, **1**, 193–201.

Stankowska-Chomicz, A. and Gawronska-Szklarz, B., 1987, Pharmacokinetics of paracetamol in ischemic cerebral apoplexy, *Polish Journal of Pharmacology and Pharmacy*, **39**, 259–265.

Stanton, B. J., Coupar, I. M. and Burcher, E., 1986, The activity of non-steroidal anti-inflammatory drugs in the rat mesenteric vasculature, *Journal of Pharmacy and Pharmacology*, **38**, 674–678.

Stanton, L. A., Peterson, G. M., Rumble, R. H., Cooper, G. M. and Polack, A. E., 1994, Drug-related admissions to an Australian hospital, *Journal of Clinical Pharmacy and Therapeutics*, **19**, 341–347.

Stark, K. L., Harris, C. and Juchau, M. R., 1989a, Influence of electrophilic character and glutathione depletion on chemical dysmorphogenesis in cultured rat embryos, *Biochemical Pharmacology*, **38**, 2685–2692.

Stark, K. L., Harris, C. and Juchau, M. R., 1989b, Modulation of the embryotoxicity and cytotoxicity elicited by 7-hyroxy-2-acetylaminofluorene and acetaminophen via deacetylation, *Toxicology and Applied Pharmacology*, **97**, 548–560.

Stark, K. L., Lee, Q. P., Namkung, M. J., Harris, C. and Juchau, M. R., 1990, Dysmorphogenesis elicited by microinjected acetaminophen analogs and metabolites in rat embryos cultured *in vitro*, *Journal of Pharmacology and Experimental Therapeutics*, **255**, 74–82.

Starkey, B. J., Loscombe, S. M. and Smith, J. M., 1986, Paracetamol (acetaminophen) analysis by high performance liquid chromatography: interference studies and comparison with an enzymatic procedure, *Therapeutic Drug Monitoring*, **8**, 78–84.

Starkey, I. R. and Lawson, A. A. H., 1978, Acute poisoning with Distalgesic, *British Medical Journal*, **2**, 1468.

Steedman, D. J., Payne, M. R., McClure, J. H. and Prescott, L. F., 1991, Gastric emptying following Colles' fracture, *Archives of Emergency Medicine*, **8**, 165–168.

Steele, C., 1974, Paracetamol toxicity in the cat, *The Veterinary Record*, **95**, 578–579.

Steele, C. M., Masson, H. A., Battershill, J. M., Gibson, G. G. and Ioannides, C., 1983, Metabolic activation of paracetamol by highly purified forms of cytochrome P-450, *Research Communications in Chemical Pathology and Pharmacology*, **40**, 109–119.

Steele, R. W., Tanaka, P. T., Lara, R. P. and Bass, J. W., 1970, Evaluation of sponging and of oral antipyretic therapy to reduce fever, *Journal of Pediatrics*, **77**, 824–829.

Steele, R. W., Young, F. S. H., Bass, J. W. and Shirkey, H. C., 1972, Oral antipyretic therapy: evaluation of aspirin-acetaminophen combination, *American Journal of Diseases of Children*, **123**, 204–206.

Steenland, N. K., Thun, M. J., Ferguson, C. W. and Port, F. K., 1990, Occupational and other exposures associated with male end-stage renal disease: a case/control study, *American Journal of Public Health*, **80**, 153–159.

Steffe, E. M., King, J. H., Inciardi, J. F., Flynn, N. F., Goldstein, E., Tonjes, T. S. and Benet, L. Z., 1990, The effect of acetaminophen on zidovudine metabolism in HIV-infected patients, *Journal of Acquired Immune Deficiency Syndromes*, **3**, 691–694.

Stegeman-Castelen, G., van Hattum, J., Koomans, H. A., de Vries, J. and van Heijst, A. N. P., 1983, Acute nierinsufficiëntie na paracetamolintoxicatie, *Nederlands Tijdschrift voor Geneeskunde*, **127**, 1052–1054.

Stein, C. M., Thornhill, D. P., Neill, P. and Nyazema, N. Z., 1989, Lack of effect of paracetamol on the pharmacokinetics of chloramphenicol, *British Journal of Clinical Pharmacology*, **27**, 262–264.

Stein, M. D., Bonanno, J., O'Sullivan, P. S. and Wachtel, T. J., 1993, Changes in the pattern of drug overdoses, *Journal of General Internal Medicine*, **8**, 179–184.

Steinhauer, H. B. and Hertting, G., 1981, Lowering of the convulsive threshold by non-steroidal anti-inflammatory drugs, *European Journal of Pharmacology*, **69**, 199–203.

Steinmetz, J. C., Lee, C. Y. and Wu, A. Y., 1987, Tissue levels of ibuprofen after fatal overdosage of ibuprofen and acetaminophen, *Veterinary and Human Toxicology*, **29**, 381–383.

Stempel, D., Simms, R. and Sullivan, T. J., 1991, Acetaminophen induced anaphylaxis, *Journal of Allergy and Clinical Immunology*, **87**, 275.

Stern, A. I., Hogan, D. L. and Isenberg, J. I., 1984a, A new method for quantitation of ion fluxes across *in vivo* human gastric mucosa: effect of aspirin, acetaminophen, ethanol, and hyperosmolar solutions, *Gastroenterology*, **86**, 60–70.

Stern, A. I., Hogan, D. L., Kahn, L. H. and Isenberg, J. I., 1984b, Protective effect of acetaminophen against aspirin- and ethanol-induced damage to the human gastric mucosa, *Gastroenterology*, **86**, 728–733.

Steru, D., Burchard, L., Choueri, H. and Lenoir, G., 1983, Action antipyrétique du paracétamol: recherche pharmacologique de la dose minimale efficace chez l'enfant, *Revue de Pédiatrie*, **19**, 305–309.

Stevens, H. M. and Gill, R., 1986, High-performance liquid chromatography systems for the analysis of analgesic and non-steroidal anti-inflammatory drugs in forensic toxicology, *Journal of Chromatography*, **370**, 39–47.

Stevens, J. C., Shipley, L. A., Cashman, J. R., Vandenbranden, M. and Wrighton, S. A., 1993, Comparison of human and rhesus monkey *in vitro* Phase I and Phase II hepatic drug metabolism activities, *Drug Metabolism and Disposition: The Biological Fate of Chemicals*, **21**, 753–760.

Steventon, G., Williams, A. C., Waring, R. H., Pall, H. S. and Adams, D., 1988, Xenobiotic metabolism in motorneuron disease, *Lancet*, **ii**, 644–647.

Steventon, G. B., Heafield, M. T. E., Waring, R. H. and Williams, A. C., 1989, Xenobiotic metabolism in Parkinson's disease, *Neurology*, **39**, 883–887.

Steventon, G. B., Heafield, M. T. E., Waring, R. H., Williams, A.C., Sturman, S. and Green, M., 1990, Metabolism of low-dose paracetamol in patients with chronic neurological disease, *Xenobiotica*, **20**, 117–122.

Stewart, J. H. and Gallery, E. D. M., 1976, Analgesic abuse and kidney disease, *Australian and New Zealand Journal of Medicine*, **6**, 498–508.

Stewart, M. J., Adriaenssens, P. I., Jarvie, D. R. and Prescott, L. F., 1979, Inappropriate methods for the emergency determination of plasma paracetamol, *Annals of Clinical Biochemistry*, **16**, 89–95.

Stewart, M. J. and Simpson, E., 1973, Prognosis in paracetamol self-poisoning: the use of plasma paracetamol concentration in a region without a poisoning treatment centre, *Annals of Clinical Biochemistry*, **10**, 173–178.

Stewart, M. J. and Watson, I. D., 1987, Analytical reviews in clinical chemistry: methods for the estimation of salicylate and paracetamol in serum, plasma and urine, *Annals of Clinical Biochemistry*, **24**, 552–565.

Stewart, M. J. and Willis, R. G., 1975, Simplified gas chromatographic assay for paracetamol, *Annals of Clinical Biochemistry*, **12**, 4–8.

Stewart, R. B., Hale, W. E. and Marks, R. G., 1982, Analgesic drug use in an ambulatory elderly population, *Drug Intelligence and Clinical Pharmacy, the Annals of Pharmacotherapy*, **16**, 833–836.

Stipon, J. P., Le Bihan, Y. and de Rotalier, P., 1983, Évaluation de l'activité antalgique de l'UP 341.01 chez des patients présentant une doleur aiguë en O.R.L, *Semaine des Hôpitaux de Paris*, **59**, 2725–2728.

Stokes, I. M., 1984, Paracetamol overdose in the second trimester of pregnancy. Case report, *British Journal of Obstetrics and Gynaecology*, **91**, 286–288.

Stolar, M. H., Siegel, F. and Morris, R. W., 1973, Influence of dosage form on antipyretic activity of acetaminophen administered intraperitoneally in the rat, *Journal of Pharmaceutical Sciences*, **62**, 338–339.

Stolley, P. D., 1991, The risks of phenacetin use, *New England Journal of Medicine*, **324**, 191–193.

Stolt, C. M. and Johnsen, S.-A., 1984, Terapeutiskt paracetamolintag orsakade akut njurinsufficiens och leverpåverkan, *Läkartidningen*, **81**, 1313.

Stramentinoli, G., Pezzoli, C. and Galli-Kienle, M., 1979, Protective role of S-adenosyl-l-methionine against acetaminophen induced mortality and hepatotoxicity in mice, *Biochemical Pharmacology*, **28**, 3567–3571.

Street, H. V., 1975, Estimation and identification in blood plasma of paracetamol (N-acetyl-p-aminophenol) in the presence of barbiturates, *Journal of Chromatography*, **109**, 29–36.

Streeter, A. J. and Baillie, T. A., 1985, 2-Acetamido-p-benzoquinone: a reactive arylating metabolite of 3'-hydroxyacetanilide, *Biochemical Pharmacology*, **34**, 2871–2876.

Streeter, A. J., Bjorge, S., Axworthy, D. B., Nelson, S. D. and Baillie, T. A., 1984a, The microsomal metabolism and site of covalent binding to protein of 3'-hydroxyacetanilide, a nonhepatotoxic positional isomer of acetaminophen, *Drug Metabolism and Disposition: The Biological Fate of Chemicals*, **12**, 565–576.

Streeter, A. J., Dahlin, D. C., Nelson, S. D. and Baillie, T. A., 1984b, The covalent binding of acetaminophen to protein. Evidence for cysteine residues as major sites of arylation *in vitro*, *Chemico-Biological Interactions*, **48**, 349–366.

Streeter, A. J., Harvison, P. J., Nelson, S. D. and Baillie, T. A., 1986, Cross-linking of protein molecules by the reactive metabolite of acetaminophen, N-acetyl-p-benzoquinoneimine, and related quinoid compounds, *Advances in Experimental Medicine and Biology*, **197**, 727–737.

Streeter, A. J. and Timbrell, J. A., 1979, The effect of dichloralphenazone pretreatment on paracetamol hepatotoxicity in mice, *Biochemical Pharmacology*, **28**, 3035–3037.

Streissguth, A. P., Treder, R. P., Barr, H. M., Shepard, T. H., Bleyer, W. A., Sampson, P. D. and Martin, D. C., 1987, Aspirin and acetaminophen use by pregnant women and subsequent child IQ and attention decrements, *Teratology*, **35**, 211–219.

Stricker, B. H. Ch., Meyboom, R. H. B. and Lindquist, M., 1985, Acute hypersensitivity reactions to paracetamol, *British Medical Journal*, **291**, 938–939.

Strom, B. L., 1994, Adverse reactions to over-the counter analgesics taken for therapeutic purposes, *Journal of the American Medical Association*, **272**, 1866–1867.

Strøm, J., Thisted, B., Krantz, T. and Bredgaard Sorensen, M., 1986, Self-poisoning treated in an ICU: drug pattern, acute mortality and short-term survival, *Acta Anaesthesiologica Scandinavica*, **30**, 148–153.

Ström, C., Forsberg, O., Quiding, H., Engevall, S. and Larsson, O., 1990, Analgesic efficacy of acetaminophen sustained release, *Journal of Clinical Pharmacology*, **30**, 654–659.

Strubelt, O., 1981, Influence of 2,4-dinitrophenol on the susceptibility of rats to hepatotoxic injury, *Toxicology Letters*, **9**, 221–224.

Strubelt, O. and Breining, H., 1980, Influence of hypoxia on the hepatotoxic effects of carbon tetrachloride, paracetamol, allyl alcohol, bromobenzene and thioacetamide, *Toxicology Letters*, **6**, 109–113.

Strubelt, O., Dost-Kempf, E., Siegers, C.-P., Younes, M., Völpel, M., Preuss, U. and Dreckmann, J. G., 1981, The influence of fasting on the susceptibility of mice to hepatotoxic injury, *Toxicology and Applied Pharmacology*, **60**, 66–77.

Strubelt, O. and Hoppenkamps, R., 1983, Relations between gastric glutathione and the ulcerogenic action of non-steroidal anti-inflammatory drugs, *Archives Internationales de Pharmacodynamie et de Thérapie*, **262**, 268–278.

Strubelt, O., Obermeier, F. and Siegers, C.-P., 1978, The influence of ethanol pretreatment on the effects of nine hepatotoxic agents, *Acta Pharmacologica et Toxicologica*, **43**, 211–218.

Strubelt, O., Siegers, C.-P. and Schütt, A., 1974, The curative effects of cysteamine, cysteine, and dithiocarb in experimental paracetamol poisoning, *Archives of Toxicology*, **33**, 55–64.

Strubelt, O., Siegers, C.-P., Völpel, M. and Younes, M., 1979, Studies on the mechanism of paracetamol-induced protection against paracetamol hepatotoxicity, *Toxicology*, **12**, 121–133.

Strubelt, O. and Younes, M., 1984, Inhibition of the carrageenan-induced rat paw edema by glutathione-depleting agents, *Agents and Actions*, **14**, 680–683.

Strubelt, O. and Younes, M., 1992, The toxicological relevance of paracetamol-induced inhibition of hepatic respiration and ATP depletion, *Biochemical Pharmacology*, **44**, 163–170.

Studenberg, S. D. and Brouwer, K. L. R., 1991, Phenacetin and acetaminophen metabolism in the isolated perfused rat liver: precursor concentration influences the selection of kinetic parameters to assess hypoxic impairment, *Drug Metabolism and Disposition: The Biological Fate of Chemicals*, **19**, 423–429.

Studenberg, S. D. and Brouwer, K. L. R., 1992, Impaired biliary excretion of acetaminophen glucuronide in the isolated perfused rat liver after acute phenobarbital treatment and *in vivo* phenobarbital pretreatment, *Journal of Pharmacology and Experimental Therapeutics*, **261**, 1022–1027.

Studenberg, S. D. and Brouwer, K. L. R., 1993a, Hepatic disposition of acetaminophen and metabolites: pharmacokinetic modelling, protein binding and subcellular distribution, *Biochemical Pharmacology*, **46**, 739–746.

Studenberg, S. D. and Brouwer, K. L. R., 1993b, Effect of phenobarbital and p-Hydroxyphenobarbital glucuronide on acetaminophen metabolites in isolated rat hepatocytes: use of a kinetic model to examine the rates of formation and egress, *Journal of Pharmacokinetics and Biopharmaceutics*, **21**, 175–194.

Styrt, B. and Sugarman, B., 1990, Antipyresis and fever, *Archives of Internal Medicine*, **150**, 1589–1597.

Subaschandran, D. V. and Balloun, S. L., 1967, Acetyl-p-aminophenol and vitamin C in heat-stressed birds, *Poultry Science*, **46**, 1073–1076.

Sugihara, J., Furuuchi, S., Nakano, K. and Harigaya, S., 1988, Studies on intestinal lymphatic absorption of drugs. I. Lymphatic absorption of alkyl ester derivatives and α-monoglyceride derivatives of drugs, *Journal of Pharmacobio-Dynamics*, **11**, 369–376.

Sugihara, N., Furuno, K., Kita, N., Murakami, T. and Yata, N., 1992, Plasma α_1-acid glyco-protein concentration in rats with chemical liver injury, *Chemical and Pharmaceutical Bulletin*, **40**, 2516–2519.

Sugimura, T., Fujimoto, T., Motoyama, H., Maruoka, T., Korematu, S., Asakuno, Y. and Hayakawa, H., 1994, Risks of antipyretics in young children with fever due to infectious disease, *Acta Paediatrica Japonica*, **36**, 375–378.

Sullivan, M. and Kenny, P., 1985, Estimation of paracetamol, *Medical Laboratory Sciences*, **42**, 118–123.

Sultatos, L. G., Vesell, E. S. and Hepner, G. W., 1978, Aminopyrine disposition: a sensitive index of acetaminophen-induced hepatocellular damage, *Toxicology and Applied Pharmacology*, **45**, 177–189.

Suma, V. and Lupone, N., 1980, Studio comparativo dell'effetto antipiretico del paracetamolo e dell'aminofenazone somministrati per via rettale, *La Clinica Terapeutica*, **95**, 297–304.

Summers, R. S. and Summers, B., 1986, Drug prescribing in paediatrics at a teaching hospital serving a developing community, *Annals of Tropical Paediatrics*, **6**, 129–133.

Sun, Y., Cotgreave, I., Lindeke, B. and Moldéus, P., 1989, The metabolism of sulfite in liver: stimulation of sulfate conjugation and effects on paracetamol and allyl alcohol toxicity, *Biochemical Pharmacology*, **38**, 4299–4305.

Sunami, K. and Hayashi, N., 1990, Prophylactic effects of acetaminophen suppository on febrile convulsions: an epidemiologic and twin study, *Japanese Journal of Psychiatry and Neurology*, **44**, 351–353.

Sundlof, S. F., 1990, Incidence and management of poisoning in companion animals, *Veterinary and Human Toxicology*, **32**, 477–478.

Sunman, W., Hughes, A. D. and Sever, P. S., 1992, Anaphylactoid response to intravenous acetylcysteine, *Lancet*, **339**, 1231–1232.

Sunshine, A., Marrero, I., Olson, N., McCormick, N. and Laska, E. M., 1986, Comparative study of flurbiprofen, zomepirac sodium, acetaminophen plus codeine, and acetaminophen for the relief of postsurgical dental pain, *American Journal of Medicine*, **80 (Suppl. 3A)**, 50–54.

Sunshine, A., Olson, N. Z., Zighelboim, I. and de Castro, A., 1993, Ketoprofen, acetaminophen plus oxycodone, and acetaminophen in the relief of postoperative pain, *Clinical Pharmacology and Therapeutics*, **54**, 546–555.

Sunshine, A., Olson, N. Z., Zighelboim, I., DeCastro, A. and Minn, F. L., 1992, Analgesic oral efficacy of tramadol hydrochloride in postoperative pain, *Clinical Pharmacology and Therapeutics*, **51**, 740–746.

Sunshine, A., Zighelboim, I., de Castro, A., Sorrentino, J. V., Smith, D. S., Bartizek, R. D. and Olson, N. Z., 1989, Augmentation of acetaminophen analgesia by the antihistamine phenyltoloxamine, *Journal of Clinical Pharmacology*, **29**, 660–664.

Surmann, P., 1980, HPLC-Bestimmung von Paracetamol im Serum unter Verwendung der elektrochemischen Detektion, *Archiv der Pharmazie*, **313**, 399–405.

Sussman, N. L., Chong, M. G., Koussayer, T., He, D.-E., Shang, T. A., Whisennand, H. H. and Kelly, J. H., 1992, Reversal of fulminant hepatic failure using an extracorporeal liver assist device, *Hepatology*, **16**, 60–65.

Sutherland, L. R., Muller, P. and Lewis, D. R., 1981, Massive cerebral edema associated with fulminant hepatic failure in acetaminophen overdose: possible role of cranial decompression, *American Journal of Gastroenterology*, **76**, 446–448.

Sutor, A. H., Bowie, E. J. W. and Owen, C. A., 1971, Effect of aspirin, sodium salicylate, and acetaminophen on bleeding, *Mayo Clinic Proceedings*, **46**, 178–181.

Sveen, K. and Gilhuus-Moe, O., 1975, Paracetamol/codeine in relieving pain following removal of impacted mandibular third molars, *International Journal of Oral Surgery*, **4**, 258–266.

Svendsen, O., Christensen, H.B., Rygaard, J. and Juul, P., 1989, Comparative study on the toxicity of acetaminophen and mercuric chloride in normal and athymic mice and rats, *Archives of Toxicology*, **Suppl. 13**, 191–196.

Svensson, C. K. and Chong, M.-T., 1989, Effect of amiodarone on the disposition of acetaminophen in the rat, *Journal of Pharmaceutical Sciences*, **78**, 900–902.

Swaan, P. W., Marks, G. J., Ryan, F. M. and Smith, P. L., 1994, Determination of transport rates for arginine and acetaminophen in rabbit intestinal tissues *in vitro*, *Pharmaceutical Research*, **11**, 283–287.

Swale, J., 1977, Elimination of interference due to ascorbic acid when detecting paracetamol in urine, *Lancet*, **ii**, 981.

Swanson, M. B. and Walters, M. I., 1982, Rapid colorimetric assay for acetaminophen without salicylate or phenylephrine interference, *Clinical Chemistry*, **28**, 1171–1173.

Sweeny, D. J. and Reinke, L. A., 1988, Sulfation of acetaminophen in isolated rat hepatocytes: relationship to sulfate ion concentrations and intracellular levels of 3'-phosphoadenosine-5'-phosphosulfate, *Drug Metabolism and Disposition: The Biological Fate of Chemicals*, **16**, 712–715.

Sweeny, D. J. and Weiner, M., 1985, Metabolism of acetaminophen in hepatocytes isolated from mice and rats of various ages, *Drug Metabolism and Disposition: The Biological Fate of Chemicals*, **13**, 377–379.

Swetnam, S. M. and Florman, A. L., 1984, Probable acetaminophen toxicity in an 18-month-old infant due to repeated overdosing, *Clinical Pediatrics*, **23**, 104–105.

Symon, D. N. K., Gray, E. S., Hanmer, O. J. and Russell, G., 1982, Fatal paracetamol poisoning from benorylate therapy in child with cystic fibrosis, *Lancet*, **ii**, 1153–1154.

Szabo, S., 1977, Acetaminophen (paracetamol) poisoning: gastrointestinal side effects of cysteamine and their possible cause and treatment, *Mayo Clinic Proceedings*, **52**, 402.

Szczeklik, A., 1986, Analgesics, allergy and asthma, *Drugs*, **32 (Suppl. 4)**, 148–163.

Szczeklik, A., 1989, Aspirin-induced asthma: new insights into pathogenesis and clinical presentation of drug intolerance, *International Archives of Allergy and Applied Immunology*, **90 (Suppl. 1)**, 70–75.

Szczeklik, A., Gryglewski, R. J. and Czerniawska-Mysik, G., 1975, Relationship of inhibition of prostaglandin biosynthesis by analgesics to asthma attacks in aspirin-sensitive patients, *British Medical Journal*, **1**, 67–69.

Szczeklik, A., Gryglewski, R. J. and Czerniawska-Mysik, G., 1977, Clinical patterns of hypersensitivity to nonsteroidal anti-inflammatory drugs and their pathogenesis, *Journal of Allergy and Clinical Immunology*, **60**, 276–284.

Szymanska, J. A., Swietlicka, E. A. and Piotrowski, J. K., 1991, Protective effect of zinc in the hepatotoxicity of bromobenzene and acetaminophen, *Toxicology*, **66**, 81–91.

Szymanska, J. A., Swietlicka, E. A., Piotrowski, J. L., Skrzypinska-Gawrysiak, M. and Sporny, S., 1992, Effects of 3-methylcholanthrene or diethyl maleate on the hepatotoxicity of acetaminophen, *Journal of Applied Toxicology*, **12**, 415–419.

Takaoki, M., Yamashita, Y., Koike, K. and Matsuda, S., 1988, Effect of indomethacin, aspirin, and acetaminophen on *in vitro* antiviral and antiproliferative activities of recombinant human interferon-α_{2a}, *Journal of Interferon Research*, **8**, 727–733.

Tal, E., Mohari, K., Koranyi, L., Kovacs, Z. and Endroczi, E., 1988, The effect of indomethacin, ibuprofen and paracetamol on the TRH induced TSH secretion in the rat, *General Pharmacology*, **19**, 579–581.

Talley, N. J., McNeil, D. and Piper, D. W., 1988, Environmental factors and chronic unexplained dyspepsia: association with acetaminophen but not other analgesics, alcohol, coffee, tea, or smoking, *Digestive Diseases and Sciences*, **33**, 641–648.

Talley, N. J., Weaver, A. L. and Zinsmeister, A. R., 1994a, Smoking, alcohol, and nonsteroidal anti-inflammatory drugs in outpatients with functional dyspepsia and among dyspepsia subgroups, *American Journal of Gastroenterology*, **89**, 524–528.

Talley, N. J., Zinsmeister, A. R., Schleck, C. D. and Melton, L. J., 1994b, Smoking, alcohol, and analgesics in dyspepsia and among dyspepsia subgroups: lack of an association in a community, *Gut*, **35**, 619–624.

Tanaka, M., Nakata, K., Takase, K. and Mita, S., 1991, The protective effect of (4R)-hexahydro-7,7-dimethyl-6-oxo-1,2,5-dithiazocine-4-carboxylic acid (SA3443), a novel cyclic disulfide on acetaminophen-induced liver injury, *Folia Pharmacologica Japonica*, **97**, 191–198.

Tange, J. D., Ross, B. D. and Ledingham, J. G. G., 1977, Effects of analgesics and related compounds on renal metabolism in rats, *Clinical Science*, **53**, 485–492.

Tarlin, L. and Landrigan, P., 1972, A comparison of the antipyretic effect of acetaminophen and aspirin: another approach to poison prevention, *American Journal of Diseases of Children*, **124**, 880–882.

Tarloff, J. B., Goldstein, R. S. and Hook, J. B., 1989a, Strain differences in acetaminophen nephrotoxicity in rats: role of pharmacokinetics, *Toxicology*, **56**, 167–177.

Tarloff, J. B., Goldstein, R. S., Mico, B. A. and Hook, J. B., 1989b, Role of pharmacokinetics and metabolism in the enhanced susceptibility of middle-aged male Sprague-Dawley rats to acetaminophen nephrotoxicity, *Drug Metabolism and Disposition: The Biological Fate of Chemicals*, **17**, 139–146.

Tarloff, J. B., Goldstein, R. S., Morgan, D. G. and Hook, J. B., 1989c, Acetaminophen and p-aminophenol nephrotoxicity in aging male Sprague-Dawley and Fischer 344 rats, *Fundamental and Applied Toxicology*, **12**, 78–91.

Tarloff, J. B., Goldstein, R. S., Silver, A. C., Hewitt, W. R. and Hook, J. B., 1990, Intrinsic susceptibility of the kidney to acetaminophen toxicity in middle-aged rats, *Toxicology Letters*, **52**, 101–110.

Tarloff, J. B., Goldstein, R. S., Sozio, R. S. and Hook, J. B., 1991, Hepatic and renal conjugation (Phase II) enzyme activities in young adult, middle-aged, and senescent male Sprague-Dawley rats, *Proceedings of the Society for Experimental Biology and Medicine*, **197**, 297–303.

Tatsuta, M. and Iishi, H., 1993, Effect of treatment with Liu-Jun-Zi-Tang (TJ-43) on gastric emptying and gastrointestinal symptoms in dyspeptic patients, *Alimentary Pharmacology and Therapeutics*, **7**, 459–462.

Tatsuta, M., Iishi, H. and Okuda, S., 1989, Gastric emptying and gastrointestinal symptoms in patients with atrophic gastritis and the effects of domperidone, *Scandinavian Journal of Gastroenterology*, **24**, 251–256.

Tatsuta, M., Iishi, H. and Okuda, S., 1990, Gastric emptying in patients with fundal gastritis and gastric cancer, *Gut*, **31**, 767–769.

Tavares, I. A., Collins, P. O. and Bennett, A., 1987, Inhibition of prostanoid synthesis by human gastric mucosa, *Alimentary Pharmacology and Therapeutics*, **1**, 617–625.

Taylor, C. J. and Betts, A. M., 1983, Non-accidental paracetamol poisoning in an eleven-month-old child, *Human Toxicology*, **2**, 317–319.

Taylor, J. P., Gustafson, T. L., Johnson, C. C., Brandenburg, N. and Glezen, W. P., 1985, Antipyretic use among children during the 1983 influenza season, *American Journal of Diseases of Children*, **139**, 486–488.

Tebbett, I. R., Omile, C. I. and Danesh, B., 1985, Determination of paracetamol, salicylic acid and acetyl salicylic acid in serum by high-performance liquid chromatography, *Journal of Chromatography*, **329**, 196–198.

Tee, L. B. G., Boobis, A. R. and Davies, D. S., 1986a, N-Acetylcysteine for paracetamol overdose, *Lancet*, **i**, 331–332.

Tee, L. B. G., Boobis, A. R., Huggett, A. C. and Davies, D. S., 1986b, Reversal of acetaminophen toxicity in isolated hamster hepatocytes by dithiothreitol, *Toxicology and Applied Pharmacology*, **83**, 294–314.

Tee, L. B. G., Davies, D. S., Seddon, C. E. and Boobis, A. R., 1987, Species differences in the hepatotoxicity of paracetamol are due to differences in the rate of conversion to its cytotoxic metabolite, *Biochemical Pharmacology*, **36**, 1041–1052.

Teicher, B. A., Holden, S. A., Ara, G., Liu, J.-T. C., Robinson, M. F., Flodgren, P., Dupuis, N. and Northey, D., 1993, Cyclooxygenase inhibitors: *in vitro* and *in vivo* effects on anti-tumor alkylating agents in the EMT-6 murine mammary carcinoma, *International Journal of Oncology*, **2**, 145–153.

Temple, A. R., 1983, Pediatric dosing of acetaminophen, *Pediatric Pharmacology*, **3**, 321–327.

Tenenbein, M., 1986, Acetaminophen poisoning, *Current Problems in Pediatrics*, **16**, 193–198.

Terblanche, J. and Hickman, R., 1991, Animal models of fulminant hepatic failure, *Digestive Diseases and Sciences*, **36**, 770–774.

Terry, S. I., Gould, J. C., McManus, J. P. A. and Prescott, L. F., 1982, Absorption of penicillin and paracetamol after small intestinal bypass surgery, *European Journal of Clinical Pharmacology*, **23**, 245–248.

Teschke, R., Stutz, G. and Strohmeyer, G., 1979, Increased paracetamol-induced hepatotoxicity after chronic alcohol consumption, *Biochemical and Biophysical Research Communications*, **91**, 368–374.

Teshima, D., Suzuki, A., Otsubo, K., Higuchi, S., Aoyama, T., Shimozono, Y., Saita, M. and Noda, K., 1990, Efficacy of emetic and United State Pharmacopoeia ipecac syrup in prevention of drug absorption, *Chemical and Pharmaceutical Bulletin*, **38**, 2242–2245.

Tesler, M. D., Wilkie, D. J., Holzemer, W. L. and Savedra, M. C., 1994, Postoperative analgesics for children and adolescents: prescription and administration, *Journal of Pain and Sympton Management*, **9**, 85–95.

Tfelt-Hansen, P. and Olesen, J., 1980, Paracetamol (acetaminophen) versus acetylsalicylic acid in migraine, *European Neurology*, **19**, 163–165.

Thankappan, T. P. and Zachariah, J., 1991, Drug-specific clinical pattern in fixed drug eruptions, *International Journal of Dermatology*, **30**, 867–870.

Thelen, M. and Wendel, A., 1983, Drug-induced lipid peroxidation in mice – V. Ethane production and glutathione release in the isolated liver upon perfusion with acetaminophen, *Biochemical Pharmacology*, **32**, 1701–1706.

Thibault, N., Peytavin, G. and Claude, J. R., 1991, Calcium channel blocking agents protect against acetaminophen-induced cytotoxicity in rat hepatocytes, *Journal of Biochemical Toxicology*, **6**, 237–238.

Thieler, H., Hottenrott, B., Marx, M., Voigt, D., Winkelmann, L., Oltmanns, U., Franke, Th. and Assmann, H., 1990, Die Analgetika-Nephropathie unter den chronischen Dialyse-Patienen im nördlichen Thüringen, *Nieren- und Hochdruckkrankheiten*, **19**, 148–157.

Thoma, J. J., McCoy, M., Ewald, T. and Meyers, N., 1978, Acetaminophen – an improved gas chromatographic assay, *Journal of Analytical Toxicology*, **2**, 226–228.

Thomas, B. H. and Coldwell, B. B., 1972, Estimation of phenacetin and paracetamol in plasma and urine by gas-liquid chromatography, *Journal of Pharmacy and Pharmacology*, **24**, 243.

Thomas, B. H., Coldwell, B. B., Zeitz, W. and Solomonraj, G., 1972, Effect of aspirin, caffeine, and codeine on the metabolism of phenacetin and acetaminophen, *Clinical Pharmacology and Therapeutics*, **13**, 906–910.

Thomas, B. H., Hynie, I. and Zeitz, W., 1980, Effect of analgesic nephropathy in women on the metabolism and excretion of ^{14}C-acetaminophen, *International Journal of Clinical Pharmacology, Therapy and Toxicology*, **18**, 26–30.

Thomas, B. H., Nera, E. A. and Zeitz, W., 1977a, Failure to observe pathology in the rat following chronic dosing with acetaminophen and acetylsalicylic acid, *Research Communications in Chemical Pathology and Pharmacology*, **17**, 663–678.

Thomas, B. H., Zeitz, W. and Beaubien, A. R., 1977b, Effect of subacute dosing and phenobarbital and 3-methylcholanthrene pretreatment on the metabolism of acetaminophen in rats, *Canadian Journal of Physiology and Pharmacology*, **55**, 77–83.

Thomas, B. H., Zeitz, W. and Coldwell, B. B., 1974, Effect of aspirin on biotransformation of ^{14}C-acetaminophen in rats, *Journal of Pharmaceutical Sciences*, **63**, 1367–1370.

Thomas, G. E., Rao, V. J. and Davis, J. H., 1983, The acetaminophen experience in South

Florida, *Journal of Forensic Sciences*, **28**, 977–984.

Thomas, J., McLean, S., Starmer, G. A. and Carroll, P. R., 1966, Paracetamol and methaemoglobinaemia, *Lancet*, **ii**, 1360.

Thomas, M., Michael, M. F., Andrew, P. and Scully, N., 1988, A study to investigate the effects of ranitidine on the metabolic disposition of paracetamol in man, *British Journal of Clinical Pharmacology*, **25**, 671P.

Thomas, S. H. L., 1993, Paracetamol (acetaminophen) poisoning, *Pharmacology and Therapeutics*, **60**, 91–120.

Thompson, D. and Eling, T., 1990, Mechanism of inhibition of prostaglandin H synthase by eugenol and other phenolic peroxidase substrates, *Molecular Pharmacology*, **36**, 809–817.

Thompson, J., Fleet, W., Laurence, E., Pierce, E., Morris, L. and Wright, P., 1987, A comparison of acetaminophen and rimantadine in the treatment of influenza A infection in children, *Journal of Medical Virology*, **21**, 249–255.

Thomson, J. S. and Prescott, L. F., 1966, Liver damage and impaired glucose tolerance after paracetamol overdosage, *British Medical Journal*, **2**, 506–507.

Thorén, T., Tanghöj, H., Wattwil, M. and Järnerot, G., 1989a, Epidural morphine delays gastric emptying and small intestinal transit in volunteers, *Acta Anaesthesiologica Scandinavica*, **33**, 174–180.

Thorén, T. and Wattwil, M., 1988, Effects on gastric emptying of thoracic epidural analgesia with morphine or bupivacaine, *Anesthesia and Analgesia*, **67**, 687–694.

Thorén, T., Wattwil, M., Järnerot, G. and Tanghöj, H., 1989b, Epidural and spinal anesthesia do not influence gastric emptying and small intestinal transit in volunteers, *Regional Anesthesia*, **14**, 35–42.

Thorgeirsson, S. S., Felton, J. S. and Nebert, D. W., 1975, Genetic differences in the aromatic hydrocarbon-inducible N-hydroxylation of 2-acetylaminofluorene and acetaminophen produced hepatotoxicity in mice, *Molecular Pharmacology*, **11**, 159–165.

Thorgeirsson, S. S., Sasame, H. A., Mitchell, J. R., Jollow, D. J. and Potter, W. Z., 1976, Biochemical changes after hepatic injury from toxic doses of acetaminophen or furosemide, *Pharmacology*, **14**, 205–217.

Thörn, S.-E., Wattwil, M. and Näslund, I., 1992, Postoperative epidural morphine, but not epidural bupivacaine, delays gastric emptying on the first day after cholecystectomy, *Regional Anesthesia*, **17**, 91–94.

Thornton, J. R. and Losowsky, M. S., 1989, Fatal variceal haemorrhage after paracetamol overdose, *Gut*, **30**, 1424–1425.

Thornton, J. R. and Losowsky, M. S., 1990, Severe thrombocytopenia after paracetamol overdose, *Gut*, **31**, 1159–1160.

Thummel, K. E., Lee, C. A., Kunze, K. L. and Nelson, S. D., 1993, Oxidation of acetaminophen to N-acetyl-p-aminobenzoquinone imine by human CYP3A4, *Biochemical Pharmacology*, **45**, 1563–1569.

Thummel, K. E., Slattery, J. T. and Nelson, S. D., 1988, Mechanism by which ethanol diminishes the hepatotoxicity of acetaminophen, *Journal of Pharmacology and Experimental Therapeutics*, **245**, 129–136.

Thummel, K. E., Slattery, J. T., Nelson, S. D., Lee, C. A. and Pearson, P. G., 1989, Effect of ethanol on hepatotoxicity of acetaminophen in mice and on reactive metabolite formation by mouse and human liver microsomes, *Toxicology and Applied Pharmacology*, **100**, 391–397.

Thun, M. J., Namboodiri, M. M., Calle, E. E., Flanders, W. D. and Heath, C. W., 1993, Aspirin use and risk of fatal cancer, *Cancer Research*, **53**, 1322–1327.

Thun, M. J., Namboodiri, M. M. and Heath, C. W., 1991, Aspirin use and reduced risk of fatal colon cancer, *New England Journal of Medicine*, **325**, 1593–1596.

Tigerstedt, I., Leander, P. and Tammisto, T., 1981, Postoperative analgesics for superficial surgery: comparison of four analgesics, *Acta Anaesthesiologica Scandinavica*, **25**, 543–547.

Tighe, T. V. and Walter, F. G., 1994, Delayed toxic acetaminophen level after initial four hour nontoxic level, *Journal of Toxicology. Clinical Toxicology*, **32**, 431–434.

Tiller, J. and Treasure, J., 1992, Purging with paracetamol: report of four cases, *British Medical Journal*, **305**, 618.

Timson, J., 1968, Paracetamol and mitosis, *Lancet*, **ii**, 1084.

Tirmenstein, M. A. and Nelson, S. D., 1989, Subcellular binding and effects on calcium homeostasis produced by acetaminophen and a nonhepatotoxic regioisomer, 3-hydroxyacetanilide, in mouse liver, *Journal of Biological Chemistry*, **264**, 9814–9819.

Tirmenstein, M. A. and Nelson, S. D., 1990, Acetaminophen-induced oxidation of protein thiols: contribution of impaired thiol-metabolizing enzymes and the breakdown of adenine nucleotides, *Journal of Biological Chemistry*, **265**, 3059–3065.

Tirmenstein, M. A. and Nelson, S. D., 1991, Hepatotoxicity after 3′-hydroxyacetanilide administration to buthionine sulfoximine pretreated mice, *Chemical Research in Toxicology*, **4**, 214–217.

Tjølsen, A., Lund, A. and Hole, K., 1991a, Antinociceptive effect of paracetamol in rats is partly dependent on spinal serotonergic systems, *European Journal of Pharmacology*, **193**, 193–201.

Tjølsen, A., Rosland, J. H., Berge, O.-G. and Hole, K., 1991b, The increasing-temperature hot-plate test: an improved test of nociception in mice and rats, *Journal of Pharmacological Methods*, **25**, 241–250.

To, E. C. A. and Wells, P. G., 1984, Rapid and sensitive assays using high-performance liquid chromatography to measure the activities of phase II drug metabolising enzymes: glucuronyl transferase and sulfotransferase, *Journal of Chromatography*, **301**, 282–287.

To, E. C. A. and Wells, P. G., 1985, Repetitive microvolumetric sampling and analysis of acetaminophen and its toxicologically relevant metabolites in murine plasma and urine using high performance liquid chromatography, *Journal of Analytical Toxicology*, **9**, 217–221.

To, E. C. A. and Wells, P. G., 1986, Biochemical changes associated with the potentiation of acetaminophen hepatotoxicity by brief anesthesia with diethyl ether, *Biochemical Pharmacology*, **35**, 4139–4152.

Tobias, J. D., Gregory, D. F. and Deshpande, J. K., 1992, Ondansetron to prevent emesis following N-acetylcysteine for acetaminophen intoxication, *Pediatric Emergency Care*, **8**, 345–346.

Todd, J. G. and Nimmo, W. S., 1983, Effect of premedication on drug absorption and gastric emptying, *British Journal of Anaesthesia*, **55**, 1189–1193.

Toghill, P. J., Williams, R., Stephens, J. D. and Carroll, J. D., 1969, Acute hepatic necrosis following an overdose of paracetamol, *Gastroenterology*, **56**, 773–776.

Tokola, R. A., 1988, The effect of metoclopramide and prochlorperazine on the absorption of effervescent paracetamol in migraine, *Cephalalgia*, **8**, 139–147.

Tokola, R. A. and Neuvonen, P. J., 1981, Absorption of effervescent paracetamol during migraine, *Acta Pharmacologica et Toxicologica*, **49 (Suppl. 1)**, 78.

Tokola, R. A. and Neuvonen, P. J., 1984, Effect of migraine attacks on paracetamol absorption, *British Journal of Clinical Pharmacology*, **18**, 867–871.

Toledo, C. F. and Borges, D. R., 1992, Doença hepática acetaminofeno-induzida: um model de hepatotoxicidade, *Revista Da Associacao Medica Brasileira*, **38**, 153–158.

Tolman, E. L., Fuller, B. L., Marinan, B. A., Capetola, R. J., Levinson, S. L. and Rosenthale, M. E., 1983, Tissue selectivity and variability of effects of acetaminophen on arachidonic acid metabolism, *Prostaglandins Leukotrienes and Medicine*, **12**, 347–356.

Tomovic, D. and Hagmann, R., 1977, Klinische Ergebnisse mit Paracetamol-Suppositorien bei Kindern, *Schweizerische Rundschau für Medizin Praxis*, **66**, 276–280.

Tompsett, S. L., 1969, The detection and determination of phenacetin and N-acetyl-p-aminophenol (paracetamol) in blood serum and urine, *Annals of Clinical Biochemistry*, **6**, 81–82.

Tone, Y., Kawamata, K., Murakami, T., Higashi, Y. and Yata, N., 1990, Dose-dependent pharmacokinetics and first-pass metabolism of acetaminophen in rats, *Journal of Pharmacobiodynamics*, **13**, 327–335.

Tongia, S. K., 1982, Paracetamol augments the sotalol induced bradycardia in man, *Indian Journal of Physiology and Pharmacology*, **26**, 97–98.

Topinka, J., Srám, R. J., Sirinjan, G., Kocisová, J., Binková, B. and Fojtiková, I., 1989, Mutagenicity studies on paracetamol in human volunteers. II. Unscheduled DNA synthesis and micronucleus test, *Mutation Research*, **227**, 147–152.

Torrado, J. J., Illum, L., Cadorniga, R. and Davis, S. S., 1990, Egg albumin microspheres containing paracetamol for oral administration. II. *In vivo* investigation, *Journal of Microencapsulation*, **7**, 471–477.

Townsend, J. C., 1983, Paracetamol and blood-glucose analysis with the YSI Analyzer, *Clinical Chemistry*, **29**, 2119.

Trautmann, M., Peskar, B. M. and Peskar, B. A., 1991, Aspirin-like drugs, ethanol-induced rat gastric injury and mucosal eicosanoid release, *European Journal of Pharmacology*, **201**, 53–58.

Tredger, J. M., O'Grady, J. G. and Williams, R., 1986a, Why patients still die after paracetamol poisoning, *British Medical Journal*, **293**, 756.

Tredger, J. M., Smith, H. M., Davis, M. and Williams, R., 1980, Effects of sulphur-containing compounds on paracetamol activation and covalent binding in a mouse hepatic microsomal system, *Toxicology Letters*, **5**, 339.

Tredger, J. M., Smith, H. M., Davis, M. and Williams, R., 1981, *In vitro* interaction of sulfur-containing compounds with the hepatic mixed-function oxidase system in mice: effects on paracetamol activation and covalent binding, *Toxicology and Applied Pharmacology*, **59**, 111–124.

Tredger, J. M., Smith, H. M., Read, R. B., Portmann, B. and Williams, R., 1985, Effects of ethanol ingestion on the hepatotoxicity and metabolism of paracetamol in mice, *Toxicology*, **36**, 341–352.

Tredger, J. M., Smith, H. M., Read, R. B. and Williams, R., 1986b, Effects of ethanol ingestion on the metabolism of a hepatotoxic dose of paracetamol in mice, *Xenobiotica*, **16**, 661–670.

Tredger, J. M., Thuluvath, P., Williams, R. and Murray-Lyon, I. M., 1995, Metabolic basis for high paracetamol dosage without hepatic injury: a case study, *Human and Experimental Toxicology*, **14**, 8–12.

Trenti, T., Bertolotti, M., Castellana, C. N., Ferrari, A., Pini, L. A. and Sternieri, E., 1992, Plasma glutathione level in paracetamol daily abuser patients. Changes in plasma cysteine and thiol groups after reduced glutathione administration, *Toxicology Letters*, **64/65**, 757–761.

Triggs, E. J., Nation, R. L., Long, A. and Ashley, J. J., 1975, Pharmacokinetics in the elderly, *European Journal of Clinical Pharmacology*, **8**, 55–62.

Tringham, V. M., Young, J. H. and Cochrane, P., 1980, Aspirin, paracetamol, diflunisal and gastrointestinal blood loss, *European Journal of Rheumatology and Inflammation*, **3**, 175–179.

Trumper, L., Girardi, G. and Elías, M. M., 1992, Acetaminophen nephrotoxicity in male Wistar rats, *Archives of Toxicology*, **66**, 107–111.

Trumper, L., Monasterolo, L. and Elías, M. M., 1993, Efectos de verapamil sobre la nefrotoxicidad de acetaminofeno, *Medicina*, **53 (Suppl.)**, 79.

Tsokos-Kuhn, J. O., 1989, Evidence *in vivo* for elevation of intracellular free Ca^{2+} in the liver after diquat, acetaminophen, and CCl_4, *Biochemical Pharmacology*, **38**, 3061–3065.

Tsokos-Kuhn, J. O., Hughes, H., Smith, C. V. and Mitchell, J. R., 1988a, Alkylating toxins and the liver plasma membrane calcium pump/calcium ATPase, *Advances in Experimental Medicine and Biology*, **232**, 151–158.

Tsokos-Kuhn, J. O., Hughes, H., Smith, C. V. and Mitchell, J. R., 1988b, Alkyation of the liver plasma membrane and inhibition of the Ca^{2+} ATPase by acetaminophen, *Biochemi-*

cal Pharmacology, **37**, 2125–2131.

Tsokos-Kuhn, J. O., Todd, E. L., McMillin-Wood, J. B. and Mitchell, J. R., 1985, ATP-dependent calcium uptake by rat liver plasma membrane vesicles: effect of alkyating hepatotoxins *in vivo*, *Molecular Pharmacology*, **28**, 56–61.

Tsuda, H., Fukushima, S., Imaida, K., Sakata, T. and Ito, N., 1984a, Modification of carcinogenesis by antioxidants and other compounds, *Acta Pharmacologica et Toxicologica*, **55 (Suppl. 2)**, 125–143.

Tsuda, H., Hasegawa, R., Imaida, K., Masui, T., Moore, M. A. and Ito, N., 1984b, Modifying potential of thirty-one chemicals on the short-term development of γ-glutamyl transpeptidase-positive foci in diethylnitrosamine-initiated rat liver, *Gann*, **75**, 876–883.

Tsuda, H., Moore, M. A., Asamoto, M., Inoue, T., Ito, N., Satoh, K., Ichihara, A., Nakamura, T., Amelizad, Z. and Oesch, F., 1988, Effect of modifying agents on the phenotypic expression of cytochrome P-450, glutathione S-transferase molecular forms, microsomal epoxide hydrolase, glucose-6-phosphate dehydrogenase and γ-glutamyltranspeptidase in rat liver preneoplastic lesions, *Carcinogenesis*, **9**, 547–554.

Tsuda, H., Sakata, T., Masui, T., Imaida, K. and Ito, N., 1984c, Modifying effect of butylated hydroxyanisole, ethoxyquin and acetaminophen on induction of neoplastic lesions in rat liver and kidney initiated by N-ethyl-N-hydroxyethylnitrosamine, *Carcinogenesis*, **5**, 525–531.

Tsui, J. C. Y. and Madsen, N. P., 1979, Species variation in sensitivity of liver glutathione levels to paracetamol *in vitro*, *Clinical and Experimental Pharmacology and Physiology.*, **6**, 172–173.

Tsuruzaki, T., Watanabe, G. and Yamamoto, M., 1982, The effects of aspirin and acetaminophen during pregnancy on chromosomal structure in rat fetuses, *Japanese Journal of Hygiene*, **37**, 787–796.

Tsutsumi, M., Takada, A. and Wang, J.-S. ., 1994, Genetic polymorphisms of cytochrome P-4502E1 related to the development of alcoholic liver disease, *Gastroenterology*, **107**, 1430–1435.

Tudhope, G. R., 1966, Comparison of flufenamic acid with aspirin and paracetamol in terms of gastrointestinal blood loss, *Annals of Physical Medicine* **(Suppl.)**, 58–61.

Tukker, J. J., Sitsen, J. M. A. and Gusdorf, Ch. F., 1986, Bioavailability of paracetamol after oral administration to healthy volunteers. Influence of caffeine on rate and extent of absorption, *Pharmaceutisch Weekblad. Scientific Edition*, **8**, 239–243.

Tulley, R. T., 1985, A fast preliminary test for acetaminophen in serum, *Clinical Chemistry*, **31**, 788–789.

Tulloch, A. L., Blizzard, L., Hornsby, H. and Pinkus, Z., 1994, Suicide and self-harm in Tasmanian children and adolescents, *Medical Journal of Australia*, **160**, 775–786.

Tuntaterdtum, S., Chaudhary, I. P., Cibull, M., Robertson, L. W. and Blouin, R. A., 1993, Acetaminophen hepatotoxicity: influence of phenobarbital and β-naphthoflavone treatment in obese and lean Zucker rats, *Toxicology and Applied Pharmacology*, **123**, 219–225.

Turek, M. D. and Baird, W. M., 1988, Double-blind parallel comparison of ketoprofen (Orudis), acetaminophen plus codeine, and placebo in postoperative pain, *Journal of Clinical Pharmacology*, **28 (Suppl. 12)**, S23–S28.

Tuso, P. J. and Nortman, D., 1992, Renal magnesium wasting associated with acetaminophen abuse, *Connecticut Medicine*, **56**, 421–423.

Tyler, D. C., Tu, A., Douthit, J. and Chapman, C. R., 1993, Toward validation of pain measurement tools for children: a pilot study, *Pain*, **52**, 301–309.

Tyson, C. A., Cohen, S. D. and Khairallah, E. A., 1991, Comparative toxicity: mechanistic studies on acetaminophen action *in vitro* and *in vivo* in various species including man, *Alternative Methods in Toxicology*, **8**, 163–170.

Tyson, C. A., Mitoma, C. and Kalivoda, J., 1980, Evaluation of hepatocytes isolated by a nonperfusion technique in a prescreen for cytotoxicity, *Journal of Toxicology and*

Environmental Health, **6**, 197–205.

Udosen, E. O., Ebong, P. E. and Ekanemessang, U. M., 1989, Hepatotoxicity evaluation in rats given a single overdose of acetaminophen (paracetamol), *Central African Journal of Medicine,* **35**, 495–496.

Udosen, E. O. and Ebong, P. E., 1991, The effect of prolonged exposure of rats to sub-lethal dose of acetaminophen, *Central African Journal of Medicine,* **37**, 126–129.

Ueno, T., Tanaka, A., Hamanaka, Y. and Suzuki, T., 1995, Serum drug concentrations after oral administration of paracetamol to patients with surgical resection of the gastro-intestinal tract, *British Journal of Clinical Pharmacology,* **39**, 330–332.

Uges, D. R. A., Bloemhof, H. and Christensen, E. K. J., 1981, An HPLC method for the determination of salicylic acid, phenacetin and paracetamol in serum, with indications; two case reports of intoxication, *Pharmaceutisch Weekblad. Scientific Edition,* **3**, 1309–1314.

Uhari, M., Hietala, J. and Viljanen, M. K., 1988, Effect of prophylactic acetaminophen administration on reaction to DTP vaccination, *Acta Pædiatrica Scandinavica,* **77**, 747–751.

Uhlig, S. and Wendel, A., 1990, Glutathione enhancement in various mouse organs and protection by glutathione *iso*-propyl ester against liver injury, *Biochemical Pharmacology,* **39**, 1877–1881.

Ullrich, D., Sieg, A., Blume, R., Bock, K. W., Schröter, W. and Bircher, J., 1987, Normal pathways for glucuronidation, sulphation and oxidation of paracetamol in Gilbert's syndrome, *European Journal of Clinical Investigation,* **17**, 237–240.

Underhill, T. J., Greene, M. K. and Dove, A. F., 1990, A comparison of the efficacy of gastric lavage, ipecacuanha and activated charcoal in the emergency management of paracetamol overdose, *Archives of Emergency Medicine,* **7**, 148–154.

Urquhart, E., 1994, Analgesic agents and strategies in the dental pain model, *Journal of Dentistry,* **22**, 336–341.

Uryvaeva, I. V. and Faktor, V. M., 1976, Resistance of regenerating liver to hepatotoxins, *Bulletin of Experimental Biology and Medicine,* **81**, 283–285.

Vaerøy, H., Abrahamsen, A., Førre, O. and Kåss, E., 1989, Treatment of fibromyalgia (fibrositis syndrome): a parallel double blind trial with carisoprodol, paracetamol and caffeine (Somadril comp) versus placebo, *Clinical Rheumatology,* **8**, 245–250.

Valbonesi, M., Garelli, S., Mosconi, L. and Cattaneo, A., 1979, Le anemie immunoemolitiche farmaco-indotte: contributo casistico, *Trasfusione del Sangue,* **24**, 108–120.

Vale, J. A. and Buckley, B. M., 1983, Asthma associated with N-acetylcysteine infusion and paracetamol poisoning, *British Medical Journal,* **287**, 1223.

Vale, J. A., Buckley, B. M. and Meredith, T. J., 1984, Deaths from paracetamol and dextropropoxyphene (Distalgesic) poisoning in England and Wales in 1979, *Human Toxicology,* **3**, 135S–143S.

Vale, J. A., Meredith, T. J., Crome, P., Helliwell, M., Volans, G. N., Widdop, B. and Goulding, R., 1979, Intravenous N-acetylcysteine: the treatment of choice in paracetamol poisoning? *British Medical Journal,* **2**, 1435–1436.

Vale, J. A., Meredith, T. J. and Goulding, R., 1981, Treatment of acetaminophen poisoning. The use of oral methionine, *Archives of Internal Medicine,* **141**, 394–396.

Vale, J. A. and Wheeler, D. C., 1982, Anaphylactoid reactions to N-acetylcysteine, *Lancet,* **ii**, 988.

Valsecchi, R., 1989, Fixed drug eruption due to paracetamol, *Dermatologica,* **179**, 51–52.

van Berge Henegouwen, G. P. and Savelkoul, T. J. F., 1994, Acetylcysteïne bij paracetamolo-verdosering: intraveneuze maar ook orale therapie, ook bij late toepassing, *Nederlands Tijdschrift voor Geneeskunde,* **138**, 1988–1992.

van Bommel, E. M. G., Raghoebar, M. and Tukker, J. J., 1991a, Kinetics of acetaminophen after single- and multiple-dose oral administration as a gradient matrix system to healthy male subjects, *Biopharmaceutics and Drug Disposition,* **12**, 355–366.

van Bommel, E. M. G., Raghoebar, M. and Tukker, J. J., 1991b, Comparison of *in vitro* and *in vivo* release characteristics of acetaminophen from gradient matrix systems, *Biopharmaceutics and Drug Disposition*, **12**, 367–373.

van Bree, J. B. M. M., Baljet, A. V., van Geyt, A., de Boer, A. G., Danhof, M. and Breimer, D. D., 1989a, The unit impulse response procedure for the pharmacokinetic evaluation of drug entry into the central nervous system, *Journal of Pharmacokinetics and Biopharmaceutics*, **17**, 441–462.

van Bree, J. B. M. M., de Boer, A. G., Danhof, M., Ginsel, L. A. and Breimer, D. D., 1988, Characterization of an 'in vitro' blood brain barrier: effects of molecular size and lipophilicity on cerebrovascular endothelial transport rates of drugs, *Journal of Pharmacology and Experimental Therapeutics*, **247**, 1233–1239.

van Bree, L., Groot, E. J. and de Vries, J., 1989b, Reduction by acetylsalicylic acid of paracetamol-induced hepatic glutathione depletion in rats treated with 4,4′-dichlorobiphenyl, phenobarbitone and pregnenolone-16-α-carbonitrile, *Journal of Pharmacy and Pharmacology*, **41**, 343–345.

van de Graaff, W. B., Thompson, W. L., Sunshine, I., Fretthold, D., Leickly, F. and Dayton, H., 1982, Adsorbent and cathartic inhibition of enteral drug absorption, *Journal of Pharmacology and Experimental Therapeutics*, **221**, 656–663.

van de Straat, R., Bijloo, G. J. and Vermeulen, N. P. E., 1988a, Paracetamol, 3-monoalkyl- and 3,5-dialkyl-substituted derivatives: antioxidant activity and relationship between lipid peroxidation and cytotoxicity, *Biochemical Pharmacology*, **37**, 3473–3476.

van de Straat, R., de Vries, J., de Boer, H. J. R., Vromans, R. M. and Vermeulen, N. P. E., 1987a, Relationship between paracetamol binding to and its oxidation by two cytochrome P-450 enzymes: a proton nuclear magnetic resonance and spectrophotometric study, *Xenobiotica*, **17**, 1–9.

van de Straat, R., de Vries, J., Debets, A. J. J. and Vermeulen, N. P. E., 1987b, The mechanism of prevention of paracetamol-induced hepatotoxicity by 3,5-dialkyl substitution, *Biochemical Pharmacology*, **36**, 2065–2070.

van de Straat, R., de Vries, J., Groot, E. J., Zijl, R. and Vermeulen, N. P. E., 1987c, Paracetamol, 3-monoalkyl- and 3,5-dialkyl derivatives: comparison of their hepatotoxicity in mice, *Toxicology and Applied Pharmacology*, **89**, 183–189.

van de Straat, R., de Vries, J., Kulkens, T., Debets, A. J. J. and Vermeulen, N. P. E., 1986, Paracetamol, 3-monoalkyl- and 3,5-dialkyl derivatives: comparison of their microsomal cytochrome P-450 dependent oxidation and toxicity in freshly isolated hepatocytes, *Biochemical Pharmacology*, **35**, 3693–3699.

van de Straat, R., de Vries, J. and Vermeulen, N. P. E., 1987d, Role of hepatic microsomal and purified cytochrome P-450 in one-electron reduction of two quinine imines and concomitant reduction of molecular oxygen, *Biochemical Pharmacology*, **36**, 613–619.

van de Straat, R., Vromans, R. M., Bosman, P., de Vries, J. and Vermeulen, N. P. E., 1988b, Cytochrome P-450-mediated oxidation of substrates by electron-transfer: role of oxygen radicals and of 1- and 2-electron oxidation of paracetamol, *Chemico-Biological Interactions*, **64**, 267–280.

van der Kraan, P. M., de Vries, B. J., Vitters, E. L., van den Berg, W. B. and van de Putte, L. B. A., 1988, Inhibition of glycosaminoglycan synthesis in anatomically intact rat patellar cartilage by paracetamol-induced serum sulfate depletion, *Biochemical Pharmacology*, **37**, 3683–3690.

van der Kraan, P. M., Vitters, E. L., de Vries, B. J., van den Berg, W. B. and van de Putte, L. B. A., 1990, The effect of chronic paracetamol administration to rats on the glycosaminoglycan content of patellar cartilage, *Agents and Actions*, **29**, 218–223.

van der Veen, J., Eissens, A. C. and Lerk, C. F., 1994, Controlled release of paracetamol from amylodextrin tablets: *in vitro* and *in vivo* results, *Pharmaceutical Research*, **11**, 384–387.

van der Wal, Sj., Bannister, S. J. and Snyder, L. R., 1982, Automated analysis of acetaminophen and caffeine in serum using the FAST-LC system: contributions to assay imprecision in procedures based on HPLC with sample pretreatment, *Journal of Chromatographic Science*, **20**, 260–265.

van der Zee, J., Mulder, G. J. and van Steveninck, J., 1988, Acetaminophen protects human erythrocytes against oxidative stress, *Chemico-Biological Interactions*, **65**, 15–23.

van Doorn, R., Leijdekkers, Ch.-M. and Henderson, P. Th., 1978, Synergistic effects of phorone on the hepatotoxicity of bromobenzene and paracetamol in mice, *Toxicology*, **11**, 225–233.

van Gossum, A., Zalcman, M., Adler, M., Peny, M. O., Houben, J. J. and Cremer, M., 1993, Anorectal stenosis in patients with prolonged use of suppositories containing paracetamol and acetylsalicylic acid, *Digestive Diseases and Sciences*, **38**, 1970–1977.

van Heijst, A. N. P., Douzeen, J. M. C. and Pikaar, S. A., 1976, Paracetamol-vergiftiging, *Nederlands Tijdschrift voor Geneeskunde*, **120**, 1151–1154.

van Heyningen, R. and Harding, J. J., 1986, Do aspirin-like analgesics protect against cataract? *Lancet*, **i**, 1111–1113.

van Kolfschoten, A. A., Dembinska-Kiec, A. and Basista, M., 1981, Interaction between aspirin and paracetamol on the production of prostaglandins in the rat gastric mucosa, *Journal of Pharmacy and Pharmacology*, **33**, 462–463.

van Kolfschoten, A. A., Hagelen, F., Hillen, F. C. and van Noordwijk, J., 1983a, The influence of paracetamol on the anti-inflammatory, the anti-pyretic and the analgesic activity of indomethacin, *Archives Internationales de Pharmacodynamie et de Thérapie*, **265**, 55–60.

van Kolfschoten, A. A., Hagelen, F. and van Noordwijk, J., 1982a, Indomethacin and paracetamol: interaction with prostaglandin synthesis in the rat stomach, *European Journal of Pharmacology*, **84**, 123–125.

van Kolfschoten, A. A., Olling, M. and van Noordwijk, J., 1985, Pharmacokinetic interactions between indomethacin and paracetamol in the rat, *Pharmaceutisch Weekblad. Scientific Edition*, **7**, 15–19.

van Kolfschoten, A. A., Zandberg, P., Jager, L. P. and van Noordwijk, J., 1982b, The influence of paracetamol on the erosive activity of indomethacin in the rat stomach, *Agents and Actions*, **12**, 247–253.

van Kolfschoten, A. A., Zandberg, P., Jager, L. P. and van Noordwijk, J., 1983b, Protection by paracetamol against various gastric irritants in the rat, *Toxicology and Applied Pharmacology*, **69**, 37–42.

van Kraaij, D. J. W., Haagsma, C. J., Go, I. H. and Gribnau, F. W. J., 1994, Drug use and adverse drug reactions in 105 elderly patients admitted to a general medical ward, *Netherlands Journal of Medicine*, **44**, 166–173.

van Miert, A. S. J. P. A. M., van der Wal-Komproe, L. E. and van Duin, C. Th. M., 1977, Effects of antipyretic agents on fever and ruminal stasis induced by endotoxins in conscious goats, *Archives Internationales de Pharmacodynamie et de Thérapie*, **225**, 39–50.

van Steveninck, J., Koster, J. F. and Dubbelman, M. A. R., 1989, Xanthine oxidase-catalyzed oxidation of paracetamol, *Biochemical Journal*, **259**, 633–637.

van Tittelboom, T. and Govaerts-Lepicard, M., 1989, Hypothermia: an unusual side effect of paracetamol, *Veterinary and Human Toxicology*, **31**, 57–59.

van Vyve, Th., Hantson, Ph., Deckers, O. and Mahieu, P., 1993, Severe acetaminophen poisoning with favorable outcome after medical treatment: report of 2 cases, *Acta Clinica Belgica*, **48**, 392–396.

van Wyk, M., Sommers, De K., Meyer, E. C. and Moncrieff, J., 1990, The mean cumulative fraction absorbed-time profiles of paracetamol as an index of gastric emptying, *Methods and Findings in Experimental and Clinical Pharmacology*, **12**, 291–294.

van Wyk, M., Sommers, De K. and Moncrieff, J., 1992, Influence of cisapride, metoclopramide and loperamide on gastric emptying of normal volunteers as measured by means of the area under the curve of the cumulative fraction absorbed-time profiles of paracetamol, *Methods and Findings in Experimental and Clinical Pharmacology*, **14**, 379–382.

van Wyk, M., Sommers, De K. and Moncrieff, J., 1993a, Effects of enhancement and antagonism of 5-hydroxytryptamine activity on the influence of metoclopramide on gastric emptying, *Digestion*, **54**, 40–43.

van Wyk, M., Sommers, De K., Moncrieff, J. and Becker, P. J., 1993b, The influence of neostigmine and metoclopramide or their combination on gastric emptying, *Current Therapeutic Research*, **54**, 300–303.

van Wyk, M., Sommers, De K., Snyman, J. R. and Moncrieff, J., 1993c, A foreshortened method of measuring liquid gastric emptying in normal volunteers, *Methods and Findings in Experimental and Clinical Pharmacology*, **15**, 61–66.

van Zyl, J. M., Basson, K. and van der Walt, B. J., 1989, The inhibitory effect of acetaminophen on the myeloperoxidase-induced antimicrobial system of the polymorphonuclear leukocyte, *Biochemical Pharmacology*, **38**, 161–165.

Vance, M. V., Selden, B. S. and Clark, R. F., 1992, Optimal patient position for transport and initial management of toxic ingestions, *Annals of Emergency Medicine*, **21**, 243–246.

Vanchieri, C., 1993, Australian study links certain analgesics to renal cancers, *Journal of the National Cancer Institute*, **85**, 262–263.

Vane, J. R., 1971, Inhibition of prostaglandin synthesis as a mechanism of action for aspirin-like drugs, *Nature*, **231**, 232–235.

Vangen, O., Doessland, S. and Lindbaek, E., 1988, Comparative study of ketorolac and paracetamol/codeine in alleviating pain in gynaecological surgery, *Journal of International Medical Research*, **16**, 443–451.

Vanherweghem, J.-L. and Even-Adin, D., 1982, Epdemiology of analgesic nephropathy in Belgium, *Clinical Nephrology*, **17**, 129–133.

Vanherweghem, J.-L., Tielmans, C., Simon, J. and Deperrieux, M., 1995, Chinese herbs, nephropathy and renal pelvic carcinoma, *Nephrology, Dialysis, Transplantation*, **10**, 270–273.

Varela-Moreiras, G., Ragel, C. and Ruiz-Roso, B., 1993, Effects of prolonged aspirin or acetaminophen administration to rats on liver folate content and distribution. Relation to DNA methylation and S-adenosylmethionine, *International Journal for Vitamin and Nutrition Research*, **63**, 41–46.

Varela-Moreiras, G., Ruiz-Rosa, B. and Varela, G., 1990, Utilización digestiva de la grasa y consumo crónico de paracetamol en ratas: influencia de dos niveles dietéticos de proteína, *Farmacia Clínica*, **7**, 51–54.

Varela-Moreiras, G., Ruiz-Roso, B. and Varela, G., 1991, Effects of long-term administration of acetaminophen on the nutritional utilization of dietary protein, *Annals of Nutrition and Metabolism*, **35**, 303–308.

Vargaftig, B. B. and Dao Hai, N., 1973, Inhibition by acetamidophenol of the production of prostaglandin-like material from blood platelets *in vitro* in relation to some *in vivo* actions, *European Journal of Pharmacology*, **24**, 283–288.

Vargas, R., Maneatis, T., Bynum, L., Peterson, C. and McMahon, F. G., 1994, Evaluation of the antipyretic effect of ketorolac, acetaminophen, and placebo in endotoxin-induced fever, *Journal of Clinical Pharmacology*, **34**, 848–853.

Vargus Busquets, M. A., Keoshian, L. A., Kelleher, R., Jervis, W. H. and Hentz, V. R., 1988, Naproxen sodium vs. acetaminophen-codeine for pain following plastic surgery, *Current Therapeutic Research*, **43**, 311–316.

Vaughan, P. A., Scott, L. D. L. and McAleer, J. F., 1991, Amperometric biosensor for the rapid determination of acetaminophen in whole blood, *Analytica Chimica Acta*, **248**, 361–365.

Velásquez-Jones, L., 1983, Intoxicación por acetaminophén en niños: grave error de prescripción médica, *Boletín Médico del Hospital Infantil de México*, **40**, 476–479.

Veltri, J. C. and Rollins, D. E., 1988, A comparison of the frequency and severity of poisoning cases for ingestion of acetaminophen, aspirin, and ibuprofen, *American Journal of Emergency Medicine*, **6**, 104–107.

Vendemiale, G., Altomare, E. and Lieber, C. S., 1984, Altered biliary excretion of acetaminophen in rats fed ethanol chronically, *Drug Metabolism and Disposition: The Biological Fate of Chemicals*, **12**, 20–24.

Vendemiale, G., Altomare, E., Trizio, T., Leandro, G., Manghisi, O. G. and Albano, O., 1987, Effect of acute and chronic cimetidine administration on acetaminophen metabolism in humans, *American Journal of Gastroenterology*, **82**, 1031–1034.

Venkataramanan, R., Kalp, K., Rabinovitch, M., Cuellar, R., Ptachcinski, R. J., Teperman, L., Makowka, L., Burckart, G. J., Van, Thiel,D. H. and Starzl, T. E., 1989, Conjugative drug metabolism in liver transplant patients, *Transplantation Proceedings*, **21**, 2455.

Ventafridda, V., De Conno, F., Panerai, A. E., Maresca, V., Monza, G. C. and Ripamonti, C., 1990, Non-steroidal anti-inflammatory drugs as the first step in cancer pain therapy: double-blind, within-patient study comparing nine drugs, *Journal of International Medical Research*, **18**, 21–29.

Venzmer, G., 1932, Eine Weltindustrie wird geboren, *Westermanns Monatshefte*, **152**, 315–318.

Verbov, J., 1985, Fixed drug eruption due to a drug combination but not to its constituents, *Dermatologica*, **171**, 60–61.

Verhagen, H., Maas, L. M., Beckers, R. H. G., Thijssen, H. H. W., ten Hoor, F., Henderson, P. Th. and Kleinjans, J. C. S., 1989, Effect of subacute oral intake of the food antioxidant butylated hydroxyanisole on clinical parameters and phase-I and -II biotransformation capacity in man, *Human Toxicology*, **8**, 451–459.

Verheggen, R. and Schrör, K., 1987, Inhibition of platelet 5-HT secretion and 5-HT induced vasoconstriction by paracetamol, *Prostaglandins in Clinical Research*, **242**, 271–276.

Verma, K. K., Jain, A. and Stewart, K. K., 1992, Flow-injection spectrophotometric determination of acetaminophen in drug formulations, *Analytica Chimica Acta*, **261**, 261 267.

Vermeulen, N. P. E., Bessems, J. G. M. and van de Straat, R., 1992, Molecular aspects of paracetamol-induced hepatotoxicity and its mechanism-based prevention, *Drug Metabolism Reviews*, **24**, 367–407.

Vernon, S., Bacon, C. and Weightman, D., 1979, Rectal paracetamol in small children with fever, *Archives of Disease in Childhood*, **54**, 469–470.

Veronese, M. E. and McLean, S., 1991, Metabolism of paracetamol and phenacetin in relation to debrisoquine oxidation phenotype, *European Journal of Clinical Pharmacology*, **40**, 547–552.

Vest, M., 1962, Vergleichende Untersuchungen über die Toxizität von Phenacetin und N-Acetyl-p-aminophenol, *Deutsche Medizinische Wochenschrift*, **87**, 2141–2147.

Vest, M., 1963, The toxicity of phenacetin and N-acetyl-p-aminophenol for infants, *German Medical Monthly*, **8**, 316.

Vest, M. F. and Streiff, R. R., 1959, Studies of glucuronide formation in newborn infants and older children: measurement of *p*-aminophenol glucuronide levels in the serum after an oral dose of acetanilid, *American Journal of Diseases of Children*, **98**, 688–693.

Vesterqvist, O. and Gréen, K., 1984, Urinary excretion of 2,3-dinor-thromboxane B_2 in man under normal conditions, following drugs and during some pathological conditions, *Prostaglandins*, **27**, 627–644.

Vial, T., Sauveur, C. and Descotes, J., 1990, Influence of acetaminophen on antipyrine kinetics in rats, *Fundamental and Clinical Pharmacology*, **4**, 79–83.

Vialatte, J., 1983, Intérêt du soluté buvable de paracétamol chez l'enfant asthmatique présentant un syndrome fébrile, *Journal des Agrégés*, **16**, 384–386.

Viallon, A., Lafond, P., Tardy, B., Zeni, F., Page, Y. and Bertrand, J. C., 1994, Perfusion tardive de N-acétylcystéine dans un cas d'intoxication au paracétamol vu au stade d'une hépatite fulminante, *Thérapie*, **49**, 144–146.

Vickers, C., Neuberger, J., Buckels, J., McMaster, P. and Elias, E., 1988, Transplantation of the liver in adults and children with fulminant hepatic failure, *Journal of Hepatology*, **7**, 143–150.

Vickers, F. N., 1967, Mucosal effects of aspirin and acetaminophen. Report of a controlled gastroscopic study, *Gastrointestinal Endoscopy*, **14**, 94–99.

Vidal, M., Bonnafous, M., Defrance, S., Loiseau, P., Bernadou, J. and Meunier, B., 1993, Model systems for oxidative drug metabolism studies: catalytic behavior of water-soluble metalloprophyrins depends on both the intrinsic robustness of the catalyst and the nature of substrates, *Drug Metabolism and Disposition: The Biological Fate of Chemicals*, **21**, 811–817.

Vignon, E., Mathieu, P., Broquet, P., Louisot, P. and Richard, M., 1990, Cartilage degradative enzymes in human osteoarthritis: effect of a nonsteroidal antiinflammatory drug administered orally, *Seminars in Arthritis and Rheumatism*, **19 (Suppl. 1)**, 26–29.

Vila-Jato, J. L., Areses, J. and Concheiro, A., 1981, Determinacion de paracetamol y oxifenbutazona en plasma por cromatografia en fase liquida de alta presion, *Bollettino Chimico Farmaceutico*, **120**, 165–171.

Vila-Jato, J. L., Blanco, J. and Alonso, M. J., 1986a, The effect of the molecular weight of polyethylene glycol on the bioavailability of paracetamol-polyethylene glycol solid dispersions, *Journal of Pharmacy and Pharmacology*, **38**, 126–128.

Vila-Jato, J. L., González, A. and Durán, R., 1986b, Estudios de distintos tipos de rellenos utilizados en HPLC: aplicación a la separación del paracetamol y sus metabolitos principales, *Ciencia e Industria Farmaceutica*, **5**, 240–245.

Villeneuve, J.-P., Raymond, G., Bruneau, J., Colpron, L. and Pomier-Layrargues, G., 1983, Pharmacocinétique et métabolisme de l'acétaminophène chez des sujets normaux, alcooliques et cirrhotiques, *Gastroentérologie Clinique et Biologique*, **7**, 898–902.

Vilstrup, H., Henningsen, N. C. and Hansen, L. F., 1977, Leverbeskadigelse efter paracetamol, *Ugeskrift for Læger*, **139**, 831–834.

Viña, J., Perez, C., Furukawa, T., Palacin, M. and Viña, J. R., 1989, Effect of oral glutathione on hepatic glutathione levels in rats and mice, *British Journal of Nutrition*, **62**, 683–691.

Viña, J., Romero, F. J., Estrela, J. M. and Viña, J. R., 1980, Effect of acetaminophen (paracetamol) and its antagonists on glutathione (GSH) content in rat liver, *Biochemical Pharmacology*, **29**, 1968–1970.

Viña, J., Sáez, G. T., Rodríguez, A., Pérez, C. and Viña, J. R., 1986, Prevention of paracetamol hepatotoxicity in rats and mice: effect of small amounts of methionine, *Journal of Clinical Nutrition and Gastroenterology*, **1**, 217–220.

Vincens, M., Ganansia, R., du Puy-Montbrun, T., Denis, J., Lugagne, F., Brule, J. and Lagier, G., 1982, Anites et anorectites nécrosantes chez des malades ayant utilisé au long cours des suppositoires associant dextropropoxyphène et paracétamol, *Thérapie*, **37**, 321–326.

Vinegar, R., Truax, J. F. and Selph, J. L., 1976, Quantitative comparison of the analgesic and anti-inflammatory activities of aspirin, phenacetin and acetaminophen in rodents, *European Journal of Pharmacology*, **37**, 23–30.

Vinegar, R., Truax, J. F., Selph, J. L. and Johnston, P. R., 1989, Pharmacological characterization of the algesic response to the subplantar injection of serotonin in the rat, *European Journal of Pharmacology*, **164**, 497–505.

Vinegar, R., Truax, J. F., Selph, J. L. and Johnston, P. R., 1990, New analgesic assay utilizing trypsin-induced hyperalgesia in the hind limb of the rat, *Journal of Pharmacological Methods*, **23**, 51–61.

Vinegar, R., Truax, J. F., Selph, J. L., Lea, A. and Johnston, P. R., 1978, Quantitative *in vivo* studies of the acute actions of anti-inflammatory drugs in the rat, *European Journal of Rheumatology and Inflammation*, **1**, 204–211.

Visen, P. K. S., Shukla, B., Patnaik, G. K. and Dhawan, B. N., 1993, Andrographolide protects rat hepatocytes against paracetamol-induced damage, *Journal of Ethnopharmacology*, **40**, 131–136.

Visen, P. K. S., Shukla, B., Patnaik, G. K., Kaul, S., Kapoor, N. K. and Dhawan, B. N., 1991, Hepatoprotective activity of picroliv, the active principle of *Picrorhiza kurrooa*, on rat hepatocytes against paracetamol toxicity, *Drug Development Research*, **22**, 209–219.

Visen, P. K. S., Shukla, B., Patnaik, G. K., Tripathi, S. C., Kulshreshtha, D. K., Srimal, R. C.

and Dhawan, B. N., 1992, Hepatoprotective activity of *Ricinus communis* leaves, *International Journal of Pharmacognosy*, **30**, 241–250.

Vivaldi, E., 1968, Effect of chronic administration of analgesics on resistance to experimental infection of the urinary tract in rats, *Nephron*, **5**, 202–209.

Volans, G. N., 1976, Self-poisoning and suicide due to paracetamol, *Journal of International Medical Research*, **4 (Suppl. 4)**, 7–13.

Volans, G. N., 1991, Antipyretic analgesic overdosage in children. Comparative risks, *British Journal of Clinical Practice*, **Suppl. 70**, 26–29.

von Moltke, L. L., Manis, M., Harmatz, J. S., Poorman, R. and Greenblatt, D. J., 1993, Inhibition of acetaminophen and lorazepam glucuronidation *in vitro* by probenecid, *Biopharmaceutics and Drug Disposition*, **14**, 119–130.

Vonen, B. and Morland, J., 1984, Isolated rat hepatocytes in suspension: potential hepatotoxic effects of six different drugs, *Archives of Toxicology*, **56**, 33–37.

Vu, D. D., Tuchweber, B., Plaa, G. L. and Yousef, I. M., 1992, Do intracellular Ca^{2+} activity and hepatic glutathione play a role in the pathogenesis of lithocholic acid-induced cholestasis?, *Toxicology Letters*, **61**, 255–264.

Waalkes, M. P. and Ward, J. M., 1989, Induction of hepatic metallothionein in male B6C3F1 mice exposed to hepatic tumor promotors: effects of phenobarbital, acetaminophen, sodium barbital and di(2-ethylhexyl) phthalate, *Toxicology and Applied Pharmacology*, **100**, 217–226.

Wade, A. G. and Ward, P. J., 1982, A double-blind comparison of meptazinol versus paracetamol and placebo in acute and chronic painful conditions presented to the general practitioner, *Current Medical Research and Opinion*, **8**, 191–196.

Wahl, K. C. and Rejent, T. A., 1978, Quantitative gas chromatographic determination of acetaminophen using trimethylanilinium hydroxide as the derivatising agent, *Journal of Forensic Sciences*, **23**, 14–20.

Wakeel, R. A., Davies, H. T. and Williams, J. D., 1987, Toxic myocarditis in paracetamol poisoning, *British Medical Journal*, **295**, 1097.

Wakuri, S., Izumi, J., Sasaki, K., Tanaka, N. and Ono, H., 1993, Cytotoxicity study of 32 MEIC chemicals by colony formation and ATP assays, *Toxicology in Vitro*, **7**, 517–521.

Wakushima, T., Murawaki, Y., Hirayama, C., kosaka, K., Tomie, K. and Morii, T., 1983, A case of acetaminophen-induced hepatitis, *Acta Hepatologica Japonica*, **24**, 1411–1415.

Walberg, C. B., 1977, Determination of acetaminophen in serum, *Journal of Analytical Toxicology*, **1**, 79–80.

Walberg, C. B., 1979, A rapid colorimetric assay for acetaminophen and experience in a large hospital, *Veterinary and Human Toxicology*, **21 (Suppl.)**, 162–164.

Waldman, R. J., Hall, W. N., McGee, H. and van Amburg, G., 1982, Aspirin as a risk factor in Reye's syndrome, *Journal of the American Medical Association*, **247**, 3089–3094.

Waldron, G., 1993, Medical messages on television: copycat overdoses coincidental, *British Medical Journal*, **306**, 1416.

Waldum, H. L., Hamre, T., Kleveland, P. M., Dybdahl, J. H. and Petersen, H., 1992, Can NSAIDs cause acute biliary pain with cholestasis? *Journal of Clinical Gastroenterology*, **14**, 328–330.

Walker, B. E., Kelleher, J., Dixon, M. F. and Losowsky, M. S., 1973, The effect of phenobarbitone pretreatment on paracetamol toxicity, *Biomedicine*, **19**, 465–468.

Walker, B. E., Kelleher, J., Dixon, M. F. and Losowsky, M. S., 1974, Vitamin E protection of the liver from paracetamol in the rat, *Clinical Science*, **47**, 449–459.

Walker, D., 1990, No effect of prostaglandin synthesis inhibition on muscle reflexes in fetal lambs, *American Journal of Physiology*, **258**, R1213–R1216.

Walker, E. M., Gale, G. R., Smith, A. B., Bowen, W. B. and Schmidt, B. J., 1989, Ketoconazole potentiation of acetaminophen toxicity, *Annals of Clinical and Laboratory Science*, **19**, 309–310.

Walker, P. C., Helms, R. A., Wall, H. P. and Jabbour, J. T., 1986, Comparative efficacy study of chewable aspirin and acetaminophen in the antipyresis of children, *Journal of Clinical Pharmacology*, **26**, 106–110.

Walker, R. J., 1991, Paracetamol, nonsteroidal antiinflammatory drugs and nephrotoxicity, *New Zealand Medical Journal*, **104**, 182–183.

Walker, R. J. and Duggin, G. G., 1988, Drug nephrotoxicity, *Annual Review of Pharmacology and Toxicology*, **28**, 331–345.

Walker, R. J. and Fawcett, J. P., 1993, Drug nephrotoxicity – the significance of cellular mechanisms, *Progress in Drug Research*, **41**, 51–94.

Walker, R. M., Massey, T. E., McElligott, T. F. and Racz, W. J., 1981, Acetaminophen-induced hypothermia, hepatic congestion, and modification by N-acetylcysteine in mice, *Toxicology and Applied Pharmacology*, **59**, 500–507.

Walker, R. M., Massey, T. E., McElligott, T. F. and Racz, W. J., 1982, Acetaminophen toxicity in fed and fasted mice, *Canadian Journal of Physiology and Pharmacology*, **60**, 399–404.

Walker, R. M., McElligott, T. F., Massey, T. E. and Racz, W. J., 1983a, Ultrastructural effects of acetaminophen in isolated mouse hepatocytes, *Experimental and Molecular Pathology*, **39**, 163–175.

Walker, R. M., McElligott, T. F., Power, E. M., Massey, T. E. and Racz, W. J., 1983b, Increased acetaminophen-induced hepatotoxicity after chronic ethanol consumption in mice, *Toxicology*, **28**, 193–206.

Walker, R. M., Racz, W. J. and McElligott, T. F., 1980, Acetaminophen-induced hepatotoxicity in mice, *Laboratory Investigation*, **42**, 181–189.

Walker, R. M., Racz, W. J. and McElligott, T. F., 1983c, Scanning electron microscopic examination of acetaminophen-induced hepatotoxicity and congestion in mice, *American Journal of Pathology*, **113**, 321–330.

Walker, R. M., Racz, W. J. and McElligott, T. F., 1985, Acetaminophen-induced hepatotoxic congestion in mice, *Hepatology*, **5**, 233–240.

Wallenstein, M. C., 1983, Effect of prostaglandin synthetase inhibitors on non-analgesic actions of morphine, *European Journal of Pharmacology*, **90**, 65–73.

Wallenstein, M. C., 1985, Differential effect of prostaglandin synthetase inhibitor pretreatment on pentylenetetrazol-induced seizures in rat, *Archives Internationales de Pharmacodynamie et de Thérapie*, **275**, 93–104.

Wallenstein, M. C., 1991, Attenuation of epileptogenesis by nonsteroidal anti-inflammatory drugs in the rat, *Neuropharmacology*, **30**, 657–663.

Wallenstein, M. C. and Mauss, E. A., 1984, Effect of prostaglandin synthetase inhibitors on experimentally induced convulsions in rats, *Pharmacology*, **29**, 85–93.

Wallenstein, S. L. and Houde, R. W., 1954, Clinical comparison of analgetic effectiveness of N-acetyl-p-aminophenol, salicylamide and aspirin, *Federation Proceedings*, **13**, 414.

Waller, D. G., Roseveare, C., Renwick, A. G., Macklin, B. and George, C. F., 1991a, Gastric emptying in healthy volunteers after multiple doses of levodopa, *British Journal of Clinical Pharmacology*, **32**, 691–695.

Waller, D. G., Usman, F., Renwick, A. G., Macklin, B. and George, C. F., 1991b, Oral amino acids and gastric emptying: an investigation of the mechanism of levodopa-induced gastric stasis, *British Journal of Clinical Pharmacology*, **32**, 771–773.

Walsh, F. X., Langlais, P. J. and Bird, E. D., 1982, Liquid-chromatographic identification of acetaminophen in cerebrospinal fluid with the use of electrochemical detection, *Clinical Chemistry*, **28**, 382–383.

Walson, P. D., 1990, Ibuprofen versus paracetamol for the treatment of fever in children, *British Journal of Clinical Practice*, **44 (Suppl. 70)**, 19–21.

Walson, P. D., Galletta, G., Braden, N. J. and Alexander, L., 1989, Ibuprofen, acetaminophen, and placebo treatment of febrile children, *Clinical Pharmacology and Therapeutics*, **46**, 9–17.

Walson, P. D., Galletta, G., Chomilo, F., Braden, N. J., Sawyer, L. A. and Scheinbaum, M. L.,

1992, Comparison of multidose ibuprofen and acetaminophen therapy in febrile children, *American Journal of Diseases of Children*, **146**, 626–632.

Walson, P. D. and Groth, J. F., 1993, Acetaminophen hepatotoxicity after a prolonged ingestion, *Pediatrics*, **91**, 1021–1022.

Walson, P. D. and Mortensen, M. E., 1989, Pharmacokinetics of common analgesics, antiinflammatories and antipyretics in children, *Clinical Pharmacokinetics*, **17 (Suppl. 1)**, 116–137.

Walt, R. P., 1995, Preventing admissions for gastrointestinal bleeding, *Lancet*, **345**, 77–78.

Walter, T., Chau, T. T. and Weichman, B. M., 1989, Effects of analgesics on bradykinin-induced writhing in mice presensitized with PGE_2, *Agents and Actions*, **27**, 375–377.

Walter-Sack, I., Lucknow, V., Guserle, R. and Weber, E., 1989a, Untersuchungen der relativen Bioverfügbarkeit von Paracetamol nach Gabe von festen und flüssigen oralen Zubereitungen sowie rektalen Applikationsformen, *Arzneimittel-Forschung*, **39**, 719–724.

Walter-Sack, I. E., de Vries, J. X., Nickel, B., Stenzhorn, G. and Weber, E., 1989b, The influence of different formula diets and different pharmaceutical formulations on the systemic availability of paracetamol, gall bladder size, and plasma glucose, *International Journal of Clinical Pharmacology, Therapy and Toxicology*, **27**, 544–550.

Walters, V., 1968, The dissolution of paracetamol tablets and the *in vitro* transfer of paracetamol with and without sorbitol, *Journal of Pharmacy and Pharmacology*, **20 (Suppl.)**, 228S–231S.

Waltman, R., Tricomi, V. and Tavakoli, F. M., 1976, Effect of aspirin on bleeding time during elective abortion, *Obstetrics and Gynecology*, **48**, 108–110.

Walton, N. G., Mann, T. A. N. and Shaw, K. M., 1979, Anaphylactoid reaction to N-acetylcysteine, *Lancet*, **ii**, 1298.

Wang, H. and Peng, R.-X., 1993, Effects of paracetamol on glutathione S-transferase activity in mice, *Acta Pharmacologica Sinica*, **14 (Suppl.)**, S41–S44.

Wang, H. and Peng, R.-X., 1994, Sodium ferulate alleviated paracetamol-induced liver toxicity in mice, *Acta Pharmacologica Sinica*, **15**, 81–83.

Wang, J., Naser, N. and Wollenberger, U., 1993, Use of tyrosinase for enzymatic elimination of acetaminophen interference in amperometric sensing, *Analytica Chimica Acta*, **281**, 19–24.

Wang, J.-J., Ho, S.-T., Hu, O. Y.-P. and Chu, K.-M., 1995, An innovative cold tail-flick test: the cold ethanol tail-flick test, *Anesthesia and Analgesia*, **80**, 102–107.

Wang, L. H., Rudolph, A. M. and Benet, L. Z., 1985, Distribution and fate of acetaminophen conjugates in fetal lambs *in utero*, *Journal of Pharmacology and Experimental Therapeutics*, **235**, 302–307.

Wang, L. H., Rudolph, A. M. and Benet, L. Z., 1986a, Pharmacokinetic studies of the disposition of acetaminophen in the sheep maternal-placental-fetal unit, *Journal of Pharmacology and Experimental Therapeutics*, **238**, 198–205.

Wang, L. H., Rudolph, A. M. and Benet, L. Z., 1990, Comparative study of acetaminophen disposition in sheep at three developmental stages: the fetal, neonatal and adult periods, *Developmental Pharmacology and Therapeutics*, **14**, 161–179.

Wang, L. H., Zakim, D., Rudolph, A. M. and Benet, L. Z., 1986b, Developmental alterations in hepatic UDP-glucuronosyltransferase. A comparison of the kinetic properties of enzymes from adult sheep and fetal lambs, *Biochemical Pharmacology*, **35**, 3065–3070.

Wang, Y. and Zhang, X. J., 1994, Cytoprotective effect of epidermal growth factor on acetaminophen-induced acute injury of hepatocytes, *Acta Physiologica Sinica*, **46**, 8–16.

Ward, J. M., Hagiwara, A., Anderson, L. M., Lindsey, K. and Diwan, B. A., 1988, The chronic hepatic and renal toxicity of di(2-ethylhexyl) phthalate, acetaminophen, sodium barbital and phenobarbital in male B6C3F1 mice: autoradiographic, immunohistochemical and biochemical evidence for levels of DNA synthesis not associated with carcinogenesis or tumor promotion, *Toxicology and Applied Pharmacology*, **96**, 494–506.

Ward, J. M., Tsuda, H., Tatematsu, M., Hagiwara, A. and Ito, N., 1989, Hepatotoxicity of agents that enhance formation of focal hepatocellular proliferative lesions (putative pre-neoplastic foci) in a rapid rat liver bioassay, *Fundamental and Applied Toxicology*, **12**, 163–171.

Ward, N., Whitney, C., Avery, D. and Dunner, D., 1991, The analgesic effects of caffeine in headache, *Pain*, **44**, 151–155.

Ward, T. S., Jablonski, H. I. and van Antwerp, J., 1992, Drug use evaluation of acetaminophen-containing products at a community hospital, *Hospital Formulary*, **27**, 947–950.

Wardle, E. N. and Williams, R., 1981, Raised serum biliverdin in hepatic necrosis, *Biochemical Medicine*, **26**, 8–11.

Ware, A. J., Upchurch, K. S., Eigenbrodt, E. H. and Norman, D. A., 1978, Acetaminophen and the liver, *Annals of Internal Medicine*, **88**, 267–268.

Warnet, J.-M., Christen, M.-O., Thevenin, M., Biard, D., Jacqueson, A. and Claude, J.-R., 1989a, Study of glutathione and glutathione-related enzymes in acetaminophen-poisoned mice. Prevention by anethole trithione pretreatment, *Archives of Toxicology*, **Suppl. 13**, 322–325.

Warnet, J.-M., Christen, M. O., Thevenin, M., Biard, D., Jacqueson, A. and Claude, J.-R., 1989b, Protective effect of anethol dithiolthione against acetaminophen hepatotoxicity in mice, *Pharmacology and Toxicology*, **65**, 63–64.

Warrander, A., Allen, J. M. and Andrews, R. S., 1985, Incorporation of radiolabelled amino acids into the sulphur-containing metabolites of paracetamol by the hamster, *Xeno-biotica*, **15**, 891–897.

Warth, H., Astfalk, W. and Walz, G. U., 1994, Schmerztherapie nach Leistenbruch- und Leis-tenhodenoperationen mit Paracetamol im Kindesalter, *Anästhesiologie Intensivmedizin Notfallmedizin Schmerztherapie*, **29**, 90–95.

Watanabe, M., 1982, The cytogenetic effects of aspirin and acetaminophen on *in vitro* human lymphocytes, *Japanese Journal of Hygiene*, **37**, 673–685.

Watanabe, Y., Tsumura, H., Sakurai, H., Haba, T., Ono, S. and Aonuma, H., 1992, Gastric emptying after pancreatoduodenectomy with total stomach preservation and selective proximal vagotomy, *Japanese Journal of Surgery*, **22**, 426–431.

Watari, N., Hanawa, N., Iwai, M. and Kaneniwa, N., 1984, Pharmacokinetic study of the enterohepatic circulation of acetaminophen glucuronide in rats, *Journal of Phar-macobiodynamics*, **7**, 811–819.

Watari, N., Iwai, M. and Kaneniwa, N., 1983, Pharmacokinetic study of the fate of acetamin-ophen and its conjugates in rats, *Journal of Pharmacokinetics and Biopharmaceutics*, **11**, 245–272.

Watcha, M. F., Ramirez-Ruiz, M., White, P. F., Jones, M. B., Lagueruela, R. G. and Ter-konda, R. P., 1992, Perioperative effects of oral ketorolac and acetaminophen in children undergoing bilateral myringotomy, *Canadian Journal of Anaesthesia*, **39**, 649–654.

Watkins, J. B., 1989, Exposure of rats to inhalational anesthetics alters the hepatobiliary clearance of cholephilic xenobiotics, *Journal of Pharmacology and Experimental Thera-peutics*, **250**, 421–427.

Watkins, J. B., Crawford, S. T. and Sanders, R. A., 1994, Chronic voluntary exercise may alter hepatobiliary clearance of endogenous and exogenous chemicals in rats, *Drug Metabo-lism and Disposition: The Biological Fate of Chemicals*, **22**, 537–543.

Watkins, J. B. and Sherman, S. E., 1992, Long-term diabetes alters the hepatobiliary clear-ance of acetaminophen, bilirubin and digoxin, *Journal of Pharmacology and Experimental Therapeutics*, **260**, 1337–1343.

Watkins, J. B., Siegers, C.-P. and Klaassen, C. D., 1984, Effect of diethyl ether on the biliary excretion of acetaminophen, *Proceedings of the Society for Experimental Biology and Medicine*, **177**, 168–175.

Watson, W. A. and McKinney, P. E., 1991, Activated charcoal and acetylcysteine absorption:

issues in interpreting pharmacokinetic data, *Drug Intelligence and Clinical Pharmacy, the Annals of Pharmacotherapy*, **25**, 1081–1084.

Weber, B. and Fontan, J.-E., 1990, Acetaminophen as a pain enhancer during voluntary interruption of pregnancy with mifepristonen and sulprostone, *European Journal of Clinical Pharmacology*, **39**, 609.

Weber, B., Fontan, J. E., Scheller, E., Debu, E., Dufour, B., Majorel, P. and Langlade, A., 1990a, Interruptions volontaires de grossesse induites par l'association mifépristone-sulprostone : essai d'antalgie par le paracétamol ou la dipropyline, *Contraception Fertilité Sexualité*, **18**, 1073–1076.

Weber, J. L. and Cutz, E., 1980, Liver failure in an infant, *Canadian Medical Association Journal*, **123**, 112–117.

Weber, M., Giffard, R., Renaud, D., Bauer, Ph., Bollaert, P. E., Royer-Morot, M. J., Larcan, A. and Lambert, H., 1990b, Intoxications aiguës par paracétamol : intérêt du traitement par N-acétyl-cystéin intraveineuse, *Annales Médicales de Nancy et de l'Est*, **29**, 275–281.

Weber, P. and Dölle, W., 1992, Isolierte Erhöhung der γ-GT, *Deutsche Medizinische Wochenschrift*, **117**, 317–318.

Webster, G. K., 1973, Pancytopenia after administration of Distalgesic, *British Medical Journal*, **3**, 353.

Webster, L. K., Tong, W. P. and McCormack, J. J., 1987, Effect of trimethoprim, paracetamol and cimetidine on trimetrexate metabolism by rat perfused isolated livers, *Journal of Pharmacy and Pharmacology*, **39**, 942–944.

Weeks, B. S., Gamache, P., Klein, N. W., Hinson, J. A., Bruno, M. and Khairallah, E., 1990, Acetaminophen toxicity to cultured rat embryos, *Teratogenesis, Carcinogenesis, and Mutagenesis*, **10**, 361–371.

Weikel, J. H., 1958, A comparison of human serum levels of acetylsalicylic acid, salicylamide, and N-acetyl-p-aminophenol following oral administration, *Journal of the American Pharmaceutical Association*, **47**, 477–479.

Weikel, J. H. and Lish, P. M., 1959, Gastrointestinal pharmacology of antipyretic-analgetic agents. II. Absorption and smooth muscle effects, *Archives Internationales de Pharmacodynamie et de Thérapie*, **119**, 398–408.

Weinberger, L. M., Schmidley, J. W., Schafer, I. A. and Raghavan, S., 1994, Delayed post-anoxic demyelination and arylsulfatase-A pseudodeficiency, *Neurology*, **44**, 152–154.

Weinberger, M., 1978, Analgesic sensitivity in children with asthma, *Pediatrics*, **62 (Suppl.)**, 910–915.

Weisburger, J. H., Weisburger, E. K., Madison, R. M., Wenk, M. L. and Klein, D. S., 1973, Effect of acetanilide and p-hydroxyacetanilide on the carcinogenicity of N-2-fluorenylacetamide and N-hydroxy-N-2-fluorenylacetamine in mice, hamsters, and female rats, *Journal of the National Cancer Institute*, **51**, 235–240.

Weise, M., Prüfer, D., Jaques, G., Keller, M. and Mondorf, A. W., 1981, β_2-Microglobulin and other proteins as parameter for tubular function, *Contributions to Nephrology*, **24**, 88–98.

Weiss, D. J., McClay, C. B., Christopher, M. M., Murphy, M. and Perman, V., 1990, Effects of propylene glycol-containing diets on acetaminophen-induced methemoglobinemia in cats, *Journal of the American Veterinary Medical Association*, **196**, 1816–1819.

Weiss, L. G., Danielson, B. G., Lööf, L., Wikström, B. and Hedstrand, U., 1987, Extrakorporeal blodbehandling vid akut fulminant leversvikt i samband med paracetamolintoxikation, *Läkartidningen*, **84**, 1559–1561.

Weiss, M. and Pang, K. S., 1992, Dynamics of drug distribution. I. Role of the second and third curve moments, *Journal of Pharmacokinetics and Biopharmaceutics*, **20**, 253–278.

Weiss, M. T. and Sawyer, T. W., 1993, Cytotoxicity of the MEIC test chemicals in primary neurone cultures, *Toxicology in Vitro*, **7**, 653–667.

Weisse, M. E., Miller, G. and Brien, J. H., 1987, Fever response to acetaminophen in viral *vs* bacterial infections, *Pediatric Infectious Disease Journal*, **6**, 1091–1094.

Welch, R. M. and Conney, A. H., 1965, A simple method for the quantitative determination of N-acetyl-p-aminophenol (APAP) in urine, *Clinical Chemistry*, **11**, 1064–1067.

Welch, R. M., Conney, A. H. and Burns, J. J., 1966, The metabolism of acetophenetidin and N-acetyl-*p*-aminophenol in the cat, *Biochemical Pharmacology*, **15**, 521–531.

Wells, P. G., 1983, Physiological and environmental determinants of phenytoin teratogenicity: relation to glutathione homeostasis, and potentiation by acetaminophen, *Progress in Clinical and Biological Research*, **135**, 367–371.

Wells, P. G., Boerth, R. C., Oates, J. A. and Harbison, R. D., 1980, Toxicologic enhancement by a combination of drugs which deplete hepatic glutathione: acetaminophen and doxorubicin (adriamycin), *Toxicology and Applied Pharmacology*, **54**, 197–209.

Wells, P. G., Ramji, P. and Ku, M. S. W., 1986, Delayed enhancement of acetaminophen hepatotoxicity by general anesthesia using diethyl ether or halothane, *Fundamental and Applied Toxicology*, **6**, 299–306.

Wells, P. G. and To, E. C. A., 1986a, Effect of diethyl ether on the bioactivation, detoxification, and hepatotoxicity of acetaminophen *in vitro* and *in vivo*, *Advances in Experimental Medicine and Biology*, **197**, 707–715.

Wells, P. G. and To, E. C. A., 1986b, Murine acetaminophen hepatotoxicity: temporal interanimal variability in plasma glutamic-pyruvic transaminase profiles and relation to *in vivo* chemical covalent binding, *Fundamental and Applied Toxicology*, **7**, 17–25.

Wells, P. S., Holbrook, A. M., Crowther, N. R. and Hirsh, J., 1994, Interactions of warfarin with drugs and food, *Annals of Internal Medicine*, **121**, 676–683.

Welty, S. E., Smith, C. V., Benzick, A. E., Montgomery, C. A. and Hansen, T. N., 1993, Investigation of possible mechanisms of hepatic swelling and necrosis caused by acetaminophen in mice, *Biochemical Pharmacology*, **45**, 449–458.

Wendel, A., 1983, Hepatic lipid peroxidation: caused by acute drug intoxication, prevented by liposomal glutathione, *International Journal of Clinical Pharmacology Research*, **3**, 443–447.

Wendel, A. and Cikryt, P., 1981, Binding of paracetamol metabolites to mouse liver glutathione S-transferases, *Research Communications in Chemical Pathology and Pharmacology*, **33**, 463–473.

Wendel, A. and Feuerstein, S., 1981, Drug-induced lipid peroxidation in mice – 1. Modulation by monooxygenase activity, glutathione and selenium status, *Biochemical Pharmacology*, **30**, 2513–2520.

Wendel, A., Feuerstein, S. and Konz, K.-H., 1979, Acute paracetamol intoxication of starved mice leads to lipid peroxidation *in vivo*, *Biochemical Pharmacology*, **28**, 2051–2055.

Wendel, A. and Hallbach, J., 1986, Quantitative assessment of the binding of acetaminophen metabolites to mouse liver microsomal phospholipid, *Biochemical Pharmacology*, **35**, 385–389.

Wendel, A. and Heidinger, S., 1980, In-vivo inhibition by copper and some Cu-complexes of paracetamol-induced lipid peroxidation in benzpyrene-pretreated mice, *Research Communications in Chemical Pathology and Pharmacology*, **28**, 473–482.

Wendel, A., Jaeschke, H. and Gloger, M., 1982, Drug-induced lipid peroxidation in mice – II. Protection against paracetamol-induced liver necrosis by intravenous liposomally entrapped glutathione, *Biochemical Pharmacology*, **31**, 3601–3605.

Wendon, J., Smithies, M., Sheppard, M., Bullen, K., Tinker, J. and Bihari, D., 1989, Continuous high volume venous-venous haemofiltration in acute renal failure, *Intensive Care Medicine*, **15**, 358–363.

Wendon, J. A., Harrison, P. M., Keays, R. and Williams, R., 1994, Cerebral blood flow and metabolism in fulminant liver failure, *Hepatology*, **19**, 1407–1413.

Werler, M. M., Mitchell, A. A. and Shapiro, S., 1992, First trimester maternal medication use in relation to gastroschisis, *Teratology*, **45**, 361–367.

Werner, C. and Wendel, A., 1990, Hepatic uptake and antihepatotoxic properties of vitamin E and liposomes in the mouse, *Chemico-Biological Interactions*, **75**, 83–92.

Wessels, J. C., Koeleman, H. A., Boneschans, B. and Steyn, H. S., 1992, The influence of different types of breakfast on the absorption of paracetamol among members of an ethnic group, *International Journal of Clinical Pharmacology, Therapy and Toxicology*, **30**, 208–213.

Wessling, A., 1987, Over-the-counter sales of drugs in Sweden 1976–1983, *European Journal of Clinical Pharmacology*, **33**, 1–6.

West, J. C., 1981, Rapid HPLC analysis of paracetamol (acetaminophen) in blood and post-mortem viscera, *Journal of Analytical Toxicology*, **5**, 118–121.

West, P. R., Harman, L. S., Josephy, P. D. and Mason, R. P., 1984, Acetaminophen: enzymatic formation of a transient phenoxyl free radical, *Biochemical Pharmacology*, **33**, 2933–2936.

Weston, M. J., Talbot, I. C., Howorth, P. J. N., Mant, A. K., Capildeo, R. and Williams, R., 1976, Frequency of arrhythmias and other cardiac abnormalities in fulminant hepatic failure, *British Heart Journal*, **38**, 1179–1188.

Weston, M. J. and Williams, R., 1976, Paracetamol and the heart, *Lancet*, **i**, 536.

Whelpton, R., Fernandes, K., Wilkinson, K. A. and Goldhill, D. R., 1993, Determination of paracetamol (acetaminophen) in blood and plasma using high performance liquid chromatography with dual electrode coulometric quantification in the redox mode, *Biomedical Chromatography*, **7**, 90–93.

Whitcomb, D. C. and Block, G. D., 1994, Association of acetaminophen hepatotoxicity with fasting and ethanol use, *Journal of the American Medical Association*, **272**, 1845–1850.

White, A. C. and Gershbein, L. L., 1985, Liver regeneration and hepatic microsomal enzyme induction by acetaminophen and derivatives, *Research Communications in Chemical Pathology and Pharmacology*, **48**, 275–289.

White, P. and Strunin, L., 1982, Post-anaesthetic dental extraction analgesia: a comparison of paracetamol, codeine, caffeine (Solpadeine) and diflunisal (Dolobid), *British Journal of Oral Surgery*, **20**, 275–280.

Whitehead, E. M., Smith, M., Dean, Y. and O'Sullivan, G., 1993, An evaluation of gastric emptying times in pregnancy and the puerperium, *Anaesthesia*, **48**, 53–57.

Whitehouse, L. W., Aubin, R. A., Swierenga, S. H. H., Mueller, R. W., Pakuts, A. P. and Lee, F., 1990, Differential susceptibility in inbred male Swiss Webster mice towards hepatotoxins which deplete glutathione, *European Journal of Pharmacology*, **183**, 1514.

Whitehouse, L. W., Paul, C. J. and Thomas, B. H., 1975, Effect of aspirin on the fate of ^{14}C-acetaminophen in guinea pigs, *Journal of Pharmaceutical Sciences*, **64**, 819–821.

Whitehouse, L. W., Paul, C. J. and Thomas, B. H., 1976, Effect of acetylsalicylic acid on a toxic dose of acetaminophen in the mouse, *Toxicology and Applied Pharmacology*, **38**, 571–582.

Whitehouse, L. W., Paul, C. J., Wong, L. T. and Thomas, B. H., 1977, Effect of aspirin on a subtoxic dose of ^{14}C-acetaminophen in mice, *Journal of Pharmaceutical Sciences*, **66**, 1399–1403.

Whitehouse, L. W., Wong, L. T., Paul, C. J., Pakuts, A. P. and Solomonraj, G., 1985, Post-absorption antidotal effects of N-acetylcysteine on acetaminophen-induced hepatotoxicity in the mouse, *Canadian Journal of Physiology and Pharmacology*, **63**, 431–437.

Whitehouse, L. W., Wong, L. T., Solomonraj, G., Paul, C. J. and Thomas, B. H., 1981, N-Acetylcysteine-induced inhibition of gastric emptying: a mechanism affording protection to mice from the hepatotoxicity of concomitantly administered acetaminophen, *Toxicology*, **19**, 113–125.

Whittington, R. M., 1977, Dextropropoxyphene (Distalgesic) overdosage in the West Midlands, *British Medical Journal*, **2**, 172–173.

Whittington, R. M. and Barclay, A. D., 1981, The epidemiology of dextropropoxyphene (Distalgesic) overdose fatalities in Birmingham and the West Midlands, *Journal of Clinical and Hospital Pharmacy*, **6**, 251–257.

Widdop, B., Medd, R. K., Braithwaite, R. A., Rees, A. J. and Goulding, R., 1975, Experimental drug intoxication: treatment with charcoal haemoperfusion, *Archives of Toxicology*, **34**, 27–36.

Wiegand, U. W., Chou, R. C., Maulik, D. and Levy, G., 1984, Assessment of biotransformation during transfer of propoxyhene and acetaminophen across the isolated perfused human placenta, *Pediatric Pharmacology*, **4**, 145–153.

Wiener, K., 1977, Paracetamol estimation: comparison of a quick colorimetric method with a standard spectrophotometric method, *Annals of Clinical Biochemistry*, **14**, 55–58.

Wiener, K., 1978, A review of methods for plasma paracetamol estimation, *Annals of Clinical Biochemistry*, **15**, 187–196.

Wiener, K., 1980, Experiences with a regional quality control scheme for salicylate and paracetamol over a period of two years, *Annals of Clinical Biochemistry*, **17**, 82–86.

Wiener, K., Longlands, M. G. and Tan, B. H. A., 1976, Interference by oxyphenbutazone in paracetamol estimation, *Annals of Clinical Biochemistry*, **13**, 452–453.

Wiens, S., Otten, J.-E. and Joos, U., 1990, Postoperativer analgetikaverbrauch, *Deutsche Zahnärztliche Zeitschrift*, **45**, 40–42.

Wilairatana, P. and Looareesuwan, S., 1994, Antipyretic efficacy of indomethacin and acetaminophen in uncomplicated falciparum malaria, *Annals of Tropical Medicine and Parasitology*, **88**, 359–363.

Wilairatana, P., Looareesuwan, S., Kaojarern, S., Vanijanonta, S. and Charoenlarp, P., 1995, Gastric emptying in acute uncomplicated falciparum malaria, *Journal of Tropical Medicine and Hygiene*, **98**, 22–24.

Wilkinson, G. S., 1976, Rapid determination of plasma paracetamol, *Annals of Clinical Biochemistry*, **13**, 435–437.

Wilkinson, K. A., Whelpton, R., Winyard, J. A. and Goldhill, D. R., 1994, Gastric emptying is delayed in patients the day after cardiac surgery, *Journal of Cardiothoracic and Vascular Anaesthesia*, **3 (Suppl. 2)**, 10.

Wilkinson, M. F. and Kasting, N. W., 1990, Central vasopressin V_1-blockade prevents salicylate but not acetaminophen antipyresis, *Journal of Applied Physiology*, **68**, 1793–1798.

Wilkinson, M. F. and Kasting, N. W., 1993, Vasopressin release within the ventral septal area of the rat brain during drug-induced antipyresis, *American Journal of Physiology*, **264**, R1133–R1138.

Wilkinson, R., James, O. F. W., Roberts, S. H., Morley, A. R. and Robson, V., 1979, Plasma renin activity during the development of paracetamol (acetaminophen) induced acute renal failure in man, *Clinical Nephrology*, **11**, 196–201.

Wilkinson, S. P., Moodie, H., Arroyo, V. A. and Williams, R., 1977, Frequency of renal impairment in paracetamol overdose compared with other causes of acute liver damage, *Journal of Clinical Pathology*, **30**, 141–143.

Will, E. J. and Tomkins, A. M., 1971, Acute myocardial necrosis in paracetamol poisoning, *British Medical Journal*, **4**, 430–431.

Willcox, D. G. A., 1985, Self poisoning: a review of patients seen in the Victoria Infirmary, Glasgow, *Scottish Medical Journal*, **30**, 220–224.

Willems, H. J. J., van der Horst, A., De Goede, P. N. F. C. and Haakmeester, G. J., 1985, Determination of some anticonvulsants, antiarrhythmics, benzodiazepines, xanthines, paracetamol and chloramphenicol by reversed phase HPLC, *Pharmaceutisch Weekblad Scientific Edition*, **7**, 150–157.

Williams, D. B., Varia, S. A., Stella, V. J. and Pitman, I. H., 1983, Evaluation of the prodrug potential of the sulfate esters of acetaminophen and 3-hydroxymethyl-phenytoin, *International Journal of Pharmaceutics*, **14**, 113–120.

Williams, F. M., Moore, U., Seymour, R. A., Mutch, E. M., Nicholson, E., Wright, P., Wynne, H., Blain, P. G. and Rawlins, M. D., 1989a, Benorylate hydrolysis by human plasma and human liver, *British Journal of Clinical Pharmacology*, **28**, 703–708.

Williams, G. M., Mori, H. and McQueen, C. A., 1989b, Structure-activity relationships in the rat hepatocyte DNA-repair test for 300 chemicals, *Mutation Research*, **221**, 263–286.

Williams, H. J., Ward, J. R., Egger, M. J., Neuner, R., Brooks, R. H., Clegg, D. O., Field, E. H., Skosey, J. L., Alarcón, G. S., Willkens, R. F., Paulus, H. E., Russell, I. J. and Sharp, J. T., 1993, Comparison of naproxen and acetaminophen in a two-year study of treatment of osteoarthritis of the knee, *Arthritis and Rheumatism*, **36**, 1196–1206.

Williams, R., 1988, Management of acute liver failure, *Postgraduate Medical Journal*, **64**, 769–771.

Williams, R., 1994, New directions in acute liver failure, *Journal of the Royal College of Physicians*, **28**, 552–559.

Williams, R. and Davis, M., 1977, Clinical and experimental aspects of paracetamol hepatotoxicity, *Acta Pharmacologica et Toxicologica*, **41 (Suppl. 2)**, 282–298.

Williams, W. R., Pawlowicz, A. and Davies, B. H., 1991, Aspirin-sensitive asthma: significance of the cyclooxygenase-inhibiting and protein-binding properties of analgesic drugs, *International Archives of Allergy and Applied Immunology*, **95**, 303–308.

Williamson, J., Davidson, D. F. and Boag, D. E., 1989, Contamination of a specimen with N-acetyl cysteine infusion: a cause for spurious ketonaemia and hyperglycaemia, *Annals of Clinical Biochemistry*, **26**, 207.

Williamson, J. M., Boettcher, B. and Meister, A., 1982, Intracellular cysteine delivery system that protects against toxicity by promoting glutathione synthesis, *Proceedings of the National Academy of Sciences of the United States of America*, **79**, 6246–6249.

Willson, R. A. and Hart, F. E., 1977, Experimental hepatic injury: the sequential changes in drug metabolizing enzyme activities after administration of acetaminophen, *Research Communications in Chemical Pathology and Pharmacology*, **16**, 59–71.

Willson, R. A., Hart, J. and Hall, T., 1991, The concentration and temporal relationships of acetaminophen-induced changes in intracellular and extracellular total glutathione in freshly isolated hepatocytes from untreated and 3-methylcholanthrene pretreated Sprague-Dawley and Fischer rats, *Pharmacology and Toxicology*, **69**, 205–212.

Willson, R. A., Winch, J., Thompson, R. P. H. and Williams, R., 1973, Rapid removal of paracetamol by haemoperfusion through coated charcoal: in-vivo and in-vitro studies in the pig, *Lancet*, **i**, 77–79.

Wilmer, J. L., Kligerman, A. D. and Erexson, G. L., 1981, Sister chromatid exchange induction and cell cycle inhibition by aniline and its metabolites in human fibroblasts, *Environmental and Molecular Mutagenesis*, **3**, 627–638.

Wilson, D. R. and Gault, M. H., 1982, Declining incidence of analgesic nephropathy in Canada, *Canadian Medical Association Journal*, **127**, 500–502.

Wilson, G., Guerra, A. J. and Santos, N. T., 1984, Comparative study of the antipyretic effect of ibuprofen (oral suspension) and paracetamol (suppositories) in paediatrics, *Journal of International Medical Research*, **12**, 250–254.

Wilson, H. T. H., 1975, A fixed drug eruption due to paracetamol, *British Journal of Dermatology*, **92**, 213–214.

Wilson, J. M., Slattery, J. T., Forte, A. J. and Nelson, S. D., 1982a, Analysis of acetaminophen metabolites in urine by high performance liquid chromatography with UV and amperometric detection, *Journal of Chromatography: Biomedical Applications*, **227**, 453–462.

Wilson, J. T., 1979, Concomitant microanalysis of salicylic acid and acetaminophen in plasma of febrile children, *Therapeutic Drug Monitoring*, **1**, 459–473.

Wilson, J. T., Brown, A. D., Bocchini, J. A. and Kearns, G. L., 1982b, Efficacy, disposition and pharmacodynamics of aspirin, acetaminophen and choline salicylate in young febrile children, *Therapeutic Drug Monitoring*, **4**, 417–180.

Wilson, J. T., Brown, R. D., Kearns, G. L., Eichler, V. F., Johnson, V. A., Bertrand, K. M. and Lowe, B. A., 1991, Single-dose, placebo-controlled comparative study of ibuprofen and acetaminophen antipyresis in children, *Journal of Pediatrics*, **119**, 803–811.

Wilson, J. T., Don Brown, R., Kearns, G. L., Eichler, V. F., Jones, E. D., Cedotal, C. J. and Gupta, N., 1990, Comparative efficacy of ibuprofen (ibu) and acetaminophen (apap) in febrile children, *European Journal of Pharmacology*, **183**, 2277–2278.

Wilson, J. T., Hinson, J. L., Johnson, V. A., Woods, T. W., Smith, I. J. and Brown, R. D., 1987, Pharmacologic factors contributing to variance in the milk to plasma ratio for acetaminophen in the goat, *Developmental Pharmacology and Therapeutics*, **10**, 60–72.

Wilson, J. T., Kasantikul, V., Harbison, R. and Martin, D., 1978, Death in an adolescent following an overdose of acetaminophen and phenobarbital, *American Journal of Diseases of Children*, **132**, 466–473.

Wilson, K., 1984, Sex-related differences in drug disposition in man, *Clinical Pharmacokinetics*, **9**, 189–202.

Wilson, S. P., Kamin, D. L. and Feldman, J. M., 1985, Acetaminophen administration interferes with urinary metanephrine (and catecholamine) determinations, *Clinical Chemistry*, **31**, 1093–1094.

Winchester, J. F., Edwards, R. O., Tilstone, W. J. and Woodcock, B. G., 1975, Activated charcoal hemoperfusion and experimental acetaminophen poisoning, *Toxicology and Applied Pharmacology*, **31**, 120–127.

Winchester, J. F., Gelfand, M. C., Helliwell, M., Vale, J. A., Goulding, R. and Schreiner, G. E., 1981, Extracorporeal treatment of salicylate or acetaminophen poisoning – is there a role? *Archives of Internal Medicine*, **141**, 370–374.

Winchester, J. F., Tilstone, W. J., Edwards, R. O., Gilchrist, T. and Kennedy, A. C., 1974, Hemoperfusion for enhanced drug elimination – a kinetic analysis in paracetamol poisoning, *Transactions of the American Society for Artificial Internal Organs*, **20**, 358–363.

Windorfer, A., 1978, Untersuchungen über Temperaturverlauf und Serumkonzentrationen von Paracetamol bei fiebernden Säuglingen nach Medikation mit Paracetamol-Suppositorien, *Pädiatrie und Pädologie*, **13**, 61–65.

Windorfer, A. and Röttger, H. J., 1974, Mikromethode zur quantitativen Bestimmung von Sedativa und Antipyretika (Aminophenazon, Diphenylhydantoin, Paracetamol, Phenobarbital, Primidone) mit der Thermo-gas-Chromatographie, *Arzneimittel-Forschung*, **24**, 893–895.

Windorfer, A. and Vogel, C., 1976, Untersuchungen über Serumkonzentrationen und Temperaturverlauf nach einer neuen oral applizierbaren flüssigen Paracetamolzubereitung, *Klinische Pädiatrie*, **188**, 430–434.

Wing, A. J., Brunner, F. P., Geerlings, W., Broyer, M., Brynger, H., Fassbinder, W., Rissoni, G., Selwood, N. H. and Tufveson, G., 1989, Contribution of toxic neuropathies to end-stage renal failure in Europe: a report from the EDTA-ERA registry, *Toxicology Letters*, **46**, 281–292.

Winick, C., 1989, A comparison of the relative safety of phenylpropanolamine, acetaminophen, ibuprofen and aspirin as measured by three compendia, *International Journal of Clinical Pharmacology, Therapy and Toxicology*, **27**, 267–272.

Winkler, E. and Halkin, H., 1992, Paracetamol overdose in Israel – 1992, *Israel Journal of Medical Sciences*, **28**, 811–812.

Winkler, E. and Halkin, H., 1993, Paracetamol overdosage in Jerusalem 1984–89, *Israel Journal of Medical Sciences*, **29**, 118.

Winnem, B., Samstad, B. and Breivik, H., 1981, Paracetamol, tiaramide and placebo for pain relief after orthopedic surgery, *Acta Anaesthesiologica Scandinavica*, **25**, 209–214.

Winter, L., Appleby, F., Ciccone, P. E. and Pigeon, J. G., 1983a, A double-blind, comparative evaluation of acetaminophen, caffeine, and the combination of acetaminophen and caffeine in outpatients with post-operative oral surgery pain, *Current Therapeutic Research*, **33**, 115–122.

Winter, L., Appleby, F., Ciccone, P. E. and Pigeon, J. G., 1983b, A comparative study of an acetaminophen analgesic combination and aspirin in the treatment of post-operative oral surgery pain, *Current Therapeutic Research*, **33**, 200–206.

Wirth, P. J., Dybing, E., von Bahr, C. and Thorgeirsson, S. S., 1980, Mechanism of N-hydroxyacetylarylamine mutagenicity in the *Salmonella* test system: metabolic activation of N-hydroxy phenacetin by liver and kidney fractions from rat, mouse, hamster, and man, *Molecular Pharmacology*, **18**, 117–127.

Witjes, W. P. J., Crul, B. J. P., Vollaard, E. J., Joosten, H. J. M. and Egmond, J. V., 1992, Application of sublingual buprenorphine in combination with naproxen or paracetamol for post-operative pain relief in cholecystectomy patients in a double-blind study, *Acta Anaesthesiologica Scandinavica*, **36**, 323–327.

Witschi, A., Reddy, S., Stofer, B. and Lauterburg, B. H., 1992, The systemic availability of oral glutathione, *European Journal of Clinical Pharmacology*, **43**, 667–669.

Witter, F. R., Woods, A. S., Griffin, M. D., Smith, C. R., Nadler, P. and Lietman, P. S., 1988, Effects of prednisone, aspirin and acetaminophen on an *in vivo* biologic response to interferon in humans, *Clinical Pharmacology and Therapeutics*, **44**, 239–243.

Wójcicki, J., Baskiewicz, Z., Gawronska-Szklarz, B., Kazmierczyk, J. and Kalucki, K., 1978, The effect of a single dose of ethanol on the pharmacokinetics of paracetamol, *Polish Journal of Pharmacology and Pharmacy*, **30**, 749–753.

Wójcicki, J. and Gawronska-Szklarz, B., 1984, Pharmacokinetics of paracetamol in patients with gastric and duodenal ulcers, *Polish Journal of Pharmacology and Pharmacy*, **36**, 59–63.

Wójcicki, J., Gawronska-Szklarz, B., Baskiewicz, Z. and Kalucki, K., 1980, Farmakokinetyka paracetamolu po doustnym podaniu pojedynczej dawki w postaci tabletek i syropu, *Acta Poloniae Pharmaceutica*, **37**, 351–354.

Wójcicki, J., Gawronska-Szklarz, B. and Kazmierczyk, J., 1977a, Wplyw atropiny na wchlanianie paracetamolu z przewodu pokarmowego ludzi zdrowych, *Polski Tygodnik Lekarski*, **32**, 1111–1113.

Wójcicki, J., Gawronska-Szklarz, B., Kazmierczyk, J., Baskiewicz, Z. and Raczynski, A., 1979a, Comparative pharmacokinetics of paracetamol in men and women considering follicular and luteal phases, *Arzneimittel-Forschung*, **29**, 350–352.

Wójcicki, J., Kazmierczyk, J. and Gawronska-Szklarz, B., 1979b, Effects of drugs altering pH and gastrointestinal tract motility on paracetamol pharmacokinetics, *Zentralblatt für Pharmazie Pharmakotherapie und Laboratoriumsdiagnostik*, **118**, 285–291.

Wójcicki, J., Kazmierczyk, J., Gawronska-Szklarz, B. and Samochowiec, L., 1979c, Effect of papaverine and atropine on pharmacokinetics of paracetamol administered orally, *Polish Journal of Pharmacology and Pharmacy*, **31**, 239–243.

Wójcicki, J., Ostrowski, M. and Gawronska-Szklarz, B., 1984, The effect of gastrectomy on pharmacokinetics of orally administered paracetamol in man, *Polish Journal of Pharmacology and Pharmacy*, **36**, 323–327.

Wójcicki, J., Rainska-Giezek, T., Gawronska-Szklarz, B. and Dutkiewicz-Serdynska, G., 1994, Effects of caffeine on the pharmacokinetics of paracetamol, *Acta Medica et Biologica*, **42**, 51–55.

Wójcicki, J., Samochowiec, L., Lawczynski, L., Sewed, G. and Olszewska, M., 1977b, A double-blind comparative evaluation of aspirin, paracetamol and paracetamol plus caffeine (Finimal) for their analgesic effectiveness, *Archivum Immunologiae et Therapiae Experimentalis*, **25**, 175–179.

Wolfe, L. S., Pappius, H. M. and Marion, J., 1976, The biosynthesis of prostaglandins by brain tissue *in vitro*, *Advances in Prostaglandin and Thromboxane Research*, **1**, 345–355.

Wollenberg, P. and Rummel, W., 1984, Vectorial release of sulfoconjugates in the vascularly perfused mouse small intestine, *Biochemical Pharmacology*, **33**, 205–208.

Wong, A. S., 1983, An evaluation of HPLC for the screening and quantitation of benzodiazepines and acetaminophen in post mortem blood, *Journal of Analytical Toxicology*, **7**, 33–36.

Wong, B. K. and Corcoran, G. B., 1987, Effects of esterase inhibitors and buthionine sulphoximine on the prevention of acetaminophen hepatotoxicity by N-acetylcysteine, *Communications in Pathology and Pharmacology*, **55**, 397–408.

Wong, B. K., Galinsky, R. E. and Corcoran, G. B., 1986a, Dissociation of increased sulfation from sulfate replenishment and hepatoprotection in acetaminophen-poisoned mice by

N-acetylcysteine steroisomers, *Journal of Pharmaceutical Sciences*, **75**, 878–880.

Wong, B. K., U, S.-W. E. and Corcoran, G. B., 1986b, An overfed rat model that reproduces acetaminophen disposition in obese humans, *Drug Metabolism and Disposition: The Biological Fate of Chemicals*, **14**, 674–679.

Wong, C.-L. and Wai, M.-K., 1981, Effects of aspirin and paracetamol on naloxone reversal of morphine-induced inhibition of gastrointestinal propulsion in mice, *European Journal of Pharmacology*, **73**, 11–19.

Wong, C.-L., Wai, M.-K. and Roberts, M. B., 1980a, The effect of aspirin and paracetamol on the increased naloxone potency induced by morphine pretreatment, *European Journal of Pharmacology*, **67**, 241–246.

Wong, H. Y., Carpenter, R. L., Kopacz, D. J., Fragen, R. J., Thompson, G., Maneatis, T. J. and Bynum, L. J., 1993a, A randomized, double-blind evaluation of ketorolac tromethamine for postoperative analgesia in ambulatory surgery patients, *Anesthesiology*, **78**, 6–14.

Wong, L. T., Solomonraj, G. and Thomas, B. H., 1976a, High-pressure liquid chromatographic determination of acetaminophen in biological fluids, *Journal of Pharmaceutical Sciences*, **65**, 1064–1066.

Wong, L. T., Solomonraj, G. and Thomas, B. H., 1976b, Metabolism of [^{14}C]paracetamol and its interactions with aspirin in hamsters, *Xenobiotica*, **6**, 575–584.

Wong, L. T., Whitehouse, L. W., Solomonraj, G. and Paul, C. J., 1980b, Effect of a concomitant single dose of ethanol on the hepatotoxicity and metabolism of acetaminophen in mice, *Toxicology*, **17**, 297–309.

Wong, L. T., Whitehouse, L. W., Solomonraj, G. and Paul, C. J., 1981, Pathways of disposition of acetaminophen in the mouse, *Toxicology Letters*, **9**, 145–151.

Wong, L. T., Whitehouse, L. W., Solomonraj, G., Paul, C. J. and Thomas, B. H., 1979, Separation and quantitation of acetaminophen and its metabolites in the bile of mice, *Journal of Analytical Toxicology*, **3**, 260–263.

Wong, S. and Gardocki, J. F., 1983, Anti-inflammatory and antiarthritic evaluation of acetaminophen and its potentiation of tolmetin, *Journal of Pharmacology and Experimental Therapeutics*, **226**, 625–632.

Wong, V., Daly, M., Boon, A. and Heatley, V., 1993b, Paracetamol and acute biliary pain with cholestasis, *Lancet*, **342**, 869.

Wood, H. C., 1931, The indispensable uses of narcotics: the therapeutic uses of narcotic drugs, *Journal of the American Medical Association*, **96**, 1140–1144.

Woodhouse, K. and Herd, B., 1993, The effect of age and gender on glucuronidation and sulphation in rat liver: a study using paracetamol as a model substrate, *Archives of Gerontology and Geriatrics*, **16**, 111–115.

Woodward, D. F. and Owen, D. A. A., 1979, Quantitative measurement of the vascular changes produced by UV radiation and carrageenin using the guinea-pig ear as the site of inflammation, *Journal of Pharmacological Methods*, **2**, 35–42.

Woolf, A. D. and Gren, J. M., 1990, Acute poisonings among adolescents and young adults with anorexia nervosa, *American Journal of Diseases of Children*, **144**, 785–788.

Woolf, A. D. and Lovejoy, F. H., 1993, Epidemiology of drug overdose in children, *Drug Safety*, **9**, 291–308.

Woollard, A. C. S., Wolff, S. P. and Bascal, Z. A., 1990, Antioxidant characteristics of some potential anticataract agents: studies of aspirin, paracetamol, and bendazac provide support for an oxidative component of cataract, *Free Radical Biology and Medicine*, **9**, 299–305.

Wootton, F. T. and Lee, W. M., 1990, Acetaminophen hepatotoxicity in the alcoholic, *Southern Medical Journal*, **83**, 1047–1049.

Wormser, U. and Ben-Zakine, S., 1990, The liver slice system: an *in vitro* acute toxicity test for assessment of hepatotoxins and their antidotes, *Toxicology in Vitro*, **4**, 449–451.

Wormser, U. and Calp, D., 1988, Increased levels of hepatic metallothionein in rat and mouse after injection of acetaminophen, *Toxicology*, **53**, 323–329.

Wormser, U., Zakine, S. B., Stivelband, E. and Eizen, O., 1990, The liver slice system: a rapid *in vitro* acute toxicity test for primary screeening of hepatotoxic agents, *Toxicology in Vitro*, **4**, 783–789.

Wortmann, D. W., Kelsch, R. C., Kuhns, L., Sullivan, D. B. and Cassidy, J. T., 1980, Renal papillary necrosis in juvenile rheumatoid arthritis, *Journal of Pediatrics*, **97**, 37–40.

Wright, C. E., Antal, E. J., Gillespie, W. R. and Albert, K. S., 1983, Ibuprofen and acetaminophen kinetics when taken concurrently, *Clinical Pharmacology and Therapeutics*, **34**, 707–710.

Wright, C. J., 1977, Analgesia following oral surgery for day patients: a clincial comparison of two analgesics, *Current Medical Research and Opinion*, **5**, 204–209.

Wright, L. A. and Foster, M. G., 1980, Effect of some commonly prescribed drugs on certain chemistry tests, *Clinical Biochemistry*, **13**, 249–252.

Wright, N. and Prescott, L. F., 1973, Potentiation by previous drug therapy of hepatotoxicity following paracetamol overdosage, *Scottish Medical Journal*, **18**, 56–58.

Wright, P. B. and Moore, L., 1991, Potentiation of the toxicity of model hepatotoxicants by acetaminophen, *Toxicology and Applied Pharmacology*, **109**, 327–335.

Wright, P. M. C., Allen, R. W., Moore, J. and Donnelly, J. P., 1992, Gastric emptying during lumbar extradural analgesia in labour: effect of fentanyl supplementation, *British Journal of Anaesthesia*, **68**, 248–251.

Wright, R. C. and Benson, R. E., 1975, Paracetamol antidote, *Anaesthesia and Intensive Care*, **3**, 163–164.

Wu, G. Y., Wu, C. H. and Rubin, M. I., 1985, Acetaminophen hepatotoxicity and targeted rescue: a model for specific chemotherapy of hepatocellular carcinoma, *Hepatology*, **5**, 709–713.

Wylie, A. S. and Fraser, A. A., 1994, Hazards of codeine plus paracetamol compounds, *British Journal of General Practice*, **44**, 376.

Wynne, H., Bateman, D. N., Hassanyeh, F., Rawlins, M. D. and Woodhouse, K. W., 1987, Age and self-poisoning: the epidemiology in Newcastle upon Tyne in the 1980s, *Human Toxicology*, **6**, 511–515.

Wynne, H. A., Cope, L. H., Herd, B., Rawlins, M. D., James, O. F. W. and Woodhouse, K. W., 1990, The association of age and frailty with paracetamol conjugation in man, *Age and Ageing*, **19**, 419–424.

Xiaodong, S., Gatti, G., Bartoli, A., Cipolla, G., Crema, F. and Perucca, E., 1994, Omeprazole does not enhance the metabolism of phenacetin, a marker of CYP1A2 activity, in healthy volunteers, *Therapeutic Drug Monitoring*, **16**, 248–250.

Xu, N., Chow, A., Goresky, C. A. and Pang, K. S., 1990, Effects of retrograde flow on measured blood volume, Disse space, intracellular water space and drug extraction in the perfused rat liver: characterization by the multiple indicator dilution technique, *Journal of Pharmacology and Experimental Therapeutics*, **254**, 914–925.

Yaksh, T. L. and Malmberg, A. B., 1993, Spinal actions of NSAIDs in blocking spinally mediated hyperalgesia: the role of cyclooxygenase products, *Agents and Actions*, **41**, 89–100.

Yamada, H., Toda, G., Yoshiba, M., Hashimoto, N., Ikeda, Y., Mitsui, H., Kurokawa, K., Sugata, F., Hughes, R. D. and Williams, R., 1994, Humoral inhibitor of rat hepatocyte DNA synthesis from patients with fulminant liver failure, *Hepatology*, **19**, 1133–1140.

Yamada, S., Murawaki, Y. and Kawasaki, H., 1993, Preventive effect of gomisin A, a lignan component of shizandra fruits, on acetaminophen-induced hepatotoxicity in rats, *Biochemical Pharmacology*, **46**, 1081–1085.

Yamada, T., 1983, Covalent binding theory for acetaminophen hepatotoxicity, *Gastroenterology*, **85**, 202–203.

Yamada, T., Ludwig, S., Kuhlenkamp, J. and Kaplowitz, N., 1981, Direct protection against acetaminophen hepatotoxicity by propylthiouracil, *Journal of Clinical Investigation*, **67**,

688–695.

Yamakawa, M., 1992, Two cases of severe liver injuries induced by acetaminophen, *Journal of Japanese Society of Internal Medicine*, **81**, 2015–2017.

Yamaki, K., Manabe, T., Yamamoto, M., Tobe, T., Kobayashi, Y., Mitani, T. and Kurono, M., 1992, Measurement of small bowel transit time in dogs with acetaminophen and indocyanine green, *Japanese Journal of Gastroenterology*, **89**, 36–41.

Yamamoto, H., 1990, Antagonism of acetaminophen-induced hepatocellular destruction by trifluoperazine in mice, *Pharmacology and Toxicology*, **67**, 115–119.

Yamamoto, R. S., Williams, G. M., Richardson, H. L., Weisburger, E. K. and Weisburger, J. H., 1973, Effect of p-hydroxyacetanilide on liver cancer induction by N-hydroxy-N-2-fluorenylacetamide, *Cancer Research*, **33**, 454–457.

Yang, S.-S., Hughes, R. D. and Williams, R., 1988, Digoxin-like immunoreactive substances in severe acute liver disease due to viral hepatitis and paracetamol overdose, *Hepatology*, **8**, 93–97.

Yasunaga, M., Matsuda, S., Murata, M., Ogino, M., Kado, Y., Shinkai, Y., Nawata, H., Handa, T., Noda, K., Fukumoto, Y., Okita, K. and Takemoto, T., 1985, Two cases of acute liver injury caused by ingesting small dose of acetoaminophen, *Acta Hepatologica Japonica*, **26**, 493–499.

Yeung, J. H. K., 1988, Effect of sulphydryl drugs on paracetamol-induced hepatotoxicity in mice, *Drug Metabolism and Drug Interactions*, **6**, 295–301.

Yeung, J. H. K., Chiu, L. C. M. and Ooi, V. E. C., 1994, Effect of polysaccharide peptide (PSP) on glutathione and protection against paracetamol-induced hepatotoxicity in the rat, *Methods and Findings in Experimental and Clinical Pharmacology*, **16**, 723–729.

Yiamouyiannis, C. A., Harris, A., Saunders, R. A., Martin, B. J. and Watkins, J. B., 1994, Paracetamol pharmacokinetics are independent of caloric intake and physical activity, *Drug Investigation*, **8**, 361–368.

Ying, Y. and Lou, Y.-J., 1993, Effects of preimplantation treatment with aspirin and acetaminophen on blastocyst and fetus in rats, *Acta Pharmacologica Sinica*, **14**, 369–372.

Yoshida, T., Taniguchi, H. and Nakano, S., 1980, Fluorometric analysis with 3-amino-2(1H)-quinolinethione. II. Fluorometric determination of p-aminophenol and acetaminophen, *Journal of the Pharmaceutical Society of Japan*, **100**, 295–301.

Younes, M., Cornelius, S. and Siegers, C.-P., 1986, Ferrous ion supported *in vivo* lipid peroxidation induced by paracetamol: its relation to hepatotoxicity, *Research Communications in Chemical Pathology and Pharmacology*, **51**, 89–99.

Younes, M., Eberhardt, I. and Lemoine, R., 1989, Effect of iron overload on spontaneous and xenobiotic-induced lipid peroxidation *in vivo*, *Journal of Applied Toxicology*, **9**, 103–108.

Younes, M., Pentz, R. and Oltmanns, D., 1979, Inhibitory and stimulatory effects on the metabolic disposition of paracetamol, *Naunyn-Schmiedeberg's Archives of Pharmacology*, **307 (Suppl.)**, R7.

Younes, M., Sause, C., Siegers, C.-P. and Lemoine, R., 1988, Effect of deferrioxamine and diethyldithiocarbamate on paracetamol-induced hepato- and nephrotoxicity. The role of lipid peroxidation, *Journal of Applied Toxicology*, **8**, 261–265.

Younes, M. and Siegers, C. P., 1980a, Inhibitory action of antidotes on the hepatotoxicity of paracetamol and its irreversible binding to rat liver microsomal protein, *Toxicology Letters*, **6**, 155.

Younes, M. and Siegers, C.-P., 1980b, Inhibition of the hepatotoxicity of paracetamol and its irreversible binding to rat liver microsomal protein, *Archives of Toxicology*, **45**, 61–65.

Younes, M. and Siegers, C.-P., 1985a, The role of iron in the paracetamol- and CCl$_4$-induced lipid peroxidation and hepatotoxicity, *Chemico-Biological Interactions*, **55**, 327–334.

Younes, M. and Siegers, C.-P., 1985b, Effect of malotilate on paracetamol-induced hepatotoxicity, *Toxicology Letters*, **25**, 143–146.

Young, W. O., Goldschmidt-Clermont, P. J., Emerson, D. L., Lee, W. M., Jollow, D. J. and Galbraith, R. M., 1987, Correlation between extent of liver damage in fulminant hepatic necrosis and complexing of circulating group-specific component (vitamin D-binding protein), *Journal of Laboratory and Clinical Medicine*, **110**, 83–90.

Yousfi, A., Garrigues, J. M., Alquier, Y., Cayrol, B., Bauret, P., Olivier, G., Brignet, J. J., Larrey, D. and Michel, H., 1993, Rectite et sténoses rectales secondaires à la prise prolongée de suppositoires à visée antagique 4 observations, *Presse Médicale*, **22**, 1930.

Yscla, A., 1988, Aceclofenac and paracetamol in episiotomal pain, *Drugs Under Experimental and Clinical Research*, **14**, 491–494.

Yurdakök, M., Çaglar, M. and Yurdakök, K., 1985, Treatment of acetaminophen poisoning with cimetidine in mice, *Hacettepe Medical Journal*, **18**, 1–5.

Yurdakök, M., Oran, O., Tekeli, T. and Erer, H., 1989, Ranitidine hepatitis potentiated by acetaminophene in mice, *Hacettepe Medical Journal*, **22**, 1–3.

Zabrodski, R. M. and Schnurr, L. P., 1984, Anion gap acidosis with hypoglycemia in acetaminophen toxicity, *Archives of Emergency Medicine*, **13**, 956–959.

Zafar, N. U., Niazi, S. and Jung, D., 1987, Influence of water deprivation on the disposition of paracetamol, *Journal of Pharmacy and Pharmacology*, **39**, 144–147.

Zand, R., Nelson, S. D., Slattery, J. T., Thummel, K. E., Kalhorn, T. F., Adams, S. P. and Wright, J. M., 1993, Inhibition and induction of cytochrome P-4502E1-catalyzed oxidation by isoniazid in humans, *Clinical Pharmacology and Therapeutics*, **54**, 142–149.

Zanoli, P., 1981, Protection of rats and mice from acetaminophen liver toxicity with 2. 4-monofurfurylidene-tetra-O-methyl sorbitol (MSF), *Rivista di Farmacologia e Terapia*, **12**, 291–299.

Zelvelder, W. G., 1961, Mededelingen van de afdeling klinisch geneesmiddelenonderzoek tno: de beoordeling van een pijnstillend middel, *Nederlands Tijdschrift voor Geneeskunde*, **105**, 1697.

Zemtsov, A., Yanase, D. J., Boyd, A. S. and Shehata, B., 1992, Fixed drug eruption to Tylenol: report of two cases and review of the literature, *Cutis*, **50**, 281–282.

Zenser, T. V. and Davis, B. B., 1984, Enzyme systems involved in the formation of reactive metabolites in the renal medulla: cooxidation via prostaglandin H synthase, *Fundamental and Applied Toxicology*, **4**, 922–929.

Zenser, T. V., Mattammal, M. B., Brown, W. W. and Davis, B. B., 1979, Cooxygenation by prostaglandin cyclooxygenase from rabbit inner medulla, *Kidney International*, **16**, 688–694.

Zenser, T. V., Mattammal, M. B. and Davis, B. B., 1978a, Differential distribution of the mixed-function oxidase activities in rabbit kidney, *Journal of Pharmacology and Experimental Therapeutics*, **207**, 719–725.

Zenser, T. V., Mattammal, M. B., Herman, C. A., Joshi, S. and Davis, B. B., 1978b, Effect of acetaminophen on prostaglandin E_2 and prostaglandin $F_{2\alpha}$ synthesis in the renal inner medulla of rat, *Biochimica Biophysica Acta*, **542**, 486–495.

Zenser, T. V., Mattammal, M. B., Rapp, N. S. and Davies, B. B., 1983, Effect of aspirin on metabolism of acetaminophen and benzidine by renal inner medulla prostaglandin hydroperoxidase, *Journal of Laboratory and Clinical Medicine*, **101**, 58–65.

Zera, R. T. and Nagasawa, H. T., 1980, N-Acetyl-DL-penicillamine and acetaminophen toxicity in mice, *Journal of Pharmaceutical Sciences*, **69**, 1005–1006.

Zezulka, A. and Wright, N., 1982, Severe metabolic acidosis early in paracetamol poisoning, *British Medical Journal*, **285**, 851–852.

Zhang, J. and Liu, G. T., 1989, Protective action of kopsinine F against experimental liver injury in mice, *Acta Pharmaceutica Sinica*, **24**, 165–169.

Zhang, Y., Hu, Y. and Wilson, G. S., 1994, Elimination of the acetaminophen interference in an implantable glucose sensor, *Analytical Chemistry*, **66**, 1183–1188.

Zhou, J. and Wang, E., 1990, Direct detection of acetaminophen in urine by liquid chromatography with electrochemical detection using dual electrodes. Preliminary application to a single dose pharmacokinetic study, *Analytica Chimica Acta*, **236**, 293–298.

Zhou, L. X., Srivastava, P. and Holtzman, J. L., 1993, Binding of 14-C-acetaminophen (AC) to mouse, hepatic, microsomal proteins, *Clinical Research*, **41**, 661A.

Zhu, C., Hirate, J., Kanamoto, I., Nakagawa, T., Adachi, I., Horikoshi, I. and Bhargava, V. O., 1991, First-pass metabolism of acetoaminophen in thyroxine treated rats, *Journal of the Pharmaceutical Society of Japan*, **111**, 40–44.

Ziemniak, J. A., Allison, N., Boppana, V. K., Dubb, J. and Stote, R., 1987, The effect of acetaminophen on the disposition of fenoldopam: competition for sulfation, *Clinical Pharmacology and Therapeutics*, **41**, 275–281.

Zieve, L., 1989, Regenerative enzyme activity of the liver after partial hepatectomy or toxic injury depressed by continuous NH_4^+ infusion, *Journal of Laboratory and Clinical Medicine*, **114**, 527–530.

Zieve, L., Anderson, W. R. and Dozeman, R., 1988, Hepatic regenerative enzyme activity after diffuse injury with galactosamine: relationship to histologic alterations, *Journal of Laboratory and Clinical Medicine*, **112**, 575–582.

Zieve, L., Anderson, W. R., Dozeman, R., Draves, K. and Lyftogt, C., 1985a, Acetaminophen liver injury: sequential changes in two biochemical indices of regeneration and their relationship to histologic alterations, *Journal of Laboratory and Clinical Medicine*, **105**, 619–624.

Zieve, L., Anderson, W. R., Lyftogt, C. and Draves, K., 1986, Hepatic regenerative enzyme activity after pericentral and periportal lobular toxic injury, *Toxicology and Applied Pharmacology*, **86**, 147–158.

Zieve, L., Dozeman, R., LaFontaine, D. and Draves, K., 1985b, Effect of hepatic failure toxins on liver thymidine kinase activity and ornithine decarboxylase activity after massive necrosis with acetaminophen in the rat, *Journal of Laboratory and Clinical Medicine*, **106**, 583–588.

Zimmerman, H. J., 1986, Effects of alcohol on other hepatotoxins, *Alcoholism: Clinical and Experimental Research*, **10**, 3–15.

Zwiener, R. J., Kurt, T. L., Ghali, F., Day, L. C. and Timmons, C. F., 1994, Potentiation of acetaminophen hepatotoxicity in a child with mercury poisoning, *Journal of Pediatric Gastroenterology and Nutrition*, **19**, 242–245.

Zwiers, A., 1993, Risicogroepen bij paracetamolintoxicaties, *Pharmaceutisch Weekblad*, **128**, 69–74.

Index

D